IMPORTANT

W9-AWN-290

png5s-4hfb-x9qf-k49e

HERE IS YOUR REGISTRATION CODE TO ACCESS MCGRAW-HILL PREMIUM CONTENT AND MCGRAW-HILL ONLINE RESOURCES

For key premium online resources you need THIS CODE to gain access. Once the code is entered, you will be able to use the web resources for the length of your course.

Access is provided only if you have purchased a new book.

If the registration code is missing from this book, the registration screen on our website, and within your WebCT or Blackboard course will tell you how to obtain your new code. Your registration code can be used only once to establish access. It is not transferable.

To gain access to these online resources

1. **USE** your web browser to go to: **www.mhhe.com/teague1e**

2. **CLICK** on "First Time User"

3. **ENTER** the Registration Code printed on the tear-off bookmark on the right

4. After you have entered your registration code, click on "Register"

5. **FOLLOW** the instructions to setup your personal UserID and Password

6. **WRITE** your UserID and Password down for future reference. Keep it in a safe place.

If your course is using WebCT or Blackboard, you'll be able to use this code to access the McGraw-Hill content within your instructor's online course.

To gain access to the McGraw-Hill content in your instructor's WebCT or Blackboard course simply log into the course with the user ID and Password provided by your instructor. Enter the registration code exactly as it appears to the right when prompted by the system. You will only need to use this code the first time you click on McGraw-Hill content.

These instructions are specifically for student access. Instructors are not required to register via the above instructions.

The McGraw-Hill Companies

Higher Education

Thank you, and welcome to your McGraw-Hill Online Resources.

ISBN-13: 978-0-07-297343-3
ISBN-10: 0-07-297343-9 t/a
Teague
Your Health Today, 1/e

REGISTRATION CODE
REGISTRATION CODE

The McGraw-Hill Companies

Higher Education

Your Health Today

CHOICES IN A CHANGING SOCIETY

This book is dedicated to our families

*To my children, Ryan and Josh, and my daughters-
in-law, Shannon and Jamie, who continuously reinforce that
family is one of nature's most precious gifts—M.T.*

*To my husband, Paul, and my daughters, Lila and
Sydda, who fill my life with laughter and balance—S.M.*

*To my wife, Jane, and my children—Daniel
and Rebecca, daughter-in-law, Courtney, and son-in-law,
Chris—the people to whom I feel closest and who
provide daily inspiration—D.R.*

Your Health Today
CHOICES IN A CHANGING SOCIETY

MICHAEL L. TEAGUE
University of Iowa

SARA L.C. MACKENZIE
University of Washington

DAVID M. ROSENTHAL
Lower East Side Harm Reduction Center

Boston   Burr Ridge, IL   Dubuque, IA   Madison, WI   New York   San Francisco   St. Louis
Bangkok   Bogotá   Caracas   Kuala Lumpur   Lisbon   London   Madrid   Mexico City
Milan   Montreal   New Delhi   Santiago   Seoul   Singapore   Sydney   Taipei   Toronto

Higher Education

Published by McGraw-Hill, an imprint of The McGraw-Hill Companies, Inc., 1221 Avenue of the Americas, New York, NY 10020. Copyright © 2007 by The McGraw-Hill Companies. All rights reserved. No part of this publication may be reproduced or distributed in any form or by any means, or stored in a database or retrieval system, without the prior written consent of The McGraw-Hill Companies, Inc., including, but not limited to, in any network or other electronic storage or transmission, or broadcast for distance learning.

This book is printed on acid-free paper.

2 3 4 5 6 7 8 9 0 VNH/VNH 0 9 8 7 6

ISBN–13 978-0-07-328495-8
ISBN–10 0-07-328495-5

Vice President and Editor-in-Chief: *Emily Barrosse*
Publisher: *William R. Glass*
Sponsoring Editor: *Christopher Johnson*
Director of Development: *Kathleen Engelberg*
Developmental Editor: *Carlotta Seely*
Marketing Manager: *Pamela S. Cooper*
Media Project Manager: *Michele Borrelli*
Technology Developmental Editor: *Julia D. Ersery*
Editorial Assistant: *Sarah B. Hill*

Production Editor: *Leslie LaDow*
Manuscript Editor: *Judith Brown*
Cover Designer: *Preston Thomas*
Interior Designers: *Caroline McGowan and Preston Thomas*
Photo Research Coordinator: *Alexandra Ambrose*
Art Editor: *Katherine McNab*
Production Supervisor: *Tandra Jorgensen*
Composition: *10.5/12 Minion by GTS-LA*
Printing: *45# Pub Matte by Von Hoffman Press*

Cover images: Row 1: © Squared Studios/Getty Images, © Royalty-Free/Corbis, © Comstock Images/Alamy, Ryan McVay/Getty Images, Brand X Pictures; **Row 2:** PhotoLink/Getty Images, Royalty-Free/Corbis, Siede Preis/Getty Images, Cartesia/Getty Images, Photodisc Collection/Getty Images; **Row 3:** John A. Rizzo/Getty Images, (Palm, Inc. Treo.™), Nancy R. Cohen/Getty Images, Getty Images, © Squared Studios/Getty Images; **Row 4:** © Squared Studios/Getty Images, © Squared Studios/Getty Images, Royalty-Free/Corbis, (no credit), © Douglas White/Corbis

Photo credits: The credits section for this book begins on page C–1 and is considered an extension of the copyright page.

Library of Congress Cataloging-in-Publication Data

Teague, Michael L., 1946-
   Your health today: choices in a changing society / Michael L. Teague, Sara L.C.
Mackenzie, David M. Rosenthal.
      p. cm.
   Includes bibliographical references and index.
   ISBN–13 978-0-07-328495-8
   ISBN–10 0-07-328495-5 (alk. paper)
      1. Health education. 2. Health promotion. I. Mackenzie, Sara L.C. II. Rosenthal,
David M. III. Title.

RA440.T43 2007
362.1—dc22

2005044392

The Internet addresses listed in the text were accurate at the time of publication. The inclusion of a Web site does not indicate an endorsement by the authors or McGraw-Hill, and McGraw-Hill does not guarantee the accuracy of the information presented at these sites.

Brief Contents

Contents

Part 1   Your Mind and Body 23

Part 2   Your Lifestyle and Health *157*

Part 4   Your Relationships and Sexuality 359

Part 5   Challenges to Your Health *443*

Part 6   Protecting Your Health *529*

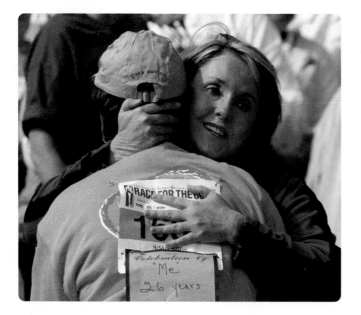

Special Features

HEALTHY PEOPLE 2010

YOU MAKE THE CALL

ADD IT UP!

TOPICS AND ISSUES OF SPECIAL INTEREST

Women's Health

Preface

The idea for *Your Health Today* arose from discussions among a health educator, a family physician, and a family therapist. Each of us—Michael Teague, Sara Mackenzie, and David Rosenthal—interacted with students in slightly different settings, and yet we all shared the belief that something more was needed to help them improve their general health. And so we started on the journey that led to this book.

Almost half of all premature deaths in the United States and Canada are caused in part by lifestyle-related behaviors. Most people want to pursue healthy lives, and most have the basic knowledge they need about healthy behaviors, yet health promotion studies show that long-term health behavior change is difficult. Why do many people find it so hard to pursue healthy behaviors? We believe there are three broad answers to this question:

1. External forces are often in opposition to healthy behaviors. Our culture offers a broad range of unhealthy choices, and advertising and the media make them look desirable. In addition, individuals are embedded in families, relationships, and communities, all of which strongly influence personal choices.

2. Many unhealthy behaviors are pleasurable, and their health consequences seem remote, unlikely, or worth the risk.

3. There is confusion about who is responsible for individual health-related behaviors and how much the government should intrude in areas of personal choice in the interest of the common good. In other words, although personal choices have health implications for individuals, these choices, increasingly, pose ethical issues and challenges faced by entire communities.

OUR GOALS

Your Health Today highlights the importance of two key factors in health—awareness and action. Both individuals and communities need to be aware of the many influences on health and balance them as they work toward better health. As authors, we hope to challenge students to think of themselves as agents of change. Individuals can make personal changes in lifestyle behaviors that impact their own health, and they can also motivate communities to make changes in response to social, political, and economic factors that impact the health of broader segments of the population.

Within the context of this broad goal, our specific goals are to

- provide accurate, up-to-date health information drawn from credible sources;

- introduce basic health concepts that students need in order to interpret health messages, understand health recommendations, and make informed decisions in a changing society;

- engage and challenge students to delve further into areas of health that are particularly relevant to them, whether because of their family, ethnic, or cultural background, their socioeconomic circumstances, or other factors;

- introduce the concept that personal health is dependent on both individual and community action;

- engage students in the ethical issues and challenges involved in promoting personal health choices at community levels; and

- empower students to become advocates for healthy lifestyle behaviors.

In short, our belief is that a personal health text needs to provide a perspective that encompasses both individual and cultural responsibility. This is why we say that personal health is "not just personal."

ORGANIZATION AND CONTENT

Your Health Today is divided into six parts. Part 1, Your Mind and Body, highlights the importance of mental health and physical health and their influence on overall well-being. Chapter 1 (Health in a Changing Society) takes a look at the many challenges involved in making informed health choices, such as evaluating health information and understanding health behavior change. Chapter 2 (Genetics) focuses on the importance of a person's family health history and its relation to health risks and health care decisions. Chapter 3 (Mental Health) addresses the balance necessary for good mental, or psychological, health, including the many influences that affect that balance. Chapter 4 (Spirituality) offers a broad view of spirituality that includes such forms of spiritual expression as volunteerism, the arts, rituals, and community and social action, in addition to organized religion. Chapter 5 (Stress) discusses how people respond to stressful events and offers practical ways of managing pressure. Chapter 6 (Sleep) focuses on this often overlooked component of good health, discussing the mechanics of sleep, how it restores us, and how to deal with sleep problems.

Part 2, Your Lifestyle and Health, highlights the connection between lifestyle choices and health. Chapter 7 (Nutrition) offers an in-depth look at nutrition that combines the latest information with its practical application, such as MyPyramid and the 2005 *Dietary Guidelines for Americans*. Similarly, Chapter 8 (Fitness) discusses the principles of physical fitness and presents physical activity as part of a lifetime approach to optimal health. Chapter 9 (Body Weight and Body Composition) considers both body weight and body composition as essential to a healthy balance. Chapter 10 (Body Image) addresses how individuals view themselves and the many influences that affect their body satisfaction.

Part 3, Your Health at Risk, addresses personal choices that may lead to health risks. Chapter 11 (Alcohol) examines issues such as binge drinking, drinking and driving, and the influence of culture and society on attitudes toward alcohol consumption. Chapter 12 (Drugs and Addictive Behavior) explores drug use, the effects of drug abuse, and issues of drug control. Chapter 13 (Tobacco) looks at smoking as a health issue that has implications for individuals and society as a whole.

Part 4, Your Relationships and Sexuality, focuses on the role that relationships and sexuality play in health. Chapter 14 (Relationships) discusses friendship, marriage, the single life, families, gay and lesbian partnerships, blended families, and other changing relationships. Chapter 15 (Sexual Health) views sexuality as a blend of biology, society, and culture, involving choices that go beyond the personal level. Chapter 16 (Reproductive Choices) addresses contraception, pregnancy, and childbirth as choices that are highly personal yet have consequences for others.

Part 5, Challenges to Your Health, highlights forces that threaten the well-being of individuals, neighborhoods, society, and our planet. Chapter 17 (Violence) examines the widespread problem of violence, from video games for children to global terrorism; the treatment of this topic separately from unintentional injury allows for greater depth of coverage. Chapter 18 (Injury) focuses on unintentional injury, emphasizing the importance of creating safe environments in the home, at work, and on campus. Chapter 19 (Environmental Issues) considers how individual efforts at conservation, such as recycling, fit into the big picture and how challenges such as global warming can be addressed.

Part 6, Protecting Your Health, explores diseases and health care choices—issues that affect all people at some time in their lives. Chapter 20 (Infectious Diseases) discusses everything from the common cold to new and emerging diseases. Chapter 21 (Cardiovascular Disease) offers the latest information on the health issues associated with cardiovascular disease, the leading cause of death for both women and men and a growing problem in children. Chapter 22 (Cancer) examines cancer in all its complexity, with researchers and health professionals working toward the same goals—more effective treatments, a better quality of life for those living with cancer, and, ultimately, a cure. Chapter 23 (Complementary and Alternative Medicine) surveys the range of options for health care—traditional approaches to medicine, complementary and alternative practices from our own and other cultures, self-care, and a blend of different methods—and discusses how to make effective choices.

Special Content

Your Health Today offers current, concise coverage of topics important to today's students in a way no other personal health book has done. Separate chapters are devoted to body image, sleep, spirituality, and genetics. Current research, important trends, and frequently asked questions are covered in depth. *Your Health Today:*

- Discusses body image for both men and women with a full chapter (Chapter 10) that emphasizes the importance of a healthy body image for overall wellness and highlights topics such as sports and body image, eating disorders, exercise disorders, and awareness and prevention of body image problems.

- Explores the importance of genetics (Chapter 2) and enables your students to make important decisions based on family health history and other relevant factors. Topics include the role of genes in personal health, ethnicity and genetic disorders, genes and behavior, genetic counseling and testing, and the social and ethical implications of genetic research.

- Covers ways in which spirituality can be experienced and expressed (Chapter 4), such as meditating and journaling, living one's values, and giving to the community. The chapter also discusses related issues, including death and dying.

- Tackles the often overlooked topic of sleep (Chapter 6) and its role in optimal wellness. Topics covered include the structure of sleep, the effect of sleep deprivation on performance, sleep disorders, and the best ways to ensure good sleep habits.

Features

- **Did You Know?** facts at the beginning of each chapter link personal behaviors with information and statistics about related health practices in the general population. This feature prompts students to think about the implications of the data—not only for themselves but for members of their family, their neighborhood, and society.

- **Challenges & Choices** boxes offer tips on changing health-related behaviors, such as quitting smoking, achieving a healthy weight, reducing stress, communicating more effectively in relationships, and choosing a heart-healthy diet. They provide ideas for getting started, dealing with setbacks, and staying motivated. The ending section, called "It's not just personal...," connects the health issue with community and societal issues.

- **Beating the Odds** boxes present profiles of three individuals and asks students who is most likely (or least likely) to have a certain health outcome. The scenarios include information on family life, personal habits, and special situations. After making their choice, students can visit the Online Learning Center to read comments by the authors.

- The **You Make the Call** feature at the end of each chapter discusses the key points of a controversial health topic, highlighting the pros and cons. Students are asked to use their critical thinking skills to evaluate the issue and take a stand. Topics include DNA profiling, smoking in public places, and same-sex marriage. To explore the topic further, students can visit the Online Learning Center and click on links.

- **Healthy People 2010** boxes highlight a key objective from the *Healthy People* initiative, showing how a selected chapter topic relates to national health objectives. Encouraging students to think about broad goals for health, this feature emphasizes national progress but also shows what work still needs to be done.

- **Highlight on Health** boxes focus on topics of special interest, background information, and practical health tips. Sample topics include vegetarian diet planning, stress and the older college student, interpreting your dreams, high-risk college drinking, the language of cancer, and global activism.

- **Consumer Clipboard** boxes equip students to evaluate health information and consumer choices and make informed decisions. By demonstrating how to think critically about health in the news and other media, this feature helps students separate fact from fiction. Topics include tattooing and body piercing, Internet dating, identity theft, alert drugs, and "superfoods."

- The **Add It Up!** feature at the end of each chapter offers students the opportunity to see how they measure up. Is their health good, or is it time to make changes for better health? Sample topics include assessing your stress level, determining your energy needs, understanding why you smoke, and estimating your HIV risk.

- The **Key Terms** boxes throughout each chapter serve as a running glossary. Each term, along with its definition, appears close to its text discussion. This aid reinforces learning in an immediate way and is also helpful for study and exam preparation.

- **Chapter Summaries** present key concepts for easy review. Students can use these summaries to determine which discussion topics will require further study.

- **Review Questions** challenge students to explain the key points of the chapter and relate that information to their own life and their health.

- The **Web Resources** list makes it easy for students to explore topics of special interest on the Internet. The accompanying brief annotations are helpful for making selections.

SUPPLEMENTS FOR INSTRUCTORS

Instructor's Resource CD-ROM (0-07-245862-3)

Organized by chapter, this instructor CD-ROM includes all the resources you need to help teach your course: Course Integrator Guide, Test Bank, Computerized Test Bank, and PowerPoint slides. The CD-ROM works in both Windows and Macintosh environments and includes the following:

- **Course Integrator Guide** This manual includes all the features of a useful instructor's manual, such as lecture outlines, suggested activities, media resources, and Web links. It also integrates the text with all the related resources McGraw-Hill offers, such as the Online Learning Center and the Resource Presentation Manager DVD-ROM.

- **Test Bank** The electronic Test Bank (Microsoft Word files) offers more than 2500 questions, including multiple choice, true-false, short answer, and matching.

- **Computerized Test Bank** The Test Bank is available with the EZ Test computerized testing software, which provides a powerful, easy-to-use way to create printed quizzes and exams. EZ Test runs on both Windows and Macintosh systems. For secure online testing, exams created in EZ Test can be exported to WebCT, Blackboard, PageOut, and EZ Test Online. EZ Test is packaged with a Quick Start Guide. Once the program is installed, you have access to the complete User's Manual, including

Flash tutorials. Additional help is available at www.mhhe.com/eztest.

- **PowerPoint slides** A comprehensive set of PowerPoint lecture slides for your course completes this package of tools. The PowerPoint presentations, ready to use in class, were prepared by a health professional. The slides correspond to the content in each chapter of *Your Health Today,* making it easier for you to teach and ensuring that your students will be able to follow your lectures point by point. You can modify the presentation as much as you like to meet the needs of your course.

Resource Presentation Manager DVD-ROM (0-07-245863-1)

This DVD-ROM is a presentation tool of videos correlated to *Your Health Today.* It is designed to help you engage students in class discussions and promote critical thinking about personal health topics. The library contains student interviews and historical health videos on body image, depression, stress, spirituality, and many other topics. Videos can be searched by chapter, topic, or media type. Once a video is located, it can be downloaded to a computer, saved to a playlist for later viewing, or simply viewed by double-clicking. For each video clip, an Instructor's Guide is available to describe the objective of the clip, provide critical thinking questions to ask before the video is shown, and suggest follow-up discussion questions.

Online Learning Center (www.mhhe.com/teague1e)

The Online Learning Center to accompany *Your Health Today,* designed with different features for instructors and for students, offers a number of special resources for instructors:

- Downloadable PowerPoint presentations
- Course Integrator Guide
- Interactive activities
- Downloadable content (for use with Classroom Performance Systems)
- Web links

Quia™ Online Wellness Workbook (0-07-301716-7)

The Online Wellness Workbook, developed in collaboration with Quia,™ offers an electronic version of assessments and quizzes compiled from the main text and its supplements. Featuring interactive assessments, self-scoring quizzes, and instant feedback for students, the Online Wellness Workbook provides you with a gradebook that automatically scores, tracks, and records your students' results and lets you review both individual and class performance. You can also customize activities and features for your course by using the activity templates provided.

SUPPLEMENTS FOR STUDENTS
Online Learning Center (www.mhhe.com/teague1e)

The Online Learning Center contains many study tools that are open to all students—those using either new or used books. These tools include:

- Self-scoring chapter quizzes
- Flashcards and crossword puzzles (for learning key terms and definitions)
- Interactive activities
- Digital audio summaries

Digital audio summaries are downloadable audio files that include overviews of key chapter topics. These 2- to 3-minute audio files are a great way to review and are easy to download. They can be used with any portable mp3 player or personal computer.

Students who have purchased new books also have access to *premium content,* which includes PowerWeb. To gain this access, students must register using the passcode that comes free with new books. Sample *premium content* includes:

- PowerWeb (with current articles and updates)
- Wellness Worksheets
- Newsfeeds
- Weekly archives
- Web links

Quia™ Online Wellness Workbook (0-07-301716-7)

Students can assess and test themselves using the interactive Online Wellness Workbook, as described under Supplements for Instructors.

OTHER RESOURCES
Daily Fitness and Nutrition Journal (0-07-302988-2)

This logbook helps students track their diet and exercise programs. It can be packaged with any McGraw-Hill textbook for a small additional fee.

NutritionCalc Plus 2.0 (http://nutritioncalc.mhhe.com)

- On-Line 2.0 (Package 0-07-321925-8; Standalone 0-07-321924-X)
- CD-ROM 2.0 (Package 0-07-319570-7; Standalone 0-07-319532-4)

NutritionCalc Plus 2.0 is a suite of powerful dietary self-assessment tools. Students can use it to analyze and monitor their personal diet and health goals. The program is based on the reliable ESHA database and has an easy-to-use interface.

PowerWeb: Personal Health

Add the Internet to your course with PowerWeb! PowerWeb: Personal Health provides students with current articles, curriculum-based materials, weekly updates with assessments, informative and timely world news, refereed Web links, research tools, student study tools, and interactive exercises. Preview the site at www.dushkin.com/powerweb.

Wellness Worksheets (0-07-297649-7)

This collection of 120 assessments is designed to evaluate health behaviors and knowledge. Categories of topics include General Wellness and Behavior Change, Stress Management, Psychological and Spiritual Wellness, Intimate Relationships and Communication, Sexuality, Addictive Behaviors and Drug Dependence, Nutrition, Physical Activity and Exercises, Weight Management, and Consumer Health. The worksheets are available online as *premium content,* or they may be packaged with the text.

Video Library

The McGraw-Hill Video Library features brief clips on a wide range of topics of interest for personal health courses. Talk with your sales representative about eligibility to receive videos.

PageOut: The Course Web site Development Center (www.pageout.net)

PageOut, available free to instructors who use a McGraw-Hill textbook, is an online program that lets you create your own course Web site. PageOut offers the following features: a course home page, an instructor home page, a syllabus (interactive and customizable, including quizzing, instructor notes, and links to the text's Online Learning Center), Web links, discussions (multiple discussion areas per class), an online gradebook, and links to student Web pages. Contact your McGraw-Hill sales representative to obtain a password.

Course Management Systems (www.mhhe.com/solutions)

McGraw-Hill's Instructor Advantage program offers customers access to a complete online teaching Web site called the Knowledge Gateway, pre-paid toll-free phone support, and unlimited e-mail support directly from WebCT and Blackboard. Instructors who use 500 or more copies of a McGraw-Hill textbook can enroll in our Instructor Advantage Plus program, which provides on-campus, hands-on training from a certified platform specialist. Consult your McGraw-Hill sales representative to learn what other course management systems are easily used with McGraw-Hill online materials.

Classroom Performance System

Classroom Performance System (CPS) brings interactivity into the classroom or lecture hall. It is a wireless response system that gives instructors and students immediate feedback from the entire class. The wireless response pads are essentially remotes that are easy to use and engage students. CPS is available for both Microsoft Windows and Macintosh computers.

Primis Online (www.mhhe.com/primis/online)

Primis Online is a database-driven publishing system that allows instructors to create content-rich textbooks, lab manuals, or readers for their courses directly from the Primis Web site. The customized text can be delivered in print or electronic (eBook) form. A Primis eBook is a digital version of the customized text (sold directly to students as a file downloadable to their computer or accessed online by a password). *Your Health Today* is included in the database.

REVIEWERS

We are grateful to the instructors and experts who reviewed the manuscript of *Your Health Today* and offered helpful suggestions. Their knowledge and insights are reflected throughout the pages of this book.

Andrea H. Abercrombie, Clemson University

Chris Adamson, University of Central Florida

Arnold E. Andersen, University of Iowa

Stan Andrews, Valdosta State University

Julianne Arient, Triton College

Charles Baffi, National Cancer Institute, Health Promotion Research Branch

Judy B. Baker, Lecturer Emeritus, East Carolina University

David Bever, George Mason University, Director of the National Center for Public Safety Fitness

Richard Blonna, William Patterson University

Todd Bowden, John Brown University

Elaine Bryan, Georgia Perimeter College

Susan Burge, Cuyahoga Community College

Virginia Burton, Alverno College

Karen Camarata, Eastern Kentucky University

Rhonda Capuano, Southern Connecticut State University

Donald G. Carter, Western Kentucky University

John M. Charles, The College of William and Mary

Amanda Collings, University of Massachusetts, Amherst

Peggy Sue Crawford, Delta College

Duane A. Crider, Kutztown University

Dick Dalton, Lincoln University

Keri S. Diez, Southeastern Louisiana University

Robert Dollinger, Florida International University

Joseph Donnelly, Montclair State University

Carla Dornsbach, Iowa State University

Leisa Easom, Georgia Southwestern State University

Maureen Eliot, Ventura College

Faye Evans, Thomas Nelson Community College

Linda Fairstein, Former Prosecutor (sex crimes), New York County District Attorney's Office, and author

Brian Findley, Palm Beach Community College

Jeanne M. Freeman, California State University, Chico

Heidi Fuller, Salem State College

Kathi Fuller, Eastern Michigan University

Stanton Gantz, University of California, San Francisco

Marilyn Gardner, Western Kentucky University

Diana Godish, Ball State University

Marilyn Grechus, Central Missouri State University

Janet Green, Los Medanos College

Mary L. Gress, Lorain County Community College

Barbara P. Hamann, Professor Emeritus, University of Wisconsin-Superior

Charlene Harkins, University of Minnesota Duluth

Jeanne Hoff, Clark College

Stephen Hohman, Ohio University

Angela Huebner, Virginia Polytechnic Institute and State University

Cathy Hunt, Henderson Community College

Kim Hyatt, Weber State University

William T. Jarvis, Professor Emeritus, Loma Linda University School of Medicine

Robert W. Jeffery, University of Minnesota

Carol L. Johnson, University of Richmond

Gary F. Kelly, Clarkson University

Cathy Kennedy, Colorado State University

Kathie Kingett, East Los Angeles College

John Kowalczyk, University of Minnesota, Duluth

Justin Laird, SUNY College at Brockport

Judith H. LaRosa, SUNY Downstate Medical Center

Joan S. Leafman, Northeastern Illinois University

Laurie Legocki, Indiana University, Bloomington

Ricki Lewis, Genetic Counselor, CareNet Medical Group, and author

Gary Liguori, North Dakota State University

Jeri M. Lloyd, Piedmont Virginia Community College

Charles F. Lynch, University of Iowa

James B. Maas, Cornell University

Priscilla MacDuff, Suffolk County Community College

C. James Maginet, Southeast Missouri State University

G. Alan Marlatt, University of Washington

Marshall Meyer, Portland Community College

Richard E. Miller, George Mason University

M. Vinson Miner, Utah Valley State College

Robert J. Moffatt, Florida State University

Rosemarie Monahan, High Point University

Susan M. Moore, Western Illinois University

Sophia Munro, Palm Beach Community College

Phyllis D. Murray, Eastern Kentucky University

Bikash R. Nandy, Minnesota State University, Mankato

Peter E. Nathan, University of Iowa

David C. Nieman, Appalachian State University

Peggy Oberstaller, Lane Community College

Michael Olpin, Weber State University

Roseann Poole, Tallahassee Community College

Lynn H. Poulson, Snow College

Bill E. Pride, University of Arizona, Emeritus

Linda L. Rankin, Idaho State University

Megan Lanee Rickard, University of Florida

Dan Ripley, Long Beach City College

Liliana Rojas-Guyler, University of Cincinnati

Pamela Rost, Buffalo State College

Robert L. Schurrer, Black Hills State University

Melinda J. Seid, California State University, Sacramento

Allen Sherman, Arkansas Cancer Research Center

Janet L. Sholes, Frederick Community College

Shannon R. Siegel, Portland Community College

Jacob M. Silvestri, Hudson Valley Community College

Carol A. Smith, Elon University

Sherman Sowby, California State University, Fresno

Darlene Staley, Portland Community College

Will Stern, Covenant College, University of Tennessee, Chattanooga

Peter Sternberg, Winona State University

Carl A. Stockton, University of North Carolina at Wilmington

Felicia D. Taylor, University of Central Arkansas

Christopher J. Tennant, California State University, Fresno

Silvea E. Thomas, Kingsborough Community College

Barbara Tyree, Valparaiso University

Karen Vail-Smith, East Carolina University

Melinda Wells Valiant, The University of Mississippi

Holly Gentry Wiley, Mississippi State University

Brenda Williams, Olivet Nazarene University

Melvin H. Williams, Old Dominion University

Royal E. Wohl, Washburn University

Jackie Wright, Cossatot Community College of the University of Arkansas

Ottley Wright, Chadron State College

Connie Zuercher, Sacramento City College

Test Bank Reviewers

We would also like to thank the following instructors, who offered helpful suggestions for developing the Test Bank to accompany *Your Health Today:*

Elaine Bryant, Georgia Perimeter College

Janet Green, Los Medanos College

Kim Hyatt, Weber State University

Gary Linguori, North Dakota State University

Susan Moore, Western Illinois University

Peggy Oberstaller, Lane Community College

Grace Pokorny, Long Beach City College

Linda Rankin, Idaho State University

ACKNOWLEDGMENTS

Many members of the McGraw-Hill Higher Education staff were instrumental in advancing *Your Health Today* from an idea to a book. In particular, we would like to acknowledge the contributions of the following individuals: Carlotta Seely, Developmental Editor, whose patience and persistence helped this book reach publication; Nicholas Barrett, Former Executive Editor, for his contagious enthusiasm and strong leadership in the middle phase of development; Kathleen Engelberg, Director of Development, who provided the creative energy essential to maintaining our vision for the book; Christopher Johnson, Senior Sponsoring Editor, who gave valuable support and guidance at key stages; Pamela Cooper, Executive Marketing Manager, whose experience and expertise helped ensure that *Your Health Today* would fit the diverse landscape for personal health courses at the college level; Vicki Malinee, Former Executive Editor, who provided invaluable support in the early stages of development; Leslie LaDow, Production Editor, who worked tirelessly and effectively to coordinate the production process; Jason Dewey, Field Publisher, who contributed good ideas and gathered market feedback; and Preston Thomas, Senior Designer, who translated the message of this book into visual form.

We would also like to thank Judith Brown for her copyediting work and our manuscript typists—Joyce Murphy, Patricia Hoback, Joy Fry, Angie Gingerich, and Anna Benyo—for their help on many drafts.

M. Teague
S. Mackenzie
D. Rosenthal

A Guided Tour of
Your Health Today

Is being healthy just a matter of exercising, eating a nutritious diet, and adopting other sensible behaviors? Or is there more to take into account? *Your Health Today* shows you not only how to make healthy lifestyle choices but also how to factor in the effects of your family upbringing, your genetic make-up, your ethnic and cultural background, and your community and society. Here are some of the features that will help you understand and integrate all these components of your personal health.

DID YOU KNOW?

"Did You Know?" facts at the beginning of each chapter link your personal behaviors with information and statistics about related health practices in the general population. You may be surprised by what you learn here.

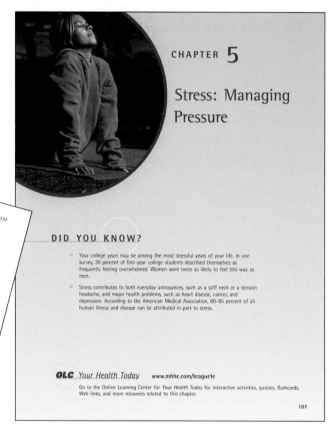

CHAPTER **5**

Stress: Managing Pressure

DID YOU KNOW?

- Your college years may be among the most stressful years of your life. In one survey, 30 percent of first-year college students described themselves as frequently feeling overwhelmed. Women were twice as likely to feel this way as men.

- Stress contributes to both everyday annoyances, such as a stiff neck or a tension headache, and major health problems, such as heart disease, cancer, and depression. According to the American Medical Association, 80–85 percent of all human illness and disease can be attributed in part to stress.

OLC *Your Health Today*   www.mhhe.com/teague1e

Go to the Online Learning Center for *Your Health Today* for interactive activities, quizzes, flashcards, Web links, and more resources related to this chapter.

107

CHALLENGES & CHOICES

"Challenges & Choices" boxes provide tips on changing health-related behaviors, such as quitting smoking, achieving a healthy weight, reducing stress, communicating with a partner about relationship issues, and choosing a heart-healthy diet. The "It's not just personal . . ." section prompts you to think beyond the level of the individual to community and societal levels.

CONSUMER CLIPBOARD

"Consumer Clipboard" boxes show you how to take a critical look at health information so that you can evaluate health and consumer choices and make informed decisions about them. These boxes will give you the confidence to take charge of your health.

BEATING THE ODDS

"Beating the Odds" boxes ask you to use the information provided in the chapter to decide which of three profiled individuals has the best chance of achieving a specific health outcome. The *OLC Web site* icon invites you to visit the Online Learning Center and read comments by the authors.

HIGHLIGHT ON HEALTH

"Highlight on Health" boxes focus on topics of special interest, such as vegetarian diet planning, consequences of high-risk college drinking, strategies for overcoming barriers to physical activity, and many more.

HEALTHY PEOPLE 2010

"Healthy People 2010" boxes in each chapter high-light a key objective from the U.S. *Healthy People* initiative and show how the personal health issues discussed in the chapter align with national health objectives.

ADD IT UP!

The "Add It Up!" feature at the end of each chapter of-fers you an opportunity to see how you measure up in the health area discussed in the chapter. Are you on the right track? Or is there room for improvement?

YOU MAKE THE CALL

The "You Make the Call" feature at the end of each chapter presents the pros and cons of a controversial topic in our society and asks you to use your critical thinking skills to evaluate the issue and take a stand. The **OLC Web site** icon directs you to the Online Learning Center, where you'll find links for further exploration.

ONLINE LEARNING CENTER

Visit the *Your Health Today* Online Learning Center (www.mhhe.com/teague1e) for resources to help you improve your grade and build a healthier lifestyle. You'll find self-quizzes, flashcards, downloadable dig-ital audio summaries, special activities, and many more study aids. You'll also have access to behavior change tools, Internet activities, and links to reliable wellness sites. A password granting access to addi-tional premium online resources is available free with each new copy of the text; these premium resources include an online wellness workbook, articles about health topics, and a daily newsfeed.

CHAPTER 1

Health in a Changing Society

DID YOU KNOW?

- If you belong to an ethnic minority group in the United States, you are part of a fast-growing segment that is expected to reach 50 percent of the population by the year 2050. Most minority populations, however, have not benefited from health gains achieved over the past 100 years to the same extent as the general population has. One of the U.S. government's health goals for the nation is to eliminate health disparities among different segments of the population.

- If you have ever researched a health issue on the Internet, you are one of more than 70 million Americans who use online technologies to access health-related material—and have to navigate a sea of health scams and false claims to find accurate, legitimate information. Consumer protection against health fraud is provided by such government agencies as the Federal Trade Commission, the Food and Drug Administration, and the U.S. Postal Service.

OLC *Your Health Today*   www.mhhe.com/teague1e

Go to the Online Learning Center for *Your Health Today* for interactive activities, quizzes, flashcards, Web links, and more resources related to this chapter.

As individuals, we are all responsible for our own health. It's up to each of us to be physically active, to eat a healthy diet, to get enough sleep, to make informed decisions about health care. Yet we do not live in a social vacuum. Our actions, thoughts, beliefs, needs, and desires are all influenced by our environment—our families and friends, the community around us, and the larger society and culture in which we live. Unfortunately, some aspects of this environment are not conducive to healthy lifestyles; in fact, they are downright antagonistic to good health. We are tempted by unhealthy foods, exposed to sedentary lifestyles, and encouraged to live fast-paced, high-stress lives.

Many of us know that certain types of behavior lead to poor health and disease—we know, for example, that eating food high in saturated fats and never exercising are linked to chronic conditions like heart disease and obesity—and common sense would suggest that we would therefore avoid such behaviors. Yet adopting healthy lifestyle behaviors requires more than having information or knowledge. Also involved is a host of other personal, community, societal, and cultural factors.

In this book we explore personal health in the context of a complex and rapidly changing society. The United States is becoming more urban, more ethnically and culturally diverse, more saturated with information, more interconnected through the mass media. Technology links us intimately with nearly every place on earth; it is commonplace today to refer to the world as a global village. So small has the planet become that a traveler can reach nearly any destination on any continent within 24 hours, and communication via cell phones, e-mail, and instant messaging over the Internet is virtually instantaneous. For good or for ill, technology has forever changed our world, giving us everything from the silicon computer chip to the keys to the human genome.

Yet just as technology promises to fulfill our every desire, we notice our unmet human needs—the needs for solitude, for a spiritual life, for supportive relationships with other people, for nutritious food, for relaxation and respite from stress, even for enough sleep. We find that periodically we have to pause and take stock of where we are and ask ourselves if we are on the right track, as individuals and as a society. And we sometimes have to make difficult choices.

A basic premise of this book is that you have the right and the responsibility to make your own health decisions; to make the best decisions, however, and to implement them, you need information, strategies, and skills. Our goals in the chapters that follow are to provide you with accurate, reliable, up-to-date information; to show you how to use proven behavior change strategies; and to help you improve your critical thinking and consumer skills. The book will guide you through a variety of health-related topics, ranging from understanding the role of your genetic heritage (Chapter 2) to making appropriate use of complementary and alternative forms of medicine (Chapter 23). Our hope is that these and all the chapters

in between will provide you with the framework and foundation for a lifetime of healthy choices and responsible decisions.

This chapter offers an introduction to key concepts and issues. We begin by defining and clarifying some health-related terminology. We then look at health issues in a multicultural society, representative approaches to the process of behavior change, and various ideas about health that have been prevalent in U.S. society over time. We end with an exploration of the challenges to maintaining good health that face you as an individual and society as a whole.

UNDERSTANDING HEALTH TERMS

People have different definitions of health. Even health professionals find it difficult to agree on a single definition. In this section we consider the meanings of the term *health* and the related concept *wellness*, along with the ideas of disease prevention, health promotion, personal health, and community health.

Health and Wellness

Traditionally, people have been considered healthy if they do not have symptoms of disease. In 1947, however, the World Health Organization (WHO) defined **health** as a state of complete physical, mental, and social well-being, not merely the absence of disease and infirmity. Physical health refers to the biological integrity of the individual. Mental health includes emotional and intellectual capabilities, or the individual's subjective sense of well-being.

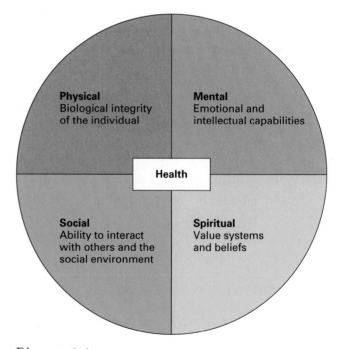

Figure 1.1   Components of health: the World Health Organization definition.

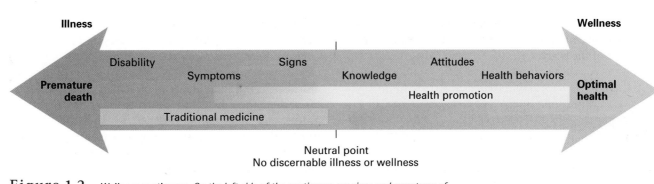

Figure 1.2   **Wellness continuum.** *On the left side of the continuum are signs and symptoms of illness and disability. On the right side are knowledge, attitudes, and behaviors that contribute to wellness.*

Source: Adapted from "Definition of Health Promotion," by M. P. O'Donnell, 1986, *American Journal of Health Promotion, 1* (1), Premier Issue. Used by permission of *American Journal of Health Promotion*.

Social health means the ability of people to interact effectively with other people and the social environment.[1]

More recently, a spiritual domain has been added to the WHO definition, reflecting the idea that people's value systems or beliefs can have an impact on their overall health. Spiritual health does not require participation in a particular organized religion but suggests a belief in (or a searching for) some type of greater or higher power that gives meaning and purpose to life. Spiritual health involves a connectedness to self, to significant others, and to the community. Figure 1.1 illustrates the components of health in the WHO definition.

Similar to this definition of health is the concept of **wellness,** which is generally defined as the process of adopting patterns of behavior that can lead to improved health and heightened life satisfaction. Although some aspects of your health are affected by factors beyond your control (such as your age, your sex, and your genes), wellness is considered to be primarily determined by the decisions you make about how to live your life. Just as several domains are included in the WHO definition of health, several dimensions are identified in the concept of wellness: physical, emotional, intellectual, spiritual, interpersonal or social, and environmental. (Some definitions also include occupational health as one of the dimensions of wellness.) A person who lacks physical symptoms of illness but who is bored, depressed, anxious, or unhappy has not achieved wellness.

Wellness may be conceptualized as a continuum (Figure 1.2). One end of the continuum represents extreme illness and premature death; the other end represents optimal health or well-being. Historically, Western medicine has focused primarily on the illness side of the continuum, treating people with symptoms of disease. This approach to medicine is referred to as *allopathic,* meaning that it attempts to treat disease with remedies that produce effects different from those caused by the disease itself. The use of drugs to cure illnesses is an example. When an individual reaches the midpoint of the continuum, representing a state in which no symptoms of disease are present, traditional Western medicine has few tools to help this individual reach a state of wellness, or optimal well-being. More recently, approaches to health have focused on the wellness side of the continuum, seeking ways to help people live their lives fully, as whole people, with vitality and meaning.[2]

Holistic Health

Wellness is similar to **holistic health,** and the two terms are sometimes used interchangeably. *Holism,* from the Greek word *holos,* means whole (person). Holistic health is also conceptualized as having several domains: physical, mental, emotional, and spiritual. When there is health in each domain, the whole person is healthy, whereas illness in any one area creates stress in the other areas.[3]

To understand holistic health better, consider the analogy of a triangle. A triangle is defined as having three sides; it does not exist if any of the three sides is missing. Similarly, if any of the domains of holistic health is missing or impaired, the person is no longer whole. Note that in traditional Western medicine, if the body seems to be in reasonably good operating condition, we assume that all is well. In holistic health, this is not the case. If the mind or the spirit is disturbed, before long the body will be affected. In many non-Western cultures, including many

KEY TERMS

health   State of complete physical, mental, social, and spiritual well-being.

wellness   Process of adopting patterns of behavior that can lead to improved health and heightened life satisfaction; wellness has several domains and can be conceptualized as a continuum.

holistic health   Health of the whole person, including physical, mental, emotional, and spiritual domains.

ethnic minority cultures represented in the United States, there is more emphasis on holistic health and not just on the health of the body.

Self-Care

A concept implicit in wellness is **self-care,** usually defined as actions taken by individuals on behalf of their own health. People are practicing self-care when they observe their own symptoms (physical, mental, or emotional), gather information and advice, make informed decisions about a course of action, and then either treat themselves or seek professional care. People practice self-care every day, whether it means putting ice on a strained muscle, taking a decongestant for a cold, doing relaxation exercises for stress, or seeking support from a clergyperson for a personal problem. Medical self-care—treating a physical problem like a headache—is sometimes distinguished from health self-care—taking action to maintain and improve health with activities related to high-level wellness.[1] Medical symptoms are experienced quite frequently—on average, individuals are faced with some symptoms of medical problems 1 out of every 3 days. Symptoms suggesting that high-level wellness has not been reached may be more subtle—for example, a person may have a low energy level or experience feelings of meaninglessness—but they may be even more pervasive than symptoms of medical problems.

In American society, adults are generally expected to be self-reliant and responsible for their own health, that is, to practice self-care. This expectation, however, assumes that all individuals have the knowledge, resources, and motivation to make and apply informed choices about health and lifestyle. It further assumes that health care resources are distributed equally across socioeconomic and cultural lines and that the values, norms, and practices of individuals match those of the mainstream culture and its health care practitioners.[1] As we will see throughout this book, these expectations and assumptions are not necessarily justified.

Disease Prevention and Health Promotion

Both disease prevention and health promotion are often thought of as activities that occur on the community or societal level, in association with programs, services, and policies, rather than as the result of personal actions. **Disease prevention** may be defined as health-protecting behaviors directed toward decreasing the probability of encountering illness. Examples of such behaviors include administering flu shots to a specific population segment, such as older adults; conducting a public health campaign to educate the public about HIV infection; removing a precancerous skin lesion before it becomes cancerous; and giving medication to someone with hypertension (high blood pressure) to prevent the development of cardiovascular disease.

Whereas disease prevention focuses on defensive actions taken to ward off specific diseases and their consequences, **health promotion** focuses on actions designed to maintain a current healthy state or advance to a more desirable state.[4] Individuals are practicing health promotion when they take time out of a busy day for a 30-minute jog or an appointment with their health care provider for a routine screening test. Communities are practicing health promotion when they build the jogging path or publicize recommendations for screening tests. Community health promotion is discussed more fully in the next section. In its broadest sense, health promotion may be conceptualized as drawing together the ideas of health, wellness, holistic health, self-care, and disease prevention.[4]

Personal Health and Community Health

Personal health refers to the actions you take and the decisions you make that affect your own individual health (and, possibly, the health of your immediate family members). It involves the lifestyle choices you make concerning your physical, mental, emotional, spiritual, and social well-being—what you eat, how much exercise you get, whether you spend time developing meaningful relationships, and so on. Over your life span, you accumulate knowledge, health beliefs, values, attitudes, and habits that shape your personal health. At the same time, as suggested earlier, there are some aspects of your personal health that you cannot control, such as your human biology (your age, sex, progression through predictable life stages and transitions, and so on), your individual genetic inheritance, and aspects of your environment. You have to take all of these factors into account when trying to understand and enhance your personal health.

Community health, in contrast, includes issues, events, and activities related to the health of a whole population or a community. Many health benefits can be attained only through the collective action of a community. **Community health promotion** refers to activities directed toward bettering the health of the public and/or activities employing resources available in common to members of the community.[5] For example, a community may decide to create bike lanes on public streets to protect cyclists, encourage people to be more physically active, and cut down on traffic and air pollution. A community may support the creation of a health clinic or a treatment center within its boundaries, or it may require builders to include green space or parks in their construction plans. The ideas of community health and community health promotion extend beyond the traditional relationship between an individual and a health care professional to involve a host of agencies, organizations, and institutions working to enhance people's health.[6] Health promotion programs can be implemented in communities through a wide range of settings (home, school, worksite, health care

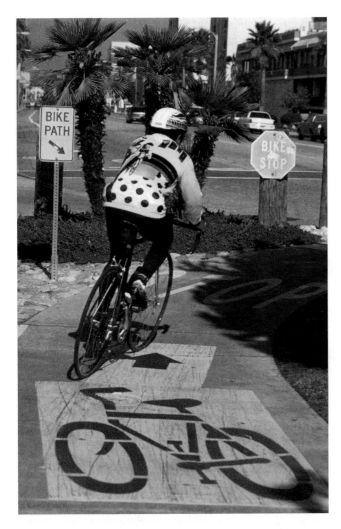

Many communities are incorporating health promotion into city planning. Having bike paths that allow people to bicycle safely to work, stores, and other locations is one example of engineering for better health.

facilities); by a wide range of techniques (health education, environmental controls, health programs); and under the auspices of a wide array of sponsors (businesses, labor unions, voluntary agencies, hospitals, public schools, self-care groups).[7]

The health and well-being of different communities can vary, depending on political, socioeconomic, and cultural factors. One community may enact a bicycle helmet law, for example, and subsequently see a reduction in head injuries and use of emergency medical services. Another community may decline to pass such a law because citizens view it as an infringement of individual rights. One community may be able to prevent the location of a toxic waste dump within its boundaries through grassroots activism and political lobbying. Another community, with a lower level of political influence or socioeconomic power, may not be able to protect itself from such environmental hazards. Clearly, a person living near a toxic dump, in a community with high levels of pollution, or in a dangerous neighborhood is not going to have the opportunity to attain the same level of wellness as someone living in a safer, healthier environment, no matter what lifestyle decisions the person makes. In other words, personal health exists within the context of community health.[6]

HEALTH IN A MULTICULTURAL SOCIETY

As a nation of immigrants, the United States has always had a diverse population. As the 21st century unfolds, the U.S. population is rapidly becoming more diverse. According to the 2000 U.S. Census, approximately 30 percent of the population currently belongs to a racial or ethnic minority group.[8] This percentage is expected to increase to 50 percent by 2050. The primary minority groups in the United States, again according the U.S. Census Bureau, are African Americans (or Black Americans), Hispanic Americans, Native Americans, Asian Americans, and Pacific Islanders.[9] There is tremendous diversity within each of these groups as well: Asian Americans, for example, include people from China, Japan, Korea, Vietnam, Laos, Cambodia, the Philippines, and other countries. (Note that diversity also refers to differences among people in age, sexual orientation, ability or disability, educational attainment, socioeconomic status, geographic location, and other characteristics.)

KEY TERMS

self-care Actions taken by individuals on behalf of their own health with respect to medical care and health care.

disease prevention Health-protecting behaviors directed toward decreasing the probability of encountering illness by active protection of the body against unnecessary stressors or by detection of illness at an early stage.

health promotion Actions designed to maintain a current healthy state or advance to a more desirable state; a guiding framework that draws together the concepts of wellness, self-care, holistic health, and disease prevention.

personal health Actions and decisions of a person that affect his or her health and possibly that of immediate family members.

community health Issues, events, and activities related to the health of a whole population or community.

community health promotion Activities directed toward bettering the health of the public and/or activities employing resources available in common to members of the community.

In this section, we consider, first, what terms such as *culture* and *ethnicity* mean and, second, what the implications are for minority populations in the United States when it comes to issues related to both personal and community health.

Understanding Cultural Terms

There are many different meanings of the term *culture,* but here the term is used in a sense articulated for a health promotion context.[10] According to this view, a **culture** is defined by five basic criteria: (1) a common language or common patterns of communication; (2) similarities in dietary practices; (3) common patterns of dress; (4) predictable socialization and relationship patterns; and (5) a common set of shared values and beliefs. As you can see in this definition, cultures help clarify acceptable and unacceptable behaviors, including health-related behaviors, in any given society.

Ethnicity refers to the sense of identity individuals draw from a common ancestry, as well as from a common national, religious, tribal, language, or cultural origin. This identity nurtures a sense of social belonging and loyalty for people of common ethnicity. It helps shape how a person thinks, relates, feels, and behaves within or outside an ethnic group. Ethnicity is often confused with **race,** a term used to describe ethnic groups based on physical characteristics, such as skin color or facial features. Although classifying people by race has been convenient for social scientists, the fact is that biologically separate and distinct races do not exist within the human species. Genetic traits are inherited individually, not in clumps, groups, or "races." Thus, it is more accurate to think of similarities and differences among people as a matter of culture or ethnicity.

In the United States we see many levels of **acculturation,** the degree to which an individual gives up the traits of one culture and adopts those of the dominant culture. In one ethnic group, or even in one family, some individuals cling to most if not all of the traits of their culture of origin; some learn to function well within both their own culture and the dominant culture (and are referred to as *bicultural*); and still others give up most of the traits of their culture of origin and adopt traits from the dominant culture (referred to as *acculturated*). Immigrants who come to the United States as adults or older adults may be more likely to retain their traditional practices; children and first-generation Americans may be more likely to be bicultural or acculturated.

Degree of acculturation, in addition to ethnic origin in general, can be a significant factor in personal health in the United States. Many people have a natural tendency to resist acculturation, holding on to traditional beliefs and rejecting mainstream health beliefs and practices. Miscommunication and misunderstanding pose significant

challenges to the promotion of healthy lifestyles among ethnic populations. In some cases, individuals may not understand or adopt behaviors that would clearly be beneficial to them, such as taking medications according to directions. In other cases, U.S. health care practitioners may misunderstand or dismiss practices that are health enhancing in another culture, such as the participation and support of the entire extended family in medical decisions and treatments. Often, the bicultural or acculturated members of an ethnic group mediate between their parents or community elders and the health care profession.

When misunderstandings occur between members of ethnic minority groups and health care practitioners, people on both sides may be guilty of **ethnocentrism,** the assumption that the beliefs and practices of one's own culture are true and correct. Standing in contrast to ethnocentrism is **ethnosensitivity,** an openness to and respect for cultural and ethnic differences in values, customs, and practices. Ethnosensitivity requires knowledge and understanding of other cultures, but it also requires awareness of one's own biases, prejudices, and stereotypes of other groups.[10]

Cultural Differences in Concepts of Illness and Health

One common and significant health-related belief in many non-Western cultures is that illness may result from an imbalance within a person or from an unbalanced or improper relationship between a person and his or her family, community, environment, or spiritual world. For example, disease may be perceived as retribution for angering a spirit by defying a family role or social custom, and a cure may involve appealing to ancestral spirits or deities who can intercede in human life. Such a view is incompatible with the Western, allopathic medical model, which is based on the idea that illness and disease are caused by organic changes in the body or by pathogens like bacteria and viruses. In the allopathic model, health care is provided by medical specialists who use drugs, vaccines, and surgery to treat and cure illness.

Although these differences are profound, some common ground exists between the two models, and in recent years Western medicine has looked with more interest at the possibility that such factors as social support, interpersonal relationships, mind-body connections, and spiritual health play some role in health and illness. This interest has led to the growing emphasis on wellness and holistic health in Western medicine, as mentioned earlier. Complementary and alternative approaches to medicine are now well known in the United States and include acupuncture, chiropractic, therapeutic massage, relaxation techniques, herbal remedies, and many other practices. The term *complementary* is used to indicate that these practices can work with Western medical practices in some cases but shouldn't supplant Western practices that have proved successful, such as using vaccines to prevent polio and smallpox, antibiotics to treat sexually transmitted infections, and surgery to remove tumors. In addition, both Western and non-Western approaches encourage individuals to adopt lifestyles that help prevent disease and promote health.

Health Concerns of Ethnic Minority Populations

Over the past 100 years, advances in medical technology, lifestyle improvements, and environmental protections have produced significant health gains for the general U.S. population. These advances, however, have not produced equal health benefits for most of the country's ethnic minority populations.[11] Morbidity and mortality rates for ethnic minority populations are disheartening. Many have higher rates of cancer, diabetes, cardiovascular disease, infant mortality, alcoholism, drug abuse, unintentional injury, and premature death than the general population does. Most also have significantly higher lifestyle risk factors, such as high-fat diets, lack of exercise, and exposure to carcinogens and other environmental toxins.

Many health problems faced by ethnic minority populations are due not to race or ethnicity but to social and economic conditions, including poverty, discrimination, and limited access to health information and resources. Reducing the health disparities that exist among different cultural and ethnic populations in the United States is a critical challenge facing society in the 21st century. Meeting this challenge will require sensitivity to and respect for the many unique cultural traditions and practices that characterize our multicultural society.[10]

MAKING HEALTH CHOICES

At the beginning of this chapter, we mentioned that even when individuals know which lifestyle choices are better for them, they often fail to make those choices. (To evaluate some of your own lifestyle behaviors, see Part 1 of the Add It Up! feature at the end of this chapter.) For example, it is nearly impossible to live in the United States and not know that smoking is bad for your health, yet millions of Americans continue to smoke. Why do people make poor choices and persist in them in the face of overwhelming evidence that their choices are incompatible with good health, a high level of wellness, and a long, vital life?

Psychologists have proposed many theory-based models for health behavior choices and change. A major assumption underlying most of these models is that people usually gravitate toward unhealthy lifestyles.

According to this assumption, most illnesses and cases of premature death are caused by unhealthy habits that people freely choose for themselves. If this is the case, then the challenge is to find ways to motivate people to change their habits and to help them overcome obstacles to change. The question is, What does it take to motivate people to change?

In this section we examine two of the more popular theories of health behavior change, the Health Belief Model and the Transtheoretical Model. We then examine some of the health behavior change strategies that have evolved from behavior change theories.

The Health Belief Model

In the 1950s, the **Health Belief Model (HBM)** was developed in an effort to understand why people failed to take advantage of disease prevention or detection programs that were accessible and low cost, such as screening for tuberculosis.[12] The model was subsequently expanded and applied to a wide range of health behaviors, including smoking, exercising, using seat belts, using sunscreen, drinking and driving, changing sexual behavior to avoid HIV infection, and many others.

KEY TERMS

culture A group's shared, distinctive pattern of living, defined by a common language, similarities in dietary practices, common patterns of dress, predictable socialization and relationship patterns, and a common set of shared values and beliefs. (Note that many other definitions of culture exist.)

ethnicity The sense of identity an individual draws from a common ancestry and/or a common national, religious, tribal, language, or cultural origin.

race Term used in the social sciences to describe ethnic groups based on physical characteristics, such as skin color or facial features; race does not exist as a biological reality.

acculturation Degree to which an individual gives up the traits of a culture of origin and adopts the traits of a dominant culture.

ethnocentrism Assumption that the beliefs and practices of one's own culture are true and correct.

ethnosensitivity Openness to and respect for cultural and ethnic differences in values, customs, and practices.

Health Belief Model (HBM) Model of behavior change that uses the constructs of health concerns, perceived threat, perceived benefits, and perceived barriers.

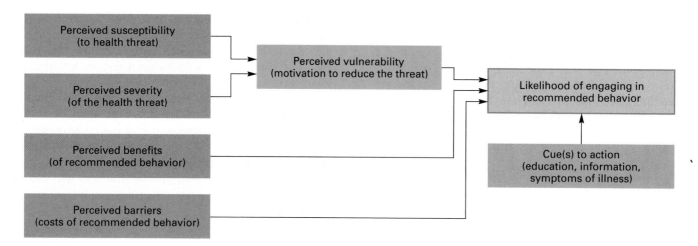

Figure 1.3   **Classic representation of the Health Belief Model.** Source: Adapted from "The Health Belief Model," by V. J. Strecher and I. M. Rosenstock, 2002, in *Health Behavior and Health Education* (3rd ed.), eds. K. Glanz, B. K. Rimer, and F. M. Lewis, San Francisco: Jossey-Bass.

According to the Health Belief Model illustrated in Figure 1.3, health behaviors are influenced by three classes of factors:

- *Health concern.* Does the individual have sufficient motivation to make health change a relevant issue?

- *Perceived threat.* Does the individual have a feeling of susceptibility to a health problem, and is the problem regarded as serious?

- *Perceived benefits and perceived barriers.* Does the individual believe that benefits will be gained from reducing the perceived threat and that these benefits will be gained at a subjectively acceptable level of personal cost?[13]

As an example, let's consider a female college student who has a sedentary lifestyle. After taking a personal health course (a *cue for action*), she starts to think about becoming more physically active. From her health course, she learned about many of the health problems associated with a physically inactive lifestyle, such as overweight, cardiovascular disease, and diabetes (*perceived threat*). She also learned that a physically active lifestyle can decrease her vulnerability to certain health problems and provide many health benefits, such as a more easily maintained body weight and a feeling of well-being (*perceived benefits*). However, she must also overcome the perceived barriers to exercise, which might include a busy schedule, a lack of information about available resources and facilities, and a set of friends who also don't exercise. According to the Health Belief Model, if she believes that she is susceptible to the threat, that the threat is serious, that the benefits outweigh the costs, and that she will be able to overcome the barriers, she is more likely to adopt a physically active lifestyle. Her decision-making process is also influenced by a host of other factors and variables, such as her personal and family background, her personality, her sense of self-responsibility,

and the actual availability of appropriate resources like jogging paths or swimming pools.

The Transtheoretical Model

Although the HBM has been one of the most frequently used models, the motivation to reduce a threat does not fully explain why a person chooses to engage or not engage in a selected behavior. When the HBM has been used as an intervention tool, the results have generally been disappointing.[14] The **Transtheoretical Model (TTM),** developed in the 1990s, has become a more useful and accepted framework for understanding health behavior change. The TTM is based on four core constructs: (1) stages of change, (2) decision balance, (3) self-efficacy, and (4) situational temptation.

Stages of Change

In this model, behavior change is seen as a transitional process that occurs in a five-stage cycle:

- *Precontemplation.* The individual has no motivation to change.

- *Contemplation.* The individual is thinking about changing a specific health behavior and intends to change it within the next six months.

- *Preparation.* The individual is planning on changing a health behavior in the immediate future, usually the next month.

- *Action.* The individual is implementing a change in health behavior and has been doing so for up to six months.

- *Maintenance.* The new behavior has been in place for more than six months.

A sixth stage, termination, occurs for some types of health behavior change, when the behavior is firmly entrenched

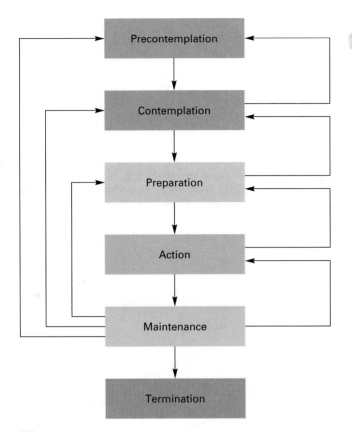

Figure 1.4   Stages of change: the Transtheoretical Model.

Source: Adapted from "The Transtheoretical Model and Stages of Change," by J. O. Prochaska, C. O. Redding, and K. E. Evers, 2002, in *Health Behavior and Health Education* (3rd ed.), eds. K. Glanz, B. K. Rimer, and F. M. Lewis, San Francisco: Jossey-Bass.

as a part of a person's lifestyle and there is zero temptation to return to the old behavior. For some types of health problems, such as alcohol addiction, few people may reach termination. The stages of change are shown in Figure 1.4. The arrows indicate how an individual moves back and forth between the stages until maintenance or termination is reached.

Several activities, or *processes of change*, have been identified as key elements of health behavior change. These processes include raising awareness about the health behavior, experiencing the negative emotions associated with the risk of not changing the behavior, developing social support systems, establishing goals and rewards, learning alternative health-related behaviors, and developing a new self-image, among others. These processes of change help people to move through the stages of change.[12]

Decision Balance

The second construct in the TTM is decision balance. People use a decision balance of pros and cons as they navigate the specific stages of change. Decisions are based on relative importance (pro) or unimportance (con) of the behavior change. Typically, con decisions are more evident in the early stages of healthy behavior change and

decrease in later stages. Pro decisions tend to be low in early stages and increase in the later stages.[13] For example, starting an exercise program might leave less time for watching TV and going out with friends (con) but might leave a person feeling better and more able to participate in sports and recreational activities (pro). In the long term, it will decrease the risk of heart disease, stroke, cancer, and premature death (pro). As long as the pros outweigh the cons, according to this view, the healthy behavior change is likely to remain in place.

Self-Efficacy

The third construct in the TTM is **self-efficacy,** adopted from the self-efficacy theory of psychologist Albert Bandura and defined as an internal state in which the person feels competent to perform a specific task. These competency feelings are called *efficacy expectations.* A person who has no trouble maintaining a healthy weight has efficacy expectations for this specific health behavior. To successfully change a behavior, he or she must have efficacy expectations about making that change. However, a sense of self-efficacy is not enough for behavior change to occur. The person must also believe that the benefits of change are of sufficient importance to balance the costs.[14] A person may have a sense of self-efficacy but still engage in an unhealthy behavior (for example, smoking cigarettes) because the outcome expectations (health risks) are not personally important at this time.

Situational Temptation

The fourth construct in the TTM is situational temptation, which occurs at each stage of change. Situational temptation decreases as the person moves from the early to later stages of change, but lapses (single slip-ups) or relapses (overall breakdown in behavior patterns) may still occur even in the maintenance stage. People are often encouraged to develop relapse prevention strategies by identifying triggers that are likely to cause relapse and practicing how they will respond. Common triggers are experiencing negative emotions, such as anger or sadness, and participating in positive social events, such as parties or celebrations. Coping skills are essential for health behaviors that are especially vulnerable to relapse.[14] Strategies and skills to deal with relapse are discussed further in the next section.

KEY TERMS

Transtheoretical Model (TTM)   Model of behavior change that uses the constructs of stages of change, decision balance, self-efficacy, and situational temptation.

self-efficacy   Internal state in which the person feels competent to perform a specific task.

Strategies for Health Behavior Change

From the health behavior change models just described, along with others, strategies have been developed to help build motivation to change. In this section we describe seven representative strategies that are used both by individuals and by programs and organizations whose goal is to facilitate behavior change.

Assessing Readiness to Change

If a person is not ready to change, undertaking a health behavior change program is pointless and even counterproductive; failure and discouragement are the likely outcomes. For this reason, a person's readiness for change needs to be assessed at the outset, and numerous assessment tools are available for this purpose. (A simple test of your own readiness for change is provided in the box "Assessing Your Stage of Change.") These tools are often coupled with a "decision balance scale" that asks the person to respond to a series of pro and con statements that apply to a given health behavior or to ask such questions as, Have you considered how your current lifestyle is affecting your health today and how it will affect your health in the future? What are the costs and benefits, short term and long term, of continuing your current health habits? Although some people can be motivated by the long-term benefits of health behavior change, such as avoiding a disease that may threaten them in 30 years, most people are more likely to be motivated by short-term benefits, such as feeling better, looking better, or increasing self-esteem.

Framing Health Messages

The HBM assumes that the likelihood of change depends on perceived benefits outweighing perceived barriers. For this reason, most health messages are framed in positive language, focusing on the benefits of change. Some messages, however, employ *gain-frame* language, which presents what a person may lose (years of life, relationships, vitality) if he or she does not adopt a given health behavior. A third type of message, using *fear appeal* language, is sometimes used to create tension designed to scare a person into changing health behavior. These scare-mongering messages are rarely successful.[14] Thus, when individuals are framing health messages to themselves to maintain or increase their motivation for change, they are more likely to be successful if they focus on the positive aspects of behavior change.

Signing a Behavior Change Contract

The most important factor influencing health behavior change is commitment to change.[14] Behavior change contracts are used to solidify commitments. Most people take a signed contract more seriously than a vague notion of "getting more exercise" or "eating less sugar." A behavior change contract is more effective if it includes short- and long-term goals, time lines, specific strategies, and,

possibly, incentives. Goals must be clearly defined, measurable, and realistic. Many people have someone sign their contract as a witness to increase their sense of commitment. Signing a behavior change contract is one of the most effective strategies for change. An example of a behavior change contract is provided in Part 2 of the Add It Up! feature at the end of this chapter.

Structuring Rewards

Another strategy for behavior change is to create incentives to support positive changes and disincentives to discourage lapses. Particularly when a goal is long term, it is useful to have rewards for short-term goals reached along the way. Individuals might reward themselves with some treat that particularly appeals to them (buying a new CD, going to a movie). More formal programs use incentives like monetary rewards, fee reductions, and public recognition. Individuals and programs sometimes also use disincentives, or *response costs*. For example, a person who fails to maintain a behavior or reach a goal might have to make a money payment. The use of incentives and disincentives to motivate change are highlighted in the You Make the Call activity at the end of this chapter.

Using Social Support

A basic assumption of most behavior change models is that people are more likely to commit to change a health behavior or maintain successful change if other people encourage them to do so. Significant others (family, friends, coworkers) are especially important in providing this social support. The use of buddy systems is an example of social support. For example, if you have a jogging partner, you're much more likely to go out every day, even in bad weather, than if you have to motivate yourself.[14]

Developing Self-Efficacy

As noted earlier, self-efficacy refers to an individual's confidence in his or her ability to take action and perform a specific task, despite any anxieties that may accompany change. Research has shown that self-efficacy can be developed in four ways: (1) mastery of a task, (2) vicarious experience acquired by observing the performance of others, (3) social persuasion from others, and (4) changing one's emotional state or reinterpreting it in a positive way.[14] Let's say that a young man wants to overcome feelings of shyness in social situations and needs to develop confidence that he can do so. His feelings of self-efficacy would increase if he was able to interact successfully in one or a few social situations (mastery of the task); if he noticed that other young men whom he knew to be shy were able to interact successfully (vicarious experience); if his friends persuaded him that he did not appear to be shy or that he would certainly be able to interact successfully (social persuasion); or if he was able to reduce his feelings of anxiety or reinterpret them as excitement (changing

Challenges & Choices

Assessing Your Stage of Change

Responding to four simple statements can help determine your readiness for behavior change as well as your stage of change for a chosen health behavior. First, choose a health area in which you think there might be room for improvement or a specific health behavior that you think you might like to change. Then answer yes or no to the following questions:

_____ 1. I solved my problem more than six months ago.

_____ 2. I have taken action on my problem within the past six months.

_____ 3. I am intending to take action in the next month.

_____ 4. I am intending to take action in the next six months.

Scoring: Answering no for all four statements means you are in the precontemplation stage. If you answered yes to statement 4 and no to the other three statements,

you are in the contemplation stage. If you answered yes to statements 3 and 4 and no to statements 1 and 2, you are in the action stage. If you answered yes to statement 2 and no to statement 1, you are in the action stage. A yes answer to statement 1 means you are in the maintenance or, possibly, the termination stage.

It's Not Just Personal . . .

Most of the leading causes of death in the United States and Canada, including heart disease, cancer, stroke, and diabetes, are considered preventable, at least in part, through lifestyle change. The lifestyle factors most frequently implicated in these diseases are diet, smoking, excessive alcohol consumption, and a sedentary lifestyle.

Source: Adapted from *Changing for Good: The Revolutionary Program That Exhibits Six Stages of Change and Shows You How to Free Yourself from Bad Habits*, by J. O. Prochaska, et al., 1994, New York: William Morrow.

one's emotional state). People can also boost their sense of self-efficacy by using specific strategies, such as practicing positive self-talk, visualizing success, and focusing on developing an internal *locus of control*—a belief that they are in control of their own lives.

Preventing Relapse

Relapse is a possibility after any behavior change. When relapse occurs, individuals need strategies to prevent feelings of loss of control. One useful approach is to be forgiving, rather than condemning, and to regard the lapse as a one-time event. In more formal settings, health promotion practitioners sometimes use programmed lapses to prepare a person for relapse situations associated with a given health behavior. The person is intentionally exposed to situations that cause a lapse and then uses self-management skills to prevent the lapse from becoming a full-blown relapse. Programmed lapses have a high risk of backfiring; therefore, they should be employed only in selective situations and under the supervision of a health professional.[14]

Limits of Health Behavior Change Theories

Behavior change theories focus on what is going on in the person's mind rather than on an interaction between the person and the environment. Although valuable, the behavior change approach does not take into account health

factors beyond the control of the individual, including genetic factors as well as socioeconomic, political, and cultural factors. In some cases, this approach can lead to a victim-blaming mentality; that is, if we assert that individuals are responsible for their own health, then we might conclude that any illness they experience is in some way their own fault. Although it is true that individuals have control over many aspects of their own health, and it is empowering for individuals to believe that this is so, there are limitations to this way of thinking.[15] Consider the two examples of poverty and racial inequality.

Poverty in and of itself is a significant risk factor for illness and premature death. One study found that an affluent person who is a heavy smoker is less likely to contract cancer than a poor person who is a heavy smoker.[15] Why? Although we could suggest a number of possible reasons—the more affluent person may have fewer other risk factors than the poorer person, for example—many researchers believe that people of progressively lower socioeconomic status have correspondingly less control over factors that affect their lives. Whether perceived or actual, the notion of control appears to significantly influence health. No matter what the mechanism, however, poverty is a factor that is largely beyond the individual's control.

Racial inequality is another factor that significantly affects health. Even after controlling for education and work experience, African Americans are exposed to more occupational and environmental hazards than whites are. For example, incinerators are placed in the neighborhoods of people of color at a rate 89 percent above the national average. Pollutants from incinerators may expose nearby residents to cancer-causing agents. Like poverty, racial inequality is largely beyond the individual's control. The implications of poverty and racial inequality as significant factors affecting health behavior choices and outcomes are troubling.[15]

Clearly, the well-being of the individual depends on both self-responsibility and a supportive culture. Supportive cultures use systematic cultural change programs that analyze health problems, set goals, develop leadership commitment, include results-oriented short- and long-term evaluation, and embrace citizen participation. A culture that is supportive of good health might, for example, have effective antismoking campaigns in place, provide young people with the information they need to make responsible decisions about sex, and ensure that people of all socioeconomic levels have access to affordable, high-quality health care. Without cultural support, it is difficult if not impossible for the individual to reach optimal wellness.[16]

HEALTH CHALLENGES IN A CHANGING SOCIETY

We are inundated with health-related information, some reliable and some not. We are immersed in a culture that overwhelms us with unhealthy but attractive options at every turn. We are confronted with perplexing ethical, social, and political issues in association with the concept of health promotion. How do we meet these challenges? This section addresses this question, but first let's consider briefly how our current ideas about health developed.

Understanding How We Got Here

We can gain a valuable perspective on ideas about health by considering the context in which our current thinking arose. Some of the ideas we have been discussing—health and wellness, personal health and community health—extend back to ancient Greece, where two contrasting views coexisted. One view, symbolized by the goddess Hygeia (from whose name we get the word *hygiene,* meaning conditions that are conducive to health), held that individuals attained health by living in harmony with the laws of nature and the environment. The other view, symbolized by the deified physician Asclepias, held that illness, disability, and premature death could be limited by human intervention, typically by people trained in medicine. Since then, the two views have surfaced and resurfaced in a kind of cyclic pattern. The first view is akin to the idea that health involves living in a healthy relationship with the environment; the second sees health as something to be restored to the individual by medical intervention.

Public Health Approach vs. Medical Intervention Approach

In the 19th and early 20th centuries in Europe and the United States, during what is called the public health era, the focus was more on the environment. Infectious diseases, the major killers in those days, were brought under control by public health efforts, including improved sanitation systems, pure water supplies, food refrigeration and pasteurization, better food delivery and distribution systems, and health education campaigns. In the early to mid-20th century, with the discovery and subsequent widespread use of antibiotics, the pendulum began to swing toward medical intervention. Improvements in health during most of the 20th century came not so much from public health measures as from medical interventions in the forms of vaccines, drugs, and surgery. This allopathic model has dominated our health care system since the 1920s.

With infectious diseases brought under control by the combination of public health measures and medical interventions, a new pattern of disease became apparent at mid-century: Chronic, degenerative illnesses such as cardiovascular disease, stroke, and cancer began to emerge as the leading causes of death. Partly in response to this trend, the health promotion movement took hold in the 1970s as a complement to allopathic medicine. Attention shifted to preventing degenerative conditions by encouraging people to adopt healthier behaviors early in life and to take personal responsibility for their health. The concepts of wellness and holistic health, as described earlier in this chapter, emerged—or reemerged—as people again began to think of health as a harmonious balance between the individual and the environment and a multidimensional construct involving physical, emotional, spiritual, and other domains.

As pointed out throughout this chapter, however, healthy behavior change on the personal level can be attained only in the framework of supportive social environments. Attempts to place responsibility for health solely on the individual have not been successful. For example, Canada implemented an action framework that emphasized individual responsibility following the publication of the Healthy Canadian Report in 1974. This plan failed miserably. In the mid-1980s, Canada restructured its plan to place a broader emphasis on social responsibility. As just one example, Canadian legislation focused directly on tobacco. Public policies and laws were passed to create smoke-free workplaces, restrictions on tobacco advertising, and bans on tobacco sponsorship of cultural and sporting events. These efforts have been more successful in promoting smoking cessation in Canada.[15]

Healthy People Initiative

The Canadian restructuring of its health plan influenced the United States in the development of its Healthy People initiative, which sets national health objectives aimed at

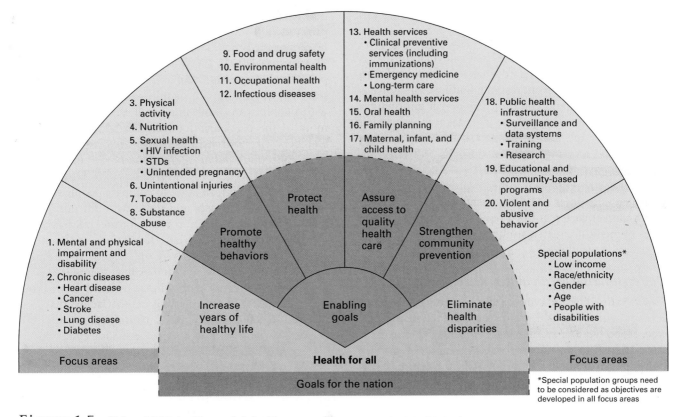

Figure 1.5   Vision of 2010: healthy people in healthy communities. Source: From *Developing Objectives for Healthy People 2010*, Washington, DC, Department of Health and Human Services, Office of Disease Prevention and Health Promotion, 1997.

improving the quality of life for all Americans.[15] The U.S. government issued the first Healthy People report in 1980 and has issued revised reports every 10 years since. The reports include broad community health goals as well as targets for improvement in individual actions, such as using safety belts in motor vehicles, engaging in regular physical activity, and maintaining a healthy weight.

The current Healthy People report, Healthy People 2010, sets two broad goals: (1) helping individuals of all ages increase life expectancy and improve their quality of life and (2) eliminating health disparities among different segments of the population (Figure 1.5). The report also reflects the growing awareness of the importance of community involvement in health issues. Most of the earlier health promotion initiatives in the United States focused primarily on personal behavioral change. Sparse attention was paid to what public health experts call "community response-ability," the ability of individuals and the community to unite to respond both to personal needs and to challenges presented by the social and political environments.[15] Community response-ability is an underlying idea in Healthy People 2010.[17] Because of the focus on both individual and societal responsibility in this book, we include examples of Healthy People objectives in every chapter, in the boxes titled "Healthy People 2010."

Healthy People 2010

OBJECTIVE AREA *Health Communication*

- Improve the health literacy of persons with inadequate or marginal literacy skills.

"Approximately 90 million adults in the United States have inadequate or marginal literacy skills. . . . Closing the gap in health literacy is an issue of fundamental fairness and equity and is essential to reduce health disparities. . . . The knowledge exists to create effective, culturally and linguistically appropriate, plain language health communications. . . . If appropriate materials exist and people receive the training to use them, then measurable improvements in health literacy for the least literate can occur."

 For more information on Healthy People 2010 objectives, visit the Web site at www.healthypeople.gov.

 For information on Canadian health objectives, visit the Health Canada Web site at www.hc-sc.gc.ca/english.

Being an Informed Consumer

A dramatic feature of 21st century society is the overwhelming amount of health-related information that is available in the media. Every day we are bombarded with news stories about current research findings, sales pitches for miracle cures, and contradictory health information about foods to avoid, supplements to take, and screening tests to have done. Part of taking responsibility for your own health is learning how to evaluate this information, sorting the reputable and credible from the disreputable and unsubstantiated—in other words, becoming an informed consumer. Your successful navigation of the health marketplace requires a basic understanding of the types of medical research studies and savvy use of health information technology.

Understanding Medical Research Studies

Scientists use different types of research studies to explore and confirm relationships between risk factors and disease. Some types of studies suggest correlations or likely associations but do not establish cause-and-effect relationships. An example is *cohort studies,* in which groups of

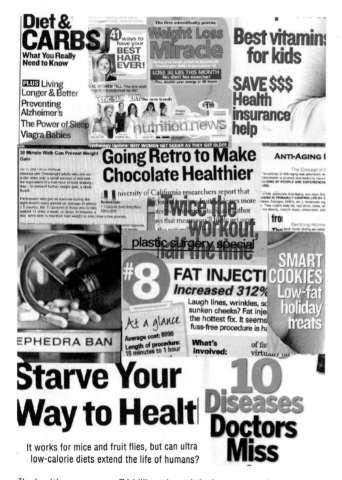

The health messages on TV, billboards, and the Internet may be dramatized, overstated, misleading, and contradictory. Evaluating these messages to distinguish fact from fiction is key to achieving health literacy.

people are studied over time, either retrospectively or prospectively. In *retrospective studies,* people are asked to recall specific behaviors from their past, such as whether they included in their diet a particular food that is hypothesized to provide protection from cancer. The researchers then compare people who developed cancer with people who didn't and see if the latter group ate more of the particular food. In *prospective studies,* researchers select a group and follow them over a period of time, collecting lifestyle, medical, and other information and noting who develops certain types of disease. They then analyze the information to compare people who developed certain diseases and those who did not and to identify factors that might account for the differences.

Both types of studies have limitations; for example, retrospective studies must rely on people's often-faulty memories, and prospective studies may follow irrelevant behaviors or measure them inconsistently. Both types may fail to sort out confounding factors (factors that confuse results), and both types, as mentioned, suggest links between variables but do not provide causal evidence.

In *clinical (experimental) studies,* researchers randomly assign matched participants to either a treatment group or a control group, apply a treatment to the first group and a *placebo* (a look-alike but ineffective treatment, such as a sugar pill) to the second, and after a period of time (usually a year or more) determine whether the treatment group has experienced a significant effect from the treatment in comparison with the control group. To be considered reliable, the same results must be obtained by other researchers replicating the study. Clinical studies are considered to establish cause-and-effect relationships, but they are often costly and time consuming.

When you read or hear about the results of a new research study in the news, ask yourself several questions about it: Was it a clinical study? If not, the results are not likely to "prove" that something is caused by something else. If it was a clinical study, were participants randomly assigned to groups? Were large enough numbers of participants used to ensure that results weren't skewed? Was it a *double-blind study*—that is, was researcher bias minimized by making sure the scientists were unaware of which group was receiving the treatment and which was receiving the placebo? Was the study sponsored by an impartial research institute or government agency, or were there sponsors who stood to benefit from the results? Has the study been replicated by other researchers? The answers to all these questions and more affect how much credence you can put in the research results.

All reputable studies contribute to the body of scientific knowledge we now have. Cohort studies are like legal arguments built on circumstantial evidence, exploring possible relationships between risk factors and disease. Clinical studies can be used to confirm these relationships in more precisely controlled ways. Both types of studies help scientists put together the "big picture" and make

HIGHLIGHT ON HEALTH

Prescription for Finding Health Information Online

Searching the multitude of sites on the Internet to find the best health information can be difficult. Although you can begin with a search engine such as Google, a more efficient approach is to go directly to one of the many Web sites that specialize in health and medicine. The following are some examples:

Centers for Disease Control and Prevention
www.cdc.gov

HealthAtoZ
www.healthatoz.com

MedFinder
www.mdchoice.com

FirstGov for Consumers
www.consumer.gov

National Health Information Center
www.health.gov

Office of Minority Health Resource Center
www.omhrc.gov

If you have a good idea of what you're looking for, you can also go directly to specific Web sites. Here are a few reliable sites:

- *www.mayoclinic.com* The Mayo Clinic site includes screening tests and consumer news.
- *www.nlm.nih.gov* The National Library of Medicine, the National Institutes of Health, and the Department of Health and Human Services operate this site, which offers searches of 4,300 biomedical journals.
- *www.healthfinder.gov* The Department of Health and Human Services site provides links to a broad selection of health-related sites on the Web, as well as publications.

Note: The Internet addresses listed above were accurate at the time of publication.

useful health recommendations. Keep in mind that scientists typically consider individual studies stepping stones in an ongoing search for answers to complex questions. Members of the lay public have a tendency to regard the results of a single study as conclusive and definitive, and many times, the media are guilty of creating or fostering this impression.[17]

Using Health Information Technology

Unlike consumers of just 10 or 15 years ago, today we have the additional challenge of sorting out and evaluating medical and health information on the Internet. More than 70 million people use online technologies for researching health issues.[18] The most common medical search is for information about a specific disease, such as depression, arthritis, or cancer. (See the box above, "Prescription for Finding Health Information Online.") The range of uses for the Internet includes everything from accessing basic health information, to scheduling online chat sessions or consultations with health care professionals, to joining online support groups formed for people struggling with similar health concerns.

The most important rule for consumers of health information on the Internet is that such information should support, not replace, a patient's relationship with his or her physician. When you do use the Internet to access health information, you need to use the same critical

thinking skills that are called for in evaluating research study results. Many Web sites provide accurate, valuable health information, and many do not. In general, you can rely on the Web sites of large, stable, nonprofit organizations such as the American Heart Association and the American Cancer Society; on the sites of government organizations and agencies like the National Institutes of Health, the Department of Health and Human Services, and the Centers for Disease Control and Prevention; and on sites associated with educational institutions such as Harvard University, the University of California at Berkeley, and Johns Hopkins University. Beware of Web sites that are trying to sell you something, that have a political agenda, or that offer health advice that does not seem to have any kind of scientific basis. Despite the tremendous potential of the Internet to provide information that used to be inaccessible, there is considerable room for error, quackery, and fraud. For advice from consumer advocates on evaluating health Web sites, see the box on the next page, "A Healthy Dose of Caution."

Although you need to take responsibility for being an informed and critical consumer of the health information you read, hear, view, and find on the Web, some protections do exist. If you have a complaint about a consumer issue, contact your local Better Business Bureau (BBB). The BBB does not provide legal advice, but it can direct consumers to the appropriate source for filing a complaint. The BBB can also serve as an intermediary in disputes between

Consumer Clipboard

A Healthy Dose of Caution

- One of the best ways to distinguish between reliable and questionable sources on the Internet is to consider who sponsors the Web page. Look for pages sponsored by well-known sources, such as medical schools, government agencies, or national organizations. Remember that Web addresses ending with .gov are sponsored by a government agency; those ending with .org, by a nonprofit organization; and those ending with .edu, by a college or university. Commercial sites—those with addresses ending with .com—can be good sources for information, but read them with some caution.

- See if the authors' names and credentials are listed. Check to see where they work and if they list board certification. Also, look for the date the site was last updated, a statement of the advertising or funding policy for the site, and information about whether data collected from individuals will remain confidential.

- Read the "Mission Statement" or "About Us" section found on most Web sites. Here you can usually gain insight into the policies and politics of the page sponsor.

- Check to see if the site features the Health on the Net Foundation (HON) emblem; these sites offer highly credible health information. You can also visit the Health on the Net Foundation site (www.hon.ch) for a comprehensive evaluation of medical and health Web sites.

- You may want to consult Quackwatch (www.quackwatch.com), a nonprofit Internet site that provides consumer advice on medical Web sites. For consumer protection, you can consult the Web sites of the FDA (www.fda.gov), which regulates food, drugs, cosmetics, and medical devices; the Federal Trade Commission (www.ftc.gov/ftc/consumer.htm), which oversees fraudulent claims in product and service advertisement; and the U.S. Postal Service (www.usps.com), which regulates products sold through the mail.

Source: Adapted from "Needed: Healthy Dose of Caution," by J. Milligan, February 14, 2000, *The Gazette*, pp. 1D, 2D; "Health Information Technology: What Every Consumer Should Know," by J. Troester, G. Bergus, and D. Rosenthal, 2000, February 8, Iowa City, IA: UI Family Care Center, University of Iowa Hospitals and Clinics.

consumers and sellers. Many other private organizations assist consumers as well. For a list of these organizations, contact the Office of Consumer Affairs in your state.

Confronting Current Health Concerns

Americans and Canadians have more health challenges than learning to be critical consumers of health information. They are also faced with lifestyle decisions that affect their own health, their children's health, and ultimately the health of the nation. Healthy People 2010 identifies the "leading health indicators" that reflect the top 10 current health concerns in the United States:[18]

- Physical activity
- Overweight and obesity
- Tobacco use
- Substance abuse
- Responsible sexual behavior
- Mental health
- Injury and violence
- Environmental quality
- Immunization
- Access to health care

As just one example, let's consider the problem of overweight and obesity.

Lifestyle Decisions: The Case of Obesity

It is generally acknowledged that Americans are currently in the midst of an obesity epidemic. More than half of the nation's adults and 25 percent of its children are classified as overweight (20 percent to 40 percent above ideal body weight) or moderately obese (40 percent to 60 percent above ideal body weight). The expanding buttocks of American citizens have forced sports stadiums, commercial airlines, and movie theaters to replace the traditional 18-inch seats with wider ones. Airlines have the added problem of redesigning pull-down trays to accommodate ever-growing bellies.[19]

Physical inactivity, combined with the abundant availability of high-calorie foods, is responsible for much of this weight gain. Surveys by the Centers for Disease Control and Prevention indicate that Americans walk 15 percent less today than they did 20 years ago. Cars account for 85 percent of travel within American cities, as compared to 45 percent in the Netherlands. Americans spend an average of 4.4 hours glued to television and computer screens every day.[15] The inactivity of children is particularly worrisome, because health habits established early in life are hard to change. Overweight and obesity are risk factors for many chronic, degenerative diseases, including heart disease and Type-2 diabetes. Because rates of overweight increased rapidly in the 1990s, we have not yet seen the full effects of this increase in rates of illness and premature death.[20] However, in 2004 the surgeon general announced that physical inactivity and poor diet are soon likely to overtake smoking as the leading preventable cause of death in the United States. Clearly, obesity has implications both for individuals and for society, and solutions must be sought at several levels.

Ethical Issues and Responsibilities for Individuals and Society

If the leading causes of death in the United States are attributable to lifestyle behaviors such as smoking, inactivity, and poor diet, as is the prevailing view, and if it is in everyone's interest to reduce the incidence of heart disease, cancer, strokes, diabetes, and other chronic conditions in our society, then what are the implications in terms of individual rights and responsibilities? If you have the fundamental right to freely choose health-related behaviors, do you also have a responsibility to make wise choices? If you make poor choices, is your resulting poor health your own responsibility? And if your poor choices lead to illness or disability, should you be held responsible for the costs to society, medical or otherwise?[15]

In this context, personal choices have ethical implications for individuals, but increasingly, ethical issues are challenges faced by entire communities. As a free society, we respect the autonomy and integrity of the individual and do not dictate to people how they must behave in many situations. People who smoke, drink, take drugs, have unsafe sex, eat unhealthy foods, and do not exercise may not share the same vision that others have of how they should live. They may be gambling that the risk of long-term health consequences is worth taking in exchange for immediate enjoyment. They may not want to (or be able to) practice the kind of self-discipline required to change a long-standing or addictive behavior. They may be tired of being told what to do.[19] For these or other reasons, they may ignore even the most carefully crafted public health message aimed at educating people about a particular unhealthy behavior. If they get sick as a result of their unhealthy lifestyles, we often try not to blame them for their illness, even when their behavior has contributed to it, and we typically do not ask people to repay society for the costs of their illnesses.

Still, these considerations raise complex ethical and moral questions about responsibility and accountability. Should people who smoke have to pay more for health insurance? Should a man who has damaged his liver through alcohol abuse have the same eligibility for a transplant as a child with liver disease? Should a woman who uses cocaine during pregnancy be held criminally liable for the health effects on her child? However we answer these questions, we cannot avoid the fact that public policies designed to promote personal health—for example, campaigns against smoking, drinking, and using drugs during pregnancy—have ethical, moral, social, and political implications.[16] In this book we discuss many of the social issues associated with health behaviors, such as needle exchange programs for drug users, state-imposed vaccination programs, and actions taken by colleges to curb binge drinking.

In the future we can expect our society to face even more complex questions, largely as a result of technological advances that have outpaced our ethics. Some of the issues we as a society will have to make decisions about include

- Pornography on the Internet and Internet addiction. Although Internet addiction is not an official medical condition, users can build up a tolerance for Internet use and need more of it to be satisfied.
- Censorship and violence in the media and the entertainment industry.
- Use of DNA technology to repair genetic disorders in the womb, replace a child who has died, or clone a human being.
- Harvesting of stem cells from embryos grown in laboratories to develop treatments for Parkinson's disease and other neurological disorders.

In addition, we need to decide to what extent we can use ethical and moral values, religious beliefs, and legal principles to help guide us through the many uncharted health issues that loom in the immediate future and, in some cases, are upon us today.

Facing the Challenge

Clearly, we have many challenges, on both the personal and the community/societal level. We need to sort healthy options from unhealthy ones in a culture that sometimes overwhelms us with choice. We need to embrace responsibility in the areas in which we have power and accept those areas that are beyond our control. We need to work to build communities and a society that provide all people with the services and resources they need to live healthy lives. These challenges can seem daunting. But on the individual level, we do have the opportunity to make a difference every day—by making thoughtful decisions that support our own health.

Throughout this book we explore the relationship between good health and a variety of lifestyle behaviors and choices. In every chapter we attempt to summarize what is known and not known about healthy and unhealthy choices. Our intent is to provide useful information that will help you understand and assess the health risks in your life. Beyond this, we want to give you the tools to change and to make a difference. As you read the chapters, reflect on your current level of wellness in that area. Is there a behavior you would like to change? First, assess your readiness to change; then develop a plan for behavior change using the tips offered throughout the book pertaining to specific types of behavior. Our hope is that applying health information to your own life in this way will empower and inspire you.

We also hope you will find ways to use this information to make better decisions involving health for your family, friends, and community. As pointed out throughout this chapter, personal and community health are intertwined; the individual cannot be truly healthy without a supportive environment. A well-informed and educated citizenry knows this and understands health not only from a personal point of view but also from a broader social and cultural perspective.

You Make the Call

Health Behavior Change: Incentives or Disincentives?

There is no doubt that healthy lifestyles make for more vital individuals and more productive workers and citizens. Inducing people to live healthier lives, however, has been difficult. Many health insurance companies have attempted to address this problem by offering incentives to people willing to undergo health screening and to adopt healthy behaviors, such as not using tobacco. Corporations have undertaken similar actions by offering incentives for workers who lower their blood pressure, have healthy cholesterol levels, wear their seat belts all the time, are physically active, maintain a healthy weight, and so on.

Some employers have gone even further, using disincentives to encourage their employees to make health behavior changes. For example, they may tell employees that if they don't stop smoking, they may lose their health insurance benefits or have to pay higher premiums. Some employers have even threatened smokers with termination of employment. Random testing for nicotine has been used by employers to ferret out noncompliance. Using a less direct approach, some employers impose health behavior goals that employees must attain in order to receive annual pay increases. Other employers have introduced hiring policies that screen out people who do not fit health behavior profiles.

The use of incentives and disincentives by employers, insurance companies, and government agencies has proven to be controversial. Do such practices unfairly discriminate against those with less control over their lives, such as the poor and disenfranchised? Should people who choose to take health risks be penalized for their actions? After all, society is more productive if its citizens are healthy, and limited health care resources can be more effectively used if they are not wasted on problems that people could have avoided if they had lived healthier lives.

Should incentives and disincentives be used to promote healthy behaviors? What do you think?

Pros

- National health care costs are skyrocketing, and individual health behaviors affect health care costs.
- The power to change health behaviors lies within each individual.
- Empirical evidence supports the relationship between health behaviors and disease.
- Insurance companies already use incentives and disincentives in their life insurance and automobile insurance plans, so it's simply a matter of extending the practice to another kind of insurance.
- Incentive systems have not usually proven effective in promoting health behavior change; therefore, disincentives are needed as well.

Cons

- An overemphasis on individual health is part of a victim-blaming mentality that does not take into account the impact of culture and racial inequality on health.
- Use of disincentives is an invasion of privacy and a violation of personal rights.
- Incentive and disincentive systems do not take into account genetic influences on health.
- The instruments used to measure personal health are usually subjective and open to interpretation.
- Incentive and disincentive systems used for health behaviors may discriminate against certain types of people.

OLC Web site For more information about this topic, visit the Online Learning Center at www.mhhe.com/teague1e.

SUMMARY

- Our fast-paced, technologically advanced society does not necessarily provide us with the best conditions for good health. Individuals need to make informed decisions about their health in the context of supportive communities.

- The World Health Organization defines health as a state of complete physical, mental, social, and spiritual well-being. Wellness, holistic health, and self-care are related concepts.

- Disease prevention includes health-protecting behaviors directed at decreasing the probability of encountering illness. Health promotion focuses on actions designed to maintain a current healthy state or advance to a more desirable state. In a broad sense, health promotion includes health, wellness, holistic health, self-care, and disease prevention.

- Personal health includes the lifestyle decisions and actions that individuals take that affect their own health, whereas community health includes activities and issues that affect communities. Community health promotion refers to activities directed toward bettering the health of the public and/or using resources available in common to members of the community.

- American society is becoming increasingly diverse, and meeting the health needs of multicultural populations requires an understanding and sensitivity to the customs, values, and beliefs of other cultures.

- Differences in cultural beliefs can impede communication between members of ethnic minority groups and health care practitioners, but differences can also be a rich source of ideas about health, such as the importance of social support and mind-body connections.

- Health behavior change theories, such as the Health Belief Model and the Transtheoretical Model, help us understand why people choose healthy and unhealthy behaviors. These theories, however, focus almost exclusively on the individual rather than on how the cultural environment influences health. Supportive cultures are complex systems that embrace both individual autonomy and social responsibility.

- A combination of public health measures and medical interventions helped bring infectious diseases under control in the first half of the 20th century, but chronic, degenerative diseases with a strong lifestyle component have emerged as the leading causes of death in the United States since then. The Healthy People initiative sets national health goals aimed at improving the quality of life for all Americans and eliminating health disparities among different segments of the population.

- People need to be critical consumers of health-related information and research studies, and they need to be savvy users of health information technology.

- Americans face numerous health challenges, both as individuals and as a society. A prime example is the current epidemic of overweight and obesity, brought on largely by physical inactivity and poor diet. Complex political, social, and ethical questions arise in the context of facing such challenges.

REVIEW QUESTIONS

1. What are the similarities among the concepts of health, wellness, holistic health, and self-care? What are the differences?

2. What are personal health and community health? How are they related?

3. What is the difference between ethnicity and race? Why is one a more accurate concept than the other?

4. According to the Health Belief Model, what are the three classes of factors that drive health behaviors?

5. Briefly explain the four core constructs of the Transtheoretical Model of behavior change.

6. Why are behavior change theories sometimes criticized as promoting a victim-blaming mentality?

7. What are the two broad goals of Healthy People 2010?

8. What are the differences between the two kinds of research studies described in the chapter? How do scientists use them to put together the "big picture"?

9. What kinds of Web sites provide reliable health information? What kinds should be avoided?

10. What ethical dilemmas and issues arise when health behaviors are promoted at the government or societal level?

WEB RESOURCES

American Cancer Society: This Web site features a wide range of information about cancer, including statistics, prevention, and treatment approaches. For those living with cancer, it offers resources such as a cancer survivors' network and support programs.
www.cancer.org

American Heart Association: With an emphasis on prevention of heart disease, this site offers publications and other resources that promote heart-healthy living. It provides easy-to-understand information on cardiac diseases and conditions. www.americanheart.org

Centers for Disease Control and Prevention: The CDC provides a national focus for disease prevention and control as well as for health promotion and education. Its Web site features health and safety topics and offers authoritative information for use in making health decisions. www.cdc.gov

U.S. Food and Drug Administration: The FDA site provides information on the many products this government agency regulates, such as food, drugs, medical devices, biologics, and cosmetics. Its news section highlights hot topics in health. www.fda.gov

National Council Against Health Fraud: With its focus on consumer protection law, the NCAHF addresses issues such as product labeling and warranties, proof of safety and effectiveness, and accountability for those who violate the law. NCAHF views health misinformation, fraud, and quackery as public health problems. www.ncahf.org

National Health Information Center: A health information referral service, NHIC is designed to connect consumers and professionals who have health questions with the organizations best suited to answer them. Its database includes 1,400 organizations and government offices offering health information. www.health.gov/nhic

National Institutes of Health: This Web site provides health information through its A–Z index, health hotlines, and databases. MEDLINEplus, a database associated with the National Library of Medicine, is a resource for finding and evaluating health information on the Web. www.nih.gov

U.S. Department of Health and Human Services: This site offers a wide range of health information on topics such as diseases and conditions, safety and wellness, drug and food information, and disasters and emergencies. Its news section includes daily updates on statements and reports by the DHHS. www.os.dhhs.gov

REFERENCES

1. Terry, P. E. (2002). Medical self-care. In M. P. O'Donnell (Ed.), *Health promotion in the workplace* (3rd ed.). New York: Delmar Thomson Learning.

2. American Holistic Medical Association. (2005). Principles of holistic medicine. www.ahha.org.

3. Travis, J. W., & Ryan, S. R. (2004). *Wellness index: A self-assessment for health and vitality.* Berkeley, CA: Ten Speed Press (Celestial Arts).

4. Goodstadt, M. S., Simpson, R. I., & Loranger, P. L. (1987). Health promotion: A conceptual integration. *American Journal of Health Promotion, 1* (3), 58–63.

5. Green, L. W., & Ottoson, J. M. (1999). *Community and population health* (8th ed.). New York: McGraw-Hill.

6. Callahan, D. (2000). Freedom, healthism, and health promotion: Finding the right balance. In D. Callahan (Ed.), *Promoting healthy behavior: How much freedom? Whose responsibility?* Washington, DC: Georgetown University Press.

7. Doyle, E., & Ward, S. (2001). *The process of community health education and promotion.* Mountain View, CA: Mayfield Publishing.

8. Centers for Disease Control and Prevention. (2004). Office of Minority Health: Racial and ethnic populations. www.cdc.gov.

9. U.S. Census Bureau. (2004). Census 2000 briefs. www.census.gov/population.

10. Huff, R. M. (1999). Cross-cultural concepts of health and disease. In R. M. Huff & M. V. Kline (Eds.), *Promoting health in multicultural populations.* Thousand Oaks, CA: Sage Publications.

11. Kline, M. V., & Huff, R. M. (1999). Moving into the 21st century: Final thoughts about multicultural health promotion and disease prevention. In R. M. Huff & M. V. Kline (Eds.), *Promoting health in multicultural populations.* Thousand Oaks, CA: Sage Publications.

12. Glanz, K. E., Rimer, B. K., & Lewis, F. M. (Eds.). (2002). *Health behavior and health education: Theory, research, and practice* (3rd ed.). San Francisco: Jossey-Bass.

13. McKenzie, J. F., & Smeltzer, J. L. (2001). *Planning, implementing, and evaluating health promotion programs.* Boston: Allyn & Bacon.

14. Wallston, K. A., & Armstrong, C. (2002). Theoretically based strategies for health behavior change. In M. P. O'Donnell (Ed.), *Health promotion in the workplace* (3rd ed.). New York: Delmar Thomson Learning.

15. Callahan, D., Koenig, B., & Minkler, M. (2000). Promoting health and preventing disease: Ethical demands and social changes. In D. Callahan (Ed.), *Promoting healthy behavior: How much freedom? Whose responsibility?* Washington, DC: Georgetown University Press.

16. Buchanan, D. R. (2000). *An ethic for health promotion.* New York: Oxford University Press.

17. Ropeik, D. L. (2002). *Risk: A practical guide for determining what's really safe and what's really dangerous in the world around you.* Boston: Houghton Mifflin.

18. U.S. Department of Health and Human Services. (2000). *Healthy people 2010* (2nd ed.). Washington, DC: U.S. Government Printing Office. www.healthypeople.gov.

19. Shaw, D. (1996). *The pleasure police.* New York: Doubleday.

20. Morkdad, A. H., Marks, J. S., Stroup, J. L., & Gerberding, J. L. (2004). Actual causes of death in the United States. *Journal of the American Medical Association, 291,* 1238–1245.

Add It Up!

EVALUATING YOUR LIFESTYLE AND PLANNING FOR CHANGE

Part 1 Scoring Your Lifestyle

For each item, indicate whether you always, sometimes, or never engage in the behavior.

Cigarette Smoking	Almost Always	Sometimes	Almost Never

If you *never smoke,* enter a score of 10 for this section and go to the next section on *Alcohol and Drugs.*

1. I avoid smoking cigarettes. — (2) — 1 — 0
2. I smoke only low tar and nicotine cigarettes *or* I smoke a pipe or cigars. — 2 — 1 — (0)

Smoking Score: 2

Alcohol and Drugs

1. I avoid drinking alcoholic beverages *or* I drink no more than one or two drinks a day. — 4 — (1) — 0
2. I avoid using alcohol or other drugs (especially illegal drugs) as a way of handling stressful situations or the problems in my life. — 2 — (1) — 0
3. I am careful not to drink alcohol when taking certain medicines (for example, medicine for sleeping, pain, colds and allergies) or when pregnant. — (2) — 1 — 0
4. I read and follow the label directions when using prescribed and over-the-counter drugs. — 2 — 1 — (0)

Alcohol and Drugs Score: 4

Eating Habits

1. I eat a variety of foods each day, such as fruits and vegetables, whole grain breads and cereals, lean meats, dairy products, dry peas and beans, and nuts and seeds. — 4 — (1) — 0
2. I limit the amount of fat, saturated fat, and cholesterol I eat (including fat on meats, eggs, butter, cream, shortenings, and organ meats such as liver). — (2) — 1 — 0

	Almost Always	Sometimes	Almost Never

3. I limit the amount of salt I eat by cooking with only small amounts, not adding salt at the table, and avoiding salty snacks. — 2 — (1) — 0
4. I avoid eating too much sugar (especially frequent snacks of sticky candy or soft drinks). — 2 — 1 — (0)

Eating Habits Score: 4

Exercise/Fitness

1. I maintain a desired weight, avoiding overweight and underweight. — (3) — 1 — 0
2. I do vigorous exercises for 15–30 minutes at least three times a week (examples include running, swimming, brisk walking). — 3 — (1) — 0
3. I do exercises that enhance my muscle tone for 15–30 minutes at least three times a week (examples include yoga and calisthenics). — 2 — 1 — (0)
4. I use part of my leisure time participating in individual, family, or team activities that increase my level of fitness (such as gardening, bowling, golf, and baseball). — 2 — (1) — 0

Exercise/Fitness Score: 5

Stress Control

1. I have a job or do other work that I enjoy. — (2) — 1 — 0
2. I find it easy to relax and express my feelings freely. — (2) — 1 — 0
3. I recognize early, and prepare for, events or situations likely to be stressful for me. — (2) — 1 — 0
4. I have close friends, relatives, or others whom I can talk to about personal matters and call on for help when needed. — (2) — 1 — 0

	Almost Always	Sometimes	Almost Never
5. I participate in group activities (such as church and community organizations) or hobbies that I enjoy.	② 2	1	0

Stress Control Score: 10

Safety

	Almost Always	Sometimes	Almost Never
1. I wear a seat belt while riding in a car.	② 2	1	0
2. I avoid driving while under the influence of alcohol and other drugs.	② 2	1	0
3. I obey traffic rules and the speed limit when driving.	2	① 1	0
4. I am careful when using potentially harmful products or substances (such as household cleaners, poisons, and electrical devices).	② 2	1	0
5. I avoid smoking in bed.	② 2	1	0

Safety Score: 9

What Your Scores Mean to YOU

Scores of 9 and 10

Excellent! Your answers show that you are aware of the importance of this area to your health. More importantly, you are putting your knowledge to work for you by practicing good health habits. As long as you continue to do so, this area should not pose a serious health risk. It's likely that you are setting an example for your family and friends to follow. Because you got a very high test score on this part of the test, you may want to consider other areas where your scores indicate room for improvement.

Scores of 6 to 8

Your health practices in this area are good, but there is room for improvement. Look again at the items you answered with a "Sometimes" or "Almost Never." What changes can you make to improve your score? Even a small change can often help you achieve better health.

Scores of 3 to 5

Your health risks are showing! Would you like more information about the risks you are facing and about why it is important for you to change these behaviors? Perhaps you need help in deciding how to successfully make the changes you desire. In either case, help is available.

Scores of 0 to 2

Obviously, you were concerned enough about your health to take the test, but your answers show that you may be taking serious and unnecessary risks with your health. Perhaps you are not aware of the risks and what to do about them. You can easily get the information and help you need to improve, if you wish. The next step is up to you.

SOURCE: U.S. Public Health Service, www.usphs.org.

Part 2 Signing a Behavior Change Contract

Signing a behavior change contract can be an effective strategy for changing a health behavior. Use this contract or adapt it to suit your own program.

I, _____ , agree to _____
       (name)   (behavior you want to change)

_____

I will begin my program on _____ , and I expect to reach my goal on _____ .
                    (date)   (date)

I will use the following tools to help me reach my goal: _____
                                         (journals, exercise buddies, social support, etc.)

When I reach my goal, I will reward myself as follows: _____
                                             (reward)

I have recruited _____ to help me reach my goal by _____
                   (name)   (helping strategies)

_____

In signing this contract, I assert my commitment to reaching my goal.

Signature _____ Date _____

Witness's signature _____ Date _____

SOURCE: Adapted from *Core Concepts in Health* (10th ed.), Wellness Worksheet 5, by P. M. Insel and T. Walton Roth, 2006, New York: McGraw-Hill.

PART 1

Your Mind and Body

If you're in good physical condition but feel stressed out all the time, are you healthy? If you're a workaholic who can't find time for fun, is your lifestyle a healthy one? In terms of your health, the connection between mind and body is real. In Part 1 we begin by exploring how your individual genetic makeup affects your health. Then we consider mental health and how to create balance in your life. In the next chapter we look at spirituality, emphasizing self-discovery and fulfillment. Then we address stress and the need to handle both the daily hassles and the unexpected challenges. This part ends with a chapter on sleep, a key element to good health that is sometimes overlooked. As you read these chapters, think about each topic in relation to the choices you make every day and how those choices affect your health.

THINK IT OVER

If you could design your own genetic makeup, what choices would you make?

Is your life in good balance, or is it a work in progress?

What does spirituality mean to you?

Are you working to prevent stress, or are you reacting to it?

Is getting a good night's sleep on your priority list?

CHAPTER 2

Genetics: You and Your Family Health History

DID YOU KNOW?

- As a human being, you are an extremely complex organism, but you do not have more genes than many simpler organisms. In fact, an individual human being has only about as many genes—20,000 to 25,000—as a mouse.

- If you are a carrier of a genetic mutation, you may not know it, but you may pass the mutation to your children. In some ethnic groups, as many as 3.7 percent of all individuals carry a gene for a particular genetic disorder.

- If you are tested for a genetic disorder, your test results may be used to make decisions about you by an employer or a health insurance company. Legislation that adequately protects individuals against discrimination based on genetic information is not yet in place in the United States or Canada.

OLC *Your Health Today*   www.mhhe.com/teague1e

Go to the Online Learning Center for *Your Health Today* for interactive activities, quizzes, flashcards, Web links, and more resources related to this chapter.

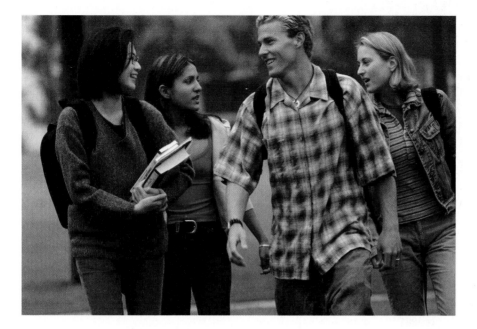

These individuals all display different facial and body features. If their parents had been able to select certain traits for them, in what ways might they look different?

It is perhaps the biggest inheritance you will ever receive. It gives you the potential to be tall or short; apple-shaped or pear-shaped; brown-eyed or blue-eyed; blonde, brunette, or bald. This inheritance may give you the athletic potential to climb to the top of the Olympic podium, grace you with a talent for languages, or require you to use a wheelchair for mobility each day. It gives you a unique bundle of strengths, vulnerabilities, and physical characteristics. It is your genetic makeup.

People have long been curious about what contribution their genetic inheritance makes to their overall makeup as individual human beings and what contribution their upbringing makes—the classic "nature versus nurture" debate. Are people the way they are—easygoing or hard-driving, musically gifted or mechanically adept, likely to live long or die young—as a result of their genetic endowment or because of experiences they have had? Today we know that there are no simple answers to such questions. In fact, we know that it does not even make much sense to pose them. Who we are as individuals is the result of a complex, ongoing interaction among our genetic inheritance, our lifestyle choices, and environmental factors of many kinds, influencing us from conception to death. This last category includes everything from our prenatal environment, to our family and community, to our ethnic or cultural group, to our society and the world at large.

What we can say definitively about genetic inheritance is that it plays a key role in establishing some of the outside parameters of what a person can be and do in his or her life. You can think of genetic inheritance as the blueprint, or starting point, for a person's life. The blueprint is filled in and actualized over the course of the person's entire life.

Genetic inheritance is also the starting point for understanding your personal health. It is important, first of all, to know what special health risks you may have, such as a predisposition for heart disease, a particular type of cancer, or even alcoholism. Because some genetic disorders appear more commonly in certain ethnic groups, you may also have some risks associated with your ethnicity. Remember, because actual outcomes are the result of the interaction of your genes and your life experiences, having a family history of a disease does not necessarily mean you will develop it yourself. Knowing that you may have such a risk factor gives you the opportunity to make informed lifestyle choices. Second, if you choose to have children, it is important to know if you are at risk for passing on a genetic disorder. Having such knowledge increases your options, especially as advancing technology improves our ability to prevent and treat such disorders.

This chapter begins with a focus on *you* as an individual—how you can explore and understand your own family health history. After taking a brief look at the basics of genetics and an overview of the Human Genome Project, we move on to a discussion of how genes influence health, from physical conditions to mental disorders to a variety of behaviors. We then consider genetic counseling, testing, and the treatment of genetic disorders. Finally, we explore the ethical, legal, and social implications of our advancing knowledge of genetics, both for individuals and for society.

YOUR FAMILY HEALTH HISTORY

When a new baby arrives, many people make comments like "he has his grandmother's nose" or "she has her father's long fingers." You do not have to be a scientist to realize that traits can be passed from one generation to the next. As with the color of your skin, hair, and eyes, some

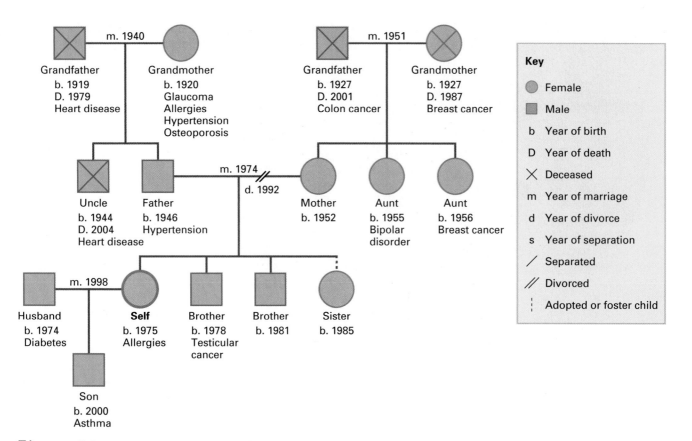

Figure 2.1   A family pedigree.

health traits are passed from one generation to the next. Your grandmother's history of colon cancer may mean you have inherited an increased risk for colon cancer from her side of the family. Your uncle's heart attack at age 40 may mean you have received an increased risk of heart disease from his side of the family. Your mother's struggles with maintaining a healthy weight may mean you have inherited an increased risk of obesity. How can you take this information and organize it in a useful way?

Creating a Genetic Pedigree

A genetic **pedigree,** also called a genogram or family health tree, is a visual representation of your family's genetic history. Creating a pedigree can help you see your family's patterns of health and illness and pinpoint any areas of special concern or risk for you. It is a first step in taking into account the genetic aspect of your health.

To construct your family pedigree, you need to assemble information concerning as many family members as you can. (A sample pedigree is shown in Figure 2.1.) The more detailed and extensive the pedigree, the easier it will be for you to see patterns. Basic information for each family member should include date of birth, major diseases, and age and cause of death for any deceased relatives. You might include additional data, such as the age of a family member when his or her disease was diagnosed,

disabilities, major operations, allergies, lifestyle habits, reproductive problems, mental health disorders, or behavioral problems. Your pedigree should include parents, siblings, grandparents, cousins, aunts, and uncles. The Add It Up! feature at the end of this chapter provides detailed instructions on how to go about putting together your own family health tree.

Gathering family health information to construct the pedigree may not be an easy process. People who are adopted at a young age may receive only a limited amount of family health history, or none at all (see the box on the next page, "Adoption and Health Information"). Relatives may be reluctant to divulge health conditions or information about family members that they consider sensitive or private. You may get more cooperation by pursuing the project as a family venture, emphasizing the importance of this information to all family members and reassuring everyone that it will remain in the family.

What Can You Learn From Your Pedigree?

Certain patterns of illness or disease suggest that the illness is more likely to be genetically linked, as in the following instances:

- An early onset of disease is more likely to have a genetic component. A family member who has a

HIGHLIGHT ON HEALTH
Adoption and Health Information

Now 47 years old, Michael has worked to control his high blood pressure through diet, exercise, and medication for the past 5 years. He often wishes he knew whether others in his biological family had high blood pressure and, if so, at what age they developed complications such as heart attacks or strokes. However, he was adopted at birth, and his parents were given little health information about his biological family.

As we learn more about the genetics of health, many people who were adopted are frustrated by their lack of knowledge of their family history. Adoption laws are designed to protect the interests of the child, biological parents, and adoptive parents. The laws vary among states and have changed greatly over the past 25 years. Fifty years ago, adoptions did not include provisions for ongoing contact or for updating of medical information. More recently, laws have been developed that increase openness of adoption and allow ways for the involved parties to communicate. The communication may occur through the agency or through an attorney. Although most states require adoption agencies to fully disclose medical information, it is often sketchy and out of date.

As adopted individuals grow older, many seek information about their biological parents or at least their biological parents' health histories. Several organizations can aid in the search for such information. For some ideas, see the Web Resources at the end of this chapter.

---

heart attack at age 35 raises more genetic concerns than does a family member who has a heart attack at age 70.

- The appearance of a disease in multiple individuals on the same side of the family is more likely to have a genetic correlation. For example, breast cancer in your mother, your mother's mother, and your mother's sister is more likely to indicate a genetic association than does breast cancer in your mother's sister and your father's grandmother.

- A family member with multiple cancers represents a greater likelihood of a genetic association. For instance, a sister with breast cancer developing independently in both breasts (rather than spreading from one to the other) raises more concern than does a sister with breast cancer in only one breast.

- The presence of disease in family members who have good health habits is more suggestive of a genetic cause than is disease in family members with poor health habits. A heart attack at age 40 in an uncle who runs 5 miles a day and maintains a healthy weight, for example, raises more concern than does a heart attack at age 40 in an overweight uncle who smokes a pack of cigarettes a day.

If you discover a pattern of illness or disease in your pedigree, you may want to consult with your physician about its meaning and implications. You may want to implement lifestyle changes, have particular screening tests, or watch for early warning signs. Again, a pattern of illness does not automatically mean that you will be affected. The main use of a pedigree is to highlight your personal health risks (such as a family history of diabetes) and strengths (such as a family tendency to be long-lived).

YOU AND YOUR GENES: THE BASICS OF HEREDITY

As you have seen, genes do not define who you are or whether you will be healthy or sick, but they do play a critical role in your overall life story. In this section we discuss the basics of genetics and genetic inheritance.

DNA, Genes, and Heredity

Our bodies are made up of about 260 different types of cells, each performing different, specific tasks. Skin cells grow into a protective sheet covering the body; nerve cells receive and transmit chemical messages; white blood cells locate and fight invading pathogens. How do they know what to do?

No matter what its function in the human body, every cell contains in its nucleus the 23 pairs of **chromosomes**

KEY TERMS

pedigree Diagram illustrating the patterns of health and illness within a family; also called a genogram or family health tree.

chromosome Gene-carrying structure found in the nucleus of a cell, composed of tightly wound molecules of DNA.

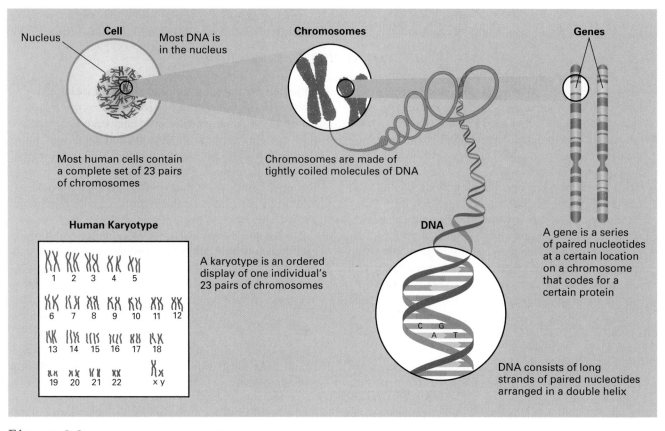

Figure 2.2   Chromosomes, genes, and DNA.

(46 chromosomes in all) that make up the human genome (the total set of an organism's or species' genes). Chromosomes are made of tightly coiled molecules of **deoxyribonucleic acid (DNA).** If we uncoiled a molecule of DNA, we would see that it is made up of two long strands arranged in a double helix—a kind of spiraling ladder structure. Each strand consists of four different chemical building blocks called nucleotide bases: adenine (A), guanine (G), cytosine (C), and thymine (T). The two strands are held together in the ladderlike structure by chemical bonds between different nucleotides; the bonds are like the rungs in the ladder. An A on one strand bonds with a T on the opposite strand, and a G on one strand bonds with a C on the opposite strand (Figure 2.2). The rungs, then, are made of A-T or C-G pairs.

Genes, the units of heredity, are segments of DNA, or specific sequential arrangements of paired nucleotides, located at precise places on the chromosomes. A gene may be thousands or millions of nucleotides long (and chromosomes may contain hundreds or thousands of genes). The arrangement of nucleotides can vary slightly at each location, resulting in alternative versions of genes; these variants are known as **alleles.** For a particular genetic trait, such as eye color, there may be two or three different alleles, producing individuals with blue eyes, brown eyes, and combinations of eye color. Similarly with blood type,

there are three alleles, called A, B, and O, resulting in individuals with types A, B, AB, and O blood.

The DNA in genes is like an instruction book for an organism, and the four bases are like a four-letter alphabet. The specific information carried by the gene is encoded by the order of the bases. Just as the letters in our 26-letter alphabet can be arranged to make thousands of words with different meanings, the bases can be arranged to make thousands of genes, each with a different message. Through a complex process, genes direct the synthesis of particular functional products, usually proteins. Proteins, structures composed of amino acids arranged in a specific order, are basically the building blocks of the body; they are required for the structure, function, and regulation of the body's cells, tissues, and organs. They give each cell instructions that enable it to perform its designated tasks. Thus, skin cells, nerve cells, and white blood cells function the way they do because the DNA in their nuclei directs them to do so.

Most of our cells contain the same full set of genes. However, cells turn on, or use, only the genes that are necessary for the function they perform. By making different proteins at different times, genes can act as switches to alter the ways a cell works, thus regulating cell function. Genes that control the rate of cell division often play a significant role in the development of cancer.

Besides protein synthesis and cell regulation, DNA has another important function: replication. DNA allows cells to divide and create new copies of themselves through the processes of mitosis and meiosis. Mitosis is simply the creation of two cells from one cell, as occurs, for example, when skin grows back over a cut. The new cells contain 23 pairs of chromosomes (46 chromosomes) just as the original cell did. Meiosis is similar to mitosis but occurs only in the cells that produce sperm and ova (egg) cells; this process includes extra steps and results in cells that contain half the normal complement of chromosomes. Thus, sperm and ova cells contain 23 chromosomes rather than 23 pairs. When a sperm and ovum combine, the resulting zygote (fertilized egg) contains 23 pairs, one set from each parent. Each ovum and each sperm contains a unique combination of the mother's or father's chromosomes; no two sperm or ova cells contain the same genes. Similarly, no two zygotes are genetically identical—nor are any two people (except identical twins, who develop from the same zygote).

Every person, then, has one set of chromosomes from the mother and one set from the father. Chromosomes 1–22 are called **autosomes,** and each pair has the same structure. Chromosome 23 is the **sex chromosome** and comes in two forms: an X and a Y. If a person receives an X from her mother and an X from her father, her sex is female (XX). If a person receives an X from his mother and a Y from his father, his sex is male (XY). It is always the father's sperm that determines the gender of an offspring.

The Human Genome Project

As noted earlier, people have long understood that traits are passed from one generation to the next. In the mid-19th century, Charles Darwin proposed that certain heritable traits are favored in a particular environment, a process he called "descent with modification." During the same time period but unknown to Darwin, an Augustinian monk named Gregor Mendel was working out the rules of inheritance by breeding garden peas. He proposed that traits are passed from parents to offspring as discrete units that retain their identity in the offspring. By the early 20th century, scientists had discovered chromosomes and genes and determined that DNA was the genetic material, and in 1953, James Watson and Francis Crick discovered the shape and structure of DNA.

By the 1980s, DNA technology and knowledge had reached such an advanced state that scientists began to think about the possibility of sequencing and mapping the location of all the genes on the 23 chromosomes in the human genome. In *genetic sequencing,* scientists determine the exact order, or sequence, of the 3 billion base pairs in the human genome. In *genetic mapping,* they determine the position of genes in relation to one another and their location on the chromosomes. In 1990, the Human Genome Project (HGP) was launched, organized as an international, collaborative research consortium of 20 groups in six countries: China, France, Germany, Great Britain, Japan, and the United States. In April 2003, the consortium announced that the sequencing of the human genome was complete.[1]

Scientists expected humans to have some 100,000 genes, given our complexity as an organism. However, they were surprised to discover that a human has only about 20,000 to 25,000 genes (the same as a mouse).[2] Genes range in size from 2,000 to 2 million base pairs. Another finding was that only about 2 percent of human DNA occurs in genes, that is, appears to code for functional products. The rest seems to contain signals and messages that are as yet not well understood.[3] The human genome might be compared to a book in which we find one sentence that makes sense followed by a page of letters that do not spell out an obvious message.

The HGP also confirmed that there are no separate biological races in the human species, as noted in Chapter 1. Although there are genes that play a role in the discrete physical characteristics associated with different groups of people in the world, these characteristics are inherited independently, not as a set. Although race remains as a sociocultural construct, it does not have a biological basis.

The HGP made its findings available for free on the Internet and encouraged researchers around the world to use the information in their own studies. Some researchers have sequenced the genomes of other species, including the laboratory mouse and rat, and others have identified specific genes on the human genome. So far, hundreds of genes have been identified, including genes that cause or contribute to such diseases as prostate cancer, breast cancer, Alzheimer's disease, and a host of others. The hope is that understanding diseases at the genetic and molecular levels will lead to the development of better diagnostic tests, treatments, and preventive strategies. It may also lead to treatments tailored to patients based on their individual genetic profiles.

The scientific implications of the HGP are vast, as are the potential applications in medicine and pharmaceuticals. There are also ethical, legal, and social implications of

KEY TERMS

deoxyribonucleic acid (DNA)   Nucleic acid molecule that contains the encoded, heritable instructions for all of a cell's activities; DNA is the genetic material passed from one generation to the next.

gene   Sequence of DNA that encode a protein or other functional product; the unit of heredity.

allele   Alternate form of a gene.

autosome   Any of the chromosomes (22 in humans) that do not contain genes that determine sex.

sex chromosome   Chromosome that include genes that determine sex.

HIGHLIGHT ON HEALTH

Sudden Death in Young Athletes

The sudden death of young athletes in sports such as basketball and football has received extensive media attention. Frequently, death occurs as a result of a rare condition called hypertrophic cardiomyopathy. This condition is an autosomal dominant disorder and has been associated with mutations in three known genes. Specific mutations are associated with differences in severity of the disease, and thus the identification of gene variants may help predict the future course for individuals.

Many different genes control the development and the function of the heart and its arteries. Heart problems can manifest themselves in young, middle, or older adulthood. Hypertrophic cardiomyopathy often appears during adolescence or early adulthood. Symptoms include breathlessness during exercise, chest pain, fainting spells, and rapid heart rate. The most telling sign, however, is a family history of hypertrophic cardiomyopathy or sudden death from an unexplained cause in an adolescent's family member. If such a history exists in your family, consider seeing a health care provider and discussing testing options to look for the condition. If you discover you are vulnerable, your physician or genetic counselor will discuss ways you can modify your lifestyle to protect yourself from future problems.

possessing such detailed genetic information about human beings. From the outset, the HGP included an ethical, legal, and social implications research program whose mission was to ensure the responsible use of genetic information. The implications of genetic research for both individuals and society are discussed in greater detail later in this chapter.

HOW DO GENES AFFECT YOUR HEALTH?

We have seen that individuals inherit one set of chromosomes from each parent and thus have two copies of each gene, one from the mother and one from the father. We have also seen that there are different versions of each gene, called alleles. An individual can inherit two identical alleles for a gene or two different alleles. If the alleles are different, one, called the dominant allele, will be expressed in the organism's appearance. The other, called the recessive allele, will not be expressed and will not have a noticeable effect on the organism's appearance. A person can inherit two dominant alleles, one dominant and one recessive allele, or two recessive alleles.

For example, there is a gene in humans for detached or attached earlobes. If a person inherits two dominant alleles for this trait, she will have detached earlobes. If she inherits one dominant and one recessive allele, she will also have detached earlobes. Only if she inherits two recessive alleles will she have attached earlobes. Some alleles code for harmless physical traits, as in this example. Others result in a disease or disability.

There are also other possible relationships between alleles, such as incomplete dominance and codominance, in which both alleles affect the organism in some way. For example, a person with one dominant and one recessive allele for a disease may not have any symptoms of the disease but have altered blood chemistry that would show up in a lab test.

The Role of Genetic Mutations

Many alleles arise as a result of changes in genes, called **mutations,** that occur during meiosis. These changes often involve alterations in the base pairs that make up a gene. For example, if one pair of nucleotides is substituted for another pair, the gene may code for a different protein or not code for anything at all. Sometimes mutations are neutral, having no apparent effect. Occasionally, they are beneficial to the organism, providing resistance or immunity to disease, for example. More often, mutations are harmful, such as when a mutation results in damage to a fetus or causes it to stop developing.

If we go back to the analogy of the alphabet, consider what happens to the following sentence when a single letter change is made: "When my brother came home, he lied." If we change one letter to a "d," it can turn the sentence into nonsense ("when my drother came home, he lied") or change the meaning entirely ("when my brother came home, he died"). Something similar can happen with DNA. For example, in sickle cell disease (discussed later in the chapter), a thymine (T) base is replaced by an adenine (A) base in the gene for hemoglobin (a protein in red blood cells). This single change at a crucial spot changes the gene's instructions and causes it to produce an altered form of hemoglobin that makes red blood cells stiff and misshapen.

Sometimes a mutation in one gene can cause a disease or disorder, called a **single-gene disorder.** At other times the mutation of several genes is required to cause a disorder, called a **polygenic disorder** (*poly* means many). Some disorders are caused by interactions among one or more genes and the environment; these are called **multifactorial disorders.** Finally, some disorders are the result

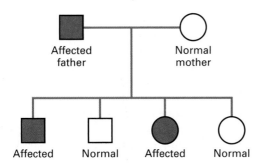

Figure 2.3   Transmission of an autosomal dominant disorder.

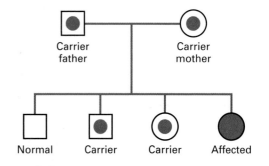

Figure 2.4   Transmission of an autosomal recessive disorder.

of alterations in entire chromosomes. We look at each of these types of genetic disorders next.

Single-Gene Disorders

Although the diseases caused by single-gene mutations are rare, there are many different ones, and so, as a group, they affect a lot of people. Keep in mind that you have two copies of each chromosome (except chromosome 23) and thus two copies of each gene. If you inherit two healthy copies of the gene—that is, two alleles that do not contain mutations—you will not get a single-gene disease. If you inherit two unhealthy copies, you will have the disease. If you inherit one healthy copy and one faulty copy, whether you acquire the disease will depend on the type of gene defect—whether it is dominant or recessive and whether it is autosomal or sex linked.

Autosomal Dominant Disorders

In an autosomal dominant disorder, the mutated gene is on one of the autosomes (chromosomes 1–22); thus, the condition occurs equally often in men and women. The mutated gene is dominant, and so only one copy is required for the disorder to be present. In other words, a person who inherits this gene will have the disorder. Hundreds of known autosomal dominant conditions exist (see the box "Sudden Death in Young Athletes"). Huntington's disease, a fatal degenerative neurological disease with symptoms appearing in middle age, is an example of a disease inherited in an autosomal dominant pattern. Individuals with an autosomal dominant disorder have a 50 percent chance of passing the condition on to each of their offspring. Figure 2.3 shows a family tree for a family with an autosomal dominant disorder.

Autosomal Recessive Disorders

In an autosomal recessive disorder, the mutated gene is again on an autosome, so men and women are equally affected, but in this case, two copies of the mutated gene are required for the disorder to be present. A person with one healthy gene and one mutated gene will not have the disorder. This person is said to be a **carrier,** because he or she carries the gene but does not show signs of the disease. Individuals carrying a mutated recessive gene have a 50 percent chance of passing the altered gene to each of their offspring. Figure 2.4 shows the possibilities of passing on an autosomal recessive disorder if both parents are carriers. There are hundreds of known autosomal recessive disorders, including sickle cell disease, Tay-Sachs disease, and cystic fibrosis.

Sex-Linked Disorders

In sex-linked disorders, the mutated gene is on the sex chromosome. Because they are almost all caused by mutations on the X chromosome, sex-linked disorders are sometimes called X-linked disorders. The Y chromosome is small and contains few genes, so it has a much lower likelihood of carrying mutations and causing a genetic disease.

Most X-linked disorders are recessive; dominant X-linked disorders are very rare. For a female to show signs of an X-linked disorder, she would need two copies of the mutated gene (since her sex chromosomes are XX). If she has only one copy, she is a carrier. For a male to show signs of an X-linked disorder, he would need to have only one mutated gene (since his sex chromosomes are XY and he has only a single copy of the X chromosome). Thus, X-linked disorders usually affect males.

KEY TERMS

mutation   Alteration in the DNA sequence of a gene.

single-gene disorder   Disease caused by a mutation within one gene.

polygenic disorder   Disease caused by mutations in several genes.

multifactorial disorder   Disease caused by the interaction of genetic and environmental factors.

carrier   A person who has one copy of an autosomal recessive mutation; this person shows no signs of the disease but may pass the disease on to his or her offspring.

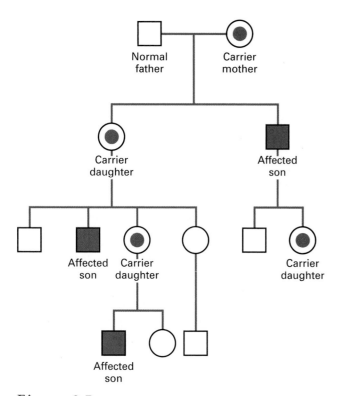

Figure 2.5   Pedigree for a family with an X-linked recessive disorder.

interactions among mutations in multiple genes. Even more common are disorders that occur as a result of the interaction of genes with environmental factors, such as tobacco smoke, pollution, and diet. These multifactorial disorders include heart disease, cancer, diabetes, schizophrenia, and a broad range of other disorders. Because so many diseases with a genetic component are multifactorial—they account for the majority of illnesses and deaths in the developed world—paying attention to the lifestyle and environmental factors that contribute to them is crucial. Figure 2.6 shows the relative contribution of genetic and environmental factors to a spectrum of common diseases.

To determine the relative contribution of genetic and environmental factors of a particular disease, researchers look at how often it occurs among family members of a person with that disease (by examining the family pedigree) compared with how often it occurs in the general population. If a disease has a genetic link, it usually occurs more frequently among first-degree relatives (mother, father, brother, or sister) of a person with the illness than in the general population. These studies are called family or familial studies. Because family members often share environmental conditions as well as genes, familial studies don't necessarily provide clear-cut evidence that disorders are genetic.

More definitive findings come from twin studies, in which researchers study how often a disease occurs among identical twins in comparison to how often it occurs among fraternal twins or siblings. Because identical twins have the same set of genes, an illness with a significant genetic contribution should occur more frequently among them than among fraternal twins (who are only as closely genetically related as any siblings).[4] A third type of study is the adoption study, in which identical twins are adopted into different families and so do not share the same environment (unlike nonadopted identical twins). Adoption studies provide strong evidence, but the conditions for this type of study occur relatively rarely.

Let's consider heart disease as an example of a multifactorial illness. Many environmental factors increase the risk for heart disease, including smoking tobacco, having a sedentary lifestyle, and being overweight. (See Chapter 21 for more details on heart disease and its risk factors.) In addition, the first-degree relatives of someone suffering

An affected man passes the mutation to all of his daughters (since he has only one X chromosome) but to none of his sons (they get his Y chromosome). A carrier mother has a 50 percent chance of passing the mutation to her daughters (they would be carriers as long as their father did not have the disease) and a 50 percent chance of passing the mutation to her sons (who would have the disease). Figure 2.5 shows a pedigree for a family with an X-linked recessive disorder, such as hemophilia, color blindness, or Duchenne muscular dystrophy.

Polygenic and Multifactorial Disorders

The disorders caused by a single-gene mutation, just described, are inherited in recognizable patterns. However, the majority of inherited disorders are not associated with a single-gene mutation. More commonly, they are polygenic disorders and diseases, those associated with

← Environmental			Genetic →
Infections	Congenital heart disease	Diabetes	Schizophrenia
Trauma, poisoning	Teratogenic defects	Neural tube defects	Coronary heart disease	Single-gene disorders

Figure 2.6   Relative contribution of environmental and genetic factors in some common disorders.

Source: Adapted from "Relative Contribution of Environment and Genetic Factors in Some Common Disorders" in *ABC of Clinical Genetics* by Helen Kingston, 2nd Impression (revised), 1997, BMJ Publishing Group. Used by permission of Blackwell Publishing.

HIGHLIGHT ON HEALTH
Down Syndrome

After the birth of their first child, Juan and Laura were surprised when the doctor said that their daughter, Julia, had facial features that were suggestive of Down syndrome. The doctor asked to have some blood work done to test Julia's chromosomes. Juan and Laura agreed to this step and anxiously awaited the results. The tests subsequently confirmed that Julia had an extra copy of chromosome 21 and had Down syndrome.

Down syndrome occurs in about 1 in every 800 live births. Risk increases with maternal age. A child with Down syndrome has characteristic facial features that include low-set ears, a flat face, protruding tongue, and extra skin on the neck. The baby will often be slightly floppy or have weaker muscle tone than usual. He or she will have developmental delays to varying degrees and may have associated congenital heart disease, bowel problems, and an increased risk for infection.

In 1965, a child with Down syndrome had a 50 percent chance of living to age 5. In comparison, a child today with Down syndrome has an 80 percent chance of survival to age 30 or beyond. The significant improvement reflects advances in medicine to correct the associated congenital abnormalities and treat infections. A range of functioning is associated with this disorder, and individuals with Down syndrome often lead satisfying and productive lives.

Source: Data from *Preventive Management of Children with Congenital Anomalies and Syndromes* (pp. 146–152), by G. N. Wilson and W. C. Cooley, 2000, Cambridge, England: Cambridge University Press.

from heart disease have a sixfold increase in risk for heart disease over that of the general population, so it is clear that there are genetic risks as well. In families with a high risk for heart disease, there may be genetic mutations that elevate cholesterol or blood pressure or that affect blood clotting.[4,5] Individuals with this kind of genetic family history need to pay even more attention to lifestyle and environmental factors than do individuals without genetic risk.

Chromosomal Disorders

Another type of inherited disorder is caused by mutations involving an entire chromosome. A chromosome may be added, lost, or altered as a result of errors during meiosis. Many chromosomal disorders lead to fetal death or death in the first year of life. Because so much genetic information is involved, individuals with chromosomal abnormalities exhibit a broad set of symptoms, called a syndrome, ranging from characteristic physical traits to developmental delays to growth abnormalities. Down syndrome and Turner syndrome are examples of chromosomal disorders.

Some chromosomal disorders are the result of an extra chromosome. In Down syndrome, for example, the individual is born with an extra copy of chromosome 21. Children with Down syndrome are developmentally impaired to varying degrees and may have other health problems. For more information on this disorder, see the box above, "Down Syndrome." In Klinefelter syndrome, a male is born with an extra

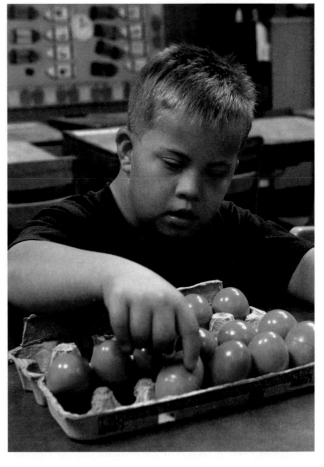

This child with Down syndrome, who has an extra chromosome, has some of the characteristic facial features of the disorder.

X chromosome (XXY). A male with Klinefelter syndrome develops some female characteristics at puberty and is sterile.[6] Males born with an extra Y chromosome (XYY) tend to be taller than average and can be prone to learning disorders.[7] They are not more violent or aggressive than other males. Females with an extra X chromosome (XXX) have no major physical problems, but they may experience early menopause, learning disorders, and other problems.[8]

Other disorders are the result of a missing chromosome. For example, females born with a missing X chromosome (XO) have Turner syndrome. These individuals are at increased risk of heart abnormalities and other physical and mental problems.[7,9] Still other disorders are caused by a chromosomal rearrangement, which can occur if a small section of DNA breaks and becomes repositioned on the same or a different chromosome.

ETHNICITY AND GENETIC DISORDERS

Because of the way different human groups have moved around the planet over the course of human evolution, often remaining isolated from other groups for hundreds of generations, some genetic patterns occur more frequently in particular groups than in others. Geneticists have used sophisticated DNA analysis to study the migration patterns of these different populations and their genetic makeup,[10] confirming that closely knit populations share genes. Thus, individuals from such populations are more likely to have the same gene variants than are individuals from other populations. Put another way, the likelihood of sharing a genetic mutation with a partner from the same ethnic group is higher than with a partner from another ethnic group. Similarly, the risk of a child receiving the same genetic mutation from both parents is higher if both parents share the same ethnic background. The result is an increased frequency of certain inherited genetic disorders within particular ethnic groups. Sickle cell disease, Tay-Sachs disease, and cystic fibrosis are examples of this type of inheritance and highlight the importance of considering ethnicity in a family pedigree.

Sickle Cell Disease

An autosomal recessive disorder, sickle cell disease primarily affects people of African descent. As mentioned earlier in this chapter, the disease is caused by a mutation in a single base pair of nucleotides in the gene that codes for a component of hemoglobin, the protein in red blood cells that carries oxygen. When a person with sickle cell disease experiences low oxygen conditions—for example, when under stress—the hemoglobin molecules clump together and cause the red blood cells to take a sickle shape rather than a circular shape. The altered red blood cells break

easily and do not flow through blood vessels smoothly, so they can clog or block the blood vessels. Because the red blood cells are not doing an adequate job of carrying oxygen throughout the body, the individual can experience weakness, fatigue, anemia, infection, organ damage, and other painful and dangerous symptoms.

About 1 in 400 African Americans in the United States has sickle cell disease, meaning that such individuals have two copies of the mutated gene.[7] About 1 in 12 African Americans is a carrier of the sickle cell gene, meaning that the affected person has one copy of the mutated gene. Carriers usually do not experience symptoms, but some evidence of the disease can be seen in their blood under laboratory conditions. The reason for the relatively high frequency of the sickle cell gene is that it confers some resistance to malaria. It is unclear exactly why, but people with sickle cell trait are less likely to die from infection with malaria than are people without sickle cell trait. In areas where malaria is a common cause of death, sickle cell trait offers a selective advantage. Thus, the prevalence of this genetic disorder in African Americans and Africans around the world can be traced back to their genetic and environmental roots.

Screening for the sickle cell gene is done by evaluating a person's hemoglobin. There is no cure for sickle cell disease, but individuals with the disorder can be treated with blood transfusions and drugs. They can also modify their lifestyles to reduce stress and practice stress management techniques.

Tay-Sachs Disease

Another autosomal recessive disorder, Tay-Sachs disease occurs in people of Ashkenazi (eastern European) Jewish ancestry about 100 times more frequently than in other populations. Between 1 in 27 and 1 in 30 people of Ashkenazi Jewish ancestry carry the mutated gene.

Tay-Sachs disease is a fatal degenerative brain disorder. In babies born with the disease, an enzyme that metabolizes certain lipids (fats) is missing, leading to the accumulation of these lipids in the brain. Brain cells are affected within a few months of birth and gradually stop functioning normally. Children with Tay-Sachs disease seldom live more than a few years.

The relationship between the alleles of the genes for this disorder is one of incomplete dominance, so that a person with only one copy of the mutated gene will not have the disease but will have half the normal level of a certain enzyme produced by the gene. Potential carriers can be identified by measuring the activity level of this enzyme, as well as through DNA analysis. The widespread use of enzyme and DNA testing has made it rare for infants in the United States and Canada to be affected by Tay-Sachs disease. In fact, the incidence of Tay-Sachs disease in the Jewish population has been reduced by more than 90 percent.[11]

Cystic Fibrosis

One of the most common genetic diseases in the United States is cystic fibrosis (CF), another autosomal recessive disorder. It occurs much more frequently in white people of European descent than in people of other ethnic backgrounds. It is thought that the gene for this disorder may have been retained in the gene pool because it confers some resistance to cholera and other diarrheal diseases.[12] CF occurs in 1 of every 3,200 live births to Caucasians and in 1 of every 3,900 live births of all Americans.

In cystic fibrosis a defective gene codes for a protein that causes the body to produce thick, sticky mucus that clogs the lungs, obstructs the pancreas, and interferes with digestion. People with cystic fibrosis have persistent coughing and shortness of breath. The majority of patients are diagnosed before the age of 3. An important part of treatment is clearing mucus from the lungs, either by physical therapy or drug therapy; lung infections can be treated with antibiotics. In the past, individuals with cystic fibrosis seldom survived childhood, but with advances in treatment, more are living into adulthood and even into their 50s and 60s. One promising treatment approach under active investigation is gene therapy, a technique discussed later in this chapter.

GENES AND MENTAL DISORDERS

We have seen that genes play a role in many physical conditions and diseases. What about mental illnesses? Do they have a genetic component as well? It is highly likely that at least some of them do. Much more research is needed in this area, but evidence suggests a genetic contribution in a number of mental disorders. In this section we look at just a few.

Schizophrenia

A severe mental disorder that appears to have a strong genetic link is schizophrenia. Symptoms include delusions (distortions in thought, not being able to determine what is real), hallucinations, disorganized speech, emotional withdrawal, and bizarre behavior. Most people who develop schizophrenia show signs by their late teens or early 20s. If a person has no signs of schizophrenia by age 30, the risk is reduced by half. After age 50, the risk is negligible.

A genetic contribution is suggested by the fact that first-degree relatives of a person with schizophrenia have a risk for the illness about 10 times higher than that of the general population.[13] Second-degree relatives (aunts, uncles, nieces, nephews) have a risk that is lower but still higher than that of the general population. The more relatives with schizophrenia a person has, the higher that person's risk for the disease.[14] A genetic link is also supported by twin studies, although these same studies also show the strong contribution of environment. Research suggests that schizophrenia is multifactorial (that is, it involves the interaction of genes and environmental factors, possibly both prenatally and postnatally). As in many other genetic disorders, some individuals may be genetically predisposed to have schizophrenia but develop the disease only in the presence of certain environmental triggers, such as stressful family dynamics or lower socioeconomic status (also a stressor).

Mood Disorders and Anxiety Disorders

Bipolar disorder and depression, known as mood disorders, also appear to have a genetic link. Bipolar disorder, sometimes referred to as manic depression, is a mood disorder with episodes of mania (characterized by euphoria, racing thoughts, excessive talkativeness, and inflated self-esteem) alternating with episodes of depression (characterized by fatigue and loss of energy, feelings of hopelessness and worthlessness, loss of interest and pleasure in daily activities, and thoughts of death or suicide). The first-degree relatives of a person with bipolar disorder have 8 to 9 times the rate of the illness experienced by the general population, and the genetic association is also supported by twin studies.[15] Again, there does not appear to be a single gene but probably several that interact with the environment. For unipolar depression (depression without manic episodes), there appears to be a moderate genetic contribution, slightly less than that for bipolar disorder. Family and twin studies show a higher risk of depression[16] and suicide among people with relatives having either of these factors.[17]

Examples of anxiety disorders include panic disorder, obsessive compulsive disorder, and generalized anxiety disorder. In panic disorder, individuals experience intense, irrational fear, and in obsessive compulsive disorder, people engage in repetitive activities that serve to suppress or neutralize anxiety. Individuals with generalized anxiety disorder are beset with excessive worries, anxieties, and related physical symptoms. Family studies and twin studies suggest a genetic link for all of these disorders.

Alzheimer's Disease

The most common form of dementia, Alzheimer's disease is marked by a gradual mental deterioration that includes loss of thinking skills and memory. The disease usually begins imperceptibly, often with a decline in alertness and interest in life. Later there is confusion, disorientation, agitation, and a loss of contact with reality. Eventually, individuals lose the ability to walk, talk, or eat. Autopsies on Alzheimer's patients reveal characteristic brain abnormalities, including deposits known as senile plaques (tangles of abnormal filaments in nerve cells) and holes in the brain tissue.

Beating the Odds

Who Is Most at Risk for Alzheimer's Disease?

A devastating neurological disorder, Alzheimer's disease is the most common cause of dementia in older adults. Although some forms of Alzheimer's disease are known to have a genetic component, as described in this chapter, lifestyle and environmental factors also play a part. Brief profiles of three people are presented here. Which person do you think is most at risk for Alzheimer's disease?

Brad, age 45, is a research scientist at a major pharmaceutical company. His father developed Alzheimer's at age 80. Brad smokes a pack of cigarettes each day, is a moderate drinker of alcohol, and considers his career stressful. He walks 2 miles to and from work each day and eats a lot of fruits and vegetables. Brad's blood pressure is high and currently untreated. His blood cholesterol level is healthy. He takes an aspirin every day because he heard it could protect him from having a heart attack.

Colleen, age 30, is a customer service agent for an airline. She has no known family history of Alzheimer's, but her mother was adopted. Colleen maintains a healthy weight by sticking to a balanced diet and daily exercise. Her blood pressure is normal but her cholesterol is high. She does not drink alcohol and quit smoking five years ago. She considers her job stressful.

Hank, age 50, is a former professional football player. He retired after two head injuries led to brain concussions at age 30. Now he teaches and coaches at a public high school. He enjoys his job and does not feel it is stressful. Hank's father developed Alzheimer's at age 70. His grandmother developed Alzheimer's at age 75. Hank maintains a healthy weight, exercises regularly, and has a diet high in fast food. His blood pressure and cholesterol are normal.

OLC Web site Visit the **Online Learning Center** at www.mhhe.com/teague1e for comments by the authors.

Alzheimer's disease affects about 10 percent of the American population over age 65 and 30 percent to 50 percent of people over age 85. In a less common form called early-onset familial Alzheimer's disease, the individual exhibits symptoms of the disease before age 60 to 65 and often before age 55.[14] Three genes are associated with early-onset familial Alzheimer's disease and are inherited in an autosomal dominant manner. Therefore, the child of an individual with one of these genetic mutations would have a 50 percent chance of early-onset familial Alzheimer's dis-

ease. Another gene, APOE, located on chromosome 19, is associated with the more common late-onset Alzheimer's disease. Mutations in this gene increase the risk of an individual developing Alzheimer's disease by two- to threefold above the background risk of 10 percent.[18]

Like so many other diseases, however, Alzheimer's is a multifactorial disorder, with both genetic and environmental contributions. One likely environmental factor is head trauma. In addition, experts now say that whatever protects your cardiovascular health probably also benefits your brain. That means controlling high blood pressure and high levels of total and LDL cholesterol ("bad cholesterol"); boosting levels of HDL cholesterol ("good cholesterol"); controlling diabetes; getting regular exercise; controlling inflammation by taking nonsteroidal anti-inflammatory drugs, such as aspirin or ibuprofen, daily; and eating a heart-healthy diet. Such a diet is rich in fruits, vegetables, whole grains, nuts, and fish. Experts also recommend that people stay physically and mentally active and remain socially involved. Investigations into the causes of Alzheimer's and research into treatments, vaccines, and cures are being aggressively pursued. To assess your ability to identify factors that may contribute to dementia, see the box "Who Is Most at Risk for Alzheimer's Disease?"

GENES AND BEHAVIOR

Is it possible that genetics plays a role in our personalities and everyday behaviors, too? We see that some people like bungee jumping and others prefer chess; some are optimists and others pessimists; some fly off the handle at any provocation while others remain placid and calm. Could these differences be part of our individual genetic endowments? And could genes influence what we eat, how much we drink, whether we use drugs, and whom we choose as sexual partners? These are complex questions, and we may never have truly definitive answers to some of them. But researchers are studying the genetic contribution to personality and behavior, looking at such characteristics as shyness, aggressiveness, sensation seeking, depression, and intelligence, to name a few.

The Role of Genes in Personality

One way to define *personality* is the sum of the mental, emotional, social, and physical characteristics of an individual. This unique, dynamic organization of characteristics influences your behavior and responses to the environment—how you communicate, react to others, and express emotions. It influences how much you exercise, study, work, play, sleep, eat, and engage in a host of other behaviors. In other words, your personality is what makes you uniquely you.

The foundation of personality is temperament, defined as a disposition that is present at birth, remains stable across the life span, and has a pervasive influence on a person's behavior. As the individual grows and develops and interacts with the environment, temperament is shaped into personality. In other words, temperament seems to be the raw material for the formation of personality. Research studies suggest that core traits of temperament are inherited.[14]

Researchers have identified three broad aspects of temperament that are observably different across individual infants: sociability, reactivity or emotionality, and activity level. Sociability is an individual's style of reaction to the environment. Some infants tend to withdraw from social contact, while others are eager to interact. Differences in sociability may account for shyness and introversion in some adults and friendliness and extraversion in others. Reactivity or emotionality is the tendency to become physiologically aroused in response to the environment. In addition to differences between individuals in how highly aroused they become, there may be differences in the tendency to experience positive emotions (happiness, joy) versus negative emotions (fear, anger). This difference may underlie optimistic versus pessimistic outlooks in adults. Finally, activity level is the amount of response to the environment an individual puts out, in terms of intensity and speed of activity. Some infants and children are highly active and others are less so; these differences persist into adult life.

Although temperament is enduring and difficult to change, it is only one piece of the infinite complexity of the individual human being. Life experiences, beginning in the prenatal environment, are inextricably bound up in a person's ultimate personality. Further, no temperament type or personality style is more desirable or worthwhile than any other. The differences we observe in infants and subsequently in children, adolescents, and adults are all part of the rich diversity of the human species.

The Role of Genes in Sexual Orientation

The origin of sexual orientation has been a controversial topic in both scientific and political arenas. Whether it should even be a topic at all is sometimes a point of contention, with some critics claiming that looking for a "cause" of homosexuality implies a negative bias. On the other hand, some people believe that homosexuality would be more accepted by society if it were shown to be biologically determined. According to this view, homosexuality would be seen not as a choice or a preference but as a genetic disposition similar to eye color or right- or left-handedness. In fact, sexual orientation seems to exist on a continuum of heterosexuality (emotional and sexual attraction to people of the other sex), bisexuality (attraction to people of both sexes), and homosexuality (attraction to people of the same sex). Homosexuality occurs in almost all cultures and in some animal species.

The data on the role of genes in sexual orientation are conflicting. A large study evaluating families, twins, and adopted individuals indicated that homosexuality, and thus sexual orientation, runs in families. This study deter-

mined that genetics accounted for half of the differences between groups.[19] In other studies, researchers have not been able to reproduce these findings. A study looking at siblings found that familial factors were important in homosexuality, with the possibility of a role of the X chromosome. This study also found that birth order (an environmental factor) appeared to affect sexual orientation, with the number of older brothers increasing the likelihood of male homosexual orientation.[20]

The X chromosome has continued to receive attention in research. A study looking at 52 gay sibling pairs, however, found no increased frequency of a suspected gene on the X chromosome. This study could not confirm a genetic predisposition toward homosexuality.[21] Like other characteristics and behaviors, sexual orientation is probably multifactorial in origin.

The Role of Genes in Addiction

Also known as dependence, addiction involves a pathological need for a substance (or activity), usually with increasing amounts of the substance required to achieve the desired effect and unpleasant withdrawal symptoms occurring without it. Addiction to alcohol and other substances is widespread in U.S. society. Although family and environmental factors play a role in addiction and dependence, there is also clearly a genetic component. Research suggests that addiction may involve genes that lead to greater sensitivity to alcohol and drugs, more motivation to use them, more craving for them, and greater loss of control despite negative consequences.

Of all forms of dependence, alcoholism has been the most widely studied. The tendency to become addicted to alcohol has been found to run in families. Familial studies show that individuals with one alcoholic parent have a higher likelihood of being alcoholics themselves, and the risks are even higher if both parents are alcoholic. When children of alcoholic parents are adopted into nonalcoholic families, their rates of alcoholism are closer to those of their biological parents than to those of their adoptive parents.

Research into the genetics of this disorder has led to the identification of two types of alcoholism, labeled Type I and Type II. Type I alcoholics are men and women who are steady drinkers; they develop alcoholism in middle age. Type II alcoholics have severe, early-onset alcoholism. Most are men who start drinking at a young age; frequently, they have antisocial tendencies. Twin and adoption studies suggest that Type II alcoholism has a greater genetic component than Type I alcoholism.[22] It is likely that multiple genes are involved.

Ironically, the only clearly identified genes with a role in alcoholism are genes that protect against it. Three gene variations have been identified that affect the way alcohol is metabolized. These genetic variations are found at higher frequencies in Asian and Southeast Asian populations. For people with these variations, even small amounts of alcohol

Challenges & Choices

Should You See a Genetic Counselor?

Genetic counselors are a source of information and education about genetic disorders. They can also provide resources, reassurance, and support. If you answer yes to any of the following questions, you may want to consider consulting a genetic counselor.

1. Do you or your partner have a genetic disorder?
2. Do you have a child, parent, or close relative with a genetic disorder?
3. Do you know or suspect that you are or might be a carrier of a specific genetic disorder (for example, based on ethnicity), or are you considering a test to determine whether you are a carrier?
4. Have you been diagnosed with a genetic disorder about which you need more information relating to features, prognosis, and treatment options?
5. Do you or your partner have an ongoing pregnancy with known genetic risks?
6. Are you planning a pregnancy and/or wish to explore options, including artificial insemination by donor and other methods of assisted reproduction, prenatal diagnosis, adoption, or pregnancy termination?
7. Do you need assistance in the care and treatment of an affected child or close relative?
8. Has a prenatal screening or diagnostic test revealed a fetal abnormality?

It's Not Just Personal . . .

Since 1970, 1.4 million individuals in the world have been voluntarily screened to see if they are carriers of the Tay-Sachs mutant gene. Prenatal testing of over 3,200 pregnancies has prevented the birth of 600 infants with this uniformly fatal disease.

Source: Data from "Population-Based Genetic Screening for Reproductive Counseling: The Tay-Sachs Disease Model," by M. Kaback, *European Journal of Pediatrics, 159* (3), pp. 5192–5195.

cause an extremely unpleasant reaction known as flushing syndrome, which includes flushing of the skin, racing heart, nausea, and headache. These effects are so uncomfortable that most people with the genetic variants do not drink.[22] It has been proposed that this genetic profile contributes to the low rate of alcoholism in Asian populations.

Environmental factors also play a critical role in the development of alcoholism, as evidenced, for example, by the fact that the great majority of children of alcoholics do not become alcoholics themselves. Environmental factors include family dynamics, psychological and personality characteristics, ethnic and cultural customs, social expectations, and a host of others. Having a genetic predisposition to alcohol or drug dependence does not relieve an individual of personal responsibility for his or her behavior, but it also does not condemn the person to a life of dependency problems.

GENETIC COUNSELING AND GENETIC TESTING

The purpose of genetic counseling is to help individuals and families understand the role of genetics in a particular disorder, evaluate their risks, learn about the diagnostic tests available, and discuss treatment options. In the past, genetic counseling typically took place after a genetic disorder was diagnosed. Today, as technology improves and expands, genetic counseling is often offered before a disorder is diagnosed. (See the box "Should You See a Genetic Counselor?" for more information on this topic.)

Unfortunately, there is a shortage of genetic counselors to assist people in this process. In 2003 the National Society of Genetic Counselors reported approximately 2,000 members. The future task of education and genetic counseling is likely to fall on primary care providers and nurses, although currently these professions have little training in this area.[23] A well-developed counseling program will be crucial as more genetic testing options become available.

Many people who see a genetic counselor and learn about their risks decide not to be tested, partly because of the potential consequences of such testing. In some cases, there is no treatment for a genetic disorder. In other cases, people are worried about privacy issues and how their genetic information may be used. Some of these issues are discussed later in this chapter.

As knowledge about genetic disorders and associations between genes and disease grows, the opportunities for genetic testing increase, as do the range and types of tests available. How these tests will be incorporated into our changing health arena remains to be seen, but many experts predict that genetic testing will become an increasingly important tool in medicine. In this section we look at the types of tests that are available.

Diagnostic Tests

When an individual shows signs of an illness, a genetic test may help confirm or exclude the possibility of certain diseases. For example, if a 35-year-old man shows symptoms of dementia, a genetic test can be performed to confirm or exclude the presence of a gene mutation associated with early-onset familial Alzheimer's disease. In this situation, when the genetic test helps to confirm a diagnosis, it is called a diagnostic test.

Predictive Tests

If an individual is currently healthy but has a family history of a genetic disorder, a genetic test may be given to assess the individual's risk for developing the disease in the future. Such predictive tests are further divided into two types: presymptomatic and predispositional. **Presymptomatic tests** are for a genetic mutation that if present will ensure the eventual development of the disorder (that is, the mutation is inherited in an autosomal dominant pattern). **Predispositional tests** are for a genetic mutation that if present increases the risk for a genetic disorder but does not ensure the development of the disorder. These tests are associated with multifactorial diseases (those involving the interaction of a gene or genes with environmental factors).

The genetic mutations associated with Alzheimer's disease serve as an example of the differences between these two types of tests. As noted earlier, three autosomal dominant genes are associated with the early-onset familial form of Alzheimer's disease. If a genetic mutation is detected in one of these genes, the individual will develop the disease. Currently, the presymptomatic test for early-onset familial Alzheimer's disease is available to siblings and offspring of an individual who has early-onset Alzheimer's disease and a known genetic mutation associated with this disease. In contrast, one gene, APOE, has so far been shown to be associated with the late-onset form of Alzheimer's disease. If a genetic mutation is detected in this gene, the individual has an increased risk of developing Alzheimer's disease but not a certainty that he or she will develop it. Until the full implications of testing are better understood and there are better interventions to delay onset or decrease symptoms of the disease, the predispositional test for APOE is currently recommended only in research settings.[18]

Another example of a predispositional genetic test is for the BRCA1 and BRCA2 gene mutations in hereditary breast and ovarian cancer, both of which are inherited in an autosomal dominant pattern. If a woman with a strong family history of breast or ovarian cancer tests positive for the BRCA1 mutation, she has a 65 percent to 85 percent risk of developing breast cancer and a 39 percent to 60 percent risk of developing ovarian cancer. If she tests positive for the BRCA2 mutation, she has a 45 percent to 85 percent risk of breast cancer and an 11 percent to 25 percent risk of ovarian cancer. In a man, the BRCA2 mutation is associated with an increased risk of breast and pancreatic cancer. Either mutation increases the risk of prostate cancer in a man.[24]

Because of their high lifetime risk of developing cancer, individuals with these mutations are urged to make certain lifestyle decisions. Women are encouraged to start medical screening for breast and ovarian cancer at age 25. They are encouraged to participate in behaviors known to decrease risk for these cancers, such as maintaining a healthy body weight, avoiding tobacco products, and if they have children, breastfeeding for a prolonged period. Other options include medications and/or surgery (to remove the breasts and ovaries) in order to further decrease the risk of cancer.

Both types of predictive tests create challenges for the individuals and families who consider them. Although a presymptomatic test, by definition, confirms the presence of a genetic mutation that will lead to a genetic disorder, it does little to predict when symptoms will appear or how severely affected the individual will be. The predispositional tests raise even more questions at this early stage of genetic knowledge, because there is less certainty about how the presence or absence of a genetic mutation will affect a person. Both types of test, but particularly predispositional tests, have implications for society and social policy, because the leading causes of disease and disability, including cancer, heart disease, and other chronic conditions, are multifactorial in origin.

Carrier Tests

If a healthy individual has a genetic mutation for a disorder that is inherited in an autosomal recessive or X-linked recessive manner, the individual is said to be a carrier, as discussed earlier. If a genetic test is available to look for that recessive gene, it is called a carrier test. A carrier test may be offered to a healthy individual who has a family member with a certain genetic disorder or who has a family member who has been identified as a carrier. Carrier tests are also offered to individuals in certain racial and ethnic groups that are known for having high carrier rates, including sickle cell disease and Tay-Sachs disease.

Prenatal Screening Tests

The most commonly practiced form of genetic testing is prenatal screening. All women who receive prenatal care

KEY TERMS

presymptomatic test   Test designed to detect a mutation that if present ensures the eventual onset of symptoms.

predispositional test   Test designed to detect a mutation that if present increases the risk of developing a disease.

Table 2.1   Common Genetic Conditions and Associated Population Groups

Ethnic Group	Inherited Disorder
Blacks of African origin	Sickle cell disease (a blood disorder)
Ashkenazi Jews	Tay-Sachs disease (a deficiency of an enzyme that metabolizes lipids)
	Breast-ovarian cancer (the BRCA1 gene)
Chinese	Thalassemia (a blood disorder)
	Lactase deficiency (a deficiency of an enzyme for digestion)
French Canadians	Familial hypercholesterolemia (high levels of blood cholesterol)
Lebanese	Familial hypercholesterolemia (high levels of blood cholesterol)
Mediterranean peoples	Thalassemia (a blood disorder)
	G6PD deficiency (a deficiency of an enzyme in blood cells)
European Caucasians	Cystic fibrosis (a deficiency of a protein in the lungs)
Scandinavians	Alpha-antitrypsin deficiency (a deficiency of an enzyme in the liver)
South African whites	Familial hypercholesterolemia (high levels of blood cholesterol)

Source: From "Genetics and Disease," by A. Beaudet, 1998, in *Harrison's Principles of Internal Medicine* (p. 389), 14th ed., by A. Fauci, et al., New York: McGraw-Hill. Used by permission.

are assessed in some manner for their risk of genetic or chromosomal diseases. If either member of a couple has a family history of a genetic disease, or if either belongs to a population with a high incidence of an autosomal recessive disease, the couple is counseled on the risks and benefits of genetic screening with a carrier test, if such a test exists (see Table 2.1). Ideally, if couples are actively planning their families, screening for known genetic disorders can occur during preconception screening. Because the risk for some genetic and chromosomal abnormalities increases with age, women over 35 are routinely offered genetic testing to evaluate the fetal chromosomes, either by amniocentesis or chorionic villus sampling. (See Chapter 16 for more details on prenatal screening.)

Although prenatal screening is commonplace today, the results can create a challenging situation for the prospective parents. For example, if they discover that they both carry a copy of the sickle cell mutation, they have a 25 percent chance that each of their children will have sickle cell disease. They may then choose not to have children, or they may decide to pursue a pregnancy and have genetic testing later to determine whether the fetus has sickle cell disease. If they find that the fetus does have sickle cell disease, they face another dilemma—whether to continue or terminate the pregnancy. Although children with sickle cell disease have many medical problems, advancing knowledge and technology is improving their quality of life and is likely to continue to do so in the future.

A similar dilemma faces prospective parents who discover through amniocentesis that their fetus has Down syndrome. Although the test tells them the fetus has an extra chromosome 21, it cannot tell them what other health problems the child may have or how functional the child will be. Many children who have a genetic disease lead

Amniocentesis is a procedure in which fluid is drawn from the amniotic sac of a pregnant woman to test for genetic disorders, birth defects, and other problems.

happy, productive lives with their own unique limitations and challenges; other children who are perfectly healthy may have a poor quality of life owing to nongenetic limitations and challenges.

Newborn Screening Tests

Newborns in the United States and Canada are routinely screened for phenylketonuria (PKU) and congenital hypothyroidism. Decisions about whether to screen for other genetic and metabolic disorders are made by individual states or provinces, usually on the basis of how often a disorder occurs in the population, whether an effective screening test exists, and whether the disorder is treatable when detected.[25]

Screening for PKU is a model of successful genetic testing. The PKU mutation is inherited in an autosomal recessive pattern. A child with two copies of the mutated gene is unable to process an amino acid called phenylalanine in the diet. If the child consumes too much phenylalanine, toxic chemicals build up that cause seizures and severe mental retardation. If the condition is detected at birth, the child is placed on a diet that restricts phenylalanine. With strict adherence to the diet and a dietary supplement, the child will grow and develop like other children. Newborn screening tests to detect PKU have become so routine that parents do not even sign a consent form to have the tests performed. In fact, parents must sign to opt out of testing.

MANAGEMENT AND TREATMENT OF GENETIC CONDITIONS

Treatments are available for a number of genetic disorders, as suggested throughout this chapter. Treatments include dietary modification, medications, environmental adaptations, and gene therapy.

Dietary Modification

Some genetic disorders can be fully or partially treated through dietary modification, whether restriction, exclusion, or supplementation.[5] Restriction is called for when a common food is toxic to a person with a genetic mutation, as in the case of phenylketonuria. For an individual with PKU, phenylalanine must be limited for life. Exclusion is required when a person has a life-threatening reaction to a particular food, as in certain food allergies. Some people are allergic to even miniscule amounts of shellfish or peanuts, and these foods have to be completely excluded from their diet. Finally, supplementation is helpful for some genetic disorders. In the case of sickle cell disease, for example, individuals are at risk for dehydration and can benefit from drinking large volumes of fluids. In cystic fibrosis, the fat-soluble vitamins A, D, E, and K are poorly absorbed, so individuals with this disorder benefit from taking vitamin supplements.

Medications

For some genetic disorders, drugs can decrease symptoms or prevent serious complications. For instance, people with hemophilia, who are missing a blood-clotting factor, can take a synthetic form of the factor. People at high risk of colon cancer owing to hereditary colon polyps can take anti-inflammatory medicines to decrease the risk. People with congenital adrenal hyperplasia (a condition in which a person cannot produce vital steroids) can take a hormone replacement to treat the disease.

Environmental Adaptations

Avoiding harmful environmental factors can be effective in managing many genetic disorders. People with albinism, for example, have an increased risk of skin cancer owing to a lack of the normal pigment in the skin, hair, and eyes, so they must avoid sun exposure more than others must. Some people have a recessive genetic disorder that makes it difficult for them to resume breathing on their own after having general anesthesia. They have to avoid certain kinds of muscle relaxant medication during surgery. Individuals with a genetic predisposition for diabetes can lower their risk for the disorder by maintaining a healthy weight. And as we saw in the case of the BRCA1 genetic mutation for breast cancer, individuals can make several lifestyle changes to avoid the environmental factors that may be associated with the disease.

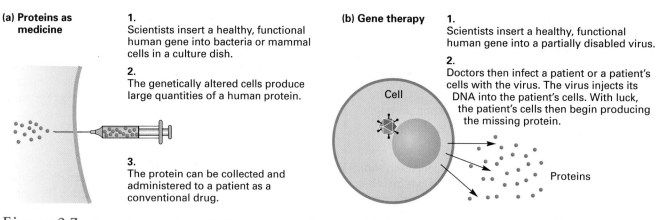

(a) Proteins as medicine

1.
Scientists insert a healthy, functional human gene into bacteria or mammal cells in a culture dish.

2.
The genetically altered cells produce large quantities of a human protein.

3.
The protein can be collected and administered to a patient as a conventional drug.

(b) Gene therapy

1.
Scientists insert a healthy, functional human gene into a partially disabled virus.

2.
Doctors then infect a patient or a patient's cells with the virus. The virus injects its DNA into the patient's cells. With luck, the patient's cells then begin producing the missing protein.

Cell

Proteins

Figure 2.7   **Harnessing a useful gene.** *Useful genes can be used to make medicinal proteins when they are grown in a lab (a) or introduced directly into the body (b).* Source: Adapted from "A Revolution in Medicine," by G. Cowley and A. Underwood, April 10, 2000, *Newsweek*, p. 61.

Gene Therapy

Although the treatments just described have helped people with genetic diseases to live better lives, they do not eliminate or cure the genetic disease. In 1972 scientists proposed replacing defective genes with healthy ones, which would treat or eliminate the cause of disease rather than simply treating symptoms of disease.[26] The healthy gene, once inserted into a cell, would provide the instructions for the cell to produce the protein that the defective gene was unable to produce.

In 1990, Ashanthi DeSilva became the first patient to receive gene therapy.[27] DeSilva suffered from a form of severe combined immune deficiency. In this disorder, a single gene codes for an enzyme that is crucial to the function of the immune system. With two defective copies of the gene, DeSilva was dangerously susceptible to even the mildest infections. To correct the defect, DeSilva received infusions of her own white blood cells, which had been given healthy genes to replace the defective genes. DeSilva became living proof that gene therapy can work. Today she is a healthy adult, although she continues to receive periodic gene therapy.

Scientists optimistically envision a future in which heart disease or cancer can be cured by injections of healthy DNA. Remember, however, that cells are microscopic and DNA is even smaller. The miniscule section of DNA that makes up the healthy gene must be collected and then somehow inserted into the cell without destroying the cell. The healthy gene then must incorporate itself into the cell's DNA in such a way as to function.

Many challenges arise during this process. First, researchers have to identify the mutations that cause a specific disease or, in the case of polygenic or multifactorial diseases, the mutations that increase risk. They then have to determine which cells within the patient need to receive a healthy copy of the gene. The protein that a gene encodes may be necessary only in certain parts of the body, or it may be vital throughout the body.

Next, researchers have to deliver the healthy gene to the cells where it is needed. One technique is to remove cells from the patient, insert the healthy gene in the cells, grow the cells in a culture dish, and then place them back into the patient. Another technique is to use a virus to carry a healthy gene into a cell that has an abnormal gene. Viruses function by injecting their genetic material into host cells and getting the host cell to incorporate the virus's genes into its own DNA and replicate the virus. Scientists can exploit a virus's ability to infect cells by putting a healthy gene into a virus. When the virus is injected into the patient, it releases the healthy, desired gene into the cells, which theoretically then start replicating the healthy gene. The gene, in turn, starts encoding the protein needed for the cell to do its job (Figure 2.7).

Gene therapy via viral transport is still in an early research stage and is not ready to be widely used, as was made tragically clear in 1999 by the death of 18-year-old Jesse Gelsinger. Gelsinger had an inherited condition that put him at risk of developing toxic levels of ammonia. He participated in a study to receive a virus that carried the corrected genetic material. Four days after the treatment, he died from an overwhelming immune response to the virus.[28] Aside from potentially fatal immune responses, other problems associated with viral transport need to be solved, including how to ensure that the healthy gene will work once it is inside the cell and how to transport a gene that is larger than a virus.

IMPLICATIONS OF GENETIC RESEARCH FOR INDIVIDUALS AND SOCIETY

Clearly, genetic research is changing the scientific, medical, and ethical landscape of the 21st century. It has conferred benefits on individuals, families, and society; at the same time, it has raised troubling issues. In this section we consider both aspects of our advancing genetic knowledge and technology.

Medical Advances and Cures

The face of medicine in particular will probably change dramatically in the next few decades, with genetic diagnosis and treatment becoming part of routine health care. Some people envision a day when the genetic pedigree or family health tree will be replaced by a personal genetic profile, created by mapping and sequencing all of an individual's genes. Physicians could then provide personalized recommendations for lifestyle choices and medical screenings based on individual risk, rather than broad public health recommendations.

Research on genes and the proteins they produce will also expand and be applied to more and more genetic diseases. Research on gene therapy for cystic fibrosis, for example, has already had some success in depositing healthy genes that produce the proteins needed for normal lung function in the damaged airway cells of CF patients. Another line of research is under way in muscle wasting diseases, such as muscular dystrophy. In the most common form of this disease, Duchenne muscular dystrophy, a defective gene leads to the absence of a protein, dystrophin, that protects muscles against the damage caused by everyday use. As muscle fibers are injured and die, patients become increasingly weak and debilitated. A similar loss of muscle occurs in natural aging but over a much longer period of time. Researchers have experimented with injecting synthetic genes that produce a muscle growth factor into muscle cells to hasten repair. Such therapies would have applications not only in curing muscular diseases but in slowing down or preventing muscle loss in older adults.

As promising as these prospects are, some gene therapies may be subject to misuse. An example is *gene doping*. Athletes wishing to build muscle and increase strength beyond what they can accomplish through training may some day be able to use the techniques developed to treat muscular dystrophy.[29] Unlike the effects of performance-enhancing drugs, gene therapy would be confined to the muscle into which the gene was injected and would be virtually untraceable. If such genetic enhancement were to become common practice, the climate of athletics and sport would undoubtedly be quite different from what it is today.

Issues in Genetic Screening and Testing

Other issues arise in the context of genetic screening and testing. The understanding of genes and genetic disorders has far outpaced treatments and cures. Most people don't want to know they have a defective gene that might cause them harm if there is nothing they can do about it. Thus, in many instances, testing is not recommended even when a defective gene can be identified, as in the case of the gene for Alzheimer's disease. In such cases, genetic information causes alarm and anxiety without, as yet, offering hope for a treatment or cure.

Further issues arise in the context of prenatal screening. Some physicians have reservations about offering tests because they feel it puts pressure on parents to consider abortion as an option. Offering prenatal screening for certain non-life-threatening conditions, such as deafness, may convey the idea that these conditions are diseases. Another issue for physicians is the concern that parents may sue them for malpractice if they fail to offer a particular screening test, especially if offering the test becomes standard practice in some states. Some genetic tests are costly for patients, but then so is caring for a disabled child, in both financial and emotional terms.

Issues of Privacy and Discrimination

Another area of concern is the possibility of discrimination based on genetic information. Individuals who undergo genetic testing may find that they are not the only ones interested in detailed genetic information about themselves; employers and health insurance companies may also be interested in that information.

Discrimination in the Workplace

Genetic testing has two potentially beneficial uses in the workplace. The first is genetic screening to determine whether an employee is at increased risk for developing a disease if exposed to specific factors in the work environment. The worker may then be relocated away from the hazardous environment. The second is genetic monitoring. Because some workplace exposures have the potential to cause genetic damage, monitoring a worker's genetic makeup for changes may help identify hazardous materials and increase worker safety. However, neither of these potential uses for genetic information has been shown to be clearly useful.[30, 31]

A disadvantage of genetic testing in the context of the workplace is the potential for discrimination. Employers may withhold promotions or refuse to hire a person on the basis of genetic information. Many such cases have been reported. For example, an employee was fired from her job after she revealed to her boss that she carried the gene for Huntington's disease. In the 8 months before her termination, she had received excellent performance reviews and promotions.[30, 31]

In theory, the 1990 Americans with Disabilities Act (ADA) may protect people in the United States from genetic discrimination. This law does protect people who have a disability because of genetic disease, as with a disability from any cause. The law also restricts when and how an employer may use an employee's medical information. Employers may collect medical information but must ensure that it is kept confidential and separate from personnel records. However, the ADA does not explicitly prohibit discrimination against an able-bodied person who is a carrier of a genetic mutation or who has a high risk of developing a disease or disability.

As noted earlier, one mandate of the Human Genome Project was to consider the ethical, legal, and social implications of possessing detailed genetic information about people. Three thousand judges received training in the fundamentals of genetics so that they would be knowledgeable regarding legal implications of new genetic information.[1] A majority of the states have proposed genetic nondiscrimination bills, and in October 2003 the U.S. Senate passed the Genetic Information Nondiscrimination Act of 2003 (s.1053). This bill is designed to protect people from discrimination based on their genetic information.[32] In Canada, human rights laws and insurance laws are believed to offer some protection against genetic discrimination. However, there remains an absence of statutes and regulations that specifically address genetic testing and information.[33]

Discrimination and Health Insurance

Genetic information is also of interest to insurance companies, who use information about risk for disease to help determine how much people will pay for health insurance. In the mid-1970s, many health insurance companies shifted from a social insurance model, in which low-risk and high-risk clients were combined in the same pool, to a casualty model, in which the cost of insurance is determined on the basis of a person's risk for getting ill.[34] For example, smoking might be a factor in a risk-rating model, and people who smoke would pay higher rates for insurance than would people who do not smoke. A person with a family history of disease might also have to pay more for insurance.

Insurance companies want to know as much as possible before contracting with a potential client because they want to be able to accurately predict the cost, or risk, of taking on a particular client. Individuals may, in turn, try to conceal disadvantageous health information. To prevent health information concealment, insurance companies can write clauses into policies that exclude preexisting conditions. Companies may also charge more for clients whose health care may be costly, or they may simply deny insurance. Companies are constrained to some degree by state laws and corporate charters that try to protect people from being denied coverage, but exclusionary policies are legal.[35]

An example of such insurance policies can be seen in the case of Jamie Stephenson, a mother of four children living in New Hampshire. Two of Stephenson's children were diagnosed with Fragile X syndrome, a genetic condition associated with developmental disability that affects approximately 1 in 1,000 males and 1 in 2,000 females. In June 1991 the Stephenson's family health insurance was canceled because of the presence of this condition.[36] Ms. Stephenson's search for coverage through other insurance agencies proved frustrating. Few companies were inclined to offer coverage, and those that would did so only with the condition that the two sons with Fragile X be excluded.

In 2003 a federal regulation known as the HIPAA Privacy Rule was added to the Health Insurance Portability and Accountability Act (HIPAA) of 1996 to address concerns over genetic testing and health insurance. It includes a provision that prohibits health insurers from using "genetic information" in evaluating an individual's eligibility. However, not everyone is reassured by the HIPAA provision. This is because insurance companies have elaborate means at their disposal for acquiring information about people. When a person applies for health insurance, he or she typically has to complete a questionnaire that contains probing family health history questions, such as the age at which family members died and specific diseases they had. Such information can be used as a substitute for genetic testing. Applicants must also sign a disclosure statement authorizing the insurance company to access all of their medical records, including physicians' notes, test results, hospital stays, and information on consultation with specialists.

In the past decade or so, health insurance companies have gone even further by amassing huge databases of personal information on applicants and policy holders. Corporations such as the Medical Information Bureau (MIB) have emerged as central storage facilities for these databases. The MIB consists of more than 700 insurance companies that share information about their policy holders. Profiles of more than 15 million policy holders are contained in the MIB databank. A person who applies for life, health, or disability insurance with one of the member groups signs a release giving the company permission to provide information to the MIB. By law, the person's privacy is not violated, because he or she voluntarily consented to the release of information. However, most companies do not give people the choice of refusing to have their records released if they want to have insurance. (See the box "Protecting Your Patient Records.")

Parental Eugenics

Yet another area of concern associated with genetic information is parental eugenics. Eugenics is the practice of selective breeding, or controlling a group's reproductive choices, in an attempt to improve the human species. A popular idea in the late 19th century, eugenics was carried to an inhumane extreme by the Nazis during World War II, and it continues to occur in troubled places around the world under the guise of ethnic cleansing.

Today we are in the midst of a new eugenics movement, based on the belief that parents have the right to decide what kind of child they want to have.[37] Prenatal screening paved the way for a new technology called preimplantation genetic diagnosis, in which an ovum is fertilized in vitro (in the laboratory) and screened for genetic diseases before being implanted in a woman's uterus. The technology is currently used when a couple is at risk for having a child with a devastating disease. As research progresses and more genes are identified; however, the same

Consumer Clipboard

Protecting Your Patient Records

On April 14, 2003, the HIPAA Privacy Rule went into effect, providing federal privacy standards to protect patients' medical records and other health information. This provision allows you to take more control of your health information. In accordance with this law, you should be able to do the following:

- Access your medical records. You should be able to see and receive copies of your medical records within 30 days. Your health care provider may charge you the cost of copying and sending the records.

- Request corrections if you identify errors in the records. You are entitled to add a statement to the record correcting errors that you find in the documentation.

- Limit the use of your medical information. Your health care provider cannot release your records to a life insurer, bank, marketing firm, or another outside business not related to your health care without your written consent.

- Request confidential communications. You may ask your health care provider to contact you only at specific locations (for example, your work site instead of your home number), and the office should comply if the request can be reasonably accommodated.

The Privacy Rule has added new layers of complexity in areas beyond patient rights, including clinical research, public health services, fund-raising by medical centers, and the compilation of vital statistics by the government. All of these endeavors rely on many sources of health information, including physician and hospital records. These effects will become clearer over the next several years.

---

technology could be used to allow parents to select the traits they want in their child—high intelligence, athletic ability, physical appearance, and so on. Although this kind of eugenics is different from the old eugenics in the sense that parents are making decisions about their children's and family's future rather than having standards imposed on them by a state, such practices may change how we as a society view qualities and flaws in appearance, personality, and the other varied dimensions of human difference.[37]

Genetics, Lifestyle Choices, and Personal Health

We conclude this chapter by reiterating the point we made at the outset: Genetics is simply the starting point of personal health. It determines potential but not outcome. Healthy genes do not guarantee a healthy life, nor does a genetic defect lead inevitably to a life of disability. Our genes are only one part of our overall wellness profile; other significant factors include individual lifestyle choices, socioeconomic factors, and sociocultural factors. If you choose to explore your personal genetics, either by completing a genetic pedigree or by having genetic tests done (for one of the reasons discussed in this chapter), keep in mind that this information is best used in helping you decide how to balance your health choices. Knowledge of your unique strengths and weaknesses, genetic and otherwise, can help you assess the risks and benefits of your actions and make the decisions that are right for you.

You Make the Call

DNA Profiling: The Ultimate Identification?

In 1983, Sir Alec Jeffries, a geneticist at the University of Leicester, England, theorized that DNA in biological materials at a crime scene—dried blood or semen, for example—could provide a means to identify the perpetrator. Jeffries' forensic DNA fingerprinting, now called profiling, helped solve a sensational murder case in England in 1987. Since then, DNA evidence has become commonplace in criminal and civil court cases.

The media hailed DNA profiling as the 20th century's greatest forensic breakthrough and predicted that it would revolutionize the investigation of violent crimes. Biotechnology firms that analyzed forensic DNA claimed that the possibility of error in DNA matching was 1 in 4 or 5 million: a virtually foolproof crime test. The perception of infallibility was dealt a blow during the O. J. Simpson murder trial in California in 1995, however. It was pointed out at the trial that in one method of DNA testing, the DQ Alpha method, the odds of two people having the same combination of DNA markers ranged from 1 in 5 to 1 in 100—a far cry from the previously claimed odds of 1 in 4 or 5 million.

Despite such claims, most scientists agree that there is only a remote possibility that two people will share the same DNA fragments unless they are identical twins. Thus, DNA profiling may offer conclusive scientific proof in criminal and civil cases. DNA information can also be used to solve crimes committed by known criminals. Blood samples from a crime scene can be compared with samples that have been taken from convicted criminals and stored in a database for such use. DNA profiling can be as useful to defendants as it is to prosecutors, since DNA evidence is as likely to establish innocence as it is to prove guilt. DNA can also be used to identify soldiers killed in war or civilians killed in accidents. DNA testing was used to help identify the remains of people killed in the World Trade Center in the terrorist attacks of September 11, 2001.

Opponents of DNA testing argue that improper collection, handling, or storage of DNA samples can contaminate evidence. DNA profiling has been disallowed in many states for this reason. The cost of DNA profiling can be prohibitive, thus giving an advantage to the prosecution, which has more resources. DNA tests may undermine the presumption of innocence that is the foundation of the justice system in democratic countries. DNA profiling could infringe upon the right of a jury to make objective decisions and call into question whether juries are needed at all in the presence of DNA evidence.

Opponents also assert that DNA profiling may violate the Fourth Amendment's protection against "unreasonable searches and seizures," interpreted as a right to privacy. DNA testing yields sensitive information about a person's health and about matters of social importance, such as paternity. Federal legislation so far has not definitively protected the rights of individuals when it comes to banking their body tissues and fluids as a source of their DNA.

Many people think DNA evidence can provide a foolproof way of identifying and convicting criminals and exonerating the innocent. Others think DNA profiling will lead to discrimination and civil rights abuses. What do you think?

Pros

- There is only a remote possibility that any two people will have identical DNA.
- DNA profiling may serve as conclusive evidence in criminal cases (establishing either guilt or innocence).
- DNA profiling can be used to track known criminals whose DNA is in a databank.
- DNA profiling can be used to identify human remains.

Cons

- The improper collection, handling, and storage of samples can contaminate DNA evidence.
- The expense of DNA profiling can lead to unequal access to the technology for different parties.
- DNA databanks may infringe on the Fourth Amendment right to privacy.

OLC Web site For more information on this topic, visit the Online Learning Center at www.mhhe.com/teague1e.

SUMMARY

- Your genetic inheritance plays an important—but not determining—role in your health. Environmental factors and behavioral choices also play important roles.
- A family health history, in the form of a pedigree or genogram, can help you see patterns of health and illness and point to problems that you may have inherited.
- Human beings have 23 pairs of chromosomes—tightly coiled molecules of deoxyribonucleic acid (DNA), which consists of four different nucleotides arranged in repeating pairs in a double helix structure. Genes are specific sequences of nucleotides that code for proteins and other functional products; they provide instructions for the work of the cells, and they are the units of heredity.
- The Human Genome Project sequenced and mapped the location of all the genes (approximately 20,000 to 25,000) on the 23 chromosomes in the human genome.
- Genes not only determine characteristics but, as a result of mutations, can cause or contribute to disease. In single-gene diseases, a change in one gene causes a disease; in polygenic diseases, changes in several genes cause disease; in multifactorial diseases, changes in one or several genes interact with environmental factors to alter the risk of disease. Most common diseases, such as heart disease, diabetes, and hypertension, are multifactorial diseases.
- A person who is a carrier for a disease has a single copy of a gene mutation and a normal copy of the gene. A carrier shows no signs of the disease but can pass the mutation to his or her children.

- Chromosomal disorders involve changes in an entire chromosome, producing a broad range of symptoms known as a syndrome. An example is Down syndrome.
- Some genetic diseases are found more often within certain ethnic groups. Examples are sickle cell disease, Tay-Sachs disease, and cystic fibrosis.
- Genes are involved in some mental disorders, such as schizophrenia, mood and anxiety disorders, and Alzheimer's disease. Genes may also play a role in personality and in some behaviors, including those associated with sexual orientation and addiction.
- Genetic counselors can help educate people about possible genetic disorders and help them weigh the pros and cons of genetic testing. People sometimes do not want to be tested, either because there is no treatment for the disease they may have or because they fear their genetic information will be used to discriminate against them.
- There are several types of genetic screening tests, including diagnostic tests, predictive tests, carrier tests, prenatal screenings, and newborn screenings.
- Genetic disorders can be managed and treated through dietary modifications, medications, and environmental adaptations. A new treatment approach, gene therapy, seeks to cure genetic disorders by inserting healthy genes into cells with defective genes. This approach, although promising, is still experimental.
- Advances in our genetic knowledge and technology have wide-ranging implications. Our knowledge of genes has thus far outpaced treatments and cures, raising more fear than hope for some. Although there are already medical benefits, there is also the possibility of misuse, as in the example of gene doping by athletes.
- Genetic information is subject to abuse by employers and health insurance companies, who may use it to discriminate against people who have or who carry genetic disorders.
- Parents may use genetic information to design the kind of children they want to have, a practice that could change society's attitudes toward certain characteristics in individuals.
- Your genetic inheritance is the starting point of your personal health. It does not relieve you of responsibility for your behavior, nor does it deprive you of your ability to exercise control over your destiny.

REVIEW QUESTIONS

1. Describe features in a family history that would suggest a genetic link to a disease.
2. Describe the relationship among chromosomes, DNA, and genes.
3. How can a genetic mutation cause a disease?
4. What are the differences between an autosomal dominant disorder and an autosomal recessive disorder?
5. What is a single-gene disease? A polygenic disease? A multifactorial disease?
6. What are the chances that a child born to parents who are both carriers for a disease will have the disease? Will be a carrier for the disease? Will not have the genetic mutation?
7. If a person has a high genetic risk for heart disease, what are some lifestyle changes he or she could make to reduce the risk?
8. If a genetic mutation causes a disease or disability, why wouldn't that mutation have been weeded out of the human genome many generations ago?
9. What are some environmental conditions that might trigger the onset of schizophrenia, depression, or Alzheimer's disease?
10. What are the different dimensions of temperament that have been observed in infants? What are some environmental conditions that could influence the development of personality?
11. What is known about the role of genetics in sexual orientation? In alcoholism?
12. What types of genetic tests are available? What is the difference between a predispositional test and a presymptomatic test?
13. What are the options for treating genetic disorders? For curing them?
14. What are some reasons that a person might not want to have a genetic test?
15. What are some advantages and some disadvantages of parental eugenics?
16. What is the role of genetics in your personal health?

WEB RESOURCES

Access Excellence Resource Center: Associated with the U.S. Department of Health and Human Services, this national educational program provides health, biology, and life sciences information. It offers answers to questions such as: What are genes? What is genetic testing? How do gene mistakes occur? www.accessexcellence.org

Gene Tests: This organization offers authoritative information on genetic testing and its use in the diagnosis and management of disease and genetic counseling. Funded by the National Institutes of Health, it promotes the appropriate use of genetic services in patient care and personal decision making. www.genetests.org

Genetics Society of America: This professional organization includes more than 4,000 scientists and educators in the field of genetics. Through its journal *Genetics,* it publishes information on advances in genetics. www.genetics-gsa.org

Gene Watch UK: Featuring developments in genetic technologies from the perspective of public interest, environmental protection, and animal welfare, this group explores topics ranging from genetically modified crops and foods to genetic testing in humans. www.genewatch.org

National Adoption Information Clearinghouse: This is a good place to start if you are looking for information about your biological parents. http: //naic.acf.hhs.gov

National Human Genome Research Institute: The leader of the Human Genome Project for the National Institutes of Health, this institute continues to do research in genetics aimed at improving human health and fighting disease. www.genome.org

National Society of Genetic Counselors: This society offers FAQs about genetic counselors, such as: What is a genetic counselor? How do I find a genetic counselor near me? What can you expect on a first visit to a genetic counselor? www.nsgc.org

REFERENCES

1. Collins, F. S., et al. (2003). The Human Genome Project: Lessons from large scale biology. *Science, 300,* 286–290.

2. International Human Genome Sequencing Consortium. (2004). Finishing the euchromatic sequence of the human genome. *Nature, 431,* 931–945.

3. Strachan, T., & Read, A. P. (2004). *Human molecular genetics* (3rd ed.). Oxford: Blos Scientific Publishers.

4. Kingston, H. (1997). *ABC of clinical genetics: Genetics of common disorders.* Margate: BMJ Publishing, Thanet Press.

5. Mulinsky, A. (2001). *Your genetic destiny.* Cambridge, MA: Perseus Publishing.

6. Gehring, W. J. (1998). *Master control genes in development and evolution: The Homeobox story.* New Haven, CT: Yale University Press.

7. Fauci, A., et al. (2005). *Harrison's principles of internal medicine* (16th ed.). New York: McGraw-Hill.

8. Pinsky, L., Erickson, R. P., & Schimke, R. N. (1999). *Genetic disorders of human sexual development.* Oxford, UK: Oxford University Press.

9. McKusick, U. A. (1998). *Mendelian inheritance in man: A catalog of human genes and genetic disorders* (12th ed.). Baltimore: Johns Hopkins University Press.

10. Tishkoff, S. A., & Verrelli, B. C. (2003). Patterns of human genetic diversity: Implications for human evolutionary history and disease. *Annual Review of Genomics and Human Genetics, 14,* 293–340.

11. Kaback, M. (2000). Population-based genetic screening for reproductive counseling: The Tay-Sachs disease model. *European Journal of Pediatrics, 159* (3), 5192–5195.

12. Thiagarajah, J. R., & Verkman, A. S. (2003). CFTR pharmacology and its role in intestinal fluid secretion. *Current Opinion in Pharmacology, 3* (6), 594–599.

13. American Psychiatric Association. (2000). *Diagnostic and statistical manual of mental disorders* (4th ed., text revision). Washington, DC: American Psychiatric Association.

14. Cowan, W. M., Kopnisky, H. L., & Hyman, S. E. (2002). The Human Genome Project and its impact on psychiatry. *Annual Review of Neuroscience, 25,* 1–50.

15. Butcher, J. M., Mineka, S., & Hooley, J. M. (2004). *Abnormal psychology* (12th ed.). Boston: Pearson/Allyn and Bacon.

16. Kendler, K. S., et al. (1992). A population-based twin study of major depression in women: The impact of varying definitions of illness. *Archives of General Psychiatry, 49,* 257–266.

17. Alec, R., Segal, N., Centerwall, B., & Robinette, C. D. (1991). Suicide in twins. *Archives of General Psychiatry, 48,* 29–32.

18. Ciarleglio, L. J., et al. (2003). Genetic counseling throughout the life cycle. *Journal of Clinical Investigation, 112* (9), 1280–1286.

19. Pillard, R. C. (1998). Human sexual orientation has a heritable component. *Human Biology, 70* (2), 347–365.

20. Bailey, J. M. (1999). A family history study of male sexual orientation using three independent samples. *Behavioral Genetics, 29* (2), 79–86.

21. Rice, G. (1999). Male homosexuality: Absence of linkage to microsatellite markers at Xq28. *Science, 284* (5414), 665–667.

22. Enoch, M. A. (1999). Genetics of alcoholism and substance abuse. *Psychiatric Clinics of North America, 22* (2), 289–299.

23. Bennett, R. L., et al. (2003). Genetic counselors: Translating genomic science into clinical practice. *Journal of Clinical Investigation, 112* (9), 1274–1279.

24. National Society for Genetic Counselors. (2004). Fact sheet for the NSAC. www.nsgc.org.

25. United States General Accounting Office Report to Congressional Requestors. (2003, March). Newborn screening. Characteristics of state programs. http://genes-r-us.uthscsa.edu.

26. Balicki, D., & Beultler, E. (2002). Gene therapy of human disease. *Medicine, 8* (1), 69–86.

27. Hubbard, R., & Wald, E. (1999). *Exploding the gene myth: How genetic information is produced and manipulated by*

scientists, physicians, employers, insurance companies, educators and law enforcers. Boston: Beacon Press.

28. Lehrman, S. (2000). Gene Letter, 1 (1). www.geneletter.com.

29. Sweeney, H. L. (2004, July). Gene doping. *Scientific American,* 63–69.

30. The National Human Genome Research Institute, Department of Health and Human Services. (1998). Genetic information and the workplace. www.nhgri.nih.gov.

31. McCunney, R. J. (2002). Genetic testing: Ethical implications in the workplace. *Occupational Medicine, 17* (4), 665–672.

32. Collins, F. (2003, October 14). Press release, National HGP Research Institute. www.genome.gov/11009127.

33. Lemmens, T. (2003). Genetics and insurance discrimination: Comparative legislative, regulatory and policy developments and Canadian options. *Health Law Journal,* Special Edition 2003: 41–86.

34. Natowitz, M. R., & Alper, J. S. (1991). Genetic screening: Triumphs, problems and controversies. *Journal of Public Health Policy, 12* (4), 475–491.

35. Stone, D. A. (1996). The implications of the Human Genome Project for access to health insurance. In T. H. Murray, M. A. Rothstein, & R. G. Murray, Jr. (Eds.), *The Human Genome Project and the future of health care.* Bloomington: Indiana University Press.

36. Winik, L. W. (1998, April 19). When you should consider a genetic test. *Parade,* 7–10.

37. Allen, G. E. (2001). Essays on science and society. Is a new eugenics afoot? *Science, 294* (5540), 59–61.

Add It Up! CREATING A FAMILY HEALTH TREE

A family health tree is a diagram of your family's health history over several generations. As such, it can provide important clues to the genes you have inherited from your parents, grandparents, and ancestors. Constructing a family health tree has three broad steps: (1) mapping the family structure, (2) recording family information, and (3) finding family relationships. Refer to the model provided in Figure 2.1 as you construct your own family health tree. You can use the template provided on the next page, or simply start with a blank piece of paper.

1. Begin with yourself and your immediate family. Draw a circle if you are female or a square if you are male, label it "Self," and indicate your current age. Draw a vertical line up from yourself and a horizontal line across it. On the left end of the horizontal line, draw a square for your father, and on the right end, draw a circle for your mother. If you have siblings, draw a horizontal line across the vertical line between you and your parents and drop lines down from it for each sibling, your brothers to the left and your sisters to the right, in order by age.

2. Now add lines to the left and right of your parents for their siblings (your aunts and uncles), as shown on the template. Continue the diagram, adding your cousins, your grandparents, your great-aunts and uncles, and as many other relatives as you can. The more generations and individuals you include, the more useful your pedigree will be.

3. Write the year that two people married on the connecting line between the two, with an "m" and the date (for example, "m1975"). If they are separated, write an "s" with the date, and draw a single slash through the line connecting them. If they are divorced, write a "d" with the date, and draw two slashes. If several divorces have taken place, write them on the opposite side of the current marriage, with the most recent closest to the spouse.

4. When placing children beneath their parents, begin with the oldest on the left. Connect adopted or foster children to their parents with a dotted line to indicate that no biological relationship exists.

5. For each person, write his or her relationship to you next to, above, or beneath the circle or square, along with the person's age or date of birth. If the person is deceased, draw an X in the circle or square and write his or her date of death (or age at death) and the cause of death. If a woman has had a miscarriage or stillbirth, indicate that with an X in a square or circle. Because some genetic conditions are more common in certain ethnic groups, include the ethnicity of each person in the oldest generation you include.

6. Now add as much health-related information as you know for each person. Include major diseases or health conditions, such as diabetes, osteoporosis, cancer, heart disease, and so on, and the person's age when diagnosed. Also include surgeries, allergies, mental health problems, and any genetic or chromosomal disorders, such as Down syndrome.

7. Once you have gathered all the information, you can analyze your family health tree. Do you see any patterns of illness or disease? Are there any special health concerns? You may want to take your family health tree to your physician or a genetic counselor for a professional opinion on your health risks. He or she may recommend that you modify certain lifestyle behaviors (such as diet or exercise) or have particular screening tests (such as an early test for cancer). You may want to have your physician keep a copy of your family health tree in your medical file for future reference. You may also want to share what you have found out, as well as your physician's recommendations, with your siblings and other family members.

Note: For a sample family health history, see "My Family Health Portrait," shown on the reverse side of this page. This template is also available online at www.hhs.gov/family/history.

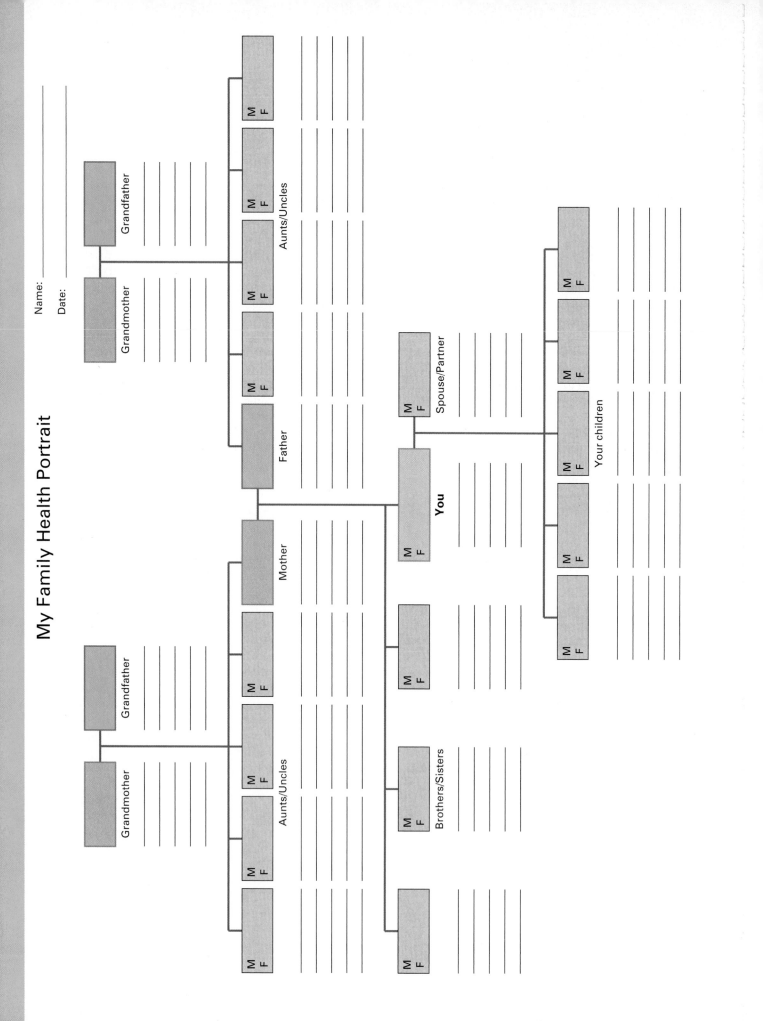

My Family Health Portrait

Name: _____

Date: _____

CHAPTER 3

Mental Health: Creating a Balance

DID YOU KNOW?

- The activities you engage in during adolescence and early adulthood—sports, academics, television watching—can have a long-term effect on your mental capabilities. Your brain is not fully developed until you reach your early 20s, and the neural connections you use the most are the ones that last.

- You can enhance your mental health by consciously working to develop such characteristics and attitudes as optimism, resilience, and a sense of self-efficacy. Optimistic people seem to enjoy better health, both physically and mentally, than pessimistic people.

- It is highly likely that you know someone with a diagnosable mental disorder. More than 20 percent of American adults—some 50 million people—experience a mental disorder in any given year. However, only about 8 million people seek treatment.

OLC *Your Health Today*   www.mhhe.com/teague1e

Go to the Online Learning Center for *Your Health Today* for interactive activities, quizzes, flashcards, Web links, and more resources related to this chapter.

Mental health encompasses several aspects of overall health or wellness. It can include the emotional, psychological, cognitive, interpersonal, and/or spiritual aspects of a person's life. Although we often think of physical health in connection with the body and mental health in connection with the mind, in practice the two are inextricably linked.

Like physical health, mental health is not simply the absence of symptoms of illness or disease. Rather, it includes the capacity to respond to challenges, frustrations, joys, and failures in ways that allow continued growth and forward movement in life. The key to mental health and happiness is not freedom from adversity in life—no one goes through life without some experience of loss, pain, guilt, or regret—but rather the ability to respond to adversity in adaptive, effective ways. A mentally healthy person is able to deal with life's inevitable bumps and bruises without becoming impaired or overwhelmed by them.

The majority of people are mentally healthy, but many experience emotional or psychological difficulties at some point in their lives. An estimated 50 percent of Americans experience some symptoms of depression during their lifetime, for example, and more than 20 percent of the American population are affected by a diagnosable mental disorder in a given year.[1] In Canada, an estimated 20 percent of the population experience a mental disorder in their lifetime.[2]

Four of the top 10 causes of disability in the United States are mental disorders: depression, bipolar disorder, schizophrenia, and obsessive-compulsive disorder.[1] The direct costs of diagnosing and treating mental disorders in the United States are estimated to exceed $69 billion annually. The indirect costs, for lost productivity in the workplace,

school, and the home because of premature death or disability, are estimated at more than $78 billion annually.[3]

In this chapter we explore mental health (also referred to as psychological health) and mental illness. We begin by exploring the characteristics of a mentally healthy person and the steps you can take to enhance your own mental health. We then take a brief look at the brain, the control center of mental activity. Following this we look at some influences on mental health and mental illness, and we examine the major mental disorders, considering first the differences between everyday emotional problems and problems for which professional treatment is needed or recommended. We close the chapter with a discussion of treatment options.

WHAT IS MENTAL HEALTH?

As noted, mental health is not just the absence of illness but also the presence of many positive characteristics and abilities. In this section we consider some of these characteristics and how they can be attained and enhanced.

Characteristics of Mentally Healthy People

Mentally healthy individuals share many characteristics. They tend to have high **self-esteem** and feel good about themselves. They respect themselves and others, but they are realistic and don't expect anyone to be perfect. They feel competent to accomplish things in their lives; they are also socially competent, demonstrating empathy and good listening skills in their interpersonal relationships. These and other traits, attitudes, and abilities indicative of

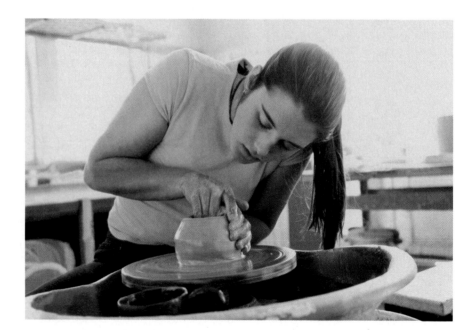

Self-actualization involves fostering your creativity. As this young woman learns the craft of pottery, she is expressing herself in a new and satisfying way.

HIGHLIGHT ON HEALTH

Characteristics of Mentally Healthy People

- They have high self-esteem and feel good about themselves.
- They are realistic and accepting of imperfections in themselves and others.
- They have a sense of control over their lives and feel capable of meeting challenges and solving problems.
- They demonstrate social competence in their relationships with others.
- They are comfortable with other people and believe they can rely on them.
- They are not overwhelmed by fear, love, or anger; they try to control irrational thoughts and levels of stress.

- They try not to respond to others' negativity or hate.
- They are optimistic; they try to maintain a positive outlook.
- They are altruistic; they help others.
- They do not fear differences and diversity.
- They have a capacity for intimacy; they do not fear commitment.
- They are creative and appreciate creativity in others.
- They take reasonable risks in order to grow.
- They bounce back from adversity.

mental health are listed in the box above, "Characteristics of Mentally Healthy People."

The Self-Actualized Person

Many of these healthy characteristics are found in the self-actualized person. The concept of **self-actualization** was developed by Abraham Maslow in the 1960s as a model of human personality development in his "hierarchy of needs" theory. Maslow proposed that once people meet their needs for survival, safety and security, love and belonging, and achievement and self-esteem, they have opportunities for self-exploration and expression that can lead them to reach their fullest human potential. According to Maslow, a self-actualized person is realistic, self-accepting, self-motivated, creative, and capable of intimacy, among other traits. Self-actualization is discussed in more detail in Chapter 4 in the context of spirituality. That chapter also includes an exercise that will let you evaluate your own progress toward self-actualization.

Optimism, Self-Efficacy, and Resilience

A key characteristic of mentally healthy people is optimism. People with an "optimistic explanatory style"—the tendency to see problems as temporary and specific rather than permanent and general—seem to have better physical and mental health than more pessimistic people do.[4] Optimistic people react to failures as things they can do something about, as challenges and opportunities for learning and growth. Pessimistic people tend to attribute failure to personal defects and react with discouragement

and a sense of defeat. (Of course, you also need to be realistic and recognize your own limitations; a person who disregards all the incoming information provided by successes and failures will end up only with more disappointment.) To assess your own optimism, see the Add It Up! feature at the end of this chapter.

Related to optimism is *self-efficacy,* the belief that you are competent to perform a particular task. In Chapter 1 we discussed self-efficacy in the context of changing a health behavior. In the context of mental health, self-efficacy refers to a general sense that you have some control over what happens in your life. Mentally healthy people have a basic belief that they can guide their own lives and when unexpected events occur, take them in stride, adapt, and move on.

This ability to bounce back from adverse events is known as **resilience,** and it is another characteristic of mentally healthy individuals. People who can respond flexibly to life's challenges and redirect their energies toward positive actions tend to be more successful in life.

KEY TERMS

self-esteem   Sense of positive regard and valuation for oneself.

self-actualization   In Maslow's work, the state attained when a person has reached his or her full potential.

resilience   Ability to bounce back from adversity.

Our lives will always have moments of adversity and vulnerability and be filled with challenging situations. Individuals who are resilient learn ways to respond to these events and situations. Resilience involves patterns of thinking, feeling, and behaving that contribute to a balanced life based on self-esteem, satisfying relationships, and a belief that life is meaningful.

Research has shown several key characteristics in resilient individuals, including the following:

- They are empathetic; they have the insight to understand other people's needs as well as the desire to make a positive difference in the lives of others.

- They are independent; they have a sense of empowerment and believe they have control over their responses, although not necessarily over their environment.

- They demonstrate initiative and creativity; they use productive coping skills.

- They have secure personal relationships; they believe they can count on the support of significant others.

- They take responsibility for their behavior; they acknowledge credit for their successes and accept responsibility for their mistakes.

- They have a sense of humor and appreciate humor in others.

We discuss resilience further in Chapter 4 as a building block of a spiritually satisfying life, and we discuss it in Chapter 5 as a quality that helps people respond effectively to stress. In both chapters, we discuss ways that you can improve your own resilience.

Emotional Intelligence

Intelligence is commonly thought of as a person's general capacity for reasoning, solving problems, and performing other mental functions accurately and efficiently. As such, intelligence can be measured by tests like the Stanford-Binet Intelligence Test, which gives a person a score referred to as an intelligence quotient (IQ). If you score above 100 on this test, you are considered to be of above-average intelligence; if you score below 100, you are considered below average.

The concept of intelligence was expanded in 1983 by psychologist John Gardner, who proposed that intelligence is not just one ability but something that can be manifested in several different areas.[5] The seven **multiple intelligences** he identified fall into three groups: Logical-mathematical and linguistic intelligences are the ones that have been traditionally valued in school. Musical intelligence, spatial intelligence, and bodily-kinesthetic intelligence are related to the arts. Interpersonal intelligence and intrapersonal intelligence involve sensitivity to and awareness of the feelings, moods, and motivations of others and oneself. Since Gardner's work was originally published, additional intelligences have been proposed.

Spiritual intelligence, for example, involves attaining a connectedness to the rest of the world, a deemphasis of self, and a level of consciousness that represents an "exemplary spiritual existence."[6]

The concept of intelligence was further expanded in 1995 by psychologist Daniel Goleman to include the idea of **emotional intelligence.** Goleman argued that such qualities as self-awareness, self-discipline, persistence, and empathy are much more important to success in life than IQ. People who are emotionally intelligent have an ability to (1) recognize, name, and understand their emotions, (2) manage their emotions and control their moods, (3) motivate themselves, (4) recognize and respond to emotions in others, and (5) be socially competent.[7] The last ability involves skills in understanding relationships, cooperating, solving problems, resolving conflicts, being assertive at communicating, and being considerate and compassionate.[6]

The significance of emotional intelligence is supported by studies showing that high scores on standardized tests such as the Scholastic Aptitude Test (SAT) and Graduate Record Exam (GRE) predict grades only for the first year of undergraduate or graduate school. They do not necessarily predict success after the first year or future success at work.[7] (See the box on the next page, "Who Has the Best Chance of Future Success?")

Whereas qualities such as resilience and optimism pertain more to internal characteristics, emotional intelligence involves how you relate to others. Like many of the other characteristics of mentally healthy people, emotional intelligence can be learned and improved. Many groups, workshops, and self-help books assist people in learning how to control impulses, manage anger, recognize emotions in themselves and others, and respond more appropriately in social situations.

Enhancing Your Mental Health

Several other factors appear to be related to the development of mental health, including a supportive social network, good communication skills, and healthy lifestyle patterns. Social support—family ties, friendships, and involvement in social activities—is one of the primary ingredients in a mentally healthy life. These social connections can provide a sense of belonging, support in difficult times, and a positive influence when you drift toward unhealthy behaviors. Social isolation, in contrast, is associated with depression and low self-esteem. The quality of the relationships is a consideration, however. Relationships that are oppressive, rigid, abusive, or psychologically unhealthy in other ways can undermine rather than enhance mental health. If you find yourself in such a relationship, take an honest look at whether you should take steps to change it.

Communication skills are necessary for negotiating relationships of all kinds. The ability to be assertive—to communicate what you want clearly and appropriately without violating other people's rights—is an important

Beating the Odds

Who Has the Best Chance of Future Success?

A multitude of factors seem to have an impact on future success—innate characteristics, personal attitudes, the support of family and friends, random opportunities. Brief profiles for three individuals are presented here. Who do you think has the best chance of success in the future?

Jamie is 25 years old and has just been laid off from her first job since graduating from college. She is unsure of what direction she would like to take in her career. Because the job market is tight, she is not feeling optimistic about her chances of getting another job. Although she has been very successful in college and her first job, she just does not feel confident right now and is worried that she will fail. Faced with this crisis, she is feeling immobilized and is not sure where to turn next. She has a supportive family, but they are not sure how to be helpful at this point. They have invited her to come home to live for a while, but she feels as if that would prove she's a failure.

Kevin is also 25, has few aspirations, and seems to be satisfied with his job and social life. He really is not interested in doing much more and believes he has gone as far as possible. He rarely has contact with his family and tries to be very self-sufficient. Overall he considers himself to be "low-maintenance" and sees the world through a pretty pessimistic lens. He believes that times are tough and he should not expect or try for much more. If he does try, he believes he will only waste his time and energy and in the end be disappointed.

Shoshana is a 24-year-old elementary school teacher. She enjoys her work and is taking classes toward a higher degree. Although she has a physical disability as a result of an auto crash when she was 16, she has tried not to let it get in the way of her aspirations. Her friends think she has unrealistic goals and sees the world through rose-colored glasses, but her parents support her in pursuing her goals. Although she continues to run into obstacles in her life, she keeps at it.

OLC Web site Visit the **Online Learning Center** at www.mhhe.com/teague1e for comments by the authors.

part of healthy communication. Another is the ability to be an effective listener. Tips on improving your communication skills are provided in Chapter 14.

Like physical health, mental health depends on a healthy lifestyle—eating well, exercising, getting enough sleep, and so on. But it is also improved by participating in activities that challenge you mentally, emotionally, socially, and physically. Consider some of the suggestions in the box on the next page, "Taking Healthy Risks."

THE BRAIN'S ROLE IN MENTAL HEALTH AND ILLNESS

Human beings have always experienced mental disturbances: descriptions of conditions called "mania," "melancholia," "hysteria," and "insanity" can be found in the literature of ancient Egypt, China, and Greece. Mental disturbances were commonly attributed to possession by demons or evil spirits, moral weakness or depravity, punishment for bad behavior, or other supernatural causes; "treatments" included imprisonment, burning at the stake, and various forms of exorcism, such as bleeding or purging.

It wasn't until the 18th and 19th centuries that advances in anatomy, physiology, and medicine allowed scientists to definitively identify the brain as the organ afflicted in cases of mental disturbance and to propose biological causes, especially damage to the brain, for mental disorders. Since then, other explanations have been proposed, involving, for example, psychological factors, sociocultural and environmental factors, and improper or inadequate learning. Debate over the roles of these various categories of causal factors continues to this day. Although it is clear that mental disorders are best understood as the result of many factors interacting in complex ways, the central role of the brain in mental health and mental illness is beyond doubt. Mental illnesses are diseases that affect the brain.[8]

KEY TERMS

multiple intelligences In Gardner's work, the many areas in which intelligence can be manifested, such as logical-mathematical, spatial, and interpersonal.

emotional intelligence In Goleman's work, the kind of intelligence that includes an understanding of emotional experience, self-awareness, and sensitivity to others.

Challenges & Choices

Taking Healthy Risks

What risks have you taken in your life? Were they healthy or unhealthy? The kind of risks that are unhealthy are those that involve potentially dangerous consequences, such as taking drugs, having unprotected sex, running away from home, or defying authority just for the sake of defiance. The kind of risks that are healthy force you to reach beyond your comfort zone to grow as a person. They can push you mentally, emotionally, and spiritually. Here are some examples of healthy risks. Try taking one today.

- Stand up for something you believe in.
- Say no to someone instead of going along.
- Confront someone who is expressing sexist or racist views.
- Run for class office.
- Run for public office.
- Address the city council on an issue you care about.

- Take up a new sport, one you've been afraid to try.
- Sign up for a marathon or cycling event to raise money for a charity, even if you don't believe right now that you can complete the event.
- Assert your right to get what you want in an intimate relationship.
- Call or talk to someone you have been admiring from afar.

It's Not Just Personal...

In 2001, cyclists riding the California AIDS Ride raised more than $11 million. In 2004, participants in the Avon Walk for Breast Cancer raised more than $30 million. Since 1998, runners, cyclists, and swimmers in the Team in Training program of the Leukemia and Lymphoma Society have raised more than $500 million. All these events are made possible by people taking risks and stretching beyond their comfort zones.

Advances in Knowledge and Understanding of the Brain

The human brain has been called the most complex structure in the universe.[9] The size of a coconut and the shape of a walnut, the color of uncooked liver and the consistency of chilled butter, this unimpressive-looking organ is the central control station for human intelligence, feeling, and creativity. It is the ultimate multitasker.

In the last 25 years, knowledge of the structure and function of the brain has increased dramatically. In fact, the 1990s have been called the "decade of the brain" because of the advances made in understanding how the brain works and how it affects emotions, relationships, attachment, addiction, and many other behaviors. Most of these discoveries have been made possible by advances in imaging technologies, such as computerized axial tomography (CAT scans), positron emission tomography (PET scans), magnetic resonance imaging (MRIs), and functional MRIs (fMRIs).

These sophisticated imaging techniques provide access to the brain without surgery, allowing researchers to see what parts of the brain are impaired when a person suffers brain damage and what parts are activated during different mental activities. They also allow researchers to discover and study the biological basis of many mental disorders, including schizophrenia and Alzheimer's disease. As scientists learn which sections of the brain control different behaviors and functions, they develop new treatments, both pharmacological and psychotherapeutic, for mental disorders.

Research has also expanded in the physiology of the brain and the function of **neurotransmitters.** These brain chemicals are responsible for the transmission of signals from one brain cell to the next. There are dozens of neurotransmitters, but four seem to be particularly important in mental disorders: norepinephrine (active during the stress response; see Chapter 5); dopamine (implicated in schizophrenia); serotonin (implicated in mood disorders); and gamma aminobutyric acid, or GABA (implicated in anxiety).[10] Neurotransmitter imbalances—for example, overproduction or delayed absorption—are believed to be involved in a variety of mental disorders. Many drugs have been developed to correct these imbalances, such as the class of antidepressants that affects levels of serotonin and includes Prozac.

The Teenage Brain

One surprise that recent brain research produced is that the brain continues to change and grow through adolescence into the early 20s. Previously, scientists thought that brain development was completed in childhood, and in fact, 95 percent of the structure of the brain is formed by the age of 6. Scientists discovered, however, that a growth spurt occurs in the **frontal cortex**—the part of the brain where such "executive" functions as planning, organizing, and rational thinking are controlled—just before puberty. During adolescence, these new brain cells are pruned and

Frontal cortex
Controls planning, organizing, rational thinking, working memory, judgment, mood modulation. Undergoes rapid growth just before puberty, followed by pruning and consolidation during adolescence.

Amygdala
Controls emotional responses and instinctual, "gut" reactions. Adolescents appear to rely more heavily on this part of the brain to interpret situations than adults do. As they mature, the center of brain activity shifts to the frontal cortex.

Corpus callosum
Relays information between the two hemispheres of the brain and is believed to play a role in creativity and problem solving. Grows and changes significantly during adolescence.

Cerebellum
Long known to be involved in motor activity and physical coordination; now understood to coordinate thinking processes, including decision making and social skills. Undergoes dynamic growth and change during adolescence.

Figure 3.1   **The teenage brain.** *Sources:* Adapted from "Adolescent Brains Are Works in Progress," by S. Spinks, 2005, Frontline, www.pbs.org; "Teenage Brain: A Work in Progress," 2001, National Institute of Mental Health, NIH Publication No. 01-4929, www.nimh.nih.gov.

consolidated, resulting in a more mature, adult brain by the early to mid-20s.

One implication of these findings is that the impulsivity, emotional reactivity, and risk-taking behavior that are more typical of adolescence than of adulthood may be caused in part by a still-maturing brain rather than (or in addition to) hormonal changes or other factors. Figure 3.1 shows the teenage brain and describes how its functions differ from those of the adult brain. Another implication is that because structural changes are taking place in the brain through adolescence and into early adulthood, the activities that teenagers engage in can have life-long effects. The brain cells and connections that are used for academics, music, sports, language learning, and other productive activities—or, alternatively, for watching television and playing video games—are the ones that are more likely to be hardwired into the brain and survive.[11]

Mental Disorders and the Brain

Although all behavior, both normal and abnormal, is mediated in some way by the brain and the nervous system, mental disorders that are caused specifically by some pathology in the brain are rare. These disorders are referred to as *cognitive disorders* and include delirium, dementia (for example, Alzheimer's disease), and various forms of amnesia. More commonly, mental disorders are caused by complex interactions of biological factors (such as neurotransmitter levels, genetics), psychological processes, social influences, and cultural factors, especially those affecting a person during early childhood. Everything that a person experiences, from a parent's approving smile to the

effects of an earthquake, happens in some way at the biological level within the individual. Thus, although evidence of mental disorders like depression or schizophrenia can be found in the brain, and although many disorders can be treated with drugs that act on the brain, neither of these facts means that mental disorders actually originate in the brain.

INFLUENCES ON THE DEVELOPMENT OF MENTAL HEALTH AND MENTAL ILLNESS

How does a person become mentally healthy or mentally ill? One model of mental illness, called the **diathesis-stress model,** proposes that a person may have a particular predisposition or vulnerability (diathesis) for an illness,

KEY TERMS

neurotransmitters   Brain chemicals that conduct signals from one brain cell to the next.

frontal cortex   The part of the brain where the executive functions of planning, organizing, and rational thinking are controlled.

diathesis-stress model   A model of mental illness in which a diathesis (a predisposition or vulnerability) exists, but a stressor (a precipitating event) is needed to trigger the onset of illness.

Healthy People 2010

OBJECTIVE AREA *Mental Health Treatment Expansion*

- For young people with mental health problems, increase the number who receive treatment.

"For many children aged 18 years and under, lifelong mental disorders may start in childhood or adolescence. For many other children, normal development is disrupted by biological, environmental, and psychosocial factors, which impair their mental health, interfere with education and social interactions, and keep them from realizing their full potential as adults. . . . Expanding effective services for children . . . will result in . . . improved educational, emotional, and behavioral development."

For more information on Healthy People 2010 objectives, visit the Web site at www.healthypeople.gov.

For more information on Canadian health objectives, visit the Health Canada Web site at www.hc-sc.gc.ca/english.

but an event (stressor) must occur to trigger the illness itself. For example, a person may have a genetic or biochemical predisposition for depression, but growing up in an abusive environment enhances the possibility that the person will someday suffer from depression. The diathesis may be something that happened in the past, such as the death of a parent in childhood; the stressor is usually something that happens in the present, such as the breakup of a relationship or the loss of a job.

Protective Factors and Risk Factors

Many factors come into play in the diathesis-stress model. **Protective factors** serve to buffer the person from threats to psychological well-being; **risk factors** increase the individual's chances for mental problems and disorders. Both protective factors and risk factors can be conceptualized as occurring in the realms of the individual, the family, and the community and environment.

Individual Factors

As you know, some characteristics of the individual are genetic in origin, such as a sociable, outgoing temperament or a predisposition for shyness or sensation seeking (see Chapter 2). Other individual factors may be the result of biochemical or hormonal factors, as in some cases of depression. Still other individual factors may result from prenatal influences; for example, a child born with fetal

alcohol syndrome (FAS) does not have the same capabilities or life chances as a healthy child. A brain injury at any age, or a medical condition that directly affects the brain, such as a stroke or a tumor, also affects mental health at the level of the individual, as do abnormalities in brain structure or function.

Whatever their origin, individual factors play a role in psychological adjustment and maladjustment. A person may be introverted or extraverted, optimistic or pessimistic, impulsive or cautious, a leader or a follower. She may believe she is highly capable and able to direct her life, or she may have an attitude of "learned helplessness." She may feel good about herself, or she may be filled with doubt and self-blame.

The characteristics that a person brings to life situations, social interactions, and interpersonal relationships strongly influence the outcome of those situations and interactions, which in turn influence the person's likelihood of maintaining psychological health or developing psychological problems. In other words, individuals are not simply affected by their environments in a one-directional way. They also shape their environment with their individual characteristics and behaviors.

Family Factors

Our family of origin has a powerful influence on what kind of people we become. We are influenced by the quality of parenting, family dynamics, and other interpersonal relationships in early childhood. If our parents provide a safe, loving environment with consistent, predictable family dynamics, we have a much better chance of becoming well-adjusted adults than if our parents are not able to provide such an early environment. Examples of protective factors include family cohesion, competent parenting, interpersonal warmth, and marital harmony. Risk factors include inadequate parenting; physical, emotional, or sexual abuse; family breakup and divorce; psychiatric disorders in parents or family members; alcohol or drug abuse in family members; and traumatic events such as the death of a parent.

Community and Environmental Factors

As noted in Chapter 1, a person has less chance of being physically healthy in an unhealthy environment, and the same is true of mental health. Schools, neighborhoods, communities, and society in general play important roles in supporting or undermining mental health. For example, an individual who grows up in a safe neighborhood, with good schools, positive adult role models, and adequate opportunities for recreation and community involvement has a better chance at achieving and maintaining mental health than someone who grows up with few positive role models in a violent or disorganized neighborhood. A person who is unemployed, undereducated, and poor is more likely to develop psychological problems than is a person with more resources, all other things being equal. Individuals

Table 3.1	Protective Factors for Mental Health
Individual Protective Factors	Active, easy, outgoing temperament
	Positive responsiveness to others
	Sense of humor
	High intelligence
	Problem-solving skills
	Emotional regulation
	Verbal/communication skills
	Self-efficacy
	Hopefulness
	Recognized talents/accomplishments
	Social skills
	Self-confidence
	Strong, positive ethnic identity
	Religious faith/affiliation/participation
	Educational aspirations
	Sense of direction or purpose
Family Protective Factors	Competent parenting
	Authoritative parenting style
	High but realistic expectations of child
	Educational attainment
	Involved in schools
	Family cohesion, marital harmony
	Socioeconomic advantages
	Religious faith/affiliation/participation
	Children have family/household duties
Community/ Environmental Protective Factors	Adequate resources for child care, health care
	Good schools
	Community cohesion, stability
	Availability of prosocial role models, norms
	Supportive friends, neighbors
	Employment opportunities
	Opportunities for involvement in community activities

Source: Adapted from "Resilience in Ecosystemic Context," by M. Waller, 2001, *American Journal of Orthopsychiatry, 71* (3), pp. 290–297.

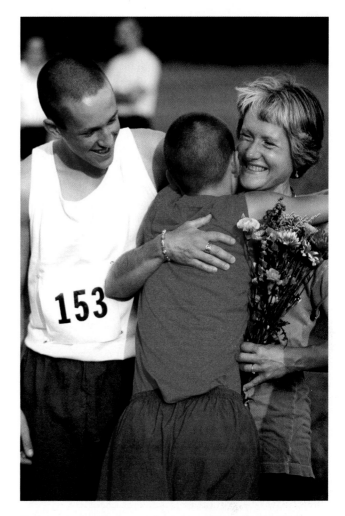

Having a strong support system is key to good mental health. This boy feels the support of a family that shares in his interests and celebrates his accomplishments.

Erikson's Theory of Psychosocial Development

Another way to think about influences on the development of mental health and mental illness is Erik Erikson's **theory of psychosocial development.** Erikson proposed that development proceeds through a series of eight life stages, each shaped by the interaction of internal, biological drives, on the one hand, and external, social and cultural forces, on the other.

KEY TERMS

protective factors   Factors that buffer a person from threats to health.

risk factors   Factors that increase the likelihood that a person will experience illness.

theory of psychosocial development   Erikson's theory that personality development proceeds through a series of eight life stages.

subjected to oppression, racism, prejudice, discrimination, or other negative cultural influences have additional obstacles to overcome. On the other hand, having a strong, positive ethnic identity, holding traditional beliefs, and participating in traditional practices are protective factors.

For an overview of protective factors and risk factors at the individual, family, and community levels, see Tables 3.1 and 3.2. The more risk factors children are exposed to, the more likely they are to develop psychiatric disorders. When sufficient numbers of protective factors are present, however, they seem to moderate the impact of those factors that place children at risk.

Table 3.2	Risk Factors for Mental Health
Individual Risk Factors	Physical health problem or disability
	Difficult temperament
	Learning problem or attention difficulty
	Poor social skills
	Poor verbal/communication skills
	Poor impulse control
	Lack of self-efficacy
	Sensation seeking
	Aggressiveness
	Antisocial tendencies
	Tolerance for deviant roles, norms
Family Risk Factors	Low parental attachment
	Poor parenting (for example, inconsistent, too many or too few rules)
	Family conflict
	Low educational attainment
	Socioeconomic disadvantages
	Isolation, lack of social connections
	Emotional disturbance/psychological problem in parent
	Physical/emotional/sexual abuse
	Parental alcohol or drug abuse
Community/ Environmental Risk Factors	Poverty
	Negative peer influence
	Neighborhood disorganization
	Poor housing
	Poor schools
	Lack of employment opportunities
	Failure to achieve at school
	Criminal activity/violence

Source: Adapted from "Resilience in Ecosystemic Context," by M. Waller, 2001, *American Journal of Orthopsychiatry, 71* (3), pp. 290–297.

According to this theory, individuals face predictable challenges, tasks, or conflicts at particular periods or stages in their lives. If they meet these challenges more or less successfully—that is, they develop an adaptive approach to the central issue—they develop "ego strengths" and continue growing in healthy ways. If they are unable to meet the challenges successfully—they develop a maladaptive approach to the central issue—their psychological, emotional, and social growth may be blocked, it may be harder to meet later challenges, and they may not reach their fullest potential.

The challenge of infancy, according to Erikson is to develop *trust,* a sense that you can rely on someone to provide for your needs and that the world is a safe place. When this challenge is successfully negotiated, you acquire the capacity for hope. The challenge of early childhood (age 18 months to 3 years) is to develop a sense of *autonomy,* the feeling that you are a separate person, can stand on your own feet, and can assert your will. This

stage is embodied by the 2-year-old shouting "No!" In the preschool years (3 to 6 years), the challenge is to develop a sense of *initiative,* the ability to take action, to plan, undertake, and attack a task. When successfully met, this challenge gives you the ability to create or discover a sense of purpose in your life.

During the school years (6 to 12 years), the challenge is to develop a sense of *industry,* the ability to produce something, to work, to demonstrate competence. The challenge of adolescence is to develop a sense of *identity,* knowledge and acceptance of your strengths and weaknesses and inklings of your future career. In early adulthood, the challenge is to develop the capacity for *intimacy,* the ability to commit to relationships and partnerships and to develop the ethical strength to abide by these commitments. In middle adulthood, the focus is on *generativity,* a concern with establishing and guiding the next generation. Finally, in older adulthood, the challenge is *integrity,* the ability to integrate your life experiences and conclude that your life is and has been meaningful.

When the challenges are not met as successfully, individuals can develop characteristics or tendencies that are not as adaptive or productive. An individual might be inclined toward mistrust rather than trust, for example; self-doubt and shame rather than autonomy; guilt rather than initiative; feelings of inferiority rather than industry; role confusion rather than a sense of identity; feelings of isolation rather than the capacity for intimacy; self-absorption and stagnation rather than generativity; and finally, a sense of despair instead of a feeling of integrity. Such psychological deficits can lead to emotional difficulties in life. For example, a person who has developed a sense of autonomy in the second stage is inclined to have high self-esteem and a sense of pride and good will toward others later in life. A person who has developed self-doubt and shame may be inclined to be self-conscious, compulsive, perfectionistic, or suspicious later in life.

This is not to say that difficulties in any particular stage doom a person to a life of unhappiness or emotional distress, and in fact, there has to be a healthy balance of qualities at every stage. For example, it is not healthy or realistic for a person to trust everyone or to be completely autonomous. However, Erikson's theory does suggest that if a person has difficulty mastering one challenge, the challenges that follow will be more difficult to negotiate. It further suggests that difficulties later in life may be traced to the stage at which the person insufficiently mastered a particular psychosocial task. This would be an area the person might benefit from addressing in psychotherapy.

MENTAL DISORDERS

Experiences of emotional pain and psychological distress are part of human life. As noted earlier, mental health is determined not by the challenges a person faces but by how the person responds to those challenges. The challenges themselves come in a range of intensities—from a lower-than-expected grade on a test to the death of a loved one—and people's responses also vary in adaptive success. In this section we consider the range, or continuum, of these responses, and then we look at some of the major mental disorders.

How Do Everyday Problems Differ from Mental Disorders?

Let's consider an experience that most people have at some point in their lives: the loss of an important love relationship. One person might respond with feelings of sadness, loneliness, and hurt for a period of time. Another person might respond with feelings of hopelessness and despair, lose interest in life, and even contemplate suicide. The first person is responding appropriately to a painful life experience. The second person shows signs of major depression, a mental disorder.

In general, a mental disorder is diagnosed on the basis of the amount of distress and impairment a person is experiencing. According to the *Diagnostic and Statistical Manual of Mental Disorders (DSM-IV-TR)*, a **mental disorder** is a pattern of behavior in an individual that is associated with distress (pain) or disability (impairment in an important area of functioning, such as school or work) or with significantly increased risk of suffering, death, pain, disability, or loss of freedom.[12] This definition is meant to be informed by clinical judgment and applied by people with professional training, but it also leaves room for interpretation. Deciding when a psychological problem becomes a mental disorder is not easy. Nevertheless, a basic premise of the *DSM-IV-TR* is that a mental disorder is qualitatively different from a psychological problem that can be considered normal, and it can be diagnosed from a set of symptoms. Let's consider a few more examples.

Some of the most common experiences that people struggle with in life and especially during the college years are feeling "down" or "blue." Feelings of sadness and discouragement can occur in response to disappointment, loss, failure, or other negative events, or they can occur for no apparent reason. Some people want to spend time alone when they feel this way, and others want to be around other people. Usually such experiences don't last too long; people recover their spirits and go on with their lives. Sometimes, however, the feelings go on for a long time and are painful and intense. In such cases, the person may be experiencing depression.

Worries, fears, and anxieties are also common during the college years. Individuals have stresses to deal with, such as grades, relationships, and learning how to live on their own without parental guidance or support. They may feel homesick and lonely, or they may have problems sleeping. A person who is naturally shy or introverted may find it difficult to make new friends, be assertive with a roommate, or find a comfortable social niche. Most people gradually make their way, learning who they are and how they want to relate to other people.

Some people, however, may develop anxiety disorders or stress-related disorders. Some people try to cope with their feelings through their eating patterns, either soothing themselves with food or asserting control over their lives by eating almost nothing. These unhealthy eating patterns can eventually develop into eating disorders. Others try to master their feelings by using alcohol or drugs, and they may go on to develop substance-related disorders.

One of our goals here is to make clear that people experience many psychological difficulties that are not a cause for alarm. Another goal is to describe some of the recognized mental disorders in ways that help you know when a person needs professional help. Far too often, people struggle with mental disorders without knowing that something is wrong or that treatments are available. They may think they are just experiencing "problems in living." They don't realize that such problems can cause unnecessary distress and impairment and that professional treatment can help.

Various chapters of this book discuss disorders that can result from psychological problems—stress-related disorders in Chapter 5, sleep difficulties in Chapter 6, eating disorders in Chapter 10, substance abuse in Chapters 11, 12, and 13. In this chapter we focus on a few of the more commonly experienced disorders—mood disorders and anxiety disorders. We also briefly touch on psychotic disorders such as schizophrenia and on the long-standing maladaptive patterns known as personality disorders.

Mood Disorders

Also called depressive disorders or affective disorders, mood disorders include major depressive disorder, dysthymic disorder, and bipolar disorder (formerly called manic depression). They are among the most common mental disorders experienced by people around the world.

People of all ages can get depressed, including children and adolescents, but the average age of onset for major

KEY TERMS

mental disorder According to the *DSM-IV-TR*, a pattern of behavior in an individual that is associated with distress (pain) or disability (impairment in an important area of functioning, such as school or work) or with significantly increased risk of suffering, death, pain, disability, or loss of freedom.

Symptoms of Depression

A person who experiences five or more of the following symptoms (including the first and second symptoms listed) for a 2-week period may be suffering from depression:

- Depressed mood, as indicated by feelings of sadness or emptiness or such behaviors as crying.
- Loss of interest or pleasure in all or most activities.
- Significant weight loss or weight gain or a change in appetite.
- Insomnia, hypersomnia, or other disturbed sleep patterns.

- Agitated or retarded (slow) body movement.
- Fatigue or loss of energy.
- Feelings of worthlessness or excessive guilt.
- Diminished ability to think, impaired concentration, or indecisiveness.
- Recurrent thoughts of death, ideas about suicide, or a suicide plan or attempt.

Source: Reprinted with permission from the *Diagnostic and Statistical Manual of Mental Disorders*, 4th ed., Text Revision (*DSM-IV-TR*), copyright © 2000, American Psychiatric Association.

depressive disorder is the mid-20s. In any one year, more than 18 million adults in the United States—about 9.5 percent of the adult population—suffer from a depressive illness.[13] Of these individuals, a significant number will be hospitalized, and many will die from suicide.[14] Women are at significantly greater risk for depression than men, experiencing depressive episodes twice as frequently. Many times, individuals get depressed following another illness, such as a stroke or heart attack, or a procedure such as an organ transplant. Women sometimes struggle with depressive symptoms following the birth of a child.

In many of these situations, people go undiagnosed and struggle with their illness for long periods of time. About two thirds of depressed individuals seek help, but many are undertreated, meaning that they don't get enough medication or they don't see a therapist on a regular basis. Many medications for depression take up to 4 weeks to begin to have an effect, and some people conclude they aren't working or stop taking them in frustration.

Mood disorders are most likely caused by a combination of genetic and environmental factors. As discussed in Chapter 2, family studies and twin studies show evidence of a moderately strong genetic link in bipolar disorder and somewhat less strong link in depression. Several genes are probably involved, interacting with the environment. There is also evidence that levels of brain chemicals and hormones are different during depressive episodes in some individuals, although it is not clear whether these changes precede or follow the onset of depression.

Major Depressive Disorder

Symptoms of **depression** include depressed mood, as indicated by feelings of sadness or emptiness or by behaviors such as crying, and a loss of interest or pleasure

in activities that previously provided pleasure. Other symptoms include fatigue, feelings of worthlessness, and a reduced ability to concentrate (see the box above, "Symptoms of Depression"). If a person experiences one or more episodes of depression (characterized by at least five of the nine symptoms listed) lasting at least 2 weeks, he or she can be diagnosed with **major depressive disorder.** In any one year, about 5 percent of the adult population suffer from this disorder.[13] Some people with major depressive disorder may become *vegetative,* meaning they have little desire to get out of bed in the morning or do daily grooming activities such as showering or brushing their teeth.

Dysthymic Disorder

Low-grade, chronic depression that goes on for 2 years or more may be diagnosed as **dysthymic disorder.** Individuals with this disorder have a generally depressed mood and may have a poor appetite, disturbed sleep patterns, low self-esteem, low energy, poor concentration and difficulty making decisions, and/or feelings of hopelessness. (Two or more of these symptoms are required for a diagnosis.) People with dysthymic disorder may have feelings of inadequacy, guilt, irritability, or pessimism.[12] The disorder usually begins in childhood, adolescence, or early adulthood and appears to have a genetic link. About 5 percent of the adult population suffer from this disorder in any given year.

Bipolar Disorder

A person with **bipolar disorder** experiences one or more manic episodes, often but not always alternating with depressive episodes. A **manic episode** is a distinct period during which the person has an abnormally elevated mood. Individuals experiencing manic episodes may be

HIGHLIGHT ON HEALTH
Symptoms of a Manic Episode

A person who experiences the following symptoms may be having a manic episode:

- A distinct period of abnormally and persistently elevated, expansive, or irritable mood lasting at least 1 week.
- During this period, three or more of the following symptoms are present:
  - Inflated self-esteem or grandiosity.
  - Decreased need for sleep.
  - More talkative than usual.
  - Flighty ideas or sense that thoughts are racing.
  - Distractability.
  - Increase in goal-directed activity or psychomotor agitation.
  - Excessive involvement in pleasurable activities with a high potential for painful consequences (such as shopping sprees, sexual indiscretions).

Source: Reprinted with permission from the *Diagnostic and Statistical Manual of Mental Disorders*, 4th ed., Text Revision (*DSM-IV-TR*), copyright © 2000, American Psychiatric Association.

euphoric, expansive, and full of energy, or, alternatively, highly irritable. They may be grandiose, with an inflated sense of their own importance and power; they may have racing thoughts and accelerated and pressured speech. They may stay awake for days without getting tired or wake from a few hours of sleep feeling refreshed and full of energy (see the box above, "Symptoms of a Manic Episode"). For the diagnosis, these symptoms have to persist for a week or more.

Individuals undergoing a manic episode typically do not know they are ill. They may travel impulsively, go on shopping sprees, make spontaneous business investments, and have indiscriminate sexual encounters. Internet shopping is particularly seductive because it can be accessed 24 hours a day and has few restrictions on purchases. After the manic episode ends, these individuals not only must deal with their depression but also have to face their credit card debt.

A manic episode usually ends when the person crashes, or loses the sense of euphoria. Many individuals with bipolar disorder cycle through periods of exhilarating highs alternating with depressive episodes or with periods of normalcy. For a description of what it's like to have this disorder, see the box on the next page, "A Brilliant Madness."

Bipolar disorder is less common than major depressive disorder or dysthymic disorder, affecting about 1 percent of the population. It occurs equally in men and women, with the average age of onset about 20. Family and twin studies offer strong evidence of a genetic component in this disorder. The disorder can be controlled with medication, but often, individuals don't take their medication because the highs are so euphoric.

Anxiety Disorders

Along with depression, anxiety disorders are the most common mental disorders affecting Americans. Almost 19 million Americans between the ages of 18 and 54—more than 13 percent of all people in this age group—have an anxiety disorder.[13,15]

Many of these disorders are characterized by a **panic attack**, a clear physiological and psychological experience of apprehension or intense fear in the absence of a real danger. Symptoms include heart palpitations, sweating, shortness of breath, possibly chest pain, and a sense that one is "going crazy." There is a feeling of impending doom or danger and a strong urge to escape. Panic attacks usually occur suddenly and last for a discrete period of time, reaching a peak within 10 minutes. Children who experience extreme anxiety, such as when being separated from

KEY TERMS

depression Mental state characterized by a depressed mood, loss of interest or pleasure in activities, and several other related symptoms.

major depressive disorder Mental disorder in which a person experiences one or more episodes of depression lasting at least 2 weeks.

dysthymic disorder Mental disorder in which a person experiences chronic, low-grade depression for 2 years or more.

bipolar disorder Mental disorder in which a person experiences one or more episodes of mania, alternating with depressive episodes or periods of normalcy.

manic episode Distinct period of time during which a person has an abnormally elevated mood.

panic attack Clear physiological and psychological experience of apprehension or intense fear in the absence of a real danger.

HIGHLIGHT ON HEALTH

"A Brilliant Madness"

Actress Patty Duke, who won an Academy Award in 1962 for her portrayal of Helen Keller in *The Miracle Worker,* suffered from bipolar disorder for 12 years before it was diagnosed. Today she is an outspoken advocate for people with mental disorders. This is an excerpt from her book *A Brilliant Madness:*

> I felt hopeless. Hopeless is really the word. I felt this was the way it was always going to be. There was nothing I could do to change it. I didn't think the phrase "I must be crazy," I really didn't think that. But I always thought there was something wrong with my character. I never talked to anyone about it. But I remember feeling so bad that I could never think the way other people did. I would hear people talking about plans, whether it was plans for two weeks from now or plans for their lives or plans for a house. I never was able to think in those terms. I almost didn't understand how you go about thinking that way. I always thought the solution was outside of me. I would have thoughts like, "If only I could meet a man like so-and-so or if only I had a home like so-and-so or if only I had children. . . ." It was always those if-onlies that were going to save me.

From *A Brilliant Madness: Living with Manic-Depressive Illness,* by P. Duke and G. Hochman, 1992, New York: Bantam Books.

a parent, usually cry, freeze, or cling. Many anxiety disorders can be effectively treated with medications and with various forms of psychotherapy.

In this section we consider panic disorder, specific phobias, agoraphobia, social phobia, generalized anxiety disorder, and obsessive-compulsive disorder. Two other kinds of anxiety disorders—acute stress disorder and posttraumatic stress disorder—are discussed in Chapter 5.

Panic disorder is characterized by recurrent, unexpected panic attacks and at least 1 month of concern about having another attack. The attacks may be triggered by a situation, or they may "come out of nowhere" (see the box "Symptoms of Panic Disorder"). Twin studies and family studies indicate a genetic contribution to this disorder. First-degree relatives of persons with panic disorder are eight times more likely to develop the disorder than the general population.[12]

A **specific phobia** is an intense fear of an activity, situation, or object, exposure to which evokes immediate anxiety. Examples of common phobias are flying, heights, specific animals or insects (dogs, spiders), and blood. Individuals with phobias realize their fear is unreasonable, but they cannot control it. Usually they try to avoid the phobic situation or object, and if they can't avoid it, they endure it with great distress. Often the phobia interferes with their life in some way. Various forms of behavioral therapy have proven effective in treating phobias. (See the section "Psychotherapy and Counseling," later in this chapter.)

Agoraphobia is characterized by anxiety about being in situations where escape may be difficult or embarrassing, or where help might not be available in case of a panic attack. Such situations may include being in a crowd, on a bus, on a bridge, in an open space, or just outside the home. Individuals with untreated agoraphobia usually try to structure their lives in such a way as to avoid these situations; in extreme situations, they may not leave their home for years.

A **social phobia** involves an intense fear of certain kinds of social or performance situations, again leading the individual to try to avoid such situations. If the phobic situation is public speaking, individuals may be able to structure their lives so as to avoid all such situations. However, some social phobias involve simply conversing with other people. This is different from shyness; individuals with this disorder experience tremors, sweating, confusion, blushing, and other distressing symptoms when they are in the feared situation. Again, they know their fear is unreasonable, and many seek treatment for the condition.

Excessive and uncontrollable worrying, usually far out of proportion to the actual likelihood of the feared event, is known as **generalized anxiety disorder.** Adults with this disorder worry about routine matters such as health, work, and money; children with the disorder worry about their competence in school or sports, being evaluated by others, and sometimes about natural disasters like earthquakes.

Obsessive-compulsive disorder is characterized by persistent, intrusive thoughts, impulses, or images that cause intense anxiety or distress. The most common obsessions are repeated thoughts about contamination, persistent doubts about having done something, a need to have things done in a particular order, aggressive impulses, and sexual imagery. To control the obsessive thoughts and images, the person develops compulsions—repetitive behaviors performed to reduce the anxiety associated with the obsession. For example, a woman might be plagued with worries about whether she turned off the oven or locked the door, and she

Symptoms of Panic Disorder

A person who experiences the following symptoms may be suffering from panic disorder:

- Recurrent, unexpected panic attacks.
- One or more of the following in the month after an attack:
  - Persistent concern about having another attack.

- Worry about what the attack means (for example, losing control, having a heart attack, going crazy).
- A significant change in behavior related to the attacks.

Source: Reprinted with permission from the *Diagnostic and Statistical Manual of Mental Disorders,* 4th ed., Text Revision, (*DSM-IV-TR*) copyright © 2000, American Psychiatric Association.

returns to the house or gets up out of bed numerous times to check.

Compulsive routines temporarily reduce the anxiety, but they become time consuming and can eventually engulf the individual. To meet the diagnostic criteria in the *DSM-IV-TR,* the obsessions and compulsions must take more than 1 hour a day and interfere significantly with the person's life. At some point during the course of the illness, the person knows that the thoughts and behaviors are unreasonable; however, he or she is unable to control them.

This disorder occurs worldwide. It usually begins in adolescence or early adulthood, but it can begin in childhood. Studies show that there is a genetic link, with first-degree relatives of someone with obsessive-compulsive disorder having a higher rate of the disorder than the general population.

Schizophrenia and Other Psychotic Disorders

A number of different disorders are included in **psychotic disorders,** which are characterized by delusions, hallucinations, disorganized speech or behavior, and other signs that the individual has lost touch with reality. **Delusional disorder,** for example, is characterized by one or more bizarre delusions persisting for at least a month. The theme of the delusion may be grandioseness (for example, the person has a great, undiscovered talent); jealousy (for example, the person's partner or spouse is unfaithful); persecution (the person is being persecuted, spied on, poisoned); erotomania (another person is in love with the person); or of an unspecified type. Another disorder, **brief psychotic disorder,** involves psychotic symptoms that last at least 1 day but less than a month. Often the episode is brought on in a vulnerable person by a specific sociocultural stressor, such as final exams or the breakup of a romantic relationship.

Schizophrenia is a particularly devastating psychotic disorder. Its characteristic symptoms are delusions, hallucinations (often voices), disorganized speech, disorganized

KEY TERMS

panic disorder Mental disorder characterized by recurrent, unexpected panic attacks and at least 1 month of concern about having another attack.

specific phobia Intense fear of a specific activity, situation, or object.

agoraphobia Disorder in which anxiety is experienced about being in situations where escape may be difficult or embarrassing, or where help might not be available in case of a panic attack.

social phobia Disorder in which intense anxiety is experienced in certain kinds of social or performance situations.

generalized anxiety disorder Mental disorder characterized by excessive and uncontrollable worrying.

obsessive-compulsive disorder Mental disorder in which a person experiences persistent, intrusive thoughts, impulses, or images that cause intense anxiety or distress (obsessions) and responds to them by performing repetitive behaviors to reduce the anxiety (compulsions).

psychotic disorders Mental disorders characterized by delusions, hallucinations, disorganized speech or behavior, and other signs that the individual has lost touch with reality.

delusional disorder Psychotic disorder characterized by one or more bizarre delusions that persist for at least a month.

brief psychotic disorder Disorder characterized by psychotic symptoms lasting at least a day but less than a month.

schizophrenia Severe psychotic disorder in which a person experiences delusions, hallucinations (often voices), disorganized speech, disorganized behavior, and sometimes a diminishing of normal functioning, for example, in speech or emotional expression.

behavior, and sometimes a diminishing of normal functioning, for example, in speech or emotional expression. The diagnosis requires that these symptoms occur actively for at least 1 month and the disturbance overall lasts at least 6 months. The symptoms are so severe that the person becomes socially, interpersonally, and occupationally dysfunctional.

The number of people reported with schizophrenia is relatively small, approximately 1–2 percent of the adult population.[16] It occurs worldwide, but it can manifest differently in different cultures because the content of delusions can be culture specific. Age of onset is usually the early 20s for men and the late 20s for women. The initial early warning symptoms include social withdrawal, a loss of interest in school or work, poor grooming, and, possibly, angry outbursts. Family members have reported that the individual with schizophrenia "gradually slipped away."[12]

As discussed in Chapter 2, schizophrenia has a strong genetic component. First-degree relatives of individuals with schizophrenia have a risk for the disorder 10 times higher than that of the general population.[12] All of the brain scanning and visualizing technologies reveal abnormalities in the brains of people with schizophrenia. Studies indicate that these abnormalities are present before the onset of symptoms, suggesting that this illness is the result of problems in brain development, perhaps even occurring prenatally.

In most cases, symptoms of the disease can be controlled with medication. Educating family members about the illness can help them better understand the cycle of the illness and the importance of medications. Another key is **case management,** an approach to treatment in which a multidisciplinary team of people is involved to ensure that all aspects of a person's life are addressed.

Personality Disorders

The disorders described thus far differ from **personality disorders,** which involve long-standing, maladaptive personality traits, defined as enduring patterns of thinking, relating, and behaving. These patterns become apparent in adolescence or early adulthood and are pervasive across most or all areas of the person's life. They are inflexible and difficult to change, and they differ markedly from what the culture expects.[12] Some 10 percent to 13 percent of the world's population are believed to suffer from a personality disorder.

Individuals with personality disorders experience varying degrees of distress and impairment, depending on the type of disorder, but they also tend to cause discomfort and disruption in the lives of those around them, including family members, friends, colleagues, and partners. Individuals with **antisocial personality disorder,** for example, demonstrate a disregard for the rights of others, often beginning in childhood. They may destroy property,

harass others, steal, and pursue criminal careers. Frequently, they deceive others for personal profit or pleasure. They are indifferent to the suffering they cause others and show no remorse. People with this pattern are sometimes referred to as *psychopaths* or *sociopaths.*

Antisocial personality disorder occurs more frequently in men than in women. Studies indicate that both genetic and environmental factors contribute to the disorder. Adopted children resemble their biological parents, but when adoptive parents have the disorder, both adopted and biological children have an increased risk for developing it.[12]

A key characteristic of individuals with **narcissistic personality disorder** is a lack of empathy—an inability or unwillingness to recognize or identify with the feelings of others. These individuals also have a grandiose sense of self-importance and a need for admiration. People with **histrionic personality disorder** always want to be the center of attention; they are theatrical, excessively emotional, and inappropriately seductive. Both of these disorders occur about equally in men and women. For a brief overview of the 10 personality disorders described in the *DSM-IV-TR,* see Table 3.3.

Mental Disorders and Suicide

A major public health concern, particularly among young people, suicide is the 8th leading cause of death among all Americans and the 3rd leading cause of death in people aged 15 to 24. In Canada, it is the 11th leading cause of death in the general population and the 2nd leading cause of death for people aged 10 to 24. The highest suicide rate in the United States occurs among white males over the age of 65. Some 30,000 Americans commit suicide annually, and an additional 500,000 attempt to kill themselves.[17]

The rate of suicide in young people has at least tripled in the past 50 years. In a national survey known as the College Health Risk Behavior Survey, a little more than 10 percent of college students reported that they had thought about suicide.[18] Nearly 7 percent had made specific plans, and approximately 1.5 percent had actually attempted to kill themselves. Among high school students, the rates are higher, with 20 percent of students reporting serious contemplation of suicide in the past year, and nearly 8 percent making an attempt.[19] Female students were significantly more likely than males to have considered suicide. About a third of those who attempted suicide had to receive some type of medical attention, often in a hospital emergency room.

Overall, women in U.S. society are more likely than men to attempt suicide, but men are four times more likely to succeed, probably because they choose more violent methods, usually a firearm. In the United States, firearms are used in 55–60 percent of all suicides. Women tend to use less violent methods for suicide, but

Table 3.3   Overview of Personality Disorders

Personality Disorder	Characteristics
Paranoid	Suspicious, mistrustful, preoccupied with doubts about loyalty of friends, on guard against attack by others.
Schizoid	Unable to form social relationships and uninterested in doing so, unable to express feelings, cold and detached in manner.
Schizotypal	Excessively introverted, impaired in social relationships and communication owing to distortions in thinking and perceiving, suspicious, superstitious.
Histrionic	Preoccupied with being the center of attention, excessively concerned with appearance, flamboyant, highly emotional, theatrical, seductive, manipulative, prone to temper tantrums if attention-seeking efforts are frustrated.
Narcissistic	Preoccupied with being admired, self-important, grandiose, lacking in empathy, exploitative, snobbish, envious of others.
Antisocial	Lacking in moral or ethical development, lacking in regard for the rights of others, deceitful, impulsive, irresponsible, without conscience or remorse.
Borderline	Unstable in sense of self, moody, impulsive, volatile in relationships, afraid of abandonment, self-destructive.
Avoidant	Extremely inhibited and introverted, insecure, hypersensitive to rejection or criticism, reluctant to enter social interactions.
Dependent	Submissive, clinging, self-effacing, indecisive, afraid of separation and abandonment.
Obsessive-compulsive	Perfectionistic, excessively concerned with maintaining order, attentive to rules and schedules, overconscientious, inflexible.

Source: From J. N. Butcher, S. Mineka, and J. M. Hooley, *Abnormal Psychology*, 12th ed. Published by Allyn and Bacon, Boston, MA. Copyright © 2004 by Pearson Education. Reprinted by permission of the publisher.

in more recent years they have begun to use firearms more frequently.

What Leads a Person to Suicide?

Most of us find it hard to understand why a person commits suicide. Many elements are involved, but someone contemplating suicide is most likely experiencing unbearable emotional pain, anguish, or despair. As many as 90 percent of those who commit suicide are suffering from a mental disorder, often depression. Studies indicate that the symptom linking depression and suicide is a feeling of hopelessness. Depression and alcoholism may be involved in two thirds of all suicides. Substance abuse is another factor; the combination of drugs and depression can be lethal. People experiencing psychosis are also at risk.

Besides mental disorders and substance abuse, other major risk factors associated with suicide are a family history of suicide, serious medical problems, and access to the means, such as a gun or pills. The most significant risk factor, however, is a previous suicide attempt or a history of such attempts (see the box on the next page, "Risk Factors for Suicide").

Sometimes, vulnerable individuals turn to suicide in response to a specific event, such as the loss of a relationship or job, an experience of failure, or a worry that a secret will be revealed. Other times there is no apparent precipitating event, and the suicide seems to come out of nowhere.

However, suicide is always a process, and certain behavioral signs indicate that a person may be thinking about suicide:

- Comments about death and threats to commit suicide.
- Increasing social withdrawal and isolation.

KEY TERMS

case management Approach to treatment of mental disorders in which a multidisciplinary team of people is involved to ensure that all aspects of a person's life are addressed.

personality disorders Disorders characterized by long-standing, maladaptive personality traits that are pervasive across most or all areas of the person's life.

antisocial personality disorder Disorder whose key characteristics are a disregard for the rights of others and a lack of remorse.

narcissistic personality disorder Disorder whose central characteristics are a lack of empathy for others and a grandiose sense of self-importance.

histrionic personality disorder Disorder characterized by theatricality, excessive emotionality, and seductiveness.

HIGHLIGHT ON HEALTH

Risk Factors for Suicide

A number of factors place adolescents at risk for suicide. The following list highlights the leading predictors.

- Suicidal thoughts
- Psychiatric disorders
- Drug and/or alcohol abuse
- Previous suicide attempts
- Access to firearms
- Recent loss or stressful situation
- Feelings of hopelessness
- Family history of suicide

- Intensified moodiness.
- Increase in risk-taking behaviors.
- Sudden improvement in mood, accompanied by such behaviors as giving away possessions. (The person may have made the decision to commit suicide.)

How to Help

If you know someone who seems to be suicidal, it is critical to get the person help. All mentions of suicide should be taken seriously. It is a myth that asking a person if he or she is thinking about suicide will plant the seed in the person's mind. Ignoring someone's sadness and depressed mood only increases the risk. Encourage the person to talk, and ask direct questions:

- Are you thinking about killing yourself?
- Do you have a plan?
- Do you have the means?
- Have you attempted suicide in the past?

If the threat does not seem to be imminent, encourage the person to get help by calling a suicide hotline or seeking counseling. Do not agree to keep the person's mental state or intentions a secret. If he or she refuses to get help or resists your advice, you may need to contact a parent or relative or, if you are a student, share your concern with a professional at the student health center. If the danger seems immediate, do not leave the person alone. Call for help or take the person to an emergency room.

If you have thought about suicide yourself, we encourage you to seek counseling. Therapy can help you resolve problems, develop better coping skills, and diminish the feelings that are causing you pain. It can also help you see things in a broader perspective and understand that you will not always feel this way. Remember

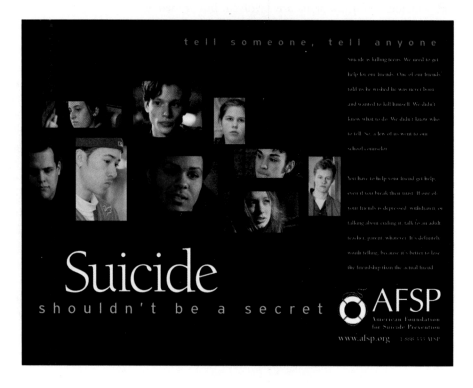

What would you do if you noticed suicidal tendencies in someone close to you?

the saying, suicide is a permanent solution to a temporary problem.

On average, every suicide leaves behind at least six people who are deeply affected by the death. Although all deaths are grieved, death by suicide can be especially difficult for loved ones to understand and accept. People dealing with the suicide of a loved one often benefit from grief counseling (see Chapter 4).

TREATING MENTAL DISORDERS

More than 250 different models of psychotherapy exist for the treatment of mental disorders, and many different drugs can be prescribed. Most of the mild and moderate mental disorders are readily treatable with therapy and, if needed, medications. In this section we consider first, several types of psychotherapy and second, the use of medications.

Whatever the nature of the problem, mental illness typically carries a social stigma that makes getting treatment problematic. Many individuals are afraid of seeking help because they fear others will see it as a sign of weakness. Some may try to pull themselves together on their own or simply tough it out. Others throw themselves into work or keep busy in an attempt to block out their feelings, not realizing that getting help might make them feel better. Sometimes, individuals who are being successfully treated for a mental disorder stop taking their medication because of this perceived social stigma. They are functioning well and feeling better, but they don't like seeing themselves as "mentally ill" or thinking that others see them that way. Unfortunately, stopping medication without medical supervision often results in a recurrence of symptoms.

Psychotherapy and Counseling

The terms *psychotherapy* and *counseling* may have different connotations, but more often than not they are used interchangeably; the term *therapy* refers to both. The key feature of most forms of **therapy** is the development of a relationship between a person seeking help (the client or patient) and a therapist, a trained and licensed professional who can provide that help. The therapeutic relationship becomes a *working alliance* (or *therapeutic alliance*) in which the two participants collaborate to resolve the problem. Most therapy models agree on the central importance of this interpersonal relationship between client and therapist.

For convenience, therapies can be grouped into broad categories reflective of underlying theories. Some commonly used categories are psychodynamic, behavioral, and cognitive-behavioral. In this section we briefly consider the characteristics and applications of these therapies. (See the box on the next page, "Counseling Services on Campus.")

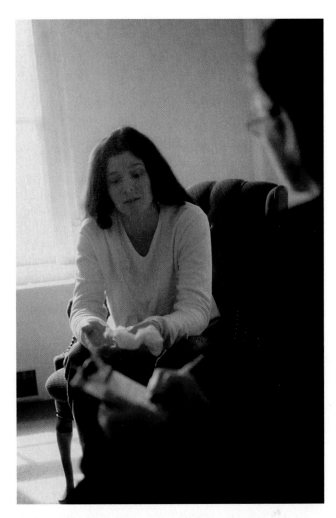

Finding a reputable counselor you can talk to comfortably is often the first step in getting your mental health in good balance.

Psychodynamic Therapies

Therapies based on the psychodynamic model are founded on theories originally developed by Sigmund Freud and subsequently adapted and modified by a host of later theorists. All these theorists believe that psychological problems arise in part from inner, often unconscious forces. Freud's method, classical psychoanalysis, is an intensive procedure for uncovering conflicts, fears, memories, and feelings from early childhood through such techniques as free association and dream interpretation. With the help of the analyst, the patient gains insight into the relationship between his or her unhealthy behaviors and the underlying, repressed conflicts that cause them, a process expected to relieve distress.

KEY TERMS

therapy Treatment for mental illness usually based on forming a therapeutic relationship or working alliance between a client and a therapist.

Consumer Clipboard

Counseling Services on Campus

You're writing papers, studying for exams, and juggling deadlines for different classes. Maybe you have a part-time job or parenting responsibilities, too. If you're feeling overwhelmed, you're not alone. Colleges and universities are reporting that the number of students who use their counseling services is currently at an all-time high. Making this choice is no longer something to hide. In fact, it's often considered the smart thing to do—an important part of taking care of your health.

Counseling services on campus vary greatly. At small schools the staff may consist of just one professional, but at large universities there is typically a team of psychologists, social workers, nurse practitioners, and usually at least one psychiatrist. At many colleges the services fall somewhere in between.

If you're feeling homesick, a chat room may be all you need to help you put things in perspective. But if you show signs of anxiety, depression, or other mental health issues, this may be the time to seek help from a professional who can offer you a variety of effective treatments. How would you describe your mental state? Are you just going through a difficult time? Or are you seriously concerned about yourself? If you're trying to decide whether you need professional help, ask yourself these questions:

- Am I feeling sad (homesick, lonely) a lot of the time?
- Am I having trouble studying for exams?
- Am I having more difficulty than usual with concentration?
- Do I have increased feelings of inadequacy?
- Am I feeling overwhelmed?
- Is this problem interfering with my everyday life?
- Have my friends and family asked if there's a problem?

- Have I lost interest in doing the things I usually like to do?
- Am I avoiding friends because of the problem?

Many colleges provide free psychological assessments, short-term counseling, and referrals. If you decide that you need help, consider these points:

- *Do I want to work with a professional counselor, or would another approach be better for me?* There may be support groups on campus that offer the chance to share your problems with peers. This may help put your problem in perspective, and it may be all the help you need. If you have ties to a religious organization, you may want to seek pastoral counseling in the local community. Either approach may be helpful as a first step.

- *Will my insurance cover mental health counseling?* Your college tuition, fees, or health insurance may cover some mental health services. However, if you choose to go off campus for counseling or treatment, those services may not be covered by your college benefits. If you are covered by health insurance through your parents, you will need to check with that insurance company about coverage.

- *Do I want my family to know that I'm undergoing counseling?* Different schools have varying policies on this matter. If you're over 18 and don't want your parents notified about your counseling, most schools will leave that up to you. If you're considered to be at risk for suicide, though, most counselors will encourage you to inform your parents about the counseling.

Source: Adapted from "The Dorms May Be Great, but How's the Counseling?" by M. Duenwald, October 26, 2004, *The New York Times*, p. D1.

More modern **psychodynamic therapies** continue to search for the origin of psychological problems and maladaptive behaviors in the client's past, particularly in early relationships and family dynamics. Through active conversation, the therapist attempts to clarify distortions and challenge defenses, helping the client gain insight. Through the therapeutic relationship, the therapist attempts to provide the client with corrective experiences.

Behavioral Therapies

Mental disorders are also treated using **behavioral therapies,** which are based on the view that problems arise from faulty learning and that new, healthy behaviors can be instilled through behavior modification and other types of training. Therapy focuses on changing the behavior in the present, not on uncovering the cause of the maladaptive behavior in the past. An example is exposure therapy for phobias and anxiety disorders. The client is exposed to the anxiety-producing stimulus at the same time that she or he practices well-rehearsed relaxation techniques, with the expectation that the anxiety will gradually dissipate. Behavioral therapies are more effective with well-defined problems, such as phobias or sexual dysfunctions, than with vague or pervasive problems like depression and personality disorders.

Cognitive-Behavioral Therapies

The **cognitive-behavioral therapies** incorporate the role of human cognition into the causes of psychological problems, focusing on how faulty and illogical thinking can influence emotions, motivation, and behavior. Therapy attempts to challenge and correct distorted thoughts and change how people think about themselves and others. This approach has gained adherents because it has proven effective in the treatment of many disorders, including depression, anxiety disorders, eating disorders, and even some personality disorders.

An Eclectic Approach

Although most therapists espouse a particular theoretical orientation, many take an eclectic approach; that is, they feel comfortable using ideas from a variety of different theories and approaches. They borrow and combine techniques and concepts depending on what seems to work best for a particular client. For example, a therapist with a psychodynamic approach may conceptualize a client's issues in terms of early needs and interpersonal relationships, but if the client is struggling with anxiety or depression, she may use cognitive-behavioral techniques to help resolve that problem and move the client forward.

Choosing Psychotherapy

What should you expect if you decide to try therapy? Typically, you will sit facing the therapist in a comfortable room. The therapist will invite you to describe the reason for your visit. You can expect to be treated with warmth, respect, and an open, accepting attitude. The therapist will try to provide you with a safe place to explore your feelings and thoughts, including those you would rather not have. Probably some questions and requests for clarification will come up, perhaps accompanied by some observations or thoughts about your story. At the end of the session, the therapist will probably propose a plan for treatment, such as a short series of sessions or a referral to another professional.

Pharmacological Treatments for Mental Disorders

Until the 1950s few effective medications for the symptoms of mental illness existed. Since that time, discoveries and breakthroughs in drug research have revolutionized the treatment of mental disorders. Today, the symptoms

of many serious disorders can be successfully treated with drugs.

The symptoms of schizophrenia and other psychotic disorders, especially delusions and hallucinations, can be treated with *antipsychotics.* Many of these drugs work by blocking the action of the neurotransmitter dopamine in the brain. Symptoms of mood disorders can be relieved with any of several different types of *antidepressants,* most of which act on the neurotransmitters serotonin and norepinephrine. The first antidepressants to be developed, in the 1950s, were a group called monoamine oxidase (MAO) inhibitors. They were followed, in the 1960s, by a group that caused fewer side effects, the tricyclics. In the 1990s another group with even fewer side effects was developed, selective serotonin reuptake inhibitors (SSRIs). Three SSRIs—Prozac, Zoloft, and Paxil—are among the most frequently prescribed drugs in the United States today. Another type of drug, lithium, is a mood stabilizer used to treat bipolar disorder.

Symptoms of anxiety disorders, including obsessive-compulsive disorder, can be reduced with antianxiety drugs (or *anxiolytics*). Benzodiazepines, the most widely used antianxiety drugs, are believed to act on the neurotransmitter GABA, which has a role in the inhibition of anxiety in the brain during stressful situations. Commonly prescribed antianxiety medications include Valium, Xanax, and Ativan. Besides the medications mentioned here, hundreds of other drugs are used to treat a wide array of symptoms and disorders.

If you seek help for a psychological problem from your physician or from a psychiatrist, your treatment is more likely to begin with medication than if you see a clinical psychologist, social worker, marriage and family counselor, school counselor, or other licensed therapist who is not also a medical doctor. Treatment is also likely to begin with medication if you are experiencing acute symptoms of depression, anxiety, or another mental disorder. Drugs

KEY TERMS

psychodynamic therapies Treatments based on the view that psychological problems arise from maladaptive behaviors developed in the client's past, particularly in early relationships.

behavioral therapies Treatments based on the view that psychological problems arise from faulty learning and that new, healthy behaviors can be instilled through behavior modification and other types of training.

cognitive-behavioral therapies Treatments that incorporate the role of human cognition into the causes of psychological problems, focusing on how faulty and illogical thinking can influence emotions, motivation, and behavior.

can help stabilize the condition so that you can make decisions and obtain benefits from psychotherapy.

The use of medications has increased dramatically in recent years. Between 1987 and 1997, for example, more people were treated for depression with drugs than with psychotherapy, even though many studies have shown that therapy can be just as effective as drugs. The use of drugs has also increased dramatically for children and adolescents diagnosed with mental disorders, a controversial issue in our society. The controversy was highlighted in 2004 when a study showed that certain antidepressants increased the risk of suicidal thinking and behavior in adolescents.[20] The FDA directed manufacturers of all antidepressants to include warnings to physicians and parents on their labels.

The increase in the use of drug treatments is due not just to improvements in the drugs themselves but also to the growing use of managed health care in the United States. Insurance companies often prefer to pay for medications, which tend to produce faster, more visible, and more verifiable results, than for psychotherapy, which may last for months or years and produce results that are less objectively verifiable. Although drugs can be extremely effective at reducing pain and misery, they treat only the symptoms of mental disorders. For understanding the root causes of problems and changing maladaptive patterns of thinking, feeling, and behaving, some form of psychotherapy is usually needed.

You Make the Call

Should Physical Illness and Mental Illness Be Treated the Same by Health Insurance Companies?

You don't have to look far to see that our society harbors deep ambivalence about mental illness. Whereas people with physical illnesses are cared for and provided with medical treatment, many people with mental illness live on the street, outcast and stigmatized. As a society we are not clear on what types of treatment programs people with mental illness ought to have, nor have we decided who is going to pay for these programs.

One of the many manifestations of this ambivalence is the way insurance companies cover mental illness. Let's consider a hypothetical situation in which you work for a company that provides you with a health insurance plan. The plan calls for a $20 copayment for a regular office visit to a physician. There is no limit to the number of visits you can make in a given year. The only requirement for coverage of the visit is that the physician be a participant in the plan. If your physician refers you to a specialist, your plan may pay a percentage of the cost.

The mental or behavioral part of your plan involves a different set of terms. Instead of a copayment of $20, you have to pay $40 for each outpatient visit. Instead of unlimited visits, you are allowed up to 30 days per calendar year for treatment of a mental illness and up to 7 days for treatment of substance abuse. For both outpatient and inpatient services you need preapproval by the insurance company. Your insurance plan further stipulates what kind of health care provider you can see. If you see a psychiatrist, your visits will be covered, but if you see a marriage and family therapist or a social worker, your visits are not covered. (Although this is not a description of a specific insurance plan, many plans have similar features.)

Why do these differences exist? Shouldn't physical and mental illnesses be treated the same? Those who oppose such an approach claim that physical illnesses can be diagnosed and treated in more or less standard, objective ways, but mental illnesses are often vague, subjective, and difficult to treat. If mental health care visits are covered equally, people will abuse the system and demand more visits than they need. Our finite health care resources should be reserved for those who truly need them, opponents argue, not wasted on the "worried well."

Opponents further argue that because of the subjective nature of treatment for mental illness, only medical doctors (M.D.s), including psychiatrists, should be covered by insurance, not the host of less well trained health care providers. If greater coverage is extended to mental health problems, insurers will end up paying for a variety of nonmedical treatments, such as marital therapy and career counseling.

Those who think physical and mental illness should be covered equally point out that the distinction between physical illnesses, with their supposedly biological causes, and mental illnesses, with their supposedly psychological causes, is no longer considered a valid one. Illnesses of all kinds are considered to have physical, mental, emotional, social, and spiritual components. The reluctance of insurance companies to cover mental illness equitably is a remnant of an outdated attitude.

Proponents also point out that in states where social workers and other kinds of therapists are covered by insurance, health care costs to insurance companies have not increased, nor has quality of treatment declined. There is no evidence that people abuse the system by demanding more visits than they need. Proponents also argue that treating problems in individuals and families proactively and preventively results in future savings both in health care costs and in costs to society.

Should physical illness and mental illness be treated the same by health insurance companies? What do you think?

Pros

○ There is no clear distinction between physical and mental illnesses. Physical illness can have psychological and behavioral causes (for example, out-of-control stress can lead to stress-related disorders and substance abuse), and mental illness can have physical, biological causes (for example, dementia can be caused by degeneration of brain cells). They should be treated the same.

○ There is no evidence that people will abuse the system if mental health visits are covered by insurance.

○ There is no evidence that including professionals such as marriage and family therapists in insurance plans results in a lower quality of care.

○ Providing preventive mental health care now reduces the cost of treatment in the future.

Cons

○ Costs to insurance companies will have to increase if mental illness is covered the same as physical illness.

○ We will have treatment "creep," and people will seek coverage for nonmedical problems such as marital conflict.

○ Finite resources will be used for the "worried well" and not for those who have the most severe problems.

○ Our society is filled with opportunists trying to sell their services and products to vulnerable individuals. Limiting insurance coverage to highly trained, licensed professionals such as psychiatrists helps to protect people and ensure effective treatment.

OLC Web site For more information about this topic, visit the Online Learning Center at www.mhhe.com/teaguele.

SUMMARY

• Mental health is not just the absence of symptoms of illness; rather it includes the capacity to respond to challenges, frustrations, joys, and failures in ways that allow continued growth and forward movement in life.

• The majority of people are mentally healthy, but many do experience symptoms of mental disorders in their lifetime. The most common mental disorders are mood disorders, especially depression, and anxiety disorders.

• Mentally healthy people have many characteristics in common, including high but realistic self-esteem, a sense of competence, and effective social skills. One conceptualization of mental health is Maslow's model of self-actualization.

• Three primary qualities of mentally healthy people are optimism, self-efficacy, and resilience (the ability to bounce back from adversity).

• Another conceptualization of mental health is Goleman's emotional intelligence—the ability to recognize, name, and express emotions, to interpret social cues, and to communicate effectively.

• Human beings have always experienced mental disorders, which are now known to be diseases that affect the brain. Advances in imaging technology have allowed scientists to visualize the brain, pinpointing the areas activated during different mental functions as well as areas affected when the brain is damaged.

• Advances have also been made in understanding neurotransmitters and in treating symptoms of mental disorders with drugs that act on neurotransmitters.

• Research has shown that the brain continues to change and develop into early adulthood, suggesting that the activities people engage in during adolescence can have a lifelong effect on the structure of their brains.

• Although mental disorders affect the brain, most are not caused by an organic problem in the brain. Rather, they are believed to be caused by complex interactions of biological, psychological, social, and cultural factors.

• The diathesis-stress model suggests that a person may have a vulnerability for an illness, but a stressor must occur to trigger the illness itself.

• Protective factors buffer the individual from threats to psychological well-being; risk factors increase the likelihood that the individual will suffer from mental problems. These factors include the genetic and biological characteristics of the individual, family factors, and social and cultural factors.

• Erikson proposed that personality development proceeds through eight life stages, each characterized by a challenge or conflict. Reasonably successful negotiation of these stages allows people to develop emotional, social, and psychological strengths and continue growing in healthy ways.

- According to the *DSM-IV-TR*, a mental disorder is a pattern of behavior in an individual that is associated with distress (pain) or disability (impairment in an important area of functioning, such as school or work) or with significantly increased risk of suffering, death, pain, disability, or loss of freedom. Mental problems exist on a continuum, but a mental disorder is qualitatively different from a more transient psychological problem.

- Mood disorders occur in people everywhere in the world. Depression is characterized by feelings of sadness or emptiness and by a loss of interest or pleasure in activities, along with several other symptoms. Low-grade, chronic depression that goes on for 2 years or more may be diagnosed as dysthymic disorder. Bipolar disorder is characterized by one or more manic episodes—periods of abnormally elevated mood—alternating with periods of depression or normal mood.

- Anxiety disorders include panic disorder, specific phobias, agoraphobia, social phobia, generalized anxiety disorder, and obsessive-compulsive disorder. In many of these disorders, individuals experience panic attacks.

- Psychotic disorders are characterized by delusions, hallucinations, disorganized speech or behavior, and other signs that the individual has lost touch with reality.

Schizophrenia affects 1–2 percent of the population worldwide.

- Personality disorders involve long-standing, maladaptive patterns of thinking, relating, and behaving that become apparent in adolescence or early adulthood and are pervasive across most or all areas of the person's life.

- Suicide is the third leading cause of death in people aged 15–24. Women are more likely to attempt suicide, but men are more willing to succeed, mainly because they use more lethal means. Up to 90 percent of those who commit suicide are suffering from a mental disorder, often depression.

- Mental disorders can be treated with psychotherapy or medications or a combination of both. Many different types of therapy are available, but among the most common are psychodynamic, behavioral, and cognitive-behavioral. Many therapists take an eclectic approach.

- The symptoms of many mental disorders can be treated with drugs. Psychoses can be treated with a variety of antipsychotics; mood disorders, with antidepressants; and anxiety disorders, with anxiolytics. Drugs treat the symptoms of illness; therapy can help a person change underlying maladaptive patterns of thinking, feeling, and behaving.

REVIEW QUESTIONS

1. What aspects of a person's life are included in mental health?

2. What are some of the characteristics of a mentally healthy person, and why do you think they contribute to mental health?

3. What are the multiple intelligences proposed by Gardner?

4. Explain what is meant by emotional intelligence and why it contributes to healthy psychological adjustment.

5. What information can scientists obtain by using advanced brain imaging techniques?

6. What is a neurotransmitter? What four neurotransmitters have been implicated in mental disorders?

7. What are two implications of the finding that the brain continues to develop into early adulthood?

8. What are the broad categories of causal factors in mental disorders?

9. What is the diathesis-stress model? What are protective factors and risk factors?

10. Name some protective factors and some risk factors at the level of the individual, the family, and the sociocultural environment.

11. What are the eight conflicts, or crises, in Erikson's model of psychosocial development?

12. What is the definition of a mental disorder?

13. Describe two situations in which an emotional or psychological difficulty might develop into a mental disorder.

14. Describe the symptoms of major depressive disorder, dysthymic disorder, and bipolar disorder.

15. Name several different anxiety disorders and describe some of their symptoms.

16. What is the typical age of onset for schizophrenia in men? In women?

17. Why do you think personality disorders are hard to treat?

18. Why do more men than women succeed in committing suicide?

19. What are the major risk factors for suicide? What are the warning signs that a person may be thinking about suicide?

20. What four questions should you ask a person who seems to be contemplating suicide?

21. Describe three commonly used types of therapy.

22. In what circumstances are you more likely to be prescribed medication for psychological difficulties than advised to seek therapy?

WEB RESOURCES

American Association of Marriage and Family Therapy: This Web site offers a variety of resources related to family therapy. In addition to books, articles, and information on family problems, it features Locate a Therapist, a service that allows you to find a reputable therapist in the United States, Canada, and overseas. www.aamft.org

American Psychiatric Association (APA): This organization offers a helpful fact sheet series and a Let's Talk Facts pamphlet series, both designed to dispel myths about mental illness. The Web site also includes information about mental health treatment and related insurance issues. www.psych.org

American Psychological Association (Help Center): This Web site features articles and information on many topics, such as work/school issues, family and relationships, and health and emotional wellness. It also offers free brochures on topics such as counseling help and the warning signs of mental problems. http://helping.apa.org

National Alliance for the Mentally Ill (NAMI): NAMI is a nonprofit organization for people affected by severe mental illness. Its Web site focuses on informing yourself about mental health issues, finding support, and taking action. www.nami.org

National Institute of Mental Health (NIMH): This division of the National Institutes of Health focuses on promoting health information to the public and sponsoring research on mental health and illness. Its authoritative information ranges from breaking news to explanations of common mental disorders. www.nimh.nih.gov

National Mental Health Association (NMHA): This organization's resource center offers brochures on mental health and referrals to treatment centers, support groups, and other national organizations. Answers to frequently asked questions about mental health are especially helpful. www.nmha.org

National Mental Health Information Center: This U.S. Department of Health and Human Services division focuses on prevention of mental illness. Topics such as youth violence and support for individuals and families dealing with HIV/AIDS are featured on its Web site. www.mentalhealth.org

REFERENCES

1. National Institute of Mental Health. (2005). Statistics. www.nimh.nih.gov.
2. Public Health Agency of Canada. (2005). A report on mental illnesses in Canada. www.phac-aspc.gc.ca.
3. Mental health: A report of the surgeon general. (2005). www.surgeongeneral.gov.
4. Seligman, M. (1998). *Learned optimism: How to change your mind and your life.* New York: Pocket Books.
5. Gardner, H. (1993). *Frames of mind: The theory of multiple intelligences.* New York: Basic Books.
6. Goleman, D. (1995). *Emotional intelligence: Why it can matter more than IQ.* New York: Bantam Books.
7. Sternberg, R. J. (1996). *Successful intelligence: How practical and creative intelligences determine success in life.* New York: Simon & Schuster.
8. Andreasen, N. (1984). *The broken brain.* New York: Harper & Row, Perennial Library.
9. Thompson, R. F. (2000). *The brain: A neuroscience primer* (3rd ed.). New York: Worth Publishers.
10. Butcher, J. N., Mineka, S., & Hooley, J. M. (2004). *Abnormal psychology* (12th ed.). Boston: Pearson/Allyn and Bacon.
11. National Institute of Mental Health. (2001). Teenage brain: A work in progress. NIH Publication No. 01-4929. www.nimh.nih.gov.
12. American Psychiatric Association. (2000). *Diagnostic and statistical manual of mental disorders* (4th ed., Text Revision [*DSM-IV-TR*]). Washington, DC: American Psychiatric Association Press.
13. National Institute of Mental Health. (2005). The numbers count: Mental disorders in America. www.nimh.nih.gov.
14. Andreasen, N. (2001). *Brave new brain: Conquering mental illness in the era of the genome.* New York: Oxford University Press.
15. National Institute of Mental Health. (2000). *Anxiety disorders.* NIH Publication No. 00-3679, Washington, DC.
16. National Alliance for the Mentally Ill. (2003). Schizophrenia fact sheet. www.NAMI.org.
17. Redfield Jameson, K. (1999). *Night falls fast: Understanding suicide.* New York: Vintage Press.
18. National College Health Risk Behavior Survey. (1997). *Morbidity and Mortality Weekly Review 46,* 1–54.
19. National Center for Health Statistics for 2001. (2005). Youth suicide. www.cdc.gov.
20. FDA. (2004). Public health advisory. Suicidality in children and adolescents being treated with antidepressant medications. www.fda.gov.

Add It Up! ASSESS YOUR OPTIMISM

Following are 24 statements about a variety of good and bad events, each followed by two different "explanations." For each statement, choose the response that more closely matches how you would explain the event. Circle the score for that answer. For now, ignore the code letters next to each question.

1. You get flowers from a secret admirer.   PvG
   - I am attractive to him/her.   ⓪
   - I am a popular person.   1 —

2. You miss an important engagement.   PvB
   - Sometimes my memory fails me.   1 —
   - I sometimes forget to check my appointment book.   ⓪

3. You host a successful dinner.   PmG
   - I was particularly charming that night.   0
   - I am a good host.   ① —

4. You and your partner have been fighting a lot.   PsB
   - I have been feeling cranky lately.   ① —
   - He/She has been hostile lately.   0

5. You run for a community office and you win.   PvG
   - I devoted a lot of time to campaigning.   ⓪ —
   - I work very hard at everything I do.   1

6. You win an athletic contest.   PmG
   - I was feeling unbeatable.   ⓪
   - I train hard.   1 —

7. You prepare a special meal for a friend and he/she barely touches the food.   PvB
   - I'm not a good cook.   ① —
   - I made the meal in a rush.   0

8. You do exceptionally well in a job interview.   PmG
   - I felt extremely confident during the interview.   ⓪ —
   - I interview well.   1

9. You fail an important test.   PvB
   - I wasn't as smart as the other people.   1 —
   - I didn't prepare for it well.   ⓪

10. You gain weight over the holidays and you can't lose it.   PmB
    - Diets don't work in the long run.   1 —
    - The diet I tried didn't work.   ⓪

11. Your boss gives you too little time to finish a project, but you finish it anyway.   PvG
    - I am good at my job.   0
    - I am an efficient person.   ① —

12. You are in the hospital and few people come to visit.   PsB
    - I'm irritable when I'm sick.   1
    - My friends are negligent about things like that.   ⓪ —

13. You save a person from choking to death.   PvG
    - I know a technique to save someone from choking.   ⓪
    - I know what to do in a crisis.   1 —

14. Your partner takes you away for a romantic weekend.   PmG
    - He/She needed to get away for a few days.   ⓪ —
    - He/She likes to explore new areas.   1

15. You were extremely healthy all year.   PsG
    - Few people around me were sick, so I wasn't exposed.   0 —
    - I made sure I ate well and got enough rest.   1 —

16. A friend says something that hurts your feelings.   PmB
    - She always blurts things out without thinking of others.   ①
    - She was in a bad mood and took it out on me.   0 —

17. A game show host picks you out of the audience to participate in the show.   PsG
    - I was sitting in the right seat.   ⓪ —
    - I looked the most enthusiastic.   1

18. They don't honor your credit card at a store.   PvB
    I sometimes overestimate how much money I have.   (1)
    I sometimes forget to pay my credit card bill.   0

19. You ask someone to dance and he/she says no.   PsB
    I am not a good enough dancer.   (1)
    He/She doesn't like to dance.   0

20. You tell a joke and everyone laughs.   PsG
    The joke was funny.   0
    My timing was perfect.   (1)

21. You are penalized for not returning your income tax forms on time.   PmB
    I always put off doing my taxes.   1
    I was lazy about my taxes this year.   (0)

22. You have a wonderful time at a party.   PsG
    Everyone was friendly.   (0)
    I was friendly.   1

23. You forget your partner's birthday.   PmB
    I'm not good at remembering birthdays.   1
    I was preoccupied with other things.   (0)

24. You buy your partner a gift and he/she doesn't like it.   PsB
    I don't put enough thought into things like that.   1
    He/She has very picky tastes.   (0)

Scoring

An optimistic or pessimistic explanatory style can be thought of as having three dimensions: personalization, permanence, and pervasiveness.

PsG   These statements assess the "personalization" dimension of optimism. When something good happens, you attribute it to something internal about yourself.

$$\frac{O}{15} \ \frac{O}{17} \ \frac{1}{20} \ \frac{O}{22} = \frac{1}{}$$

1 0 1 0 = 2

PmG   These statements assess the "permanence" dimension of optimism. When something good happens, you attribute it to something permanent about people.

$$\frac{1}{3} \ \frac{O}{6} \ \frac{O}{8} \ \frac{O}{14} = \frac{1}{}$$

1 1 0 0 = 2

PvG   These statements assess the "pervasive" dimension of optimism. When something good happens, you attribute it to a characteristic you have across most situations.

$$\frac{O}{1} \ \frac{O}{5} \ \frac{1}{11} \ \frac{O}{13} = \frac{1}{}$$

1 0 1 1 = 3

For each of these optimism scores, 4 = very optimistic; 3 = moderately optimistic; 2 = average; 1 = moderately pessimistic, 0 = very pessimistic.

PsB   These statements assess the "personalization" dimension of pessimism. When something bad happens, you attribute it to something internal about yourself.

$$\frac{1}{4} \ \frac{O}{12} \ \frac{1}{19} \ \frac{O}{24} = \frac{2}{}$$

1 0 1 0 = 2

PmB   These statements assess the "permanence" dimension of pessimism. When something bad happens, you attribute it to something permanent about people.

$$\frac{O}{10} \ \frac{1}{16} \ \frac{O}{21} \ \frac{O}{23} = \frac{1}{}$$

1 0 0 0 = 1

PvB   These statements assess the "pervasive" dimension of pessimism. When something bad happens, you attribute it to a characteristic you have across most situations.

$$\frac{O}{2} \ \frac{1}{7} \ \frac{O}{9} \ \frac{1}{18} = \frac{2}{}$$

0 1 1 1 = 3

For each of these three pessimism scores, 4 = very pessimistic; 3 = moderately pessimistic; 2 = average; 1 = moderately optimistic, 0 = very optimistic.

Now you can compute your overall scores. First add your three G (good event) scores to get your total G score:

$$\frac{1}{PmG} + \frac{1}{PvG} + \frac{1}{PsG} = \frac{3}{Total\ G\ score}$$

2 3 2 = 7

11 to 12	Very optimistic; you have an "optimistic explanatory style" toward life in general
8 to 10	Moderately optimistic
5 to 7	Average
2 to 4	Moderately pessimistic
0 to 1	Very pessimistic

Now add your three B (bad event) scores to get your total B score:

$$\frac{1}{PmB} + \frac{2}{PvB} + \frac{2}{PsB} = \frac{5}{Total\ B\ score}$$

1 3 2 6

11 to 12	Very pessimistic; you have a "pessimistic explanatory style" toward life in general
8 to 10	Moderately pessimistic
5 to 7	Average
2 to 4	Moderately optimistic
0 to 1	Very optimistic

Now subtract your B score from your G score to get your total score:

$$\frac{5}{\text{Total G}} - \frac{3}{\text{Total B}} = \frac{2}{\text{Total score}}$$

8 to 12	Very optimistic across all areas of your life
3 to 7	Moderately optimistic
2 to −2	Average
−3 to −7	Moderately pessimistic
−8 to −12	Very pessimistic across all areas of your life

If your scores are more in the pessimistic range than the optimistic range, try cultivating some of the characteristics of mentally healthy people described in this chapter. You might also consider some of the strategies for building a spiritual life suggested in Chapter 4, such as keeping a gratitude journal, and some of the stress management and relaxation techniques detailed in Chapter 5. Developing a more optimistic outlook is worth the effort!

SOURCE: From *Learned Optimism* by Martin E. P. Seligman. Copyright © 1991 by Martin E. P. Seligman. Used by permission of Alfred A. Knopf, a division of Random House, Inc.

Spirituality: Finding Meaning in Life and Death

DID YOU KNOW?

- If you have ever said a prayer when facing a health crisis, you belong to the one-third of Americans who use prayer, in addition to conventional medical treatments, for health concerns. Hundreds of studies have demonstrated a relationship between religious involvement and spirituality, on the one hand, and better health outcomes, on the other.

- Individuals can cultivate spiritual wellness by turning inward—by practicing meditation, writing in a journal, or developing rituals to sanctify everyday experiences. They can also cultivate spiritual wellness by turning outward—by participating in community projects, engaging in social activism, or incorporating environmental values into their lives.

OLC *Your Health Today*   www.mhhe.com/teague1e

Go to the Online Learning Center for *Your Health Today* for interactive activities, quizzes, flashcards, Web links, and more resources related to this chapter.

Someone once said that the longest journey is the journey inward. The spiritual journey is deeply personal and individual. It may begin as a yearning for connection with what is universal and timeless or a belief in a power operating in the universe that is greater than oneself. It often involves a search for meaning and purpose or a desire for a more intense participation in life. Many people now believe that spiritual health enhances their psychological and physical well-being, and they pursue spiritual wellness as one of the important dimensions of total wellness.

It seems that all people in all times have experienced spiritual aspirations. Worldwide, there are more than 20 major religions and thousands of other forms of spiritual expression. In the spirit of modern genetics, some scientists have been searching for a biological basis for human spirituality—a gene or genes that would account for our spiritual experiences and yearnings—and one researcher, Dean Hamer of the National Cancer Institute, believes he has found such a gene.[1] No matter what the role of biology, however, spiritual experience and expression are clearly the product of complex interactions between individuals and their cultures.

In this chapter we explore spirituality as a broad expression of human thought, feeling, and aspiration that takes many forms and appears in various guises. We begin by considering what is included in the concept of spirituality, and we present a variety of approaches to building a spiritual life. We then examine several ways in which spirituality can be cultivated and expressed in everyday life, and we review the effects of spirituality on physical and mental health. We also look at different forms of community involvement that offer avenues for connectedness beyond our individual lives. Finally, we explore the topics of dying, death, and bereavement, arguably the greatest challenges and greatest opportunities for spiritual growth that any of us will ever face. Our hope is that the chapter will inspire you to explore your own spirituality and deepen your sense of meaning and purpose in life.

WHAT IS SPIRITUALITY?

Because spirituality may involve a different path for each individual, it has been defined in many ways. In health promotion literature, **spirituality** is commonly defined as a person's connection to self, significant others, and the community at large. Many experts also agree that spirituality involves a personal belief system or value system that gives meaning and purpose to life. For some individuals this personal value system may include a belief in and reverence for a higher power, which may be expressed through an organized religion. For others the spiritual dimension is nonreligious and centers on a personal value system that may be reflected in activities such as volunteer work. In either case, spirituality provides a feeling of participation in something greater than oneself and a sense of unity with nature and the universe.

In this section, we explore spirituality in the context of everyday life. As you read, you might want to ask yourself such questions as: Do I have strong and satisfying relationships with family, friends, and people in my community? What are my values, and how do they guide my decisions? Do I have a meaningful purpose in life? These questions are central to your spiritual journey; they will recur throughout your life.

Maintaining Connectedness

As noted, spirituality involves connectedness to self, to others, and to a larger purpose. Connectedness to self includes developing self-awareness and self-esteem. Building these attributes is an incremental process in which you develop a reservoir of inner strengths through such practices as becoming more compassionate, or learning to be a better listener.

Spirituality also includes being responsible for yourself and taking charge of your life. Your spiritual health affects your capacity for love, compassion, joy, forgiveness, altruism, and fulfillment. It can be an antidote to stress, cynicism, anger, fear, anxiety, self-absorption, and pessimism. When you learn to handle life in general with more resilience and balance, you are able to make the best of whatever you may face.

Connectedness with significant others through positive relationships is also essential to spiritual health and growth. Healthy relationships involve a balance between closeness and separateness and are characterized by mutual support, respect, good communication, and caring actions. Overall, having strong personal relationships seems to improve self-esteem and gives greater meaning to life.[2]

Connectedness to and participation in the community includes enjoying constructive relationships at school, in the workplace, or in the neighborhood. When individuals join together to achieve shared goals, both they and society as a whole benefit. Several studies have demonstrated links between social connectedness and positive outcomes for individual health and well-being.[3] Evidence shows that social participation and engagement are related to the maintenance of cognitive function in older adulthood and to lowered mortality rates. In general, the size of a person's social network and his or her sense of connectedness are inversely related to risk-related behaviors such as alcohol and tobacco consumption, physical inactivity, and behaviors leading to obesity.[4] Community involvement is discussed in more detail later in this chapter.

Developing a Personal Value System

Another aspect of spirituality involves developing a personal **value system,** a set of guidelines for how you want to live your life. *Values,* the criteria for judging what is good and bad, underlie moral principles and behavior. Your value system shapes who you are as a person, how you make decisions, and what goals you set for yourself. When you develop a way of life that makes sense and enables you to navigate the world effectively, the many choices you face each day become much less complex and easier to handle. Your value system becomes your map, providing a structure for decision making that allows flexibility and the possibility of change.

Finding Meaning and Purpose in Life

Why am I here? This question has been asked by people all over the world, in all eras, and at all stages of life. For children, the answer may be simply to have fun and learn. For teens, it may involve developing and enjoying new relationships. For young adults, the focus might be career and family. Those in middle age may see their purpose as caring for others. Older adults might turn their energy toward creating a safer and healthier planet.

The search for meaning and purpose in life becomes especially important in adulthood. According to psychologist Abraham Maslow, people are always striving to meet their needs (as briefly noted in Chapter 3). His hierarchy of needs theory, developed in the 1960s, suggests that only after our most basic needs are met (such as survival needs) can we proceed toward higher goals. In Maslow's theory, needs are conceptualized as a pyramid, with physiological needs forming the base and higher levels consisting, in ascending order, of safety and security, love and belongingness, self-esteem, and finally self-actualization (Figure 4.1). Self-actualization is the state in which we

achieve our fullest human potential. Those who reach this level achieve a state of transcendence, a sense of well-being that comes from finding purpose and meaning in life.[5] To assess your own progress toward self-actualization, try the Add It Up! feature at the end of this chapter.

BUILDING A SPIRITUAL LIFE

The quest for self-fulfillment often begins with the question, Who am I? The answer to this question begins with self-exploration. What are your abilities and talents, your interests and passions? What are your core values and guiding principles? Finding the answers to these questions will help you build a spiritual life, one in which you have a better idea of who you are. In this section we consider several approaches to self-exploration that can help people broaden and deepen their self-knowledge and self-awareness.

Practicing Mindfulness

Many times we are unaware of the thoughts going through our heads. We may be thinking about what someone said to us, how someone behaved toward us, how we might have done things differently. We repeat the same thoughts and patterns of thinking as a matter of habit, and over time they become stronger and more powerful. Unless we make a conscious effort to be aware of this old "tape," we typically continue to relive our past experiences, even if they are negative. We filter new experiences through our habitual way of seeing the world and end up reacting to our own expectations instead of what may really be in front of us. In this way, we miss opportunities for positive change.

Mindfulness is the practice of living fully in the moment, concentrating on what is happening right now. By learning to be conscious of your thoughts as they pass by—observing them, not judging them—you develop your ability to control and stop habitual, impulsive, or undesirable reactions. You become more capable of responding in a "thoughtful" and "mindful" way rather than becoming overwhelmed with negative emotions or self-criticism.[6] As

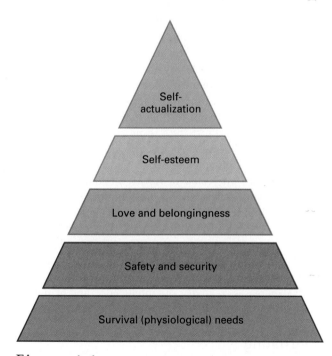

Figure 4.1 **Abraham Maslow's hierarchy of needs.** Source: Maslow, Abraham H., Frager, Robert D. (Ed.), Fadiman, James (Ed.), *Motivation and Personality*, 3rd ed., copyright © 1987. Adapted by permission of Pearson Education, Inc., Upper Saddle River, NJ. New York: Harper & Row.

KEY TERMS

spirituality The experience of connection to self, others, and the community at large, providing a sense of purpose and meaning.
value system Set of criteria for judging what is good and bad that underlies moral decisions and behavior.
mindfulness Awareness and acceptance of living fully in the moment.

Challenges & Choices

Learning to Meditate

Meditation is an ancient technique with modern adaptations. Various forms of meditation have been developed, but their common goals are to calm the mind, raise awareness, and increase attention to what is happening in the present moment. Here are some guidelines for a type of meditation in which you focus on your breathing:

- Sit in a comfortable place—on a pillow on the floor or in a chair, for example—in a quiet room where you won't be disturbed. Close your eyes.
- Breathe deeply. Feel the breath as it enters your nostrils and fills your chest and abdomen; then release it.
- Focus your attention on your breathing and awareness of the moment. Try to be silent and still.
- Remain passive and relaxed as your thoughts come and go, noticing them without getting caught up in them. At first, your mind will fill with memories, worries, and random thoughts. Let go of the thoughts and feelings and return to the

awareness of breath. Eventually, you will be able to concentrate for longer periods of time, and these periods of concentration may be accompanied by feelings of great tranquility.

Meditate for brief periods of time each day. Start out with 5 minutes and gradually build up to 15 minutes or more. Make a commitment to continue meditating for 3 months; you will not experience any changes or benefits unless you practice. Experiment until you find a place, time, and approach that works for you. If you would like more information about techniques, contact a meditation center, consult a teacher or book, search online, talk with more experienced meditators, or listen to a tape.

It's Not Just Personal . . .

People all over the world, of all spiritual and secular persuasions, practice meditation. Types of meditations include transcendental, mindfulness, mantra (chanting), zazen (sitting), walking, and chakra, among many others.

---

you learn to focus on the present moment, you can be more in touch with your life as it is happening.

When people learn to live fully in the moment, they sometimes experience a phenomenon known as **flow**, a feeling of being completely absorbed in an activity and a moment. In this state, people forget themselves, lose track of time, and feel as if they have become one with what they are doing. Writers describe times when words seem to come through them; athletes refer to being "in the zone." The feeling can happen to anyone, whether engrossed in a hobby, involved in a heated debate about politics, communing with nature in a quiet setting, or taking the last shot in a tied basketball game. Flow has been described as one of the most enjoyable and valuable experiences a person can have.[7] When you learn to be mindful and live in the moment, you are more likely to experience flow in your daily activities.

Mindfulness is celebrated by the noted Vietnamese monk Thich Nhat Hanh in these words:

> Our true home is in the present moment.
> To live in the present moment is a miracle.
> The miracle is not to walk on water.
> The miracle is to walk on the green Earth in the present moment,
> To appreciate the peace and beauty that are available now.[8]

Meditation

One way of quieting the mind is to practice **meditation.** Over time, with practice, you can slow your racing thoughts, not only while you are meditating but also while engaged in your routine daily life. There are many ways to meditate, but all of them involve introspection and, ultimately, self-exploration and self-discovery. The goal is to relax your body, let your feelings and thoughts come and go as they will, and just "be." Some people are able, with practice, to go beyond thoughts, ego, self, and personality to reach "pure consciousness."

If you are interested in trying meditation as a way to deepen your self-knowledge and build a spiritual life, follow the guidelines in the box "Learning to Meditate." Although meditation may not appeal to everyone, the practice can offer many benefits. It is widely used in stress management and stress reduction programs. Proponents claim that meditation provides deep relaxation, promotes health, increases creativity and intelligence, and brings inner happiness and fulfillment.

Journaling

Another approach to building a spiritual life is **journaling.** As you record your feelings, thoughts, breakthroughs, and desires in a private journal, you will begin to understand yourself more clearly. Whether you write about a loss or a triumph, a remembrance from childhood, a struggle with disease, or any of an infinite number of experiences, you can use daily writing as a path to deeper knowledge of yourself.

Researcher and psychologist James Pennebaker has found that writing about emotional upheavals can improve physical and mental health. He suggests writing about any of the following:

- Something that you are thinking or worrying about too much.
- Something that you are dreaming about.
- Something that you feel is affecting your life in an unhealthy way.
- Something that you have been avoiding for days, weeks, or years.[9]

The more honest you are, the better. Don't censor yourself as you write; just let your thoughts flow. Try to move beyond the superficial telling to asking yourself, Why am I feeling this way?

In *Writing to Save Your Life*, journalist and professor Michele Weldon describes her growth through journaling as both difficult and rewarding:

> You need to call to your words, beckon them, listen for them, and offer them a safe place to arrive. If there is too much confusion and noise, the words inside you will retreat, like fish that see your wiggling feet in the splashing water and sense the bait is a trap. Writing is not passive, and it doesn't happen without you, to you, or in spite of you. When I have done writing that is raw and honest, I am exhausted and energized at the same time, the way you feel after running or walking a mile very fast. It takes energy and concentration and a commitment to the Big Idea.[10]

Journaling is an effective way to learn about who you are and where you have been. It can give you the courage to recognize and pursue your passion. Listening to your inner dialogue may offer you a sense of peace and a positive outlook on your experiences. Writing can bring up unresolved issues in your life, help you reach understanding and forgiveness, show you how to find closure, and allow you to move on. In some cases, journaling can be painful, stirring up emotions that may be difficult to handle on your own. If you find yourself in such a situation, consider contacting a professional for counseling.[11]

Experiencing Retreat

Spiritual **retreat** and personal growth retreat are both names for a place of refuge, seclusion, or privacy or an activity in which you can create quiet space for raising your personal spiritual awareness. Retreats may involve solitude or group withdrawal for meditation, prayer,

Journal writing offers a way to explore your feelings, understand yourself, and discover what is important to you.

exploration, or study. They are intended to reenergize your life and restore your zest for living. A spiritual retreat might offer a balance of activities that encourage growth, foster learning, and restore energy, so that when you return to your normal surroundings, you may live life to the fullest in a loving and purposeful way.

KEY TERMS

flow Pleasurable experience of complete absorption and engagement in an activity.

meditation Technique for quieting the mind by focusing on a word, an object (such as a candle flame), or a process (such as breathing).

journaling Approach to self-exploration in which a person writes feelings and experiences in a journal as an aid to personal growth.

retreat Period of seclusion, solitude, or group withdrawal for prayer, meditation, exploration, or study.

Challenges & Choices

Enhancing Your Spirituality

How can you begin to deepen and enhance your spirituality? Here are a few ways to initiate the process.

- Think of three activities or rituals that might deepen your connection to yourself or others. You might consider taking a quiet walk in the park, going on a retreat, tutoring a child in a local school, keeping a gratitude journal, practicing mindfulness, delivering Meals on Wheels to an elderly neighbor, gardening, listening to a new piece of music, drawing or painting, or doing any other activity that feels meaningful to you. Now schedule time to do one of these three things this week.

- Practice random acts of kindness with the intention of improving someone else's day, even if it means giving up a little something for yourself. Try smiling at the people you pass on the street, bringing coffee to your colleagues, letting someone into your lane on the highway, or helping a stranger struggling with packages. Instead of rushing to take care of yourself, slow down and take care of those around you.

- Think about a person in your life who you feel has wronged you or with whom you are angry. It might be a parent, a sibling, a partner, a roommate. Can you find it in your heart to forgive this person at this time? To do so, you might need to talk with the person, or you may simply be able to do the internal emotional work on your own. Even when hurts are deep and real, the process of forgiving is a healing one. If you can forgive, you will release the energy locked up in your anger or resentment and enhance your capacity for love.

It's Not Just Personal . . .

Most people are aware of the moral imperative to forgive that is embedded in many faith traditions, but they also acknowledge the difficulty of doing so. In a Gallup poll reported by the Campaign for Forgiveness (www.forgiving.org), 94 percent of Americans surveyed said it was important to forgive others. However, only 48 percent said they usually try to forgive.

Many kinds of facilities offer retreats, workshops, and programs for spiritual growth, but you can use your home for a retreat as well. Set aside a weekend and plan to give up all social events, phone calls, errands, television, newspapers, Internet, and all nonessential housework. Then prepare for exploration. You might meditate, journal, draw, write poetry, take walks to enjoy the beauty of nature, listen to music, read—whatever you want to do that you find deepening and centering. At their best, retreats stimulate the mind, enhance self-awareness, and refresh the spirit. They provide food for the body, mind, and spirit. For more ideas on retreats and other forms of self-exploration, see the box above, "Enhancing Your Spirituality."

Experiencing the Arts

Scholar and mythologist Joseph Campbell once asserted, "The goal of life is rapture. Art is the way we experience it. Art is the transforming experience." Experiencing the arts—whether sculpture, painting, music, poetry, literature, theater, storytelling, dance, or some other form—is another way to build a spiritual life. Some people are moved by the solemn works of Bach or Mozart, others by the elegant jazz of John Coltrane, and still others by the intricate ragas of Ravi Shankar. Some people experience rapture while viewing the sculptures of Michelangelo, others while watching a Shakespearean tragedy, still others while enjoying a Balanchine ballet. Experiencing great art can inspire you, through felt experience, to think about the purpose of life and the nature of reality.[12] By engaging your heart, mind, and spirit, art can give you fresh insights, challenge preconceptions, and trigger inner growth.

When you enjoy and appreciate the arts, you embrace diverse cultures past and present and frequently discover in them the universal themes of human existence—love, loss, birth, death, isolation, community, continuity, change. When you express yourself creatively, you may be able to experience a spiritual connection between your inner core and the natural world beyond yourself. Both experiences—art appreciation and artistic expression—can be transforming. If the visual or performing arts are not part of your life right now, try to schedule time to visit a museum or attend a concert. Make notes or sketches in a journal reflecting on your experiences. Doing so may stimulate new spiritual connections in your life.

Living Your Values

The approaches described so far can help you discover who you are by promoting self-exploration. It is also important to bring your deepest beliefs and intentions into the world, that is, to live your values. Can you articulate what is most important to you in life? Are you living and acting in accordance with it? Try writing a "purpose statement" that will remind you of who you truly are and why you believe you are here on earth. Then ask yourself, Do I stay "on purpose" in my daily interactions and activities? Commit your purpose statement to memory, and read or recite it daily. It may be "to live and learn" or "to know my higher being and teach and express love."

Adopting a new habit, such as putting your best intentions into practice, takes time and work, as does changing an old or destructive habit. Ingrained habits, whether overeating, nail biting, procrastinating, or personalizing all situations, can be as difficult to break as substance addictions.[13] Experts say that you have to continue to take action for 60 to 90 days to make a behavior change stick. As Aristotle understood almost 2,500 years ago, "We are what we repeatedly do. Excellence is not an act, then, but a habit."

One way to create new habits is to develop **rituals**—routines or practices, often symbolic, that you follow regularly. Building rituals, such as "an early bedtime, a daily run, a diet low in sugar, a morning meditation, a ritual walk in the park, an inspirational photograph—even an uncluttered desk or Daytimer," can, over time, effect life-transforming changes.[13] In addition, rituals may sanctify everyday experiences, investing them with spiritual significance. Later in this chapter we discuss daily rituals specifically designed to enhance your spiritual life.

Another way to change an old habit or build a new one is through supportive relationships. Anyone who has had a workout buddy, attended Alcoholics Anonymous, or prayed with a group on retreat is familiar with the powerful effect of acting in concert with others. In a 2-year study of 200 people who made New Year's resolutions, psychologist John Norcross found that those individuals most likely to persist beyond 6 months were those with social support.[13]

SPIRITUALITY AND HEALTH
Spirituality in Everyday Life

Spiritual wellness is one dimension of total wellness, as described in Chapter 1. Spiritual wellness includes the ability to

- Examine personal beliefs and values.
- Search for meaning and purpose in life.
- Make connections with other people.
- Appreciate natural forces in the universe.

Your ability to develop spiritual wellness lies in the choices you make every day on your own behalf. If you react out of habit or fixed attitudes, you may not be using your choices wisely to create wellness in your life. In this section we discuss some daily behavior choices that will promote your spiritual health and help you to live your values more consistently.

Your Physical Health

Over the ages, various spiritual traditions have thought of the human body as the temple of the spirit. It is certainly true that if you neglect or abuse your body, it is difficult if not impossible to reach wellness. Consider how your daily physical routine affects your health. How can you better respect your body? Exercise regularly and get plenty of rest. Keep your energy high by selecting a well-balanced diet. Do not abuse alcohol or drugs, and avoid tobacco products. If you participate in sexual activity, be responsible and keep yourself safe. Actively participate in your health care decisions.

As with any behavior change, improving your physical wellness requires not just inspiration, but practice, practice, practice. Think about ways to incorporate "training rituals" in your life to create daily rhythms and build physical energy: a brisk walk every morning before school or work, a quick swim at lunch, a day a week working at home, a yoga break or a healthy snack in midafternoon. Remember that your environment is powerful in shaping your behavior too. Clear junk foods out of your pantry, pack a protein bar, nuts, or a piece of fruit in your backpack or briefcase, and always keep a water bottle within arm's reach.

Your Mental and Emotional Health

Spiritual health overlaps with psychological (mental and emotional) health in numerous ways. Feeling that you are part of something greater in the universe can help you handle many daily challenges. It provides perspective on what is really important and helps you find creative ways to deal with problems. It also helps you maintain a positive outlook and sense of humor. Spiritual health includes recognizing your feelings and expressing them appropriately as well as taking responsibility for your behavior and accepting what you cannot change. Spiritual wellness gives you hope for the future.

Communication skills are valuable in connecting to others in an emotionally healthy way. Active listening is a way of paying attention to the feeling behind what someone else is saying. It means not arguing or passively

KEY TERMS

ritual   Procedure or routine, often symbolic, that is regularly followed.

agreeing with the other person but opening your heart to the feeling the person is trying to express. The healing elements of listening are *compassion*—a sympathetic understanding of another person's distress—and *empathy*—the ability to "walk in someone else's shoes," to understand from the inside what someone else is experiencing.[14] It take practice to learn how to listen with compassion and empathy.

Another communication skill that fosters emotional connection is acceptance of another person's experience. A good listener conveys this idea: "I believe this is what you are trying to communicate, and I hear you. I accept and acknowledge what you're saying. I might not feel the way you do, but I can understand that this is your feeling."[14]

Many people enhance their mental and emotional health by cultivating the art of relaxation. Taking time to relax on a regular basis—even if it is only a few moments—is vital to maintaining a positive psychological outlook and keeping stress under control. A variety of relaxation techniques can be done almost anytime, anywhere, in a matter of moments. Chapter 5 provides detailed descriptions of several relaxation techniques.

Praying, listening to soothing music, or taking a few moments to be alone can also help you relax. Stretching, closing your eyes and counting to 10, or simply finding something to laugh about, may also prove beneficial. Some people find that a hobby such as gardening, weaving, jogging, painting, or arranging flowers helps them relax and tune in to their spiritual side. The key is to find relaxation exercises that are effective for you and to practice them regularly.

Building Resilience

One of the greatest challenges to spiritual wellness is stress. As discussed in detail in Chapter 5, any events that upset our daily lives—including negative events such as the death of a spouse and positive ones such as getting married—create stress. You cannot avoid stress in your life, but you can learn to manage it in a healthy way.

The ability to bounce back from adversity, as discussed in Chapter 3, is known as resilience. It is not just an aptitude that we are born with but a skill that anyone can learn and develop. Parents and educators can even instill a resilient mind-set in children, fostering hope, strength, and optimism.[15] In Chapter 3, we listed several characteristics of resilient individuals. In addition, resilient people tend to hold religious or spiritual beliefs. Possessing strong personal values provides a foundation for coping and fosters growth through faith, hope, and love. (See the box "Understanding Your Personal Values.")

Resilience is particularly well developed in some trauma survivors, such as those who lived through concentration camps or natural disasters, patients with serious illnesses, or people from troubled homes.[16] Tour de France cycling champion and cancer survivor Lance Armstrong has often said that cancer was the best thing that ever happened to him:

> There's no great sense of foreboding, no premonition, you just wake up one morning and something's wrong in your lungs, or your liver, or your bones. But near-death cleared the decks, and what came after was a bright, sparkling awareness: time is limited, so I better wake up every morning fresh and know that I have just one chance to live this particular day right, and to string my days together into a life of action, and purpose. If you want to know what keeps me on my bike, riding up an alp for six hours in the rain, that's your answer.[17]

Even though their ordeals were painful, resilient people often look back on them as bringing positive changes into their lives. By developing qualities of resilience, we become better able to deal with an unpredictable world and more flexible in facing the unknown.

Resilience often means developing new abilities simply to get through an unfamiliar and stressful experience. Along with the new skills comes the psychological confidence associated with doing something new and being successful. Just as *negative scripts*—repetitive, self-defeating ways of thinking and behaving—can lead to hopelessness, depression, and anxiety, *positive scripts* can help you not only survive stressful experiences but also surpass your previous level of functioning. A resilient mind-set will help you shrug off harsh self-criticisms and negative self-images. Especially during difficult times, you need to focus on building your assets rather than expending time and energy on fixing your perceived deficits.

Adversity often causes resilient individuals to look to deeper meaning and purpose in life. They may become more aware of and interested in spiritual pursuits. Faith and resilience sometimes go hand in hand. Even if you have a terminal illness, you do not know what the next moment will bring, in terms of relationships, healing, and forgiveness. The resilience of the human spirit is enormous.

Finding Joy in Everyday Things

Sometimes we are trying so hard to reach our big goals that we miss daily opportunities to appreciate ordinary things. In our pursuit of happiness we often overlook simple pleasures that are right in front of us. Joy is an attitude, a state of mind that can be developed and nurtured.

Today, take the time to notice, appreciate, and delight in all the good things your life has to offer. Try keeping a gratitude journal by your bed. Each evening jot down five things for which you are grateful that day. They can range from the concrete to the abstract, from fresh strawberries to a more relaxed attitude about money to an appreciation of simply being alive. Document all of the valuable things you accomplished. Include progress you made toward your goals, random acts of kindness, occasions when you replaced negative reactions with positive ones, and new behaviors. It can be hard to do at first, but it will

Challenges & Choices

Understanding Your Personal Values

Many people are unaware of their core values and the guiding principles by which they live their lives. We seldom actually think through our values until we are faced with a difficult choice, and even then we may make a choice without being aware of our values. At times we may even compromise those values because we feel pressured or powerless.

For inspiration we can look to people who took a stand and stood up for their values despite enormous pressure to conform and foreseeable negative consequences. Sherron Watkins, former vice president for corporate development at Enron, blew the whistle on that company's accounting practices, leading to the uncovering of widespread financial misdeeds in many American corporations. Julia Bonds, winner of the Goldman Environmental Prize, took on the coal mining industry to fight mountain removal in West Virginia. Erin Brockovich initiated the investigation of California residents' exposure to toxic chromium 6. And, of course, Rosa Parks sparked the civil rights movement when she refused to sit in the back of the bus.

In each of these individuals' actions, we can see a belief in core values and a set of guiding principles derived from them. What do you think they are? How would you articulate your own core values? Consider the following list of major life values:

achievement	financial	integrity	service
autonomy	well-being	learning	spirituality
compassion	freedom	love	status
creativity	health	personal	
education	home	growth	
family	honesty	prestige	

Which of these (or others) are most important and meaningful to you? What guiding principles can you derive from them? How can you embody them in your life?

It's Not Just Personal . . .

Societies as well as individuals operate from core values and principles. Some core values of American society, as expressed in such documents as the Declaration of Independence and the U.S. Constitution, include life, liberty, the pursuit of happiness, justice, popular sovereignty, the common good, truth, diversity, and patriotism. How do your personal values line up with these societal values?

become easier as you make a habit of looking for good in yourself and your day.

With the awareness that comes from an appreciation of all the good that goes unnoticed every day, the "ordinary" moments of your life become imbued with meaning and deserving of profound respect. Your daily inventory of positive behaviors will train you to focus on your thoughts and actions, which in turn fosters change and develops persistence. Individuals who keep gratitude journals on their own and families or other groups who keep and discuss their gratitude journals together express the same sentiments: their attitudes have been more positive, they are able to find the good in tough situations, and they are more aware of what makes them happy.[18]

Creating Balance

In our fast-paced society, the lines dividing work, personal life, and family frequently blur, and it can be hard to balance competing priorities. We are conditioned to think that doing more will lead to greater success. A more successful strategy is to prioritize the important things and delegate or forego the rest.

Another approach to creating balance is to view your life from a broader perspective. In his book *Seven Habits of Highly Effective People,* Stephen Covey suggests, "Begin with the end in mind." As an exercise, try writing your own obituary or viewing your life as if from your funeral, looking back at your life experiences and reflecting on what was important. What did you accomplish? What did you want to accomplish but didn't? What were the happy moments? What were the sad times? What would you do again, and what would you not do again? Did you live out your deepest values?

If you are like many people, you may find that doing this exercise means focusing more on the relationships built over a lifetime than on material possessions accumulated. It means recognizing and acknowledging those around you who are responsible for making your success possible. It also means taking time to enjoy the fruits of your labor and sharing those fruits with others.

Health Benefits of Spirituality

People have always believed in the ability of divine power to heal. In the cultures of ancient Egypt, Greece, and Rome, religious ceremonies were conducted by priests to cure disease. According to a CBS News poll, 80 percent of Americans believe that prayer holds the power to heal,[19] and according to a 2004 study, one-third of Americans use

Making time for hobbies is one way of keeping your life—and your mental health—in balance.

prayer, in addition to conventional medical treatments, for health concerns.[20] The connection between spirituality and health is gaining serious attention from the medical and scientific communities. Hundreds of studies have been conducted on spirituality and health over the last 15 years. More than half the nation's medical schools now offer courses on spirituality and medicine, whereas only three did 20 years ago. The National Institutes of Health plans to spend millions of dollars over the next several years on "mind-body" medicine.[21] The pursuit is not without its skeptics, however, and the connection between spirituality and health remains an area of controversy and debate.

Physical Effects of Spirituality

Can prayer cure cancer or slow its progression? Can it lower blood pressure? Does spirituality speed healing after accidents or help people recover from surgery? Do religious people live longer?

There are no definitive answers to these questions, but a majority of 350 studies of physical health and 850 studies of mental health suggest a direct relationship between religious involvement and spirituality, on the one hand, and better health outcomes, on the other.[22] Research has found that religious involvement and spirituality are associated with lower blood pressure, decreased

risk of substance abuse, less cardiovascular disease, less depression, less anxiety, enhanced immune function, and longer life.[23] Meditation and prayer in combination with traditional medical treatments are reported to relieve medical problems such as chronic pain, depression, anxiety, insomnia, and premenstrual syndrome.[24] There are enough positive results to spur further inquiry.

This does not mean that scientists would go so far as to say that spirituality causes wellness or that illness is due to a lack of spirituality. Such questions are basically beyond the power of science to answer; that is, it is difficult to use scientific methods to answer what are essentially metaphysical questions. New research into the spirituality-health connection focuses on finding, eliminating, and understanding other factors that might affect their relationship.

One of the most consistent research findings is that spiritually connected persons stay healthier and live longer than those who are not connected.[23] An important reason for this outcome is that people who are religious or spiritually connected generally have healthier lifestyles. They smoke less, drink less alcohol, have better diets, exercise more, and are more likely to wear seat belts and to avoid drugs and unsafe sex. However, these factors don't account for all of the health-related benefits of religious and spiritual commitment. Studies find that the positive differences in death rates persist even after controlling for factors such as age, health, habits, demographics, and other health-related variables.[23]

Another explanation for better health among people who are spiritually involved is that they react more effectively to health crises. People who are religious or spiritual seem to be more willing than those who are not spiritually connected to alter their health habits, to be more proactive in seeking medical treatment, and to be more likely to receive the support of others. They benefit from their connectedness to the community. People who have strong ties to a religious group or another community segment may receive help and encouragement from that community in times of crisis. Friends may transport them to the doctor and to church, shop for them, prepare meals, arrange child care, and encourage them to get appropriate medical treatment.[25]

Mental Effects of Spirituality

People who are spiritually involved tend to enjoy better mental health as well as physical health. One reason may be that religious people tend to be more forgiving, and recent research has linked forgiveness with lower blood pressure, less back pain, and overall better personal health.[26]

In addition, highly spiritual people benefit from their connectedness to themselves and their beliefs. Spiritual practices such as meditation, prayer, and worship seem to promote positive emotions such as hope, love, contentment, and forgiveness, which can result in lower levels of anxiety. This in turn may help to minimize the *stress response*—the body's response to stressors. As explained in Chapter 5, the stress response includes the release of the hormones cortisol and epinephrine (adrenaline), which suppress certain aspects of immune functioning and are thought to produce a number of other undesirable effects, including weight gain, menopausal symptoms, and inflammation.[27–29] Many studies have shown that prayer and certain relaxation techniques, such as meditation, yoga, and hypnotherapy, reduce the secretion of these body chemicals and their harmful side effects.

Depression may also be mediated by spiritual involvement. Some studies indicate that people who are religiously involved suffer less depression and recover faster when they are depressed. Spiritual involvement appears to be associated with less anxiety and anxiety-related disorders. Religious people are also less likely to consider suicide.[21]

Studies have shown that spiritual connectedness appears to be associated with high levels of **health-related quality of life,** the physical, psychological, social, and spiritual aspects of a person's daily experience. Spiritual connectedness is especially important when a person is coping with serious health issues such as cancer, HIV infection, heart disease, limb amputation, or spinal cord injury.[23] This positive relationship persists even as physical health declines with serious illness.[30]

An Alternative View

Although the majority of studies indicate that spiritual connectedness has health benefits, many studies have found no relationship between health and spirituality. Some researchers have even suggested that spirituality can have negative outcomes for physical and mental health. For example, several studies indicate that when people experience a spiritual conflict in association with a health crisis, there is a negative impact on their health status.[23,31–34] It seems that the connection between spirituality and health can have both positive and negative implications.

SPIRITUALITY AND COMMUNITY INVOLVEMENT

As mentioned earlier, spirituality involves connectedness to the community, which in turn promotes recognition of the interdependence of all people and, indeed, all living things. Not only are we accountable for our own personal development, we are also entrusted with gifts and talents to be shared with others. Many believe that people can develop their spirituality by participating in their communities in a positive way. Unpaid work directly promotes community well-being through the services provided, whether that means caring for an elderly relative or working on a community project. It also has indirect benefits

by building the social networks that contribute to optimal well-being.

Service Learning

One way that people can connect classroom activities to community service and community building is through **service learning.** The purpose of integrating community service with academic study is to enrich learning, teach civic responsibility, and strengthen communities. Students are encouraged to take a positive role in their community, such as by tutoring, caring for the environment, or conducting oral histories with senior citizens. Participation offers opportunities to master new skills, build self-esteem, and enhance self-image. All of these activities are meant to teach people how to extend themselves beyond their enclosed world, taking a risk to get involved in the lives of others. In this way they learn about caring and taking care of—two particularly important concepts for personal growth. Researchers have commented on the current trend in the generation dubbed the "Millennials" (born in 1982 and later) to forge a new youth ethic of teamwork and civic purpose.[35] For more on spirituality among young adults, see the box on the next page, "Who Has the Best Chance to Explore Spirituality?"

Volunteering

Volunteering is another way to be connected with other people, and may confer health benefits as well. While helping others, volunteers may experience the euphoric feelings that athletes often describe as being "in the zone," mentioned earlier in this chapter. This "runner's high" has been called a "helper's high" when it is applied to a volunteering experience.[36]

Not all kinds of volunteering have the same effect, however. One-on-one contact and direct involvement significantly influence the effect of volunteering on the volunteer.[37] Working closely with strangers appears to increase the potential health benefits of the experience. Liking the volunteer work, performing it consistently, and having unselfish motives further increase the feelings of helper's high and the health benefits associated with it.[35] Simply donating money or doing volunteer work in isolation does not seem to have the same positive effect. In addition, mandated volunteer work, which many

KEY TERMS

health-related quality of life Physical, psychological, social, and spiritual aspects of a person's daily experience.

service learning Form of education that combines academic study with community service.

Beating the Odds

Who Has the Best Chance to Explore Spirituality?

A person's experiences in the family while growing up play a role in spiritual development and activity later in life. More specifically, parenting styles can support or discourage individual spiritual exploration. Presented here are profiles of three young men who all grew up in the same neighborhood. Which of the three do you think will feel most comfortable integrating spirituality into his life? What part will spirituality likely play in each of their lives as they raise children of their own? Who do you think has the best chance to make decisions about his own spirituality and values?

Abraham attended a religious school and followed his parents' instructions to adhere to religious teachings without questioning them. Now that he has reached young adulthood, Abraham is not certain that he wants to be as devout as his parents wish. His parents insist, though, that he must practice his religion faithfully by following all the traditional rituals and teachings. The result has been many arguments at home. With few hobbies or other interests, Abraham has learned to take the path of least resistance to avoid any conflicts.

Ali spends a lot of time with his family. They discuss profound issues, such as the purpose of life and the different ways in which people demonstrate their spirituality. Although Ali's parents are devout in their beliefs, they value knowledge and discussion and believe that if they model their beliefs, Ali will follow in their path. They have encouraged him to volunteer in a local mentoring program and to spend time learning about different cultures. Ali has many hobbies and does well in school, where he is known for asking many questions.

José's parents don't belong to an organized religion. They describe themselves as being spiritual, however, and often mention a higher being. They believe in traditional healing practices and alternatives to modern medicine. José is not interested in his parents' beliefs about traditional healing or what he thinks of as their old-country values. In school, where he is a good student, and with his friends, José discusses ideas about power and relationships that his parents would consider disrespectful. José and his parents often clash over their different cultures. José tries to explain his beliefs to his parents, but they think that he'll only get into trouble if he doesn't follow their belief system.

OLC Web site Visit the **Online Learning Center** at www.mhhe.com/teague1e for comments by the authors.

believe has a teaching benefit, may diminish the positive benefits of volunteerism for both the giver and the receiver. It has been suggested that individuals must *choose* to volunteer in order to gain the most significant health benefits.

Just as the high of helping may create enjoyable immediate benefits, the calm of helping may result in significant long-term health benefits. For example, volunteering may reduce the negative health effects of living with high levels of stress for long periods of time. Those who have experienced a helper's high have noted specific improvements in their physical well-being. These improvements included a reduction in arthritis pain, lupus symptoms, asthma attacks, migraine headaches, colds, and episodes of the flu. Volunteering may even result in longer life for the volunteer.[38,39]

Social Activism and the Global Community

Some people connect with their communities—local, national, and global—through social activism. A social cause, such as overcoming poverty or fighting illiteracy, can unite people from diverse backgrounds for a common good. Many people find it meaningful to participate in global citizenship by joining organizations such as those described in the box "Global Activism."

If you are interested in social activism, look for ways to participate through your school, your religious community, or broader groups you locate on the Internet. When you volunteer for such an organization, you commit yourself to building a foundation for a better world, making a contribution through service to others, and creating opportunities for mutual understanding. Many people have the opportunity to experience an "adventure in service" and to become directly involved in waging peace or conserving the environment. A week or two of working hand in hand with people of different backgrounds can persuade even the most cynical that we can all make a difference.

How is spirituality related to community involvement? Some claim that when we attend to our inner life, we nurture our compassionate responses to human need and develop a passion for social justice. Others believe

HIGHLIGHT ON HEALTH
Global Activism

Many organizations help individuals put their values into practice in the world. Here are a few:

- Amnesty International is a worldwide movement of people who campaign for internationally recognized human rights—physical and mental integrity, freedom of conscience and expression, and freedom from discrimination.

- Doctors Without Borders delivers emergency aid to victims of armed conflict, epidemics, and natural and human-made disasters and to others who lack health care owing to social or geographical isolation. Each year, more than 2,500 volunteer doctors, nurses, other medical professionals, logistics experts, water/sanitation engineers, and administrators provide medical aid in more than 80 countries.

- Greenpeace focuses on the most crucial worldwide threats to the planet's biodiversity and environment. Greenpeace has been campaigning against environmental degradation since 1971, bearing witness in a nonviolent manner.

- The Earth Charter Initiative is an international organization dedicated to building a sustainable world based on respect for nature, universal human rights, economic justice, and peace. A basic premise of the Earth Charter is that these attributes must be cultivated at the local community level before they can emerge at the national and global levels.

that contributing to community welfare and striving for justice are the ways to a rich inner life.

Some people turn away from social activism because they think it's "just politics." We hear news stories that use catchphrases associating traditional values with the religious right and social justice with the liberal left. Any action can be cloaked in the guise of religiosity, and distinguishing politics with a religious flavor from the practice of authentic spiritual values can be difficult. The former is designed to manipulate people's feelings for political gain; the latter has no hidden agenda or ulterior motive. The question for the individual is, How can I best put my faith into action while respecting the beliefs of others? Some social activists have transcended their religious and social conditioning and become universal spiritual beings, ready to serve all. Both Mahatma Gandhi and the Reverend Martin Luther King, Jr., developed an integrated worldview and worked to create global community.

Spiritual Rituals and Ceremonies

In virtually all cultures, faith and its accompanying belief system provide individuals and groups with rituals and practices that foster the development of a sense of community. Rituals and ceremonies feed our spirits, making them richer and deeper. Modern culture tends to downplay the importance of the rites of passage that mark our transition from one life stage to another, but they are as important as ever. Baptisms, bar mitzvahs and bat mitzvahs, marriages, and funerals are familiar ceremonies that help us mark important milestones and provide social support. Hispanic families mark their daughters' 15th birthday with a traditional "quince" (*quinceañera*) coming-of-age celebration. Birth or adoption ceremonies, divorce and separation rituals, and initiation ceremonies can also help us with transitions, both psychologically and spiritually.

Researchers have noticed a trend among the Millennial generation to embrace group activities and traditional rituals more than their mostly baby boomer parents have. These young people seem more spiritual and less individualistic than their parents. Their renewed interest in tradition is combined with a hunger for intimacy, a desire and ability to organize themselves, and great interest in group activities that help others, rather than individual spirituality.[35]

Even if you don't want to participate in group rituals, you can create your own private spiritual rituals. Choose a time when you will not feel rushed and a place where you will not be disturbed. Think about what inspires you and use it to create a sanctuary for yourself. If you are inspired by nature, use flowers, pictures of beautiful places, or natural objects like seashells or gem stones. If you follow a particular religious tradition, you might want to use a symbol of your faith or a picture of a spiritual guide. Some people like to light a candle or burn incense. Some find it helpful to listen to recordings of chanting, sacred music, prayer bells, or natural sounds like the wind in trees or waves breaking on a beach.

Once you have created a sacred space, you might meditate, breathe deeply, pray, recall memories of a deceased loved one, ponder a difficult situation in your life, or simply see what feelings come up. Spend some time

A christening ceremony, through which this infant becomes a member of a religious group, may be the first of many rituals that have great significance for family, friends, and the entire congregation.

there every day, starting with just 10 minutes or so. At first you may resist, feeling bored or lonely, but if you persist, you may find yourself becoming calmer and more centered in your life and your spirituality deepening.

Nature and the Environment

The impulse that propels people to the mountains or seashore for their holidays is the same impulse that drives pilgrims to sites of religious importance—the need to reconnect with the natural world. Many cultures in history, including many Native American cultures, did and do have a strong spiritual connection to nature or "Mother Earth." These cultures promote reverence for the universe, which results in a strong spiritual connection to nature.

Some people experience a sense of connectedness to the whole of nature, the environment, and the cosmos and describe this sense of connection as an energy or spirituality that manifests itself in the natural world. One person might feel the need to get away to pristine areas to feel connected, while another connects daily when experiencing the wonder of nature in her own garden. Many people say the feeling of being close to nature energizes and strengthens them; interacting with animals may evoke the same spiritual response.

Some people combine ecological, ethical, and spiritual interests and beliefs into what has been called *eco-spirituality.* They might participate in retreats or periods of reflection to deepen their connections to the earth. They may advocate respect for the sacredness of creation and the concept of tending (caring for, nurturing, and participating in nature). Daily activities that incorporate environmental values might include recycling, composting,

and walking or riding a bike instead of driving. As with volunteerism and social activism, when you are environmentally active, the benefits flow back to you, sustaining your spirituality and adding meaning to life.

DEATH AND DYING

Death and dying have great spiritual significance for people of all cultures. When someone you love dies, the experience is extremely personal, yet it is one that you also share with others. Life and death are part of the cycle of existence and, when death occurs in old age, part of the natural order of things. Many report that because of their personal faith, they do not fear death, since they know that their lives have had meaning within the context of a larger plan. When death occurs in an untimely fashion, however—when someone dies in childhood or in the prime of life—people often find it senseless and look for explanations through spiritual insight.

Stages of Dying and Death

In 1969 Elisabeth Kübler-Ross published *On Death and Dying,* one of the first books to propose a set of stages that people go through when they believe they are in the process of dying.[40] The five stages are (1) denial and isolation, (2) anger, (3) bargaining, (4) depression, and (5) acceptance. Over time, further study has shown that these stages are not linear—individuals may experience them in a different order or may return to stages they have already gone through—nor are they necessarily universal—individuals may not experience some stages at all.

Many believe that life is full of transitions, with death being the last. A shared sense of mortality can be the basis for feeling connected with other human beings. When we recognize our fragility, our sense of the preciousness of time and life may enhance our appreciation of each minute and every encounter. Recently, health care professionals have begun to describe ways to *live* with an illness rather than simply looking at the diagnosis as the point at which one begins to prepare for death. As medical care has improved, many individuals diagnosed with cancer or HIV infection have recovered or lived with the disease for many years. The critical thing to remember is that one need not go on a "death watch" after a diagnosis; usually, there is time to repair relationships, to build memories, and to review one's life. The dying person and family and friends may find comfort and strength in talking through the process with each other, with health care workers, or with a spiritual advisor.

Research has found that terminally ill persons derive strength and hope from spiritual and religious beliefs. In fact, terminally ill adults report significantly greater religious involvement and depth of spiritual perspective than do healthy adults. Studies suggest that, unrelated to belief in an afterlife, religiously involved people at the end of life are more accepting of death than those who are less religiously involved. In addition, religious involvement and spirituality are associated with less death anxiety.[23]

Hospice Care

The word *hospice* comes from the Latin word *hospitum*, meaning guesthouse. Originally, the term described a

Hospice is a program designed to help people approach death with comfort and dignity.

place of shelter for weary and sick travelers, often returning from religious pilgrimages. Today, **hospice** is a program intended for people who no longer respond to cure-oriented medical treatment. Hospice is not a place but a concept of care. Eighty percent of this type of care is provided in the patient's home, a family member's home, or a nursing home.[41] Hospitals sometimes provide or assist with hospice.

The goal of hospice is to improve the quality of a patient's last days by providing comfort and enhancing dignity. Terminally ill patients typically receive symptom and pain relief and emotional and spiritual support. In addition to this **palliative care,** hospice programs offer support for family members who might need comfort as they care for their loved one. Volunteers often provide support by cooking, cleaning, and being available when people need to talk. According to the Hospice Foundation of America, more than 95,000 people volunteer for

KEY TERMS

hospice   Program that provides care for the terminally ill and their loved ones.

palliative care   Care that focuses on relieving pain and making a patient comfortable, while recognizing that a cure may not be possible.

hospice annually, providing more than 5 million hours of care.[41]

Healthy Grieving

Grief is a natural reaction to loss. The grief associated with death is familiar to most of us, but we may grieve many kinds of losses throughout our lives: divorce, relocation, traumatic experiences, loss of health and mobility, and even expected life transitions such as having the last child leave home. Grief is often expressed by feelings of sadness, loneliness, anger, and guilt. These feelings are part of the process of healing, since we do not begin to feel better until we have acknowledged and felt sorrow over our loss.

Even though grief is expected following loss, it can affect your health. Physical symptoms of grief may include crying and sighing, aches and pains, sleep disturbances, headaches, lethargy, reduced appetite, and stomach upset. The intense emotions you feel at the time of a loss can have a negative impact on immune system functioning, reducing your ability to fight off illness. Studies have shown that surviving spouses may have increased odds for heart disease, cancer, depression, alcoholism, and suicide.[42,43] Everyone has higher risk for disease after the loss of a loved one, but those who are more resilient may cope with the loss better.

Bereavement after the loss of a loved one typically involves four phases. The first, numbness and shock, usually occurs immediately after the loss and lasts for a brief period. Phase two, feelings of separation, occurs when you start to miss the person. In this phase you might begin to find yourself having conversations with the person who has died as if he or she were still there. There is a void, something is missing, and you feel that loss. The third phase is disorganization; you might feel easily distracted and have difficulty concentrating. This period can last for a longer time than we realize or anticipate. Some of us might describe ourselves as being lethargic or simply "not the same" for a long time after the death of a loved one. We may be able to function, but we are still grieving and have not yet reached the last phase of our bereavement. That phase, called reorganization, marks the time when we begin to adjust to our loss. While we might see reminders of our loved one for the rest of our lives, our feelings will not have the same intensity as the emotions we experienced while we were grieving.

If you experience the death of a loved one, it is important to take care of yourself while you are grieving. There is no right or wrong way to grieve and no specific timetable. Friends who suggest that it's time to move on need to understand that you are on your own journey and cannot be rushed. You need to give yourself permission to feel the loss and take time to heal. Some people seem to cope better if they talk about the death rather than inter-

nalizing their feelings. During the grieving process it is vital that you eat a balanced diet, exercise regularly, drink plenty of fluids, and get enough rest. Keeping a journal and talking about the person who has died can also be part of the healing process. Finally, you should not hesitate to ask friends for support, since having a nurturing social network is particularly helpful in coping with loss.

If intense grief persists for more than a year, or if you find yourself losing or gaining weight or not sleeping, consult a health professional to get a treatment referral. Treatment options might include support groups, family therapy, individual counseling, or a psychiatric evaluation.

Spiritual Beliefs and Rituals

Beliefs about death and rituals for marking the loss of loved ones vary across cultures. In some cultures, mourners have wakes and parties that last for days; in others, they sing and play music; in still others, they cover mirrors so they cannot see what they look like during times of grief.

Many rituals that surround death and dying are actually for the living, to help people cope with the loss of a loved one. When a Muslim dies, he or she is washed, usually by a family member, wrapped in a clean white cloth, and buried with a simple prayer, preferably the same day. Muslims consider this one of the final services they can do for their relatives and an opportunity to remember their own brief existence on earth. In Japanese Buddhist traditions, close family members prepare the body of their loved one for burial or cremation. Traditionally, family and friends "visit" with the deceased for two days. There is prayer, burning of incense, and gifts.

In many Hispanic communities, a wake is held in the home of the deceased or at a funeral parlor for at least one day before the funeral. Rituals include lighting candles and blessing the dead and their resting places. *Luto,* or mourning, is marked by wearing black, black and white, or dark clothing, and by subdued behavior. Following the funeral, many Hispanics pray for the soul of the loved one for a *novena,* a set period of time for prayer.

In Jewish culture, following burial, mourners experience a week of intense mourning called *shiva,* at the end of which they symbolically return to the life of the living. At one year, in the unveiling ritual, a marker is placed on the grave, signifying an end to the grieving period. This ritual helps family and friends mark their loss while giving them permission to move ahead with their own lives. Annual markers of the death allow mourners to continue integrating the loss into their lives.

Rituals around death help mourners move through the emotional work of grieving. When a person has been important to us, we never forget that person or lose the relationship. Instead, we find ways of "emotionally

Consumer Clipboard

Considering Organ Donation

Have you ever noticed that on the reverse side of your driver's license there's an option for organ donation? You may have told yourself you'd think about that decision later. Although every day 70 people in the United States receive an organ transplant, 16 people die because of a shortage of donated organs, so it's worth thinking about now. Let's look at some of the commonly asked questions about organ donation so you'll have the facts you need to consider when making this commitment.

- *Who can be an organ donor?* If you're in good physical condition, you can be an organ donor. Age doesn't matter, but if you're younger than 18, you'll need the consent of a parent or guardian. You don't even need to be a U.S. citizen. Resident aliens are eligible to donate organs.

- *Which organs are most commonly transplanted?* Transplant procedures commonly involve the kidneys, cornea, heart, liver, lung, pancreas, and bone marrow, but successful transplantation of other organs has been done on a limited basis.

- *What if I have a preexisting medical condition—can I still donate?* Determination of suitability for donation is made at the time of donation. Organs are tested for infectious diseases, including HIV. The final decision is based on a combination of factors, including the donor's general health and the urgency of need of the recipient.

- *Are there any negative consequences for the donor?* Donating an organ will not disfigure your body. Organ removal involves a standard surgical procedure. You can still have a funeral, including an open-casket service.

- *Who pays for organ donation?* All costs associated with organ or tissue donation are paid for by the recipient, not the donor. This is usually done through the recipient's insurance plan.

- *How are organs distributed for donation?* Patients are matched to organs based on several factors, such as blood and tissue type, medical urgency, time on the waiting list, and geographical location. Being wealthy or famous is not a factor.

- *Are there any special considerations for minorities in organ donation?* Successful organ transplantation is commonly associated with having cells that are a good genetic match. Therefore transplantation is enhanced by matching of organs between members of the same ethnic and racial group.

- *If I decide to become an organ donor, what do I need to do?* Simply indicate that you intend to be an organ and tissue donor on your driver's license. Carry an organ donor card with you at all times. Another step, though, is to discuss your decision with family members and loved ones, because your family may be asked to sign a consent form before the donation can be carried out. It's also a good idea to record your wishes about organ donation in legal documents related to end-of-life decisions.

Today more than 87,000 people are waiting for the gift of life. Think about it. . . .

Sources: Adapted from U.S. Government Advisory Committee on Organ Transplantation, 2005, www.organdonor.gov; "The Ultimate Gift: 50 Years of Organ Transplants," by L.K. Altman, 2004, Dec. 21, *New York Times*, p. F1.

relocating" the deceased person in our lives, keeping our bonds with them while moving on. How do you think the rituals of your culture facilitate this process? Which ones are personally meaningful to you?

End-of-Life Decisions

Although the achievements of modern medicine prolong and enhance life for many, they have also contributed to difficult conditions associated with dying. Costly technology may keep people alive, but frequently they are isolated from meaningful relationships with others. They exist with little or no hope for recovery. Many people dread a situation at the end of their lives in which they or those they trust will have no say in decisions about their treatment.

In this context, patients should be informed of their right to make decisions about medical treatments. Then they should make known their preferences for health care. They can do this through the use of formal legal documents that grant a **durable power of attorney for health care (DPOAHC)** to someone they trust to make decisions if they become unable to do so. These directives, which may be called *living wills* or *advance directives,* must be tailored to each specific situation and location, since laws vary. The directives may cover any issue the patient considers important.

A common concern is whether palliative nutrition and hydration should be continued at the very end of life and whether life-sustaining treatment should be withdrawn when there is no hope of recovery. These decisions should be made in supportive consultation with family members, close friends, a spiritual advisor, and health care professionals. Such decisions must take into account the patient's values, the most common ones being family and interpersonal relationships, spiritual beliefs or religion, and independence.[44,45]

Some medical practices and public policies foster humane treatment and dignity for those who are dying; others open the door to abuse. Some decisions about dying are morally acceptable to most people, and others go beyond morally acceptable limits. Proposals to expand end-of-life choices and to legalize physician-assisted death have sparked renewed interest in these old questions.

Beyond medical decisions, there are also practical concerns to take care of at the end of life. People need to let their loved ones know whether they want to be buried or cremated, whether they want to donate their organs (see the box, "Considering Organ Donation"), what kind of funeral or memorial service they prefer, and who will administer their financial and legal affairs, among other issues. There are also profound emotional issues to work through, including the grief of both the dying person and the loved ones who will be left behind.

Life after Death

Belief in an afterlife is a tenet of most faith traditions. Although some investigators say no proof of life after death exists, other researchers argue that there is empirical evidence from those who have been contacted by loved ones after they have died and from individuals who have been resuscitated following a near-death experience.[46,47] It would be comforting to know that there is some afterlife and that we will be reunited with our loved ones in another state of existence. However, such comforts cannot be provided by science; they remain in the realm of faith and belief.

***

Spirituality is an important, but often overlooked, part of life. Whether you choose to explore spirituality through mindfulness, volunteer work, the arts, an organized religion, an environmental group, or an ethical society, this dimension promises to enrich your life in many ways. By building strong and healthy relationships, developing a personal value system, and living a meaningful life, you can enhance your overall wellness and enjoy the profound rewards of a spiritual life.

KEY TERMS

durable power of attorney for health care (DPOAHC) Formal legal power to make health care decisions for someone who is no longer able to do so for himself or herself.

You Make the Call

Does Spirituality Improve Your Health?

Kevin Burke was not a religious person, and when he was employed as a social worker at San Francisco General Hospital in the 1980s, he was discouraged from discussing religious beliefs with patients. He did notice, however, that several patients seemed to have better outcomes because of their spirituality.

Years later, Burke studied the effects of religion and spirituality on mental health. Before going on to join the University of Minnesota faculty, Burke interviewed critically ill elderly people for his doctoral dissertation at the University of Chicago. He asked 131 patients for their views on religion and spirituality as part of a study of personality structure. His study showed that "religion"—as

measured by church attendance, denomination, and satisfaction with religious life—had no bearing on mental health. But patients who reported that they felt a "closeness to God," which Burke defined as spirituality, fared much better, according to a standard research tool, the RAND Medical Outcome Survey.

Does spirituality really make a difference in keeping you healthy, in helping you cope with an illness, or in the outcome of a health crisis? Some people claim that "faith heals," but how do we know if it's true? Both skeptics and believers now can refer to medical studies that explore the relationship between recovery from an illness and psychosocial factors such as social support, religion, and spirituality.

In one study, Paul S. Mueller, M.D., and colleagues reviewed much of the research to date on the use of prayer for improving health. Mueller concluded that although the relationship between religion/spirituality and health seems valid, currently there is no way to establish its real effect. He suggests that the link is complex, involving psychological, behavioral, and biological factors.

In another study, groups of varying denominations around the world prayed for a group of heart patients to recover. In this pilot study, called the MANTRA project, 150 heart patients were randomly assigned to one of five groups. One group received standard, high-tech cardiac care, while each of the other groups also received one of four *noetic* therapies: imagery, stress relaxation, touch therapy, and off-site intercessory prayer (prayer by others).

The study found that patients receiving the noetic therapies had better outcomes and fewer complications than those who received standard care alone. The intercessory prayer group had more than a 50 percent reduction in complications. The project director reported that intercessory prayer has also shown promising results in preliminary studies with patients with HIV infection and couples dealing with infertility: "The human spirit obviously has at least a potential role both in how we get sick and how we recover in every organ system."

Another study, conducted at Dartmouth Medical School, focused on the role religion might play in the health and recovery of elderly people. Researchers studied 232 patients over 55 years of age who had open-heart surgery. The study showed that those who derived at least some strength and comfort from their religious faith were three times as likely to survive the surgery as those who did not. Patients who took part in any community activity were also three times as likely to survive the surgery as those who did not. Those who were both believers and joiners were nine times as likely to survive.

The Dartmouth study found that feelings of comfort and support from one's faith were more important to health than religious activity. For instance, if people attended church two or three times a week but did not derive any support or comfort from their faith, they were not likely to reap significant benefits. Similarly, participation in organized groups was found to have significantly more benefits than just visiting friends and relatives.

Some scientists, such as Columbia University professor Richard P. Sloan, challenge the faith-medicine connection, maintaining that "even in the best studies, the evidence of an association between religion, spirituality, and health is weak and inconsistent." Sloan and his colleagues have published papers in the medical journals *The Lancet* and *The New England Journal of Medicine* attacking faith and healing research for weak methodologies and soft thinking: "We believe," they wrote, "that it is premature to promote faith and religion as adjunctive medical treatments."

The debate on spirituality and health continues. Given the difficulty of putting spirituality through rigorous scientific testing, some people claim that we will never be able to pinpoint or prove the precise effect that faith has on healing. Others argue that, with a growing body of evidence pointing to positive health effects from religious and spiritual beliefs, it is irresponsible to keep spirituality out of the clinic. What do you think?

Pros

- Research shows that most people have a spiritual life.
- Research also indicates that most patients want their spiritual needs assessed and addressed.
- Most studies have found a direct relationship between religious involvement and spirituality and better health outcomes.
- Supporting a patient's spirituality may enhance coping and recovery from illness.

Cons

- Research does not show that religious people do not get sick or that illness is caused by lack of religious faith.
- Research also does not indicate that spirituality is the most important health factor.
- If spirituality were accepted as having a role in recovery and healing, physicians would have to prescribe religious activities, which would be intrusive and potentially offensive to many patients.
- Other factors can be used to explain the association between spirituality and better health outcomes.

OLC Web site For more information on this topic, visit the Online Learning Center at www.mhhe.com/teaguele.

SOURCES: Data from "Integrative Noetic Therapies as Adjuncts to Percutaneous Intervention During Unstable Coronary Syndromes: Monitoring and Actualization of Noetic Training (MANTRA) Feasibility Pilot," by M. Krucoff, et al., *American Heart Journal, 142* (5), 760–769; "How Religion Influences Morbidity and Health: Reflections on Natural History, Salutogenesis and Host Resistance," by J. S. Levin, 1996, *Social Science Medicine, 43,* 849–864; "Religious Involvement, Spirituality, and Medicine: Implications for Clinical Practice," by P. S. Mueller, D. J. Plevak, and T. A. Rummans, 2001, *Mayo Clinic Proceedings, 76* (12), 1189–1191; "Lack of Social Participation or Religious Strength and Comfort as Risk Factors for Death After Cardiac Surgery in the Elderly," by T. E. Oxman, D. H. Freeman, Jr., and E. D. Manheimer, 1995, *Psychosomatic Medicine, 57* (1), 5–15; "Spirituality Helps Patients Deal With Pain," by S. Scott, 2001, *Akron Beacon Journal;* "Religion, Spirituality and Medicine," by R. Sloan, et al., 1999, *The Lancet, 325,* 664–667; "Should Physicians Prescribe Religious Activities?" by R. Sloan, et al., 2000, *New England Journal of Medicine, 342,* 1913–1916.

SUMMARY

- Spirituality can be thought of as a person's connection to self, significant others, and the community at large, accompanied by a personal belief system or value system that gives meaning and purpose to life. Spirituality provides a feeling of participation in something greater than oneself and a sense of unity with nature and the universe.

- Psychologist Abraham Maslow proposed that after human beings meet their needs for survival, safety and security, love and belonging, and achievement and self-esteem, they strive for self-actualization, a state in which the individual fulfills her or his highest human potential.

- Building a spiritual life involves self-exploration and self-awareness. Paths to such a state include the practice of mindfulness, meditation, journaling, spiritual retreat, experiencing the arts, living your values, and creating rituals.

- Spirituality can be embedded in daily life through practices that promote physical health, such as exercising and eating well. Spirituality is also promoted by the same habits that enhance mental and emotional health, such as learning to communicate with compassion and empathy and using relaxation techniques to control stress.

- Other behaviors that promote spirituality are developing resilience, finding joy in everyday things, and creating balance by viewing your life from a broader perspective.

- Interest is growing in the connection between spirituality and health, although the pursuit is not without its skeptics.

- Many studies have supported a relationship between religious involvement and spirituality, on the one hand, and better health outcomes and greater longevity, on the other. Explanations for this relationship include healthier lifestyles, more effective responses to health crises, and social support.

- There is also a positive relationship between spiritual involvement and mental health, perhaps as a result of spiritual attitudes and practices that reduce anxiety and stress, protect against depression, and discourage suicide. Spiritual connectedness is related to high levels of health-related quality of life.

- Community involvement is another expression of spirituality. Examples include service learning, volunteering, social activism, participating in ceremonies and rituals, and connecting with nature and the environment.

- Death and dying have spiritual significance for people of all cultures and offer opportunities for spiritual growth.

- Elisabeth Kübler-Ross identified five stages of dying: denial, anger, bargaining, depression, and acceptance. The stages are not linear or necessarily universal.

- Hospice is a concept of care for people who can no longer benefit from cure-oriented medical treatment.

- Grief is an experience of intense sadness and loneliness following a loss. It can be experienced physically, emotionally, mentally, and spiritually. Rituals around death can help mourners move through the grieving process.

- Patients can make decisions in advance about their preferences for health care at the end of life. One way is to grant a durable power of attorney for health care to someone they trust to make treatment decisions if they are unable to do so.

- Questions about life after death cannot be answered by science; they remain in the realm of faith and belief.

REVIEW QUESTIONS

1. How is spirituality defined in a health context?
2. What are some examples of connectedness?
3. What are values, and what role do they play in a spiritually conscious life?
4. What are some qualities of a self-actualized person?
5. What is mindfulness? What is flow?
6. Describe three ways to cultivate a more spiritual life.
7. How can good communication skills enhance spiritual wellness?
8. What is resilience in the context of spiritual wellness?
9. What are some of the effects of spiritual involvement on physical health? On mental health?
10. How can service learning and volunteering affect spiritual growth?
11. What is eco-spirituality?
12. How have attitudes toward terminal illnesses changed in recent years?
13. What is palliative care?
14. What are the typical four phases of bereavement?
15. What values are most commonly taken into account in a patient's end-of-life decisions?

WEB RESOURCES

American Meditation Institute for Yoga Science and Philosophy: As an introduction, this Web site describes a systematic procedure for meditation. For those interested in learning meditation, the organization advocates finding a qualified teacher for personal instruction.
www.americanmeditation.org

A Campaign for Forgiveness Research: This organization is dedicated to promoting forgiveness around the world as a way of improving the human condition. The site features myths and truths about forgiveness and offers ways to make forgiveness a part of your life.
www.forgiving.org

Hospice Foundation of America: Focusing on hospice as a concept of care, this site describes the growth of the hospice movement and explains its goals. Hospice is presented as a unique source of comfort for patients and families facing death.
www.hospicefoundation.org

Journaling: This site offers an introduction to journaling as a way of keeping healthy. It includes links to other journaling sites that feature further information and resources such as journaling tools and software.
www.healthierliving.org

Organ Donation: This official U.S. government Web site for organ donation and transplantation describes the myths and facts associated with organ donation. It features a donor card that you can sign and carry.
www.organdonor.gov

Religious Society of Friends (Quakers): For anyone interested in learning about Quakers and the issues of peace and silence promoted by this religious group, this is a helpful resource. The site offers reference material, informational articles, and essays on Quakerism.
www.quakerinfo.com

REFERENCES

1. Kluger, J. (2004, October 25). Is God in our genes? *Time,* 62–72.

2. Blieszner, R., & Ramsey, J. L. (2003, December). *Spiritual resiliency in later life: Implications for family educators and practitioners* (Report, Vol. 48, F7–F9). Minneapolis, MN: National Council on Family Relations.

3. Donovan, N., & Halpern, D. (2002). *Life satisfaction: The state of knowledge and implications for government.* UK Cabinet Office: Strategy Unit.

4. Berkman, L. F., & Glass, T. (2000). Social integration, social networks, social support, and health. In L. F. Berkman & I. Kawachi (Eds.), *Social epidemiology.* Oxford, UK: Oxford University Press.

5. Maslow, A. (1970). *Motivation and personality* (2nd ed.). New York: Harper & Row.

6. Kabat-Zinn, J. (1993). Mindfulness meditation: Health benefits of an ancient Buddhist practice. In D. Goleman & J. Gurin (Eds.), *Mind/body medicine.* Yonkers, NY: Consumer Reports Books.

7. Csikszentmihalyi, M. (1998). *Finding flow: The psychology of engagement with everyday life.* New York: Basic Books.

8. Ellsberg, R. (Ed.). (2001). *Thich Nhat Hanh: Essential writings.* Maryknoll, NY: Orbis Books.

9. Pennebaker, J. W. (1997). *Opening up: The healing power of expressing emotion.* New York: Guilford Press.

10. Weldon, M. (2001). *Writing to save your life: How to honor your story through journaling.* Center City, MN: Hazelden Publishing, Health Communications, Inc.

11. DeSalvo, L. A. (2000). *Writing as a way of healing: How telling our stories transforms our lives.* Boston: Beacon Press.

12. Beckett, W. (1993). *The mystical now: Art and the sacred.* New York: Universe Publishing.

13. Butler, K. (2003, September/October). Living on purpose. *Psychotherapy Networker.*

14. Kahn, H. (2000). Achieving love and intimacy through group support. WebMD live events transcript archive. http://my.webmd.com.

15. Brooks, R., & Goldstein, S. (2001). *Raising resilient children.* New York: McGraw-Hill.

16. Wolin, S. J., & Wolin, S. (1993). *The resilient self: How survivors of troubled families rise above adversity.* New York: Villard.

17. Armstrong, L., & Jenkin, S. (2003). *Every second counts.* New York: Random House.

18. R.E.A.D.: Road to reading project. (2000). Reading Enhancement and Development. www.roadtoreading.org.

19. CBS News Poll, April 20–21, 1998.

20. McCaffrey, A. M., Eisenberg, D. M., Legedza, A. T. R., Davis, R. B., & Phillips, R. S. (2004). Prayer for health concerns: Results of a national survey on prevalence and patterns of use. *Archives of Internal Medicine, 164,* 858–862.

21. Kalb, C. (2003, November 10). Faith and healing. *Newsweek.*

22. Koenig, H. G. (2000). Religion, spirituality, and medicine: Application to clinical practice. *Journal of American Medical Association, 284,* 1708.

23. Mueller, P. S., Plevak, D. J., & Rummans, T. A. (2001). Religious involvement, spirituality, and medicine: Implications for clinical practice. *Mayo Clinic Proceedings, 76* (12).

24. Benson, H., & Klipper, M. (2000). *The relaxation response.* New York: HarperTorch.

25. Strawbridge, W. J., et al. (2001). Religious attendance increases survival by improving and maintaining good health behaviors, mental health, and social relationships. *Annals of Behavioral Medicine, 23,* 68–74.

26. Campaign for Forgiveness Research. (1999–2001). www.forgiving.org.

27. Koenig, H. G., McCullough, M. E., & Larson, D. B. (2001). *Handbook of religion and health.* Oxford, UK: Oxford University Press.

28. Larson, D. B., Swyers, J. P., & McCullough, M. E. (1998). *Scientific research on spirituality and health: A report based on the scientific progress in spirituality conferences.* Rockville, MD: National Institute for Healthcare Research.

29. Seybold, K. S., & Hill, P. C. (2001). The role of religion and spirituality in mental and physical health. *Current Directions Psychological Science, 10,* 21–24.

30. Brady, M. J., et al. (1999). A case for including spirituality in quality of life measurement in oncology. *Psychooncology, 8,* 417–428.

31. Pargament, K. I. (1997). *The psychology of religion and coping: Theory, research, practice.* New York: Guilford Press.

32. Pargament, K. I., et al. (2001). Religious struggle as a predictor of mortality among medically ill elderly patients. *Archives of Internal Medicine, 161,* 1881–1885.

33. Fitchett, G., et al. (1999). The role of religion in medical rehabilitation outcomes: A longitudinal study. *Rehabilitation Psychology, 44,* 1–22.

34. Koenig, H. G., Pargament, K. I., & Nielsen, J. (1998). Religious coping and health status in medically ill hospitalized older adults. *Journal of Nervous Mental Disorders, 186,* 513–521.

35. Howe, N., & Strauss, W. (2000). *Millennials rising: The next great generation.* New York: Vintage Books.

36. Luks, A. (1988, October). Helper's high. *Psychology Today,* 39–42.

37. Hafen, B. Q., et al. (1996). *Mind/body health: The effects of attitudes, emotions and relationships.* Boston: Allyn and Bacon.

38. House, J. S., Landis, K. R., & Umberson, P. (1988). Social relationships and health. *Science, 241,* 540–545.

39. Luks, A., & Payne, P. (1992). *The healing power of doing good: The health and spiritual benefits of helping others.* New York: Fawcett, Columbine.

40. Kübler-Ross, E. (1997). *On death and dying.* New York: Simon & Schuster Adult Publishing Group.

41. Hospice Foundation of America. (2003). What is hospice? www.hospicefoundation.org.

42. Can you die of a broken heart? (2002, January). *Harvard Mental Health Letter.*

43. Zamora, D. (2003). Death from a broken heart. www.WebMd.com.

44. Gesensway, D. (1998, May). Talking about end-of-life issues. *ACP Observer.*

45. Oliver, S. L. (1998). *What the dying teach us: Lessons on living.* Binghamton, NY: The Haworth Press.

46. Braude, S. (2003). *Immortal remains: The evidence for life after death.* Lanham, MD: Rowman & Littlefield.

47. Evidence of "life after death" (2000, October 23). BBC News. http://news.bbc.co.uk.

Add It Up! CHARACTERISTICS OF THE SELF-ACTUALIZING PERSON

How do we live to our fullest potential and become everything that we are capable of becoming? Dr. Abraham Maslow called the person who is in the process of developing his or her full potential "self-actualizing." For Maslow, self-actualized living is the ultimate achievement in the development of the human personality. Listed here are 15 characteristics of self-actualizing people. After carefully reading the descriptions, rate yourself on each characteristic on a scale from 1 to 10.

SCORE

1. Reality-based perceptions: Self-actualizing people have a more efficient perception of reality and a more comfortable relationship with it. They have an ability to detect the phony and the inaccurate in both people and things.

1   2   3   4   5   6   7   8   9   10   _____

2. Acceptance: Self-actualizing people have the ability to accept themselves, other people, and nature as they are. They are not defensive, enjoy living, and are genuine.

1   2   3   4   5   6   7   8   9   10   _____

3. Spontaneity: Self-actualizing people behave with spontaneity, simplicity, and naturalness. They are serene and characterized by lack of worry.

1   2   3   4   5   6   7   8   9   10   _____

4. Problem-centered: Self-actualizing people focus on problems and people outside themselves. They are not self-centered and often choose to help others. This involvement is sometimes seen as a mission in life.

1   2   3   4   5   6   7   8   9   10   _____

5. Need for privacy and downtime: Self-actualizing people enjoy solitude and aloneness.

1   2   3   4   5   6   7   8   9   10   _____

6. Autonomy and independence: Self-actualizing people act independently of culture and environment. They are capable of doing things for themselves and making decisions on their own. They believe in who and what they are.

1   2   3   4   5   6   7   8   9   10   _____

7. Sense of wonder and appreciation: Self-actualizing people experience a continuing freshness of appreciation about the world. They tend to have rich emotional reactions, are intensely alert and alive to things around them, and live the present moment to the fullest.

1   2   3   4   5   6   7   8   9 · 10   _____

8. Periodic peak experiences: Most self-actualizing people have had profound spiritual experiences, although not necessarily religious in character. These are referred to as peak experiences.

1   2   3   4   5   6   7   8   9   10   _____

9. Identification with all of humankind: Self-actualizing people have deep empathy and compassion for others.

1   2   3   4   5   6   7   8   9   10   _____

10. Deep relationships: Self-actualizing people have profound and meaningful interpersonal relationships with a few people. They tend to select friends who exhibit self-actualizing characteristics.

1   2   3   4   5   6   7   8   9   10   _____

11. Democratic values: A self-actualizing person does not discriminate against others, being virtually unaware of differences in social class, race, or color. He or she respects everyone as potential contributors to his or her knowledge, merely because they are human beings.

1   2   3   4   5   6   7   8   9   10   _____

12. Strong ethical sense: Self-actualizing persons are highly ethical. They clearly distinguish between means and ends and subordinate means to ends. They follow their own set of internal moral values.

1   2   3   4   5   6   7   8   9   10   _____

13. Sense of humor: The self-actualizing person has a philosophical, unhostile sense of humor. He can laugh at himself but does not make jokes that will hurt others.

1   2   3   4   5   6   7   8   9   10   _____

14. Creativeness: The self-actualizing person has greatly increased, original creativeness that carries over into everything he or she does.

1   2   3   4   5   6   7   8   9   10   _____

15. Independence from culture and environment: Self-actualizing people are autonomous and have an ability to transcend the environment rather than just coping. They are capable of making decisions on their own.

1   2   3   4   5   6   7   8   9   10   _____

16. Aware of imperfections: Self-actualizing people are aware of the fact that they are not perfect, that they are as human as the next person, and that there are constantly new things to learn and new ways to grow.

1   2   3   4   5   6   7   8   9   10   _____

TOTAL _____

Scoring: What are your strengths in moving toward being a self-actualizing person? What are your weaker characteristics? Why? What might you do to make your score higher on any given characteristic? The highest possible total is 160 points. How close are you?

SOURCE: Reprinted with permission from "Characteristics of a Self-Actualizing Person: An Evaluation Instrument," by R. Boyum, Ed.D. University of Wisconsin Counseling Services. www.uwec.edu/counsel/pubs/chars.htm.

CHAPTER 5

Stress: Managing Pressure

DID YOU KNOW?

- Your college years may be among the most stressful years of your life. In one survey, 30 percent of first-year college students described themselves as frequently feeling overwhelmed. Women were twice as likely to feel this way as men.

- Stress contributes to both everyday annoyances, such as a stiff neck or a tension headache, and major health problems, such as heart disease, cancer, and depression. According to the American Medical Association, 80–85 percent of all human illness and disease can be attributed in part to stress.

OLC *Your Health Today*   www.mhhe.com/teague1e

Go to the Online Learning Center for *Your Health Today* for interactive activities, quizzes, flashcards, Web links, and more resources related to this chapter.

Stress is a fact of life; we experience varying levels of stress throughout the day as our bodies and minds continually adjust to the demands of living. We often think of stress as negative, as an uncomfortable or unpleasant pressure—for example, to complete a project on time, to deal with a traffic ticket, to care for a sick parent. But stress can also be positive. When we get a promotion at work or when someone throws us a surprise birthday party, we also experience stress.

Surveys have consistently found that 90 percent of all American adults experience high stress levels about one or two times a week. More than half of American women say they are excessively distressed much or most of the time.[1] Such statistics only reinforce the need to manage the stress in our lives and to reduce its negative impact on our well-being. When excessive stress is unavoidable, having a repertoire of stress management techniques to fall back on is invaluable.

This chapter begins with an exploration of stress and the physiology of the stress response, distinguishing acute stress from chronic stress. We then look at the wide-ranging effects of stress on health and disease and consider the factors that lead different people to respond differently to the same stressors. Next we examine the myriad sources of stress, from major life transitions to petty daily hassles and from worry about grades to societal conditions such as racism and discrimination. Finally, we describe several effective ways of reducing and managing stress.

WHAT IS STRESS?

The term *stress* is often used in different ways, so we begin this chapter with some definitions. Events or agents in the environment that cause us stress are called **stressors.** They can range from being late for class to having a close friend die, from finding a parking space to winning the lottery. Your reaction to these events is called the *stress response;* this concept is discussed at length in the next section. Stressors disrupt the body's balance and require adjustments to return to normal. **Stress** can be defined as the general state of the body, mind, and emotions when an environmental stressor has triggered the stress response.

Different people respond differently to stressors, depending on such variables as personality factors, past experiences, overall level of wellness, and different ways of thinking about the stressful event. These variables can be thought of as mediating the stress response, making the same situation stressful for one person and not stressful for another. For example, one person may find public speaking exciting and asking someone for a date excruciating. Another person may be terrified of public speaking and relaxed about asking for a date. We discuss such differences later in the chapter.

Because there is so much variation in individual responses to stressors, stress may be thought of as a transaction between an individual and a stressor in the environment, mediated by personal variables that include the person's perceptions and appraisal of the event.[2] When faced with a stressor, people evaluate it without necessarily realizing they are doing so: Is it positive or negative? How threatening is it to my well-being, my self-esteem, my identity? Can I cope with it or not? When you appraise an event as positive, you experience *eustress,* or positive stress. When you appraise it as negative, you experience *distress.*

The Stress Response

Regardless of the nature of the stressor and the individual's appraisal of it, all stressors elicit the **stress response** (also known as the **fight-or-flight response**), a series of physiological changes that occur in the body in the face of a threat. All animals, it appears—humans included—need sudden bursts of energy to fight or flee from situations they perceive as dangerous.

The fight-or-flight response is orchestrated primarily by two body systems, the nervous system and the endocrine system. The nervous system, consisting of the brain, spinal cord, and peripheral nerves, has two parts, the somatic nervous system and the autonomic nervous system. The somatic nervous system controls voluntary, conscious actions; the **autonomic nervous system** controls involuntary, unconscious functions, such as breathing, heart rate, and digestion. The autonomic nervous system, in turn, has two branches. The **sympathetic branch** is responsible for initiating the fight-or-flight response—that is, for activating the body's organs in response to a threat. The **parasympathetic branch** is responsible for turning off the stress response and returning the body to normal. The other body system primarily responsible for the stress response, the endocrine system, is the complex network of glands and tissues that produce and release hormones and other chemical messengers in the body.

To understand the physiology of the stress response, imagine that you are walking down a street at night in an unfamiliar city, and a stranger suddenly appears out of a doorway and demands your money. This challenge elicits a biological and biochemical process that begins in the brain and quickly spreads through the autonomic nervous system. Hormones are released, creating a cascade of effects throughout the body organs and systems.

First, within the brain, the cerebral cortex sends a message to the **hypothalamus,** a part of the brain that activates and coordinates the autonomic nervous system and other major functions of the body. The hypothalamus stimulates the pituitary gland, which releases hormones that in turn stimulate the adrenal glands to release **corticoids,** hormones that include **epinephrine** (adrenaline). Functions that are not critical in the moment—digestion, reproduction, growth, tissue repair, and the immune

Scalp The scalp tightens so that hair appears to stand up	**Brain-center** Neurotransmitters in the brain activate amygdala, triggering an emotional response to the stressor, such as fear or anger
Eyes Pupils dilate to sharpen vision	**Brain-front** Neurotransmitters suppress activity in the frontal cortex of the brain (concerned with short-term memory, inhibition, and rational thought), allowing quick reactions to take over
Ears Hearing becomes sharper	
Mouth Salivation decreases as fluids are diverted from nonessential functions	
Heart Heart rate increases, heart beat becomes stronger	**Stomach, intestines** Digestion in the stomach slows or stops
Blood vessels Blood pressure increases, clotting time decreases	**Adrenal glands** Adrenal glands release hormones that cause physiological and metabolic changes
Lungs Breathing rate increases, lungs take in more oxygen	
Liver Liver converts glycogen to glucose for instant energy	**Large muscles, legs** Muscle tension in the large muscles increases to prepare body for action
Sweat glands Perspiration increases to cool the body	
	Hands and feet Extremities become cold as blood is directed away from skin and toward large muscles

Figure 5.1   The stress response: changes in the body.

system's ability to fight infection—are all inhibited in the interest of preparing you to deal with an emergency.

Your heart rate, breathing rate, muscle tension, metabolism, and blood pressure all increase. Your hands and feet get cold as blood is directed away from your extremities into the larger muscles that can help you run or fight. Your pupils dilate to sharpen your vision, your hearing becomes sharper, your lungs take in more oxygen, and your liver begins to convert glycogen to glucose for instant energy to fuel your muscles (Figure 5.1). All this happens in an instant.

The challenge that elicits this chain of events does not have to be an actual threat or danger, as noted earlier. You may be about to go on stage, walk down the aisle, or run for the gold in an Olympic event. No matter what the challenge, your body reacts by becoming more aroused and alert. You may be able to do things you would not have believed possible as a result of your acute concentration. As noted in Chapter 4, some people who play sports experience this effect as "being in the zone."

The Relaxation Response

When a stressful event is over—you decide the situation is no longer dangerous, or you complete your task—the parasympathetic branch of the autonomic nervous system takes over, turning off the stress response.[3] Heart rate, breathing, muscle tension, and blood pressure all decrease.

KEY TERMS

stressor   Event or agent in the environment that causes stress.

stress   The general state of the body, mind, and emotions when an environmental stressor has triggered the stress response.

stress response or **fight-or-flight response**   Series of physiological changes that activate body systems, providing a burst of energy to deal with a perceived threat or danger.

autonomic nervous system   Part of the nervous system that controls involuntary, unconscious functions.

sympathetic branch   Branch of the autonomic nervous system responsible for activating the stress response.

parasympathetic branch   Branch of the autonomic nervous system responsible for deactivating the stress response.

hypothalamus   Part of the brain that activates and coordinates the autonomic nervous system and other major functions of the body.

corticoids   Hormones released by the adrenal cortex.

epinephrine   Hormone secreted by the adrenal glands that activates and stimulates the body systems; also known as *adrenaline*.

The body returns to **homeostasis,** a state of stability and balance in which functions are maintained within a normal range. The term **relaxation response** has been used to describe this process, and we discuss it in more detail later in this chapter.

Acute Stress and Chronic Stress

The fight-or-flight response is part of our evolutionary biology, and as such it served an important function for our ancestors. No doubt they were often on guard, watching their surroundings or preparing to respond to a particular threat. Today, most of us do not live in such dangerous environments, but this innate response to threat is still essential to our survival, warning us when it is time to fight or flee. Although the fight-or-flight response requires a great deal of energy, our bodies are equipped to deal with short-term, **acute stress** as long as it does not happen too often and as long as we can relax and recover afterward.

A problem occurs, however, when the stress response occurs repeatedly or when it persists without being turned off and replaced by the relaxation response. In these instances, the stress response itself becomes damaging. Many people live in a state of **chronic stress,** in which stressful conditions are ongoing and the stress response continues without resolution. When a person experiences stress for long periods, the effects of the stress response can linger, multiply, and intensify, ultimately damaging the ability to function. The stress response increases the likelihood that the person will become ill or, if already ill, that her or his defense system will be overwhelmed by the disease. Prolonged or severe stress has been found to weaken the immune system, strain the heart, damage memory cells in the brain, and contribute to physical illnesses such as heart disease, arthritis, and diabetes. Sources of chronic stress include everything from financial worries, relationship concerns, and loneliness to poverty, crowding, and discrimination. In these situations, reducing and managing levels of stress are critical.

Clearly, the stress response process is a double-edged sword. It allows you to protect yourself from danger and helps you survive, yet it can damage your body and impair your health. As noted earlier, the stress response is an inefficient process; mobilizing the body's resources requires a great deal of energy, which is why you often feel so tired after a stressful event. If your stress response is activated too frequently, you expend so much energy that you tire more readily and feel generally fatigued. In this state, you are more vulnerable to illness and disease, a topic we turn to next.

STRESS AND YOUR HEALTH

Researchers have been looking at the relationship between stress and disease for the last 50 years. One of the first scientists to develop a broad theory of stress and disease was Hans Selye,[4] who in turn drew from the work of Walter Cannon. Early in his career, Selye studied the effects of an ovarian extract on the body. During his experiments, he had a difficult time injecting his lab rats with the extract, mishandling them and sometimes accidentally dropping them on the floor. He then had to chase them around the lab. He later realized that the physiological changes he observed in the rats could not have been due to the extract; instead, he theorized, they were a result of the stress the rats experienced because of his poor technique.

Selye made the distinction we described earlier between stress, a state of the body, and stressors, the external situations to which organisms respond, and he developed the ideas of eustress and distress. He also realized that different individuals might respond to stressors differently, depending on what they brought to the situation. How they perceived the event was critical to what followed.

The General Adaptation Syndrome

Selye developed what he called the **General Adaptation Syndrome (GAS)** as a description and explanation of the physiological changes that he observed and that he believed to be predictable responses to stressors by all organisms. The process has three stages: alarm, resistance, and exhaustion. In the first, alarm, the individual experiences the fight-or-flight response. During this stage, there is a reduction in immune system functioning, which will be temporary if the stress is over quickly. The person in this stage is often more susceptible to infection and disease. During the second stage, resistance, the body works overtime to cope with the added stress. At this point the body is working hard to stay at a peak level to be prepared to handle difficult, intense situations. The last stage, exhaustion, is reached when the body can no longer keep up with the demands of stress (Figure 5.2). Without a period of rest and relaxation, the immune system breaks down, and the body is vulnerable to serious stress-related disorders.

Figure 5.2   General Adaptation Syndrome. *Selye's model describes the physiological response to stress. In the alarm stage, the body's fight-or-flight response is activated, accompanied by reduced immune system functioning. In the resistance stage, the body uses energy to adjust to the continued stress. After prolonged exposure to stress, the body may become totally depleted, leading to exhaustion, illness, and even death.*

Homeostasis   Alarm   Resistance   Recovery

Exhaustion

HIGHLIGHT ON HEALTH
Symptoms of Stress

Cognitive Symptoms
  Anxious thoughts
  Fearful anticipation
  Poor concentration
  Memory problems
Emotional Symptoms
  Feelings of tension
  Irritability
  Restlessness
  Worries
  Inability to relax
  Depression
Behavioral Symptoms
  Avoidance of tasks
  Sleep problems
  Difficulty in completing work or school assignments
  Fidgeting
  Tremors
  Grinding teeth
  Strained facial expression
  Clenched fists

Crying
Changes in drinking, eating, or smoking behaviors
Physiological Symptoms
  Stiff or tense muscles
  Sweating
  Tension headaches
  Feeling faint
  Feeling of choking
  Difficulty swallowing
  Stomachache, nausea, or vomiting
  Diarrhea or constipation
  Frequent or urgent urination
  Heart palpitations
  Social Symptoms
  Social withdrawal, or need to be with people most or all of the time
  Change in the quality of relationships

Source: "Between Mind and Body: Stress, Emotions, and Health," by K. Pelletier, 1993, in *Mind-Body Medicine: How to Use Your Mind for Better Health* (p. 24), edited by D. P. Goleman and J. Gurin, Yonkers, NY: Consumer Reports Books.

Symptoms of Stress

Since the time of Selye's work, researchers have concluded that almost every system in the body can be damaged by stress[1] (see the box "Symptoms of Stress"). According to the American Medical Association, stress plays a role in 80–85 percent of all human illness and disease.[5] For example, stress-triggered changes in the lungs increase the symptoms of asthma and other respiratory conditions. Stress appears to inhibit tissue repair, which increases the likelihood of bone fractures and is related to the development of osteoporosis (porous, weak bones). Stress can lead to sexual problems, including failure to ovulate and amenorrhea (absence of menstrual periods) in women and sexual dysfunction and loss of sexual desire in both men and women. Overall, if the stress response fails to shut down, a person is at risk for a variety of medical problems. In the next sections we look at how stress affects several different body systems.

Stress and the Immune System

Selye observed that stress affects the immune system, the body's elaborate defense system against infection and illness. Since Selye's time, research has definitively shown that stress decreases immune function. One study demonstrated a strong relationship between levels of psychological stress and the possibility of infection by a common cold virus. Other studies have found that both brief and long-term stressors have an impact on the function of the immune system.[6] Stressors as diverse as taking exams, experiencing major life events, and providing long-term care for someone with Alzheimer's disease affect the immune system.

KEY TERMS

homeostasis   State of stability and balance in which body functions are maintained within a normal range.
relaxation response   Series of physiological changes that calm body systems and return them to normal functioning.
acute stress   Short-term stress, produced by the stress response.
chronic stress   Long-term, low-level stress in which the stress response continues without resolution.
General Adaptation Syndrome (GAS)   Selye's classic model used to describe the physiological changes associated with the stress response. The three phases are alarm, resistance, and exhaustion.

One way of protecting your health against stress is to build time for relaxing and enjoyable activities into your days.

A growing area of study, **psychoneuroimmunology,** looks at the relationships among the nervous system, the endocrine system, and the immune system.[7] Research findings from this field confirm that stress can increase the body's susceptibility to diseases by affecting the functioning of the immune system.[8] Some studies have demonstrated the relationship between stress, immune function, disease outcome, and longevity. For example, those with fewer social relationships (and thus fewer resources to provide buffers against stress) seem to have shorter life expectancies.[6] On the other hand, stress reduction techniques and support groups appear to have a positive impact on people with cancer.[9]

Studies have also found that individuals vary dramatically in their psychological responses to stressful events. Cognitive factors such as negative expectancies, self-blame, and psychological inhibition appear to be related to poorer immune function and may have an effect on health. Scientists still do not fully understand why the stress response suppresses immune function or whether there is an evolutionary explanation for this suppression.

Stress and the Cardiovascular System

As we have seen, the stress response causes heart rate to accelerate and blood pressure to increase. When heart rate and blood pressure do not return to normal, as in low-level chronic stress, the person can experience elevated levels for long periods of time. Chronic hypertension (high blood pressure) makes blood vessels more susceptible to the development of atherosclerosis, a disease in which arteries are damaged and clogged with fatty deposits. Both hypertension and atherosclerosis increase the risk of heart attack and stroke. Chronic stress may exacerbate the development of heart disease in individuals with other risk factors, such as a sedentary lifestyle, a diet high in saturated fat, or a smoking habit. Chronic stress can also contribute to migraine headaches, which often result from narrowing and expansion of the carotid artery, the main artery leading to the brain.

Sudden severe stress can cause heart failure in some people who do not have heart disease. The condition, called *stress-induced cardiomyopathy,* is believed to occur when the heart muscle is temporarily "stunned" by a huge burst of adrenaline and cannot contract properly. The condition is reversible and causes no permanent heart damage, but it resembles a heart attack and requires medical treatment. Ninety-five percent of those experiencing the condition are women, and most are middle-aged.[10]

Stress and the Gastrointestinal System

Some 66 percent of people surveyed in one study reported that stress affected their gastrointestinal functioning, with most describing diarrhea as their most significant problem.[11] Another 49 percent of those who were surveyed reported that stress caused some type of abdominal pain.[12] Although not conclusive, evidence suggests that gastrointestinal problems can be stress related. More specifically, conditions such as acid reflux, indigestion, and stomach pain all seem to be more common in people who have higher levels or more frequent occurrences of stress.

For a long time, stress was commonly believed to cause stomach ulcers. Research suggests, however, that ulcers may be caused or exacerbated by a bacterial infection that irritates the stomach lining. While not causing ulcers, stress may contribute to their development. People in stressful occupations seem more likely to have ulcers, and people who experience their lives as stressful seem to develop more ulcers than those who report lower levels of stress.[13]

Stress and Mental Health

Both acute stress and chronic stress can contribute to psychological problems and the development of psychological illnesses, including anxiety disorders and depression (see Chapter 3). In acute stress disorder, for example, a person develops symptoms after experiencing a severely traumatic event, such as an assault, a serious accident, or a natural disaster. Symptoms can include a feeling of numbness, a sense of being in a daze, amnesia, flashbacks, increased arousal and anxiety, and impairment in functioning. If such symptoms appear 6 months or more after the traumatic event, the person may have post-traumatic stress disorder, a condition characterized by a sense of numbness or emotional detachment from people, repeated reliving of the event through flashbacks and/or nightmares, and avoidance of things that might be associated with the trauma. Years may pass after the trauma before symptoms of post-traumatic stress disorder appear.[14] An example of a less severe stress-related disorder is adjustment disorder, in which a response to a stressor (such as anxiety, worry, social withdrawal) continues for a longer period than would normally be expected. The stressor in this case could be losing a job, getting divorced, retiring, or other life event.

Low-level, unresolved chronic stress can be a factor in psychological problems as well. Stress can diminish wellness and reduce the ability to function at the highest level even without an identifiable disorder. Symptoms such as irritability, impatience, difficulty concentrating, excessive worrying, insomnia, and forgetfulness, like physical symptoms, can be addressed with stress management techniques.

MEDIATORS OF THE STRESS RESPONSE

We have noted throughout this chapter that different people respond differently to stressors. Consider the example of John and Donald. John had a pilot's license and had flown a small airplane many times, so when he was flying on a small commuter plane in rough weather, he was relaxed and able to chat and laugh. His colleague Donald had never flown on a small plane before, and on the same flight he got frightened and felt out of control. His heart raced and he began to sweat profusely. As the plane bumped along, he thought he might be having a heart attack, while John continued to enjoy the flight.

Both men were in the same situation, but their subjective experiences were very different. Among the factors that may play a role in these differences are past experiences and overall level of wellness. Also critical are personality traits, habitual ways of thinking, and inborn or acquired attitudes toward the demands of life. In this section, we consider these last three categories.

Responding to Stress: Personality Factors

Some of the difference between John's and Donald's reactions to the bumpy flight might have come from inborn personality traits. Perhaps John is more easygoing and flexible, more able to take things in stride. Maybe Donald feels a greater need to be in control, or maybe he reacts more intensely to perceived threats. Personality differences contribute to how people respond to stressful situations.

In the 1970s, two cardiologists, Meyer Friedman and Ray Rosenman, described and named the **Type A behavior pattern.**[15] Type A individuals tend to be impulsive, need to get things done quickly, and live their lives on a time schedule. Type As seem to be guided by the perception that they are responsible for everything that goes on in their lives; they are hard driving, achievement oriented, and highly competitive, "keeping score" in situations that others might consider trivial. They tend to be impatient, selfish, easily angered, and hostile. They set unrealistic goals and are easily bored. They may display pressured

KEY TERMS

psychoneuroimmunology   Field of study that focuses on the relationships among the nervous system, endocrine system, and immune system.

Type A behavior pattern   Set of personality traits originally thought to be associated with risk for heart disease. Type A individuals are hard driving, competitive, achievement oriented, and quick to anger; further research has identified hostility as the key risk factor in the pattern.

Challenges & Choices

Stress and Your Job

Stress affects every aspect of modern life, including how you earn a living. When you are exploring careers, don't forget to take into account the levels of stress that people in those occupations typically experience. Then try to match your own preferences, coping style, and ability to handle stress with an appropriate occupation. Remember that boredom can be as stressful for some people as danger is for others! Here are some tips on finding a job with the right amount of stress for you:

- If you are not comfortable with high levels of stress, don't choose a job with tight deadlines (for example, newspaper reporter) or life-or-death responsibilities (for example, emergency medical technician).

- If you have high security needs, don't choose an occupation that might depend on the marketplace or tenuous funding.

- Look for an occupation or position that allows you to have both responsibility and control. The most stressful positions are those in which people have important decision-making responsibilities but do not have control over how results are achieved.

- Visit a workplace where you think you might like to work to see how you respond to the environment. Do you find it too quiet or too loud? Too boring or too chaotic? Too slow paced or too fast paced?

- Interview someone working in an occupation you are interested in. Ask about pressure, deadlines, responsibility, control, management style, interpersonal relationships. Are people generally happy and satisfied, or is there dissatisfaction, frustration, and burnout?

- Be realistic about your own abilities. Allow yourself room to grow, but try not to set yourself up for disappointment or failure. That will lead only to more stress.

It's Not Just Personal . . .

It is generally thought that job stress has increased over the past 20 years, especially in industrialized countries such as the United States and Canada. However, increased awareness could account for this: Workers are more aware of on-the-job stress and report problems, such as repetitive motion injuries and poor workstation ergonomics, more frequently.

speech, rapid eye blinking, and jerky, repetitive body movements. Some estimates are that more than 40 percent of the population of the United States might be Type As and possibly half of all men.

Individuals who fit this description are prime candidates for stress-related illnesses. The relationship between Type A personality traits and heart disease has been known for some time. More recently, there have been indications that a Type A personality can mean increased risk for a number of other diseases, including peptic ulcers, asthma, headaches, and thyroid problems.

However, not all the characteristics of this personality seem to be harmful. Many Type As are achievement oriented and successful and yet remain healthy. According to recent research, a key culprit is **hostility,** defined as an ongoing accumulation of irritation and anger. Hostile individuals are generally cynical toward others, frequently express anger, and display aggressive behaviors.[16] The at-risk hostile person demonstrates an inability to trust others, gets angry easily, is unable to laugh, and reacts with a great deal of intensity to minor errors. Research has indicated that hostility, by itself, is related to coronary heart disease, and it may also contribute to premature death.

Friedman and Rosenman also described a constellation of personality traits they labeled Type B. In contrast to the Type A personality, the Type B personality is less driven and more relaxed. Type Bs do not have the aggressiveness, competitiveness, or sense of time urgency seen in Type As. They are more easygoing and less readily frustrated. All other things being equal, Type Bs are less susceptible to coronary heart disease. However, their personalities do not necessarily mean that they experience less stress in their lives. For example, if a Type B ends up in a Type A job, he or she may become overwhelmed by the competitiveness and pace needed to be successful.[15] (See the box "Stress and Your Job" for tips on matching your personality to your job.)

A third type of personality, Type C, has also been described. Type Cs are individuals who suppress their emotions and "bottle things up." They tend to respond to stress by giving up, becoming helpless and hopeless. They don't believe they can overcome their problems and so don't try to change, frequently becoming depressed in the process. Some researchers have suggested a relationship between the Type C personality and risk for cancer. These individuals can benefit from interventions that reinforce their sense of control over their lives and their ability to overcome problems.

Much less research has been done on Type B and C personalities than on the Type A personality. Overall, Type As appear to have the greatest risk of developing stress-related illnesses. However, all types of personalities can benefit from practicing the stress management techniques described at the end of this chapter.

Responding to Stress: Cognitive Factors

We noted earlier that how you think about an event has a lot to do with whether you experience it as a stressor. Until you decide that it is actually a threat and/or beyond your ability to cope, it remains merely a potential stressor. In the case of John and Donald, John remained calm because he did not think the bumpy flight was a threat. Donald thought his life was in danger, if not from the flight itself, then from a heart attack. No wonder he experienced a full-blown stress response!

Experts have identified specific cognitive mediators of the stress response. They suggest that people create their own distress with illogical thinking, unrealistic expectations, and negative beliefs.[2] For example, a person may think she has to be perfect—get straight As, always be caring and compassionate, never make a mistake—in order to be a worthy human being. If she gets a B or lets a friend down, she will experience much more stress than if she had more realistic expectations about herself and was more self-forgiving. Her ideas can transform a relatively neutral event into a stressor.

Other common illogical ideas and unrealistic expectations are "life should be fair," "friends should be there when you need them," "everyone I care about has to love and approve of me," and "everything has to go my way." When everyday experiences don't live up to these ideas, people who hold them end up feeling angry, frustrated, disappointed, or demoralized. They may experience misunderstandings, breakdowns in communication, and relationship conflicts as a result of such assumptions. With a more realistic attitude, they can take things in stride and reduce the frequency and intensity of the stress response. This doesn't mean you should have unrealistically low expectations. When your expectations are too low, you may experience underachievement, depression, resignation, and lowered self-esteem. The goal is a realistic balance.

People also increase their level of stress when their thinking has a negative bias. They may overgeneralize, believing, for example, that one job rejection means no one will ever hire them. They may pick out the one negative aspect of an overall positive experience and focus only on that. They may be pessimistic, expecting the worst in every situation. They may think they are the center of the universe and thus responsible for a friend's bad mood. Such ideas can turn relatively minor and innocuous events and situations into stressors.

Responding to Stress: Resilience and Hardiness

In Chapters 3 and 4 we discussed the quality of resilience, the ability to bounce back from adversity and overcome a problem. Resilient people may have some innate advantages over others, but healthy responses to stress can also be learned and acquired through education and practice. (See the box "Who Will Handle Stress Best?")

Research has led to a better understanding of resilient or stress-resistant people. As noted in Chapter 3, they appear to share an optimistic explanatory style and assume troubles are temporary rather than permanent.[17] The consequences of each event are seen as related to only that event and not generalized into a universal self-evaluation. Stress-resistant people also seem to focus on immediate issues and explain their struggle in positive and helpful ways. For example, a poor grade on one exam might motivate the stress-resilient person to study harder, using the grade as motivation. A person who is not so resilient may react to a poor grade by feeling like a failure and giving up. The stress-resistant person makes choices about his or her responses and tries to gain some wisdom from each challenge. Many of the protective factors for mental health described in Chapter 3, such as social skills and a sense of humor, also serve to enhance resilience and resistance to stress.

Another line of research has developed the concept of **hardiness,** an effective style of coping with stress. Researchers have studied people who were exposed to a great deal of stress but never seemed to become ill as a result.[18,19] They argue that if negative psychological traits such as hopelessness and defensiveness can intensify the effects of stressors, then positive ways of coping may buffer the body from their effects. They call this style *hardiness* and have suggested that people high in hardiness are more resistant to illness.

These researchers found three particular traits in those who stayed healthiest. The first is called *challenge*. Individuals who perceive the demands of living as a challenge rather than a threat typically responded to change with excitement and energy. A second trait is *commitment*. People are considered hardier if they participate in and are committed to meaningful activities. The third trait is *control,* the individual's ability to gain important information, to make decisions, and have a sense of being in control. Having a sense

KEY TERMS

hostility Ongoing accumulation of irritation and anger.

hardiness Effective style of coping with stress, characterized by a tendency to view life events as challenges rather than threats, a commitment to meaningful activities, and a sense of being in control.

Beating the Odds

Who Will Handle Stress Best?

Innumerable factors contribute to a person's overall level of stress and vulnerability to illness. Brief profiles of three men are presented here. Who do you think will be best able to handle stress and least likely to experience a stress-related disorder?

Jason, 35, is a frustrated writer who is currently tending bar. Although he makes enough money to support himself, he is not satisfied at his job and spends most of his time trying to write or find a job as a full-time writer. He is close to his parents and siblings and has a great deal of self-confidence. He works evenings at the bar and tries to freelance during the day, but he never feels as if he has enough time to write. His sleep patterns are poor—he averages 4 hours of sleep a night. He has a very small support system of friends and does not have a significant other. Jason's mother has a history of feeling overwhelmed in stressful situations.

Fred is a 40-year-old physician who travels a great deal and spends little time with his family. He works long hours but appears to like his work seeing patients at the hospital. He feels young, works out on a regular basis at the hospital gym, and generally takes good care of himself. Although he says he would like to spend more time with his children, his behavior suggests he is happy with the way things are. His family seems to be supportive of his intense work situation and usually accommodates his needs. However, his wife describes herself as often feeling "stressed out," since she takes care of the kids and also works outside of the home. She enjoys their lifestyle, but she is beginning to think that money may not buy happiness. Fred appears to be unaware of her feelings.

Hector is a 27-year-old case manager at a social services agency who just started a new job. He enjoys his work and is thinking about returning to school to get a graduate degree. He is concerned, however, that if he returns to school, he will not have enough time to be with his significant other, get married, and start a family. Although he has had episodes of depression, he claims he has never felt better in his life. He believes that since he has met the other challenges in his life, he is in a good position to do well.

OLC Web site Visit the **Online Learning Center** at www.mhhe.com/teague1e for comments by the authors.

---

of control may be especially critical in avoiding illness and responding to stressful situations. In sum, these researchers found that people who demonstrate an ability to see life as a challenge, who are committed to what they do, and who believe they are in control tend to do better.

SOURCES OF STRESS

Are our lives more stressful than the lives of people living a century ago? Some people think so. They point to our harried lifestyle and fast pace, punctuated by e-mails, faxes, call waiting, escalating demands of the workplace, and more recently, threats to security. However, every era has its stressors. Our ancestors' lives may have depended on whether their crops got enough rain or their farm animals were able to resist disease. In many cases, the sources of stress for our ancestors may have been every bit as harsh as they are for us. Still, we do live stressful lives, and some of our stressors are unique to our times. They include not just life changes and transitions but time pressure, technology, and terrorism.

Life Events

Can stressful life events make people more vulnerable to illness? Thomas Holmes and Richard Rahe, medical researchers at the University of Washington, observed that individuals frequently experienced major life events before the onset of an illness. They proposed that life events—major changes and transitions that force the individual to adjust and adapt—may precipitate illness, especially if several such events occur at the same time.[20] Holmes and Rahe studied patients' medical records and developed a scale of stressful life events based on ratings by outside experts. The scale made it possible to create a stress score, or profile, for an individual and compare it to the onset of illnesses.

From this work they developed the Holmes-Rahe Social Readjustment Scale, a list of life events that require the individual to adjust and adapt to change. They assigned point scores to the events, rating stressfulness in terms of "life change units." The higher a person's score on the scale, the more likely that person is to experience symptoms of illness. The most stressful event on this scale is the death of a spouse, followed by such events as divorce, separation, a personal injury, and being fired from a job. Many stressful events are not necessarily negative, such as marriage, pregnancy, and "outstanding personal achievement." The key is change—the individual must adapt and adjust to these events, seeking to restore balance or create a new balance. Less stressful events on the scale include moving, going on

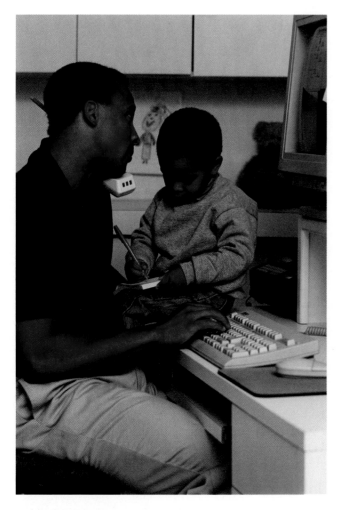

Juggling the demands of parenthood, school, and work is common but can be a source of chronic stress.

vacation, experiencing a change in sleeping habits, and dealing with a minor violation of the law.

An adaptation of the Social Readjustment Scale for college students, the Student Stress Scale, is presented in the Add It Up! feature at the end of this chapter. Fill it out to find out what your stress level is and how likely you may be to experience stress-related health problems in the near future.

Daily Hassles

Major life events contribute to illness for many people, but surprisingly, everyday hassles can also cause health problems. In fact, daily hassles are related to subsequent illness and disease to a greater degree than are major life events.[7] Daily hassles include such interactions with the environment as arguments, car problems, deadlines, traffic jams, long lines, money worries, and so on. Maybe your printer breaks and you can't get an assignment in on time, or you lose your wallet, or your plumbing backs up, or your group project partners don't do their work. All of these events can lead to a state of chronic, low-level stress, especially if they pile up and you don't have a period of recovery.

Although daily hassles often occur in the absence of major life events, life events are usually accompanied by daily hassles. For example, a person who is newly divorced may face innumerable hassles associated with moving to a new home, dealing with financial problems, settling legal and custody issues, and working out child care arrangements.[21] For some ideas on reducing the number and impact of daily hassles, see the box "Planning for Less Stress."

Time Pressure, Overload, and Technostress

As noted earlier, the modern world presents us with some unique stressors that our ancestors didn't have to face. These stressors may make our lives more difficult, although they don't necessarily mean we have to experience the stress response more intensely or frequently.

Time Pressure

In New York City the time between a traffic light turning green and a car honking has been referred to as a "New York second." Most of us experience some degree of time pressure in our lives, although our impatience may not be as intense as the New York driver's. Many people find that they have more and more to do, despite time-saving devices, and want to compress more activity, more experience, more living into less and less time. Multitasking is common—people talk on the phone while driving, answer e-mail while eating lunch, take laptops on vacation. They read headlines and listen to sound bites; they don't have time for anything more. They surf through TV channels and Web sites, get impatient waiting for elevators, and become enraged at slow drivers on the road. The rush to do things quickly and use time well ultimately increases levels of stress.

Overload

Many people do not see their overstuffed schedules as a problem. Instead, they go to time management classes to learn how to squeeze more activities into the time they have. Although planning and good use of time are effective stress management techniques, there are limits to how much a person can do. Many times the solution is not to use time more effectively but to do less. Many "stressed out" people are not poor stress managers; they are simply overloaded with responsibilities. Their stress arises from an overbooked schedule or a greater number of commitments than they can reasonably handle.

Most of us are familiar with the feeling of wondering why we ever agreed to take on yet one more responsibility. Despite a looming thesis deadline, for example, you agree to organize the holiday party or participate in another extracurricular activity. You may assume too many responsibilities because you don't want to be perceived as unsupportive, selfish, or lazy. In these cases, learning to be more

Challenges & Choices

Planning for Less Stress

We often don't recognize what we do on a daily basis that increases our stress levels. For example, going without meals, procrastinating when papers are due, and doing without sleep are personal patterns that generate stress and make us more vulnerable to illness. Planning is a great antidote to stress. Here are a few things you can try if you want to plan for less stress:

- Set a deadline for your next class paper a week before it is due.
- Hand in a draft before your paper is due and ask your instructor for feedback.
- Keep a journal of your daily activities and try to change one behavior that increases stress, such as skipping breakfast.
- Close your eyes at least once a day and listen to some music.

- Keep a schedule. People who are more organized tend to have lower levels of stress and feel more in control of their lives.
- Ask one or two people in a class to form a study group with you and try to spend at least one night a week studying with them. After a few hours of reviewing, take a break and reward yourself with some positive social time.

It's Not Just Personal...

Some people choose unhealthy ways to deal with stress, such as drinking alcohol and smoking tobacco. Smoking is considered the leading preventable cause of death in the United States, and alcohol plays a part in 10 of the top 13 causes of death. This is just one reason to choose stress management techniques such as planning ahead and taking time to relax rather than less healthy approaches.

assertive and say no to others' requests is the best way to handle time management issues. If you find that your schedule is too full, evaluate how you spend your nonworking, nonsleeping hours, and try to identify things you can cut. Ask yourself if each commitment is a genuine obligation for you. Opening up your schedule will not only help you reduce stress but give you more time for yourself and more energy to deal with your remaining commitments.

Technostress

Like time pressure and overload, technostress is a familiar source of stress for many of us. The term *technostress,* coined in 1984, is defined as a "modern disease of adaptation caused by an inability to cope with new computer technologies."[22] Although it may be premature to define technostress as an illness, few would deny the negative effect that modern technology can have on people, directly and indirectly.

Most new technologies are designed to save time and improve life, but they can also be sources of stress. We feel pressure to learn them and master them; once they are widely accepted, we find we are expected to use them to get more done in less time. Further, they often let us down at critical moments, as anyone can attest who has broken into a sweat when a computer crashes or a PowerPoint presentation fails to work as expected.

With each new technological innovation—e-mail, the Internet, voice mail, DVDs, mp3 players, camera phones, and on and on—we are faced with the choice of mastering it or ignoring it. Learning a new technology can

be both fun and frustrating, as well as time consuming. Choosing to ignore a new technology can raise the fear of being left behind in a fast-paced world. Both are stressful.

Job Pressure

Occupational pressures and stressors appear to be the leading source of stress for American adults, and job pressure contributes to many stress-related illnesses. High levels of job stress increase a person's risk of cardiovascular disease[1] and may be related to the incidence of back pain, fatigue, muscular pain, and headaches. The costs are high in terms of dollars and worker performance, seen in accidents, absenteeism, turnover, reduced levels of productivity, and insurance costs. People who struggle with stressful jobs and high levels of hostility are at particularly high risk.

Many of the stressors just described (time pressure, overload, technostress) apply to the work setting. Jobs can also be stressful because they are too complex or difficult, too easy, boring, repetitive, unsafe, or environmentally stressful (noisy, too hot or cold, and so on). What seems to make a job particularly stressful is the combination of a great deal of responsibility and a lack of control over how to fulfill that responsibility.[2] Some of the most stressful occupations are law enforcement, teaching, and health care.

At the same time, many people thrive in highly stressful occupations. For example, journalists work under tight deadlines and other stressful conditions, yet certain people appear well matched to that profession. As we have seen, many factors, including inborn personality traits, past

Challenges & Choices

Are You a Workaholic?

Do you get up early no matter how late you go to bed? Do you work on weekends and holidays? Do you find vacations hard to handle? Do you find it difficult to do nothing? Do you work while you eat? Do you always carry a cell phone so your office can reach you?

If you answered yes to most of these questions, you may be a workaholic. You would probably benefit from learning how to make use of leisure time and from practicing some of the relaxation techniques described in this chapter. Here are some additional tips on keeping your life in balance:

- Take time to think about your goals in life. Are you spending your time advancing the things that are really important to you? Remember that you have more control over your life than you may realize.

- Find something you enjoy doing and place it in your schedule.

- Leave all electronic devices off at least one day every weekend.

- Find something you might like to do when you are ready to retire.

- Do some volunteer work with a human service organization.

It's Not Just Personal . . .

At their extremes, workaholism and work stress can place a heavy burden on the heart. The Japanese even have a word for sudden death due to overwork, *karoushi*. According to the American Institute of Stress, several studies are now suggesting that job-related stress is as great a threat to health as smoking or not exercising.

experiences, and different ways of perceiving and managing stress, have an influence on such variations. When you are thinking about career options, the key is to choose an occupation that matches your preferred stress levels.

Workaholism

A current trend in the workplace is toward longer and longer hours on the job. Over the course of the past century many jobs have become physically easier, but expectations have grown that people will work more, especially since the 1970s. Managers and professionals seem to work the longest days and are subject to associated stresses.[23] Although they have more control of their time (a factor associated with lower levels of stress), they spend more time working. They bring work home and thus never really leave the job. Some employers encourage workers to spend even more time at work by offering sleeping rooms, free dinners, and laundry service. The effect is to create the idea that work is the place to be. As a result, many people who want to be successful become workaholics, never taking a break from work. For more on this phenomenon, see the box "Are You a Workaholic?"

Burnout

Sometimes, when workers experience too much frustration on the job over an extended period of time, they experience a syndrome called burnout. **Burnout** is an adverse, work-related stress reaction with physical, psychological, and behavioral components. It appears to be

linked to absenteeism, low morale, high turnover, and physical illness. The symptoms of burnout include increasing discouragement and pessimism about work; a decline in motivation and job performance; irritability, anger, and apathy on the job; and physical complaints.[24] For more on job burnout and what you can do about it, see the box "How Can You Avoid Burnout?"

Burnout can have a negative impact on everyone in the workplace.[25] It can be contagious, infecting all the workers in a particular setting. Additionally, when someone has become apathetic about his or her job, other workers often have to take up the slack. Incidents of "office rage" have occurred, in which disgruntled employees or ex-employees have expressed their frustrations with violence.[26] These incidents are rare, but many employees experience chronic anger on the job. Some of this anger may result from job insecurity, as companies seek to increase productivity by downsizing, laying off workers following corporate mergers, and moving factories to other countries. Adapting to a global economy is yet another source of stress in many people's everyday lives.

KEY TERMS

burnout Adverse work-related stress reaction with physical, psychological, and behavioral components.

Challenges & Choices

How Can You Avoid Burnout?

An excessive workload and frequent frustration on the job can lead to job burnout. If you find yourself in this situation, be aware of the signs of burnout and take steps to care for yourself. The signs of burnout include the following:

- Not eating, or skipping meals.
- Feeling fatigued, irritable, and overwhelmed on a regular basis; feeling that there is always something else you have to do.
- Feeling that there is no time for rest.
- Finding you've lost your sense of humor.
- Withdrawing from friends and people you work with; wanting to be alone.
- Feeling that you cannot take a vacation; if you do, you will only be more overwhelmed by work or school when you get back.
- Not trusting that others will support you.
- Using drugs or alcohol to get "rest" and numb yourself.
- Feeling trapped in your position, unable to discuss the situation with others around you.

Stop and think about some specific things you can do to care for yourself. Here are some examples:

- Do something physical away from work. For example, set a non-work-related goal based on doing something you enjoy.

- Examine the consequences of "finding your voice." Should you speak up or remain silent? Sometimes the solution to job stress is being more assertive about what you can and cannot do.
- Decide if this is the workplace for you. Make a list of what attracts you to the position you currently have and what its disadvantages are. Then do a cost-benefit analysis. What will happen to you over the next few years if you continue to work there? What will happen if you don't? Decide where you have to draw the line.
- Try to exercise more control over what happens in your life.
- Seek professional help if you can't find the answers on your own.

It's Not Just Personal . . .

Burnout and other stress-related problems are costly to business. According to the *Toronto Globe and Mail*, Canadian businesses lose approximately $12 billion every year to stress-related disorders. According to on-line sources, American businesses lose an estimated $200–$300 billion dollars per year.

College Stress

College students experience a great deal of life change, and some studies even suggest that the college years may be the most stressful time in people's lives.[27,28] Many college students are free of the constraints of their parents' home for the first time, and they must replace them with their own structures and routines. They may have opportunities to put off homework, go out on school nights, and participate in sexual adventures their parents would not have allowed. They also have to find time to do the laundry, shop, and take care of many other routine chores. Considering these changes and the effects of stress, it should not be surprising that colds, mononucleosis, and sexually transmitted diseases are familiar on college campuses.

Besides the effect of this major life transition, common sources of stress for college students include school work and grades, sleep deprivation, worries about money, relationship concerns, and uncertainty about their futures. The pressure of college may be growing even more intense, particularly for young women. In a survey published in 2000, 30 percent of first-year students described themselves as frequently feeling overwhelmed. Women were nearly twice as likely to feel this way as men.[29] Rising tuition costs also appear to affect stress levels of many students. A record number of students say they have to work to afford college, and again, women in greater numbers describe themselves as feeling the pressure to work. Concern about the economy and being successful also has an impact on students. For nontraditional students, who are usually older, there can be additional stressors. For more on this topic, see the box "Stress and the Older College Student."

Colleges usually offer resources to help students deal with stress, and at some major universities 40 percent of all undergraduates visit the counseling center. However, a sign that not enough students are getting the help they need is the fact that suicide is the second leading cause of death on college campuses. Many universities are averaging one

Stress and the Older College Student

Although all college students have to deal with such stressors as completing administrative tasks, finding time to study, and getting assignments in on time, older college students have to deal with some stressors that younger students may not have. Some of the stressors older students report are listed here:

- Trying to balance work, family, and school can be difficult.
- The financial cost of college added to the cost of supporting oneself or one's family can make a budget very tight.

- Socializing with friends and family often has to be restricted when school deadlines loom.
- Older college students may have doubts about their ability to do well in school.
- Older students may find they have to miss their children's activities because of school or work obligations, and this can cause additional stress, sadness, and frustration.

suicide per year.[30] More effort must be made to reach and educate students about stress reduction and stress management techniques, including time management, relaxation techniques, exercise, and good nutrition.

Families, Relationships, and Interpersonal Issues

Family can be your greatest source of support, but they can also be a source of stress. A family is a system, a complex network of interactions and relationships, and a change that affects one family member will affect all family members. For example, if one person is suffering from depression, alcoholism, or cancer that illness disrupts the system and forces everyone to adjust and adapt. The same

is true if one person is having financial problems or difficulties on the job.

Families have to continuously adapt to a series of life changes and transitions. The birth of a baby places new demands on parents and siblings, and families must adapt as a teenager moves through adolescence to adulthood and leaves home. A family may be disrupted by death or divorce; and in fact, a growing number of children spend part of their lives in single-parent households, blended family units, or stepfamily systems created by cohabitation. Learning to deal with these changes can create opportunities for families to become stronger and more resilient, or families may become weakened and less able to cope.

Studies have identified a number of protective factors that make families resilient across the life cycle. These

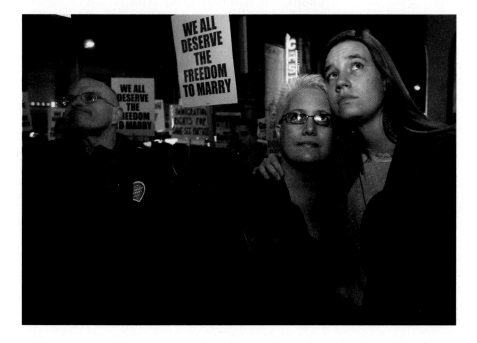

Gay men and lesbians face stressors that heterosexuals don't have to deal with, including discrimination, social inequities, and homophobia. Such stressors can also affect the relationship of the partners.

HIGHLIGHT ON HEALTH
Factors That Make Families Resilient

Accord: Balanced family relationships that allow conflict resolution and reduce chronic strain.

Celebrations: Commemoration of birthdays, religious occasions, and other special events.

Communication: Sharing beliefs and emotions with family members.

Financial management: Money management skills and satisfaction with economic status.

Hardiness: Family members' sense of control over their lives, commitment to family, and confidence that the family will survive no matter what.

Health: Physical and psychological well-being of family members.

Leisure activities: Similarities and differences in preferences for how to spend free time.

Personality compatibility: Acceptance of a partner's traits, behaviors, general outlook, and dependability.

Support network: Positive aspects of relationships with in-laws, relatives, and friends.

Time and routines: Family meals, chores, togetherness, and other routines contributing to continuity and stability in family life.

Traditions: Honoring holidays and important family experiences carried across generations.

Source: Adapted from H. I. McCubbin et al. "Families Under Stress: What Makes them Resilient?" Journal of Family & Consumer Sciences (Fall 1997), Table 1. Family Protective Factors Across the Family Life Cycle, p. 5.

factors are associated with the family's ability to manage transitions and changes over time and with family harmony and balance. For more detail, see the box "Factors That Make Families Resilient."

Whether with family members or not, relationships with significant others are frequently stressful. Even in the best of circumstances, difficulties arise when two people, each with different histories, personalities, needs, and ways of doing things, try to get along with each other on a daily basis. Some of the difficulties in couple relationships spring from different expectations, many of them unspoken and some even unconscious. We simply expect the other person to do things the way we've always done them or seen them done. Many experts agree that the key to a successful relationship is not finding the perfect partner but being able to communicate effectively with the partner you have. Whereas poor communication skills can cause interactions to escalate into arguments and fights (or deteriorate into cold silences), thoughtful communication and conflict resolution techniques can resolve issues before they become problems.

Anger

Sometimes the source of stress is within the individual. Unresolved feelings of anger and hostility can be extremely stressful. People who are prone to anger (Type A personalities) may be more likely to have a heart attack than their calmer counterparts who take annoyances and frustrations in stride. In a study of nearly 13,000 people, those who had the highest anger scores also had the greatest risk of suffering a heart attack or sudden cardiac death.

When compared with the least angry people in the study, the members of the angriest group were nearly three times as likely to have an acute or fatal heart attack over the course of the 6 years. One reason for this is that a sudden and sustained elevation in blood pressure and heart rate (such as during an argument) raises the risk for a heart attack. The angriest individuals were also twice as likely as the least angry ones were to develop heart disease.[31]

The idea that blowing off steam, or venting anger, is a positive way to deal with this difficult emotion is generally not the case. Releasing anger in an uncontrolled way often reinforces the feeling and may cause it to escalate into rage.[2] Venting creates anger in the person on the receiving end and hurts relationships. Suppressing anger or turning it against oneself is also unhealthy, lowering self-esteem and possibly fostering depression.

If you are a person who responds to life events and daily hassles with anger, you can benefit greatly from examining your emotions and taking action to change your behavior. A first step in reducing your risk is identifying the things in your life that upset you. Then try to find ways either to avoid them or to reduce their impact on you. If you find yourself in a situation in which you are getting angry, take a time-out, remove yourself from the situation physically, and do some deep breathing and muscle relaxation exercises (see the section "Relaxation Techniques" at the end of this chapter). Examine the situation and think about whether your reaction is logical or illogical and whether you could see it another way. Look for absurdity or humor in the situation. Put it in perspective. If you cannot avoid the situation or reduce your reaction, try some of the stress management strategies described later in this chapter.

Financial Worries

In a survey of 30,000 college students, one in three students indicated that his or her financial situation was causing physical and/or mental stress.[32] Many of us experience financial stress because our income is not equal to our expenditures. The stress that accompanies budget difficulties can result in short tempers, arguments, and even illness. Familiar sources of financial stress are fear of running short of money before the end of the month, carrying too much debt, reduced employment or unemployment, no savings to cover medical emergencies, and unexpected home or car repairs.

One of the best ways to relieve financial stress is to plan ahead. Being willing to follow a budget and make the lifestyle changes necessary to live within available funds may be the key to relief from financial stress. Simplifying your life, shedding those items and events that you can live without, can be liberating. Having some savings is reassuring, and experts recommend that people put money in a savings account every month before they use their money any other way, in effect "paying themselves" first. That money is then available if an emergency arises. Finding ways to ensure financial peace of mind is an excellent stress reduction technique.

Illness and Caregiving

Illness and disease are sources of stress, at the same time that stress can cause illness and disease.[6] It's a vicious cycle. Everyday stressors often cause muscle tension and pain, and chronic stress compromises the immune system. The resulting health problems, in turn, become stressors. Stress management techniques can help break this stress-tension-pain-illness-stress cycle.

Caring for a loved one who is sick is also highly stressful. A study of parents caring for children with cancer showed that chronic stress compromises the immune system.[33] Although the study did not establish direct links between stress and any specific health problem, it revealed a process by which stress can cause abnormalities in the immune system, changes that could leave caregivers more vulnerable to allergies, heart disease, and a host of other health problems. The findings suggest a pathway through which stress can influence medical conditions that involve excessive inflammation, as is the case in heart disease, respiratory infections, rheumatoid arthritis, and many common diseases of adulthood. The good news found by the researchers was that social support reduced the effects on the immune system of caring for a child with cancer, perhaps by helping the parents deal with the economic, work, and family disruptions caused by the disease and its treatment.

Societal Issues

Intolerance, prejudice, discrimination, injustice, poverty, pressure to conform to mainstream culture—all are common sources of stress for members of modern society. Exposure to racism and homophobia, for example, can cause distrust, frustration, resentment, negative emotions such as anger and fear, and a sense of helplessness and hopelessness. Experiencing racism has been associated with both physical and mental health-related symptoms, including hypertension, cardiovascular reactivity, depression, eating disorders, substance abuse, and violence. Similar effects are seen in lesbians, gay males, bisexuals, and transgendered individuals when they are the targets of prejudice and homophobia.[34] These individuals often have higher rates of school-related problems, substance abuse, criminal activity, prostitution, running away from home, and suicide than do their nongay peers.

Trauma

The effect of emotionally traumatic experiences has received a great deal of study. Examples of traumatic events range from sexual assault to airplane crashes to natural disasters to terrorist attacks. The Holocaust, the Vietnam War, the bombing of the federal building in Oklahoma City in 1999, and the attacks of September 11, 2001, are frequently cited as traumatic events of the highest order. Most people are not equipped to deal effectively with events of this magnitude. They overwhelm individuals' ability to cope and destroy any sense of control, connection, or meaning. They shake the foundations of beliefs about the safety and trustworthiness of the world.

Some people react to extreme trauma by developing post-traumatic stress disorder (PTSD), as described earlier in this chapter. Although the triggering event may be overwhelming, often it alone is not sufficient to explain the occurrence of PTSD in certain individuals. At the same time, many people who are exposed to a traumatic event never develop PTSD. For example, fewer than 40 percent of those with war zone experience in Vietnam developed PTSD.[35] Again, this is evidence of the role of mediating factors in the individual experience of stress.

MANAGING STRESS

The effects of unrelieved stress on the body and mind can range from muscle tension to a pervasive sense of hopelessness about the future, yet life without stress is unrealistic if not impossible. The solution is to find ways to manage stress. In this section we offer a number of ways to do that.

Choosing an Approach to Stress Management

There are many different ways to manage stress, but not all of them appeal to everyone. What works for someone else may not be helpful or comfortable for you. For example, some individuals can remain silent and feel comfortable

Consumer Clipboard

Selecting a Stress Management Approach

If you're looking for ways to manage your stress level, the options range from ancient relaxation techniques to modern "miracle" pills. Some methods have research to back up their effectiveness and safety, but others don't. Before you commit your time and money, educate yourself about stress-relieving practices and products.

With its roots in the Stone Age and similarities to modern Hinduism, yoga is a popular and respected approach to relaxation and well-being. Through prescribed positions and mental exercises, it offers a quiet and calm approach to stress relief. Many YMCAs and recreation centers offer yoga lessons at reasonable rates. Gyms and yoga studios tend to be more expensive. As you work through the classes, assess yourself: How do you feel mentally and physically after class? Do you notice a change in your response to stressful events? Do you have a stronger sense of control over your life?

T'ai chi is a form of Chinese martial arts that dates back to the 14th century. Central to this method is the concept of *qi*, or life energy, and practicing t'ai chi is said to increase and promote the flow of *qi* throughout the body. T'ai chi combines 13 postures with elements of other stress-relieving techniques, such as exercise, meditation, and deep breathing. Research has shown that t'ai chi is beneficial in combating stress, although exactly how it works is unclear. You can take t'ai chi classes in a group setting, although these are not as widely available as yoga classes. Using instructional videos to learn t'ai chi is another option.

Certain dietary supplements are advertised as anti-stress aids, but, like other supplements, they aren't reg-ulated by the FDA. Research on their effectiveness and safety is often weak or nonexistent. The herbal supplement kava kava, for example, is advertised as relieving anxiety and stress, but it may also cause severe liver damage. The hormone supplement DHEA is also promoted as relieving stress, since in its natural state it counteracts cortisol in the body. However, it isn't clear whether taking DHEA in supplement form produces the same effect. B-complex vitamins are often advertised as stress-busters because stress saps the body of B vitamins. But if you're not deficient in this vitamin, taking more of it won't help you. Similarly, zinc, which supports the immune system, is promoted as a stress reliever, but any direct connection between taking supplemental zinc and stress relief has not been proved. Before taking any dietary supplement for stress relief, check with your health care professional.

If you're coping with the death of a parent or adjusting to the drug addiction of a close friend, you might benefit from joining a support group. Such groups provide an open, safe environment for you to discuss your problems with counselors and others who have had, or are going through, similar experiences. To find out about support groups near you, go to www.211.org, which has listings of various support groups in major U.S. cities, or check your phone directory for local listings.

Sources: "Health Benefits, Tai Chi Linked," April 2004, *Tufts e-News;* "Yoga in San Diego," by Maya Kroth, April 2005, *SignOn SanDiego.com* (Union Tribune).

with meditation, while others need a more active stress reduction method and might choose exercise. As you review the methods described in the following pages, consider how they might fit with your personality and lifestyle. Experiment with a few methods—and try something new—before you settle on something you think will work for you. (See the box "Selecting a Stress Management Approach.") Whatever methods you choose, we recommend practicing them on a regular basis. They will become second nature to you and part of your everyday life. They will be available during stressful moments and may even be activated naturally. Remember that skills can be improved and beliefs can be modified—which means that you have the power to manage most stressful moments.

Sometimes stressful events and situations are overwhelming, and your resources and coping abilities are insufficient to support you. These times call for professional help. Don't hesitate to visit your college counseling center or avail yourself of other resources if you find that you need more support.

Stress Reduction Strategies

Any activity that decreases the number or lessens the effect of stressors is a stress reduction technique. Although you might not think of avoidance as an effective coping strategy, sometimes protecting yourself from unnecessary stressors makes sense. For example, try not listening to the news for a few days. You'll find that world events continue as always without your participation. If certain people in your life consistently trigger negative feelings in you, try not seeing them for a while. When you do see them, you may have a better perspective on your interpersonal dynamics. If you have too many activities going on in your life, assert your right to say no to the next request for your time. Downscaling and simplifying your life are effective ways of alleviating stress.

In addition to these simple techniques, two powerful stress reduction strategies are practicing time management and bolstering your social support system.

Time Management

One of the most difficult tasks of adult life is using time well—finding a balance between the things you have to do and the things you want to do. Sometimes people spend time in a frenzy of activity but end up achieving little. Often they spend time on the wrong tasks and never get to the things that matter. They may be overcommitted and overscheduled; they may procrastinate, or always be running late. All of these time-related behaviors and outcomes are stressful.

Time management is the topic of seminars and books, and some experts have devoted their entire careers to helping people learn how to manage their time. Here, we focus on two key points: planning and prioritizing. In time management, it has been noted that typically 80 percent of unfocused effort generates only 20 percent of results. The remaining 20 percent of effort produces 80 percent of results. In other words, people spend most of their time on the wrong tasks. You may be focusing on the wrong tasks if you're spending time on things you are not very good at or the tasks are taking much longer than you expected. You may be focusing on the right tasks if you're engaged in activities that advance your overall purpose in life; if you're doing things you have always wanted to do or that make you feel good about yourself; or if you're working on tasks you don't like, but you're doing them knowing they relate to the bigger picture.[36]

To make sure you focus on the things that matter to you, think about your goals in life and what you want to achieve. Are they worthy of your time? Obviously, you need time for sleeping, working, studying, and so on, but remember to allow yourself time for maintaining wellness through such activities as relaxing, playing, and spending time with family and friends. A global picture of your goals and priorities provides a framework and perspective that can give you a sense of control and reduce stress.

When you want to manage your time on the everyday level, keep a daily "to do" list and prioritize the items on it. Write the items down, because it's stressful to just keep them in your head! As you look at the list, assign each task a priority. Is it something you must get done today, such as turning in a paper? Is it something you would like to get done, such as catching up on the week's reading? Is it something that can wait until tomorrow, such as buying a new pair of jeans? Then organize the items into these three categories. Complete the tasks in the first category first, before moving on to tasks in the other two categories. This approach will help you be more purposeful, organized, and efficient about the use of your time, giving you more of a sense of control in your life.

In the course of evaluating your goals and prioritizing your daily tasks, you may find that you have too many commitments, an issue discussed earlier in the chapter. Try thinking about this issue in terms of your commitments to yourself: How can you best honor and take care of yourself? If you are stressed out because you are breaking your commitments, you have three choices: Don't make the commitments (lower your expectations), keep the commitments (get busy and work efficiently to wrap them up), or reframe

Time management is an effective stress prevention strategy. Are you budgeting your time well and meeting or beating your deadlines?

the commitments (constantly review and make intelligent choices about what you can and should be doing at any particular moment). Trying to do more than you have time for and doing the wrong things in the time you have are stressful. Managing your time well is a key to reducing stress.

Social Support

Another key to reducing stress, just as it is a key to mental health (Chapter 3) and to a meaningful spiritual life (Chapter 4), is social support. Numerous studies show that social support decreases the stress response hormones in the body. Dr. Dean Ornish points out that people who have close relationships and a strong sense of connection and community enjoy better health and live longer than do those who live in isolation. People who suffer alone suffer a lot.[37]

Many of us lack the sense of belonging and community that were provided by the extended family and closer-knit society of our grandparents' day. You may have to consciously create a social support system to overcome isolation and loneliness and buffer yourself from stress. The benefits make the effort worthwhile. They include a shoulder to lean on and an ear to listen when you need support. Communicating about your feelings reduces stress and helps you to work through problems and feel better about yourself.

The best way to develop a support system is to give support to others, establishing relationships and building trust. Cultivate a variety of types of relationships. Stay in touch with your friends, especially when you know they're going through a hard time, and keep your family ties strong. Find people who share your interests and pursue activities together, whether it's hiking, dancing, or seeing classic movies. You may want to join a group with a goal that interests you, such as a church group, a study group, or a book club. Try to get involved with your community and participate in activities that benefit others. Maintain and improve your communication skills—both listening to other people's feelings and sharing your own. When you have a network of relationships and a community to belong to, you will be able to cope with the stress of life more effectively. And when you need support, you will have a connection that can be reciprocated comfortably.

Maintaining a Healthy Lifestyle

A healthy lifestyle is an essential component of any stress management program. A nutritious diet helps you care for your body and keep you at your best. Experts recommend emphasizing whole grains, vegetables, and fruits in the diet and avoiding excessive amounts of caffeine. Getting enough sleep is also essential for wellness, as are opportunities for relaxation and fun.

Exercise is probably the most popular and most effective "stress buster" available. It has a positive effect on both physical and mental functioning and helps people withstand stress. Regular exercisers are also less likely to use smoking, drinking, or overeating as methods for reducing

their levels of stress.[38] A growing body of evidence suggests that regular exercise is the best thing you can do to protect yourself from the effects of stress. All of these components of a healthy lifestyle—nutrition, sleep, exercise, and more—are discussed in detail in separate chapters in this book.

Relaxation Techniques

If you are in a state of chronic stress and the relaxation response does not happen naturally, it is in your best interest to learn how to induce it. Relaxation techniques seem to have an effect on a number of physiological functions, including blood pressure, heart rate, and muscle tension. Here we describe just a few of the many techniques that have been developed.

Deep Breathing

One relaxation tool that is simple and always available is breathing. When you feel yourself starting to experience the stress response, you can simply remember to breathe deeply. As you learn to be aware of breathing patterns and practice slowing that process, your mind and body will begin to relax. Breathing exercises have been found to be effective in reducing panic attacks, muscle tension, headaches, and fatigue.

To practice deep breathing, inhale through your nose slowly and deeply through the count of 10. Don't just raise your shoulders and chest; allow your abdomen to expand as well. Exhale very slowly through your nose and concentrate fully on your breath as you let it out. Try to repeat this exercise a number of times during the day even when you're not feeling stressed. Once it becomes routine, you can use it to help you relax before an exam or in any stressful situation.

Progressive Relaxation

Progressive muscle relaxation was developed by Edmund Jacobson in 1929 as a tool to reduce stress.[39] The technique is based on the premise that deliberate muscle relaxation will block the muscle tension that is part of the stress response, thus reducing overall levels of stress. Progressive relaxation has provided relief when used to treat such stress-related symptoms as neck and back pain and high blood pressure.

To practice progressive muscle relaxation, find a quiet place and lie down in a comfortable position without crossing your arms or legs. Maintain a slow breathing pattern while you tense each muscle or muscle group as tightly as possible for 10 seconds before releasing it. Begin by making a fist with one hand, holding it, and then releasing it. Notice the difference between the tensed state and the relaxed state, and allow your muscles to remain relaxed. Continue with your other hand, your arms, shoulders, neck, and so on, moving around your entire body. Don't forget your ears, forehead, mouth, and all the muscles of your face. If you take the time to relax your body this way, the technique will provide significant relief from stress. You will also find that once your body learns the process, you will be able to relax your muscles quickly on command during moments of stress.

Meditation

Research indicates that meditation can help people deal with a variety of medical problems, including chronic pain and symptoms of stress. Sitting quietly, undisturbed by the distractions of life, induces the relaxation response and provides a respite from stress.[40] There is nothing magical about meditation; it is primarily a learned technique for calming the mind and relaxing the body. Its effectiveness, however, depends on commitment and practice. If you are interested in trying meditation, refer to Chapter 4 for a more detailed discussion.

Visualization

Also called *guided imagery*, visualization is the mental creation of visual images and scenes. Because our thoughts have such a powerful influence on our reactions, simply imagining a relaxing scene can bring about the relaxation response.[41] Visualization can be used alone or in combination with other techniques such as deep breathing and meditation to help reduce stress, tension, and anxiety.

To try visualization, sit or lie in a quiet place. Imagine yourself in a soothing, peaceful scene, one that you find particularly relaxing—a quiet beach, a garden, an alpine meadow. Try to visualize all you would see there as vividly as you can, scanning the scene. Bring in your other senses; what sounds do you hear, what scents do you smell? Is the sun warm, the breeze gentle? If you can imagine the scene fully, your body will respond as if you were really there. Commercial tapes are also available that use guided imagery to promote relaxation, but because imagery is personal and subjective, you may need to be selective in finding a tape that works for you.

Yoga

The ancient practice of yoga is rooted in Hindu philosophy, with physical, mental, and spiritual components. It is a consciously performed activity involving posture, breath, and body and mind awareness. In the path and practice of yoga, the aim is to calm the mind, cleanse the body, and raise awareness. The outcomes of this practice include a release of mental and physical tension and the attainment of a relaxed state.

The most widely practiced form of yoga in the Western world is hatha yoga. The practitioner assumes a number of different postures, or poses, holding them while stretching, breathing, and balancing. They are performed slowly and gently, with focused attention. Yoga stretching improves flexibility as well as muscular strength and endurance. However, for yoga to be effective, the poses have to be performed correctly. If you are interested in trying yoga, we recommend that you begin by taking a class with a certified instructor. There are also commercial videos that can get you started.

Biofeedback

Biofeedback is a kind of relaxation training that involves the use of special equipment to provide feedback on the body's physiological functions. You receive information about your heart rate, breathing, skin temperature, and other autonomic nervous system activities and thus become more aware of exactly what is happening in your body during both the relaxation response and the stress response. Once you have this heightened awareness, you can use relaxation techniques at the first sign of the stress response in daily life. Biofeedback can be used to reduce tension headaches, chronic muscle pain, hypertension, and anxiety.[42] If you are interested in trying biofeedback, check with your school to see if the special equipment and training are available.

We have provided just a sampling of relaxation techniques; there are many others, including massage, t'ai chi ch'uan, and hypnosis. Many people develop their own relaxation strategies, such as listening to soothing music, going for walks in a beautiful natural setting, or enjoying the company of a pet. Whatever your preferences, learn to incorporate some peaceful moments into your day, every day. You will experience an improved quality of life today and a better chance of avoiding stress-related illness in the future.

You Make the Call

Should Stress Reduction Programs Be Covered by Health Insurance?

Imagine this scene: You lead a stressful, complex life, and lately you have been experiencing a lot of anxiety. You find it hard to unwind at the end of the day and even harder to fall asleep. You've been feeling tense and nervous, and you realize it's time to get a better handle on your stress level. So the next time you see your regular physician, you mention that you sometimes feel overwhelmed by the stress in your life. Your physician's first response is to offer some medication you could take to reduce anxiety. You're not sure you want to take drugs, though, so you ask if she can recommend some other approach, such as a stress management program. She says there are such programs, and in fact the clinic has a biofeedback training program, but it is not covered by your health insurance plan. She also mentions yoga classes and meditation groups—again, not covered by your insurance plan.

This is a fairly common scenario in many medical offices. Physicians often advise their patients to quit smoking, lose weight, exercise more, and engage in other health promotion activities that will improve their overall quality of life and reduce their effects on the health care system later in their lives. Numerous programs exist that help people make these difficult lifestyle changes. Some are commercial programs, and some are part of health promotion activities offered by clinics, hospitals, and other health care facilities. Most of them are not covered by health insurance.

The health promotion industry argues that getting people involved in taking care of their own health can result in improved quality of life and a reduction in overall health care costs. Recently, with overweight and obesity identified as major health problems for the nation, some have suggested that health insurance companies cover the cost of weight loss programs. Given the cost to the nation of stress-related illnesses, injuries, and accidents, a similar case can be made for the coverage of stress reduction programs.

Insurance companies argue that their mandate is to pay medical expenses for people who are sick, not cover the cost of health promotion activities for people who are well. They also argue that most health promotion programs have not been proven effective by broad-based, high-quality research; most have not been studied at all. Without a research base, they cannot distinguish an effective stress reduction program from an ineffective one.

Decisions about these issues will affect public policy concerning coverage of health promotion and wellness activities in the future. What do you think?

Pros

○ Participation in a stress reduction program can improve a person's quality of life.

○ Individuals in such programs may get sick less often and may be at lower risk for chronic diseases such as cancer and heart disease. They may use the health care system less frequently.

○ Such programs may contribute to a reduction in overall health care costs for the nation.

Cons

○ Health insurance should cover only treatments for illness.

○ Health promotion/stress reduction programs have not been proven to be effective.

○ It is a slippery slope: If we cover these programs, where will it stop?

OLC Web site For more information on this topic, visit the Online Learning Center at www.mhhe.com/teague1e.

SUMMARY

- Stress is an everyday part of our lives, something we experience as our bodies and minds continually adjust to the demands of living.

- Stressors are events or agents in the environment that cause stress.

- Individuals respond differently to stressors, depending on such variables as past experiences, personality traits, and how they perceive or appraise the stressors. Stress can be thought of as a transaction between an individual and an event, mediated by personal variables.

- If you perceive a stressor as positive, you experience eustress. If you perceive it as negative, you experience distress.

- During the stress response, the body goes through physiological changes that prepare you to fight or flee. The sympathetic branch of the autonomic nervous system activates the stress response; the parasympathetic branch deactivates it and initiates the relaxation response.

- The body is equipped to handle acute stress if it doesn't occur too often; it is not so well equipped to handle chronic stress.

- Hans Selye developed the General Adaptation Syndrome, a description of the body's response to stressors over time. He proposed that stress affects the immune system and can lead to illness and disease.

- Stress also affects the cardiovascular system, the digestive system, and just about every other part of the body and mind.

- Some personality patterns seem to place people at greater risk for stress-related illness, including heart disease. Individuals with Type A personality traits, especially anger and hostility, are at greater risk than are the more relaxed Type Bs.

- Such cognitive factors as illogical thinking, unrealistic expectations, and negative beliefs can make events more stressful than they need to be.

- The qualities of resilience and hardiness seem to protect people from the negative effects of stress.

- Major life events are a common source of stress in life, making people more vulnerable to symptoms of illness and disease. When daily hassles pile up, people also become more vulnerable to illness.

- Other sources of stress include time pressure, the pressures of work and school, relationships, financial worries, illness, societal issues, and major traumatic events.
- Because chronic stress can impair health, part of maintaining wellness is learning how to reduce and manage stress.
- Two effective approaches to reducing stress are learning how to manage your time and maintaining a social support system.

- Maintaining a healthy lifestyle—eating well, exercising, getting enough sleep, avoiding tobacco and drugs—is a critical aspect of overall stress management.
- Relaxation techniques include deep breathing, progressive relaxation, meditation, visualization, yoga, and biofeedback.
- Responses to stress are individual and so are ways to manage stress. Every person needs to discover and develop approaches to stress management that can be used effectively over a lifetime.

REVIEW QUESTIONS

1. What is the difference between stress and stressors?
2. What physiological changes occur in the body when the stress response is activated? What is the purpose of each of these changes?
3. What physiological changes occur in the body when the relaxation response is initiated?
4. Why is chronic stress hard on the body?
5. Describe and explain the General Adaptation Syndrome.
6. Describe some common symptoms of stress in the body and mind.
7. Why are personal variables like personality traits important in mediating the stress response?
8. What are some differences between individuals with Type A and Type B behavior patterns? What are the characteristics of people with the Type C behavior pattern?

9. How can patterns of thinking affect a person's response to a stressor in the environment? Give examples of an illogical thought and a negative belief.
10. Describe some characteristics of a person who is resilient and of a person who is hardy. How might these characteristics protect people against the health effects of stress?
11. What are some examples of major life events? How might they contribute to a person's vulnerability to illness?
12. Describe some sources of stress listed in the chapter. Why do they contribute to chronic stress?
13. Describe two approaches to stress reduction, and explain why they work.
14. Describe three relaxation techniques, and explain why they lower stress levels.

WEB RESOURCES

American Institute of Stress: This organization is a clearinghouse for information on all stress-related topics. Its monthly newsletter, *Health and Stress,* presents the latest advances in stress research and related health issues.
www.stress.org

American Psychological Association: Offering a variety of psychological topics, this site presents current information on stress. Its news section, quick links, and consumer help center are helpful features.
www.apa.org

Harvard Mind-Body Medical Institute: Highlighting the work of Herbert Benson, M.D., author of *The Relaxation Response,* this organization presents information on mind/body basics and wellness. It offers ways to deal with stress in everyday life.
www.mbmi.org

Medical Basis for Stress: This site presents practical approaches to dealing with stress in all aspects of life. It offers tips related to

nutrition and exercise, checklists to keep you on track, and rules to live by to reduce your stress level.
www.teachhealth.com

National Institute of Mental Health (NIMH): This organization takes a scientific approach to various mental health topics, including stress. Its breaking news feature and its highlights section are of particular interest.
www.nimh.nih.gov

National Institute for Occupational Safety and Health (NIOSH): A valuable resource for information about stress at work, this site focuses on understanding the influence of organizations and psychosocial factors on stress, illness, and injury. It also aims to find ways of redesigning jobs to create safer and healthier workplaces.
www.cdc.gov/niosh/topics/stress

REFERENCES

1. Hafen, B. Q., Karren, K. J., Frandsen, K. J., & Smith, N. L. (1996). *Mind/body health: The effects of attitudes, emotions, and relationships.* Boston: Allyn & Bacon.

2. Blonna, R. (2005). *Coping with stress in a changing world* (3rd ed.). New York: McGraw-Hill.

3. Benson, H. (1993). The relaxation response. In D. P. Goleman & J. Gurin (Eds.), *Mind-body medicine: How to use your mind for better health* (pp. 233–257). Yonkers, NY: Consumer Reports Books.

4. Selye, H. (1956). *The stress of life.* New York: McGraw-Hill.

5. Stress: It is deadly. (2005). Holisticonline.com.

6. Kiecolt-Glaser, J. K., et al. (2002). Psychoneuroimmunology: Psychological influences on immune function and health. *Journal of Consulting and Clinical Psychology 70,* 537–547.

7. Segerstrom, S. C., & Miller, G. E. (2004). Psychological stress and the human immune system: A meta-analytic study of 30 years of inquiry. *Psychological Bulletin, 130* (4), 610–630.

8. Everly, G. S., & Lating, J. M. (2002). *A clinical guide to the treatment of the human stress response* (2nd ed.). Amsterdam: Kluwer Academic Publishers.

9. National Institute of Mental Health Fact Sheet. Facts on cancer and depression. (2002). www.nimh.nih.gov.

10. Wittstein, I. S., et al. (2005). Neurohumoral features of myocardial stunning due to sudden emotional stress. *New England Journal of Medicine, 352* (6), 539–548.

11. Girdano, D. A., Dusek, D. E., & Everly, G. S., Jr. (2005). *Controlling stress and tension* (7th ed.). San Francisco: Benjamin Cummings.

12. Whitehead, W. E. (1993). Gut feelings: Stress and the GI tract. In D. P. Goleman & J. Gurin (Eds.), *Mind-body medicine: How to use your mind for better health* (pp. 161–176). Yonkers, NY: Consumer Reports Books.

13. Greenberg, J. S. (2006). *Comprehensive stress management* (9th ed.). New York: McGraw-Hill.

14. American Psychiatric Association. (2000). *Diagnostic and statistical manual of mental disorders* (4th ed., Text Revision [*DSM-IV-TR*]). Washington, DC: American Psychiatric Association Press.

15. Friedman, M., & Rosenman, R. H. (1982). *Type A behavior and your heart.* New York: Fawcett Books.

16. Williams, R. (1989). *The trusting heart: Great news about type A behavior.* New York: Random House.

17. Seligman, M. (1998). *Learned optimism: How to change your mind and your life.* New York: Pocket Books.

18. Kobasa, S. O. (1984, September). How much stress can you survive? *American Health,* 71–72.

19. Maddi, S. (2002). The story of hardiness: Twenty years of theorizing, research and practice. *Consulting Psychology: Practice & Research, 54* (3), 175–185.

20. Holmes, T., & Rahe, R. (1967). The social readjustment rating scale. *Journal of Psychosomatic Research,* 11, 213–218.

21. Weinberger, M., Heines, S. L., & Tierney, W. M. (1987). In support of hassles as a measure of stress in predicting health outcomes. *Journal of Behavioral Medicine, 10* (1), 19–32.

22. Brod, C. (1984). *Techno Stress: The human cost of the computer revolution.* Boston: Addison-Wesley.

23. Gleick, J. (2000). *Faster: The acceleration of just about everything.* New York: Vintage Books.

24. Pines, A. M. (1993). Burnout, an existential perspective. In W. B. Schaufeli, C. Maslach, & T. Marek (Eds.), *Professional burnout: Recent developments in theory and research.* Philadelphia: Taylor & Francis.

25. Posig, M., & Kickul, J. (2003). Extending our understanding of burnout: Test of an integrated model in nonservice occupations. *Journal of Occupational Health Psychology, 8* (1), 3–19.

26. Janicak, C. A. (2003). Regional variations in workplace homicide rates. www.bls.gov.

27. Greenberg, J. (1984). A study of the effects of stress on the health of college students: Implications for school health education. *Health Education, 15,* 11–15.

28. Greenberg, J. (1981). A study of stressors in the college student population. *Health Education, 12,* 8–12.

29. Reisberg, L. (2000, January 18). Students' stress is rising, especially among young women. *Chronicle of Higher Education,* A49–A52.

30. Gose, B. (2000, February 25). Elite colleges struggle to prevent student suicides. *Chronicle of Higher Education,* A54–A55.

31. Williams, J. E., et al. (2000, May). Anger proneness predicts coronary heart disease risk. *Circulation, 101,* 2034–2039.

32. Lyons, A. (2003). Economic downturns impact health. http://web.aces.uiuc.edu.

33. Miller, G. E. (2002, November). Chronic psychological stress and the regulation of pro-inflammatory cytokines: A glucocorticoid-resistance model. *Health Psychology, 21,* 6.

34. Meyer, I. H. (2003). Prejudice, social stress, and mental health in lesbian, gay and bisexual populations: Conceptual issues and research evidence. *Psychological Bulletin, 129* (5), 674–697.

35. Shay, J. (1996, July/August). Shattered lives. *Family Therapy Networker,* pp. 46–54.

36. Vaccaro, P. (2000, September). The 80/20 principle of time management. *Family Practice Management.*

37. Ornish, D. (1998). *Love and survival: 8 pathways to intimacy and health.* New York: Harper Perennial.

38. Sacks, M. H. (1993). Exercise for stress control. In D. P. Goleman & J. Gurin (Eds.), *Mind-body medicine: How to use your mind for better health* (pp. 315–327). Yonkers, NY: Consumer Reports Books.

39. Jacobson, E. (1974). *Progressive relaxation: A physiological and clinical investigation of muscular states and their significance in psychology and medical practice* (3rd ed.). Chicago: University of Chicago Press.

40. Kabat-Zinn, J. (1990). *Full catastrophic living: Using the wisdom of your body and mind to face stress, pain, and illness.* New York: Delta.

41. Davis, M., McKay, M., & Eshelman, E. R. (2000). *The relaxation and stress reduction workbook* (5th ed.). Oakland, CA: New Harbinger Publications.

42. Schwartz, M., & Andrasik, F. (Eds.). (2003). *Biofeedback: A practitioner's guide* (3rd ed.). New York: Guilford Publications.

Add It Up!   STUDENT STRESS SCALE

This adaptation of the Holmes-Rahe Social Readjustment Scale has been modified to apply to young adults. If you have experienced any of the events listed here in the last 12 months, check that item.

1. Death of a close family member _____ 100
2. Death of a close friend _____ 73
3. Divorce between parents _____ 65
4. Jail term _____ 63
5. Major personal injury or illness _____ 63
6. Marriage _____ 58
7. Firing from a job _____ 50
8. Failure of an important course _____ 47
9. Change in health of a family member ✓ 45
10. Pregnancy _____ 45
11. Sex problems _____ 44
12. Serious argument with close friend _____ 40
13. Change in financial status _____ 39
14. Change of major ✓ 39
15. Trouble with parents _____ 39
16. New girlfriend or boyfriend _____ 37
17. Increase in workload at school ✓ 37
18. Outstanding personal achievement _____ 36
19. First quarter/semester in college _____ 36
20. Change in living conditions ✓ 31

21. Serious argument with an instructor _____ 30
22. Lower grades than expected ✓ 29
23. Change in sleeping habits _____ 29
24. Change in social activities _____ 29
25. Change in eating habits ✓ 28
26. Chronic car trouble _____ 26
27. Change in the number of family get-togethers _____ 26
28. Too many missed classes _____ 25
29. Change of college ✓ 24
30. Dropping of more than one class _____ 23
31. Minor traffic violations _____ 20

TOTAL _____

Scoring

Now total your points. A score of 300 or more is considered high and puts you at risk for developing a serious stress-related health problem. A score between 150 and 300 is considered moderately high, giving you about a 50-50 chance of developing a stress-related health problem. Even a score below 150 puts you at some risk for stress-related illness. If you do have an accumulation of stressful life events, you can improve your chances of staying well by practicing stress management and relaxation techniques, as described in this chapter.

SOURCES: Adapted from "The Social Readjustment Rating Scale," by T. E. Holmes and R. H. Rahe, 1967, *Journal of Psychosomatic Research, 11,* 213; *Core Concepts in Health,* 4th ed., by P. M. Insel and W. T. Roth, 1985, Palo Alto, CA: Mayfield.

CHAPTER 6

Sleep: Renewal and Restoration

DID YOU KNOW?

- If you sometimes have trouble falling asleep, you're not alone. Some 40 million Americans report that they have a chronic sleep problem, and another 20 to 30 million report intermittent sleep problems. Sleep deprivation and sleep disorders cost Americans an estimated $100 billion per year in lost productivity, medical expenses, sick leave, and property and environmental damage.[1]

- If you do not get enough sleep on a regular basis, you may find yourself feeling drowsy behind the wheel of your car. More than half of all Americans say they sometimes drive while drowsy, and nearly one in five say they have actually fallen asleep at the wheel.

OLC *Your Health Today*   www.mhhe.com/teague1e

Go to the Online Learning Center for *Your Health Today* for interactive activities, quizzes, flashcards, Web links, and more resources related to this chapter.

Do you frequently feel sleepy in the afternoon? Do you often drop off while watching television? Does it take only a couple of minutes to fall asleep after you get into bed? If you answered yes to these questions, you are probably experiencing sleep deprivation. And you are not alone. According to the 2003 Sleep in America Poll[2] conducted by the National Sleep Foundation (NSF), many Americans are not sleeping enough to sustain optimum health. Most adults need about 8 hours of sleep each night,[3] although there is some variation across individuals. More than two-thirds of the poll's respondents—adults aged 18 to 54—reported sleeping less than 8 hours on weekdays, and nearly one-third said they slept less than 7 hours. On average, the respondents reported sleeping about 6 ½ hours on weekdays and 7 ½ hours on weekends.

Many people are unaware of the vital role that adequate sleep plays in good health. In this chapter we explore the importance of sleep and the negative effects of sleep deprivation. We also examine the nature of sleep—the cyclic rhythms of sleeping and waking that we experience every 24 hours and the complex structure of sleep itself. We then consider some of the more common sleep problems and disorders, and we conclude the chapter with a number of tips and strategies for strengthening sleep habits and improving the quality of sleep.

SLEEP AND YOUR HEALTH

Sleep is commonly understood as a period of rest and recovery from the demands of wakefulness. It can also be described as a state of unconsciousness or partial consciousness from which a person can be roused by stimulation (as distinguished from a coma, for example). All mammals and birds sleep, but scientists aren't sure about whether other organisms experience sleep as we understand it. It appears that the smaller a mammal or bird is, the more sleep it requires: A cat sleeps about 14 hours a day, a monkey about 9, a horse only about 2 ½ hours.[4] As noted, humans require, on average, 8 hours of sleep a night.

We spend about one-third of our lives sleeping, a fact that in itself indicates how important sleep is. In this section we consider the positive health effects of sleep and the negative consequences of sleep deprivation.

Health Effects of Sleep

Research indicates that getting adequate sleep is critical to the maintenance of good health. During the deepest stages of sleep, restoration and growth take place. Proteins and hormones that repair organs and organ systems are released, blood supply to the muscles is increased, body temperature is lowered to conserve energy, metabolic activity slows to facilitate tissue growth and repair, and the secretion of growth hormone reaches its peak. Growth hormone stimulates the growth and repair of the body's tissues and helps to prevent certain types of cancer. Natural immune system moderators also increase during deep sleep to promote resistance to viral infections. When sleep time is deficient, a breakdown in the body's health-promoting processes can occur.[3,5–7]

Sleep Deprivation

Most of us know what it feels like when we don't get enough sleep—we feel drowsy, our eyes burn, we find it hard to pay attention. The effects of **sleep deprivation** can be much more serious than this, however. Studies have shown that individuals with severe sleep deprivation (staying awake for 19 to 24 hours, for example) score worse on performance tests and alertness scales than do people with a blood alcohol content (BAC) of 0.1 percent—legally too drunk to drive.

A sleep-deprived driver can be as dangerous on the road as a drunk driver. Alertness, reaction time, and coordination are all affected by lack of sleep, sometimes with fatal consequences.

Sleep deprivation has effects in all domains of functioning. Heightened irritability, lowered anger threshold, frustration, nervousness, and difficulty handling stress are some of the emotional effects. Reduced motivation may affect school and job performance, and lack of interest in socializing with others may cause relationships to suffer. Performance of daily activities is affected, as is the brain's ability to learn new material. Reaction time, coordination, and judgment are all impaired. The body is more susceptible to infections, and pain can intensify because of the physical and mental consequences of poor sleep quality. Individuals who are sleep deprived may experience microsleeps—brief episodes of sleep lasting a few seconds at a time—which increase their risk of being involved in accidents.[5,8,9–12]

Recent research has indicated that women who sleep only 6 hours a night have an 18 percent higher risk of heart attack than do women who sleep 8 hours a night. Other studies found that people who sleep less than 8 hours a night have a higher incidence of hormone-mediated conditions, including diabetes and thyroid disorders. There may also be an association between lack of sleep and being overweight, although the mechanism for this connection is still unknown. It could be that the more hours a person is awake, the higher that person's caloric needs are; or it could be that lack of sleep disrupts regulation of body temperature and more calories are needed to correct it. Other possible explanations are that lack of sleep leads to hormonal irregularities, which in turn contribute to overweight, or that being awake more hours simply offers more time for eating.[13,14]

How can you tell if you are getting enough sleep? A prime symptom of sleep deprivation is daytime drowsiness. Thirty-seven percent of adults report that daytime drowsiness is a problem, and nearly 10 percent report experiencing daytime drowsiness a few days a week.[3] If you feel alert during the day, you are probably getting enough sleep. If you are sleepy in sedentary situations such as reading, sitting in class, or watching television, you may be sleep deprived. Another measure of sleep deprivation is how long it takes you to fall asleep at night. A well-rested person will need 15 to 20 minutes to fall asleep.[3] If you fall asleep the instant your head hits the pillow, there is a good chance that you are sleep deprived.

Sleep Debt

Each of us maintains a sleep bank account. The hours that you sleep are deposits to this account; the hours of wakefulness are withdrawals. As noted, most adults need to deposit 8 hours of sleep each night to meet the demands of 16 hours of wakefulness. Deposits of less than 8 hours cause a **sleep debt.**[15]

Your sleep debt accumulates over time, so that sleeping 1 hour less than you need every night for a week, for example, feels to your body like staying up all night. College students are especially vulnerable to building up a sleep debt, such as by pulling an all-nighter to prepare for an exam. (See the box "Alert Drugs: Prescription for an All-Nighter?") Many college students and others who build up a sleep debt during the week—night-shift workers and airline personnel, for example—try to cancel the debt by sleeping more on the weekends. This "solution," however, can actually worsen sleep deprivation during the week by disrupting sleep structure.[3,16,17] Getting the same sufficient amount of sleep each night strengthens sleep structure.

WHAT MAKES YOU SLEEP?

Sleep and waking generally occur in accordance with **circadian rhythms,** daily 24-hour cycles of physiological and behavioral functioning. Over the course of this daily period, your body undergoes rhythmic changes that help you move from waking to sleep and back to waking.

Circadian rhythms are maintained primarily by two tiny structures in the brain, the *suprachiasmatic nuclei* (SCN), located directly behind the optic nerve in the hypothalamus. This internal "biological clock" controls body temperature and levels of alertness and activity. These controls are active in the daytime, increasing wakefulness, and inactive at night, allowing the body to relax and sleep. They are also less active in the early afternoon. In addition, the SCN control the release of certain hormones. They signal the pineal gland to release **melatonin,** a hormone that increases relaxation and sleepiness, and they signal the pituitary gland to release growth hormone during sleep, to help repair damaged body tissues.

Also important in maintaining circadian rhythms are external, environmental cues, especially light. Neurons in the SCN monitor the amount of light entering the eyes, so that as daylight increases, the SCN slow down the secretion of melatonin and begin to be more active.[11] This

KEY TERMS

sleep Period of rest and recovery from the demands of wakefulness, experienced by all mammals and birds; a state of unconsciousness or partial consciousness from which a person can be roused by stimulation.

sleep deprivation Lack of sufficient time asleep, a condition that impairs physical, emotional, and cognitive functioning.

sleep debt The difference between the amount of sleep attained and the amount needed to maintain alert wakefulness during the daytime, when the amount attained is less than the amount needed.

circadian rhythms Daily 24-hour cycles of physiological and behavioral functioning.

melatonin A hormone that increases relaxation and sleepiness, released by the pineal gland during sleep.

Consumer Clipboard

Alert Drugs: Prescription for an All-Nighter?

When an exam is coming up or a paper is due, most college students reach for coffee, Mountain Dew, or Red Bull to help them stay awake. But a growing number of students are turning to prescription drugs to keep them going without sleep.

Ritalin is commonly prescribed for individuals with attention deficit hyperactivity disorder (ADHD). Although a stimulant, this drug produces a calming effect on those with ADHD. For those without ADHD, Ritalin offers a way to stay awake for long hours. Students can get extra pills from their friends with ADHD. Adderall is another stimulant used to treat patients with ADHD. It helps students stay awake for up to 48 hours straight but costs more than Ritalin.

Both Ritalin and Adderall have a downside, though. They increase the heart rate and elevate blood pressure. An overdose can be dangerous, even fatal. Anyone with heart problems should avoid these drugs. They can also be addictive—both physically and psychologically—and the long-term effects are still unknown. In January 2005, Canada took Adderall off the market because it was linked to 12 reports of death. Although still on the market in the United States, Adderall is currently being viewed with increased caution.

Recently, students have been turning to another drug to stay awake and alert. Provigil is classified as a wakefulness-promoting agent. It is used to combat daytime sleepiness in individuals with narcolepsy. Provigil targets a specific area of the brain, the hypothalamus, and therefore doesn't produce the "wired" feeling that Ritalin and Adderall do. Students are finding that they can stay awake for an additional 10 to 15 hours with very few side effects. Although not physically addictive, Provigil can cause psychological dependence. Long-term use may also cause sleep deprivation and weaken the immune system.

With the use of these drugs estimated at about 7 percent of college students in the United States and increasing, college administrators are concerned. Some colleges are offering time management workshops to teach students how to avoid the late-night syndrome. Some campus doctors won't prescribe these drugs for students. There's also the issue of illegality to consider. Taking someone else's prescription drug is a felony offense. Still, many students who use these drugs are sold on their benefits. Besides keeping them awake, they say, the drugs help them focus better, giving them an extra edge. Experts warn that the health risks are just not worth it. Their "prescription" for study aids? Get organized so you don't have to pull an all-nighter. Otherwise, stick with coffee or tea.

Sources: Data from "Seven Percent of College Students Have Used Prescription Stimulants for Nonmedical Purposes," 2005, www.news-medical.net; "Staying Alert With Drugs," by N. Sowti, 2005, www.ucfnews.com; FDA information sheets on Ritalin, Adderall, and Provigil, "FDA Public Advisory for Adderall and AdderallXR," "Statement on Adderall," U.S. Food and Drug Administration, 2005, www.fda.gov.

process keeps your sleep/wake cycles generally synchronized with the changing lengths of day and night. The process is sensitive to artificial light as well as natural light, and even relatively dim lights in the evening (for example, from a lamp or a computer screen) may delay your biological clock from inducing sleepiness.

The biological clock operates even without the cues of daylight or darkness, though not in perfect synchrony with a 24-hour day. Without the stimulation of light and dark, human beings would have a daily cycle several minutes longer than 24 hours. Every morning your body resets your biological clock to adjust to the next 24-hour period.[3] Your body easily tolerates a 1-hour adjustment. However, when bedtimes and awakening times differ greatly from their established norms, the adjustment is more difficult. Working night shifts and flying across several time zones, for example, can play havoc with your biological clock.[12,18] (See the box "Dealing With Jet Lag.")

Another factor plays a role in cycles of sleep and waking: your body's need for a certain amount of sleep every 24 hours for recovery from the work of the day. Some experts believe that recovery involves the chemical *adenosine,* which accumulates in the body's cells during the day as a waste product of cellular activity. When levels of adenosine get too high, the brain gets the signal that it's time to slow down and go to sleep. Another way of saying this might be that sleep debt accumulates throughout the day until it triggers your biological clock to induce sleepiness.[3,19] During sleep, adenosine levels decrease, a process that helps your body feel refreshed and restored. The brain and body structures that are involved in producing sleep and wakefulness are shown in Figure 6.1.

Challenges & Choices

Dealing With Jet Lag

When you fly across multiple time zones, your body's internal wake/sleep cycle gets out of sync with the day/night cycle of your environment, a condition called *jet lag*. Common symptoms of jet lag include headache, fatigue, lethargy, irritability, depression, inattentiveness, and slow mental reactions. Less common symptoms include nausea, earache, and loss of appetite. If you have to fly long distances, use these strategies to reduce symptoms of jet lag:

- Select a flight that allows early evening arrival and stay up until 10:00 p.m. local time.

- If you must sleep during the day in your new location, take a short nap—no longer than 2 hours—in the early afternoon. Set an alarm so you don't oversleep.

- Anticipate the time change by getting up and going to bed earlier or later several days before a trip.

- Avoid alcohol or caffeine at least 3 to 4 hours before bedtime.

- When you arrive at your destination, avoid heavy meals.

- Avoid heavy exercise near bedtime. Light exercise earlier in the day is fine.

- Use earplugs and blindfolds to dampen noise and block light while sleeping.

- Go outside in the sunlight whenever possible. Daylight is a powerful regulator of your biological clock; staying indoors worsens symptoms of jet lag.

It's Not Just Personal . . .

It has been estimated that nearly half of all U.S. business travelers suffer from travel-related sleep difficulties. Another category of jet lag sufferers are elite athletes traveling to other continents for the Olympics.

Source: "Taking the Air out of Jet Lag," The National Sleep Foundation, 2002, www.sleepfoundation.org.

Retina (eye)
The job of the retina at the back of the eye is to sense changes in light levels during daytime and night. Once nerves in the retina are stimulated, the signal is sent through the optic nerve to the hypothalamus.

Suprachiasmic nuclei (SCN)
These two tiny neural structures are located in the hypothalamus and function as a master biological clock. By monitoring levels of light entering the eyes and managing body temperature, hormone release, and metabolic rate, the SCN control falling asleep and awakening.

Pineal gland
Regulated by the SCN, the pineal gland releases melatonin, a hormone that elicits drowsiness and sleep.

Pituitary gland
Also regulated by the SCN, the pituitary gland releases growth hormone during sleep to help repair damaged body tissues.

Pons
Located in the brain stem, the pons is active during REM sleep, when it signals nerves in the spine to immobilize the body to prevent movement during dreams.

Figure 6.1   Brain structures involved in sleep and waking.

THE STRUCTURE OF SLEEP

Researchers study sleep through *polysomnography,* the monitoring and measuring of several different physiological functions, including electrical activity in the brain, eye movement, and body movement, while their subjects are asleep. Studies have revealed that sleep consists of distinct stages in which muscle relaxation and nervous system arousal vary, as do types of brain waves and levels of neural activity. The brain cycles into two main states of sleep: non-rapid eye movement (NREM) sleep, divided into four stages, and rapid eye movement (REM) sleep.

NREM Sleep

You spend about 75 percent of your sleep time in **non-rapid eye movement sleep.** During this state, your brain activity slows considerably. When you are awake and alert, your brain produces electrical activity called *beta brain waves,* which are fast and low voltage. When you close your eyes to sleep, beta brain waves give way to slower *alpha brain waves.* You usually remain in the alpha brain wave state for several minutes. Then you enter a four-stage NREM sleep process that cycles throughout the night.

Stage 1 NREM

This stage is a transitional, light sleep—a relaxed or half-awake state. Your brain activity slows and produces mixed-frequency waves consisting of alpha and *theta brain waves.* You are falling asleep in this stage. Your heart rate slows and stabilizes, and your breathing becomes shallow and rhythmic. This stage may last from 10 seconds to 10 minutes and is sometimes accompanied by visual imagery. You may experience a sensation of falling and jerking awake for a moment as your muscles relax. You have a general awareness of your external environment. People awakened in stage 1 often deny that they were asleep.[15,19]

Stage 2 NREM

In stage 2, your brain's activity slows further, producing slower theta waves. These theta waves intermingle with *sleep spindles,* beta waves that display little bursts of brain activity. Sleep spindles represent a cascade of calcium into the motor cortex of the brain. You stop moving in bed about 7 ½ minutes before the sleep spindles appear. This lack of movement decreases muscle tension and brain stem stimulation so that sleep is induced. Stage 2 lasts about 10 to 20 minutes and represents the beginning of actual sleep. You are no longer consciously aware of your external environment. People awakened in stage 2 readily admit that they were asleep.[15,19]

Stages 3 and 4 NREM

These stages are also called *slow-wave sleep.* Stage 3 consists of a combination of theta and *delta brain waves.* Delta waves are very low frequency and high voltage.

Theta brain waves usually disappear within 5 to 15 minutes as you enter stage 4 (deep sleep). Your blood pressure drops, your heart rate and respiration slow, and the blood supply to your brain is minimized. If you were suddenly awakened during stage 4, you would feel momentarily groggy. You usually spend about 20 to 40 minutes at a time in deep sleep, and most of your deep sleep takes place in the first third of the night.[15,19]

REM Sleep

Rapid eye movement sleep begins about 70 to 90 minutes after you have fallen asleep. As you enter this stage, your breathing and heart rate increase, and brain wave activity becomes more like that of a waking state. REM sleep is characterized by noticeable eye movements, usually lasting between 1 and 10 minutes. During this period you are most likely to experience your first dream of the night. Although dreams may occur in all stages of sleep, they generally happen in REM sleep. Your eyes may dart around as though you are watching your dreams unfold.[3,15,20]

When you dream, there are periods when you have no muscle tone and your body cannot move, except for your eyes, diaphragm, nasal membranes, and erectile tissue (such as penis or clitoris).[3] This state is referred to as *REM sleep paralysis.* The pons, a mass of nerve fibers located at the base of the brain, is responsible for immobilizing the body during REM sleep by sending signals to the nerves in the spine (see Figure 6.1). If you were not immobilized, there is a danger that you would act on—or act out—your dreams. REM sleep is sometimes called *paradoxical sleep,* because the sleeper appears peaceful and still but is in a state of physiological arousal.

What Are Dreams?

People in every part of the world have long been interested in dreams, and the interpretation and meaning of dreams have been used in some cultures to guide both personal and community decisions. In many such cultures, dreams are seen as coming from outside the dreamer, from a supernatural source such as a dead ancestor or a divinity.

Probably the best known theory of dreams in Western culture is that of Sigmund Freud, who believed that the purpose of dreaming was the gratification of unconscious desires. By dreaming about them in disguised, symbolic form while we are sleeping, we fulfill wishes we would find unacceptable during waking life. At the opposite pole is a theory proposed in the 1970s that dreams are the product of random neural activity that goes on during REM sleep. Our memories and emotions provide stories that make some "sense" out of this neural activity, producing dreams. According to this theory, dreams have little or no meaning.[3]

Many people believe that dreams do have some meaning and relevance to daily life, often reflecting changes or shifts in emotions. By examining your dreams, according

HIGHLIGHT ON HEALTH
Interpreting Your Dreams

In her book *The Universal Dream Key,* Patricia Garfield identified 12 dream themes that commonly occur in every culture. Dream themes often represent changes in a person's daily life, particularly emotional shifts. Many dreams are negative in tone, conveying underlying difficult feelings. The following are the five most common negative dream themes and their associated feelings.

Dream Theme	Associated Feelings
1. Being chased or attacked	Threatened, harassed, anxious, fearful, emotionally hurt
2. Falling or drowning	Insecure, overwhelmed, helpless, hopeless, disconnected, without social support
3. Lost or trapped	Anxious, confused, helpless, uncertain
4. Naked or inappropriately dressed in public	Exposed, vulnerable, awkward, unencumbered, concealing weakness
5. Accidentally injured, ill, or dying	Fearful of impending physical risk, fearful of losing a loved one, without control, emotionally hurt, wishing someone would go away

Other dream themes include natural disasters, poor performance, having difficulty with a vehicle or with transportation, losing property or having damaged property, having difficulty operating a telephone or machine, and being menaced by an evil spirit. Children tend to dream more about animals, men more about sex, and women more about family and friends. Aggression is more likely to be physical (punching, chasing) in men's dreams and social or verbal (insulting, rejecting) in women's dreams.

Many people feel they can gain insight into their inner worlds by thinking about and interpreting their dreams. If you are interested in interpreting your dreams, try keeping a dream journal. Keep it by your bedside and remind yourself about it before you go to sleep. As soon as you awake and remember a dream, write it down in the journal. You may want to keep your eyes closed while you write so you can continue to be in the world of the dream and remember its details. Even if you don't remember any dreams at first, just having the journal by the side of your bed and reminding yourself may set the stage for better dream recall.

After you write down the dream, ask yourself what associations you have to its various elements. What pieces of your previous day or week might be showing up in the dream? What themes do you notice, and how do they relate to what's going on in your life? Are you trying to solve a problem in your dreams or work through a difficult situation or emotion? For more insight, try coming back to a dream during the day and thinking about it in a less direct, more intuitive way. If you are interested in pursuing dream interpretation, many books on the subject are available in bookstores and online.

Source: *The Universal Dream Key,* by P. Garfield, 2001, New York: HarperCollins.

to this view, you may gain insight into the mental and emotional processes you are applying to problems or events in your life. For more on working with your dreams, see the box "Interpreting Your Dreams."

REM Sleep and the Brain

REM sleep appears to give the brain the opportunity to "file" important ideas and thoughts in long-term storage, that is, in memory. Scientists speculate that because it is inefficient to store every piece of information in a file, we organize information into networks of associated ideas already in the brain during REM sleep. This reorganization and consolidation may account for the fact that we are able to solve problems in our dreams. Scientists further believe that creative and novel ideas are more likely to flourish during REM sleep, because we have easier access to memories and emotions. Because ideas are filed in long-term storage during REM sleep, memory may be impaired if sleep time is insufficient. As a result of such memory impairment, the ability to learn new skills is also

KEY TERMS

non-rapid eye movement (NREM) sleep   Type of sleep characterized by slower brain waves than are seen during wakefulness as well as other physiological markers; divided into four stages of increasingly deep sleep.

rapid eye movement (REM) sleep   Type of sleep characterized by brain waves and other physiological signs characteristic of a waking state but also characterized by reduced muscle tone, or sleep paralysis; most dreaming occurs during REM sleep.

Figure 6.2   One night's sleep cycles.

impaired. Performance in learning a new skill does not improve until an individual has had 6 hours of sleep; performance improves even more after 8 hours of sleep.[3,21,22]

The importance of REM sleep to the brain is demonstrated by what is called the **REM rebound effect.** If you get inadequate sleep for several nights, you will have longer and more frequent periods of REM sleep when you have a night in which you can sleep longer.[22]

Sleep Cycles

After your first REM period, you cycle back and forth between REM and NREM sleep stages. These cycles repeat themselves about every 90 to 110 minutes until you wake up. Typically, you experience four or five sleep cycles each night. After the second cycle, however, you spend little or no time in NREM stages 3 and 4 and most of your time in NREM stage 2 and REM sleep (Figure 6.2). After each successive cycle, the time spent in REM sleep doubles, lasting from 10 to 60 minutes at a time.[3,15,20]

Changes in Sleep Across the Life Span

The sleep cycle changes across the life span, with children and young adolescents experiencing large quantities of NREM stages 3 and 4 sleep (deep sleep). Sleep needs are constant across adulthood, but as people get older, high-quality sleep may become more elusive as a result of changes in sleep structure, medical conditions, and lifestyle choices.

As people age, they may experience changes in the voltage and frequency of brain waves, frequent shifts in the sleep stages, and more nighttime awakenings. In later life, adults experience less deep sleep and REM sleep and more NREM stage 1 sleep and wakefulness.[3] The production of melatonin and growth hormone declines with age, and the body temperature cycle may become irregular. All of these changes decrease total nighttime sleep.[23] Medical conditions also affect sleep in older adults. Sleep is disrupted by such conditions as arthritis, heartburn, osteoporosis,

Parkinson's disease, heart and lung diseases, dementia, incontinence, and cancer, as well as by some of the drugs used to treat these conditions. Additionally, sleep disorders are more common in middle and later life (see the next section).

However, many healthy older individuals have few or no sleep problems.[24] Some experts believe sleep problems are caused more by lifestyle choices—changes in diet, lack of exercise, decreased mental stimulation, daytime naps, and going to bed too early—than by biological changes. Older adults who maintain healthy lifestyle practices may still be able to get a good night's sleep.

Gender Differences in Sleep

There are also some gender differences in sleep, beginning as early as 6 months of age. Although the structure of sleep is essentially the same for men and women, women tend to have more slow-wave sleep (NREM stages 3 and 4) than men do and to experience more insomnia. Men have more REM periods. Men begin to experience a decrease in slow-wave sleep in their 20s. This decline does not begin for women until their 30s and progresses more slowly. The typical woman in her 50s has the slow-wave sleep pattern of a 20-year old man.[19,25] For more on sleep differences between men and women, see the box "Gender and Sleep Habits."

SLEEP DISORDERS

Because many sleep disorders are undiagnosed or not reported to physicians, many people who are chronically exhausted may not know why. Sleep disorders can be divided into dyssomnias and parasomnias.

Dyssomnias

Sleep disorders associated with difficulty in falling asleep or staying asleep or with excessive sleepiness—the timing, quality, and quantity of sleep—are labeled **dyssomnias.**

- Women are more likely than men are to report having daytime sleepiness at least a few times a week.
- Women are more likely than men to have symptoms of insomnia at least a few times a week.
- More men than women report snoring or having pauses in their breathing at least a few times a week, but men and women are almost equally likely to experience symptoms of restless legs syndrome.
- Men and women are about equal in their use of over-the-counter and prescription sleep medications.

They are also about equal in their use of products to help them stay awake and alert.

- On weekdays, women tend to get less sleep than they need in order to feel alert. Men tend to get more than they need.
- On weekends, men and women get about the same amount of sleep.

Source: Adapted from 2005 Sleep in America Poll, Executive Report, National Sleep Foundation, 2005, www.sleepfoundation.org.

The more common dyssomnias are insomnia, sleep apnea, narcolepsy, and restless legs syndrome.

Insomnia

In a poll conducted by the National Sleep Foundation (NSF), 58 percent of adults reported experiencing one or more symptoms of **insomnia**—defined as difficulty falling or staying asleep—at least a few nights a week. About 5 percent of these people were younger than 30, and 35 percent were older than 65.[2] Clinical symptoms of insomnia include (1) taking longer than 30 minutes to fall asleep, (2) experiencing five or more awakenings per night, (3) sleeping less than a total of 6 ½ hours as a result of these awakenings, and/or (4) experiencing less than 15 minutes of deep/slow-wave sleep.[26] These symptoms must persist for at least 1 month before insomnia may be clinically diagnosed, according to the American Psychiatric Association's *Diagnostic and Statistical Manual of Mental Disorders* (*DSM-IV-TR*).

According to the NSF, insomnia can be caused by stress, anxiety, medical problems, poor sleep environment, noisy or restless partners, and schedule changes (due to travel across time zones or shift work, for example).[2] For adult women, more than half of whom report symptoms of insomnia during any given month, additional causes may include depression, headaches, effects of pregnancy, premenstrual syndrome, menopausal hot flashes, and overactive bladder. Often the person with insomnia has become distressed by his or her inability to fall asleep, which increases arousal and makes it even harder to fall asleep. In time, the bedroom, bedtime, or sleep itself becomes associated with frustration instead of relaxation, and a vicious cycle sets in.

Chronic insomnia is difficult to treat, but individuals may be able to break the cycle and experience relief through such approaches as improving their sleep habits and sleeping environment and using relaxation techniques such as deep breathing and massage. See the section "Getting a Good Night's Sleep" later in this chapter for more strategies and tips on dealing with insomnia.

Sleep Apnea

Also known as breathing-related sleep disorder, **sleep apnea** is a condition characterized by periods of nonbreathing during sleep. Some health experts estimate that almost 40 percent of the U.S. population have some form of sleep apnea and that half of those afflicted may have a severe condition. In other words, millions of Americans stop breathing while they are asleep almost every night. The condition occurs in all ethnic, age, and socioeconomic groups, although men are more at risk for developing sleep apnea than women are.[2,27,28]

Scientists have distinguished two main types of sleep apnea, central sleep apnea and obstructive sleep apnea. In **central sleep apnea,** a rare condition, the brain fails to

KEY TERMS

REM rebound effect Increase in the length and frequency of REM sleep episodes that are experienced when a person sleeps for a longer time after a period of sleep deprivation.

dyssomnia Category of sleep disorder in which the timing, quality, and/or quantity of sleep are disturbed.

insomnia Sleep disorder characterized by difficulty falling or staying asleep.

sleep apnea Sleep disorder characterized by periods of nonbreathing during sleep; also known as breathing-related sleep disorder.

central sleep apnea Rare form of sleep apnea in which the brain fails to regulate the diaphragm and other breathing mechanisms correctly.

regulate the diaphragm and other breathing mechanisms correctly. In **obstructive sleep apnea,** by far the more common type, the upper airway is obstructed during sleep.[3] Individuals with obstructive sleep apnea are frequently overweight and have an excess of bulky soft tissue in the neck and throat. When the muscles relax during sleep, the tissue can block the airway (Figure 6.3).

Normally, the airway is open during sleep.

When the muscles of the soft palate, tongue, and uvula relax, they narrow the airway and cause snoring.

If these structures collapse on the back wall of the airway, they close the airway, preventing breathing. The efforts of the diaphragm and chest cause the blocked airway to become even more tightly sealed. For breathing to resume, the sleeper must rouse enough to cause tension in the tongue, which opens the airway.

Figure 6.3   Obstructive sleep apnea.

In obstructive sleep apnea, the individual stops breathing many times during sleep, often for as long as 60 to 90 seconds. The person's breathing pattern is usually characterized by periods of loud snoring (when the airway is partially blocked), alternating with periods of silence (when the airway is completely blocked), punctuated by sudden loud snores or jerking body movements as the person awakens for a few seconds and gasps for air. The individual is usually not aware of this pattern of snoring and gasping, although bed partners and other members of the household often are. The chief complaint of those with obstructive sleep apnea is daytime sleepiness, not nighttime awakening.

Obstructive sleep apnea is a potentially dangerous condition; occasionally, it is even fatal. It is frequently seen in association with high blood pressure, and it can increase the risk of heart disease and stroke. Oxygen saturation of the blood decreases and levels of carbon dioxide rise when a person stops breathing, increasing the likelihood that heart and blood vessel abnormalities may occur. If sufficient oxygen is not delivered to the brain, death may occur during sleep.[3,27,29]

In children, sleep apnea is usually associated with enlarged tonsils; symptoms include snoring, bedwetting, unusual sleeping positions, and daytime sleepiness. In adults, obstructive sleep apnea occurs most often in overweight, middle-aged men, although it becomes almost equally common in women after menopause. It is associated with larger neck circumferences (greater than 17 inches in men and 16 inches in women). People with the disorder often smoke, use alcohol, and/or sleep on their backs. There is sometimes a family history of sleep apnea, suggesting a genetic link. (See the box "Who Is at Greatest Risk for Sleep Apnea?")

Individuals with the disorder are usually described as restless sleepers and may have great difficulty awakening. In addition to daytime sleepiness, symptoms can include frequent nightly urination, heavy sweating, raspy throat, esophagus problems, reduced sex drive, erectile dysfunction, irritability, morning headaches, and problems with memory, attention, and concentration.[30]

If sleep apnea is not severe, it can be addressed with a variety of behavioral strategies. They include losing weight, forgoing alcoholic nightcaps or sedatives, avoiding allergens, not smoking, using a nasal decongestant spray, using a firm pillow and mattress, and not sleeping on the back. In addition, adjustable mouthpieces are available that extend the lower jaw, adding room to the airway. They are expensive, however, and may not be covered by health insurance.[3,31]

In cases of severe sleep apnea, one treatment option is continuous positive airway pressure (CPAP). A small, comfortable mask is fitted over the nose to hold the air passage open. The mouth is uncovered. Through the mask, a CPAP machine gently blows slightly pressurized air into the patient's nose. Other treatment options include surgery

Beating the Odds

Who Is at Greatest Risk for Sleep Apnea?

Sleep apnea is a serious condition that can be associated with high blood pressure, heart disease, and stroke; it can even cause death. Most people who suffer from sleep apnea do not realize they have it. They feel perpetually tired during the day, unaware that they are suffocating at night. Although there seems to be a genetic component to sleep apnea, there are also associated behavioral and lifestyle factors. Below are brief profiles of three people. Which person do you think is most at risk for sleep apnea?

Daniel, a 22-year-old college student, has a size 17 collar. He snores and often complains about being tired during the day despite sleeping 8 hours or more. Daniel is not overweight and does not drink alcohol. He smokes and often uses over-the-counter sleep medications to help him sleep. Daniel has high blood pressure and a family history of sleep apnea.

Sally, age 23, is pregnant. Although not a habitual snorer, she is experiencing chronic snoring during her pregnancy. She was 30 pounds overweight before she became pregnant but has not gained an excessive amount of weight since. She has a collar size of 14. Sally does not use sleep medications, alcohol, or tobacco. Her father and brother have sleep apnea. Sally often has morning headaches and daytime drowsiness.

Richard is 70 years old and resides in a nursing home. He is a chronic snorer. His collar size is 16, and he weighs 10 pounds less than his ideal weight. Richard drinks a glass of wine each day and uses sleeping medication, but he does not smoke. He has a thyroid problem and borderline high blood pressure. He complains about daytime drowsiness but does not suffer from morning headaches.

OLC Web site Visit the **Online Learning Center** at www.mhhe.com/teague1e for comments by the authors.

---

to cut away excess tissue at the back of the throat and a new technique called *samnoplasty* that involves shrinking tissue in the back of the throat with radio-frequency energy.[3,32]

Narcolepsy

The neurological disorder **narcolepsy** is characterized by frequent, irresistible "sleep attacks," in which the individual unintentionally falls asleep in inappropriate situations, such as while driving a car. A person with narcolepsy expe-

---

Healthy People 2010

OBJECTIVE AREA *Respiratory Disease*

- Increase the proportion of persons with symptoms of obstructive sleep apnea whose condition is medically managed.

"Persons with excessive daytime sleepiness, loud snoring, and other signs associated with obstructive sleep apnea [need to] seek medical evaluation . . . and receive followup medical care for long-term management of their condition."

 For more information on Healthy People 2010 objectives, visit the Web site at www.healthypeople.gov.

For more information on Canadian health objectives, visit the Health Canada Web site at www.hc-sc.gc.ca/english.

---

riences excessive daytime sleepiness, falls asleep for 10 to 20 minutes, and awakes feeling refreshed. Within 2 to 3 hours, however, the person once again feels sleepy.

Other symptoms of narcolepsy are cataplexy, sleep-related hallucinations, and sleep paralysis. *Cataplexy* is a sudden loss of muscle tone, usually lasting from a few seconds to a few minutes. The person may drop something he or she is holding or even fall to the ground but does not lose consciousness. Cataplexy is often triggered by a strong emotion, such as surprise. Sleep-related hallucinations occur when an episode of REM sleep, with its associated vivid dreams and muscle paralysis (sleep paralysis), intrudes during the transition from sleep to waking. Such dreams have a hallucinatory quality and often incorporate elements of the environment, such as the furnishings of the room. Other symptoms of narcolepsy include automatic behavior (repeatedly performing a single function such as speaking in a meaningless manner) and fragmented nighttime sleep.[26]

Narcolepsy affects about 3 to 6 people in 10,000. Nearly 80 percent of cases of narcolepsy are not diagnosed. A person who has a relative with narcolepsy has a

KEY TERMS

obstructive sleep apnea   The more common type of sleep apnea, in which the upper airway is obstructed during sleep.

narcolepsy   Sleep disorder characterized by frequent, irresistible "sleep attacks."

3 percent chance of developing this disorder—a risk 60 times greater than that of someone with no family history of narcolepsy. If a person has one parent with narcolepsy, the odds are 1 in 20 that the person will have the disorder. Narcolepsy occurs as early as age 3 but usually does not begin until puberty, which suggests that maturation of the brain may play an important role in onset.[3,26]

There is no cure for narcolepsy, but symptoms may be reduced by taking a 10- to 20-minute nap every 2 hours throughout the day, avoiding alcohol and sleeping pills, and getting sufficient sleep on a regular basis. Stimulant medications such as amphetamines have been used to treat pervasive daytime sleepiness. Different medications, usually antidepressants that retard REM sleep, are used for treating cataplexy, sleep paralysis, and hallucinations.[3,33]

Restless Legs Syndrome

As the name suggests, **restless legs syndrome (RLS)** is a sleep disorder characterized by disagreeable sensations in the limbs, usually the legs. These uncomfortable and sometimes painful feelings, such as creeping, tingling, or burning, create an almost irresistible urge to move the legs. Discomfort is relieved by vigorously stretching and crossing the legs and, sometimes, walking about for a short time. The symptoms and the individual's responses to them can delay and disturb sleep, leading to daytime sleepiness. Sleep experts estimate that about 4 percent of the population have this syndrome.[26]

In some cases, RLS is a central nervous system disorder; in other cases, a cause cannot be found. RLS is more prevalent among women; pregnant women; and people who have rheumatoid arthritis, iron-deficiency anemia, or kidney failure with dialysis.[26] Taking iron and vitamin E supplements may help reduce RLS symptoms. Avoiding late-night alcohol and engaging in moderate exercise are also encouraged.

Other Dyssomnias

Two other kinds of dyssomnia are hypersomnia and circadian rhythm disturbances. **Hypersomnia** is characterized by excessive daytime sleepiness despite an adequate amount of sleep at night. Individuals with this disorder may require up to 12 hours of sleep a night. They have great difficulty waking up, a condition referred to as *sleep drunkenness,* and they sometimes carry out routine activities during the day without awareness or recall (automatic behavior). In some cases of hypersomnia there is a family history of the disorder and evidence of nervous system dysfunction.[3]

In **circadian rhythm sleep disorder,** the person's internal sleep/wake cycle is out of sync with the sleep/wake demands of the environment. In one subtype of this disorder, individuals seem unable to delay or advance their internal clocks to match the clock time of their occupations or of society in general. In the delayed phase type, individuals naturally go to sleep later at night than is commonly accepted and have a hard time getting up in the morning. In the advanced phase type, people fall asleep early in the evening and wake up early in the morning. In another subtype, known as *jet lag type,* there is a discrepancy between the person's internal clock and the sleep/wake cycle of the time zone to which the person has traveled. Most people have more difficulty adjusting to eastward travel than westward travel, that is, more trouble advancing their sleep/wake cycles than delaying them. Finally, a subtype known as *shift work type* occurs when the person's internal clock is mismatched with the requirements of night-shift work. These individuals often get insufficient sleep because of disturbances, such as noise and light, during the hours in which they try to sleep. Female shift workers may experience reproductive problems, such as irregular menstrual cycles, difficulty getting pregnant, and premature births. It is not clear why these effects occur, but suspected factors are sleep deprivation and changes in exposure to light. In general, circadian rhythm disturbances are not disorders except in the context of environmental demands and to the extent that they cause the individual distress.[3,26]

Parasomnias

Whereas dyssomnias involve the timing, quality, or quantity of sleep, **parasomnias** involve physiological functioning or behavior during sleep. Body systems become activated as if the person were awake, usually during specific stages of sleep; that is, some parasomnias occur during NREM sleep, and others occur during REM sleep. Parasomnias include sleepwalking disorder, nocturnal eating disorder, nightmare disorder, REM behavior disorder, and teeth grinding, among others.

Sleepwalking Disorder

People with **sleepwalking disorder** rise out of an apparently deep sleep and act as if they are awake. They do not respond to other people while in this state, or, if they do, it is with reduced alertness. For example, they may answer a question or acquiesce to a request to return to bed, but they do so automatically, often with a blank stare. Sleepwalking takes place during slow-wave (stages 3 and 4) NREM sleep and therefore usually occurs during the first third of the night's sleep. Episodes typically last less than 10 minutes.[3] If sleepwalkers are awakened, they are often confused for several minutes; if they are not awakened, they may return to bed and have little or no memory of the episode the next day.

Many examples of sleepwalking have been chronicled by the American Sleep Disorders Association and other groups. In one case, a woman awoke in a grocery store to find herself wheeling a grocery cart containing 56 boxes of cornflakes. Another woman drew a map of the United States on her bathroom wall while she slept. Although some sleepwalking incidents are humorous, others have proved fatal, as in the case of a man in the back of a moving trailer who sleepwalked out the door and was killed on the highway.[31]

Sleepwalking usually begins between the ages of 5 and 12 and disappears in most cases during adolescence. It rarely starts in adulthood; adults who sleepwalk usually did so as children. Although there may be a genetic link to sleepwalking, most sufferers do not have a family history of this disorder. Episodes may be brought on by excessive sleep deprivation, fatigue, stress, illness, and the use of sedatives.[3,26]

Nocturnal Eating Disorder

A person with **nocturnal eating disorder** rises from bed during the night and eats and drinks while asleep. The person may consume bizarre concoctions but has no memory of these experiences in the morning. Fifty percent of people suffering from this disorder binge eat without awakening. Even if they awaken, they continue to compulsively eat a wide assortment of food. Although they may binge up to six times a night, they do not experience indigestion or feelings of fullness after the binge.[3,34]

Episodes of nocturnal eating disorder may be triggered by episodes of sleepwalking or of obstructive sleep apnea. There does not seem to be a relationship between this disorder and daytime eating disorders, such as anorexia or bulimia, although both are more common in women than in men. The disorder has been treated with a variety of medications, including antidepressants, as well as with behavioral and psychotherapeutic interventions. To date, however, success has been limited, and there is no consensus on treatment.[35,36]

Distinct from nocturnal eating disorder is a newly identified sleep disorder, **night eating syndrome,** in which affected persons are awake while they are eating. These people binge late at night, have difficulty falling asleep, repeatedly awaken during the night and eat again, and then eat very little the next day. Some people with night eating syndrome consume more than 50 percent of their daily calories at night. Sleep experts estimate that the syndrome's frequency is about 1.5 percent in the general population and up to 10 percent among obese people seeking treatment for their weight. Treatments include medications and behavior management techniques.[35]

Nightmare Disorder

A person with **nightmare disorder** experiences vivid, often frightening dreams during REM sleep. Nightmares commonly occur in the middle to late part of the sleep night, when REM sleep periods become longer. They may be accompanied by sleep talking and body movements. Typically, the dreamer awakens from the nightmare, is fully alert, and can recount the dream, which usually involves imminent danger or threat.

About 50 percent of very young children experience nightmares, beginning between the ages of 2 and 5. Although nightmares typically disappear completely by age 7, they can continue into adulthood. Only about 1 percent of the adult population experiences recurrent nightmares, but adults who do should consult a sleep specialist.[3,26,37]

Nightmare disorder is different from *sleep terror disorder,* or *night terrors*. In this disorder, the individual awakens from deep NREM sleep, usually with a scream or cry, and is difficult to orient. The person does not remember a dream or nightmare but is physiologically aroused, with rapid breathing, pounding heart, sweating, skin flushing, and other signs of extreme fear. Sleep terror disorder is seen in both children and adults and occurs more often when there is a family history of the disorder, indicating a genetic link.

REM Behavior Disorder

In **REM behavior disorder,** which occurs most often in older adults,[26] the inhibition of muscle movement that normally occurs during REM sleep does not take place. As a result, individuals get up and act out their dreams, often

KEY TERMS

restless legs syndrome (RLS)   Sleep disorder characterized by disagreeable sensations in the limbs, usually the legs.

hypersomnia   Sleep disorder characterized by excessive daytime sleepiness despite an adequate amount of sleep at night.

circadian rhythm sleep disorder   Condition in which a person's internal sleep/wake cycle is out of sync with the sleep/wake demands of the environment.

parasomnia   Category of sleep disorder in which physiological functioning or behavior during sleep is disturbed.

sleepwalking disorder   Sleep disorder in which a person rises out of an apparently deep sleep and acts as if awake.

nocturnal eating disorder   Sleep disorder in which a person rises from bed during the night and eats and drinks while asleep.

night eating syndrome   Condition in which a person eats excessively during the night while awake.

nightmare disorder   Sleep disorder in which a person experiences vivid, often frightening dreams during REM sleep.

REM behavior disorder   Sleep disorder in which muscle movement is not inhibited during REM sleep, allowing the person to move around while dreaming.

injuring themselves in the process. They are easily awakened and can recount the dream they were having. The disorder can occur as a result of Parkinson's disease, brain stem damage, alcoholism, or the use of hallucinogenic drugs. Sleep experts recommend that the bedroom be structured for safety to protect the individual from injury.[3] In addition, medications have been shown to be effective in treating the disorder.

Teeth Grinding

Nearly 9 in 10 people grind or clench their teeth during sleep, a condition known as *bruxism*. About 1 in 20 do so chronically. Stress is often a cause; symptoms include headache, damaged or sensitive teeth, and pain in the temporomandibular joint (TMJ) in the jaw. Frequent teeth grinding is most commonly found in 10- to 20-year-olds. It is also more common in children with mental retardation and cerebral palsy.[2,19,26] Individuals who grind their teeth can be fitted with a plastic tooth guard by their dentist to protect their teeth.

Evaluating Your Sleep

You don't have to have a sleep disorder to experience sleep difficulties; nearly everyone experiences some kind of

Some people who experience insomnia watch TV to fill the wakeful late-night hours, but this actually works against their problem. Reading a book, with soft lighting used, is a better approach to inducing sleep.

sleep problem at one time or another. Some sleep problems are temporary or situational and resolve on their own, but others are serious enough to warrant further investigation.

How can you tell if you have a sleep problem? First, get a sense of your general level of daytime sleepiness by taking the **sleep latency** test (a measure of how long it takes you to fall asleep) in Part 1 of the Add It Up! feature at the end of this chapter. Next, check to see if you have any symptoms of a sleep disorder by completing Part 2 of the Add It Up! feature. Then take a look at the various behavior change strategies in the next section of the chapter and make any appropriate improvements. Of course, the most basic recommendation is to make sure you are getting enough hours of sleep every night. If you still experience a sleep problem after following these recommendations, you may want to consult your physician. If the problem is serious enough, your physician, in turn, may refer you to a sleep clinic or lab or a sleep disorder specialist.

If you are referred to a sleep clinic or lab, you may be asked to monitor your sleeping habits at home by keeping a sleep diary for a week or more. You will record the times you go to bed, awaken during the night, and wake up in the morning, as well as what and when you eat in the evening; any alcohol, tobacco, or drugs you consume; and so on. Alternatively, you may be evaluated at the lab. You may take a **Multiple Sleep Latency Test (MSLT),** in which you lie down in a dark room and are told not to resist sleep. This test, repeated five times during the day, measures sleep latency as an index of daytime sleepiness.

You will also sleep at the lab at night. While you are sleeping, electrodes attached to your head and jaw will monitor and record your brain waves, eye movements, and muscle tension. Other instruments will record various physiological characteristics to evaluate air flow, respiratory effort, heart rate, blood oxygen content, limb muscle activity, snoring, body positions, and sometimes esophageal pressure and esophageal pH. From these measurements, clinicians assess sleep latency, sequence of sleep stages, time spent in sleep stages, frequency and duration of awakenings, and other features of sleep and waking patterns. If it turns out that you do have a sleep disorder, the clinicians will advise you on treatment and management options.

GETTING A GOOD NIGHT'S SLEEP

We have seen that getting enough sleep is essential to optimal functioning and that sleep deprivation is a major problem for many adults, including many college students. What is the best way to ensure healthy sleep patterns over the course of the life span? In this section we provide several strategies and tips that will help you get a good night's sleep.

It's easy to get in the habit of staying up late at night to study for an exam or finish a paper. Instead, plan ahead for deadlines and follow a routine that allows you to get at least 8 hours of sleep every night.

Establishing Good Sleep Habits

Several habits and behaviors concerning when and where you sleep and what you do before you sleep can help you sleep better and solve sleep problems.

Maintain a Regular Sleep Schedule

Try to get about 8 hours of sleep every night, 7 days a week. With a regular sleep schedule, you fall asleep faster and awaken more easily, because you are psychologically and physiologically conditioned for sleep and waking. Only about 10 percent of undergraduates report that they get 8 hours or more of sleep on weekdays. However, 70 percent get 8 or more hours on weekends, meaning that most students have an irregular sleep schedule.[7] As noted earlier in this chapter, such a schedule throws off your internal biological clock and disrupts the structure of sleep.

Create a Sleep-Friendly Environment

Your bedroom should be a comfortable, secure, quiet, cool, and dark place for inducing sleep. Your mattress should be hard enough to allow you to get into a comfortable sleep position. If it is too hard, however, it may not provide an adequate cushion to prevent painful pressure on your body.[3]

Noise can reduce restful sleep. Research on people who live near airports has found that excessive noise may jog individuals out of deep sleep and into a lighter sleep. Street noises have a similar effect. If it isn't possible to eliminate noise, try creating *white noise,* a monotonous and unchanging sound such as that of an air conditioner or a fan. Noise generators that create soothing sounds such as falling rain, wind, and surf have been proven effective in protecting sleep.[15,31]

Temperature is important too. You sleep best when the temperature is within your specific comfort zone. A temperature below or above that zone often causes fragmented sleep or wakefulness. The ideal is usually 62° F to 65° F. Generally, temperatures above 75° F and below 54° F cause people to awaken.[3,15]

Finally, don't expect to get a good night's sleep if you cannot assume a recumbent body position, such as when taking a long airplane flight at night. Research has shown that people sleeping in an upright position have poorer quality sleep than those sleeping in a horizontal position. The amount of slow-wave sleep a person experiences in a sitting position is almost zero. If you fall asleep while standing up, your body begins to sway so that you quickly awaken. Perhaps the brain operates in a similar fashion when you are sleeping in a seated position. With your body mainly upright, your brain may interpret this position as not sufficiently safe to allow deep sleep.[3,15]

Avoid Caffeine, Nicotine, and Alcohol

Caffeine, a stimulant, disrupts sleep, whether it comes in coffee, tea, chocolate, or soda. It enters your bloodstream

KEY TERMS

sleep latency   Amount of time it takes a person to fall asleep.

Multiple Sleep Latency Test (MSLT)   Test of sleep latency, administered as an index of daytime sleepiness and usually given five times in a sleep clinic.

quickly, reaches a peak in about 30 to 60 minutes, and may take up to 6 hours to clear your blood system. A single cup of coffee may double the amount of time it takes an average adult to fall asleep. It may also reduce the amount of slow-wave or deep sleep by half and quadruple the number of nighttime awakenings.[15] Avoiding caffeine intake 6 to 8 hours before going to bed may improve sleep quality.

Like caffeine, nicotine is a stimulant that can disrupt sleep. People who smoke a pack of cigarettes a day have been shown to have sleep problems. Brain wave pattern analysis indicates that they do not sleep as deeply as nonsmokers. Smoking also affects the respiratory system by causing congestion in the nose and swelling of the mucous membranes lining the throat and upper airway passages. These physiological factors increase the likelihood of snoring and aggravate the symptoms of sleep apnea. They also decrease oxygen uptake, which leads to more frequent awakenings.[3,15,38]

Alcohol has been shown to induce sleepiness and to reduce the amount of time it takes to fall asleep, but it causes poorer sleep and restlessness later in the night. Because alcohol is a depressant, it prevents REM sleep from occurring until most of the alcohol has been absorbed. After absorption, vivid dreams are more likely. Sleep experts call this an *alcohol rebound effect,* in which the body seems to be trying to recover REM sleep that was lost earlier. Alcohol is also more likely to cause twitching and body movements that interfere with sleep.[15,39,40]

Get Regular Exercise but Not Close to Bedtime

Regular exercise during the day or early evening hours may be beneficial for sleep. Exercising within 3 hours of going to bed, however, is not recommended, because exercise stimulates the release of adrenaline and elevates core body temperature. It takes 5 to 6 hours for body temperature to drop enough after vigorous exercise for drowsiness to occur and deeper sleep to take place.[15,39,40]

Manage Stress and Establish Relaxing Bedtime Rituals

Stress increases physiological arousal and can adversely affect sleep patterns. Stress management and reduction techniques, such as those described in Chapter 5, can be used to help induce sleepiness. For example, keep a worry book by your bedside and record bothersome thoughts and problems in it that keep you awake at night. Once you've written them down, tell yourself you'll work on them during daylight hours, and then let go of them. Use your notes to focus energy and attention on these problems over the course of the next few days.

It can also be helpful to develop a bedtime ritual, such as reading, listening to soothing music, or taking a warm (but not too hot) bath; your mind and body will come to associate bedtime with relaxation and peacefulness. Avoid stressful or stimulating activities before bedtime, such as working or paying bills, and dim the lights to let your internal clock know that drowsiness is appropriate. Experiment until you find a method of calming down and relaxing at bedtime that works for you.

If you do have a hard time falling asleep, don't stay in bed longer than 30 minutes. Get up, leave the room, and listen to soothing music or read until you feel sleepy.

Avoid Eating Too Close to Bedtime

Try not to eat heavy meals within 3 hours of bedtime, particularly meals with high fat content. When you are lying down, the force of gravity cannot assist the movement of food from the stomach into the small intestine to complete digestion, and you may experience acid indigestion, or heartburn. Also avoid caffeinated beverages, citrus fruits and juices, tomato-based products, and pasta sauce, because these foods can temporarily weaken the esophageal sphincter. When weakened, this sphincter allows stomach contents to move back into the esophagus, a condition known as acid reflux. If this is a problem for you, you can also try raising the head of your bed 6 to 8 inches, which will allow gravity to help empty stomach contents into the small intestine. Tilting the bed is more effective than elevating the upper body with pillows. For those who are overweight, moderate weight loss may reduce discomfort, because excessive stomach fat can cause abdominal pressure that contributes to heartburn.[15]

Be Smart About Napping

The typical North American adult takes one or two naps a week, and about a third of adults nap more than four times a week. On the other hand, about a fourth never take a nap. If you are a napper, sleep experts recommend naps of only 15 to 45 minutes, which can be refreshing and restorative. If you nap longer than 45 minutes, your body is able to enter stage 4 deep sleep. It is more difficult to awaken from this stage, and you are more likely to feel groggy.[3,31]

If you know you will be going to bed later than usual, you may want to take a "preventive nap" of 2 to 3 hours. Research suggests that people who take preventive naps increase their alertness by about 30 percent over that of people who do not nap. Napping 15 minutes every 4 hours until you attain 2 hours of preventive napping is also recommended. This short nap strategy has been effectively used by physicians and law enforcement officers, who must perform in emergency situations for long hours.[31]

Consider Your Bed Partner

Snoring is a major disrupter of partners' sleep, and body movement during sleep can also be a problem for partners.

Challenges & Choices

Tips to Reduce Snoring

Loud snoring means your throat is narrowing and your breathing is becoming strained. The narrower your throat during inhalation, the more strenuously your diaphragm must pull down to obtain air. The result is a stronger vibration of tissues and a louder snore. Here are some tips for reducing snoring:

- Avoid alcohol before bedtime.

- Try nasal sprays to help reduce nasal tissue congestion and "Breathe Right" strips to widen nostrils.

- Use a humidifier to increase moisture in a heated bedroom and reduce nasal tissue congestion.

- Obtain an adjustable mouth piece that extends the lower jaw to widen the airway.

- Have someone roll you onto your side if you are snoring. Sleeping on your back increases the chance of snoring.

- Alternatively, make a "snoreball" by placing a tennis ball in a sock and pinning it to your back. The ball will cause discomfort if you turn over onto your back while you are asleep and you will roll back onto your side.

- Lose weight if necessary.

It's Not Just Personal . . .

Snoring is a key sign of obstructive sleep apnea, a sleep disorder that can increase the seriousness of other diseases. For example, an estimated 38,000 deaths a year occur as a result of cardiorespiratory illnesses caused or exacerbated by obstructive sleep apnea.

Source: Adapted from *Overcoming Sleep Disorders: A Natural Approach*, by B. O'Hanlon, 2000, Freedom, CA: The Crossing Press.

Men tend to thrash around in bed more than women do, and older couples tend to move in less compatible ways than do younger couples. A mattress with low motion transfer may help prevent sleep disruption caused by a partner's movement. Sleep can also be disrupted if a partner has a different sleep schedule or has a sleep disorder. If your partner's sleep habits create a problem for you, encourage your partner to improve his or her sleep habits or to see a sleep disorder specialist (see the box "Tips to Reduce Snoring"). As a last resort, you or your partner may have to sleep in a different bed or room.

Using Sleep Aids

Because sleep is so influential in your daily functioning, and because sleep problems are so common, it should not be surprising that many people resort to sleep aids of one kind or another to help them get a good night's sleep. About 15 percent of adults use a prescription sleep medication and/or an over-the-counter sleep aid to help them sleep a few nights a week.[41]

Prescription Medications

Safe and effective sleep medications are those that can be taken at higher doses, are not addictive, do not produce serious side effects, and wear off quickly so you are not drowsy the next day. Sleep experts disagree about whether today's sleep medications meet these criteria.[3] No sleep medication should be used over a long period without physician consultation.

Before the 1970s, most medications prescribed for sleep problems were barbiturates. They depressed the central nervous system enough to produce unconsciousness; at high doses they could cause death.[3] In the 1970s, physicians began prescribing benzodiazepine drugs, such as Valium and Librium, which were developed to treat anxiety. They have fewer side effects than barbiturates, and at higher doses, they induce sleep. However, they are addictive. Today, the most frequently prescribed, longer acting benzodiazepine sleep medications are Restoril, Dalmon, and Doral. These drugs induce sleep but suppress both deep sleep and REM sleep. Their effects can last from 3 to 24 hours, and daytime side effects include decreased memory and intellectual functioning. People quickly build tolerance to long-lasting benzodiazepines, which lose their effectiveness after 30 nights of consecutive use. Like Valium and Librium, they are addictive. There are some shorter acting benzodiazepines on the market that do not suppress deep sleep and REM sleep.[40]

A new category of sleep medications is the imidazopyridines. They are not addictive and do not cause side effects or drowsiness the next day when taken as directed. The National Sleep Foundation considers these drugs the best prescription sleeping aids.[40]

There are also drugs designed to make people more alert despite sleep deprivation, as many college students

Challenges & Choices

Safety Precautions With Sleeping Pills

Sleeping pills can be useful for treating transient or short-term insomnia. They should be discontinued once the cause of the disorder has been eliminated. Recommended maximum duration of use is 4 weeks. To use sleeping medications safely, follow these guidelines:

- Use sleeping medications in the smallest effective dose, for the shortest possible time.
- Read the drug labels and instructions. Never take more than the recommended dose, and don't take more than one prescription or over-the-counter remedy unless advised to do so by your physician.
- Don't drink alcohol while using sleep medications.
- Don't take sleeping pills if you are pregnant. The FDA has not approved any sleep medications for use during pregnancy, and pregnant

women who use them put their babies at risk for addiction.

- Do not drive after taking sleeping medication, since these substances generally impair your motor control responses by causing drowsiness.
- Consult your physician before taking sleeping pills. These medications may mask an underlying sleep disorder.

It's Not Just Personal . . .

Insomnia can be more than an annoyance. The National Institutes of Health estimates the direct costs of insomnia—including the cost of sleeping pills and other treatments for insomnia—to be nearly $14 billion annually.

Source: Adapted from *Power Sleep*, by J. B. Maas, 1998, New York: Villard Books/Random House.

and long-haul truck drivers know. As noted earlier in the chapter, Provigil is a new, FDA-approved "pep pill" that treats excessive daytime sleepiness and its attendant fatigue and low energy. The effectiveness of this drug in improving alertness has led to its broader use, for example, by medical residents and by pilots flying missions in Afghanistan and Iraq. Concerns have been raised about Provigil, however, because of its potential side effects for some people, which include reduced vigilance, interference with concentration and memory, and increased irritability.

Over-the-Counter Medications

Nonprescription, or over-the-counter (OTC), medications can be useful for treating transient or short-term insomnia, such as may occur under conditions of great stress or trauma. They should be discontinued once the cause of the problem has been eliminated, ideally within 2 weeks. The recommended maximum use is 4 weeks.

Many over-the-counter sleep products contain antihistamine, a type of drug developed to treat allergies. The effects of antihistamines are general throughout the body; besides drowsiness, they cause dehydration, agitation, and constipation. Additionally, you can quickly develop tolerance of antihistamines, and when you stop taking them, you may experience **rebound insomnia**—insomnia that is worse than what you experienced before you started taking the medication.[40] Rebound insomnia can be avoided by gradually reducing the dose. For more information on OTC sleep medications, see the box "Safety Precautions With Sleeping Pills."

Complementary and Alternative Products and Approaches

Complementary and alternative products and approaches to sleep problems include herbal products, dietary supplements, and aromatherapy. The herbal product most commonly used for insomnia is valerian, which has a tranquilizing or sedative effect. Hops is another product currently receiving attention as a possible sleep aid. Both are widely available in health food stores. Herbal products can interact with other medications and drugs, including caffeine and alcohol; it is strongly recommended that you consult with your physician before trying any herbal remedies.

Melatonin is a dietary supplement that has been marketed as a sleep aid, but health experts are divided on its effectiveness. As noted earlier in this chapter, melatonin is a hormone naturally secreted by the pineal gland in response to darkness. It lowers body temperature and causes drowsiness. Most experts agree that the 3-milligram dose of synthetically produced melatonin available in health food stores is too high and that a dose of 0.1 milligram is as effective as a higher dose.[40,41] Potential side effects, interactions with drugs, and long-term health effects of melatonin supplements have not been extensively studied. Caution is advised, because some studies have reported increased risk of heart attack, infertility, fatigue, and depression with melatonin use.

In aromatherapy, certain essential oils, such as jasmine and lavender, are used to induce relaxation and sleepiness. Aromatherapists believe these oils relieve insomnia by reducing stress, enhancing moods, and easing respiratory or muscular problems, but no strong scientific evidence supports these claims.[41] Aromatherapy oils may be applied to the skin by full body massage, or a drop may be placed on the wrist or at the base of the throat so the scent is inhaled during sleep. Scented sprays can be used on bed linens, but aromatherapy candles should not be used when you are sleeping. Aromatherapy products are generally available in health food stores; if you are interested in trying this approach, however, it is recommended that you consult a trained aromatherapist before making any purchases.

∗∗∗

As noted, it is not surprising that people go to great lengths to get enough high-quality sleep. Nothing is so refreshing and restorative as a good night's sleep, giving us a fresh perspective and renewed energy for facing the demands of the day. Shakespeare called sleep the "balm of hurt minds, chief nourisher in life's feast." Sleep, he wrote, "knits up the ravell'd sleeve of care." Conversely, almost nothing is so distressing as being unable to avail ourselves of the respite provided by sleep. Chronic sleep deprivation can interfere with physical, emotional, and cognitive functioning and leave us fatigued, depressed, and more susceptible to illness and disease. As with so many other facets of lifestyle, good sleep habits and practices, established early in life, can help you maintain wellness in both younger and older adulthood.

KEY TERMS

rebound insomnia   Insomnia that occurs after a person stops taking sleep medication and that is worse than it was before the medication was started.

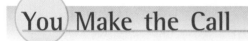

You Make the Call

Should Medical Residents Work Fewer Hours?

Imagine this scenario: You are about to undergo major surgery. As you are wheeled into the operating room, you notice that your surgeon is finishing off a beer. Several empty beer cans are littered nearby. No one seems to think anything of it.

Ridiculous? Yes. However, the American Medical Student Association suggests something similar happens every day in American hospitals. Residents—new physicians who have just graduated from medical school—may work up to 120 hours a week, sometimes in 36-hour shifts for several weeks at a time. They may be required to stay awake all night every third night for the duration of their residency and specialty training, which last from 3 to 7 years. This level of sleep deprivation has been shown to be comparable to being legally intoxicated.

Common sense suggests that significant sleep deprivation impairs cognitive and motor functions and that these impairments endanger patient health. One study found that 41 percent of medical residents attributed their most serious medical error in the previous year to exhaustion. About one in three patients died from these physician mistakes. More than 10 percent of medical residents indicate that sleep deprivation is an almost daily occurrence. Studies consistently show that well-rested physicians outperform sleep-deprived physicians in tests of visual stimulation, concentration, and memory. Furthermore, many residents report feelings of anger, resentment, and depression and reduced feelings of kindness, compassion, and empathy because of sleep deprivation.

Why is sleep deprivation allowed and even required in hospitals and the medical training system? The main reason seems to be tradition: Some regard residency training as a rite of passage that tests a physician's ability to endure difficult situations. They claim that rigorous and systematic exposure to the realities of a physician's life are essential for ensuring adequate preparation. This aspect of the medical resident training system has remained virtually unchanged for more than a century.

Another reason for the practice is that pressures to reduce health care costs have intensified the hourly workloads of medical residents. If this practice were reversed, additional nurses and physician assistants would have to cover the loss of resident hours, increasing labor costs by millions of dollars. Some also argue that more frequent handoffs of patient care from one physician to another would increase rather than decrease medical errors.

Because of concerns about sleep deprivation and medical errors, the Accreditation Council for Graduate Medical Education (ACGME) has called for limiting the medical resident workweek to 80 hours and shifts to no more than 24 hours. Residents would be entitled to up to 10 hours of rest before shifts. Because the ACGME accredits the nation's teaching hospitals, failure to meet the accreditation standards could result in the loss of a hospital's accreditation. In 2005, legislation was introduced in Congress that would make the ACGME's recommendations law and limit medical residents to an 80-hour workweek. The American Medical Association has endorsed the legislation, but some physicians oppose it, citing tradition, cost, and other concerns. What do you think?

Pros

◎ Medical residents are inexperienced, overworked, and sleep deprived, making them prone to medical errors that can lead to injury and even death. A 2001 study by the Institute of Medicine estimated that nearly 98,000 hospitalized patients die each year and more than 1 million are injured as a result of medical errors, many of which are associated with chronic sleep deprivation.

◎ Sleep-deprived physicians are less able to provide compassionate care for their patients.

◎ Evidence from the trucking and aviation industries supports limits on shift length as an effective safety measure for employees and the public.

Cons

◎ Long work hours are needed to sufficiently train medical residents. If work hours are cut, an added

year of resident training may be needed. The financial implications for residents are enormous.

◎ If additional nurses and physician assistants are used to cover the loss of resident hours, labor costs to hospitals and the medical system will increase by millions of dollars.

◎ Clinical evidence linking sleep deprivation to medical errors is insufficient. The trucking and aviation industries are not comparable to hospital settings.

◎ More frequent handoffs of patient care between physicians will increase rather than decrease medical errors. Cross-coverage, a system in which a fresh resident covers patients for several other residents at night, is increasingly used in U.S. hospitals. A Harvard study reported that the covering residents were six times more likely to make serious medical errors than were the fatigued residents.

OLC Web site For more information about this topic, visit the Online Learning Center at www.mhhe.com/teague1e.

SOURCES: "Physician Work Hours and Patient Safety," by C. A. Czeisler, October 10, 2003, presentation at the First Sleep and Health Gala Benefit Dinner, Washington, DC; "Through the Physician's Eyes: Optional Work Scheduling for Residents," by A. Heins, 2003, American Medical Association, www.ama-assn.org; "Sleepy Residents: More ZZZ's Needed for New MDs?" 2003, ABCNews.go.com; "Medical Residency: An Exercise in Sleep Deprivation," by S. Turner, 2003, *George Street Journal*, www.brown.edu; "Practice With Sleep Makes Perfect: Sleep-Dependent Motor Skill Learning," by M. P. Walker, T. Brakefield, A. Morgan, J. Hobson, & R. Stickgold, 2002, *Neuron, 35,* 205–211.

SUMMARY

- Sleep, a period of rest and recovery experienced by all mammals and birds, is essential for all domains of functioning. Adults need about 8 hours of sleep every night, but many adults do not get that many hours.

- Adequate sleep is critical to good health. Restoration of body systems, in particular the immune system, occurs during sleep, as do the growth and repair of tissues and cells.

- Sleep deprivation causes impairments in physical, emotional, and cognitive functioning, especially memory, learning, and performance. It has been associated with impaired immune system functioning, disrupted growth and development, and accidents, among other effects. Accumulated hours of sleep deprivation are known as sleep debt.

- Cycles of sleep and waking are regulated primarily by an internal biological clock located in the hypothalamus, but they are also influenced by environmental stimuli such as light.

- Scientists have discovered that sleep is a complex state characterized by cycling changes in brain wave activity, eye movement, and body movement. During the course of a night's sleep, a person cycles through a five-stage sleep process several times.

- About 75 percent of sleep time is spent in non-rapid eye movement (NREM) sleep, which is divided into four progressively deeper stages of sleep. Stage 1 is a light sleep; deep sleep occurs in stages 3 and 4.

- During REM sleep, physiological functioning becomes almost as active as during waking, but muscle movement is inhibited. REM provides an opportunity for filing important ideas and thoughts in long-term memory. Most dreams occur during REM sleep.

- The structure of sleep changes over the life span, with older adults experiencing less deep sleep and more wakefulness. There are also gender differences in sleep, with women experiencing more slow-wave sleep and more insomnia and men experiencing more REM sleep.

- Sleep disorders are divided into dyssomnias, problems associated with the quantity, quality, and/or timing of sleep, and parasomnias, problems associated with behavior or physiological functioning during sleep.

- Dyssomnias include insomnia, sleep apnea, narcolepsy, restless legs syndrome, hypersomnia, and circadian rhythm sleep disorder.

- Parasomnias include sleepwalking, nocturnal eating disorder, nightmares, REM behavior disorder, and teeth grinding.

- Evaluation of sleep usually includes measurement of time needed to fall asleep (sleep latency), sequence of sleep stages and time spent in sleep stages, frequency and duration of awakenings, and daytime drowsiness.
- Many sleep problems can be resolved by establishing good sleep habits and implementing other behavioral and environmental changes.

- Sleep medications include prescription drugs, over-the-counter products, and complementary and alternative approaches. The best sleep medications are those that can be safely taken at higher doses, are not addictive, do not produce serious side effects, and wear off quickly.

REVIEW QUESTIONS

1. What are some of the health benefits of adequate sleep? What are some of the impairments that accompany sleep deprivation?
2. Why is it ineffective to try to catch up on missed sleep by "sleeping in" on the weekends?
3. Why would a person have difficulty adjusting to the time difference after traveling through several time zones?
4. Describe the four stages of NREM sleep. How do they differ from REM sleep?
5. What is meant by *paradoxical sleep*?
6. What differences in sleep have been identified between men and women?
7. How do medical conditions and physical changes associated with aging affect sleep in middle and later life?
8. What is the difference between a dyssomnia and a parasomnia?
9. What are some of the causes of insomnia?
10. What are the two main types of sleep apnea? What are the health effects of sleep apnea?
11. What are some treatment approaches to narcolepsy?
12. Why are most forms of circadian rhythm sleep disorders not really disorders in the same sense that sleep apnea and narcolepsy are?
13. What is the difference between nocturnal eating disorder and night eating syndrome?
14. What is the difference between nightmare disorder and sleep terror disorder?
15. What are some questions you would ask to determine whether a person had a sleep disorder?
16. What are some questions you would ask to determine whether a person was getting enough sleep?
17. Briefly describe four recommendations for good sleep practices.

WEB RESOURCES

American Academy of Sleep Medicine: This professional organization focuses on the advancement of sleep medicine and sleep research. Its Web site offers links to several sleep resources, such as journals and other sleep organizations. www.aasmnet.org

American Sleep Apnea Association: This organization focuses on increased understanding of sleep apnea disorders. It is dedicated to reducing injury, disability, and death from sleep apneas and to enhancing the well-being of those affected by this common disorder. www.sleepapnea.org/asaa.html

National Sleep Foundation: From the basics of getting a good night's sleep to understanding sleep problems and disorders,

this site offers helpful information. It features interactive sleep quizzes, brochures, and a variety of tools for better sleep. www.sleepfoundation.org

SleepNet: If you want to locate a sleep lab, take a sleep test, understand sleep terms, and learn about sleep disorders, this site is the place to visit. It highlights various sleep problems, offering clear explanations, and features related readings. www.sleepnet.com

Sleep Research Society: This scientific society is dedicated to scientific investigation on all aspects of sleep and its disorders. It promotes the exchange of knowledge pertaining to sleep. www.sleepresearchsociety.org

REFERENCES

1. National Sleep Foundation. (2005). Facts and stats. www.sleepfoundation.org.

2. National Sleep Foundation. (2003). 2003 Sleep in America Poll, Executive Report. www.sleepfoundation.org.

3. Dement, W. C., & Vaughn, C. (1999). *The promise of sleep.* New York: Delacorte Press/Random House.

4. Passer, M. W., & Smith, R. E. (2004). *Psychology: The science of mind and behavior* (2nd ed.). New York: McGraw-Hill.

5. Cauter, E. V., Leproult, R., & Plat, L. (2000). Age-related changes in slow wave sleep and REM sleep and relationship with growth hormone and cortisol levels in healthy men. *Journal of American Medical Association, 284* (7), 861–868.

6. Office of Communications and Public Affairs. (2003). Stanford research builds link between sleep, cancer progression. http://mednews.stanford.edu/news_releases_html/2003.

7. Balachandran, D. D., Ewing, S. B., Murray, B. S., LeBleau, L., & Mulligan, S. M. (2002). Human host response during chronic partial sleep deprivation. *Sleep, 25*, A107.

8. Baylor, G. W., & Carallero, C. (2001). Memory sources associated with REM and NREM dream reports throughout the night: A new look at the ???? of sleep. *Sleep, 24* (C2),165–170.

9. Gilyatt, P. (1999, March 19). Sleep may play a bigger role in learning and memory. *Harvard Medical School Focus.*

10. Garbarino, S., Nobili, L., Beelke, M., et al. (2001). The contributing role of sleepiness in highway vehicle accidents. *Sleep, 24* (2), 203–210.

11. Von Dongen, P. A., Maislin, G., Mullington, J. M., & Dinges, D. F. (2003). The cumulative cost of additional wakefulness: Dose-response effects on neurobehavioral functions and sleep physiology from chronic sleep restriction and total sleep deprivation. *Sleep, 26* (2), 117–126.

12. Akerstedt, T. G., Fredlung, P., Jansson, B., & Gillberg, M. (2001). A prospective study of fatal accidents and sleep disturbances, fatigue, work stress, and work hours. *Sleep, 24*, A123.

13. Special Supplement to the Tufts University Health & Nutrition Letter. (2004, October). Boston.

14. Vorona, R. D., Winn, M. P., Babineau, T. W., Eng, B. P., Feldman, H. R., & Ware, J. C. (2005). Overweight and obese patients in a primary care population report less sleep than patients with a normal body mass index. *Archives of Internal Medicine, 165* (1), 25–30.

15. Coren, S. (1996). *Sleep thieves.* New York: Free Press Paperbacks/Simon & Schuster.

16. Sejnowski, T. J., & Desteyhe, A. (2000). Why do we sleep? *Brain Research, 886,* 208–223.

17. National Sleep Foundation. Sleep and the traveler. (2002). www.sleepfoundation.org/publications.

18. Hughes, R. J., Sack, R. L., Lewy, A. J. (1998). The role of melatonin and circadian phase in age-related sleep maintenance insomnia: Assessment in a clinical trial of melatonin replacement. *Sleep, 1,* 52–68.

19. Walsleben, J. A., & Baron-Faust, R. (2000). *A woman's guide to sleep.* New York: Three Rivers Press/Crown Publishing Group.

20. Drummond, S., Kuchinsky, A., Solamat, J. S., Brown, G. G., & Gillin, S. C. (2002). Effects of cognitive demands on cerebral response to total sleep deprivation. *Sleep, 25*, A88.

21. Fosse, R., Stickgold, R., & Hobson, J. A. (2001). The mind in REM sleep: Reports on emotional experience. *Sleep, 24* (8), 947–956.

22. Peigneux, P., Laureys, S., Delbeuck, X., & Maquet, P. (2001). Sleeping brain, learning brain: The role of sleep in memory systems. *Neuroreport, 12*, 11A–124A.

23. Ferreni, A. F., & Ferreni, R. L. (2000). *Health in the later years.* New York: McGraw-Hill.

24. Giraudo, G. G., Rinaldi, P. A., Dolso, P., & Brotini, S. (2001). Sleep disturbances in the elderly: A population study of the subjects over 85 years old. *Sleep, 24*, A235, A236.

25. Ehlers, C. L., & Kupfer, D. I. (1997). Slow wave sleep: Do young adult men and women age differently? *Journal of Sleep Research, 6,* 211–215.

26. Chokroverty, S. (1999). *Sleep disorders medicine: Basic science, technical considerations, and clinical aspects* (2nd ed.). Boston: Butterworth-Heinemann.

27. Hypopnea in sleep-disordered breathing in adults. (2001). Position paper. *Sleep, 24* (4), 469–470.

28. National Sleep Foundation. Women and sleep. (2003). www.sleepfoundation.org.

29. National Sleep Foundation. Sleep apnea. (2002). www.sleepfoundation.org/publications.

30. Larie, P., & Hoffstein, L. (2001). Sleep apnea syndrome: A possible contributing factor to resistant hypertension. *Sleep, 35* (6), 721–725.

31. Maas, J. B. (1998). *Power sleep.* New York: Villard Books/Random House.

32. Practice parameters for the use of laser-assisted uvulopalatoplasty: An update for 2000. (2001). Position paper. *Sleep, 24* (5), 603–619.

33. Practice parameters for the treatment of narcolepsy: An update for 2000. (2001). Position paper. *Sleep, 24* (4), 451–456.

34. Yaeger, J. (1999). Nocturnal eating syndromes: To sleep, perchance to eat. *Journal of American Medical Association, 282* (7), 689–692.

35. Birketredt, G. S., & Stunkard, A. (1999). Behavioral and neuro-endocrine characteristics of night-eating syndrome. *Journal of American Medical Association, 282* (7), 657–663.

36. Schenk, C. H., & Mahowald, M. W. (1994). Review of nocturnal sleep-related eating disorders. *International Journal of Eating Disorders, 15* (4), 343–356.

37. Levin, R. (1994). Sleep and dreaming characteristics of frequent nightmare subjects in a university population. *Dreaming: Journal of the Association for the Study of Dreams, 4,* 127–137.

38. Wetter, D. W., & Young, T. B. (1994). The relation between cigarette smoking and sleep disturbance. *Preventative Medicine, 23,* 328–334.

39. Vein, A. M., et al. (1991). Physical exercise and nocturnal sleep in healthy humans. *Human Physiology, 17,* 391–397

40. National Sleep Foundation. Sleep aids. (2002). www.sleepfoundation.org/publications.

41. O'Hanlon, B. (2000). *Overcoming sleep disorders: A natural approach.* Freedom, CA: The Crossing Press.

Add It Up! EVALUATING YOUR SLEEP

Part 1 How sleepy are you?

The Epworth Sleepiness Scale is an informal sleep latency test that can help you evaluate how sleepy you are during the day, a key symptom of many sleep disorders. To evaluate your daytime sleepiness, use the scale from 0 to 3 to rate how likely you would be to doze off in the situations listed here.

> 0 = would never doze
>
> 1 = slight chance of dozing
>
> 2 = moderate chance of dozing
>
> 3 = high chance of dozing

Situation	Chance of Dozing
Sitting and reading	1
Watching television	2
Sitting inactive in a public place (for example, a theater or a meeting)	0
Riding in a car for an hour without a break	1
Lying down in the afternoon	3
Sitting and talking to someone	0
Sitting quietly after lunch (when you have had no alcohol)	2
Sitting in a car stopped in traffic	3
TOTAL	12

Interpretation:

0–8   You are probably not suffering from excessive daytime sleepiness.

9–14   You need to think seriously about getting more sleep.

15+   You should probably consult your physician, describing all your sleep-related symptoms.

Part 2 Do you have symptoms of a sleep disorder?

Ask yourself the following questions:

- Do you have trouble falling asleep three nights a week or more?
- Do you wake frequently during the night?
- Do you wake up too early and find it difficult to get back to sleep?
- Do you wake up unrefreshed?
- Do you snore loudly?
- Are you aware of gasping for breath or not breathing while you are sleeping, or has anyone ever told you that you do this?
- Do you feel sleepy during the day or doze off watching TV, reading, driving, or engaged in daily activities, even though you get 8 hours of sleep a night?
- Do you have nightmares?
- Do you feel unpleasant, tingling, creeping sensations in your legs while trying to sleep?

If you answer yes to any of these questions, it is possible that you are suffering from a sleep disorder. The first step to take is to make sure you have good sleep habits and practices, as described in the chapter. If you are doing everything you can to ensure a good night's sleep, consult your physician. He or she may refer you to a sleep disorder specialist.

SOURCE: Part 1: Adapted from National Sleep Foundation, 2002, www.sleepfoundation.org; Epworth Sleepiness Scale developed by Dr. Murray Johns. Used by permission of Dr. Johns. Part 2: Adapted from National Sleep Foundation, 2004, www.sleepfoundation.org.

PART 2

Your Lifestyle and Health

Chapter 7   Nutrition: Healthy Food Choices
Chapter 8   Fitness: Physical Activity for Life
Chapter 9   Body Weight and Body Composition: The Healthy Balance
Chapter 10   Body Image: Viewing Yourself

As you learned in Part 1, your health is influenced by many factors, both personal and environmental, that relate to your mind and body. In Part 2 we explore the lifestyle issues that are instrumental in shaping your health. We begin with nutrition, showing how the food choices you make every day have a direct influence, either positive or negative, on your health status. Next we consider physical fitness and the approaches you can take—at any age—to improve your fitness level. Then we turn to body weight and body composition, an important part of optimal health. Part 2 ends with a chapter on body image, which addresses how the media, culture, and family and friends influence your view of yourself. As you read these chapters, think about your lifestyle and habits. Is your lifestyle today a healthy one? Or is it time for improvement?

THINK IT OVER

Do you think there's a message for you in the maxim "You are what you eat"?

Where does physical fitness fall in your list of priorities?

Have you been the same weight for most of your adult life, or is your weight increasing over time?

If you could change one thing about your appearance today, what would it be?

CHAPTER 7

Nutrition: Healthy Food Choices

DID YOU KNOW?

- The convenience, price, and tasty flavors of burgers, fries, and shakes place them among the most popular food choices available. Half the money spent on restaurant food in the United States goes for fast food.

- Current sugar consumption in the United States averages out to 32 teaspoons— nearly three quarters of a cup—per person per day. Increased consumption of sugar, notably in soft drinks, is thought to be linked to the rise in overweight and obesity among Americans.

- If you eat organically grown foods, you are probably not protecting your health any more than you would if you ate conventionally grown foods. However, you are supporting agricultural practices that sustain the environment and benefit the health of the planet.

OLC *Your Health Today* www.mhhe.com/teague1e

Go to the Online Learning Center for *Your Health Today* for interactive activities, quizzes, flashcards, Web links, and more resources related to this chapter.

If you live to age 80, you will have consumed more than 86,000 meals and nearly 63 tons of food. If you follow a diet that is nutritionally beneficial, this food will help you stay energetic, lean, and healthy, supporting your attainment of overall wellness. If your diet is inadequate or harmful—for example, if burgers and fries show up on your daily menu more often than not—your quality of life when you are older may be seriously compromised. In other words, what you eat today has a direct effect on how healthy you will be later in life.

Unfortunately, healthy eating can be a challenge in a culture that promotes the consumption of fast foods and convenience foods in shopping malls, sports arenas, airports, and college dining halls. The media constantly bombards us with ads for foods and meals that undermine our health. Supermarkets devote entire aisles to chips and soft drinks. As consumers, we may find it difficult or impossible to find a healthy snack—an apple, for example, or a glass of milk—when we're out in public. What's worse, many people have acquired a taste for the high-calorie, full-fat, heavily salted foods so plentiful in our environment. People living in low-income communities have an even harder time finding healthy food (see the box below, "Low-Income Communities and Healthy Food"). The result, as noted throughout this text, is a high incidence of overweight and lifestyle-related chronic illnesses among Americans.

Choosing a healthy diet in this culture is possible, however, and in this chapter, we provide you with the tools you need to do so. We begin with a brief explanation of the different sets of nutritional guidelines you need to know about, followed by a description of the nutrients required in a healthy diet. We then explore in more detail the tools that are available to guide your dietary choices, and we discuss how you can use them to create your own healthy diet. We then consider a number of current consumer concerns, and we close with a discussion of several issues in food safety and technology. Throughout the chapter, we offer specific suggestions and tips for improving your diet and thus safeguarding your long-term wellness.

UNDERSTANDING NUTRITIONAL GUIDELINES

Decisions about the best foods to eat are influenced by personal tastes, experiences, and habits; by family and cultural traditions; by lifestyle and budget; and by the availability of different foods. With all these factors playing a part in decision making, you also need knowledge—current and accurate information about the food choices that are most likely to promote health and prevent disease.

As discussed in Chapter 1, society has a vital interest in the good health of its citizens. A natural outcome of this is that both governmental and nongovernmental organizations support scientific research in nutrition and have developed several different kinds of guides to healthy eating. In this section we briefly describe some of these guides; later in the chapter we discuss ways to apply them to your daily food decisions.

HIGHLIGHT ON HEALTH

Low-Income Communities and Healthy Food

Studies have shown that different neighborhood and community environments significantly affect eating practices. In low-income neighborhoods, fast-food outlets and small food markets dominate the retail food landscape, providing consumers with less healthy foods, at higher prices. In affluent neighborhoods, where supermarkets predominate, low-fat and whole-grain foods are much more readily available, along with diverse fruit and vegetable choices. One study found that supermarkets were four times more likely to be located in affluent than low-income communities. The result is that residents of low-income neighborhoods do not have the same access to healthy foods as residents of high-income neighborhoods.

All communities are equally entitled to healthful, affordable, accessible food choices. Supermarket chains may be reluctant to locate stores in low-income communities because of insufficient space for large stores,

negative stereotypes of the environment, and the challenge of marketing to diverse cultural populations. Federal, state, and local financial incentives, such as loan guarantees and reduced property taxes for supermarkets and small stores that provide healthy foods, may help overcome these barriers. Stores also need assistance with zoning approval and building permits. Neighborhood and community groups can help create healthier and more equitable food landscapes in their communities by becoming actively involved with city government and development.

Sources: "Improving the Nutritional Resource Environment for Healthy Living Through Community-Based Participatory Research," by D. C. Sloan, et al., 2003, *Journal of General Internal Medicine, 2,* 568–575; *Food Fight,* by K. D. Brown, 2004, New York: McGraw-Hill; "The Effect on Dietary Quality of Participation in the Food Stamp and WIC Programs," by P. E. Wilde, P. E. McNamara, and C. K. Rannex, 2000, *Food Assistance and Nutrition Research Report,* No. 9. USDA.

Beating the Odds

Who Will Meet the Food Court Challenge Best?

Eating well on a college campus can be a challenge. Many college food courts offer a limitless selection of foods, including fast foods loaded with calories, fat, sodium, and sugar. The typical student diet may look more like an inverted food pyramid, driven by late-night munching, ordering in, overconsumption of alcohol, and careless eating habits. The challenge to students is to navigate the abundance of choices and find those foods that lead to healthy nutrition. Experts suggest that students (1) arrive at the food court before they are very hungry; (2) walk through the entire food court before making selections; (3) make fruit and vegetables the major portion of food selections; (4) sit far away from the food that is being served; and (5) do not go back for seconds. Brief profiles of three people are presented here. Who do you think makes the best choices for a healthy lunch?

Joni, a relatively sedentary 30-year-old student, is ravenously hungry by lunchtime because she did not eat breakfast. She makes her food selections from the salad bar and dessert section. She creates a salad from lettuce, fresh vegetables, grated cheese, hard-boiled eggs, and walnuts, and she tops it with a generous portion of salad dressing. She adds servings of potato salad and macaroni salad on the side. Her choice of dessert is a 5-ounce brownie, and her beverage is a 10-ounce glass of 2 percent milk. She sits close to where the food is served.

Andy is a 19-year-old student who is very active in sports. Andy skipped breakfast and had an iced raspberry fruit and oatmeal cereal bar from a vending machine at 10:00 a.m. For lunch he chooses a quarter-pound cheeseburger, french fries, and water. Andy has a slice of fat-free apple pie for dessert. He sits far away from where the food is served.

Sandy, a 22-year-old graduate student, is moderately active. She regularly eats breakfast, usually a bagel with fat-free cream cheese and an 8-ounce glass of orange juice. She chooses a hot turkey sandwich, a small order of pasta, and a salad with a moderate amount of low-fat dressing. Her choice of beverage is a 12-ounce Diet Coke. Sandy has a frozen yogurt for dessert. She sits close to where the food is served.

***OLC* Web site** Visit the **Online Learning Center** at www.mhhe.com/teague1e for comments by the authors.

In 1997 the National Academies' Food and Nutrition Board introduced the **Dietary Reference Intakes (DRIs),** a set of recommendations designed to promote optimal health and prevent both nutritional deficiencies and chronic diseases like cancer and cardiovascular disease. The DRIs, developed by American and Canadian scientists, encompass four kinds of recommendations. The **Estimated Average Requirement (EAR)** is the amount of nutrients needed by half of the people in any one age group, for example, teenage boys. Nutritionists use the EAR to assess whether an entire population's normal diet provides sufficient nutrients. It is used in nutrition research and as a basis on which recommended dietary allowances are set. The **Recommended Dietary Allowances (RDAs)** are based on information provided by the EAR and represent the average daily amount of any one nutrient an individual needs to protect against nutritional deficiency. If there is not enough information about a nutrient to set an RDA, an **Adequate Intake (AI)** is provided. The **Tolerable Upper Intake Level (UL)** is the highest amount of a nutrient a person can take in without risking toxicity.

In 2002 the Food and Nutrition Board introduced another measure, the **Acceptable Macronutrient Distribution Range (AMDR).** These ranges represent intake levels of essential nutrients that provide adequate nutrition and that are associated with reduced risk of chronic disease. If your intake exceeds the AMDR, you increase your risk of chronic disease. For example, the AMDR for dietary fat for adult men is 20–35 percent of the calories consumed in a day. A man who consumes more than 35 percent of his daily calories as fat increases his risk for chronic diseases.

Whereas the DRIs are recommended intake levels for individual nutrients, the ***Dietary Guidelines for Americans,*** published by the U.S. Department of Agriculture (USDA) and the U.S. Department of Health and Human Services, provide scientifically based diet and exercise recommendations designed to promote health and reduce the risk of chronic disease. The **USDA Food Guide Pyramid** was designed to translate the *Dietary Guidelines* and the DRIs into healthy food choices. The *Dietary Guidelines,* first published in 1980 and revised every 5 years, are the cornerstone of U.S. nutrition policy. The Food Guide Pyramid, released in 1992 and revised in 1996, became the most widely publicized and used nutritional tool in the country. Many alternative pyramids were developed for different populations and kinds of diet (for example, young children, vegetarians). Comparable Canadian documents are Canada's Food Guide to Healthy Eating and the Food Guide Rainbow, currently undergoing revision.

In 2005 new *Dietary Guidelines* were published, and the Food Guide Pyramid was replaced by the **USDA MyPyramid.** We discuss all these nutritional guidelines later in the chapter. To assess your current knowledge of nutritional recommendations in general, take a minute to read the three profiles in the box "Beating the Odds: The Food Court Challenge." Which of these college students do you think has the healthiest diet?

One other set of standards—the Daily Values—is in common use. Also developed by the USDA, the **Daily Values** are used on food labels and indicate how a particular food contributes to the recommended daily intake of major nutrients in a 2,000-calorie diet. We explain Daily Values in more detail later in the chapter in the discussion of food labels.

Before we explore healthy diets, we take a look at the major nutrients that make up our diet. For each nutrient, we include general recommendations for intake based either on the DRIs or the AMDRs.

TYPES OF NUTRIENTS

As you work, play, and engage in the daily activities of your life, your body is powered by energy produced from the food you consume. Your body needs the **essential nutrients**—water, carbohydrates, proteins, fats, vitamins, and minerals—contained in these foods, but not only to provide fuel. They also build, maintain, and repair tissues; regulate body functions; and support the communication among cells that allows you to breathe, move, think, see, hear, smell, and taste—in short, to be a living, sensing human being.

These nutrients are referred to as "essential" because your body cannot manufacture them; they must come from food or from nutritional supplements. People who fail to consume adequate amounts of an essential nutrient are likely to develop a nutritional deficiency disease, such as scurvy from lack of vitamin C or beri-beri from lack of vitamin B1. Nutritional deficiency diseases are seldom seen in developed countries because most people consume an adequate diet. A varied and balanced diet usually provides all the essential nutrients.

The essential nutrients are often divided into macronutrients and micronutrients. We need large quantities of **macronutrients;** they provide energy and perform important functions like building new cells and facilitating chemical reactions. Macronutrients include water, carbohydrates, protein, and fat. We need only small amounts of **micronutrients;** their role generally is to help

KEY TERMS

Dietary Reference Intakes (DRIs) An umbrella term for four sets of dietary recommendations: Estimated Average Requirement, Recommended Dietary Allowances, Adequate Intake, and Tolerable Upper Intake Level; designed to promote optimal health and prevent both nutritional deficiencies and chronic diseases.

Estimated Average Requirement (EAR) The population-wide average nutrient requirements used in nutrition research and as a basis for setting RDA values.

Recommended Dietary Allowance (RDA) The average daily amount of any one nutrient an individual needs to protect against nutritional deficiency.

Adequate Intake (AI) The recommended amount of a nutrient if there is not enough information to set an RDA.

Tolerable Upper Intake Level (UL) The highest amount of a nutrient a person can take in without risking toxicity.

Acceptable Macronutrient Distribution Range (AMDR) Intake ranges that provide adequate nutrition and that are associated with reduced risk of chronic disease.

Dietary Guidelines for Americans Set of scientifically based recommendations designed to promote health and reduce the risk for many chronic diseases through diet and physical activity.

USDA Food Guide Pyramid Set of practical recommendations for daily food choices in five major food groups, based on the DRIs; superseded in 2005 by MyPyramid.

USDA MyPyramid The new set of practical recommendations for daily food choices developed to accompany the 2005 *Dietary Guidelines for Americans.*

Daily Values Set of dietary standards used on food labels to indicate how a particular food contributes to the recommended daily intake of major nutrients in a 2,000-calorie diet.

essential nutrients Chemical substances used by the body to build, maintain, and repair tissues and regulate body functions. They cannot be manufactured by the body and must be obtained from foods or supplements.

macronutrients Essential nutrients that the body needs in large amounts—water, carbohydrates, proteins, and fats.

micronutrients Essential nutrients that the body needs in small amounts—minerals and vitamins.

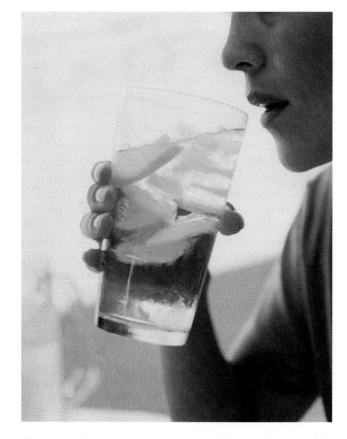

The amount of water you need every day depends on many factors, such as your activity level, environmental conditions, and the kinds of foods you eat. Making a habit of drinking water throughout the day is one way of getting enough of this essential nutrient.

regulate body functions. Minerals are inorganic micronutrients; vitamins are organic micronutrients.

When food is *metabolized*—chemically transformed into energy and wastes—it fuels our bodies. The energy provided by food is measured in kilocalories, commonly shortened to *calorie*. One **kilocalorie** is the amount of energy needed to raise the temperature of 1 kilogram of water by 1 degree centigrade. The more energy we expend, the more kilocalories we need to consume. We get the most energy from fats, 9 calories per gram of fat. Carbohydrates and protein provide 4 calories per gram. In other words, fats provide more calories than do carbohydrates or proteins, a factor to consider when planning a balanced diet that does not lead to weight gain.

We turn now to a closer look at the essential nutrients—water, carbohydrates, proteins, fats, minerals, and vitamins.

Water—The Unappreciated Nutrient

We need water to digest, absorb, and transport nutrients. Water provides a medium in which biochemical reactions can occur, helps regulate body temperature, dilutes wastes to make them less toxic, carries waste products out of the body, cushions body cells, and lubricates our moving parts. Water is such an integral part of our lives that we are rarely conscious of its importance.[1] You can live without the other nutrients for weeks, but you can survive without water for only a few days. You lose an amount of water equal to about 4 percent of your body weight each day in exhaled air, perspiration, urine, and feces.

When your body is healthy, the right fluid balance—the right amount of fluid inside and outside each cell—is maintained. Fluid balance is essential to life. When a cell has too little water inside, it shrivels and dies; when it contains too much water, it bursts. Fluid balance is maintained through the action of substances called **electrolytes,** mineral components that carry electrical charges and conduct nerve impulses. Electrolytes include sodium, potassium, and chloride. Sweat contains electrolytes, but heavy sweating usually does not cause electrolyte deficiency. Water alone, in combination with a balanced diet, replaces electrolytes lost daily through sweat.[2]

How much water should you drink every day? Your water needs vary according to the foods you eat, the temperature and humidity in your environment, your activity level, and other factors. Adults generally need 1 to 1.5 milliliters of water for each calorie spent in the day. If you expend 2,000 calories a day, you require 2 to 3 liters—8 to 12 cups—of fluids.[3] Heavy sweating increases your need for fluids. You obtain fluids not only from the water you drink but also from the water in foods, particularly fruits such as oranges and apples. Caffeinated beverages and alcohol are not good sources of your daily fluid intake because of their dehydrating effects, although some recent research suggests that the water in such beverages may offset these effects to some extent.[3]

Carbohydrates—Your Body's Fuel

Carbohydrates are the body's main source of energy.[3] They fuel most of the body's cells during daily activities; they are used by muscle cells during high-intensity exercise; and they are the only source of energy for brain cells, red blood cells, and some other types of cells. Athletes in particular need to consume a high-carbohydrate diet to fuel their high-energy activities. Fiber, a nondigestible form of carbohydrate, helps maintain gastrointestinal health.

Carbohydrates are the foods we think of as sugars and starches. They come almost exclusively from plants (the exception is lactose, the sugar in milk). Plants are complex food factories that make glucose, a sugar they later convert to starch, by acquiring water and nutrients from the soil, carbon dioxide from the air, and energy from the sun (the process of photosynthesis). As plants grow, they also make various vitamins, minerals, and chemicals and some protein and fat. Most of the carbohydrates and other nutrients we need come from grains, seeds, fruits, and vegetables.[2]

Simple Carbohydrates

Carbohydrates are divided into simple carbohydrates and complex carbohydrates. In **simple carbohydrates,** each molecule is composed of either one or two sugar units. Six simple carbohydrates (sugars) are important in nutrition: glucose, fructose, galactose, lactose, maltose, and sucrose. Glucose, the main source of energy for the brain and nervous system, is found primarily in honey, molasses, fruits, syrups, and vegetables. Fructose, or fruit sugar, is found mostly in fruits, honey, and table sugar, as well as in some vegetables. Galactose is one of two single sugars that together make up milk sugar, or lactose.

The other three simple carbohydrates—lactose, maltose, and sucrose—all contain glucose. Lactose (milk sugar) is formed by the combination of glucose and galactose. Maltose (malt sugar, which appears wherever starch is digested in the body) is formed by the combination of two units of glucose. Sucrose (table sugar) consists of fructose and glucose. Sugars are absorbed into the bloodstream and travel to body cells, where they can be used for energy. Glucose also travels to the liver and muscles, where it can be stored as **glycogen** (a complex carbohydrate) for future energy needs.

When you eat a food containing large amounts of simple carbohydrates, sugar enters your bloodstream quickly, giving you a burst of energy or a "sugar high." It is also absorbed into your cells quickly, leaving you feeling depleted and craving more sugar. Foods containing added sugar, such as candy bars and sodas, have an even more dramatic effect. Consumption of sugar has been linked to the epidemic of overweight and obesity in the United States and to the parallel increase in the incidence of diabetes, a disorder in which body cells cannot use the sugar circulating in the blood.

Complex Carbohydrates

The type of carbohydrates called **complex carbohydrates** are composed of multiple sugar units and include starches and dietary fiber. **Starches** come in a variety of textures, flavors, and molecular structures and occur in grains, vegetables, and some fruits. Most starchy foods also contain ample portions of vitamins, minerals, proteins, and water. Starches must be broken down into single sugars in the digestive system before they can be absorbed into the bloodstream to be used for energy or stored for future use.

The complex carbohydrates found in whole grains are often refined or processed to make them easier to digest and more appealing to the consumer, but the refining process removes many of the vitamins, minerals, and other nutritious components found in the whole food. Refined carbohydrates include such foods as white rice, white bread and other products made from white flour, pasta, and sweet desserts. Like sugar, refined carbohydrates can enter the bloodstream quickly and just as quickly leave you feeling hungry again. Whole grains (such as whole wheat, brown rice, oatmeal, and corn) are preferred because they provide more nutrients, slow the digestive process, and make you feel full longer. The consumption of whole grains is associated with lowered risk of diabetes, obesity, heart disease, and some forms of cancer.[4]

The RDA for carbohydrates is 130 grams for males and females from the age of 1 to 70 years. Pregnant and lactating women require more (175 and 210 grams per day,

KEY TERMS

kilocalorie   Amount of energy needed to raise the temperature of 1 kilogram of water by 1 degree centigrade; commonly shortened to *calorie.*

electrolytes   Mineral components that carry electrical charges and conduct nerve impulses.

simple carbohydrates   Easily digestible carbohydrates composed of one or two units of sugar.

glycogen   The complex carbohydrate form in which glucose is stored in the liver and muscles.

complex carbohydrates   Carbohydrates that are composed of multiple sugar units and that must be broken down further before they can be used by the body.

starch   A complex carbohydrate found in many plant foods.

respectively). The AMDR for carbohydrates is 45 percent to 65 percent of daily energy intake, which amounts to 225 to 325 grams in a 2,000-calorie diet (even though only about 130 grams per day are enough to meet the body's needs). In the typical American diet, carbohydrates do contribute about half of all calories, but most of them are in the form of simple sugars or highly refined grains. Instead, carbohydrates should come from a diverse spectrum of whole grains and other starches, vegetables, and fruits.[5] The Food and Nutrition Board recommends that no more than 25 percent of calories come from added sugars, and many health professionals recommend only 10 percent.[3]

Dietary fiber, a complex carbohydrate found in plants, cannot be broken down in the digestive tract. A diet rich in dietary fiber makes stools soft and bulky. They pass through the intestine rapidly and are expelled easily, helping to prevent hemorrhoids and constipation.[6] Some foods contain **functional fiber,** natural or synthetic fiber that has been added to increase the healthful effects of the food. **Total fiber** refers to the combined amount of dietary fiber and functional fiber in a food.

Dietary fiber that dissolves in water, referred to as viscous fiber (or sometimes as soluble fiber), is known to lower blood cholesterol levels and can slow the process of digestion so blood sugar levels remain more even. Foods containing viscous fiber include oat bran, many fruits, and legumes (such as peas, beans, peanuts, soybeans). Dietary fiber that does not dissolve in water (sometimes called insoluble fiber)—contained in such food sources as wheat bran and psyllium seed—passes through the digestive tract essentially unchanged. Because it absorbs water, insoluble fiber helps you feel full after eating and stimulates your intestinal wall to contract and relax, serving as a natural laxative. Some scientists speculate that the increased water content of high-fiber stools dilutes any carcinogens that may be present (from food, additives, and so on), although this theory remains unproven.[6,7]

The RDAs for fiber are 25 grams for women aged 19 to 50 and 38 grams for men aged 14 to 50 (or 14 grams of fiber for every 1,000 calories consumed). For people over 50, the RDA is 21 grams for women and 30 grams for men.[5] The typical American diet provides only about 14 or 15 grams of fiber a day. If you want to increase the fiber in your diet, it is important to do so gradually. A sudden increase in daily fiber may cause bloating, gas, abdominal cramping, or even a bowel obstruction, particularly if you fail to drink enough liquids to easily carry the fiber throughout the body.[2]

Fiber is best obtained through diet. Pills and other fiber supplements do not contain the nutrients found in high-fiber foods.[2] Excessive amounts of fiber (generally 60 grams or more per day) can decrease the absorption of important vitamins and minerals such as calcium, zinc, magnesium, and iron.[3] Fruits, vegetables, dried beans, peas and other legumes, cereals, grains, nuts, and seeds are the best sources of dietary fiber.

Protein—Nutritional Muscle

Your body uses **protein** to build and maintain muscles, bones, and other body tissues. Proteins also form enzymes that in turn facilitate chemical reactions, making it possible for antibodies to help fight illness and disease, for hemoglobin to transport oxygen, and for hormones to regulate many body functions. Proteins are constructed from 20 different amino acids. Amino acids that your body cannot produce on its own, nine in all, are called **essential amino acids;** they must be supplied by foods. Those that can be produced by your body are called nonessential amino acids.

Food sources of protein include both animals and plants. Animal proteins (meat, fish, poultry, milk, cheese, and eggs) are usually a good source of **complete proteins,** meaning they are composed of ample amounts of all the essential amino acids. Vegetable proteins (grains, legumes, nuts, seeds, and other vegetables) provide **incomplete proteins,** meaning they contain small amounts of essential amino acids or some, but not all, of the essential amino acids. If you do not consume sufficient amounts of the essential amino acids, body organ functions may be compromised.

People who eat little or no animal protein may not be getting all the essential amino acids they need. One remedy is to eat plant foods with different amounts of incomplete proteins. For example, beans are low in the essential amino acid methionine but high in lysine, and rice is high in methionine and low in lysine. In combination, beans and rice form **complementary proteins.** Eating the two together at one meal or over the course of a day provides all the essential amino acids.[3] The matching of such foods is called **mutual supplementation.**

The AMDR for protein is 10 percent to 35 percent of daily calories consumed.[5] The need for protein is based on body weight: The larger your body, the more protein you need to take in. A healthy adult typically needs 0.8 grams of protein for every kilogram (2.2 pounds) of body weight, or about 0.36 grams for every pound.[8] At the upper end of the AMDR range, the percentages provide a more than ample amount of protein in the diet. Growing children and pregnant or lactating women have a higher than average RDA, since building new tissue requires more protein.

Fats—A Necessary Nutrient

Fats are a concentrated energy source and the principal form of stored energy in the body. The fats in food provide essential fatty acids, play a role in the production of other fatty acids and vitamin D, and provide the major material for cell membranes. They transport the fat-soluble vitamins (A, D, E, and K) and assist in their absorption; they affect the texture, taste, and smell of foods; stimulate appetite; and contribute to feelings of fullness. Fats provide an emergency reserve when we are sick or our food intake is diminished. Fats also serve as a shock absorber to protect body organs, and they insulate the body membranes.

Fats, or lipids, are composed of fatty acids. Nutritionists divide these acids into three groups—saturated, monounsaturated, and polyunsaturated—on the basis of their chemical composition. **Saturated fats** remain stable (solid) at room temperature; **monounsaturated** fats are liquid at room temperature but solidify somewhat when refrigerated; **polyunsaturated fats** are liquid both at room temperature and in the refrigerator. Liquid fats are commonly referred to as oils.

Saturated fatty acids are found in animal sources, such as beef, pork, poultry, and whole-milk dairy products. They are also found in certain tropical oils and nuts, including coconut and palm oil and macadamia nuts. Monounsaturated and polyunsaturated fatty acids are found primarily in plant sources. Olive, safflower, peanut, and canola oils, as well as avocados and many nuts, contain mostly monounsaturated fat. Corn and soybean oils contain mostly polyunsaturated fat, as do many kinds of fish, including salmon, trout, and anchovies.

Saturated fats pose a risk to health because they tend to raise blood levels of **cholesterol,** a waxy substance that can clog arteries, leading to cardiovascular disease. More specifically, saturated fats raise blood levels of low-density lipoproteins (LDLs), known as "bad cholesterol," and triglycerides, another kind of blood fat. Unsaturated fats, in contrast, tend to lower blood levels of LDLs, and some unsaturated fats (monounsaturated fats) may also raise levels of high-density lipoproteins (HDLs), known as "good cholesterol." [9]

Cholesterol is needed for several important body functions, but too much of it circulating in the bloodstream can be a problem. The body produces it in the liver and also obtains it from animal food sources, such as meat, cheese, eggs, and milk. It is recommended that no more than 300 milligrams of dietary cholesterol be consumed per day. The effects of cholesterol on cardiovascular health are discussed in detail in Chapter 21.

Another kind of fatty acid, **trans fatty acid,** is produced through **hydrogenation,** a process whereby liquid vegetable oils are turned into more solid fats. Food manufacturers use hydrogenation to prolong a food's shelf life and change its texture. Peanut butter is frequently hydrogenated, as is margarine. With some hydrogenation, margarine becomes semisoft (tub margarine); with further hydrogenation, it becomes hard (stick margarine). (See the box on the next page, "Butter or Margarine?")

Trans fatty acids (or trans fats) are believed to pose a risk to cardiovascular health similar to or even greater than that of saturated fats, because they tend to raise LDLs and lower HDLs. Foods high in trans fatty acids include baked and snack foods like crackers, cookies, chips, cakes, pies, and doughnuts, as well as deep-fried fast foods like french fries. A single large (5-ounce) order of french fries contains 4 grams of trans fatty acids; an 8-ounce order of onion rings contains 10 grams. In packaged foods, the phrase "partially hydrogenated vegetable oil" in the list of ingredients provides a clue to the presence of trans fats.

KEY TERMS

dietary fiber   A complex carbohydrate found in plants that cannot be broken down in the digestive tract.

functional fiber   Natural or synthetic fiber that has been added to food.

total fiber   Combined amount of dietary fiber and functional fiber in a food.

protein   Essential nutrient made up of amino acids, needed to build and maintain muscles, bones, and other body tissues.

essential amino acids   Amino acids that the body cannot produce on its own.

complete proteins   Proteins composed of ample amounts of all the essential amino acids.

incomplete proteins   Proteins that contain small amounts of essential amino acids or some, but not all, of the essential amino acids.

complementary proteins   Proteins that in combination provide essential amino acids.

mutual supplementation   The nutritional strategy of combining two incomplete protein sources to provide a complete protein.

fats   Also known as lipids, fats are an essential nutrient composed of fatty acids and used for energy and other body functions.

saturated fats   Lipids that are the predominant fat in animal products and other fats that remain solid at room temperature.

monounsaturated fats   Lipids that are liquid at room temperature and semisolid or solid when refrigerated.

polyunsaturated fats   Lipids that are liquid at room temperature and in the refrigerator.

cholesterol   A waxy substance produced by the liver and obtained from animal food sources, essential to the functioning of the body but a possible factor in cardiovascular disease if too much is circulating in the bloodstream.

trans fatty acids   Lipids that have been chemically modified through the process of hydrogenation so they remain solid at room temperature.

hydrogenation   Process whereby liquid vegetable oils are turned into more solid fats.

Challenges & Choices

Butter or Margarine?

For many years, health-conscious consumers chose margarine rather than butter, knowing that the saturated fat in butter increased their risk for heart disease. But in 1993, researchers at Harvard University concluded that the trans fatty acids contained in margarine might actually increase the risk for heart disease more than the saturated fat in butter does. Consumers were left uncertain which was the better—or worse—choice.

Although trans fat and saturated fat can both contribute to heart disease, margarine is still considered healthier than butter. The American Heart Association offers the following advice:

- Choose margarine over butter, but choose soft or liquid margarine over stick margarine. The harder the margarine, the more saturated and trans fat it contains.

- When buying margarine, look for one that contains at least twice as much polyunsaturated as saturated fats. Margarine made from canola, safflower, sunflower, and corn oils are the preferred choices.

- For baking, use a stick margarine that lists monosaturated or polyunsaturated fats as the first ingredients.

- Avoid products that list hydrogenated or partially hydrogenated oil as an ingredient, since they are high in trans fatty acids.

- Reduce your use of butter or margarine by using herbs, spices, and low-fat ingredients to enhance taste; for example, try dipping French bread in olive oil rather than spreading it with butter or margarine.

It's Not Just Personal . . .

The American Heart Association recommends limiting consumption of saturated and trans fats to no more than 10 percent of total daily calories—in a 2,000-calorie diet, about 22 grams. Doing so helps you avoid high levels of cholesterol and overweight, two major risk factors in cardiovascular disease—the leading cause of death for Americans.

Sources: "Foods That Harm, Foods That Heal," 1997, Reader's Digest Association; *Nutrition: Concepts and Controversies*, by F. Sizer and E. Whitney, 2003, Belmont, CA: Wadsworth/Thomson Learning.

Unlike trans fats, two kinds of polyunsaturated fatty acids—omega-3 and omega-6 fatty acids—provide health benefits. **Omega-3 fatty acids,** which contain the essential nutrient alpha-linolenic acid, help slow the clotting of blood, decrease triglyceride levels, improve arterial health, and lower blood pressure. They may also help protect against autoimmune diseases such as arthritis.[10] **Omega-6 fatty acids,** which contain the essential nutrient linoleic acid, are also important to health, but nutritionists believe that Americans consume too much omega-6 in proportion to omega-3.[11] They recommend increasing consumption of omega-3 sources—fatty fish like salmon, trout, and anchovies; vegetable oils like canola, walnut, and flaxseed; and dark-green leafy vegetables—and decreasing consumption of omega-6 sources, mainly corn, soybean, and cottonseed oils.

How much of your daily caloric intake should come from fat? The AMDR is 20 percent to 35 percent.[5] It is recommended that Americans get about 30 percent of their calories from fats and only about one third of that (10 percent) from saturated fats. Most adults need only 15 percent of their daily calorie intake in the form of fat, whereas young children should get 30 percent to 40 percent of their calories from fat to ensure proper growth and brain development, according to the American Academy of Pediatrics. A tablespoon of vegetable oil per day is recommended for both adults and children.[3] No recommendation has been set for trans fat, but it should be avoided as much as possible.

These recommendations are designed to help improve cardiovascular health and prevent heart disease. On average, fat intake in the United States is about 34 percent of daily calorie intake.[3] You can limit your intake of saturated fat by selecting vegetable oils instead of animal fats, reducing the amount of fat you use in cooking, removing all visible fat from meat, and choosing lean cuts of meat over fatty ones and poultry or fish over beef. Limit your consumption of fast-food burgers and fries, since these foods are loaded with both saturated and trans fats.

To determine what levels of fat, protein, and carbohydrate intake are recommended for your age and body weight, and to determine your individual goals within the ranges, see the Add It Up! feature at the end of this chapter.

Minerals—A Need for Balance

Minerals are naturally occurring inorganic substances that are needed by the body in relatively small amounts.

Minerals are important in building strong bones and teeth, helping vitamins and enzymes carry out many metabolic processes, and maintaining proper functioning of most body systems. Magnesium, for example, is critical to the transmission of nerve impulses; iodine is needed for thyroid function; iron is a component of hemoglobin; and potassium and sodium both play a role in nerve function and the regulation of water balance in the body.

Our bodies need 20 essential minerals. We need more than 100 milligrams daily of each of the six *macrominerals*—calcium, chloride, magnesium, phosphorous, potassium, and sodium. We need less than 100 milligrams daily of each of the *microminerals,* or *trace minerals*—chromium, cobalt, copper, fluorine, iodine, iron, manganese, molybdenum, nickel, selenium, silicon, tin, vanadium, and zinc. Other minerals are present in foods and the body, but no requirement has been found for them.

A varied and balanced diet provides all the essential minerals your body needs, so mineral supplements are not recommended for most people.[12] (Exceptions are listed in the next section.) You should take mineral supplements only on a physician's recommendation.[3] These insoluble elements that we obtain from the soil through the plants we eat can build up in the body and become toxic if consumed in excessive amounts.

Iron provides an illustration of this need for balance. If your body is deprived of iron, you cannot make enough hemoglobin for new blood cells, resulting in anemia. Too much iron, however, damages tissue and organs, including the heart. Women of childbearing age need from 15 to 18 milligrams each day and 27 milligrams daily during pregnancy.[5] Men over age 18 need 8 milligrams of iron daily. Children's intake of iron should be monitored, because iron supplements are the number-one cause of fatal accidental poisonings among children under the age of 3.[13]

Vitamins—Small but Potent Nutrients

Vitamins are organic substances needed by the body in small amounts. They serve as catalysts for releasing energy from carbohydrates, proteins, and fats; they aid chemical reactions in the body; and they help maintain components of the immune, nervous, and skeletal systems. Vitamin A, for example, helps to maintain healthy vision and skin; Vitamin D promotes the absorption of calcium; and Vitamin B_{12} is needed for synthesis of blood cells.

Your body needs at least 11 specific vitamins: A, D, E, K, C, and the B-complex vitamins—thiamin (B_1), riboflavin (B_2), niacin, B_6, folic acid, and B_{12}. Biotin and pantothenic acid are part of the vitamin B complex and are also considered important for health. Choline, another B vitamin, is not regarded as essential.

Four of the vitamins, A, D, E, and K, are fat soluble (they dissolve in fat), and the rest are water soluble (they dissolve in water). The fat-soluble vitamins can be stored in the liver or body fat, and if you consume larger amounts than you need, you can reach toxic levels over time. Excess water-soluble vitamins are excreted in the urine and must be consumed more often than fat-soluble vitamins. Most water-soluble vitamins do not cause toxicity, but vitamins B_6 and C can be stored to some extent and can build to toxic levels if taken in excess. Excessive niacin can be toxic to the liver. Toxicity usually occurs only when these substances are taken as supplements.

More than half the people in the United States take vitamin and mineral supplements. The food supplement industry markets these products as a kind of insurance against nutritional deficiencies. They also claim that supplements decrease stress, prevent or manage disease, replace lost nutrients caused by food processing, or slow the effects of aging. As noted earlier, however, supplements can cause toxicity, lead to life-threatening situations induced by misguided self-therapy, and engender a false sense of security in people whose diets are deficient.[3,14]

Specific groups for whom vitamin and/or mineral supplements may be recommended include

- People with nutrient deficiencies.
- People with low energy intake (less than 1,200 calories per day).
- Individuals who eat only foods from plant sources.
- Women who bleed excessively during menstruation.
- Individuals whose calcium intake is too small to preserve strength.
- People in certain life stages (infants, older adults, women of childbearing age, and pregnant women).

Taking supplements to enhance your energy level or athletic performance or to make up for perceived inadequacies in your diet is not recommended.[3] Instead, try to adopt a healthy diet that provides needed nutrients from a variety of foods. Many foods provide, in one serving, the

KEY TERMS

omega-3 fatty acid Polyunsaturated fatty acid that contains the essential nutrient alpha-linolenic acid and that has beneficial effects on cardiovascular health.

omega-6 fatty acid Polyunsaturated fatty acid that contains linoleic acid and that has beneficial health effects.

minerals Naturally occurring inorganic micronutrients, such as magnesium, calcium, and iron, that contribute to proper functioning of the body.

vitamins Naturally occurring organic micronutrients that aid chemical reactions in the body and help maintain healthy body systems.

Table 7.1	Overview of Recommended Daily Intakes
Nutrient	**Recommended Daily Intake**
Water	1–1.5 ml per calorie spent; 8–12 cups of fluid
Carbohydrates	AMDR: 45–65% of calories consumed
Added sugars	No more than 10–25% of calories consumed
Fiber	14 g for every 1,000 calories consumed; 21–25 g for women, 30–38 g for men
Protein	AMDR: 10–35% of calories consumed; 0.36 g per pound of body weight
Fat	AMDR: 20–35% of calories consumed
Saturated fat	No more than 10% of calories consumed
Trans fat	As little as possible
Minerals	
6 macrominerals	More than 100 mg
14 trace minerals	Less than 100 mg
Vitamins	
11 essential vitamins	Varies

same amounts of nutrients found in a vitamin supplement pill. If at certain times in your life you are not able to eat a healthy, balanced diet, taking a vitamin-mineral supplement that provides 50 percent to 150 percent of the RDA or AI for each of the nutrients may be prudent.[14] This range reflects the percentages usually found in foods and is compatible with the body's metabolism.

For a concise overview of recommended daily intakes of the macronutrients and micronutrients, see Table 7.1.

Other Substances in Food: Phytochemicals

Scientists are currently exploring a range of nutrients and non-nutrients in foods that may have valuable health benefits. One promising area of research is **phytochemicals,** substances that are naturally produced by plants to protect themselves against viruses, bacteria, and fungi. In the human body, phytochemicals may keep body cells healthy, slow down tissue degeneration, prevent the formation of carcinogens, reduce cholesterol levels, protect the heart, maintain hormone balance, and keep bones strong.[15] Three important types of phytochemicals are antioxidants, phytoestrogens, and phytonutrients.

Antioxidants

Every time you take a breath, you inhale a potentially toxic chemical that could damage your cell DNA.[4] This chemical is oxygen, which makes up about 21 percent of air. If you breathed 100 percent oxygen over a period of days, you would go blind and suffer irreparable damage to your lungs. The reason for this destructive effect is that the process by which oxygen is metabolized in the body produces unstable molecules, called **free radicals,** which react with other molecules in the body and damage cell structures and DNA. The production of free radicals can also be increased by exposure to certain environmental elements, such as cigarette smoke and sunlight, and even by stress. Free radicals are believed to be a contributing factor in aging, cancer, heart disease, macular degeneration, and other degenerative diseases.[12]

Antioxidants are substances in foods that neutralize the effects of free radicals by preventing their formation, reducing the damage they cause, or repairing tissues they have damaged. Antioxidants are found primarily in fruits and vegetables, especially brightly colored ones (yellow, orange, and dark green), and in green tea, which is brewed from unfermented tea leaves. Vitamins E and C are antioxidants, as are some of the precursors to vitamins, such as beta carotene. Most nutritionists do not recommend supplements as a source of antioxidants because of the potential toxic effects of vitamin megadoses.[15] The best source is whole foods.

Phytoestrogens and Phytonutrients

Phytoestrogens are plant hormones similar to human estrogens but less potent. Research suggests that some phytoestrogens may lower cholesterol and reduce the risk of heart disease. Other claims—that they lower the risk of osteoporosis and some types of cancer and reduce menopausal symptoms like hot flashes—have not been supported by research.

Phytoestrogens have been identified in more than 300 plants, including vegetables of the cabbage family such as brussels sprouts, broccoli, and cauliflower. (These are called *cruciferous* vegetables, because they have cross-shaped blossoms.) Phytoestrogens are also found in plants containing lignins (a woody substance like cellulose), such as rye, wheat, sesame seed, linseed, and flax seed; and in soybeans and soy products. Foods containing phytoestrogens are safe, but, as with all phytochemicals, research has not established the safety of phytoestrogen supplements.[3,16]

Phytonutrients are substances extracted from vegetables and other plant foods and used in supplements. For example, lycopene is an antioxidant found in tomatoes that may inhibit the reproduction of cancer cells in the esophagus, prostate, or stomach.[17] A group of phytochemicals known as *bioflavonoids* are believed to help maintain capillaries, inhibit the formation of blood clots, enhance the action of vitamin C, act as antioxidants and natural antibiotics, and help prevent cancer and heart disease.[3] They are found in many brightly colored fruits and vegetables, such as apricots, blackberries, and citrus fruits.

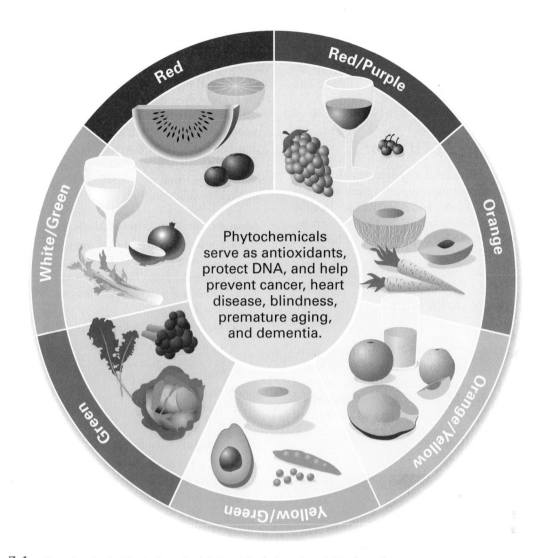

Figure 7.1   The color wheel of foods. *An optimal diet contains fruits and vegetables from all seven groups.*
Source: Adapted from *What Color Is Your Diet?* by D. Heber, 2001, New York: HarperCollins.

To date, the FDA has not allowed foods containing phytochemicals to be labeled or marketed as agents that prevent disease. According to the National Academy of Science, the evidence that phytochemicals prevent cancer, heart disease, diabetes, or Alzheimer's disease is in the "promising-but-not-conclusive" stages. Nutritionists and organizations with an interest in the health of the general population, such as the American Heart Association, do not recommend taking phytochemical supplements. Instead, they recommend that people eat a balanced diet containing a variety of fruits, vegetables, and whole-grain products.[18] National campaigns such as "Reach for It" in Canada and "Eat 5 a Day" in the United States encourage consumers to select fruits and vegetables high in phytochemicals.

Because different fruits and vegetables contain different phytochemicals, a color-coded dietary plan has been developed that helps you take full advantage of all the beneficial phytochemicals available. An optimal diet contains fruits and vegetables from seven categories, as shown in Figure 7.1. The phytochemical sulforaphane,

KEY TERMS

phytochemicals   Substances that are naturally produced by plants to protect themselves against viruses, bacteria, and fungi and that provide health benefits in the human body.

free radicals   Unstable molecules that are produced when oxygen is metabolized and that react with other molecules in the body and damage cell structures and DNA.

antioxidants   Substances in foods that neutralize the effects of free radicals.

phytoestrogens   Plant hormones similar to human estrogens that may lower cholesterol and reduce the risk of heart disease.

phytonutrients   Substances extracted from vegetables and other plant foods and used in supplements.

for example, is found in the green group, cruciferous vegetables; it has cancer-fighting properties. Lutein and zeaxanthin are found in the yellow-green group; they are important in maintaining vision and the structure and function of the eye.

PLANNING A HEALTHY DIET

Knowing your daily nutritional requirements in grams and percentages is not enough; you also need to know how to translate DRIs, RDAs, and AMDRs into healthy food choices and appealing meals. In this section we look at several tools that have been created to help you do that.

The 2005 *Dietary Guidelines for Americans*

The *Dietary Guidelines* published in 2005 represent a synthesis of current information and knowledge about nutrition, presented as general recommendations for diet and physical activity. The guidelines are designed to address two major concerns: the role of poor diet and a sedentary lifestyle in the major causes of disease and death in the

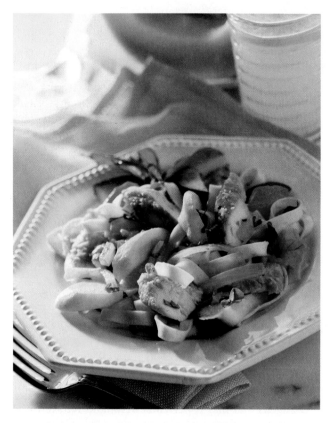

To lower your risk of developing a chronic disease like cancer, choose meals that include chicken or fish, at least two vegetables, whole-grain bread or pasta, and fruit.

United States, and the role of these same factors in the increase in overweight and obesity in this country. MyPyramid was developed as a graphic, readily accessible educational tool to help people apply the guidelines and the DRIs to their daily meal planning.

For each of the nine guidelines in the document, key recommendations are made both for the general population and for specific population groups, such as people over 50, people who need to lose weight, women of childbearing age, and so on. The nine dietary guidelines address the following areas.[19]

Adequate Nutrients Within Calorie Needs

- Consume a variety of nutrient-dense foods and beverages within and among the basic food groups while choosing foods that limit the intake of saturated and trans fats, cholesterol, added sugars, salt, and alcohol.
- Meet recommended intakes within energy needs by adopting a balanced eating pattern, such as the USDA Food Guide or the DASH Eating Plan.

Weight Management

- To maintain body weight in a healthy range, balance calories from foods and beverages with calories expended.
- To prevent gradual weight gain over time, make small decreases in food and beverage calories and increase physical activity.

Physical Activity

- Engage in regular physical activity and reduce sedentary activities.
  - To reduce the risk of chronic disease in adulthood, engage in at least 30 minutes of moderate-intensity physical activity, above usual activity, at work or home on most days of the week.
  - To help manage body weight and prevent gradual weight gain, engage in at least 60 minutes of moderate- to vigorous-intensity activity on most days of the week.
  - To sustain weight loss in adulthood, participate in at least 60–90 minutes of daily moderate-intensity activity.
- Achieve physical fitness by including cardiovascular conditioning, stretching exercises for flexibility, and resistance exercises or calisthenics for muscle strength and endurance.

Food Groups to Encourage

- Consume a sufficient amount of fruits and vegetables—2 cups of fruit and 2½ cups of vegetables—without exceeding energy needs.

- Choose a variety of fruits and vegetables each day; in particular, select from five vegetable subgroups (dark green, orange, legumes, starchy vegetables, and other vegetables) several times a week.
- Consume 3 or more ounce-equivalents of whole-grain products per day, with the rest of the recommended grains coming from enriched or whole-grain products.
- Consume 3 cups of fat-free or low-fat milk or equivalent milk products.

Fats

- Consume less than 10 percent of calories from saturated fats and less than 300 mg/day of cholesterol, and keep trans fatty acid consumption as low as possible.
- Keep total fat intake between 20 and 35 percent of calories, with most fats coming from sources of polyunsaturated and monounsaturated fatty acids, such as fish, nuts, and vegetable oils.
- When selecting and preparing meat, poultry, dry beans, and milk or milk products, make choices that are lean, low fat, or fat free.
- Limit intake of fats and oils high in saturated and/or trans fatty acids, and choose products low in such fats and oils.

Carbohydrates

- Choose fiber-rich fruits, vegetables, and whole grains often.
- Choose and prepare foods and beverages with little added sugars or caloric sweeteners.
- Reduce the amount of dental caries by practicing good oral hygiene and consuming sugar- and starch-containing foods and beverages less often.

Sodium and Potassium

- Consume less than 2,300 mg of sodium per day (approximately 1 tsp of salt).
- Choose and prepare foods with little salt. At the same time, consume potassium-rich foods, such as fruits and vegetables.

Alcoholic Beverages

- Those who choose to drink alcoholic beverages should do so sensibly and in moderation—defined as the consumption of up to 1 drink per day for women and up to 2 drinks per day for men.
- Alcoholic beverages should not be consumed by some individuals, such as pregnant women, and they should be avoided by individuals engaging in activities that require attention, skill, or coordination.

Food Safety

- To avoid microbial foodborne illnesses:
  - Clean hands, food contact surfaces, and fruits and vegetables. Meat and poultry should *not* be washed or rinsed.
  - Separate raw, cooked, and ready-to-eat foods while shopping, preparing, or storing foods.
  - Cook foods to a safe temperature to kill microorganisms.
  - Chill (refrigerate) perishable food promptly and defrost foods properly.
  - Avoid raw (unpasteurized) milk or any products made from unpasteurized milk, raw or partially cooked eggs or foods containing raw eggs, raw or undercooked meat and poultry, unpasteurized juices, and raw sprouts.

The USDA Food Guide (MyPyramid) and the DASH Eating Plan

A basic premise of the guidelines is that recommended diets should provide all the nutrients needed for health and growth (so that supplements are not needed). As noted in the first guideline, two eating plans that show how to integrate dietary recommendations into daily food choices are the USDA Food Guide (presented graphically as MyPyramid) and the DASH Eating Plan. The DASH Eating Plan was originally developed to reduce high blood pressure. (DASH stands for Dietary Approaches to Stop Hypertension.)

Both of these plans are based on the familiar food groups (grains, vegetables, fruit, milk, meat and beans), although the DASH plan also has a nuts, seeds, and legumes group. Unlike the previous Food Guide Pyramid, which provided a range of servings for each food group, these plans give specific serving recommendations for several different calorie levels—4 levels in the DASH Eating Plan (1,600, 2,000, 2,600, and 3,200) and 12 levels in the Food Guide (ranging from 1,000 to 3,200 calories). This allows consumers to identify the recommended number of servings on the basis of their activity level. A table of estimated calorie requirements is provided for three levels of physical activity—sedentary, moderately active, and active—broken down by age group and gender (Table 7.2). Samples of the Food Guide and the DASH plan at the 2,000-calorie level are shown in Table 7.3.

The USDA has created a general MyPyramid graphic as well as specific MyPyramid graphics for each of the 12 different calorie levels in the Food Guide. The general graphic includes short statements summarizing important points from the guidelines, such as "Eat more orange vegetables like carrots and sweet potatoes," as well as recommendations about physical activity and

Table 7.2 Estimated Calorie Requirements at Three Activity Levels, by Age and Gender

Gender	Age (years)	Sedentary	Moderately Active	Active
Child	2–3	1,000	1,000–1,400	1,000–1,400
Female	4–8	1,200	1,400–1,600	1,400–1,800
	9–13	1,600	1,600–2,000	1,800–2,200
	14–18	1,800	2,000	2,400
	19–30	2,000	2,000–2,200	2,400
	31–50	1,800	2,000	2,200
	51+	1,600	1,800	2,000–2,200
Male	4–8	1,400	1,400–1,600	1,600–2,000
	9–13	1,800	1,800–2,200	2,000–2,600
	14–18	2,200	2,400–2,800	2,800–3,200
	19–30	2,400	2,600–2,800	3,000
	31–50	2,200	2,400–2,600	2,800–3,000
	51+	2,000	2,200–2,400	2,400–2,800

Activity Level*

*Sedentary: A lifestyle that includes only the light physical activity associated with typical day-to-day life.

Moderately active: A lifestyle that includes physical activity equivalent to walking about 1.5 miles per day at 3–4 miles per hour, in addition to the light physical activity associated with typical day-to-day life.

Active: A lifestyle that includes physical activity equivalent to walking more than 3 miles per day at 3–4 miles per hour, in addition to the light physical activity associated with typical day-to-day life.

Source: 2005 Dietary Guidelines for Americans, USDA, February 4, 2005, www.health.gov/dietaryguidelines.

limits on fats, sugars, and sodium (Figure 7.2, on p. 174). The 12 different MyPyramid graphics include specific recommendations for number of serving from each group, allowance for oils, and extra calories available per day. They are available at www.MyPyramid.gov.

Both the Food Guide (MyPyramid) and the DASH plan differ significantly from current eating patterns in the United States. Specifically, they encourage more consumption of whole grains ("Make half your grains whole"), vegetables, legumes, fruits, and low-fat milk products and less consumption of refined grain products, total fats (especially cholesterol and saturated and trans fats), added sugars, and calories. Both plans emphasize foods high in **nutrient density**—proportion of vitamins and minerals to total calories. Especially in a lower calorie diet, the goal is that all the calories consumed provide nutrients (as opposed to the "empty calories" in sodas, sweets, and alcoholic beverages). Otherwise, you reach your maximum calorie intake without having consumed the nutrients you need. If you choose nutrient-dense foods from each food group, you may have some calories left over—your discretionary calorie allowance—that can be consumed as added fats or sugars, alcohol, or other foods. At the 2,000-calorie level, your discretionary calorie allowance is 267 calories (see Table 7.3). It is also notable that the new MyPyramid includes recommendations for daily physical activity and focuses on maintaining a healthy weight through a balance of physical activity and food.

Recommendations for Specific Population Groups

As noted earlier, the 2005 Dietary Guidelines for Americans include recommendations, where relevant, for specific population groups, including children and adolescents, older adults, pregnant and breastfeeding women, overweight adults and children, and people with chronic diseases or special medical problems. For example, women of childbearing age and women in the first trimester of pregnancy are advised to consume adequate synthetic folic acid daily in addition to eating foods rich in folate. Individuals with hypertension, African Americans, and middle-aged and older adults are advised to consume no more than 1,500 milligrams of sodium per day. Specific recommendations for the consumption of fat-free or low-fat milk or equivalent milk products are given for children aged 2 to 8 and 9 and older.

Table 7.3   Sample USDA Food Guide and DASH Eating Plan at the 2,000–Calorie Level

Food Groups and Subgroups	USDA Food Guide Amount	DASH Eating Plan Amount	Equivalent Amounts
Fruit Group	2 cups (4 servings)	2 to 2.5 cups (4 to 5 servings)	½ cup equivalent is • ½ cup fresh, frozen, or canned fruit • 1 med fruit • ¼ cup dried fruit • USDA: ½ cup fruit juice • DASH: ¾ cup fruit juice
Vegetable Group • Dark green vegetables • Orange vegetables • Legumes (dry beans) • Starchy vegetables • Other vegetables	2.5 cups (5 servings) 3 cups/week 2 cups/week 3 cups/week 3 cups/week 6.5 cups/week	2 to 2.5 cups (4 to 5 servings)	½ cup equivalent is • ½ cup of cut-up raw or cooked vegetable • 1 cup raw leafy vegetable • USDA: ½ cup vegetable juice • DASH: ¾ cup vegetable juice
Grain Group • Whole grains • Other grains	6 ounce-equivalents 3 ounce-equivalents 3 ounce-equivalents	7 to 8 ounce-equivalents (7 to 8 servings)	1 ounce-equivalent is • 1 slice bread • 1 cup dry cereal • ½ cup cooked rice, pasta, cereal • DASH: 1 oz dry cereal (½–1¼ cup depending on cereal type—check label)
Meat and Beans Group	5.5 ounce-equivalents	6 ounces or less meat, poultry, fish 4 to 5 servings per week nuts, seeds, and dry beans	1 ounce-equivalent is • 1 ounce of cooked lean meats, poultry, fish • 1 egg • USDA: ¼ cup cooked dry beans or tofu, 1 Tbsp peanut butter, ½ oz nuts or seeds • DASH: 1½ oz nuts, ½ oz seeds, ½ cup cooked dry beans
Milk Group	3 cups	2 to 3 cups	1 cup equivalent is • 1 cup low-fat/fat-free milk, yogurt • 1½ oz of low-fat or fat-free natural cheese • 2 oz of low-fat or fat-free processed cheese
Oils	24 grams (6 tsp)	8 to 12 grams (2 to 3 tsp)	1 tsp equivalent is • DASH: 1 tsp soft margarine • 1 Tbsp low-fat mayo • 2 Tbsp light salad dressing • 1 tsp vegetable oil

Discretionary Calorie Allowance
• Example of distribution:
  Solid fat
  Added sugars
	267 calories
	
	18 grams
	8 tsp
		
		~2 tsp (5 Tbsp per week)
			1 Tbsp added sugar equivalent is
			• DASH: 1 Tbsp jelly or jam
			• ½ oz jelly beans
			• 8 oz lemonade

Source: 2005 *Dietary Guidelines for Americans*, USDA, February 4, 2005, www.health.gov/dietaryguidelines.

Because eating habits are generally learned in childhood, this is the time to teach children to make healthy food choices. A key element is helping them listen to internal rather than external cues for eating. Children are especially vulnerable to advertisements for junk food and

KEY TERMS

nutrient density   The proportion of nutrients to total calories in a food.

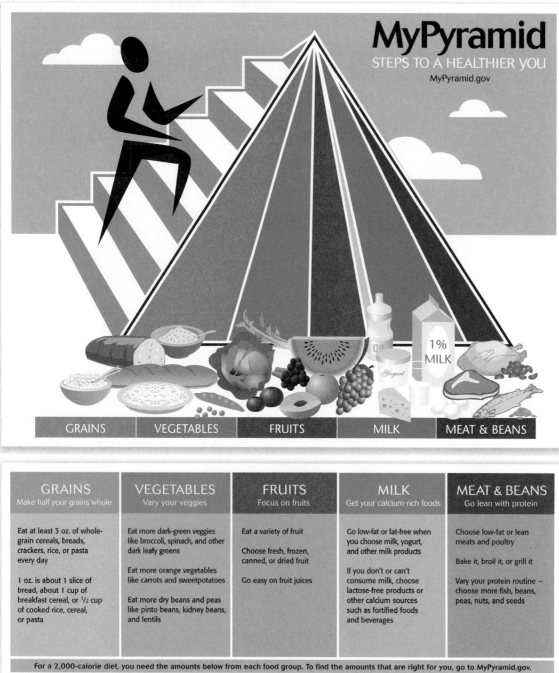

GRAINS	VEGETABLES	FRUITS	MILK	MEAT & BEANS

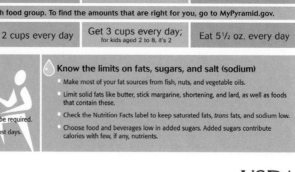

GRAINS Make half your grains whole	VEGETABLES Vary your veggies	FRUITS Focus on fruits	MILK Get your calcium-rich foods	MEAT & BEANS Go lean with protein
Eat at least 3 oz. of whole-grain cereals, breads, crackers, rice, or pasta every day 1 oz. is about 1 slice of bread, about 1 cup of breakfast cereal, or ½ cup of cooked rice, cereal, or pasta	Eat more dark-green veggies like broccoli, spinach, and other dark leafy greens Eat more orange vegetables like carrots and sweetpotatoes Eat more dry beans and peas like pinto beans, kidney beans, and lentils	Eat a variety of fruit Choose fresh, frozen, canned, or dried fruit Go easy on fruit juices	Go low-fat or fat-free when you choose milk, yogurt, and other milk products If you don't or can't consume milk, choose lactose-free products or other calcium sources such as fortified foods and beverages	Choose low-fat or lean meats and poultry Bake it, broil it, or grill it Vary your protein routine — choose more fish, beans, peas, nuts, and seeds

For a 2,000-calorie diet, you need the amounts below from each food group. To find the amounts that are right for you, go to MyPyramid.gov.

Eat 6 oz. every day	Eat 2½ cups every day	Eat 2 cups every day	Get 3 cups every day; for kids aged 2 to 8, it's 2	Eat 5½ oz. every day

Find your balance between food and physical activity
- Be sure to stay within your daily calorie needs.
- Be physically active for at least 30 minutes most days of the week.
- About 60 minutes a day of physical activity may be needed to prevent weight gain.
- For sustaining weight loss, at least 60 to 90 minutes a day of physical activity may be required.
- Children and teenagers should be physically active for 60 minutes every day, or most days.

Know the limits on fats, sugars, and salt (sodium)
- Make most of your fat sources from fish, nuts, and vegetable oils.
- Limit solid fats like butter, stick margarine, shortening, and lard, as well as foods that contain these.
- Check the Nutrition Facts label to keep saturated fats, *trans* fats, and sodium low.
- Choose food and beverages low in added sugars. Added sugars contribute calories with few, if any, nutrients.

MyPyramid.gov
STEPS TO A HEALTHIER YOU

U.S. Department of Agriculture
Center for Nutrition Policy and Promotion
April 2005
CNPP-15

USDA

USDA is an equal opportunity provider and employer.

Figure 7.2 The USDA MyPyramid. *Released in 2005, this chart emphasizes whole grains, a variety of vegetables, and a balance between food and physical activity. Specific pyramids for 12 different calorie levels are available at www.MyPyramid.gov.* Source: U.S. Department of Agriculture, Center for Nutrition Policy and Promotion, April 2005.

Challenges & Choices

Establishing Healthy Nutrition Practices in Childhood

The childhood years are important for establishing healthy nutrition practices. Here are some tips for ensuring healthy eating in children:

- Check out the USDA's MyPyramid for Kids (MyPyramid.gov), based on MyPyramid but adapted for kids. It shows a girl running up the stairs of the pyramid to remind kids to be physically active every day. It includes tips for families and nutrition advice children can understand.

- Make sure children eat a filling, nutritious breakfast. When they don't, they often fill up later on sugary and high-fat snack foods.

- Serve small portions; they are more appealing in general and are less daunting if the food is not a favorite one.

- Do not follow the "clean your plate" dictum. Forcing children to eat when they are full may predispose them to obesity. Let them be guided by their sensations of hunger and fullness.

- Provide healthy snacks—whole or sliced fruit, yogurt, raw vegetables, low-fat cheese.

- Include children in food preparation; it can help them develop an appreciation for healthy food.

- Provide a good model of healthy eating practices; children like to imitate adults they care about.

It's Not Just Personal . . .

Healthy People 2010 reports that 11 percent of girls and 12 percent of boys aged 6 to 11 are overweight or obese. Included in this group are 15 percent of African American children, 17 percent of Mexican American children, and 10 percent of white children. Equal numbers of overweight and obese children come from lower income and higher income families.

Source: Adapted from *Nutrition Concepts and Controversies,* by F. Sizer and E. Whitney, 2003, Belmont, CA: Wadsworth/Thomson Learning.

---

fast food, and these external cues can override natural appetite regulators like sensations of being hungry and being full. For some tips on helping children eat well, see the box above, "Establishing Healthy Nutrition Practices in Childhood.")

Other Eating Plans

The 2005 *Dietary Guidelines for Americans* and the recommended eating plans are flexible enough to be adapted for a variety of food preferences, including ethnic diets—those that are typical of particular cultures or geographic locations—and vegetarian diets. The term *diet* in this context includes the concepts of *cuisine,* a particular style of preparing food, and *food way,* the food habits, customs, beliefs, and preferences of a certain culture.[20]

Pyramids have been developed for ethnic diets, including the traditional Asian diet, the traditional Latin diet, and the Mediterranean diet. The Mediterranean pyramid was developed from the diet typical of the region in southern Europe, including Italy and Greece. Rates of cardiovascular disease and some kinds of cancer are lower in these countries than in Northern Europe and North America,[3] so experts have been interested in investigating whether this diet includes healthier food choices.

Like MyPyramid, the Mediterranean pyramid emphasizes grains, fruits, and vegetables, but it also recommends daily servings of beans, legumes, and nuts and foods that are high in protein, fiber, and fats. In addition, it encourages the use of olive oil over other oils. Although rates of heart disease and cancer are lower in Mediterranean countries, the prevalence of stroke is almost double that in the United States. This puzzle may be explained by lifestyle factors other than diet, such as smoking and level of physical activity.[3]

Planning a Vegetarian Diet

People choose to follow a vegetarian diet for a number of reasons, including ethical or religious beliefs, health concerns, and environmental awareness. There are at least four types of vegetarians:

- Vegans eat no animal products and abstain from wearing wool, silk, and leather.

- Lacto-vegetarians eat no meat, poultry, seafood, or eggs but do eat dairy products.

- Lacto-ovo-vegetarians eat no meat, poultry, or seafood but do eat dairy products and eggs.

- Semivegetarians eat no red meat but do eat small amounts of poultry and fish, along with eggs and dairy products.

The 2005 *Dietary Guidelines for Americans* provide some direction for vegetarian choices, and several pyramids

Figure 7.3   Food Guide Pyramid **for vegetarian meal planning.** Source: Data from "Vegetarian Diets: Position of ADA," 1997, *Journal of the American Dietetic Association, 97,* 1317–1321.

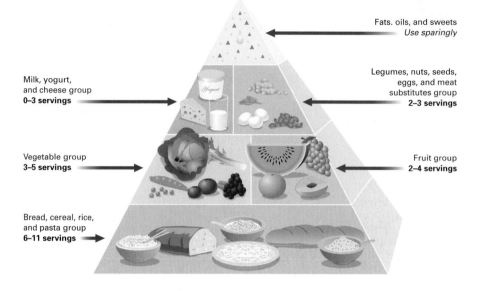

Fats. oils, and sweets
Use sparingly

Milk, yogurt, and cheese group
0–3 servings

Legumes, nuts, seeds, eggs, and meat substitutes group
2–3 servings

Vegetable group
3–5 servings

Fruit group
2–4 servings

Bread, cereal, rice, and pasta group
6–11 servings

have been developed for vegetarian diets; one is shown in Figure 7.3. The vegetarian pyramid has a bread, cereal, rice, and pasta group at the base and vegetable and fruit groups above that. It also has a milk, yogurt, and cheese group but allows 0–3 servings to accommodate those vegetarians who do not eat dairy products. Instead of a meat, fish, and poultry group, it has a dry beans, nuts, seeds, eggs, and meat substitutes group. This group includes soy products (for example, tofu, tempeh), legumes, and peanut butter. Vegetarians using this pyramid should also adopt the recommendations included in the 2005 *Dietary Guidelines for Americans* (such as making sure foods in the bread group are whole grain).

Vegetarian diets may offer protection against obesity, heart disease, high blood pressure, diabetes, digestive disorders, and some forms of cancer, particularly colon cancer,[21] depending on the type of vegetarian diet followed. Despite the potential benefits of vegetarian diets, however, vegetarians need to make sure that their diets provide the energy intake and food diversity needed to meet dietary guidelines.[5] (See the box "Vegetarian Diet Planning.")

Understanding Food Labels

Like MyPyramid, food labels on packaged foods can be helpful in making healthy diet decisions. Whereas MyPyramid gives you information about the overall components of a healthy diet, food labels can help you apply these principles to specific foods and your daily diet.

The Nutrition Education and Labeling Act of 1990 (NELA) required nutrition labeling for most foods and allowed labels to contain health claims approved by the Food and Drug Administration (FDA).[22] Labeling of meat and poultry products is regulated by the USDA, whose regulations are similar to those of the FDA. Although fresh meat, poultry, fish, and produce are exempt from the labeling law, many food producers voluntarily label their products.

The standardized food label (see Figure 7.4 on p. 178) shows how the food fits into a 2,000-calorie-a-day diet that includes no more than 65 grams of fat (30 percent of total calories). The top of the label lists serving size and number of servings in the container. The second part of the label gives the total calories and the calories from fat. A quick calculation will tell you whether this food is relatively high or low in fat. Look for foods with no more than 30 percent of their calories from fat. The next part of the label shows how much the food contributes to the Daily Values established for important nutrients, expressed as a percentage. The bottom part of the label, which is the same on all food labels, contains a footnote explaining the term "% Daily Value" and shows recommended daily intake of specified nutrients in a 2,000- and a 2,500-calorie diet.

Packaged foods frequently display food descriptors and health claims, which are also regulated by the FDA to help consumers know what they are getting. For example, the term *light* can be used if the product has one-third fewer calories or half the fat of the regular product; *low-fat* can be used if the product has 3 grams of fat or less per serving; and *fat-free* can be used if a product has less than 0.5 fat grams per serving. To find out more about common nutritional claims, see the Web Resources at the end of this chapter.

Putting It All Together

The 2005 *Dietary Guidelines for Americans,* the Food Guide and DASH Eating Plan, MyPyramid, and the food label provide you with the information you need to make

HIGHLIGHT ON HEALTH
Vegetarian Diet Planning

Vegetarian diets can be healthy if they are carefully designed to include adequate amounts of all the essential nutrients. Vegetarians, especially vegans, need to pay careful attention to the following nutrients:

- **Protein** Some vegetarians can get their protein from dairy products, eggs, fish, or poultry. Vegans can get all the essential and nonessential amino acids by eating a variety of plant foods—whole grains, legumes, seeds and nuts, and vegetables—and consuming foods from two or more of these categories over the course of a day. Soy protein provides all the essential amino acids and can be the sole protein source in a diet.

- **Iron** Nonvegetarians get much of their iron from red meat and eggs. Good plant sources of iron are prune juice, dried beans and lentils, spinach, dried fruits, molasses, brewer's yeast, and enriched products, such as enriched flour. Cooking in iron cookware (cast iron pans) also provides iron in the diet.

- **Vitamin B$_2$, riboflavin** Good sources of this vitamin are dairy products, nutritional yeast, leafy green vegetables (collard greens, spinach), broccoli, mushrooms, and dried beans.

- **Vitamin B$_{12}$** This vitamin is found naturally only in animal sources, especially meat and dairy products, so it is particularly important for vegans to make sure it is present in their diets. It can be found in some fortified (not enriched) breakfast cereals, fortified soy beverages, some brands of

nutritional (brewer's) yeast, and other foods (check the labels), as well as vitamin supplements.

- **Vitamin D** This vitamin is found in eggs, butter, and fortified dairy products. Sunlight transforms a provitamin into a substance that the body can use to make vitamin D. Vegans who don't get much sunlight may need a vitamin D supplement (but supplementation should not exceed the RDA).

- **Calcium** Calcium is plentiful in dairy products, molasses, leafy green vegetables like kale and mustard greens, broccoli, tofu and other soy products, and some legumes. (The calcium in some foods, including spinach, chocolate, and wheat bran, is poorly used in the body.) Studies show that vegetarians absorb and retain more calcium from foods than nonvegetarians do.

- **Zinc** Good plant sources of this essential mineral are legumes, whole grains, soy products, peas, spinach, and nuts. It is also abundant in dairy products and shellfish. Take care to select supplements containing no more than 15–18 milligrams of zinc. Supplements containing 50 milligrams or more may lower HDL ("good") cholesterol in some people.

- **Calories** Plant foods have fewer calories than animal foods, so vegetarians should make sure they are consuming enough calories to meet their bodies' energy needs.

Source: Adapted from "Vegetarian Diets," American Heart Association, 2004, www.americanheart.org.

healthy food choices. Additional resources, such as food pyramids and guidelines for vegetarian diet planning, can be used to supplement your knowledge. Remember to eat nutrient-dense foods and to stay within your calorie needs. Eat a variety of foods from all the food groups, consume them in moderation, and strive for overall balance. Favor whole grains and fresh, whole vegetables and fruits. Limit the amount of saturated fat, trans fat, and cholesterol in your diet by choosing fish, poultry, and lean meats. Use low-fat or nonfat dairy products and vegetable oils (olive oil, safflower oil) rather than animals fats (butter, lard). Limit the amount of added sugar you consume in candy, soda, fruit drinks, and sweet desserts, and choose foods with less salt. Making such healthy choices improves your chances of living longer, maintaining a healthy weight, avoiding chronic diseases, and having a higher quality of life as you get older.

CURRENT CONSUMER CONCERNS

The topics discussed so far in this chapter represent the basics of nutrition and dietary planning, but what you are likely to read and hear more about are consumer issues and concerns, such as the problems associated with high-sodium diets or fast foods. In this section we look at five such consumer concerns: soft drinks, high-sodium diets, food allergies and food intolerances, convenience foods, and fast foods.

Overconsumption of Soft Drinks

Americans consume an average of 25 pounds of sugar per person each year, about 32 teaspoons daily. To visualize this consumption, imagine pouring three quarters of a cup of sugar on your foods and into your beverages every

Figure 7.4   Nutrition Facts panel on a food label.

Serving sizes, stated in both household and metric measure, reflect the amounts that different people actually eat.

The nutrients required on the nutrient panel are those considered most important to the health of today's consumers.

The Daily Values are based on daily diets of 2,000 and 2,500 calories. Individuals should adjust these values to fit their own calorie intake. (Moderately active people consume about 15 calories per day for each pound of body weight.)

Calories from fat are shown to help consumers meet dietary guidelines, which recommend that people get no more than 30% of calories from fat.

% Daily Value shows how a food fits into the overall daily diet. You may want to limit your intake of fat, cholesterol, sodium, and sugar and make sure you get enough fiber, protein, vitamins, and minerals.

Nutrition Facts

Serving Size 1/2 cup (114g)
Servings per Container 4

Amount per Serving

Calories 260   Calories from Fat 120

	% Daily Value*
Total Fat 13g	**20%**
Saturated Fat 5g	**25%**
Trans Fat 0.5g	
Cholesterol 30mg	**10%**
Sodium 660mg	**28%**
Total Carbohydrate 33g	**11%**
Dietary Fiber 9g	**36%**
Sugars 2g	
Protein 5g	

Vitamin A 4%	•	Vitamin C 2%
Calcium 15%	•	Iron 4%

*Percent Daily Values are based on a 2,000 calorie diet. Your daily values may be higher or lower depending on your calorie needs:

		Calories	2,000	2,500
Total Fat	Less than		65g	80g
Sat Fat	Less than		20g	25g
Cholesterol	Less than		300mg	300mg
Sodium	Less than		2,400mg	2,400mg
Total Carbohydrate			300g	375g
Dietary Fiber			25g	30g

Calories per gram:
Fat 9 • Carbohydrate 4 • Protein 4

day. Sugar is believed to promote and maintain obesity, cause and aggravate diabetes, increase the risk of heart disease, and cause dental decay and gum disease. It should be noted, however, that scientific evidence suggests that moderate levels of sugar (no more than 10 percent of total calories) pose no health risk.[3,5,23,24]

Much of this sugar comes from soft drinks. For adults, these beverages represent the fifth largest contributor of daily calories, about 6 percent of calories consumed. For teenagers, they account for 8–9 percent of calories consumed daily. Consumption of soft drinks doubled from the mid-1970s to the mid-1990s and increased further in the decade that followed. Some experts attribute the surge in overweight and obesity among American children and adults largely to the increase in the consumption of soft drinks.

Equally important is the decreased consumption of milk, which is a major source of calcium, protein, vitamin A, and vitamin D, as well as decreased consumption of orange juice and other fruit juices. Soft drinks contain about the same number of calories as milk and juice but none of the nutrients. Diet soft drinks don't contain sugar, but like regular soft drinks, they fill you up without providing any nutrients (Figure 7.5). Teenage girls are believed to be getting 40 percent less calcium than they need, during a pe-

riod of life when they should be building bone mass.[3] Soft drinks also contain relatively high levels of caffeine, which is mildly addictive and can lead to nervousness, irritability, insomnia, and bone demineralization. Nutritionists recommend limiting soft drinks in the diet and drinking low-fat milk and water instead.

High-Sodium Diets

Another current concern is the amount of sodium consumed in our diets. Sodium is an essential nutrient, but we need only about 500 milligrams per day—about 1/10 of a teaspoon. Although many foods contain sodium, we get most of our sodium—about 90 percent—from salt (which is made up of sodium and chloride). The recommended upper limit for salt is 2,400 milligrams per day, about 1 teaspoon, and the 2005 *Dietary Guidelines for Americans* recommend no more than 2,300 milligrams per day.

Salt may be a factor in causing hypertension (high blood pressure) in some "salt-sensitive" people; hypertension is both a form of cardiovascular disease and a risk factor for stroke, another type of cardiovascular disease. Even people who are not salt sensitive can benefit from reducing the salt in their diets.[3]

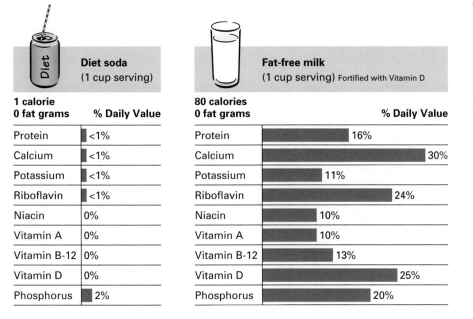

Diet soda (1 cup serving)		Fat-free milk (1 cup serving) Fortified with Vitamin D	
1 calorie 0 fat grams	% Daily Value	80 calories 0 fat grams	% Daily Value
Protein	<1%	Protein	16%
Calcium	<1%	Calcium	30%
Potassium	<1%	Potassium	11%
Riboflavin	<1%	Riboflavin	24%
Niacin	0%	Niacin	10%
Vitamin A	0%	Vitamin A	10%
Vitamin B-12	0%	Vitamin B-12	13%
Vitamin D	0%	Vitamin D	25%
Phosphorus	2%	Phosphorus	20%

Figure 7.5 Diet soda vs. fat-free milk. *Diet soda has virtually no nutritional value, but it has replaced milk in the diets of many Americans, including adolescent and young adult women, who need calcium to build bone mass. Milk is one of the best sources of calcium, protein, potassium, and many other nutrients.*

Many packaged foods, convenience foods, and fast foods are heavily salted, primarily to enhance flavor, and therefore contain very high levels of sodium. An order of buffalo wings, for example, has 1,800 milligrams of sodium, and an order of cheese fries has about 4,000 milligrams.[25] Canned soups, lunch meats, pickles, soy sauce, teriyaki sauce, catsup, mustard, salad dressing, and barbecue sauce are also high in sodium.

You can reduce the amount of salt in your diet by emphasizing whole foods, like grains, vegetables, and fruits, which are naturally low in sodium. Remove the salt shaker from your table, and don't use salt in cooking. When buying packaged foods, read the labels to check for salt content, and look for descriptors such as "reduced sodium" or "low sodium." Highly salted food is an acquired taste; if you use less salt, you will gradually rediscover the natural taste of the food.

Food Allergies and Food Intolerances

Food allergies occur when the immune system overreacts to specific proteins in food; they affect about 7 percent of children and 2 percent of adults. More than 200 food ingredients can cause an allergic reaction, but eggs, peanuts, and milk account for 75 percent of food allergies.[3] Other common allergenic foods are fish, shellfish, wheat products, corn, fruits, and chocolate.

Typical symptoms of allergic reactions include skin rash, nasal congestion, hives, nausea, and wheezing. Most children eventually outgrow food allergies, except for allergies to peanuts, nuts, and seafood.[3] Generally, people suffer temporary discomfort from allergic reactions to food, but approximately 30,000 people each year in the United States have an *anaphylactic shock* reaction to a

food they have eaten—the throat swells enough to cut off breathing.[2] A person experiencing this type of allergic reaction needs immediate medical attention.

Most food reactions are not caused by allergies, however; most are caused by food intolerances.[3] These are less severe than allergies and can be triggered by almost any food. The most common culprits are lactose, sulfur-containing additives in preservatives (used, for example, in dried fruits and red wine), and monosodium glutamate (a flavor enhancer). Lactose intolerance, a condition that results from an inability to digest the milk sugar lactose, is especially prevalent (see the box on the next page, "Lactose Intolerance").

There is no treatment or cure for food allergies or intolerances. If you experience these reactions, the best you can do is avoid the offending food.[3] This is not always easy to do, however, because labels don't always disclose allergens in flavoring agents, and trace amounts can cause a reaction.

Nutritional Value of Convenience Foods

Packaged foods that require little or no preparation, known as convenience foods,[2] include ready-to-eat breakfast cereals, frozen baked goods, and prepackaged heat-and-serve meals. Most of these foods do not have the same nutrient content as home-cooked foods, and the majority contain more sugar, sodium, and fat.[26] They also cost more than fresh foods. Nutritionists recommend using fresh foods as often as possible.

Energy bars are a newer type of convenience food. People who have busy schedules or who follow intense exercise regimens often find these foods convenient for attaining daily nutrient needs. Some products claim to have all the

HIGHLIGHT ON HEALTH
Lactose Intolerance

About 75 percent of the world's people suffer from lactose intolerance—difficulty digesting lactose, the sugar in milk. The condition is common among many Asians, African Americans, Middle Easterners, South Americans, and people from eastern, central, and southern Europe. People with lactose intolerance lack the enzyme lactase, which breaks lactose into glucose and galactose. When they consume milk or milk products, undigested lactose passes into their intestinal tract. As bacteria in the intestinal tract consume the undigested lactose, wastes are produced that cause gas, cramps, and nausea.

Lactose intolerance affects people to different degrees. Very few people are severely intolerant to lactose.

Many can tolerate a cup or two of milk a day, and some can tolerate lactose-reduced milk. Lactose-intolerant children and women, especially, need to find alternative sources of calcium. "Predigested" milk products, such as yogurt or buttermilk, as well as lactose-free cheese and enzyme-treated milk, are potential sources. Over-the-counter products are also available that help people digest lactose by replacing the missing enzymes. Other sources of calcium include green leafy vegetables, tofu, fortified orange juice and bread, and fish with bones, such as sardines or anchovies.

Source: *Nutrition Concepts and Controversies,* by F. Sizer and E. Whitney, 2003, Belmont, CA: Wadsworth/Thomson Learning.

amino acids, antioxidants, dietary fiber, and other nutrients needed to meet 100 percent of the RDAs. However, many of these products are high in calories, and they don't provide the balanced nutrition of whole foods. For more on this type of convenience food, see the box below, "Energy Bars."

Fast Foods—Making Smart Choices

By fast foods, we mean ready-to-eat foods sold by commercial establishments such as McDonald's, KFC, Wendy's, Taco Bell, Burger King, and others. For every $10 paid for restaurant food in the United States, almost $5 is spent at fast-food establishments.[27] The quick service, convenience, and relatively low cost of fast food make it popular North American fare. But fast foods—burgers, fries, shakes, and so on—are a minefield of high calories, saturated and trans fats, cholesterol, and sodium.

We recommend limiting visits to fast-food restaurants as much as you can, but when you do go, make smart selections by following these tips: Don't order unnecessarily large servings; standard size orders are already very large. In 1955, an order of McDonald's fries contained

HIGHLIGHT ON HEALTH
Energy Bars

To many consumers, a food advertised as supplying energy means that it makes a person feel energetic. But to nutritionists, energy simply means calories, so any food with calories is an energy food. This distinction has not stopped food companies from marketing energy bars as a tool to help you run farther, faster, or longer; to give you an energy boost; or to replace a meal when you are too busy to eat.

Different energy bars promise different results. High-carbohydrate, low-fat bars are designed to keep athletes from running out of glucose during long sporting events. Bars with a 40-30-30 ratio of carbohydrate to protein to fat are recommended in the bestselling diet book *The Zone*. High-protein bars are intended for people who want bigger muscles. And supplement bars made from soy products contain phytoestrogens, which the manufacturers claim reduce the risk of breast and prostate cancer.

Most energy bars are low in saturated fat and trans fatty acids and contain up to 5 grams of fiber. They are better for you than are candy bars or other snack foods high in saturated fat, trans fatty acids, and sugar. However, even healthier alternatives are whole foods like fruits and vegetables, with their abundant vitamins, minerals, and phytochemicals. If you do buy energy bars, check the labels for calories, total fat, saturated fat, protein, carbohydrate, and fiber, and choose the healthiest products.

Source: "Bar Exam: Energy Bars Flunk," by B. Liebman and D. Schardt, December 10–12, 2000, *Nutrition Action Health Letter.*

Challenges & Choices

Healthy Strategies When Ordering Pizza

Some people claim pizza is healthy because it draws from several different food groups; others point out that it is very high in sodium, calories, and saturated fat. The Center for Science in the Public Interest suggests that you follow some basic strategies to get the healthiest pizza possible:

- Select the right toppings. Choose vegetables (mushrooms, bell peppers, tomatoes, onions) as often as possible. If you want meat toppings, chicken and ham are lower in calories and fat than pepperoni, pork, sausage, or beef.

- Select no-cheese or half-cheese pizza if your pizzeria has it as an option.

- Skip the hidden cheese. Make sure your order, especially if it is stuffed-crust pizza, does not come with extra cheese.

- Avoid multimeat pizzas like pepperoni, salami, and sausage. More meat means more calories, fat, and sodium.

- Order a salad to help you eat fewer slices of pizza.

- Avoid side dishes at pizzerias. Buffalo wings, for example, have 50 calories each and bread sticks 100 calories each.

It's Not Just Personal . . .

Two slices of a 14-inch deep-dish cheese pizza have about 675 calories—about a third of the recommended daily total in a 2,000-calorie diet—and 35 grams of fat. Americans consume more than 3 billion pizzas a year, and one of every six restaurants in the United States is a pizzeria.

Source: "What a Pizza Delivers," June 2002, *Nutrition Action Health Letter*, pp. 3–9.

roughly 200 calories; today, a large order has 610. Choose grilled meat (such as a grilled chicken sandwich) rather than fried or deep fried (such as a breaded chicken sandwich). Finally, choose low-calorie items such as salads with low-fat dressing.[27]

Pizza is another fast food loaded with calories and fat. For help in making wise choices at the pizzeria, see the box above, "Healthy Strategies When Ordering Pizza."

FOOD SAFETY AND TECHNOLOGY

Well-informed consumers can make smart personal choices about soft drinks, sodium, and fast foods, but they also face larger issues over which they may have less control and choice. These issues involve food safety and the use of technology to modify the food supply. Although the FDA is charged with monitoring the safety of the U.S. food supply, consumers, too, need to learn to distinguish between safe and unsafe foods and understand key elements of food safety, including food additives, organic and natural foods, functional foods, food-borne illness, and genetically modified foods.

Food Additives

Many substances are added to food to maintain or improve nutrient value, aid in food preparation, and/or improve taste or appearance.[3] Currently, about 2,800 different additives are approved by the FDA, which requires that they be effective, detectable, measurable, and safe. No additives receive permanent approval; all are reviewed periodically.

Additives include antimicrobial agents, antioxidants, artificial colors, artificial flavors and flavor enhancers, texture and stability enhancers, and nutrients. Questions about the safety of additives are continually raised[28]; we consider here just one topic, artificial sweeteners.

Artificial sweeteners enable people to enjoy a sweet taste in foods and beverages without consuming sugar. One sweetener, saccharin, was associated with bladder cancer in animal studies in 1977. The FDA proposed banning it, but withdrew the proposal because of public opposition. The FDA has set the acceptable daily intake (ADI) for saccharin at 5 milligrams per kilogram (2.2 pounds) of body weight,[3] and excessive consumption is probably not safe.

Another sweetener, aspartame, has undergone rigorous study. It is marketed as Nutrasweet, Equal, and Spoonful. Many products contain it, including Diet Pepsi and Diet Coke. In the United States, the ADI of aspartame is 50 milligrams per kilogram of body weight; in Canada, it is 40 milligrams per kilogram.[3] This means a 150-pound person would have to consume 97 packets of Equal or 20 cans of diet soft drinks a day to exceed the ADI. The typical person consumes less than 5 milligrams of aspartame per kilogram of body weight per day.[29] Aspartame contains phenylalanine and should be avoided by people with phenylketonuria (PKU), an inherited metabolic disorder (see Chapter 2). Generally, artificial sweeteners are considered safe.[3] Still, they should be consumed only in moderation and as part of a well-balanced diet.

Organic Foods

Plant foods labeled "organic" are grown without synthetic pesticides or fertilizers,[2] and animal foods labeled organic are from animals raised on organic feed without antibiotics or growth hormone. Organic foods appeal to health- and environment-conscious consumers who want to protect their own health, the health of farm workers, and the health of the planet's soil and water. Organic foods are more expensive than foods grown using conventional methods, however, and consumers cannot always determine exactly how some foods were grown.

In 2002 the USDA issued regulations standardizing the use of terms related to organic foods on the labels of certain meat and poultry products. The label "100% organic" means that all contents are organic; "organic" means that contents are at least 95 percent organic; "made with organic ingredients" means the contents are at least 70 percent organic. Food manufacturers who comply with the USDA standards can place the seal "USDA Organic" on their labels.

Although it seems that organic foods ought to be healthier and safer than foods grown conventionally, no research has demonstrated that this is the case. Conventional food products do contain pesticide residues that can be toxic at high doses, but research has not documented ill effects from them at the levels found in foods, nor is there any evidence that people who consume organic food are healthier than those who don't.[3] What has been documented is that organic farming is beneficial to the environment (see the box "Organic Agriculture and the Environment").

A disadvantage of organic foods is that they may place consumers at higher risk of contracting foodborne illnesses. If you purchase organic food, buy only the amount you need immediately, store and cook the food properly, and wash organic produce thoroughly before eating it.[3]

Organic foods are different from "natural" foods. The descriptor "natural" usually means that the food was produced with minimal processing and contains no additives or artificial ingredients. Proponents of natural foods claim that they are healthier and safer than other foods; critics argue that the U.S. food supply is already the safest and most nutritious in the world. Critics also point out that the term *natural* has no clear definition and that natural foods cost more than conventional foods.[30] To be a smart consumer, check labels of packaged foods for ingredients and nutrients, and choose more whole foods—vegetables, fruits, and grains—which are always "natural."

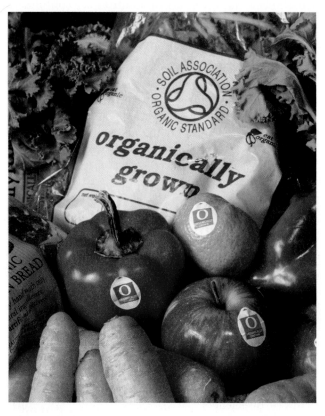

Organic foods are often more expensive than conventional foods. Do you think it's worth it to buy organically grown produce?

Functional Foods

The term **functional foods** is applied to foods that do more than provide nutrients; they may also help prevent chronic diseases and provide other health benefits.[31] Since almost every natural food is functional in some way, scientists have struggled with how to distinguish these health-promoting foods.[3] The term is most commonly used to describe foods to which ingredients have been added to improve their health benefits. For example, food companies sell margarine spreads with added plant stanol esters, substances that have been found to lower blood levels of cholesterol. Other functional foods include cereals with added vitamins and minerals, orange juice with added calcium, and various foods with added soy protein or fiber. The FDA allows functional foods to make research-based health claims on their labels, such as "Proven to significantly reduce cholesterol" or "Reduces the risk of heart disease." (For a discussion of foods that offer extra nutritional benefits naturally, see the box on p. 184, "Superfoods—A Nutritional Boost?")

The FDA does not have full regulatory authority over herbs, however, nor does it review general claims like "Boosts energy" or "Enhances mood." Foods touted as "liquid vitamins" or sold under names such as "St. John's Wort Tortilla Chips," or "Kava Kava Corn Chips" should be viewed with some skepticism. Claims that herbally fortified foods improve memory, lift moods, melt away

HIGHLIGHT ON HEALTH
Organic Agriculture and the Environment

Conventional industrialized agriculture relies on chemical fertilizers, synthetic pesticides, energy from fossil fuels, and large quantities of water to produce the food consumed by most people in the developed world. Unfortunately, this type of agriculture has a significantly harmful impact on air, soil, water, and energy resources and on biodiversity (the variety of plant and animal species on earth). To meet these challenges, environmentalists propose a greater use of organic agricultural practices. Organic agriculture is based on several principles:

- **Biodiversity**   A diverse mix of crops promotes a balanced ecosystem and supports the beneficial organisms that help in pest management.

- **Integration**   Farms that raise both crops and livestock benefit from their interdependence; for example, crops are raised that feed the livestock, and manure from the livestock replenishes the soil for the crops.

- **Sustainability**   Organic farms protect environmental resources rather than depleting them.

- **Natural plant nutrition**   Soils are maintained so they can provide plants with the minerals,

vitamins, antibiotics, and other substances they need; natural fertilizers are used to replace nutrients in the soil.

- **Natural pest management**   Pests are repelled by healthy, well-nourished plants. Insect outbreaks occur as a result of imbalances in the ecosystem, often the result of overuse of pesticides.

- **Integrity**   Farmers ensure that products are organically grown through such practices as buffer strips between organically grown and conventionally grown crops.

Although organic agriculture is often associated with small farms, large commercial farming enterprises are putting more and more of their fields under organic cultivation. As this happens, consumers will benefit from lower prices, and, more importantly, the planet will benefit from more environmentally sound farming practices.

Sources: *Living in the Environment,* by G. T. Miller, 2004, Belmont, CA: Wadsworth/Thomson Learning; "What Is Sustainable Agriculture?" National Sustainable Agriculture Information Service, 2005, www.attra.org.

pounds, or soothe joint pain are not supported by scientific evidence.[31] As a consumer, be aware of the following cautions when considering herbally enhanced functional foods:

- Labels on functional foods rarely detail the amount of nutrient or botanical ingredient contained in the product. Furthermore, many claims on labels are not supported by solid research and are often misleading.

- Functional foods rarely have enough beneficial herbal ingredients to improve health. Some of the most common herbal ingredients—gingko (used to improve memory), ginseng (used to improve memory and immune function), Echinacea (used to boost immunity and protect against colds), St. John's wort (used to treat depression), and kava kava (used to reduce anxiety)—are effective only when taken in large amounts.

- Functional foods can be expensive and may contain few nutrients overall, especially for the calories they provide. Nutritionists recommend eating a wide range of foods containing a variety of nutrients and non-nutrients rather than relying on herbally enhanced functional foods.

Foodborne Illnesses

Data from the Centers for Disease Control and Prevention (CDC) suggest that Americans contract foodborne illnesses at a rate of one illness per person per year. Foodborne illnesses may be caused by food intoxication or by food infection; both types are commonly referred to as *food poisoning.*

Food intoxication occurs when a food is contaminated by natural toxins or by microbes that produce toxins. Botulism is an example of food intoxication. The botulism bacterium thrives in the absence of oxygen (as in a can or vacuum-packed container), in low-acidic conditions, and at 40° F to 120° F. When food has been

KEY TERMS

functional foods   Foods that may help prevent disease, usually because health-promoting ingredients have been added to them.

food intoxication   A kind of food poisoning in which a food is contaminated by natural toxins or by microbes that produce toxins.

Consumer Clipboard

Superfoods—A Nutritional Boost?

"Polymeals" and "superfoods" are two different approaches to healthy eating. What they have in common is a focus on eating certain natural foods that offer outstanding nutritional benefits.

In 2004 Dr. Oscar H. Frank and his colleagues at the University Medical Center in The Netherlands reported on the combined results of various studies showing the effects of the polymeal on the health of men and women. The polymeal ingredients were wine, fish, dark chocolate, fruits and vegetables, almonds, and garlic. Each food was eaten on a daily basis (except for fish, which was eaten 4 times a week) and in specific amounts. The researchers found that eating 100 grams of dark chocolate daily reduced blood pressure and that a dose of garlic and almonds a day lowered cholesterol levels. The overall results showed that the polymeal decreases the risk of heart disease by 76% and significantly increases life expectancy. The most dramatic results were among men. Men who followed the polymeal approach lived 6.6 years longer than those who didn't. Women who ate polymeals also lived significantly longer than those who didn't—almost 5 years longer.

That same year Dr. Steven Pratt, an ophthalmologist at Scripps Memorial Hospital in La Jolla, California, reported on dramatic improvement among his patients with macular degeneration, a leading cause of blindness. After comparing the common foods among the world's healthiest diets, Pratt recommended that these patients modify their diets to focus on 14 key foods. These "superfoods" are beans, blueberries, broccoli, oats, oranges, pumpkin, salmon, soy, spinach, tea (green or black), tomatoes, turkey, walnuts, and yogurt. "Sidekick" choices have similar, though lesser, benefits. So if broccoli isn't your favorite vegetable, you can choose brussels sprouts, cabbage, kale, turnips, cauliflower, collards, bok choy, mustard greens or Swiss chard to get lots of folate, fiber, calcium, and vitamin C. If you don't like blueberries, substitute purple grapes, cherries, and other berries. They're low in calories and loaded with nutrition, including carotenoids, fiber, folate, and vitamins C and E.

Polymeals and superfoods aren't the answer to all your nutritional needs. They must be eaten in the context of an overall healthy diet—lots of fruits and vegetables, protein, nuts and seeds, whole grains, high-calcium foods, and healthy fats. The refreshing thing about them is that they don't involve gimmicks, high prices, or warnings—just great nutritional value.

Sources: "Superfoods Everyone Needs" by Gina Shaw, 2004, http://aolsvc.health.webmd.aol.com; "Eat 'Supermeals' to Protect Heart: Experts" by Allison Cook, 2004, http://abcnews.go.com.

---

contaminated with this bacterium and then improperly prepared or stored, the bacterium releases a dangerous and potentially fatal toxin. Warning signs of botulism poisoning are double vision, weak muscles, difficulty swallowing, and difficulty breathing.[3] Immediate medical treatment is needed.

Food infections are caused by disease-causing microorganisms, or pathogens, that have contaminated the food. Although most foods are safe, some are more commonly contaminated than others; they include ground beef, chicken, turkey, salami, hot dogs, ice cream, lettuce, cantaloupe, and apple cider. Between 4,000 and 9,000 Americans die every year from food infection.[32]

Common Food Pathogens

Three of the most common pathogens that cause food infection are Escherichia coli (E. coli), salmonella, and campylobacter. E. coli occurs naturally in the intestines of humans and animals. Raw beef, raw fruits and vegetables, and unpasteurized juices are the foods most commonly contaminated by it. One strain, E. coli 015-H7, is especially dangerous because it can cause hemolytic uremic syndrome (HUS), which can lead to kidney failure, a potentially fatal condition. E. coli is a hearty microbe, thriving in moist environments for weeks and on kitchen countertops for days. It can survive on the skin, on clothing, in lakes and pools, and at temperatures below freezing and up to 160° F.[3] The CDC estimates that E. coli 015-H7 causes nearly 20,000 illnesses each year in the United States and kills 250 to 500 people.[33] Young children and older adults are particularly at risk.

Salmonella enteritis can contaminate raw eggs, poultry and meat, fruit and vegetables, and other foods. Eggs containing salmonella enteritis are the number-one cause of food poisoning outbreaks in the nation. An estimated

1 of every 10,000 eggs laid each year contains salmonella enteritis.[32] The enteritis bacterium multiplies inside eggs that are not properly refrigerated to an internal temperature of 45° F. The best way to prevent salmonella enteritis infection is to thoroughly cook eggs, chicken, and other foods to kill the bacterium. Avoid eating raw or undercooked eggs, such as in raw cake batter or cookie dough, salad dressings, and eggnog.[34]

Campylobacter occurs in raw or undercooked poultry, meat, and shellfish, in unpasteurized milk, and in contaminated water. Campylobacter and salmonella together cause 80 percent of the illnesses and 75 percent of the deaths associated with meat and poultry practices.[35] Campylobacter bacteria from contaminated poultry can spread when packaged juices spill onto kitchen surfaces and other foods; it can also be spread by hand.[34]

Food poisoning causes flu-like symptoms such as diarrhea, abdominal pain, vomiting, fever, and chills. More serious complications can include rheumatoid arthritis, kidney or heart disease, meningitis, HUS, and death. Some symptoms are cause for immediate medical attention: (1) bloody diarrhea or pus in the stool, (2) fever that lasts more than 48 hours, (3) faintness, rapid heart rate, or nausea when standing up suddenly, and/or (4) a significant drop in the frequency of urination.[34]

Protecting Yourself from Foodborne Illness

According to national data, more than 40 percent of all reported food poisoning incidents are associated with food eaten in restaurants, delicatessens, and cafeterias. Only about 20 percent are attributed to food eaten at home.[36] Although community health experts are responsible for monitoring sanitation practices in public eating establishments, consumers can actively support licensing requirements and inspections to ensure cleanliness, proper waste disposal, and correct refrigeration and food storage practices. If you suspect that a public eating establishment is the source of a food poisoning incident, you should also call your local health department.

Even though a smaller percentage of food poisoning cases occur at home, the best defense against foodborne illness is the use of safe food practices in your own kitchen. Review the recommendations given in the Dietary Guidelines for food safety, and see the additional guidelines illustrated in Figure 7.6.

When traveling to countries outside the United States, you may want to take additional precautions. Use bottled water (even for brushing your teeth), avoid ice, and take along disinfectant tablets in case you have to use water that isn't safe. Avoid raw fruit and vegetables unless you boil or peel them yourself. You may want to ask your physician for medication to take with you in case you become ill.[34]

Food Irradiation

The food industry and the government, particularly the USDA and the FDA, are also interested in preventing foodborne illness, and many regulations are in place to ensure that the food supply is safe. A relatively new approach to safety is **food irradiation,** a process in which food is passed through a chamber containing radioactive rods with powerful gamma rays. These eliminate almost all microbiological threats, with the exception of the pathogens that cause botulism, hepatitis, and bovine spongiform encephalitis (mad cow disease).

The American Dietetic Association Scientific Position on food irradiation is that it is an effective way to protect consumers from foodborne illness.[37] There is disagreement, however, on the safety of irradiation. One fear is that radiation may destroy nutrients and cause people to develop nutrient deficiencies. The FDA argues that the loss of nutrients is minimal. Another fear is that the health effects of irradiated foods are not completely understood. Some studies have found chromosomal abnormalities, impaired fertility, and depressed immune responses in animals on diets containing irradiated foods, although research on humans has not produced the same findings.

A third fear is that radioactive substances used to irradiate food may endanger food plant workers, the general population, and the environment. Food industrialists who support food irradiation advocate strict safety regulations and enforcement to limit radiation exposure.[3]

Genetically Modified Foods

Farmers, scientists, and breeders have long been tinkering with the genetic makeup of plants and animals to breed organisms with desirable traits, a process known as selective breeding. Compared to modern techniques, however, selective breeding is an old technology, slow and imprecise. Using biotechnology to produce **genetically modified (GM) organisms** is a faster and more refined process. Genetic modification involves the addition,

KEY TERMS

food infection A kind of food poisoning in which a food is contaminated by disease-causing microorganisms, or pathogens.

food irradiation Process that exposes food to gamma rays to destroy contaminants.

genetically modified (GM) organisms Organisms whose genetic makeup has been changed to produce desirable traits.

Wash your hands for 20 seconds with hot, soapy water before and after handling food, especially raw meat. If you have cuts on your hands, wear rubber gloves.

Wash raw produce carefully.

Clean sponges and dish towels regularly in a bleach solution.

Clean the counter with a bleach solution or commercial cleaning agent.

Keep separate cutting boards for foods that will be eaten raw (for example, salad ingredients) and poultry, meat, and seafood. Clean cutting boards after each use.

Refrigerate foods as soon after purchasing them as possible, and defrost meat and poultry in the refrigerator or the microwave, not at room temperature.

Keep the refrigerator cold, 40°F or lower. Refrigerate leftovers no more than 2 hours after serving (1 hour if room temperature is near 90°F).

Cook food to an internal temperature of 160°F, and hold cooked foods at 140°F or hotter until served.

Don't eat raw batter or cookie dough. Uncooked foods with raw eggs carry a salmonella risk.

Figure 7.6   Food safety in the kitchen.

deletion, or reorganization of an organism's genes in order to change that organism's protein production. Research on genetic modification in agriculture has focused on three areas: (1) new strains of crops and animals with improved resistance to disease and pests (for example, corn plants that resist blights); (2) strains of microorganisms that produce specific substances that occur in small amounts or not at all in nature (for example, bovine somatotropin, a growth hormone used in cattle to produce more meat); and (3) crops that resist destruction by herbicides (for example, soybean plants that can survive herbicides used to kill weeds). Many crops have already been genetically modified, and 60 percent of processed foods currently sold in supermarkets contain one or more GM ingredients.[38]

Proponents of GM crops and animals envision an overpopulated world with increasing demands for food and a significant loss of farmland in which to produce that food. To meet these looming needs, they say, we must develop new agricultural technologies that increase crop and animal productivity and support food growers and producers economically while not harming the environment. They see genetic modification as a promising agricultural technology that may meet these potentially conflicting needs, and many in the food and biotechnology industries have hailed the benefits of GM organisms.[38]

On the other hand, a growing number of consumers, animal rights supporters, national consumer watchdog organizations, and environmentalists have expressed concerns about GM foods. They fear that agriculture driven by biotechnology without restraint will destroy natural ecosystems, create new viruses, increase cruelty to animals, and reduce biodiversity.[38]

The safety of food products produced by biotechnology is assessed by the FDA's new National Center for Food Safety and Technology. To date, the center has held that GM foods do not require any special safety testing—nor do they have to be labeled as GM foods—unless they differ significantly from foods already in use.[3, 38] Consumer advocacy groups have called for all foods containing GM ingredients to be labeled. One of their concerns is that genetic material may be added to a product from a source that causes allergic reactions, such as would be the case if genes from peanuts were added to GM soybeans. Another is that people with religious objections to certain foods might unknowingly consume them in GM foods[3]; for example, a person maintaining a kosher kitchen might purchase a food containing genes normally found in pork.

The American Dietetic Association and many other scientific organizations support the FDA position on GM foods, citing the potential benefits. For biotechnology in agriculture to achieve the objectives of ensuring safe, abundant, and affordable food, however, it must be accepted by the public. Surveys suggest that consumers are not well informed about this technology, but they are cautiously optimistic about its potential benefits in food production and processing.[28]

***

North Americans enjoy the safest and most nutritious food supply in the world. We also enjoy immense choice in what we eat. With choice comes responsibility—the responsibility to be informed, to make wise decisions, to consume foods that promote health and prevent disease. After reading this chapter, you have sufficient information to make nutrition choices that support your own lifelong health and, by extension, the well-being of society at large. We encourage you to make those healthy choices!

You Make the Call

Junk Food in Schools

Have you been on the campus of a public school in the United States lately? If you have, you might have been surprised to see the names of soft drinks splashed prominently across buildings, fast food served in the cafeteria, and vending machines stationed at strategic spots, filled with candy, sweet desserts, and high-sodium snack foods. School campuses are as much a part of the junk-food advertising and sales scene as any shopping mall or city street.

How did junk foods get a foothold on school campuses? In recent years, many school districts were hit hard by cuts in local and state funding; to adjust to reduced revenue, they made cutbacks everywhere they could—in sports, extracurricular activities, art and music, even library hours. When students and parents objected, they turned to corporate offers. Some schools have signed exclusive contracts with soft drink companies to stock soda machines or with fast-food chains to provide school lunches. Others have accepted partnerships with corporations allowing corporate advertising on school buses, school walls, book covers, and teaching materials. In exchange, schools receive funds that allow them to offer both academic and extracurricular programs that would otherwise be unavailable.

The benefits to food companies are clear. U.S. food manufacturers produce enough food to provide a per capita average intake of 3,800 calories per day, up from 3,300 in 1970. Since most people do not consume 3,800 calories, food manufacturers must either make other products or get consumers to eat more. Children are relentlessly targeted, since nutrition practices tend to be established early in life.

Parents and health experts are fighting the explosion of junk-food sales in schools, and lawmakers have tried to limit such sales. By 2002, 10 states had restricted junk-food sales, and similar legislation was pending in 16 other states. Health experts point out that only 2 percent of American youth comply with all the recommendations of the USDA *Dietary Guidelines for Americans,* and 16 percent do not meet any of the recommendations. Fewer than 15 percent of children eat the recommended servings of fruit; fewer than 20 percent consume the recommended servings of vegetables; fewer than 25 percent eat the recommended servings of grain; and only 30 percent consume the recommended servings of dairy products. Teenagers drink twice as much soda as milk.

Nutritionists also point to the current rates of overweight and obesity in children and adolescents, which are linked to overconsumption of high-fat, high-sugar foods. Nearly 4.7 million youths ages 16 to 17, for example, are overweight or obese. Diseases associated with excess weight include Type-2 diabetes, heart disease, high blood pressures, stroke, and colon cancer. Overweight and obesity are among the 10 leading preventable causes of death.

For their side, corporate junk-food makers argue that individual self-control is the remedy for obesity, not legislation to curb sales. Parents have the primary responsibility for ensuring healthy nutrition practices in their children, according to this view. Fast-food corporations also note that changes in the American family, such as an increase in the number of working parents and single parents and an associated decrease in the amount of supervision children receive, have produced a generation of children who are self-indulgent and who have not learned self-discipline. Food manufacturers say they are simply providing foods that children want.

The corporations also argue that parents are responsible for making sure schools are adequately funded to meet students' academic and extracurricular needs. These programs and activities are now being funded by pizza and candy sales, vending machine operations, and contracts with soft drink companies. Corporate-school partnerships are a valuable social service, according to these corporations.

Finding an appropriate balance among corporate profits, the urgent demand of schools for revenue, and the health of children has become a dilemma. Some people feel that by depending on revenue from partnerships with corporations, schools have put children's health at risk. Should junk food continue to be part of the scene at public schools? What do you think?

Pros

- Parents are responsible for teaching their children good nutrition habits and monitoring what they eat.
- Parents are also responsible for ensuring that schools receive adequate funding, whether from government or corporate sources.
- The changing American family has produced children with little self-discipline; the food industry is simply giving them what they want.

- Food manufacturers are providing a valuable service by financing school programs, sports, and extracurricular activities that parents and students demand.

Cons

- Children in the United States do not consume nutritious foods in quantities sufficient to promote health and prevent illness. They do consume enough unhealthy foods to be overweight and at risk for chronic diseases.
- Food manufacturers have to create desires and needs for their products because more food is produced per capita in the United States than is needed for good health. The family cannot compete with the powerful forces of the food and advertising industries.
- Nutrition education is an important part of the school curriculum. Corporate partnerships cause schools to push junk foods at the same time that they are supposedly teaching children about healthy food choices.

OLC Web site For more information on this topic, visit the Online Learning Center at www.mhhe.com/teague1e.

SOURCES: "American Children's Diets Not Making the Grade, by L. Biing-Hwan, J. Guthrie, and E. Frazio; 2001, *Food Review, 24* (2), 8–17; "Promoting Healthy Eating Behaviors: The Role of School Environments," by A. Gallagher, October 23, 2002, speech, Healthy Eating Environments Conference, USDA, www.fns.usda.gov; "Policy Implications and Strategies for Change," by M. Nestle, October 23, 2002, speech, Healthy Eating Environment Conference, USDA, www.fns.usda.gov; "Fighting Big Fat," by P. Tyre, August 5, 2002, *Newsweek,* 38–39; *Healthy People 2010* (2nd ed.), 2000, U.S. Dept. of Health and Human Services.

SUMMARY

- Society has a stake in the good health of citizens; therefore, governments commonly develop nutritional guidelines and recommendations.
- The Dietary Reference Intakes (DRIs) are designed to promote optimal health and prevent both nutritional deficiencies and chronic diseases such as cancer and cardiovascular disease. They include four sets of guidelines, the Estimated Average Requirement (EAR), the Recommended Dietary Allowances (RDAs), the Adequate Intake (AI), and the Tolerable Upper Intake Level (UL).
- The Acceptable Macronutrient Distribution Range (AMDR) represents intake levels of essential nutrients that provide adequate nutrition and that are associated with reduced risk of chronic disease.
- The USDA Food Guide Pyramid, a set of practical recommendations for daily food choices in five major

food groups, has been superseded by the USDA Food Guide, which exemplifies the pattern of eating recommended in the 2005 *Dietary Guidelines for Americans;* it is graphically depicted in the new MyPyramid.

- The Daily Values, used on food labels, indicate how a particular food contributes to the recommended daily intake of major nutrients in a 2,000-calorie diet.
- Essential nutrients are those that the body cannot manufacture and must get from foods or supplements. The macronutrients include water, carbohydrates, protein, and fats. The micronutrients are minerals and vitamins.
- The body needs water to digest, absorb, and transport nutrients, maintain proper fluid balance in the cells and tissues, regulate body temperature, and perform other essential bodily functions. People need to consume an average of 8 to 12 cups of fluid a day.

- Carbohydrates are the body's main source of energy. Simple carbohydrates consist of one or two units of sugar per molecule; complex carbohydrates consist of multiple sugar units. Most carbohydrates, including starches and dietary fiber, come from plant sources. The AMDR for carbohydrates is 46 percent to 65 percent of daily energy intake (calories consumed). No more than 25 percent of these calories should come from simple carbohydrates.

- The body needs protein to build, maintain, and repair tissues and regulate body functions. Complete proteins, derived primarily from animal sources, contain all the essential amino acids; incomplete proteins, primarily from plant sources, do not. The AMDR for protein is 10 percent to 35 percent of daily energy intake.

- Fats, or lipids, are made of fatty acids; they are a concentrated energy source and perform other essential bodily functions. Saturated fats are found mainly in animal products; monounsaturated and polyunsaturated fats are found mainly in plant products. Saturated fats can raise blood levels of cholesterol and contribute to cardiovascular disease.

- Trans fat, produced during the process of hydrogenation, is believed to contribute even more than saturated fats do to cardiovascular disease. Omega-3 and omega-6 fatty acids contribute to cardiovascular health. The AMDR for fat is 20 percent to 35 percent of daily energy intake. No more than 10 percent of these calories should come from saturated fats.

- Minerals are inorganic micronutrients needed to build bones and teeth, help vitamins and enzymes carry out metabolic processes, and maintain proper functioning of most body systems. The body needs 20 essential minerals.

- Vitamins are organic micronutrients needed to help release energy from other nutrients, aid in chemical reactions, and maintain components of the immune, nervous, and skeletal systems. The body needs 11 to 13 essential vitamins. Vitamins A, D, E, and K are fat soluble; the rest are water soluble. Most people do not need mineral or vitamin supplements.

- Phytochemicals are substances found in plants that provide health benefits when consumed. They include antioxidants, phytoestrogens, and phytonutrients.

- The 2005 *Dietary Guidelines for Americans* represent a synthesis of current information and knowledge about nutrition, presented as general recommendations for diet and physical activity. The guidelines are designed to address the role of poor diet and a sedentary lifestyle in (1) the major causes of disease and death in the United States and (2) the increase in overweight and obesity in this country.

- The 2005 *Dietary Guidelines for Americans* are illustrated in two recommended eating patterns: the USDA Food Guide and the DASH Eating Plan. Both plans give serving recommendations for several different calorie (activity) levels.

- MyPyramid graphically represents the USDA Food Guide recommendations; it comes in a general version as well as 12 different versions specific to calorie patterns.

- It is particularly notable that the 2005 *Dietary Guidelines for Americans* and MyPyramid emphasize physical activity, managing weight through a balance of activity and food, eating nutrient-dense foods, and consuming half of all grains as whole grains.

- Food labels can help you determine how a food fits into your overall diet by showing what percentage of the Daily Value of various nutrients it provides. Food labels and food descriptors are regulated by the FDA.

- Current consumer concerns include consumption of soft drinks, high-sodium diets, food allergies and intolerances, convenience foods, and fast foods. Soft drinks contribute large amounts of sugar to the diet and are implicated in the current epidemic of overweight in the United States.

- Many processed foods contain large amounts of sodium, which can elevate blood pressure in some people; nutritionists recommend that sodium consumption be reduced.

- Some children and adults are allergic to eggs, peanuts, milk, and other foods, but most food reactions are intolerances. The only way to avoid an allergic reaction is to avoid an offending food.

- Convenience foods usually have less nutritional value than home-prepared foods do. Similarly, fast foods are overloaded with calories, saturated and trans fats, and sodium.

- Other consumer issues involve food safety and technology. Food additives are substances added to food to maintain or improve nutrient value, aid in food preparation, and/or improve taste or appearance; their safety is monitored by the FDA.

- National standards have been developed to regulate organic foods—those raised without synthetic pesticides or fertilizers, antibiotics, or growth hormones. These foods have not proven to be healthier than conventional foods, but organic agriculture is better for the environment.

- Functional foods are usually defined as foods to which ingredients have been added to improve their healthful effects, such as margarine with added plant stanol esters.

- Foodborne illnesses cause thousands of deaths in the United States every year. The most common food pathogens are E. coli, salmonella enteritis, and campylobacter. Although most food-poisoning incidents are associated with public eating establishments, safe food practices at home are recommended.

- Food irradiation is a method of destroying most food pathogens, but it is not fully accepted by the public.
- Genetic modification is the altering of a plant's or an animal's genetic makeup to produce desirable traits, such as resistance to disease or production of particular substances. About 60 percent of processed foods in supermarkets contain one or more genetically modified ingredients.

REVIEW QUESTIONS

1. Explain the differences among the four sets of standards that make up the DRIs.
2. What are the essential macronutrients and the essential micronutrients?
3. What functions does water perform in the body?
4. What is the difference in metabolism between simple and complex carbohydrates?
5. Why is dietary fiber unlike other carbohydrates? What role does it play in the body's functioning?
6. What is a complementary protein?
7. Why are fats important in the diet?
8. What are the AMDRs for carbohydrates, protein, and fats?
9. Under what circumstances might a person need a vitamin or a mineral supplement?
10. What are the effects of antioxidants in the body?
11. Describe the areas addressed by the nine guidelines in the 2005 *Dietary Guidelines for Americans.*
12. Describe the serving recommendations for the five food groups at the 2,000-calorie level.
13. What are the Daily Values?
14. Describe some of the nutritional problems associated with consumption of soft drinks and with high-sodium diets.
15. What are some of the functions of food additives? What are some concerns associated with them?
16. What is the difference between organic foods and natural foods?
17. Explain what functional foods are.
18. What three pathogens are the most common causes of foodborne illness? What food practices can individuals adopt in their own kitchens to lower their risk of contracting a foodborne illness?
19. What arguments are made for and against genetic modification of foods?

WEB RESOURCES

American Dietetic Association: This organization focuses on healthy living, addressing obesity and overweight, aging, complementary care and dietary supplements, safe and nutritious food supply, and human genome and genetics as key topics. www.eatright.org

American Heart Association: Delicious Decisions is an online booklet featuring chapters on enjoying eating, shopping for food, recipes, eating out, and staying fit for a lifetime. www.deliciousdecisions.org

Center for Science in the Public Interest: This advocacy organization focuses on nutrition and health, food safety, alcohol policy, and sound science. Its Web site features press releases, health tips, and articles on food-related topics. www.cspinet.org

FDA Center for Food Safety and Applied Nutrition: This resource offers a wide range of information—from food and nutrition topics in the news to legal issues related to food safety. http://vm.cfsan.fda.gov

Food Allergy and Anaphylaxis Network: Featuring information on common food allergens, ways to manage food allergies, allergy-free recipes, and FAQs, this site offers practical approaches to living with food allergies. www.foodallergy.org

Food Safety: This is an excellent resource for food news and safety alerts, consumer advice, and topics related to children and teens. It also offers information on reporting illnesses and submitting product complaints. www.foodsafety.gov

National Cancer Institute: This site offers easy approaches to making "eat 5 to 9 a day for better health" a part of your daily routine. It discusses the reasoning behind eating fruits and vegetables, serving sizes, and the color guide. http://5aday.nci.nih.gov

National Dairy Council: Offering nutrition and product information on dairy products, this site features education materials, recipes, health tips, and weight management issues. www.nationaldairycouncil.org

Nutrition.gov: A gateway to reliable information on nutrition, healthy eating, food safety, and physical activity, this site provides access to a wide range of information from the U.S. government. www.nutrition.gov

The Partnership for Food Safety: This site features information on the four-step approach to fighting bacteria, safe food-handling practices, seasonal cooking, children's issues, and safety tips. www.fightbac.org

U.S. Pharmacopeia: This organization sets standards for the quality and safety of drugs for humans and animals. Its site offers information on drugs, dietary supplements, and patient safety. www.usp.org

The Vegetarian Resource Group: This site features information on vegetarian nutrition, vegetarian recipes, food ingredients, and the vegan approach to eating. It addresses topics related to teens, families, and children. www.vrg.org

REFERENCES

1. Kleiner, S. M. (1999). Water: An essential but overlooked nutrient. *Journal of the American Dietetic Association, 99* (2), 200–206.

2. Reader's Digest. (1997). *Foods that harm, foods that heal.* Pleasantville, NY: Reader's Digest Association.

3. Sizer, F., & Whitney, E. (2003). *Nutrition: Concepts and controversies.* Belmont, CA: Wadsworth/Thomson Learning.

4. Willett, C. W. (2001). *Eat, drink and be healthy.* New York: Simon & Schuster.

5. *Dietary reference intakes for energy, carbohydrate, fiber, fat, fatty acids, cholesterol, protein, and amino acids (macronutrients).* (2002). Washington, DC: National Academy Press.

6. Anderson, J. W., Smith, B. M., & Gustafson, J. (1994). Health benefits and practical aspects of high-fiber diets. *American Journal of Clinical Nutrition, 59,* S1242–S1247.

7. Slattery, M. L., Curtin, K. P., Edwards, S. L., & Schaffer, D. M. (2004). Plant foods, fiber and rectal cancer. *American Journal of Clinical Nutrition, 79,* 274–281.

8. U.S. Department of Agriculture. (2005). 2005 *Dietary guidelines for Americans.* www.health.gov/dietaryguidelines.

9. American Society for Clinical Nutrition/American Institute of Nutrition Task Force. (1996). Position paper on trans-fatty acids. *American Journal of Clinical Nutrition, 63,* 663–670.

10. DeWailly, E., Blanchet, C., Gingras, S., Lemieux, S., & Holub, B. J. (2002). Cardiovascular disease risk factors and N-3 fatty acids status in the adult population of James Bay Cree. *American Journal of Clinical Nutrition, 76* (1), 85–92.

11. Kark, J. D., Kaufmann, N. A., Binka, F., Goldberger, N., & Berry, E. M. (2003). Adipose tissue n-6 fatty acids and acute myocardial infarction in a population consuming a diet high in polyunsaturated fatty acids. *American Journal of Clinical Nutrition, 77* (4), 796–802.

12. Tribble, D. L. (1999). Antioxidant consumption and risk of coronary heart disease: Emphasis on vitamin C, E, and B-carotene. American Heart Association, *Circulation, 99,* 591–595.

13. Schumann, K., Borch-Johnsen, B., Hentze, M. W., & Marx, J. M. (2002). Tolerable upper intakes for dietary iron set by the U.S. Food and Nutrition Board. *American Journal of Clinical Nutrition, 76* (3), 499–500.

14. Morris, C. D., & Carson, S. (2003). Routine vitamin supplementation to prevent cardiovascular disease: A summary of the evidence for the U.S. Preventive Services Task Force. *Annals of Internal Medicine, 139* (1), 56–70.

15. The antioxidant responsive element (ARE) may explain the protective effects of cruciferous vegetables on cancer. (2003). *Nutrition Reviews, 61* (7), 250–254.

16. Munro, I. C., et al. (2003). Soy isoflavones: A safety review. *Nutrition Reviews, 61* (1), 1–33.

17. Giovannucci, E. (1999). Tomatoes, tomato-based products, lycopene and cancer: Review of the epidemiogic literature. *Journal of the National Cancer Institute, 91,* 317–331.

18. Nuovo, J. (1999). AHA statement on antioxidants and coronary disease. *American Family Physician, 59* (10).

19. USDA. (2004). Q&As, revision of the Food Guidance System. www.usda.gov.

20. Trichopoulou, A., & Lasiou, P. (1997). Healthy traditional Mediterranean diet: An expression of cultures, history, and lifestyle. *Nutrition Reviews, 55,* 383–389.

21. Sabate, J. (2003). The contribution of vegetarian diets to health and disease: A paradigm shift. *American Journal of Clinical Nutrition, 78* (3), 502–507.

22. Rolfes, S. R., DeBruyne, L. K., & Whitney, E. N. (1998). *Life span nutrition: Conception through life.* Belmont, CA: Wadsworth.

23. USDA. (1996, March 3–4). Sugar and sweetener. *Situation and Outlook Report.*

24. Jacobson, M. F. (n.d.). *Liquid candy: How soft drinks are harming Americans' health.* Washington, DC: Center for Science in the Public Interest.

25. High blood pressure: The end of an epidemic. (2000, December 3–9). *Nutrition Action Healthletter.*

26. Guthrie, J. F., Biing-Hwan, L., & Frazo, E. (2002). Role of food prepared away from home in the American diet, 1997–98 versus 1994–96: Changes and consequences. *Journal of Nutrition Education and Behavior, 34* (3), 140–150.

27. Jacobson, M. F., & Fritschner, S. (1998). *The fast food guide.* New York: Workman Publishing.

28. Biotechnology and the future of food. (1995). Position statement of the American Dietetic Association. *Journal of the American Dietetic Association, 95,* 1429–1432.

29. Use of nutritive and nonnutritive sweeteners. (1998). Position of the American Dietetic Association. *Journal of the American Dietetic Association, 98,* 581–687.

30. Barrett, J., Jarvis, W. T., Kroger, M., & London, W. M. (1997). *Consumer health: A guide to intelligent decisions.* Dubuque, IA: Brown & Benchmark.

31. Taylor, C. L. (2004). Regulator's framework for functional foods and dietary supplements. *Nutrition Reviews, 62* (2), 55–59.

32. Centers for Disease Control and Prevention: Incidence of foodborne illnesses. (1999). Preliminary data from the foodborne disease active surveillance network (food net). *Morbidity and Mortality Weekly Report, 48* (9), 189–194.

33. U.S. Food and Drug Administration Center for Food Safety and Applied Nutrition. (1998). Foodborne pathogenic microorganisms and natural toxins handbook ("The Bad Bug Book"). http://vm.cfsan.fda.gov.

34. Fox, N. (1999). *It was probably something you ate.* New York: Penguin Books.

35. Altekruse, S. F., et al. (1999). Campylobacter jejuni—an emerging foodborne pathogen. *Emerging Infectious Diseases.*

36. Greene, L. W., & Ottoson, J. M. (2001). *Community and population health.* Dubuque, IA: WCB/McGraw-Hill.

37. Food irradiation. (2000). *Journal of the American Dietetic Association, 100,* 246–253.

38. Brown, K. (2001). Seeds of concern. *Scientific American, 284* (4), 60–61.

Add It Up!

CALCULATING YOUR RECOMMENDED INTAKE OF FAT, PROTEIN, AND CARBOHYDRATE

Many nutritional recommendations are given as percentages of total daily calories. How do these percentages translate into grams of fat, protein, and carbohydrate in your daily diet? And what individual goals do you want to set for yourself?

Begin by multiplying your body weight in pounds by 15; this will give you an estimate of your recommended daily calories. For example, if you weigh 150 pounds, you need 2,250 calories per day, if your weight is stable. Then complete the following calculations.

Calculation for Fat

The Acceptable Macronutrient Distribution Range (AMDR) set by the Food and Nutrition Board for fat is 20–35% of total daily calories. Many nutritionists, however, recommend that no more than 30% of daily calories come from fat and no more than 10% come from saturated fat. In the average American diet, 34% of calories come from fat.

Step 1: To determine the maximum number of calories you should consume from fat per day, multiply your recommended daily calories by .30. *607.5*

Calories from fat

Step 2: To calculate the grams of fat you should consume per day, divide your calories from fat by 9 (the number of calories in a gram of fat). *67.5*

Grams of fat

Step 3: To determine the maximum number of calories you should consume from saturated fat, multiply your recommended calorie intake by .10. To determine the grams of saturated fat you should consume per day, divide by 9. *202.5*

Calories from saturated fat

22.5

Grams of saturated fat

Example: In a 2,250-calorie diet, the recommended intake is no more than 675 calories from fat (2,250 × .30), or 75 grams of fat (675/9), and no more than 225 calories from saturated fat (2,250 × .10), or 25 grams of saturated fat (225/9).

Calculation for Protein

The AMDR for protein is 10–35% of total daily calories. The RDA is 56 grams for men and 46 grams for women. The average American consumes 100 grams of protein daily.

Step 1: To determine the minimum number of calories you should consume from protein, multiply your recommended daily calories by .10. _____

Minimum calories from protein

Step 2: To calculate your recommended minimum intake of protein in grams, divide your minimum calories from protein by 4 (the number of calories in a gram of protein). _____

Minimum grams of protein

Step 3: To determine your maximum intake of calories from protein, multiply your recommended daily calories by .35. To determine your maximum intake of protein in grams, divide by 4. _____

Maximum calories from protein

_____

Maximum grams of protein

Example: In a 2,250-calorie diet, the recommended intake ranges from 225 calories from protein (2,250 × .10), or about 56 grams of protein (225/4), to about 787 calories from protein (2,250 × .35), or about 195 grams of protein (225/4).

Alternative method 1: A healthy adult typically needs 0.8 grams of protein for every kilogram (2.2 pounds) of body weight, or about 0.36 grams for every pound.

Step 1: Enter your body weight in pounds. _____

Pounds

Step 2: Multiply by 0.36. _____

Recommended grams of protein

Example: A person weighing 150 pounds would need 54 grams of protein per day.

Alternative method 2: A rough estimate of recommended protein intake can be obtained by dividing your body weight by 3.

Step 1: Enter your body weight in pounds   _____
                                                                    Pounds

Step 2: Divide by 3.   _____
                              Recommended grams of protein

Example: A person weighing 150 pounds would need 50 grams of protein per day.

Calculation for Carbohydrate

The AMDR for carbohydrate is 45–65% of total daily calories, but many nutritionists recommend about 55%. The RDA is 130 grams for both men and women.

Step 1: To determine the minimum recommended number of calories from carbohydrates, multiply your recommended daily calories by .45.   _____

Minimum calories from carbohydrates

Step 2: To calculate your recommended minimum intake of carbohydrate in grams, divide your minimum calories from carbohydrates by 4 (the number of calories in a gram of carbohydrate).   _____

Minimum grams of carbohydrate

Step 3: To determine the maximum recommended intake of calories from carbohydrates, multiply your recommended daily calories by .65. To determine your maximum intake of carbohydrates in grams, divide by 4.

_____

Maximum calories from carbohydrate

_____

Maximum grams of carbohydrate

Example: In a 2,250-calorie diet, the recommended intake ranges from about 1,012 calories (2,250 × .45), or 253 grams of carbohydrate, to 1,462 calories (2,250 × .65), or about 365 grams of carbohydrate. In a 2,250-calorie diet with 55% of calories from carbohydrates, intake would be about 1,237 calories, or 309 grams of carbohydrates.

Summary of Your Recommended Intakes and Individual Goals

To set your own goals, decide how you want to distribute your calories within the ranges, based on your preferences (for example, 25% fat, 30% protein, 45% carbohydrate).

Fat: Recommended maximum intake: 30% of total daily calories

Your goal: _____ % = _____ grams per day

Saturated fat: Recommended maximum intake: 10% of total daily calories

Your goal: _____ % = _____ grams per day

Protein: AMDR: 10–35% of total daily calories

Your goal: _____ % = _____ grams per day

Carbohydrate: AMDR: 45–65% of total daily calories

Your goal: _____ % = _____ grams per day

SOURCES: *Nutrition: Concepts and Controversies,* by F. Sizer and E. Whitney, 2003, Belmont, CA: Wadsworth/Thomson Learning; *Dietary Reference Intakes for Energy, Carbohydrate, Fiber, Fat, Fatty Acids, Cholesterol, Protein, and Amino Acids (Macronutrients),* 2002, Washington, DC: National Academy Press.

CHAPTER 8

Fitness: Physical Activity for Life

DID YOU KNOW?

- Every hour that you spend in vigorous physical activity is repaid, on average, with two additional hours of life expectancy. Expending 2,000 calories a week in moderate physical activity is optimal for attaining greater longevity.

- If you walk 10,000 steps a day, you will expend between 300 and 400 calories and cover about 5 miles. The 10,000 Steps Program, a nationwide initiative sponsored by the Shape Up America! program, is motivating people to get moving and helping them keep their weight under control.

OLC *Your Health Today*   www.mhhe.com/teague1e

Go to the Online Learning Center for *Your Health Today* for interactive activities, quizzes, flashcards, Web links, and more resources related to this chapter.

Being physically active is a natural state for human beings, and good health depends on it. Our bodies are designed to move, stretch, and exert force against resistance; when we don't use them for these purposes, they deteriorate. Our culture does not provide many natural opportunities for physical activity, however; in fact, we are often encouraged to just sit back and be entertained. Although numerous organizations have set exercise guidelines designed to promote health and fitness, the fact is that most people don't exercise. Of all those adults who hear the message about exercise, 20 percent become believers and 80 percent tune it out. According to the U.S. Surgeon General, at least 50 percent of American adults do not get enough physical activity for health benefits.[1]

The good news is that there are simple and enjoyable ways to build physical activity into your lifestyle to take advantage of its many health benefits. Becoming more active does not have to be punishing, nor do you have to belong to a health club or buy home fitness equipment to improve your well-being. With planning and commitment, you can enhance the quality of your life with daily physical activity.

In this chapter we explore how and why to make physical activity a lifelong pursuit. We begin with the benefits of physical activity and exercise and then present guidelines for how much exercise you need. We continue with the components of health-related fitness and ways to improve your health through daily moderate physical activity. We end with special considerations in exercise and physical activity, including health and safety considerations, the impact of environmental conditions, and exercise for special populations.

WHAT IS FITNESS?

In Chapter 1 we discussed the concept of *wellness*. In this chapter we look at the related concept of *fitness* and the role it plays in overall good health and well-being. In the context of fitness, you are considered to be in good health if you have sufficient energy and vitality to accomplish daily living tasks and leisure-time physical activities without undue fatigue. **Physical activity**—activity that requires any type of movement—is an important part of good health. Any kind of physical activity is better than no activity at all, and benefits increase as the level of physical activity increases, up to a point. Too much physical activity can make you susceptible to injury. **Exercise** is structured, planned physical activity, often carried out to improve fitness.

Physical fitness, in general, is the ability of the body to respond to the physical demands placed upon it. When we talk about *fitness,* we are really talking about two different concepts: skill-related fitness and health-related fitness.[2] **Skill-related fitness** refers to the ability to perform specific skills associated with various leisure activities or

sports. Components of skill-related fitness include agility, speed, power, balance, coordination, and reaction time. **Health-related fitness** refers to the ability to perform daily living activities (like shopping for groceries) and other activities with vigor.[2] The components of health-related fitness are cardiorespiratory fitness, musculoskeletal fitness, and body composition. Musculoskeletal fitness, in turn, includes muscular strength, muscular endurance, and flexibility.

Benefits of Physical Activity and Exercise

Why should you be physically active? Your answers to this question may include having fun, looking good, feeling good, controlling body weight, relieving stress, learning a new leisure skill, or improving performance in sport activities. Beyond these excellent answers, however, is another reason to be physically active: People who are active are healthier than those who are not.[3] There are benefits in the domains of physical, cognitive, psychological, emotional, and spiritual health, among others. An overview of the health benefits associated with physical activity is presented in Figure 8.1.

Physical Benefits of Exercise

One major benefit can be seen in the fact that people with moderate to high levels of physical activity have a lower mortality rate than do those who are sedentary—in other words, they live longer. A study of more than 17,000 Harvard graduates showed that every hour spent in vigorous physical activity as an adult is repaid with two hours of additional life expectancy. Physical activity and exercise are associated with improved functioning in just about every body system, from the cardiorespiratory system to the skeletal system to the immune system. A sedentary lifestyle, on the other hand, has been associated with 28 percent of deaths from the leading chronic diseases, including cancer, heart disease, osteoporosis, diabetes, high blood pressure, and obesity.[4–11] For more information on these benefits, see the Web Resources at the end of this chapter.

Cognitive Benefits of Exercise

Although there is no compelling evidence that short-term exercise training significantly improves cognitive functioning,[12] some research has suggested positive effects. For example, evidence suggests that fit individuals process information more quickly than do less fit individuals of the same age. Other research has shown that aerobic fitness may prevent or slow down the loss of cognitive functions associated with advancing age.[13] Endurance exercises have also been shown to temper the ability of the central nervous system to inhibit unwanted or undesirable responses to environmental stimuli.[12] This regulatory efficiency is probably due to improved blood circulation to

Figure 8.1   Health benefits of physical activity.

the brain, nerve cell regeneration, and changes in the synthesis of neurotransmitters. However, generalizations about the influence of exercise on cognitive performance must be viewed with caution. Improvements as a result of physical activity may have more to do with overall feelings of well-being than with specific cognitive functions. (For some tips on maintaining cognitive functions, see the box "Jogging Your Memory.")

Psychological and Emotional Benefits of Exercise

Moderate-to-intense levels of physical activity have been shown to influence mood, decrease the risk of depression and anxiety, relieve stress, and improve overall quality of life.[14] Biological explanations for these effects include body warming, increased blood flow to the brain, regulation of stress hormones, and the action of brain chemicals. However, such biological explanations have not been well supported by the research literature.[15] For example, many people experience feelings of euphoria—sometimes called "runner's high"—after intense aerobic exercise as a result of the release of endorphins (particular brain chemicals that produce a sense of well-being). These brain chemicals do not come from the part of the brain that influences mood, however, so it is unlikely that they are responsible for the improvement in mood associated with exercise.

Better explanations for the improved sense of psychological and emotional well-being associated with physical activity are improved self-esteem, improved quality of sleep, more opportunities for social interaction, and more effective physiological responses to stress. As noted in Chapter 5, the stress response, also known as the fight-or-flight response, includes increases in heart rate, respiration rate, blood pressure, release of stress hormones, and nervous system activity. The magnitude of these increases—referred to as an individual's "cardiovascular reactivity" to stress—can be mitigated by exercise. If you are physically fit, your body is conditioned to react more calmly to stressful situations. Exercise can also help you deal with

KEY TERMS

physical activity   Activity that requires any type of movement.

exercise   Structured, planned physical activity, often carried out to improve fitness.

physical fitness   Ability of the body to respond to the physical demands placed upon it.

skill-related fitness   Ability to perform specific skills, such as agility, speed, and coordination, associated with various sports and leisure activities.

health-related fitness   Ability to perform daily living activities with vigor.

Challenges & Choices

Jogging Your Memory

Have you ever walked to another room and forgotten what you went there for? Found you didn't have a clue where you put your car keys? Or where you parked your car? If you have, the problem is probably not that you're losing your mind; it's much more likely that you are distracted, preoccupied, or overly busy. Some experts believe that memory problems are becoming more common because people are under more stress, are more sleep deprived, and are struggling to absorb a huge volume of information on a daily basis. If you want to preserve or improve your memory, try some of these simple mental exercises:

- Turn off the television and do mental exercises, such as crossword puzzles or brain teasers, to keep your mind active and alert.

- Take turns brushing your teeth with your non-dominant hand, including opening and squeezing the tube of toothpaste. Do the same thing when you floss your teeth. This activity will exercise the opposite side of your brain and activate a whole new range of neuron connections in another part of your brain.

- Vary your routine, such as by taking a different route to class or work. New behavior activates larger areas of your brain than habitual behavior.

- Scramble the location of familiar objects to stimulate your visual and sensory brain areas. Wear your watch on your other wrist, for example, or move the items on your desk to different locations. These changes take your brain off "automatic pilot" and force it to work harder.

- Participate in aerobic activities and be physically active in your daily life. Activity improves blood flow throughout your body, including to your brain.

It's Not Just Personal . . .

Mental exercises may help prevent or slow the advance of Alzheimer's disease. According to the Alzheimer's Association (www.alz.org), research has shown that keeping the brain active by reading, writing, taking classes, playing games, and doing puzzles may build a reserve of brain cells and neural connections. It may even contribute to the generation of new nerve cells.

---

stressful situations by providing a temporary distraction, increasing your feelings of control or commitment, and providing a sense of success in doing something that is important to you. Thus, exercise improves your ability to handle stress by providing both physical and mental buffers.

Spiritual Benefits of Exercise

When you exercise, you are taking charge of your life and taking care of yourself. Exercising and being physically active give you the opportunity to connect with yourself, with other people, and with nature in deep and immediate ways. As you jog through a park, cycle on a bike path, hike in a natural area, or cross-country ski on a wilderness trail, you may find yourself feeling refreshed and reinvigorated both by a sense of physical well-being and by the natural scene around you. Thus, exercise enhances your feelings of self-esteem and mastery as well as your connection to yourself and something beyond yourself.

Guidelines for Physical Activity and Exercise

As with nutrition and other aspects of health and wellness, every society has an interest in the physical fitness of

its citizens. In 1996 the U.S. Surgeon General released the *Physical Activity and Health Report,* summarizing the importance of health-related fitness. The report had these major conclusions:

- People who are usually inactive can improve their health and well-being by becoming even moderately active on a regular basis.

- Physical activity need not be strenuous to confer health benefits.

- Greater health benefits can be achieved by increasing the amount (duration, frequency, or intensity) of physical activity.[16]

The surgeon general's report established two kinds of exercise guidelines. First, significant health benefits can be obtained by participating in moderate-intensity physical activity, such as brisk walking or raking leaves, for 30 minutes on most, if not all, days of the week. Second, additional health benefits can be received by participating in more vigorous activities, 20 to 30 minutes in duration, two to five times a week. The second guideline is based on the 1990 fitness recommendations of the American College of Sports Medicine (ACSM) that call for aerobic exercise (cardiorespiratory endurance exercise) three to five times a week, plus multiple sets of strength training

HIGHLIGHT ON HEALTH

Guidelines for Vigorous Exercise

Dimension	Lower Limit	Upper Limit
Frequency	3 days a week	5 days a week
Intensity	55% of maximal heart rate	90% of maximal heart rate
Time	20 minutes per session	60 minutes per session
Type	Aerobic activity, using large muscles of the body, for example, running, cycling, swimming	Aerobic activity, using large muscles of the body, for example, running, cycling, swimming

Source: Adapted from *ACSM Fitness Book,* American College of Sports Medicine, 2003, Champaign, IL: Human Kinetics.

(muscle training) exercises two times a week (see the box "Guidelines for Vigorous Exercise").[17]

Another way to think about the surgeon general's report is in terms of unstructured activities (physical activity) and structured activities (exercise). Unstructured activities may include such activities as washing your car, gardening, running errands on foot, or walking to class. Structured activities include moderate activities of longer duration (walking at a brisk pace for 30 minutes) or more vigorous activities of shorter duration (running for 15 to 20 minutes).[17]

Research suggests that death rates decline as physical activity increases from 500 to 3,000 calories per week.[18] This benefit plateaus at about 3,000 calories. Thus, health experts have generally concluded that 2,000 calories of physical activity per week is optimal for attaining the benefit of longevity. The duration of the exercise is less important than the total amount of calories expended in physical activity.[19] Three 10-minute exercise sessions are comparable to one 30-minute session. Exercise intensity, however, does have an effect on health benefits. (Duration and intensity are discussed in more detail in the next section.) Light exercises (bowling, household chores) do not reduce death rates. Moderate physical activities (golf, dancing) are beneficial for reducing death rates, and vigorous physical activity (jogging, lap swimming) are more beneficial.[16]

The National Academies' Institute of Medicine (IOM) has issued guidelines for vigorous exercise that are more strenuous than are those given in the surgeon general's report. The primary goal of the surgeon general's recommendation is to reduce the risk of chronic disease in the future. IOM recommendations focus on weight control in the present. Research suggests that 60 minutes of physical activity each day are necessary for maintaining body weight and avoiding excess weight gain.[19] This recommendation is particularly important for children, now that 25 percent of America's children are defined as overweight.[13] Inactivity among children has significantly

contributed to increases in chronic diseases, especially Type-2 diabetes (adult onset).[13]

As described in Chapter 7, the 2005 *Dietary Guidelines for Americans* recommends 30 minutes of moderate-intensity physical activity above usual activity on most days of the week to reduce the risk of chronic disease; 60 minutes of moderate- to vigorous-intensity activity on most days of the week to manage body weight and prevent gradual weight gain; and 60–90 minutes of daily moderate-intensity activity to sustain weight loss in adulthood. The guidelines recommend that children get 60 minutes of physical activity on most, preferably all, days of the week as well (see Chapter 7).

Many graphic models have been developed to illustrate recommendations for exercise and physical activity. The one shown in Figure 8.2 provides an overview of recommendations for the various components of fitness. We turn to a more detailed discussion of these components next.

COMPONENTS OF HEALTH-RELATED FITNESS

As noted earlier in the chapter, the components of health-related fitness are cardiorespiratory fitness, musculoskeletal fitness (muscular strength, muscular endurance, and flexibility), and body composition. Fitness training programs can improve each of these components and help you experience health benefits. These benefits can also be experienced without necessarily adhering to a rigorous or strenuous exercise program.[16]

The key to fitness training is the body's ability to adapt to increasing demands by becoming more fit—that is, as a general rule, the more you exercise, the more fit you become. The amount of exercise, called *overload,* is significant, however. If you exercise too little, your fitness level won't improve. If you exercise too much, you may be susceptible

Figure 8.2
Exercise and physical activity pyramid.

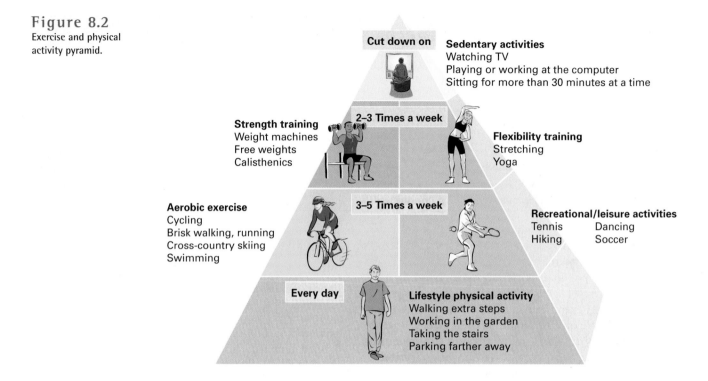

to injury. When you are designing an exercise program, you need to think about four different dimensions of your exercise sessions that affect overload: frequency (number of sessions per week), intensity (level of difficulty of each exercise session), time (duration of each exercise session), and type (type of exercise in each exercise session). You can remember these dimensions with the acronym FITT.

Cardiorespiratory Fitness

Cardiorespiratory fitness is the ability of the heart and lungs to efficiently deliver oxygen and nutrients to the body's muscles and cells via the bloodstream. This should be at the heart of any fitness program. It is developed by activities that use the large muscles of the body in continuous movement, such as jogging, running, cycling, swimming, cross-country skiing, and aerobic dance.

Cardiorespiratory Training

Benefits of cardiorespiratory training are an increase in the oxygen-carrying capacity of the blood, improved extraction of oxygen from the bloodstream by muscle cells, an increase in the amount of blood the heart pumps with each heartbeat, and increased speed of recovery back to a

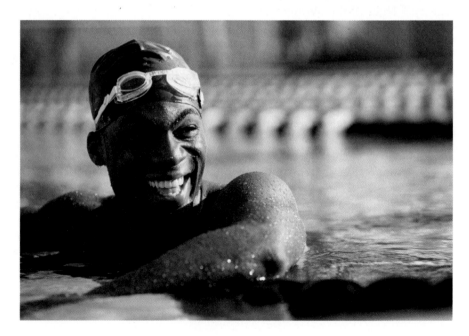

Swimming offers excellent cardiorespiratory benefits with a low risk of injury. Through daily workouts, this swimmer is improving the oxygen-carrying capacity of his blood and decreasing his resting heart rate and resting blood pressure.

HIGHLIGHT ON HEALTH

Calculating Your Target Heart Rate Zone Using the Heart Rate Reserve Method

Follow these steps to calculate your target heart rate zone:

1. To determine your resting heart rate (RHR), take your pulse at the carotid (neck) or radial (wrist) artery while you are at rest. Use your middle finger or forefinger or both when taking your pulse; do not use your thumb, since it has a pulse of its own. Take your pulse for 15 seconds and multiply by 4.

2. To determine your maximum heart rate (MHR), subtract your age from 220.

3. To determine your THR objective, use the maximal **heart rate reserve (HRR)** formula, which is considered the most accurate method. Heart rate reserve is the difference between your maximum heart rate and your resting heart rate. The THR is usually 60 percent to 80 percent for young adults and 55 percent to 70 percent for older adults. Here is the HRR formula:

$$THR = X\% (MHR - RHR) + RHR.$$

Example: Serena is 20 years old and just starting a cardiorespiratory training program. Her THR goal is 60 percent to 80 percent, and she has a resting heart rate of 70. For a 60 percent threshold, the THR would be calculated as follows:

$$0.6 (200 - 70) + 70 =$$
$$0.6 (130) + 70 = 78 + 70 = 148$$

For an 80 percent threshold, the THR would be calculated as follows:

$$0.8 (200 - 70) + 70 =$$
$$0.8 (130) + 70 = 104 + 70 = 174$$

Thus, Serena's THR is between 148 and 174.

---

resting level after exercise. Cardiorespiratory training improves muscle and liver functioning and decreases resting heart rate, resting blood pressure, and heart rate at any work level. The average resting heart rate of a fit person, for example, ranges from 55 to 65 beats per minute. A person who is not fit has to work 20 percent to 30 percent harder just to meet the minimal energy needs for everyday activities. In a day, that totals 28,000 more heartbeats for the unfit heart compared to a fit heart. In one year, the unfit heart has experienced approximately 10,512,000 extra beats of unnecessary workload.

How do you go about developing a cardiorespiratory training program to improve your level of fitness? Start by using the FITT acronym (frequency, intensity, time, and type of activity).

Frequency   In general, you must exercise at least twice a week to experience improvements in cardiorespiratory functioning. The ideal frequency for training is three times per week. Interestingly, several studies have suggested that running four or five times per week provides either no greater benefits or only slightly greater benefits than running three times per week.[16] Exercising five or six times a week is appropriate if weight control is a primary concern.[20] After age 40, however, people exercising five or six times a week should change exercises from day to day, because muscles can't mend as quickly after use with advancing age. Additional time is needed for recuperation.[17]

Intensity   A certain level of vigor in exercise is necessary to condition the cardiorespiratory system, but finding the right level of intensity can be tricky. If you are a runner, for example, and you run too slowly, it may take you forever to experience any effect. If you run too fast, you may tire too quickly and have to stop before you reach your goal. The in-between point at which you are stressing your cardiorespiratory system for optimal benefit but not overdoing it is called the **target heart rate zone (THR)**. The most accurate way to calculate your THR, the heart rate reserve method, is shown in the box "Calculating Your Target Heart Rate Zone Using the Heart Rate Reserve Method." The ACSM recommends that people set their THR at 55 percent to 90 percent of their MHR—that

KEY TERMS

cardiorespiratory fitness   Ability of the heart and lungs to efficiently deliver oxygen and nutrients to the body's muscles and cells via the bloodstream.

heart rate reserve (HRR)   Difference between maximum heart rate and resting heart rate.

target heart rate zone (THR)   Range of exercise intensity that allows you to stress your cardiorespiratory system for optimal benefit without overloading the system.

is, that they exercise at 55 percent to 90 percent of their maximum heart rate.

Time   Generally, exercise sessions should last from 15 to 60 minutes; 30 minutes is a good average to aim for. Duration and intensity of exercise have an inverse relation with each other, so that a shorter, higher intensity session can give your cardiorespiratory system the same workout as a longer, lower intensity session, all other things being equal. For example, you can achieve significant cardiorespiratory improvements by exercising from 5 to 10 minutes at a 90 percent THR intensity level. This practice, however, is not advisable for older adults or sedentary people. It is used primarily by those interested in elite athletic competition.[21]

Type of Activity   As noted earlier, cardiorespiratory fitness is developed through aerobic exercise—steady-state exercise that demands an uninterrupted output from working muscles for at least a 12-minute period. There are two types of aerobic exercise: (1) exercises that require sustained intensity with little variability in heart rate response, such as running and rowing, and (2) exercises that involve "stop and go" activities and do not maintain continuous exercise intensity, such as basketball, soccer, and tennis. Stop and go activities usually have to be done for a longer period of time than do sustained intensity activities to confer cardiorespiratory benefits. Both types of activity can be part of a cardiorespiratory training program.

Training Progression

To receive the maximum benefit from exercise, you need to adjust your level of activity by altering duration and intensity every so often. As a general rule, it takes people between the ages of 20 and 29 two weeks to adapt to a cardiorespiratory activity workload. Older people need to add 10 percent to adaptation time for each decade after age 30. A 20-year-old, for example, can expect to adjust activity workload every 2 weeks. A 70-year-old would adjust workload about every 3 weeks (40 percent longer is about 6 days). After you have obtained a satisfactory level of cardiorespiratory fitness and are no longer interested in increasing your conditioning workload, you can maintain your fitness level by continuing the same level of workout.

Developing Your Own Program

To develop your own regular cardiorespiratory training program, start out slowly to avoid injury and gradually build up your endurance. If you have any known medical conditions, or if you have been sedentary and are over the age of 40, see your physician for a checkup before starting. To ensure that you will stick with your program, select activities that you enjoy and that are compatible with the constraints of your schedule, budget, and lifestyle. Whether you choose running, swimming,

cycling, a team sport, or another aerobic activity, try to build sessions of at least 30 minutes duration into your schedule three times a week. If you make these sessions part of your life, they can be the foundation of a lasting fitness program.

Muscular Strength and Endurance

Health-related fitness also includes muscular strength and muscular endurance. Benefits of improved muscular fitness are increased lean body mass, which helps prevent obesity; increased bone mineral density, which prevents osteoporosis; improved glucose metabolism and insulin sensitivity, which prevents diabetes; and decreased anxiety and depression, which improves quality of life.[22] Muscular fitness improves posture, prevents or reduces low back pain, enables you to perform the tasks of daily living with greater ease, and helps you to look and feel better.[23]

Muscular fitness has two main components: muscular strength and muscular endurance. **Muscular strength** is the capacity of the muscle to exert force against resistance. It is primarily dependent on how much muscle mass you have. Your muscular strength is measured by how much you can lift, push, or pull in a single, all-out effort. **Muscular endurance** is the capacity of the muscle to exert force repeatedly over a period of time, or to apply and sustain strength for a period lasting from a few seconds to a few minutes.

Strength Training

Muscular strength and endurance are developed by strength training, also known as weight training or resistance training. This is a type of exercise in which the muscles exert force against resistance, such as free weights (dumbbells, barbells) or exercise resistance machines.

Types of Muscle Action   Different types of exercise produce different types of muscle action. If force is exerted against an immovable object or without producing movement, the type of muscle contraction that occurs is known as **isometric.** Placing your hand on a wall and pushing against it as hard as you can is an isometric exercise. So is contracting the muscles of your abdomen. If there is no movement, it is an isometric exercise.

If force is applied with movement, the type of muscle contraction is known as **isotonic.** Using free weights, using weight machines, and using the weight of the body, as in calisthenics (sit-ups, pull-ups, push-ups, and so on), are all forms of isotonic exercise, and all seem to be equally effective in developing muscular fitness. The only advantage of weight training machines over free weights appears to be safety.[24]

A third type of muscle contraction occurs in **isokinetic** exercise, which involves machines or other kinds of equipment that regulate the speed by which the muscles can be shortened. Isokinetic exercises are also called accommodating-resistance exercise. They are not performed as often as isotonic exercises because the equipment is less commonly available. However, isotonic and isokinetic programs are considered comparable for their effects on muscle strength and size.

Intensity and Duration: The Strength-Endurance Continuum   The same exercises develop both strength and endurance, but their intensity and duration vary. To develop strength, you need to exercise at a higher intensity (greater resistance or more weight) for a shorter duration; to develop endurance, you need to exercise at a lower intensity for a longer duration. Duration is measured in terms of repetitions—the number of times you perform the exercise (for example, lift a barbell). If you lift a heavy weight a few times (for example, 1 to 5 repetitions), you are developing strength. If you lift a lighter weight more times (for example, 20 repetitions), you are developing endurance.

To develop strength, begin by choosing a weight you can lift about 8 times and gradually build to 12 times. Do just one set of these repetitions at first and increase to three sets, allowing your muscles to recover between sets. When you can do three sets of 12 repetitions, increase the weight. To develop endurance, do more repetitions at a lower weight.

Frequency and Type of Activity   Two to three resistance training sessions a week are sufficient for building muscle strength and endurance. The primary muscle groups targeted in resistance training are the deltoids (shoulders), pectorals (chest), triceps (back of upper arms), biceps (front of upper arms), quadriceps (front of thighs), hamstrings (back of thighs), gluteus maximus (buttocks), and abdomen. Other areas to exercise are the upper back, the lower back, and the calves. Whether you choose free weights or weight machines, try to exercise every muscle group during your strength training sessions.

When you participate in one activity or sport to improve your performance in another, or when you use several different types of training for a specific fitness goal, you are **cross training.** For example, you might lift weights, run, and cycle on different days of the week. Two key advantages of cross training are that you avoid the boredom of participating in the same exercise every day and you reduce the risk of overuse injuries. You can also cross train by using different types of resistance training equipment— free weights and machines—on different days.

Breathing and Safety   Oxygen flow is vital for preventing muscle fatigue and injury during resistance training. Inhale when your muscles are relaxed and exhale when you initiate the lifting or push-off action. Never hold your breath while performing resistance exercises. For more on safe lifting, see the box "Safety Tips for Weight Training."

Gender Differences in Muscle Development   The amount of muscle that can be developed in the body differs by gender. Muscle mass growth is influenced by the male sex hormone testosterone, and although women do produce this hormone, they do so at levels that are only about 10 percent of the levels seen in men. Women can increase muscle mass through strength-training programs, but the increase will be less than that achieved by men.[23] There is also a wide range of individual variability in both men and women. Regardless of gender, some people can make significantly more improvements than others can.[24]

Training for Muscular Power

In addition to strength training, there are many other ways of developing the physical capabilities of the body. You can train for muscular power by performing any exercise faster. The amount of work that can be performed in a given period of time is known as **muscular power.** Power is determined by the amount and quality of muscle; it requires great strength and the ability to produce that strength quickly.

One type of exercise program developed specifically for muscular power is *plyometrics,* a program that trains muscles to store energy and then immediately release that energy in the opposite direction.[25] It uses jumping, hopping, and bounding movements for lower body power development and swinging, quick-action push-offs for upper body power development.

If you are interesting in seeing how plyometrics works, try jumping in place and then consciously forcing

KEY TERMS

muscular strength   Capacity of a muscle to exert force against resistance.

muscular endurance   Capacity of a muscle to exert force repeatedly over a period of time.

isometric   Type of muscle contraction that occurs when force is exerted against an immovable object or without producing movement.

isotonic   Type of muscle contraction that occurs when force is exerted against a movable object or with movement.

isokinetic   Type of muscle contraction that occurs when force is exerted at a constant rate and through the same range of motion by special isokinetic exercise equipment.

cross training   Participation in one sport to improve performance in another, or use of several different types of training for a specific fitness goal.

muscular power   Amount of work performed by muscles in a given period of time.

Challenges & Choices

Safety Tips for Weight Training

Follow these guidelines when you work out with weights:

- Warm up by gently stretching, jogging, or lifting light weights.
- Do not hold your breath or hyperventilate. As you are lifting, breathe rhythmically.
- To protect your back, hold weights close to your body. Do not arch your back. Weight belts may prevent arching.
- When using resistance training machines, always check to make sure the pins holding weights are in place. When using free weights, make sure collars are tight.

- Lift weights with a slow, steady cadence through a full range of motion. Do not jerk the weights to complete a repetition.
- Always use a spotter when working out with free weights.

It's Not Just Personal...

Men typically experience significant strength loss beginning in their early 50s, but women may begin to experience strength loss as early as their 20s. Preserving strength and preventing strength loss are important factors in maintaining a high quality of life with age.

---

yourself to jump in the opposite direction as you land. This action forces your quadriceps, the large muscle in front of your thighs, to stretch like a rubber band and then recoil as you land. When you quickly jump again, some of the upward force is due to a recoil action, which has two effects: (1) You can jump higher because you are combining the elastic recoil with the force production of your quadriceps muscles; and (2) over time your quadriceps muscles will learn to produce force quicker on the rebound. Both of these actions increase your power to perform that movement.[25]

Core-Strength Training

Another type of training is **core-strength training,** also called functional strength training, which conditions the body torso from the neck to the lower back. The objectives of core-strength training are to lengthen the spine, develop balance, reduce the waistline, prevent back injury, and sculpt the body without bulking it up. Scientific evidence in support of these claims is sparse. Exercise experts, however, argue that training programs increase muscle mass, and metabolic expenditure provides health benefits.[26]

Probably the most popular core-body training program being taught in health clubs today is Pilates ("pi-**lah**-teez"), an exercise system developed in the 1920s by physical trainer Joseph Pilates. The exercises, performed on special apparatus, are based on the premise that the body's "powerhouse" is in the torso, particularly the abdomen. Exercises are taught by trained instructors and are tailored to the individual. A runner, for example, may have very strong quadricep muscles but need more

hamstring flexibility. A dancer may have great muscle flexibility but need joint strengthening.

Many other core-body training programs are currently popular. They use a variety of equipment and focus on aspects of physical development such as proper spine alignment, spinal flexibility, the development of long, lean muscles, and improved balance and agility. The fundamental premise is the development of a "tall spine," pulling the naval into the back of the spine. Remember that there will always be fads and gimmicks on the market; be sure to use your critical thinking skills when investigating any commercial product, whether an exercise system, a particular type of equipment, or a health club.

Gaining Weight and Muscle Mass Safely

There are basically three reasons why people want to gain weight: improve appearance, improve health, or improve performance. Gaining weight simply by eating more is not a productive strategy, because the weight gain will be nearly all fat, and extra fat does not improve appearance, health, or performance. The goal is to increase muscle tissue with little or no increase in body fat stores. The healthy way to attain such a gain in muscle tissue is through physical activity, particularly strength training, combined with a high-calorie diet. Some people, especially athletes, attempt to gain muscle tissue by using drugs, dietary supplements, or protein supplements. Most of these substances are expensive and ineffective; some are dangerous, and some are illegal.

Drugs and Dietary Supplements   People who use performance-enhancing drugs and dietary supplements

Table 8.1	Selected Performance-Enhancing Drugs and Dietary Supplements and Their Effects	

Substance or Dietary Supplement	Effects	Side Effects
Anabolic steroid, testosterone	Promotes muscle growth by improving ability of muscle to respond to training and improving recovery.	Masculinization of females; feminization of males; acne; mood swings; sexual dysfunction.
Human growth hormone	Promotes muscle growth.	Widened jaw line and nose, protruding eyebrows, buck teeth; increased risk of high blood pressure, congestive heart failure.
Ephedrine	Boosts energy, promotes weight loss (stimulates metabolism).	High blood pressure; irregular heartbeat; increased risk of stroke and heart attack.
Androstenedione (Andro)	Promotes muscle growth.	Decreased good cholesterol (HDL); increased levels of estrogen, promotes breast enlargement in men; increased risk of pancreatic cancer; may significantly increase testosterone levels in women (little known about Andro effects in women).
Dehydroepion-Drosterone (DHEA)	May promote muscle growth.	Body hair growth; liver enlargement; aggressive behavior; long-term health effects not known.
Creatine monohydrate	May increase performance in brief high-intensity exercises; promotes increased body mass when used with resistance training.	Diarrhea; dehydration and muscle cramping; muscle tearing; long-term health effects not known.
Chromium picolinate	May build muscle tissue, facilitate burning of fat, and boost energy.	Large doses increase chromium buildup and may cause liver damage and other health problems; long-term health effects not known.

Sources: "The Physiological and Health Effects of Oral Creatine Supplementation," American College of Sports Medicine, 2000, *Medicine and Science in Sports and Exercise, 32,* 706–717; "Dietary Supplements and the Promotion of Muscle With Resistance Exercise," by R. B. Kreider, 1999, *Sports Medicine, 27,* 97–110; "How Effective Is Creatine?" by C. Nelson, 1998, *Sport Medicine Digest, 73,* 73–81; *The Ergogenic Edge: Pushing the Limits of Sports Performance,* by M. H. Williams, 1998, Champaign, IL: Human Kinetics.

may enhance their athletic performance by building bigger muscles, but they also may be heading for health problems that can shorten their lives. Unfortunately, any discussion of the risks and benefits of these substances is clouded by a lack of scientific data. Scientists often don't know who is using them, what the effects of different doses are, how long they can be taken before causing side effects, or what happens when they are taken with other drugs.[27] An overview of some of the major performance-enhancing drugs and dietary supplements, along with their possible benefits and side effects, is shown in Table 8.1.

Protein Supplements   The sports and fitness industry is experiencing a boom in powdered protein products, canned liquid products high in protein and calories, and special foods high in protein content.[28] The protein in these commercial supplements is from natural protein sources, such as soy protein, eggs, milk, or chicken. Other substances, such as purified amino acids, are often added to these mixtures. Commercial protein supplements are expensive and do not carry all the nutrients of natural

fuels. They can serve as a convenient adjunct to a balanced diet for people who are too busy to obtain enough protein in their diet, but most Americans, including athletes, get more than enough protein their diets. Further, weight gain supplements are useless without activity and offer no special benefits.[28]

Training Programs for Weight Gain   The best way to gain muscle tissue, as noted earlier, is through a weight training program combined with a high-calorie diet. Gaining a pound of muscle and fat requires consuming about 3,000 extra calories.[29] To build muscle, you need to

KEY TERMS

core-strength training   Strength training that conditions the body torso from the neck to the lower back.

consume 700–1,000 calories a day above energy needs or take in sufficient calories to support both the added activity energy requirements and the formation of new muscle.[28] A gain of a half pound to a pound a week is a reasonable goal.

Your primary exercise activity to gain muscle should be weight training. The bulk-up method was designed specifically to increase muscle mass.[28] Six to 10 different exercises are used to stress major muscle groups of the body, including the chest, back, shoulders, arms, stomach, and calf. Three to five sets of each exercise are done. As noted earlier, you should start with a resistance you can manage for 8 repetitions and gradually progress to 12 repetitions. After you can do 12 repetitions, increase the resistance and return to 8 repetitions.[28]

Flexibility

Another component of musculoskeletal fitness is **flexibility,** the ability of joints to move through their full range of motion. Flexibility is needed in everyday tasks—from getting out of bed in the morning to bending over to pick up a child—and in recreational activities—from table tennis to kayaking. Good flexibility helps you maintain posture and balance, makes movement easier and more fluid, and lowers your risk of injury. It is a key factor in preventing low back pain and injury.

Flexibility is affected by factors that you cannot change, such as genetic heritage, gender, and age, and by factors that you can change, such as physical activity patterns. A common misconception is that women are naturally more flexible than men, but this assumption is not supported by the research literature.[15] Another common misconception is that flexibility declines steadily once a person reaches adulthood. Flexibility does seem to be highest in the teenage years, and aging is accompanied by

a shortening of tendons and an increased rigidity in muscles and joints. However, there is also strong evidence that much of the flexibility lost as a result of aging can be reduced by stretching programs.[21]

Types of Stretching Programs

Medical and fitness experts agree that stretching the muscles attached to the joints is the single most important part of an exercise program designed to promote flexibility, reduce muscle tension, and prevent injuries. Stretching serves not just as a preface (warm-up) and epilogue (cool-down) to exercise programs; it is a vital workout component in itself. However, stretching done incorrectly can cause more harm than good. Thus, understanding the right stretching techniques and progressing gradually are keys to a successful program. Four different kinds of stretching are used: (1) passive stretching, (2) static stretching, (3) ballistic stretching, and (4) proprioceptive neuromuscular facilitation.

Passive Stretching   In **passive stretching,** a partner applies pressure to your muscles, typically producing a stretch beyond what you can do on your own. If you can totally relax your muscle fibers, the use of pressure by another person can help prevent the problem of partial contraction of muscle fibers. In active stretching, by contrast, you stretch a muscle by contracting the opposite muscle; for example, you stretch the triceps muscle in the back of your upper arm by contracting the biceps muscle in the front of your upper arm.

Passive stretching provides a more intense stretch than active stretching, and it is often used by physical therapists. There is a danger, however, of forcing a stretch beyond the point of normal relaxation of the muscles and

Although some flexibility is lost through aging, performing stretching exercises regularly can help to counterbalance this change.

tendons, causing tearing and injury. For this reason, passive stretching should be limited to supervised medical situations and persons who cannot move by themselves.[30]

Static Stretching   In **static stretching,** you stretch until you feel tightness in the muscle and then hold that position for a set period of time without bouncing or forcing movement. After you have held the stretch for 30 seconds to 60 seconds, the muscle tension will seem to decrease, and you can stretch farther without pain. Static stretching lengthens the muscle and surrounding tissue, reducing the risk of injury. Because it is done slowly, it affords greater control and better positioning of the muscle. Static stretching is the kind of stretching done in hatha yoga and is the type recommended for general fitness purposes.

Ballistic Stretching   In **ballistic stretching,** the muscle is stretched in a series of bouncing movements designed to increase the range of motion. As you bounce, receptors in the muscles, called *muscle spindles,* are stretched. The muscle spindles sense the rapid stretching and initiate a reflex response to contract the muscles to prevent overstretching. Ballistic stretching is used by experienced athletes, but because it can increase vulnerability to muscle pulls and tears, it is not recommended for most people.

Proprioceptive Neuromuscular Facilitation   In **proprioceptive neuromuscular facilitation (PNF)** stretching, your body's reflex responses are used to enhance muscle relaxation and increase joint range of motion.[31] It is usually done with a partner. The technique involves contracting, relaxing, and stretching the muscles of opposite muscle groups, alternating muscle contractions and static stretching in the same muscle. To experience one PNF stretching technique, sit with your right leg extended in front of you. Wrap a rolled-up towel around your right foot and hold both ends of the towel with your hands. Exert force against the towel with the ball of your foot to contract your calf muscles for about 5 seconds. Relax your calf muscle for a few seconds. Now wrap the towel around the toes of your right foot and gently pull them toward you, holding the stretch in your calf muscle for about 30 seconds. The combination of contracting, relaxing, and stretching the muscle allows you to stretch farther.

Developing Your Own Flexibility Program

Stretching can be part of your warm-up for your cardiorespiratory or resistance training program as long as these stretches are gentle, slow, and steady. You will experience the greatest improvement in flexibility, however, if you do your stretching exercises after your other exercise, when your muscles are warm and less likely to be injured by stretching. For guidelines on developing your own flexibility training program, see the box "Tips for Stretching."

Body Composition

The final component of health-related fitness we consider here is **body composition**—the relative amounts of fat and fat-free mass in the body. Fat-free mass includes muscle, bone, water, body organs, and other body tissues. Body fat includes both fat that is essential for normal functioning, such as fat in the nerves, heart, and liver, and fat stored in fat cells, usually located under the skin and around organs. The recommended proportion of body fat to fat-free mass, expressed as *percent body fat,* is 21–35 percent for women and 8–24 percent for men.

The relative amount of body fat has an effect on overall health and fitness. Too much body fat is associated with overweight and obesity and with a higher risk for chronic diseases like heart disease, diabetes, and many types of cancer. Too much body fat impairs movement and activity and places individuals at significantly greater risk for premature death. A greater amount of fat-free mass, on the other hand, gives the body a lean, healthy appearance. The heart and lungs function more efficiently without the burden of extra weight. Because muscle tissue uses energy at a higher metabolic rate than does fat tissue, the more muscle mass you have, the more calories you can consume without gaining weight.

We discuss body composition in detail in Chapter 9 on body weight. Here, the basic message is that you can control body weight, trim body fat, and build muscle tissue by incorporating more physical activity into your daily life. Use the stairs rather than taking the elevator, walk or ride your bike rather than driving, and if you drive, park your car at the far end of the parking lot. Beyond such simple steps to increase physical activity, plan to incorporate regular exercise into your life as well. You will see improvements not only in your body composition but also in many other areas of your life.

KEY TERMS

flexibility   Ability of joints to move through their full range of motion.

passive stretching   Stretching with the assistance of a partner, providing a stretch beyond what an individual can do himself or herself.

static stretching   Stretching in which the individual stretches and holds it without bouncing or forcing movement.

ballistic stretching   Stretching that includes dynamic action (bouncing).

proprioceptive neuromuscular facilitation (PNF)   Stretching that uses the body's reflex responses to enhance muscle relaxation and joint range of motion.

body composition   Relative amounts of fat and fat-free mass in the body.

Challenges & Choices

Tips for Stretching

Flexibility improves according to the principle of specificity—that is, to improve flexibility in specific joints and their associated muscle groups, you have to stretch those specific muscle groups. The following are some guidelines for stretching:

- To improve flexibility, you have to stretch beyond your normal range of motion. Stretch until you feel a mild to moderate tension, and then hold that position. Gradually increase the time you hold the stretch from 10 seconds to 60 seconds over several months. Repeat the stretch three times.

- There are hundreds of exercises that improve flexibility. Select exercises that work the muscles associated with the major joint areas in the body: the neck; the shoulders, upper back, and chest; the triceps and biceps; the torso; the hip; the quadriceps; the hamstring; the inner thigh; the outer thigh; the lower back; the buttocks; the calf; and the ankle.

- While you are building fitness, do stretching exercises at least 5 days a week. When you have reached your desired level of fitness, you can maintain flexibility by stretching 2 or 3 days a week.

- Exercises that cause an increased curvature in the lower back area, such as the plow posture in hatha yoga, should be avoided. These exercises hyperextend your back and can cause serious injury. Avoid stretches that put excessive strain on the knees, spine, or neck.

It's Not Just Personal . . .

Four out of five adults experience significant lower back pain sometime during their life; lower back pain is the most frequent cause of lost work days in adults under the age of 45. A program of stretching and strengthening exercises can improve lower back health and reduce the risk of lower back pain and injury.

IMPROVING YOUR HEALTH THROUGH MODERATE PHYSICAL ACTIVITY

As noted earlier, exercise does not have to be vigorous to provide health benefits. There are many simple, easy, and enjoyable ways to use physical activity to obtain health benefits. The surgeon general's report suggests that adults engage in 30 minutes of moderate physical activity on most, preferably all, days of the week, expending about 150 calories a day (about 1,000 calories a week) in physical activity *beyond* the calories used in customary, everyday tasks of living. They can be expended in several different activities over the course of the day, such as walking to the grocery store, gardening, cleaning the house, climbing stairs, and so on. Becoming more physically active has many health benefits, including better control of body weight, improved body composition, more stamina, and higher self-esteem. We consider here three ways to increase your physical activity—daily activities, walking, and the 10,000 Step Program.

Making Daily Activities More Active

How do you spend most of your time? You may be surprised at how much time you spend being inactive. To find out exactly, use a personal time sheet to record all of your activities on a typical day. The more specific you can be, the better. At the end of the day, add up the minutes you spent being active (doing laundry, walking to class, for example) and how many minutes you spent being inactive (watching television, playing a computer game, driving, riding public transportation, for example). After determining your time spent in activity versus inactivity, look at the sedentary activities in your day. How can you make them more active? Try getting up to change the TV channel instead of using the remote, or walk around, stretch, or do sit-ups during commercials. Ride your bike to class instead of taking the bus, take the stairs instead of the elevator at the library, or walk around while checking your cell phone messages.

You can also turn light activity into moderate activity by cranking up the intensity. For example, if you are cleaning your apartment or home, play some fast dance music and try to keep up with it. When you are standing in line, stretch or do isometric exercises (for example, contract and relax your abdominal muscles). Increase your pace while cycling, walk briskly instead of strolling, take the stairs two at a time. Why is it important to move from light to moderate activities? Consider that an order of french fries contains about 400 calories. If you are sitting and watching television, it will take you 308 minutes, or more than 5 hours, to use up that many calories. If you are walking briskly or jogging slowly, it will take you about

Moderate physical activity is key to physical fitness. A hobby such as gardening may not be strenuous, but it involves stretching, tones muscles, and burns calories.

an hour. If you are doing line dancing, it will take you about 42 minutes. If you are running at a 9-minute-mile pace, it will take you about 17 minutes.[3]

Walking for Fitness

Walking is the most popular physical activity in North America,[32] and it has many health benefits. Results from the Harvard Nurses Health Study indicate that women who walk 1 hour a week have half the risk of cardiovascular disease experienced by those who are sedentary. Women who do moderate or vigorous physical activity at least 4 hours a week reduce their risk of premature death by 25 percent to 35 percent.[33] Thus, as with other activity, increasing the pace and/or duration of walking results in greater health benefits. (For some guidelines, see the box "Tips on Walking for Fitness.")

The quest to expend more calories in less time has led many people to use exercise tools like hand weights and elastic resistance cords to increase the intensity of their physical activity while walking. Many of these tools can also increase upper body strength.

The 10,000 Steps Program

Experts at the Shape Up America! program (founded in 1994 by former U.S. Surgeon General C. Everett Koop) set out to determine whether the recommended expenditure of 150 calories per day in moderate physical activity was high enough to help people manage their weight and avoid weight gain after weight loss. They found that this recommendation was not high enough for weight management but that people *could* control their weight if they walked 10,000 steps each day.[34] There are roughly 2,000 walking steps in a mile, so 10,000 steps is equivalent to about 5 miles.

Walking 10,000 steps expends between 300 and 400 calories, depending on body size and walking speed—well above the recommended 150 calories a day. Walking 10,000 steps a day 5 days a week expends the optimal 2,000 calories per week recommended for preventing premature death. Thus, although more research is needed, the 10,000 Steps Program appears to set a reasonable goal for healthy children and adults. Two concerns are that (1) this goal may be too high for people with disabilities and chronic health problems and (2) the goal may be perceived as a threshold value, leading people to think that steps below that threshold have no health benefit, which is not the case.[35] Still, the 10,000 Steps Program is proving to be a powerful motivator, helping people move from sedentary and light activity levels to moderate activity levels.[34]

Steps are counted with a step counter (or pedometer), a pager-sized device worn on the belt or waistband. Step counters record the number of steps you take based on your body's movement, so they should be centered over the right or left hipbone. Step counters that convert activities into calories expended are not accurate, because they do not factor in activity intensity.

If you are interested in trying the 10,000 Steps Program and using a step counter, first determine how many steps you typically take each day. Record the number of steps you take every day for 7 days. Most inactive people take between 2,000 and 4,000 steps a day. Then, to set a reasonable goal, plan to increase this number by about 500 steps at a time. If you typically take 5,000 steps a day, set a goal of 5,550 steps. Once you achieve 5,550 steps, raise your goal by 500 steps, and continue until you reach 10,000 steps.[35]

Although the 10,000 Steps Program is designed to facilitate weight management, you can benefit from it even

Challenges & Choices

Tips on Walking for Fitness

A sedentary lifestyle can kill you, and a moderate activity such as walking can be life saving. Walking can lower your risk for heart disease, help you lose weight, prevent diabetes, and provide many other health benefits.

If you have been completely sedentary, begin a walking program with as little as 10 minutes a day. Gradually work up to 30 minutes a day, most days of the week, as recommended by the surgeon general. If you want to lose weight by walking, you will need to walk from 45 to 60 minutes a day, most days of the week. To improve your cardiovascular functioning, walk briskly (at a pace of 4–4.5 mph). The following are some guidelines for getting the most out of walking:

- Schedule your daily walk as you would an appointment. Plan it for a time of day when you're most likely to make it a permanent habit.
- Increase your walking time gradually. Don't increase duration by more than 10 percent to 20 percent a week.
- After you have walked for a couple of weeks, focus on quicker steps. As you do so, bend your arms 90 degrees at the elbow and move them when you walk. Moving your arms increases your caloric expenditure. Pushing vigorously off your toes at the end of every step will help you increase your walking pace.

- Choose comfortable footwear. Shoes that squeeze your toes or let your heel slip are likely to cause foot problems, such as blisters and bunions. Replace your shoes after you have used them to walk 300 miles to 500 miles.
- Stretch at the end of your walk or after warming up. Adding 4 minutes of stretching to your daily walking habit can have a beneficial effect on your muscles, joints, and bones.
- Don't ignore or exercise through pain. If the pain is severe, see a physician. Pain that is not serious should be treated by rest, ice, compression, and elevation; massage may also help. Discontinue walking up or down hills if doing so causes pain.

It's Not Just Personal...

Although walking can be done by almost anyone almost anywhere, studies have shown that people walk more if there is a park, trail, school track, or other facility nearby. They also walk more if they have a destination, such as a hardware store or grocery store, within walking distance. Some experts argue that more businesses and recreational facilities need to be located in residential areas to encourage people to make walking trips from home.

---

if you don't have a weight problem. It is an easy, painless way to add physical activity to your day and to move from light to moderate activity levels.

SPECIAL CONSIDERATIONS IN EXERCISE AND PHYSICAL ACTIVITY

Physical activity is an essential component of healthy living for everyone, everywhere. However, special considerations have to be taken into account to ensure health and safety in exercise and physical activity, to accommodate the effects of certain environmental conditions, and to make exercise appropriate for particular populations.

Health and Safety Precautions

Injuries and illness associated with exercise and physical activity are usually the result either of excessive exercise or of improper techniques. In this section we look at several

considerations related to health and safety: proper warm-up and cool-down; fatigue, overtraining, and overexertion; soft tissue injury; and the female athlete triad.

Warm-Up and Cool-Down

Proper warm-up before exercise helps to maximize the benefits of a workout and minimize the potential for injuries. Muscles contract more efficiently and more safely when they have been properly warmed up. Warming up decreases muscle viscosity, susceptibility to injury, and the likelihood of heart rate abnormalities (irregular heartbeat) that may be provoked by sudden strenuous exertion. Warming up also elevates the pulse rate, raises body temperature, and allows muscle fibers to be slowly stretched in preparation for the vigorous phase of the workout, all of which help prevent injury. Stretching exercises increase the amount of oxygen-laden blood reaching the performance muscle sites.

Suggested warm-up activities include light calisthenics, walking or slow jogging, and gentle stretching of the specific muscles to be used in the activity. You can also do

Healthy People 2010

OBJECTIVE AREA *Physical Activity in Adults*

- Reduce the proportion of adults who engage in no leisure-time physical activity.
- Increase the proportion of adults who engage regularly, preferably daily, in moderate physical activity for at least 30 minutes per day.

"Because the highest risk of death and disability is found among those who do no regular physical activity, engaging in any amount of physical activity is preferable to none. Physical activity should be encouraged as part of a daily routine. . . . Increases in daily activity to ensure a weekly expenditure of 1,000 calories would have significant individual and public health benefit for [coronary heart disease] prevention and deaths from all causes, especially for persons who are sedentary."

 For more information on Healthy People 2010 objectives, visit the Web site at www.healthypeople.gov.

For more information on Canadian health objectives, visit the Health Canada Web site at www.hc-sc.gc.ca/english.

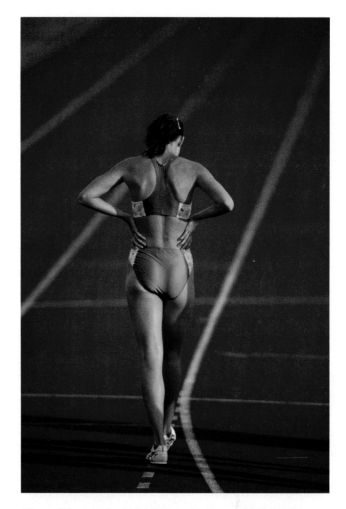

After a vigorous workout, blood may pool in the extremities, briefly depriving the heart and brain of oxygen, which can cause a feeling of faintness. To avoid this, continue the activity at a much lower intensity rather than stopping abruptly.

a low-intensity version of the activity you are about to engage in, such as hitting tennis balls against a wall before a match. Your warm-up should last from 5 to 10 minutes.

A minimum of 5 minutes to 10 minutes should also be devoted to cool-down, depending on environmental conditions and the intensity of the exercise program. Pooling of blood in the extremities may temporarily disrupt or reduce the return of blood to the heart, momentarily depriving your heart and brain of oxygen. Fainting or even a coronary abnormality may result. If you continue the activity at a lower intensity, the blood vessels gradually return to their normal smaller diameter, and muscle massage assists proper return of blood flow.

Walking, mimicking the exercise at a slower pace, and stretching while walking are all excellent cool-down activities. Never sit down, stand in a stationary position, or take a hot shower or sauna immediately after vigorous exercise.

Fatigue, Overtraining, and Overexertion

Fatigue is a complex phenomenon but is generally defined as an inability to continue exercising at a desired level of intensity. The cause of fatigue may be psychological—for example, depression can cause feelings of fatigue—or physiological, as when you work out too long or too hard,

do an activity you're not used to, or become overheated or dehydrated. Sometimes fatigue occurs because the body cannot produce enough energy to meet the demands of the activity. In this case, consuming enough complex carbohydrates to replenish the muscle stores of glycogen may solve the problem (see Chapter 7). Athletes need to eat a high-carbohydrate diet to make sure they have enough reserve energy for their sport.

Chronic fatigue—a continual state of exhaustion—is typically caused by overtraining.[36] Overtraining affects both the body and mind. Physically, overtraining makes a person excessively tired and more susceptible to illnesses like colds. Mentally, overtraining can cause irritability, chronic anger, and even depression. Ignoring symptoms of overtraining can be costly, because recovery may take several months. Elite athletes typically avoid overtraining by employing strategies that maximize physical conditioning without weakening the body. For example, they may adjust the intensity, frequency, and duration of physical activity by alternating short, intense exercise bouts with less intense activities of longer duration. For recreational pursuits, taking days off between exercise sessions and alternating types of activity can reduce the risk of overtraining.

Overexertion occurs when an exercise session has been too intense. Warning signs of overexertion include (1) pain or pressure in the left or midchest area, jaw, neck, left shoulder, or left arm during or just after exercise; (2) sudden nausea, dizziness, cold sweat, fainting, or pallor (pale, ashen skin); and (3) abnormal heartbeats, such as fluttering, rapid heartbeats or a rapid pulse rate immediately followed by a very slow pulse rate. If you experience any of these symptoms, consult a physician before exercising again.

Soft Tissue Injury

Injuries to soft tissue (muscles and joints) include tears, sprains, strains, and contusions; they usually result from a specific activity incident, such as a fall on the basketball court or a cycling crash. Some injuries, known as overuse injuries, are caused by the cumulative effects of motions repeated many times. Tendinitis and bursitis are examples of overuse injuries.

Soft tissue injuries should be treated according to the R-I-C-E principle: rest, ice, compression, and elevation. Immediately stop doing the activity, apply ice to the affected area to reduce swelling and pain, compress it with an elastic bandage to reduce swelling, and elevate it to reduce blood flow to the area. Do not apply heat until all swelling has disappeared. When you no longer feel pain in the area, you can gradually begin to exercise again. Don't return to your full exercise program until your injury is completely healed.

The Female Athlete Triad

Some athletes are susceptible to a condition called the **female athlete triad,** a set of three interrelated disorders: disordered eating patterns, often accompanied by excessive exercising; **amenorrhea** (cessation of menstruation); and premature **osteoporosis** (reduced bone density).[37] The syndrome usually begins when young athletes engage in unhealthy eating behaviors, such as fasting or extreme dieting, to lose weight or attain a lean body appearance. (Body weight and body image are discussed in detail in Chapters 9 and 10.) These behaviors often develop into full-blown eating disorders, such as anorexia nervosa and bulimia nervosa, which require medical treatment and can cause severe illness and even death. Low body weight and low body fat, in combination with excessive exercise and psychological stress, can reduce levels of estrogen and other hormones to a level so low that the menstrual cycle is interrupted. Lack of menstrual periods, even for a few months, can lead to bone loss and premature osteoporosis. Often the first sign of decreased bone density is an exercise-related stress fracture.[38]

Why are some women susceptible to the female athlete triad? Possible risk factors include young age; pressure to excel at a selected sport; focus on attaining or maintaining an "ideal" body weight or body fat percentage; participation in endurance sports; competition judged on aesthetic appeal (such as ballet or figure skating); sports requiring clothing that reveals body contouring (such as cheerleading); sports emphasizing a prepubertal body type (such as gymnastics); dieting at a very young age (through calorie restriction, diet pills, or laxatives); and unsupervised diets.[39]

Although the triad includes some conditions unique to women, men are becoming more vulnerable to eating disorders associated with weight-regulated sports, such as wrestling and endurance sports. Anorexia nervosa coupled with excessive exercise has been correlated with small testes and osteoporosis in men. Both male and female athletes need to understand the importance of good eating habits and moderation in exercise, as well as the dangers of eating disorders, which can cause long-term, life-threatening illness.[38]

Effects of Environmental Conditions on Exercise and Physical Activity

Certain environmental conditions require adjustment of physical activity and exercise workload. Environmental conditions of particular concern are altitude, heat and cold, and air pollution.

Altitude

Traveling too quickly to elevations above 6,000–8,000 feet causes altitude sickness, or acute mountain sickness (AMS), in about 7 percent of men and 22 percent of women.[40] Symptoms of AMS include cough, headache, difficulty breathing, rapid heartbeat, general malaise, weakness and nausea, loss of appetite, and difficulty sleeping. These symptoms occur as the body adjusts to the lower oxygen content of the air, which probably results in accumulation of carbon dioxide in body tissues and leakage of fluids into the brain. It is not clear why men and women are affected differently.

AMS can affect performance levels and health,[41] but after about 10 days to 14 days, the body begins to acclimate and make adjustments that are permanent. The muscles become more efficient at extracting oxygen from the air, which reduces the workload on the heart. After 4 weeks to 8 weeks, the body produces more red blood cells to compensate for the thinner air.

If you are going to be in a situation that puts you at risk for AMS, the best prevention strategy, besides acclimation, is adjustment of physical activity workload and nutrition.[42] Your initial activity should be less intense and shorter in duration than your activity at lower altitudes. To prevent dehydration, increase your fluid intake from

Table 8.2   Heat-Related Disorders

Heat Disorder	Cause	Symptoms	Treatment
Heat cramps	Excessive loss of electrolytes in sweat; inadequate salt intake.	Muscle cramps.	Rest in cool environment; drink fluids; ingest salty food and drinks; get medical treatment if severe.
Heat exhaustion	Excessive loss of electrolytes in sweat; inadequate salt and/or fluid intake.	Fatigue; nausea; dizziness; cool, pale skin; sweating; elevated temperature.	Rest in cool environment; drink cool fluids; cool body with water; get medical treatment if severe.
Heat stroke	Excessive body temperature.	Headache; vomiting; hot, flushed skin (dry or sweaty); elevated temperature; disorientation; unconsciousness.	Cool body with ice or cold water; give cool drinks with sugar if conscious; get medical help immediately.

Source: Adapted from *Nutrition for Health, Fitness and Sport*, 7th ed., (p. 341), by M. H. Williams, 2005, New York: McGraw-Hill.

water, instant fruit drinks, reconstituted powdered milk, hot chocolate, and soup. To prevent glycogen depletion, eat small, frequent meals, and consume at least 60 percent of your calories from carbohydrates, since they are better tolerated than fat is at higher altitudes.[40]

Heat and Cold

Exercising in excessive heat and exercising in excessive cold both put a strain on the body. Heat disorders can be caused by impaired regulation of internal core temperature, loss of body fluids, and loss of electrolytes (Table 8.2).[28] In response to heat stress, the blood vessels expand, and sweating increases in an effort to cool the body. Problems develop when these two responses falter. The circulatory system attempts to regulate both body temperature and blood pressure at the same time. When heat stress is excessive, blood pressure is considered more important than is regulation of body temperature, which becomes impaired.[28]

Two strategies for preventing excessive increases in body temperature are skin wetting and hyperhydration. Skin wetting involves such practices as sponging or spraying the head or body with cold water. This strategy cools the skin but has not been shown to effectively decrease core body temperature.[28] Hyperhydration is the practice of taking in extra fluids shortly before participating in physical activity in a hot environment.[43] This practice is recommended by the ACSM and may improve cardiovascular function and temperature regulation during physical activity in conditions of excessive heat.[44]

If you are going to be exercising in very hot conditions, you can hyperhydrate by drinking a pint of water (16 ounces) when you get up in the morning, another pint 1 hour before your activity, and a final pint 15 minutes to 30 minutes before exercising. Plan to consume from 4 to 8

ounces of fluid every 15 minutes during your exercise. After exercise, consume 24 ounces of water for every pint you lose.[28]

Exercising in the cold also poses challenges. Symptoms of **hypothermia** (dangerously low body temperature) include shivering, feelings of euphoria, and disorientation. Core body temperature influences how severe these symptoms are and whether the hypothermia is considered mild, moderate, or severe. In mild hypothermia, core body temperature drops to between 97 and 95 degrees Fahrenheit; in moderate hypothermia, it is between 95 and 90 degrees; and in severe hypothermia, it is below 90 degrees. Caution is called for when exercising in cold and windy conditions.[28] Dress in several thin layers of clothes and wear a hat and mittens. If cold air bothers your throat, breathe through a scarf. Exercise at midday whenever possible, and plan out-and-back workouts heading into the wind on the way out. Finally, tell someone your route and when you expect to be back.

KEY TERMS

female athlete triad Condition involving three related disorders: eating disorders, amenorrhea, and premature osteoporosis.

amenorrhea Abnormal absence of menstrual periods.

osteoporosis Disease characterized by bone loss and reduced bone density.

hypothermia Low body temperature, a life-threatening condition.

Air Pollution

If you live and exercise in a large city, air pollution can be a concern. Pollution can have an irritating effect on the airways leading to your lungs,[45] causing such problems as coughing, wheezing, and shortness of breath. To minimize the effect of air pollution, exercise early in the morning before motor vehicle pollution has its greatest impact. If possible, exercise in areas with less motor vehicle traffic, such as parks. Pay attention to smog alerts, and move your exercise indoors when air pollution is severe.

Exercise for Special Populations

In this section we look briefly at special exercise considerations for children and adolescents, people with disabilities, and older adults.

Exercise for Children and Adolescents

A national survey by the Centers for Disease Control and Prevention (CDC) reported that 63 percent of American adolescents have two or more of the five key risk factors related to chronic disease. One of those five risk factors is a sedentary lifestyle.[37] To obtain the direct and indirect health benefits of fitness, the surgeon general recommends that children get 60 minutes of exercise a day.

Although children need exercise, they are not miniature adults, so they should not be expected to perform at the same level as adults. They have important anatomical differences, such as smaller hearts, lungs, and blood volumes.[37] The cardiovascular system does not fully mature until late in the teen years. This means that children's hearts deliver less oxygen to working muscles. Additionally, the musculoskeletal and reproductive systems are rapidly maturing and are vulnerable to lifelong damage.[46]

A serious concern is the incidence of sudden death in adolescents engaged in strenuous physical activities and competitive sports programs. About 12 young athletes die each year from fatal heart disease while participating in vigorous sports.[36] Most of these deaths are thought to be caused by congenital heart defects, such as an abnormally enlarged heart, that go undetected until an incident occurs. (See Chapter 2 for more on congenital heart disease in young athletes.) Health insurance companies usually will not cover sophisticated screening for heart defects for children, since the tests have not proven to be cost effective.[37]

New guidelines issued by the American Heart Association (AHA) urge parents, coaches, and physicians to be vigilant for symptoms that may indicate a heart defect.[46] These symptoms include fainting episodes, sudden chest pain during exercise or at rest, high blood pressure, and irregular or high heart rate at rest or during exercise. The AHA also recommends that a family history of heart disease or unexplained death be considered in evaluating whether children should be involved in vigorous physical

activity.[37] For more information on vigorous physical activity guidelines for children and adolescents, see the Web Resources at the end of this chapter.

Exercise for Persons With Disabilities

Physical activity and exercise are especially beneficial for persons with disabilities and chronic health problems. Immobility or inactivity may aggravate the original disability and increase the risk for secondary health problems, such as heart disease, osteoporosis, arthritis, and metabolic disorders like diabetes. The American College of Sports Medicine (ACSM) stresses the importance of physical activity for people with disabilities for two reasons: (1) to counteract the detrimental effects of bed rest and sedentary living patterns and (2) to maintain optimal functioning of body organs or systems.[14]

Not too long ago, regular physical activity was missing in the lives of many people with disabilities.[37] The reasons for this absence included lack of knowledge about the importance of physical activity to healthy living, limited access to recreation sites and difficulty with transportation to and from these sites, and a low level of interest. Fortunately, this situation is changing. Laws have strengthened the rights of persons with disabilities and fostered their inclusion in programs and facilities providing physical activity opportunities. Increased visibility and positive images of people with disabilities engaging in physical activity, such as in the Special Olympics and wheelchair basketball, have also helped raise awareness. To further increase their participation in physical activity, people with disabilities need to have access to equipment, need to be prepared to learn new skills, and must draw on support networks that promote such activity.[37]

Exercise for Older Adults

Over a typical lifetime, **functional capacity,** the physical and mental ability to perform everyday tasks, gradually declines. From age 30 onward, organ systems decline in functional capacity about .5 percent to .75 percent each year. Eventually, declines in functional capacity leave older adults more susceptible to the chronic diseases that plague later life, such as arthritis, heart disease, and osteoporosis, and have a detrimental effect on the performance of everyday activities.[47] Simply climbing a flight of stairs or taking a stroll may be exhausting. Some of the declines associated with increasing age are described in the box "Functional Capacity in the Older Body."

Although age remodels everything from bones to brain cells, physical activity is an effective antidote against many of these remodeling effects. Studies show that functional capacity does not decline as sharply in people who are physically active.[47] Further, it is never too late to become more active. The ACSM has concluded that older adults generally respond to increased physical activity and receive health and fitness benefits similar to those of young

HIGHLIGHT ON HEALTH
Functional Capacity in the Older Body

Muscles   Muscle mass declines progressively after age 40. There is a fairly minimal loss of strength in the 40s and 50s, but by the 60s and 70s, people have lost from 10 to 20 percent of total body strength, and by the 80s, they have lost from 30 to 40 percent. Hand-grip strength declines 45 percent by age 75.

Bones   Men lose 3 percent of their skeletal weight per decade, and women lose 8 percent per decade. The total reduction in mineral density throughout life is about 15 percent in men and 30 percent in women.

Joints   There is some loss of flexibility as people age, which restricts mobility. Some common forms of arthritis begin in the 30s and progress each decade.

Brain   Aging doesn't cause a significant loss of mental function until the 80s. About 5 percent of people over age 65 have Alzheimer's disease, which progressively destroys brain function.

Teeth   Tooth enamel becomes more prone to cracks, gums may recede, and old fillings tend to disintegrate, inviting decay. Oral health problems are a primary cause of poor diets in late life.

Ears   As children, we can hear sounds reaching as high as 20,000 Hertz (Hz). This ability is reduced to 15,000 Hz in the 30s (the sound of a cricket), 12,000 Hz in the 50s ("silent" dog whistle), 10,000 Hz in the 60s (upper range of a songbird), and 6,000 Hz in the 70s (high notes on a pipe organ).

Eyes   Structural changes in the eye beginning after age 40 affect the ability to focus properly on close objects, impair depth perception and night vision, diminish peripheral vision, increase sensitivity to glare, and decrease the ability to distinguish between blue and green colors.

Lungs   Maximum breathing capacity begins declining at age 20 and falls almost 40 percent by age 65. The overall effect is a reduced level of oxygen in the blood that causes a form of oxygen starvation in the tissues.

Heart   By age 65, people have lost from 30 to 40 percent of the aerobic power they had at age 20.

Coronary arteries begin accumulating plaque during childhood and begin clogging arteries about age 50.

Taste and smell   In later adulthood, more molecules of certain substances are needed on the tongue to recognize the flavor (salt, sweet, sour, bitter). The ability to taste food is also closely related to the ability to smell. The ability to discriminate among odors remains fairly constant until age 65, when a noticeable decrease occurs for some people.

Touch: pressure, pain, heat, cold   The hands lose sensitivity to touch as people age, and they become less able to perceive changes in heat and cold.

Pancreas   Ability to metabolize glucose declines with age, which appears to accelerate degeneration of vital organs, especially after age 60. By age 70, nearly 20 percent of men and 30 percent of women have abnormal glucose tolerance levels that increase their risk for developing diabetes.

Reproductive system   For men, sperm count declines with age and fertility sharply drops after age 65. For women, menopause typically occurs at about age 50 but can begin as early as 35 or as late as 55. At age 30, the normal menstrual cycle is 28 to 30 days. By age 40, the cycle period has shrunk to 25 days and several years later to 23 days. After age 35, the ova are more defective genetically. If fertilization occurs, the babies are at higher risk for birth defects.

Urinary system   Bladder muscles weaken and the kidneys become less efficient. One third of people over 65 experience incontinence. An enlarged prostate makes urination difficult for many men.

Skin   Skin loses flexibility and firmness, sags, and forms wrinkles. Men do not wrinkle as quickly as women because they have more sebaceous glands and thicker skin. The skin of African American women and men absorbs sunlight better and experiences less damage from sun exposure than does the skin of white women. Sweat glands do not function as effectively in later life, making it more difficult to adjust to hot environments.

adults.[21] These benefits include improvements in cardiorespiratory endurance, lean body mass, muscular strength and endurance, flexibility, balance, postural stability, motor agility, and mental and psychological functioning. Regular supervised physical activity can also enhance the quality of life for adults who are very old and frail.[21]

KEY TERMS

functional capacity   Physical and mental ability to perform everyday tasks.

PHYSICAL ACTIVITY FOR LIFE

We all know we should be physically active, but many of us do not act on that knowledge. The most significant drop in physical activity occurs in the last few years of high school and the first year of college.[3] The decline accelerates again after college graduation. Forty percent of men and 30 percent of women continue to participate in various physical activities in young adulthood.[1] Certain key factors help people make physical activity a lifetime pursuit. In this section we consider a few of them—commitment to change, an understanding of your fitness personality, and social and community support.

Making a Commitment to Change

Every year many of us make New Year's resolutions, vowing to lose weight, eat healthier foods, or get more exercise. Yet we often fail to follow through with our resolutions, in part because behavior change is so difficult. In Chapter 1 you learned about the Transtheoretical Model, a theory about how people change their behavior (see Figure 1.4). The model includes five stages that most people go through when adopting new habits: (1) precontemplation (not even thinking about change); (2) contemplation (thinking about change in a general way but not acting on it); (3) preparation (deciding when, where, and how to adopt a new habit); (4) action (consistently practicing the new habit for up to 6 months); and (5) maintenance (maintaining the new habit for 6 months or more).[3] For some behaviors, there is a sixth stage, termination, when the behavior has become part of the person's lifestyle and there is no temptation to return to the old behavior.

Let's consider exercise in terms of the Transtheoretical Model. In the precontemplation and contemplation stages, the biggest challenges for most people are barriers to exercise.[48] Common barriers to active lifestyles cited by adults are inconvenience, lack of self-motivation, lack of time, fear of injury, the perception that exercise is boring, lack of social support, and lack of confidence in one's ability to be physically active. (To find out what your barriers are, see the Add It Up! feature at the end of this chapter.) If you are in the precontemplation or contemplation stage and feel overwhelmed by these or other barriers, see the box "Strategies for Overcoming Barriers to Physical Activity."

In the preparation stage, self-assessment is critical. Ask yourself these four questions: (1) What physical activities do I enjoy? (2) What are the best days and times for me to participate in physical activities? (3) Where is the best place to pursue these activities? and (4) Do I have friends and/or family members who can join in my physical activities? In making specific preparations, you need to take into account your current level of fitness and your previous experiences in various physical activ-

ities. This information about yourself will help you develop an exercise program that you can commit to and maintain.

In the action stage, a key component is goal setting. Your goals should be based on the benefits of physical activity, but they should also be specific and reasonable. Achievable and sustainable goals are essential for exercise compliance. Include both short-term and long-term goals in your plan, and devise ways to measure your progress. Build in rewards along the way.

When you have been physically active almost every day for at least 6 months, you are in the maintenance stage. One key to maintaining an active lifestyle is believing that your commitment to physical activity can make a difference in your life. People who establish a personal stake in physical activity are more likely to maintain an active lifestyle. Another key is having a social support network consisting of family members and/or friends who share your enthusiasm for physical activity. When exercise has become entrenched as a lifelong behavior—when it's as much a part of your day as eating and sleeping—you are in the termination stage.

Which stage are you in right now? If you are in an early stage, you probably do not have sufficient commitment to follow through on an exercise plan. To make any change, you must want to change. Work on overcoming barriers and gaining more information about the health benefits of physical activity and the problems associated with a sedentary lifestyle. Knowledge is one of the best predictors of a commitment to healthy living.[49] Being a mentor to friends and family members can also help you become or stay motivated to make exercise a lifelong habit. Remember, the more active you are, the more health benefits you will receive. (See the box "Who Is Most Likely to Become More Physically Active?")

Discovering Your Fitness Personality

Different people enjoy different types of activity and exercise. If you are doing an activity you don't really like, your interest and motivation will soon flag. Research in human dynamics suggests that how we move physically is closely correlated with our general behavior patterns. In other words, people have distinct "fitness personalities."[50] Four broad types of movement personalities have been identified: racer, stroller, dancer, and trekker.

- *Racer.* Competitive, aggressive, easily bored, loves to develop skills and strategy; will train for a marathon, tennis match, long-distance bike ride; may like martial arts classes, racquet sports, race-walking clubs.

- *Stroller.* Social, friendly, supportive, relaxed; works best if there's a buddy to exercise and chat with; needs a social network to get involved in exercises;

HIGHLIGHT ON HEALTH

Strategies for Overcoming Barriers to Physical Activity

Lack of time

- Identify available time slots. Monitor your daily activities for 1 week. Identify at least three 30-minute time slots you could use for physical activity.
- Add physical activity to your daily routine: Walk or ride your bike to work or shopping, organize school activities around physical activity, walk the dog, exercise while you watch TV, and park farther away from your destination.
- Make time for physical activity. Walk, jog, or swim during your lunch hour; take fitness breaks instead of coffee breaks.
- Select activities requiring minimal time, such as walking, jogging, or stair climbing.

Social influence

- Explain your interest in physical activity to friends and family. Ask them to support your efforts.
- Invite friends and family members to exercise with you. Plan social activities involving exercise.
- Develop new friendships with physically active people. Join a group, such as the YMCA or a hiking club.

Lack of energy

- Schedule physical activity for times in the day or week when you feel energetic.
- Convince yourself that if you give it a chance, physical activity will increase your energy level; then, try it.

Lack of willpower

- Plan ahead. Make physical activity a regular part of your daily or weekly schedule and write it on your calendar.
- Invite a friend to exercise with you on a regular basis, and write the dates on both your calendars.
- Join an exercise group or class.

Fear of injury

- Learn how to warm up and cool down to prevent injury.
- Learn how to exercise appropriately considering your age, fitness level, skill level, and health status.
- Choose activities involving minimum risk.

Lack of skill

- Select activities requiring no new skills, such as walking, climbing stairs, or jogging.

- Exercise with friends who are at the same skill level as you are.
- Find a friend who is willing to teach you some new skills.
- Take a class to develop new skills.

Lack of resources

- Select activities that require minimal facilities or equipment, such as walking, jogging, jumping rope, or calisthenics.
- Identify inexpensive, convenient resources available in your community (such as community education programs, park and recreation programs, worksite programs).

Weather conditions

- Develop a set of regular activities that are always available regardless of weather (indoor cycling, aerobic dance, indoor swimming, calisthenics, stair climbing, rope skipping, mall walking, dancing, or gymnasium games).
- Think of outdoor activities that depend on weather conditions (cross-country skiing, outdoor swimming, outdoor tennis) as "bonuses"— extra activities possible when weather and circumstances permit.

Family obligations

- Trade babysitting time with a friend, neighbor, or family member who also has small children.
- Exercise with your children. Go for a walk together, play tag or other running games, get an aerobic dance or exercise tape for kids (there are several on the market) and exercise together. You can spend time together and still get your exercise.
- Hire a babysitter and look at the cost as a worthwhile investment in your physical and mental health.
- Jump rope, do calisthenics, ride a stationary bicycle, or use other home gymnasium equipment while the kids are busy playing or sleeping.
- Try to exercise when the kids are not around (during school hours or their nap time).
- Encourage exercise facilities to provide child care services.

Source: "Physical Activity for Everyone: Making Physical Activity Part of Your Life," Centers for Disease Control and Prevention, 2005. www.cdc.gov.

Beating the Odds

Who Is Most Likely to Become More Physically Active?

Barriers to physical activity can arise from many sources—lack of knowledge, lack of motivation, lack of experience, lack of opportunities, and so on. At the same time, people find ways to overcome these barriers every day. Brief profiles of three people are presented here. Which person do you think is most likely to become more physically active?

Ryan is 20 years old and works as a forklift operator for a large transportation corporation. He dropped out of high school after 10th grade and is pursuing a high school equivalency degree. He was very active in school sports before dropping out but now spends his free time hanging out with friends, watching television, and playing video games. He is slightly overweight and often feels tired and bored. Ryan's company has an on-site fitness center that is free to employees, but Ryan has never used it.

Juan is a 30-year-old graduate student in business management. He works 20 hours a week as a graduate assistant and carries 12 semester hours of classes. Juan has diabetes and is moderately overweight. He has never been physically active, nor has his wife, who works full time as a computer programmer. They share parenting responsibilities for their two children, ages 5 and 8, who are both very active in the many recreational opportunities provided by the university and the city. Juan's physician recently told him that if he didn't start an exercise regimen to help manage his diabetes, he was going to experience serious health problems. Juan doesn't see how he can add one more thing to his busy schedule, but he also doesn't want to jeopardize his health or his ability to provide for his family.

Susan is a 25-year-old nurse. She works 40 hours a week and is pursuing a graduate degree in social work at night. Susan was on the swim team in college, but now her lifestyle is quite sedentary. She has gained 25 pounds since college, a fact that causes her great distress. Many of her friends belong to gyms and hiking groups, and they encourage her to join them. Usually she feels too tired and stressed out to exercise, but she has begun to think about establishing some weight loss and physical activity goals for herself.

OLC Web site Visit the **Online Learning Center** at www.mhhe.com/teague1e for comments by the authors.

---

may enjoy ballroom dancing, aerobics classes, or other kinds of group exercise.

- *Dancer.* Lively, enthusiastic, energetic, extroverted, loves variety in exercise; doesn't do well with goal-oriented activities; may buy exercise equipment but is unlikely to use it every day; needs to do something different daily—in-line skating one day, swimming the next, yoga the next.

- *Trekker.* Disciplined, highly organized, very efficient, reliable; enjoys working out alone; can buy a treadmill and use it every day; is very likely to be getting enough exercise to impact health.

Although you are likely to identify with characteristics of more than one movement personality, many people find that one type stands out for them. If this is the case for you, try to choose activities accordingly so you are tapping into movements that are natural and enjoyable to you. Experimenting with new movements is also a good idea. The more enjoyment and satisfaction you get from movement in your life, the more likely you are to pursue it.

Using Social and Community Support

A network of friends, coworkers, and family members who understand the benefits of exercise and join you in your activities can make the difference between a sedentary and an active lifestyle. In one survey, two out of every five respondents cited the encouragement of a spouse or significant other as the most important motivator to exercise.[3]

Family and friends are not enough, however; activity-friendly communities are also instrumental in promoting physical activity. Many communities have paths, trails, sidewalks, and safe streets that encourage people to become physically active. There are community programs that encourage parents to walk their children to school, that promote "mall walking" (walking at shopping malls), and that sponsor biking and walking days.

Consumer Clipboard

Reengineering Communities for Physical Activity

Can living in the suburbs be hazardous to your health? This may sound like an exaggeration, but think about the different activity patterns of a suburbanite and an urbanite. The suburbanite drives to work, takes a car to get to the grocery store, and drives to the nearest state park on the weekend. In contrast, the urbanite walks to a bus or subway stop to get to work, walks to the stores in the neighborhood, and rollerblades to a local park on the weekends. It's no wonder that a 2003 study of over 200,000 adults in 445 U.S. counties found that people living in areas with less sprawl tended to walk more, weigh less, and have lower blood pressure than did those living in areas with more sprawl. How communities are set up actually does make a difference—forcing people who live in the suburbs to use their car to get around while people living in the city find it easy to get to places by walking.

The New Urbanism movement, founded in the late 1980s, is dedicated to combating sprawl in the United States by changing the way communities are designed. This consortium of architects, builders, politicians, and citizens is rethinking the way cities emerge and expand. With 500 projects completed or underway, it is promoting communities built with open land and highways at the outer edges, with increasingly dense development of mixed-use neighborhoods (housing with commercial, civic, and recreational areas near the center). Instead of having suburban-style cul-de-sac streets, these neighborhoods have streets set in a grid-shape to allow for walking routes and easy access to stores, schools, and offices. With so many places of interest nearby, it's easy to turn off the TV, leave the car in the garage, and get active.

That's a good plan for new communities, but what about existing ones? Older communities are growing

in both density and area—with buildings going up and borders pushing out. One "solution" has been to build sprawling, maze-like subdivisions along the perimeter of these areas. Residents still have to use cars to get to most places, though. But all new growth doesn't have to be this way. Aggie Village, a 12-acre New Urbanism community, was built on the fringe of downtown Davis, California, and includes single-family houses, duplexes, shops, open spaces, and bicycle trails that connect it to the nearby campus of the University of California at Davis.

What can you do to encourage community planning that promotes physical activity? In existing communities, you can advocate for new growth designed around public transportation hubs and for bicycle lanes incorporated into new and redeveloped streets. As a citizen and taxpayer, you can vote on local growth measures and become active in local chapters of organizations such as New Urbanism and Smart Growth America. Taking political action can work. In 2002, for example, New Jersey voters and antisprawl lobbyists were rewarded with an executive order against sprawl by their governor, which preserved open areas and focused expansion and redevelopment on existing urban and suburban areas.

When making personal choices about where to live and work, look at a map of the immediate area and think about how communities you're considering are planned. How close are recreational areas? What types of places are within a 10-minute walking radius of home and work? Will living in this community help to make you more active and physically fit?

Sources: "New Jersey Is Running Out of Open Land It Can Build On," by L. Mansnerus, May 2003, *Wired New York Forum.* "Relationship Between Urban Sprawl and Physical Activity, Obesity and Mortality," by R. Ewing et al., Sep. 2003, *American Journal of Health Promotion,* (18:1) pp. 47–57. "Smartcode: A Comprehensive Form-Based Planning Ordinance," by A. Duany, *Newurbanism.org.*

Many communities are also passing laws and instituting public policies that encourage physical activity (see the box "Reengineering Communities for Physical Activity"). One example is restricting motor vehicle traffic to downtown centers and building pedestrian malls accessible only to people on foot, on bicycles, or in wheelchairs. Another is changing building codes so that stairways can be designed to be more convenient and usable than elevators or escalators are. A third is requiring that parking lots be located at a greater distance from buildings so that people have to walk farther.[51] The Centers for Disease Control and Prevention has initiated the Active Community Environments Initiative (ACES) project to promote and support social environments that encourage active lifestyles.[52]

***

Take a few minutes and reflect on the kinds of physical activity you enjoy. It could be dancing, hiking, snowboarding, swimming, basketball, or yoga. Why do you enjoy these activities? What are the barriers you encounter when pursuing these activities? How do you overcome these barriers? The key message of this chapter is that physical activity is a natural, enjoyable, sometimes thrilling, frequently challenging part of human life. It is a part of life that children instinctively embrace but that adults may have lost touch with living in a fast-paced, sedentary culture. We encourage you to get up, get moving, and get back in touch with the lifelong pleasures of physical activity.

You Make the Call

Is "Fitness for Life" Physical Education the Right Direction?

Elementary school students juggle balls, rings, and pins. Middle school students propel push scooters through an obstacle course lined with balloons, hoops, nets, rings, and mats. High school students play a modified version of volleyball with a rubber chicken. All of these activities are part of a kinder, gentler physical education promoting fitness for life. Today's physical education classes bear little resemblance to the competitive, military-style fitness classes of the past.

As early as the mid-1700s, Benjamin Franklin argued that schools needed to provide running, leaping, wrestling, and swimming activities for children. Physical education in schools, however, did not become a national priority until the 1950s, when a much-publicized study reported that 58 percent of American children could not pass a muscular fitness test, compared with only 9 percent of Austrian, Italian, and Swiss youth. In 1956 the Eisenhower administration established the President's Council on Youth Fitness (changed to the President's Council on Physical Fitness and Sports in the Johnson administration) and developed the President's Youth Fitness Test. The test consisted of a series of fitness skills, including pull-ups, sit-ups, the standing long jump, the shuttle run, the 50-yard dash, the softball throw, and the 600-yard run.

The President's Youth Fitness Test conferred an official status on school physical education (PE) programs, and fitness levels greatly improved throughout the 1960s. But, beginning in the early 1970s, a series of events reversed the status of school PE programs. In 1972, the federal law known as Title IX established the right of girls to the same physical education opportunities as boys, which led to coed PE classes except in cases where contact sports like football and basketball were being played. Although equal rights were served, PE classes changed to accommodate the different physical capabilities of males and females and the coed population.

A second event was a national decline in reading and math scores, which led to the redirection of funds supporting PE into academic programs. Physical education classes grew so large that logistical and equipment problems became common. School boards and local and state governments have continued to slash funds for PE programs over the past three decades (despite concerns over a youth obesity crisis). Although PE has declined in importance, competitive sports have become a priority in many school districts. As a result of these and other changes, PE programs have become oriented more toward leisure activities and fitness for life skills and less toward exercise, physical fitness, and sports skills.

Some physical educators say that fitness for life and leisure activities do not meet the health-related physical fitness demands of youth. They are calling for a return to physical education programs that place a premium on physical fitness activities. Proponents of the kinder, gentler type of physical education say that a wellness orientation promotes lifelong physical activity and teaches students self-discipline. What do you think?

Pros

- A focus on fitness for life and leisure activities encourages cooperation over competition and movement over intimidation, thus contributing to students' healthy development and eliminating the terrors that old-fashioned PE classes held for many students.

- Physical fitness is more than cardiorespiratory fitness and weight management; PE classes also need to provide students with relief from stress, opportunities for socialization, and ways to enhance self-esteem.

- Leisure activities such as Frisbee golf, Tae-Bo, and kickboxing are enjoyable activities that students will pursue throughout their lives.

- School fitness centers that provide various cardiovascular machines and weight training equipment are used by students before and after school. Wellness-oriented physical education facilitates this use.

Cons

- Fitness scores on the President's Youth Fitness Test have dropped significantly in the past decade.

- In light of current concerns about overweight and obesity among American children and teenagers, a return to the rigorous physical education programs of the past would seem to make sense.

- The orientation toward fitness for life and leisure activities makes physical education seem trivial and irrelevant, both to students and to the public.

About 26 percent of high school students in the United States have a daily PE class; 40 percent of high school students are enrolled in PE of any kind; and 75 percent of high school seniors get no physical education at all.

- As further evidence of the decline in status of physical education, only seven states require elementary schools to employ a certified physical education instructor; in all the other states, classroom teachers are responsible for physical education.

OLC Web site For more information about this topic, visit the Online Learning Center at www.mhhe.com/teague1e.

SOURCES: Active Community Environments Initiative (ACES) Project, Centers for Disease Control and Prevention, 2000, www.cdc.gov; "Gym Class Struggle," by A. Singer, April 24, 2000, *Sports Illustrated*, 82–96; "Adolescent Participation in Sports and Adult Physical Activity," by T. Tammelin, S. Nayha, A. P. Hills, and M. R. Jarvelin, 2003, *American Journal of Preventive Medicine, 24* (1), 22–28.

SUMMARY

- Physical fitness is the ability of the body to respond to the physical demands placed upon it. Skill-related fitness is the ability to perform specific skills associated with leisure activities and sports. Health-related fitness is the ability to perform daily living activities with vigor.

- Physical activity and exercise confer benefits in the physical, cognitive, psychological, and spiritual domains. Overall, people who are active are healthier and live longer than do people who are inactive.

- The surgeon general's report established two kinds of exercise guidelines: (1) for significant health benefits, at least 30 minutes of moderate activity on most, if not all, days of the week, expending 150 calories a day; and (2) for additional health benefits, from 20 to 30 minutes of vigorous activity two to five times a week.

- American College of Sports Medicine (ACSM) guidelines call for aerobic exercise three to five times a week and strength training exercise two times a week.

- Research shows that 60 minutes of physical activity a day are needed for weight loss and weight management.

- Four dimensions of exercise affect the amount of overload (stress) provided by an exercise session: frequency, intensity, time, and type of activity (FITT).

- Cardiorespiratory fitness is the ability of the heart and lungs to efficiently deliver oxygen and nutrients to the body's muscles and cells. It is developed by activities that use the large muscles of the body in continuous movement, such as running, cycling, and swimming.

- Musculoskeletal fitness consists of muscular strength, muscular endurance, and flexibility. Muscular strength

is the capacity of the muscles to exert force against resistance. Muscular endurance is the capacity of the muscles to exert force repeatedly over a period of time. Both are developed by weight training, also known as strength training or resistance training. Muscular power is the amount of work performed by muscles in a given period of time.

- The only safe way to gain muscle mass and weight is through weight training combined with a high-calorie diet.

- Flexibility is the ability of joints to move through their full range of motion. Stretching the muscles attached to joints is the best way to increase flexibility. Four kinds of stretching are used: passive, static, ballistic, and PNF.

- Body composition is the relative proportion of body fat and fat-free mass in the body. The recommended percentage of body fat for women is 21–35 percent and for men, 8–24 percent.

- Engaging in moderate physical activity, defined as activity that expends 150 calories a day or 1,000 calories a week, can provide health benefits, including greater longevity. Increasing the intensity of daily activities, walking, and participating in the 10,000 Steps Program are some ways to get more moderate activity into your life.

- Health and safety considerations in exercise and physical activity include properly warming up and cooling down, avoiding fatigue, treating injuries, and eating properly. The female athlete triad is a set of three interrelated conditions—disordered eating patterns and excessive exercise, amenorrhea, and premature osteoporosis.

- Physical activity workloads may need to be adjusted to certain environmental conditions, including altitude, heat and cold, and air pollution.

- Special adjustments should be made in exercise programs for children, people with disabilities, and older adults.

- Three approaches to making physical activity a lifelong pursuit are understanding the stage of change you are currently in, selecting activities that match your general patterns of behavior, and drawing on social and community support.

REVIEW QUESTIONS

1. Explain the difference between skill-related fitness and health-related fitness. What are the components of health-related fitness?

2. What are the best explanations for the positive effects of exercise on psychological functioning?

3. Briefly describe the two kinds of exercise guidelines included in the U.S. Surgeon General's *Physical Activity and Health Report* of 1996.

4. How many minutes of physical activity are necessary each day to facilitate weight loss and weight management?

5. What are the four dimensions you need to take into account when designing an exercise session? How are they interrelated?

6. Explain how to calculate your target heart rate zone.

7. List some of the benefits of muscular fitness.

8. What is the difference between muscular strength and muscular endurance? How do you train for each of them?

9. What is muscular power, and how can it be developed? What is core-strength training?

10. Describe some of the disadvantages and dangers of performance-enhancing drugs and dietary supplements used by athletes.

11. Describe the differences among the four stretching techniques discussed in the chapter.

12. Describe several ways to increase the amount of physical activity in your life and to turn light activity into moderate activity.

13. Explain the physiological effects of warming up before exercise and cooling down afterwards. What are some appropriate warming up and cooling down activities?

14. What are the symptoms of overexertion that require a physician's attention?

15. Explain the R-I-C-E approach to treating soft tissue injuries.

16. Explain the female athlete triad.

17. What are some of the physiological adjustments the body makes to high altitude over time?

18. What are two techniques used to prevent excessive increases in body temperature during exercise in hot weather?

19. What are two special concerns when children and adolescents are engaged in exercise?

20. What is functional capacity? Describe some of the changes in functional capacity that occur with aging.

21. List some barriers to exercise that people experience and some ways to overcome them.

22. What are some ways that communities can promote physical fitness?

WEB RESOURCES

Aerobics and Fitness Association of America: In addition to training and certification of fitness professionals, this organization offers information on exercise, health and safety, lifestyle, and nutrition.
www.afaa.com

American College of Sports Medicine: ACSM presents various health and fitness topics, with expert commentary and tips for maintaining a lifestyle of physical fitness, through its e-newsletter and brochures.
www.acsm.org

American Council on Exercise: This site offers health and fitness information, including core stability training, healthy recipes, fitness fact sheets, and what to look for in a health club.
www.acefitness.org

American Heart Association: Just Move: This site features an assessment for matching your fitness type to your lifestyle and an online exercise diary. Highlighting the benefits of exercise, it offers guidelines for physical activity for children and adolescents.
www.justmove.org

Health Canada: This organization features Canada's Physical Activity Guide and offers specialized physical activity guides for children and youth and for older adults.
www.hc-sc.gc.ca

National Center for Chronic Disease Prevention and Health Promotion: Look here for CDC recommendations on physical activity, information on measuring physical activity intensity, and strength training for older adults.
www.cdc.gov/nccdphp/dnpa

The National Center on Physical Activity and Disability: This site features information on lifetime sports, competitive sports, and exercise/fitness for individuals with disabilities.
www.ncpad.org

President's Council on Physical Fitness and Sports: This advisory council offers a challenge to people of all abilities and fitness levels to make physical activity part of their everyday life, featuring programs for kids, teens, adults, and seniors that use "presidential awards" for motivation.
www.fitness.gov

Shape Up America! Fitness Center: This site features a variety of ways to improve your fitness and lose weight, offering assessment tools, tips on motivation, and ways to design an improvement program that matches your individual needs and goals.
www.shapeup.org/fitness.html

REFERENCES

1. U.S. Department of Health and Human Services. (2005). Fact sheet: Physical activity and health. http://fitness.gov.

2. Corbin, C. B., & Pangrazi, R. (2000). *Definitions: Health fitness and physical activity.* President's Council on Physical Fitness and Sports, 3 (9), 1–8.

3. Blair, S. N., Dunn, A. L., Marcus, B. H., Carpenter, R. A., & Jaret, P. (2001). *Active living everyday.* Champaign, IL: Human Kinetics.

4. Blair, S. N., Kohl, H. W., Barlow, C. E., et al. (1995). Changes in physical fitness and all-cause mortality: A prospective study of healthy and unhealthy men. *Journal of the American Medical Association, 273,* 1093–1098.

5. Evenson, K. R., Stevens, J., Cai, J., Thomas R., & Thomas, O. (2003). The effect of cardiorespiratory fitness and obesity on cancer mortality in men and women. *Medicine and Science in Sports and Exercise, 35* (2), 270–277.

6. Schnohr, P., Scharling, H., & Jensen, J. S. (2003). Changes in leisure-time physical activity and risk of death: An observational study of 7,000 men and women. *American Journal of Epidemiology, 158* (7), 639–644.

7. Schnirring, L. (2003). Getting patients moving: Is activity promotion paying off? *The Physician and Sportsmedicine, 31* (2), 19, 46.

8. Miller, L. E., Nickols-Richardson, S. M., Ramp, W. K., et al. (2004). Bone mineral density in postmenopausal women: Does exercise training make a difference? *The Physician and Sportsmedicine, 32* (2), 18–24.

9. Kang, H. S., Gutin, B., Barbeau, P., et al. (2002). Physical training improves insulin resistance syndrome markers in obese adolescents. *Medicine and Science in Sports and Exercise, 34* (12), 1920–1927.

10. Wilmore, J. H. (2003). Aerobic exercise and endurance: Improving fitness for health benefits. *The Physician and Sportsmedicine, 3* (5), 45–51.

11. Jakicic, J. M., Marcus, B. H., Gallagher, K. I., Napolitano, M., & Lang, W. (2003). Effect of exercise duration and intensity on weight loss in overweight, sedentary women: A randomized trial. *Journal of American Medical Association, 290* (1), 1377–1379.

12. Gauvin, L., Spence, S. C., & Anderson, S. (1999). Exercise and psychological well-being in the adult population: Reality or wishful thinking? In J. Rippe (Ed.), *Lifestyle medicine.* Malden, MA: Blackwell Science.

13. U.S. Preventive Services Task Force. (2000). *Guide to clinical prevention services* (3rd ed.). Alexandria, VA: International Medical Publishing.

14. Trine, M. R. (1999). Physical activity and quality of life. In J. Rippe (Ed.), *Lifestyle medicine.* Malden, MA: Blackwell Science.

15. Jackson, A. W., Morrow, J. R., Hill, D. W., & Dishman, R. K. (2004). *Physical activity for health and fitness.* Champaign, IL: Human Kinetics.

16. American College of Sports Medicine. (2003). *ACSM Fitness Book* (3rd ed.). Champaign, IL: Human Kinetics.

17. American College of Sports Medicine. (1998). Position stand: The recommended quality and quantity of exercise for developing and maintaining cardiorespiratory and muscular fitness, and flexibility in health adults. *Medicine and Science in Sports and Exercise, 30,* 975–991.

18. Paffenbarger, R. S., Jr., Hyde, R. T., Hyde, A. L., et al. (1993). The association of changes in physical activity level and other lifestyle characteristics with mortality among men. *New England Journal of Medicine, 328,* 538–545.

19. Murphy, M., Nevill, A., Neville, C., Biddle, S., & Hardman, A. (2002). Accumulating brisk walking for fitness, cardiovascular risk, and psychological health. *Medicine and Science in Sports and Exercise, 34* (9), 1468–1474.

20. Larew, K., Hunter, G. R., Larson-Meyer, D. E., Newcomer, B. R., McCarthy, J. P., & Weinsier, R. L. (2003). Muscle metabolic function, exercise performance, and weight gain. *Medicine and Science in Sports and Exercise, 35* (2), 230–236.

21. American College of Sports Medicine. (1998). Position stand: Exercise and physical activity for older adults. *Medicine and Science in Sports and Exercise, 30,* 992–1008.

22. Pollock, M. L. (1999). Symposium: Resistance training for health and diseases. *Medicine and Science in Sports and Exercise, 31,* 10–45.

23. American College of Sports Medicine. (2002). Position stand: Progression models in resistance training for healthy adults. *Medicine and Science in Sports and Exercise, 34* (3), 64–380.

24. Kraemer, W. J., & Ratamess, N. A. (2004). Fundamentals of resistance training: Progression and exercise prescription. *Medicine and Science in Sports and Exercise, 36* (4), 674–688.

25. Hunter, J. P., & Marshall, R. N. (2002). Effects of power and flexibility training on vertical jump technique. *Medicine and Science in Sports and Exercise, 34* (3), 478–486.

26. Sorgen, C. (2003, November 11). Your way to a stronger body. WebMD Feature. http://content.health.msn.com.

27. Williams, M. H. (1998). *The ergogenic edge: Pushing the limits of sports performance.* Champaign, IL: Human Kinetics.

28. Williams, M. H. (2005). *Nutrition for health, fitness and sport* (7th ed.). New York: McGraw-Hill.

29. Grandjean, A. (1999). Nutritional requirements to increase lean mass. *Clinics in Sports Medicine, 18,* 623–632.

30. Thacker, S. B., Gilchrist, J., Stroup, D. F., & Kimsey, D. Jr. (2004). The impact of stretching on sports injury risk: A systematic review of the literature. *Medicine and Science in Sports and Exercise, 36* (3), 371–378.

31. Rowlands, A. V., Marginson, V. F., & Lee, J. (2003). Chronic flexibility gains: Effect of isometric contraction during proprioceptive neuromuscular facilitation stretching techniques. *Research Quarterly for Sport and Exercise, 74* (1), 47–51.

32. Fenton, N. (2001). *The complete guide to walking for health, weight, and fitness.* Guilford, CT: Lyons Press.

33. Oguma, Y., & Shinoda-Tagawa, T. (2004). Physical activity decreases cardiovascular disease risk in women: Review and meta-analysis. *American Journal of Preventive Medicine, 26* (5), 407–418.

34. 10,000 Steps Program. (2003). Shape Up America. www.shapeup.org.

35. Tudor-Locke, C. E., & Myers, A. M. (2001). Methodological considerations for researchers and practitioners using pedometers to measure physical ambulatory patients. *Research Quarterly for Exercise and Sport, 72* (1), 1–12.

36. Hawley, C. J., & Schoene, R. B. (2003). Overtraining syndrome: A guide to diagnosis, treatment and prevention. *The Physician and Sportsmedicine, 31* (6), 25–31.

37. Nieman, D. C. (1998). *The exercise-health connection.* Champaign, IL: Human Kinetics.

38. Cobb, K. L., Bachrach, L. K., Greendale, G., et al. (2003). Disordered eating, menstrual irregularity, and bone mineral density in female runners. *Medicine and Science in Sports and Exercise, 35* (5), 719–722.

39. Putukian, M. (1998). The female athlete triad. *Clinics in Sports Medicine, 17* (4), 675–696.

40. Eberle, S. G. (2000). *Endurance sports nutrition.* Champaign, IL: Human Kinetics.

41. Antol, J. D. (1999). High-altitude acclimatization and illness. In J. Rippe (Ed.), *Lifestyle medicine.* Malden, MA: Blackwell Science.

42. Schneider, M., Bernacsch, D., Weymann, J., Holle, R., & Bartsch, P. (2002). Acute mountain sickness: Influence of susceptibility, pre-exposure, and ascent rate. *Medicine and Science in Sports and Exercise, 34* (12), 1863–1867.

43. Schnirring, L. (2003). New hydration recommendations: Risk of hyponatremia plays a big role. *The Physician and Sportsmedicine, 31* (7), 15–18.

44. American College of Sports Medicine. (1996). Position stand: Heat and cold illness during distance running. *Medicine and Science in Sports and Exercise, 28,* i–x.

45. Linn, S. W., & Gong, H. (1999). Air pollution exercise, nutrition, and health. In J. Rippe (Ed.), *Lifestyle medicine.* Malden, MA: Blackwell Science.

46. Trost, S. G., & Pate, R. R. (1999). Physical activity in children and youth. In J. Rippe (Ed.), *Lifestyle medicine.* Malden, MA: Blackwell Science.

47. American Council for Exercise. (1998). *Exercise for older adults: ACE's guide for fitness professionals.* Champaign, IL: Human Kinetics.

48. Rhodes, R. E., Jones, L. W., & Courneya, K. S. (2002). Extending the theory of planned behavior in the exercise domain: A comparison of social support and subjective norm. *Research Quarterly for Sport and Exercise, 73* (2), 187–192.

49. Rafferty, A. P., Reeves, M. J., McGee, H. B., & Pirarnik, J. M. (2002). Physical activity patterns among walkers and compliance with public health recommendations. *Medicine and Science in Sports and Exercise, 34* (81), 1255–1261.

50. Jordan, P. (1999). *The fitness instinct.* Emmaus, PA: Rodale Press.

51. Hirschhorn, J. S. (2004). Zoning should promote public health. *American Journal of Health Promotion, 18* (3), 258–260.

52. Singer, A. (2000, April 24). Gym class struggle. *Sports Illustrated,* 82–96.

Add It Up! WHAT KEEPS YOU FROM BEING MORE ACTIVE?

People give many different reasons when asked why they don't get more exercise. To find out what the major barriers to exercise and physical activity are in your life, complete the following quiz. Indicate how likely you are to consider the following statements a barrier by using this key: Very likely = 3, Somewhat likely = 2, Somewhat unlikely = 1, Very unlikely = 0.

1. My day is so busy now, I just don't think I can make the time to include physical activity in my regular schedule.

2. None of my family members or friends like to do anything active, so I don't have a chance to exercise.

3. I'm just too tired after work to get any exercise.

4. I've been thinking about getting more exercise, but I just can't seem to get started.

5. I'm getting older so exercise can be risky.

6. I don't get enough exercise because I have never learned the skills for any sport.

7. I don't have access to jogging trails, swimming pools, or bike paths.

8. Physical activity takes too much time away from other commitments like home, work, and family.

9. I'm embarrassed about how I will look when I exercise with others.

10. I don't get enough sleep as it is. I just couldn't get up early or stay up late to get some exercise.

11. It's easier for me to find excuses not to exercise than to go out and do something.

12. I know of too many people who have hurt themselves by overdoing it with exercise.

13. I really can't see learning a new sport at my age.

14. It's just too expensive. You have to take a class or join a club or buy the right equipment.

15. My free times during the day are too short to include exercise.

16. My usual social activities with family or friends do not include physical activity.

17. I'm too tired during the week and I need the weekend to catch up on my rest.

18. I want to get more exercise, but I just can't seem to make myself stick to anything.

19. I'm afraid I might injure myself or have a heart attack.

20. I'm not good enough at any physical activity to make it fun.

21. If we had exercise facilities and showers at work, I would be more likely to exercise.

Scoring

Enter your individual scores for each statement on the following lines. For example, enter your scores for statements 1, 8, and 15 on the first three lines, and add each group of three scores. Barriers to exercise and physical activity fall into the seven categories shown. A score of 5 or above in any category indicates that this is a significant barrier for you. For ideas on how to overcome these and other barriers, see the box "Strategies for Overcoming Barriers to Physical Activity" on p. 217.

	1	+	8	+	15	=	Lack of time
	2	+	9	+	16	=	Social influence
	3	+	10	+	17	=	Lack of energy
	4	+	11	+	18	=	Lack of willpower
	5	+	12	+	19	=	Fear of injury
	6	+	13	+	20	=	Lack of skill
	7	+	14	+	21	=	Lack of resources

SOURCE: Barriers to Being Active Quiz, 2003, Centers for Disease Control and Prevention, www.cdc.gov.

CHAPTER 9

Body Weight and Body Composition: Achieving a Healthy Balance

DID YOU KNOW?

- More than half of all Americans are overweight, and one fifth are obese. Obesity is one of the leading preventable causes of death for Americans, second only to tobacco use.

- If you have tried the Atkins diet or joined Weight Watchers, you are one of 80 million Americans who go on a diet every year. The diet industry takes in about $40 billion a year.

- Individual serving sizes have increased dramatically over the past 40 years. A typical cookie used to have about 65 calories; now it can have up to 500. A hot dog used to have 150 calories; now it can have 350. A specialty meal at a fast-food restaurant can contain 1,300 calories, more than half the daily caloric requirement for most people.

OLC *Your Health Today*   www.mhhe.com/teague1e

Go to the Online Learning Center for *Your Health Today* for interactive activities, quizzes, flashcards, Web links, and more resources related to this chapter.

Obesity is an increasingly worrisome problem in the United States. Half of all Americans meet the criteria for overweight, and one fifth meet the criteria for obesity. **Overweight** is defined as body weight that exceeds the recommended guidelines for good health; **obesity** is body weight that greatly exceeds the recommended guidelines. In 1991, 4 states reported a prevalence rate of obesity greater than 15 percent, and no states reported a prevalence greater than 20 percent. Ten years later, all 50 states reported a prevalence rate of obesity greater than 15 percent, 31 states reported a prevalence between 20 and 24 percent, and only 4 states reported a prevalence of less than 25 percent.[1] If these trends continue, all Americans could be overweight within a few generations.

The Centers for Disease Control and Prevention (CDC) has determined that no sex, age, state, racial group, or educational level is spared from the problem of overweight, although the problem is worse for the young and the poor. A recent report indicated that 64 percent of children between 6 and 19 years of age are overweight.[2] This trend is a concern because research shows that a child who is obese at age 12 has odds of 4 to 1 against maintaining a normal weight later. A person who is obese at age 18 faces odds of 28 to 1 against maintaining a normal adult weight.[3]

Overweight and obesity are associated with serious health problems. Obese people are four times as likely as people with a healthy weight to die before reaching their expected life span. They have an increased risk for high blood pressure, diabetes, elevated cholesterol levels, coronary heart disease, stroke, gallbladder disease, osteoarthritis (a type of arthritis caused by wear and tear on the joints), sleep apnea (interrupted breathing during sleep), lung problems, and certain cancers, such as uterine, prostate, and colorectal.[4,5] The CDC attributes 400,000 deaths in the United States each year to overweight, a number not too far behind the 435,000 deaths attributed to smoking.[6]

In this chapter, we examine this current trend toward overweight and obesity in the United States. We begin by considering what is meant by healthy body weight and healthy body composition. We then look at the factors that influence weight, including genetics and lifestyle, and we discuss energy balance as the key to weight management. Next, we consider whether fad diets, medical options, and other approaches successfully address weight issues, and we briefly discuss the nondiet movement as an alternative to the current obsession with thinness. We close with a look at factors that contribute to maintaining a healthy weight and body composition for life.

WHAT IS A HEALTHY BODY WEIGHT?

How much should you weigh? The answer to this question depends on who is asking and why. If you are a 16-year-old varsity wrestler getting ready for your compe-

tition weigh-in, your coach and the wrestling weight classes may influence your weight goals. If you are an 18-year-old girl comparing yourself with the fashion models you see daily in magazines, your goals may be determined by a media-generated cosmetic ideal. If you are a 50-year-old woman wondering whether you should be concerned about the 25 pounds you gained last year, you may be more interested in health goals for weight and fitness.

There is no ideal body weight for each person, but there are ranges for a healthy body weight. A healthy body weight is defined as (1) a weight within an acceptable range on a height-weight table or an acceptable body mass index (explained in the following sections); (2) a fat distribution that is not a risk factor for illness; and (3) the absence of any medical conditions (such as diabetes or hypertension) that would suggest a need for weight loss.[7] There are no known health advantages in losing weight if you meet all these criteria. If you don't meet them, you may need to lose weight.

In this section, we examine several different ways to evaluate weight and overweight: height-weight tables, body mass index, body fat percentage, and body fat distribution.

Height-Weight Tables

If we consider a person weighing 200 pounds and a person weighing 130 pounds, we cannot determine whether either is of healthy weight, underweight, overweight, or obese without more information. If we also know that both people are 5 feet 3 inches tall, we are likely to assume that the person who weighs 200 pounds is overweight or obese. In this sense, a height-to-weight ratio provides useful information, although the standards associated with height-weight tables have changed over time. Every 5 years the Metropolitan Life Insurance Company provides healthy weight charts. Currently these charts are not used as much as another measure, the body mass index. For more information about weight-height tables, see the Web Resources at the end of this chapter.

Body Mass Index

Body mass index (BMI) is a single number that represents height-to-weight ratio. BMI is used to estimate the health significance of body weight (you can check your BMI in Table 9.1). Researchers disagree about exactly what the cutoff BMI for being overweight should be. In classic studies, if they considered the relationship between BMI and the relative risk of death, there appeared to be a significant increase in risk of death above a BMI of somewhere between 25 and 27 and below a BMI of 18.5 (Figure 9.1). Based on this information, obesity guidelines established by the National Institutes of Health (NIH) set a healthy weight BMI as 18.5 to 25, overweight as a BMI of at least 25, and obesity as a BMI of at least 30.[8] A recent study raises further questions, as it found the risk of death asso-

Table 9.1 Body Mass Index (BMI)

Find your height in the lefthand column and look across the row until you find the number that is closest to your weight. The number at the top of that column identifies your BMI. The darkest shaded area represents healthy weight ranges.

BMI	18	19	20	21	22	23	24	25	26	27	28	29	30	31	32	33	34
Height																	
4'10"	86	91	96	100	105	110	115	119	124	129	134	138	143	148	153	158	162
4'11"	89	94	99	104	109	114	119	124	128	133	138	143	148	153	158	163	168
5'0"	92	97	102	107	112	118	123	128	133	138	143	148	153	158	163	168	174
5'1"	95	100	106	111	116	122	127	132	137	143	148	153	158	164	169	174	180
5'2"	98	104	109	115	120	126	131	136	142	147	153	158	164	169	175	180	186
5'3"	102	107	113	118	124	130	135	141	146	152	158	163	169	175	180	186	191
5'4"	105	110	116	122	128	134	140	145	151	157	163	169	174	180	186	192	197
5'5"	108	114	120	126	132	138	144	150	156	162	168	174	180	186	192	198	204
5'6"	112	118	124	130	136	142	148	155	161	167	173	179	186	192	198	204	210
5'7"	115	121	127	134	140	146	153	159	166	172	178	185	191	198	204	211	217
5'8"	118	125	131	138	144	151	158	164	171	177	184	190	197	203	210	216	223
5'9"	122	128	135	142	149	155	162	169	176	182	189	196	203	209	216	223	230
5'10"	126	132	139	146	153	160	167	174	181	188	195	202	209	216	222	229	236
5'11"	129	136	143	150	157	165	172	179	186	193	200	208	215	222	229	236	243
6'0"	132	140	147	154	162	169	177	184	191	199	206	213	221	228	235	242	250
6'1"	136	144	151	159	166	174	182	189	197	204	212	219	227	235	242	250	257
6'2"	141	148	155	163	171	179	186	194	202	210	218	225	233	241	249	256	264
6'3"	144	152	160	168	176	184	192	200	208	216	224	232	240	248	256	264	272
6'4"	148	156	164	172	180	189	197	205	213	221	230	223	246	254	263	271	279
6'5"	151	160	168	176	185	193	202	210	218	227	235	244	252	261	269	277	286
6'6"	155	164	172	181	190	198	207	216	224	233	241	250	259	267	276	284	293

Underweight (<18.5)   Healthy Weight (18.5–24.9)   Overweight (25–29.9)   Obese (≥30)

Source: Adapted from "Obesity Part 1. Pathogenesis," by G. A. Bray and D. S. Gray, 1998, *Western Journal of Medicine, 149,* 429–441.

ciated with BMI increased somewhere above a BMI of 30 and below a BMI of 18.5.[9]

Critics of the NIH BMI guidelines argue that healthy weight increases as we age and BMI does not take this into account. Others strongly disagree, saying that the healthy weight range is the same for adults at age 60 as at age 30. Another criticism of BMI is that it refers to height and weight measurements and not to *body composition,* the proportion of fat to other tissues, such as muscle and bone. In fact, muscle tissue is heavier than fat, and muscular people may be above the healthy range for BMI without having any known increased risk of health problems.

KEY TERMS

overweight Body weight that exceeds the recommended guidelines for good health, as indicated by a body mass index of 25 to 29.

obesity Body weight that greatly exceeds the recommended guidelines for good health, as indicated by a body mass index of more than 30.

body mass index (BMI) Measure of body weight in relation to height.

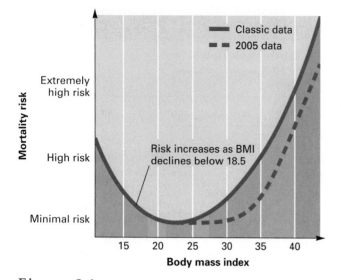

Figure 9.1 **BMI and mortality risk.** *The solid line shows the traditional relationship between risk of death and BMI. The dotted line reflects the results of a 2005 study that suggests that the risk of death may not increase until BMI exceeds 30.*

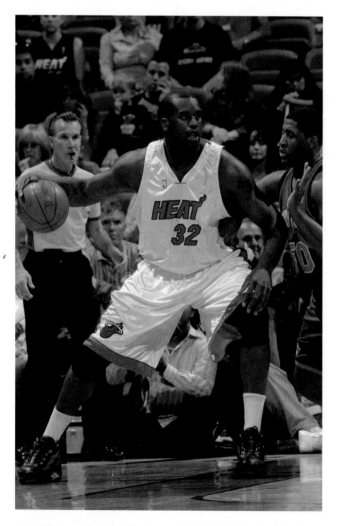

Basketball star Shaquille O'Neal has a BMI of 31.6, which puts him in the obese range, yet he is in top physical condition. Since a high proportion of his body weight is in muscle tissue rather than fat, his body composition must be considered in relation to his body weight.

Body Fat Percentage

Body composition is measured in terms of percentage of body fat, as noted in Chapter 8. There are no clear, accepted guidelines for healthy body fat ranges, although ranges of 12 percent to 20 percent have been used for men and 20 percent to 30 percent for women.[10] In general, body fat percentage increases with age and body mass index. At each level of BMI, differences exist for ethnic groups. For example, for any BMI, on average, African American men have a slightly lower body fat percentage than white men do, and Asian men have a slightly higher body fat percentage than do white men.[11] Differences also exist for gender, with women, on average, having 10 percent to 12 percent more body fat than men have.[12]

Some people may need less body fat. Many athletes, for example, find that a lower body fat percentage is better for their performance. The lower healthy range may be from 5 to 10 percent for male athletes and from 15 to 20 percent for female athletes. Still other people may need higher levels of body fat. During early pregnancy, women need extra body fat to support fetal growth. Hormones cannot be produced below a certain body fat threshold. Infertility, lack of menstruation, depression, and abnormal appetite are associated with a body fat level below a person's threshold needs.[7]

Because body fat percentage is considered an important component in judging the need for weight reduction, it may be measured as part of a physical examination. There are several different ways to measure body fat: skinfold measurement, immersion, electroimpedance, and the Bod Pod. These methods are described in the box "Body Fat Measuring Techniques."

Body Fat Distribution

Research has shown that not only the amount but also the distribution of body fat is important in determining your health risk. **Waist-to-hip ratio** is one way to judge the location of body fat. If you are apple shaped, you carry your fat mainly around and above the waist. This abdominal fat is considered more "active" than fat carried on the hips and thighs, a disadvantage because it breaks down more easily and enters the bloodstream more readily. A large abdominal circumference (more than 40 inches for a man, more than 35 inches for a woman) is associated with high cholesterol levels and higher risk of heart disease, stroke, diabetes, hypertension, and some types of cancer.

You can calculate your waist-to-hip ratio by dividing your waist measurement by your hip measurement. For men, a ratio of less than 0.80 (pear shape) is considered low risk, 0.81 to 0.99 is considered moderate risk, and 1.00 or more (apple shape) is considered high risk. For women, a ratio of less than 0.70 (pear shape) is considered low risk, 0.71 to 0.89 is considered moder-

HIGHLIGHT ON HEALTH
Body Fat Measuring Techniques

Skinfold Test

Calipers, a special kind of tong, are used to measure the folds of skin and fat in several locations around your body, such as your upper arm and your abdomen. The readings are used to calculate your body fat percentage. This method is not considered to be a precise way of determining body fat percentage, but it is often used because it is relatively cheap and easy to perform.

Immersion

Immersion is the most accurate way to measure your body fat. You are first weighed on land and then weighed again underwater. Because fat is more buoyant than muscle, a formula can be used to calculate your body fat percentage from your dry weight and your weight underwater.

Electroimpedence

This technique measures the electrical resistance (impedance) to a weak electrical current passed through your body. Electrodes are attached to your arms and legs. Fat tissue resists electrical flow more than muscle does, so your percentage of body fat can be calculated from the measured resistance. This is an expensive test that is not readily available to everyone.

Bod Pod

The Bod Pod, an egg-shaped chamber that you sit in, is a relatively new invention. The chamber is closed, and the air that your body displaces is measured. Because muscle is denser than fat, your weight and the air displacement in the Bod Pod can be used to calculate your percentage of body fat. This method appears to be as accurate as immersion, but it's more convenient because you don't have to get wet. However, it is not available to everyone.

ate risk, and 0.9 or more (apple shape) is considered high risk.

Obese men tend to accumulate abdominal fat (apple shape), whereas obese women tend to accumulate fat on the hips and thighs (pear shape). However, women have a change in body fat distribution at the onset of menopause, with fat shifting to the abdomen. This shift coincides with an increased risk of heart disease for women. Obesity experts suggest working toward maintaining a healthy weight and healthy body fat distribution, rather than focusing on losing weight, since it is much easier to put on weight than to take it off and keep it off.

WHAT FACTORS INFLUENCE YOUR WEIGHT?

There is no simple answer to why Americans are getting fatter. Many factors contribute to this trend, both personal and environmental. You may look to other family members, for example, and think that it is your genes that make you overweight. Unless you are adopted, however, the people who gave you your genes also taught you how to eat. In addition, they probably raised you in a culture similar to their own. Separating genetic factors (nature) from family behaviors and culture (nurture) is difficult. In this section we consider genetics, gender and age, food environments, lifestyle factors, dieting, and stress as factors that can contribute to overweight.

Genetic Influences on Weight

If both your parents are obese, you have an 80 percent chance of becoming obese. The risk shrinks to 10 percent if neither parent is obese. Even adopted children tend to be similar in weight to their biological parents. Twin studies support a genetic tendency toward obesity (see Chapter 2). These findings have led researchers to search for genes associated with obesity. It appears that for most people, obesity is a multifactorial disease; that is, as explained in Chapter 2, it results from a complex interaction between multiple genes and the environment. Each gene may increase a person's susceptibility to obesity, and together they greatly increase that susceptibility.

There are some rare conditions in humans in which a single gene can cause obesity, and by looking closely at these conditions, we are able to understand how genetics can influence weight.[13] Genes that can cause obesity have been isolated in animals. The most publicized is the *ob* gene in mice. The *ob* gene provides the genetic instruction

KEY TERMS

waist-to-hip ratio　Ratio between the circumference of the waist and the circumference of the hips, used as a measure of overweight and obesity.

Even though these siblings have a similar genetic makeup, their bodies are not alike. What other factors may be responsible for the differences you see here?

for **leptin,** a protein released by fat cells when increased energy stores are present. Leptin acts in the hypothalamus to decrease appetite and increase energy expenditure and, as such, helps in food regulation. Humans have this same gene. A child born with a mutation in the *ob* gene has low levels of leptin or none at all. As a result, the child has an insatiable appetite, eats huge amounts of food, and develops severe obesity at a young age. A few such children have been treated with injections of leptin and have been able to reduce food intake and weight.[13]

Other proteins have also been found to influence appetite and energy expenditure. Some proteins act at brain centers that signal when to start and finish eating. The centers may monitor external cues for food, such as smells and sights, or internal cues, such as body fat stores, glucose level, levels of amino acids and free fatty acids, stomach fullness, and basal metabolic rate. (We discuss basal metabolic rate later in this chapter.) In these centers, serotonin, norepinephrine, and other neurotransmitters are thought to interact in a complex way. Other proteins act on the fat tissues and appear to increase basal metabolic rate and decrease fat stores. An increased understanding of the complex roles of these body chemicals may lead to new treatments for obesity.

Except in the rare cases of a single gene mutation, genetics alone is not the culprit. Cross-cultural studies support the assertion that genetics does not completely explain obesity. As groups of people move from one country to another, they may change their weights but not their genes (at least for the first few generations).[14] Examples of this can be found within the United States. The Pima Indians in the American Southwest have a significant obesity problem and 20 times more diabetes than do whites in the Southwest. When American Pima Indians are compared with Mexican Pima Indians, the results are startling. The average American Pima woman has a BMI of 35.5, compared with the average Mexican Pima woman's BMI of 25.1. The average American Pima man has a BMI of 30.8, compared with the average Mexican Pima man of 24.8.

Japanese immigrants to the United States have a similar pattern. Among Japanese men from 45 to 49 years of age, the percentages of obesity are 4 percent in Japan, 12 percent in Hawaii, and 14 percent in California. Genes are slow to change, requiring generations and hundreds of years. Environmental influences, such as abundant food and a sedentary lifestyle, can produce such effects in a much shorter period. Although genetics is a factor in obesity, it doesn't deserve all the blame. Culture and individual behaviors are also important.

Weight Differences Due to Gender and Age

When it comes to weight, men and women are not created equal. Studies indicate that men and women have different patterns of weight gain over the course of a lifetime. Normal changes with aging affect when, where, and why we gain weight. Understanding the phases of life when significant weight changes often occur can help you to control weight gain.

Most of us develop our eating patterns from our families during childhood. (Researchers believe that poor childhood eating habits are a major cause of the recent surge in overweight and obesity.) There are several crucial

Challenges & Choices

Tips for Eating Out

Many people eat a healthy diet at home but have less success in restaurants, college dining halls, and food courts. Try these tips to maintain control the next time you eat out.

- Increase the proportion of plant-based foods in your diet. Take larger servings of vegetables and fruits and smaller servings of meat, cheese, and eggs.
- Include two vegetables in your meal or a vegetable and a salad.
- Choose whole wheat bread, brown rice, or whole-grain cereals. Whole-grain foods are more filling.
- Have fresh fruit or yogurt for dessert instead of cake or ice cream.
- Drink water instead of soda or juice.
- Control your portion size by taking smaller servings. Don't go back for seconds.

- Eat slowly and savor the taste of your food.
- Stop eating when you first feel full rather than waiting until you feel stuffed.
- Share large portions or take some home for another meal. Don't feel obligated to eat everything on your plate.
- Don't skip meals—you'll only be inclined to eat quickly and to eat more at the next meal.

It's Not Just Personal . . .

Eating out has become a way of life. Americans consume about 30 percent of their calories in restaurants and spend almost half of every food dollar on food eaten outside the home. The restaurant industry is one of the nation's largest businesses.

Source: Data from "The Way We Eat Now," by C. Lambert, May–June 2004, *Harvard Magazine*.

times in your life when you may change these patterns. When you leave home for the first time for college or to live independently, you will be exposed to different opportunities and challenges. College presents the unique challenges of dormitory cafeterias, changing class schedules, and different work demands (see the box "Tips for Eating Out"). Students may find new stresses associated with being away from home, assignment deadlines, exams, and increased potential for alcohol consumption and parties. Each of these challenges requires students to assess how, when, and why they eat in light of new situations. When you start living with other people, either in a marriage or a shared housing situation, you will be influenced by the eating patterns of others.

During puberty, boys and girls undergo significant hormone changes that alter their respective body compositions. Female hormones begin preparing girls for childbearing with increases in body fat, especially on the hips, buttocks, and thighs. Before puberty, a girl of a healthy weight will have approximately 12 percent body fat. After puberty, the healthy range can increase to up to 25 percent body fat. In contrast, a boy's hormones in late adolescence are geared more toward muscle development. Before puberty, a boy of healthy weight has approximately 12 percent body fat; after puberty, he levels out at approximately 15 percent body fat. In addition to experiencing the hormonal influences of puberty on body composition, the average adolescent girl is less physically active than are her male peers, an additional pressure toward increased body fat percentage. Although this situation is changing, boys overall tend to remain more active through adolescence and early adulthood.[15]

Between the ages of 20 and 40, both men and women gain weight, but the reasons appear to be different. Marriage is common in this age group and appears to correlate with men's weight gain. Married men weigh more than do men who have never been married or were previously married but are currently unmarried. For women, these are the years in which pregnancy typically occurs. Weight gain is a normal part of pregnancy. The majority of women will lose this weight within a year of delivery. However, about 15 percent to 20 percent of women continue to maintain the weight gain a year after delivery, partly as a result of changes in lifestyle associated with childrearing.[16]

As people enter their 50s, weight remains an issue. Both women and men can have potentially serious problems with weight gain. Men tend to see an increase in abdominal fat. Women in their late 40s and early 50s undergo significant hormonal changes. During perimenopause (the 5- to 7-year period before menstruation stops), estrogen and progesterone levels fall. These decreases can cause such symptoms as hot flashes, mood swings, headaches, and sleep disturbance. Testosterone also begins to exert a stronger influence. Women produce testosterone at low levels throughout life, but during menopause, with the

KEY TERMS

leptin A protein produced by fat cells, under the direction of a particular gene, that causes decreased appetite and increased energy expenditure.

HIGHLIGHT ON HEALTH
Poverty and Obesity

The highest rates of obesity are found among groups that also have the highest rates of poverty. Both obesity and poverty are complex problems, and there is a strong inverse correlation between them. In other words, the less well off you are economically, the more likely you are to be obese. You may also be more likely to have other serious health conditions. Poor nutrition is probably the key: People with low incomes are more likely to eat highly processed, high-fat foods and less likely to eat fruits and vegetables. Energy-dense (high-calorie) foods made from processed grains and loaded with added sugar and fat may be the lowest-cost option for consumers.

Physical activity is another factor linked to income. For example, low-income housing is often located in areas of a community that are less safe, so residents may be less likely to be active outside. They may prefer that their children play indoors rather than in the schoolyard or on the streets. They may be less likely to walk to work or school or to go for walks around the neighborhood. If people are worried about personal safety, they are less likely to think about building exercise into their daily routines. Thus, they are less likely to expend the energy needed to balance the calories they consume in food. In such cases, it is clear that obesity is a societal issue.

Sources: "Poverty and Obesity: The Role of Energy Density and Energy Costs," by A. Drewnowski and S. E. Specter, 2004, *American Journal of Clinical Nutrition, 79* (1), 6–16; "Obesity Is an Environmental Issue," by W. Carlos Poston and J. P. Foreyt, 1999, *Atherosclerosis, 146,* 201–209.

decrease in estrogen and progesterone levels, testosterone has a comparatively greater effect. This change may help explain the redistribution of fat deposits toward the abdomen and away from the hips, a more typically male pattern.

At the age of 60 and beyond, weight tends to decline. This loss can be attributed to a number of causes, including decreased calorie needs, less muscle tissue, and less body mass. These changes give older adults thinner limbs. During these years, weight-bearing exercise, such as walking, becomes critical to maintain body mass and bone strength.

Food Environments and Their Influences on Weight

For many people in the United States, hunger is rare. Fortunately, owing to an abundant food supply and low cost of food, income level in the United States is not strongly associated with the quantity of food intake.[17] (However, poverty is associated with the *quality* of food intake—see the box "Poverty and Obesity."[18]) Therefore, food has taken on new meanings and is no longer just for sustenance. It plays a role in entertainment and is used as a cure for boredom, a mechanism for coping with failure, or a reward for accomplishment. Restoring the link between appetite and hunger is an important step in attaining and maintaining a healthy body composition. Becoming aware of your food requirements and your food environment will help you make conscious choices about when and why you eat.

Eating Out

In the 1950s eating out was a rare event; today it has become a part of daily life. Forty-eight percent of adults report eating out daily. Twenty-one percent of households use some form of take-out food or food delivery service daily.[17] This trend is most likely related to the increased number of dual-career households, single-parent households, and the convenience and accessibility of fast foods. No matter what its cause, we need to evaluate this trend more closely. Studies show that increased use of fast food is associated with increased weight gain. Foods served in restaurants and fast-food outlets tend to be higher in fat and total calories and lower in fiber than are foods prepared at home.[17]

Food Choices

What you eat can be as important as how much you eat. Healthy foods provide the body with the nutrients it needs. Some food choices are considered empty calories because they provide energy but little else of nutritional value. The biggest offender is soft drinks. The rate of soft drink consumption in America has skyrocketed, as noted in Chapter 7. Average annual consumption increased from 34 gallons per person to 44.4 gallons per person in a 10-year period, while milk consumption declined from 31 gallons per person to 24 gallons per person in the same period.[17] Added sugars now make up 16 percent of the average American's total calorie intake.

Fast-food restaurants have attempted to offer options that are lower in fat and calories than traditional options are, and many fast-food restaurants list salads, baked potatoes, and soups as options. These items tend to be less popular than less nutritious choices are, and many of them have been discontinued owing to low sales.[17]

Supersized Meal Portions

Serving size has steadily increased both inside and outside the home. The largest increases in serving size have occurred in fast-food restaurants and may be due to "supersized" pricing strategies.[19] Serving sizes of other foods have increased as well. Bagels and muffins used to weigh 2–3 ounces; now the standard is 4–7 ounces. In 1916 Coca-Cola was sold in 6.5-ounce bottles; in 1950 it was offered in 10- and 12-ounce bottles; now it is common to find Coke in 20- or 32-ounce bottles.[17]

The impact of supersizing on the caloric bottom line is dramatic. A typical McDonald's Value Meal provides you with 1,340 calories, more than half the daily caloric requirement for most people. In addition, fast foods are low in protein and high in saturated fats, sodium, and sugar. Another problem with supersized portions is that we all have trouble estimating serving size. (See Figure 9.2 for some visual images of portion sizes.) The larger a portion of food, the worse we become at estimating how much we are eating.

Lifestyle Influences on Weight

Modern labor-saving devices first appeared in the late 18th century during the Industrial Revolution. Washing machines replaced scrubbing clothes by hand. Dishwashers replaced standing at the sink to do dishes. Electronic garage door openers have even relieved us of the task of getting out of our cars and bending over to lift the door. The television remote control completes the true image of a couch potato. Before the mid-1900s, most of the population would never have considered exercise to be a necessity for health, because their daily lives involved regular physical activity. Our current lifestyle has become so mechanized, however, that

many of us can go through a regular day spending almost no energy on physical activity. In addition, 60 percent of adults engage in little or no leisure-time physical activity.[17] Three inventions in particular have created this lifestyle: the automobile, the television, and the computer.

The Automobile

Automobiles have literally changed the way we live our lives. They bring great freedom but also decrease our physical activity. Surveys show that 25 percent of all trips in the United States are less than 1 mile, and yet 75 percent of these trips are taken by car. Less than 30 percent of children living within a mile of their school walk to school.[20] Automobile use significantly decreases the use of walking and bicycling for transportation. Increased time spent in the car each day increases the risk of obesity.[21]

Safety and community structure are factors likely to influence transportation style. Communities designed with centralized shopping, reliable public transportation, and safe trails promote walking and bicycle riding.[17] Consider the typical suburbanite on a typical workday: She gets up and gets in her car in a garage (opening and closing the door with an automatic door opener); drives a 20- to 45-minute commute to work (maybe with a quick detour to the drive-through lane of a fast-food restaurant for a high-fat, high-calorie breakfast); parks in a covered lot at work; takes the elevator to the office; and sits at the computer all day, only to reverse the path at night. Should we be surprised that we are out of shape and gaining weight? People who live in communities that are designed in a way

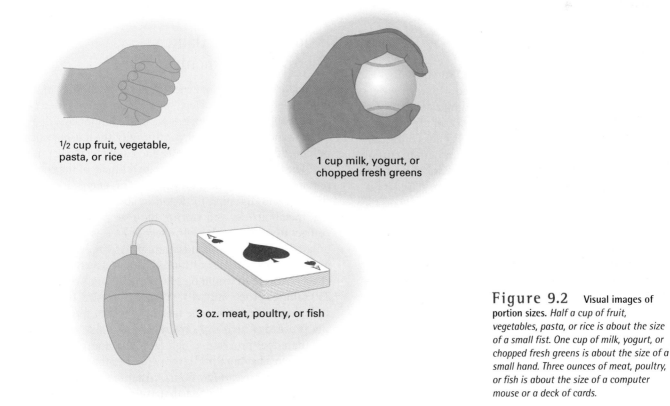

½ cup fruit, vegetable, pasta, or rice

1 cup milk, yogurt, or chopped fresh greens

3 oz. meat, poultry, or fish

Figure 9.2   **Visual images of portion sizes.** *Half a cup of fruit, vegetables, pasta, or rice is about the size of a small fist. One cup of milk, yogurt, or chopped fresh greens is about the size of a small hand. Three ounces of meat, poultry, or fish is about the size of a computer mouse or a deck of cards.*

that is less favorable for walking (no sidewalks, nowhere to walk) have an increased risk of obesity compared with people who live in more walkable communities.[21]

Television

The average American man watches 29 hours of television per week, and the average American woman watches 34 hours per week.[22] Studies have found an association between television watching and overweight in children and youth.[23] Television viewing is considered by many to be one of the most easily modifiable causes of obesity in childhood.

Television is thought to influence obesity patterns in two ways. First, sitting in front of the television takes minimal energy. The time spent there is time that could be spent performing a more energy-expending activity. Second, television viewing appears to alter patterns of eating. Food intake is increased during viewing in response to food advertisements that promote high-energy, high-fat foods. Candy, snacks, packaged foods, soft drinks, and alcohol are the most commonly advertised items; fruits and vegetables are shown the least.[17] In addition, people often eat mindlessly while watching TV, oblivious of how much they are consuming.

Computers

Another opportunity for children and adults to spend hours in a sedentary activity is provided by computers. Talking to friends, playing games, and ordering items online, from groceries to cars, are just a few computer activities that would previously have involved some physical activity. A recent survey found that people find time to use the Internet by reducing the time they spend watching television, working, and exercising.[24]

Dieting and Obesity

Contributing to the obesity trend is the "yo-yo dieting" effect, or **weight cycling.** People frustrated with their weight often turn to fad diets in hopes of finding a solution. Fad diets do not consist of realistic food plans that can be maintained for a lifetime. People who follow fad diets drastically alter their eating patterns as part of the program, cutting calories and altering the balance of carbohydrates, proteins, and fats. They may lose weight initially, but most find it difficult to maintain the harsh restrictions and thus go off the diet and return to their previous eating patterns (usually a higher caloric intake). With rapid weight loss on a highly restrictive diet, the body can enter starvation mode, with a physiological response of decreased basal metabolic rate. When a person goes off the restrictive diet, he or she rapidly gains back the weight lost and sometimes gains even more before the body's metabolism readjusts.

The Stress Response

One of the health consequences of stress is that it affects eating patterns, which can lead to significant weight abnormalities. In response to stress, our bodies release several hormones (see Chapter 5), including **adrenaline** (also called epinephrine) and cortisol. Fat cells have receptors for both hormones, and they both release fatty acids and triglycerides in response to stress as well as increase the amount of circulating glucose.

These responses are vital in enabling the body to handle acute stress, especially physical stress. They give you the energy to run away or fight if you are being threatened. But when stress is chronic, the constant presence of these hormones can lead to problems. They can influence fat deposits, increasing the amount of fat deposited in the abdomen. Abdominal fat, as explained earlier, is more closely associated with heart disease risk. The stress response also affects eating patterns. Adrenaline is an appetite suppressant, whereas cortisol stimulates the appetite.

THE KEY TO WEIGHT CONTROL: ENERGY BALANCE

The relationship between the calories you take in and the calories you expend is known as **energy balance.** If you take in more calories than you use through metabolism and movement (a negative energy balance), you store these extra calories in the form of body fat, your body's main reserve for potential energy. If you take in fewer calories than you need (a positive energy balance), you draw on body fat stores to provide energy. Energy in must equal energy out in order to maintain your current weight. If you adjust one or the other side of the equation, you will gain or lose weight (Figure 9.3).

Estimating Your Daily Energy Requirements

In Chapter 7 we discussed energy intake, the calories-in side of the energy equation. Here, we are more interested in energy expenditure, the calories-out side. Components of energy expenditure include physical activity, the thermic effect of food, adaptive thermogenesis, and basal metabolic rate.

The **thermic effect of food** is an estimate of the energy required to process the food you eat. This energy is used in chewing and digesting food and in absorbing, transporting, metabolizing, and storing the energy and nutrients you get from it. The thermic effect of food is generally estimated at 10 percent of energy intake. If, for example, you ingested 2,500 calories of food during a day, the thermic effect of this food would be 250 calories—you would burn 250 calories processing what you ate. Meal size, frequency, and composition affect the thermic effect of food. Generally, processing high-carbohydrate foods burns more calories than does processing high-fat foods, and processing a meal eaten all at once burns more calories than when foods are consumed over a few hours.[7] **Adaptive thermogenesis** takes into account the fact that your baseline energy ex-

Figure 9.3   Balancing calories in with calories out.

penditure varies with changes in the environment, such as in response to cold, or with physiological events, such as trauma, overeating, and changes in hormonal status.

Basal metabolic rate (BMR) is the rate at which the body uses energy to maintain basic life functions, such as digestion, respiration, and temperature regulation. About 70 percent of energy consumed is used for these basic metabolic functions, with the brain accounting for about 20 percent, the liver for 20 percent, the heart 10 percent, the kidneys 10 percent, and digestion 7 percent to 10 percent.[25] BMR is affected by several factors, including age, gender, and weight (Table 9.2). Ten percent to 30 percent of the calories consumed each day are used for physical activity.

You can estimate your daily energy expenditure by considering (1) the energy spent on basal metabolic rate, (2) the energy spent on physical activities, and (3) the thermic effect of food. The effects of adaptive thermogenesis on basal metabolic rate are not usually taken into account except in extreme situations, such as severe injury or prolonged illness. To estimate your daily energy expenditure, complete the Add It Up! activity at the end of this chapter.

After the age of 25, BMR decreases by 2–3 percent per decade. Percentage of body fat, on the other hand, commonly increases with age, also by 2–3 percent per decade.[10] The change in body composition is caused by a combination of hormonal changes that affect metabolism and a decline in general physical activity. By the age of 65, if you have not taken measures to preserve lean tissue (muscle), the number of calories expended on basal metabolism will have decreased significantly from the num-ber of calories expended on basal metabolism at age 25. Endurance and strength-building activities can help counter this trend and preserve lean muscle tissue.

Adjusting Your Caloric Intake

Dietary guidelines recommend that if you are trying to lose weight, a reasonable weight loss of 1 pound to 2 pounds per week is a healthy goal. Because a pound of

KEY TERMS

weight cycling   Repeated cycles of weight loss and weight gain as a result of dieting; sometimes called yo-yo dieting.

adrenaline   Stress hormone that suppresses ap-petite, among other effects.

energy balance   Relationship between caloric in-take (in the form of food) and caloric output (in the form of metabolism and activity).

thermic effect of food   Estimate of the energy re-quired to process the food you eat.

adaptive thermogenesis   Adjustments in energy use in response to changes in the external environ-ment and to internal physiological events.

basal metabolic rate (BMR)   Rate at which our bodies use energy for basic life functions, such as breathing, circulation, and temperature regulation.

Challenges & Choices

Calculating Your Fat Budget

How much fat can you eat in a day as part of a healthy diet? The calculation is simple:

1. First, take your ideal daily caloric intake, starting with the exact intake that you would need to balance your daily energy expenditure. (Calculate this number in the Add It Up! activity at the end of the chapter.) If you are trying to lose weight, you can further reduce the number so you have an energy deficit. Because safe weight loss doesn't exceed 2 pounds per week and it takes a deficit of about 3,500 calories to lose a pound of fat, don't decrease your total intake by more than 500–1,000 calories per day or below a threshold of about 1,000 calories per day.

    Ideal calorie intake: _____

2. Now, multiply your ideal caloric intake by your desired percentage of calories from fat (for example, 0.2 for 20 percent or 0.3 for 30 percent of calories from fat). The American Heart Association and American Dietetic Association both currently recommend no more than 30 percent of calories from fat and no more than a third of those from saturated fat.

    Desired fat calories: _____

3. Divide by 9 (the number of calories in a gram of fat). This is your daily fat budget in grams.

    Daily fat grams: _____

Use this number and the information on fat labels to plan your daily menu. You can go over on some days as long as your intake over several days averages out to no more than your daily budget.

It's Not Just Personal . . .

Although most experts recommend limiting fats to 30 percent of calories consumed—in a 2,000-calorie diet, about 66 grams of fat—many Americans consume 40 percent of their calories from fat—in a 2,000-calorie diet, about 88 grams of fat.

body fat stores about 3,500 calories, you will need to decrease your total calorie intake for the week by 3,500 calories in order to lose 1 pound per week. Weight loss beyond these guidelines tends to include loss of lean tissue like muscle. Additionally, diets too low in calories may not provide enough nutrients.

Reducing your intake of fat is also important. A high fat intake leads to higher caloric intake and is linked with obesity. As discussed in Chapter 7, fat contains 9 calories per gram, and carbohydrates and proteins contain only 4 calories per gram, so calorie intake is considerably higher if you eat a gram of high-fat food compared to a gram of low-fat food (see the box "Calculating Your Fat Budget"). Excess energy intake encourages fat storage. High-carbohydrate foods also have a greater thermic effect than high-fat foods do. Thus, it takes more energy to process a high-carbohydrate diet, and less of the food's energy is available for storage as fat.[7]

Table 9.2   Factors Affecting Basal Metabolic Rate

Factor	Effect on BMR
Age	BMR decreases 2–3% per decade after age 25.
Height	Tall, thin people have higher BMRs.
Growth	Children and pregnant women have higher BMRs.
Stress	Stresses from disease and medications can raise BMR.
Environmental temperature	Heat and cold raise BMR.
Fasting/starvation	Lower BMR.
Malnutrition	Lowers BMR.
Smoking	Raises BMR.
Caffeine	Raises BMR.
Body composition	Lean tissue turns toward fat at a 2–3% rate per decade after age 25, lowering BMR.

QUICK FIXES FOR OVERWEIGHT AND OBESITY

Time is a major issue for most Americans, and few of us feel we have extra time to devote to nutrition and exercise. Most of us would love a quick and easy way to stay at a healthy body weight. You can find the latest recommendations for losing 30 pounds quickly by reading magazines and diet books, but do these fads work? Are they healthy? Are they worth the money?

The Diet Industry

The diet industry has done an excellent job of catering to the hopes of people who want to lose weight. From self-help books, to celebrity diets, to "fat farms," to pills, there is something to appeal to everyone. Americans pay an estimated $40 billion for the diet industry's quick fixes.[26] Two prominent players in this field are fad diets and weight management organizations.

Fad Diets

Every year, "new and improved" fad diets seduce consumers despite the fact that their safety and effectiveness are often unproven. No matter what the latest title, fad diets follow a pattern of altering the balance of carbohydrates, protein, and fat with the goal of promoting weight loss.

Perhaps the most famous of recent fad diets is the Atkins diet, developed by Dr. Robert Atkins. A detailed description of this diet is provided in the book *Dr. Atkins' New Diet Revolution,* which was on the *New York Times* bestseller list for more than 100 weeks. The Atkins diet advocates eating all the fat and protein you want while severely limiting carbohydrates. Less extreme low-carbohydrate diets, such as the South Beach diet, have grown in popularity as enthusiasm for the Atkins diet has waned, particularly after the death of Dr. Atkins in 2003 and the bankruptcy of his company in 2005.

The premise behind low-carbohydrate diets is that cutting down on carbohydrates will decrease blood sugar levels, which will in turn cause the pancreas to produce less insulin. With less insulin available, the body is forced to burn fat reserves for energy, thus leading to a weight loss. Opponents argue that cause and effect have been reversed: Excess insulin is caused not by eating too many carbohydrates but by being too fat. They propose that people lose weight on low-carbohydrate diets simply because they are cutting out an entire food group and thus reducing their total caloric intake. Evidence supports the fact that weight loss occurs with a low-carbohydrate diet if total calories are also restricted.[27]

Low-carbohydrate diets remain a popular choice in the United States, but the jury is still out on both their short-term effects (safe weight loss) and their long-term effects (weight maintenance and healthy food choices). Many dietitians and physicians are critical of fad diets in general and instead encourage monitoring energy balance and eating a balanced diet that emphasizes complex carbohydrates.

Weight-Management Organizations

Weight-management organizations offer dietary advice, support groups, exercise counseling, stress management education, and other services. Some of these organizations are associated with hospitals or university wellness

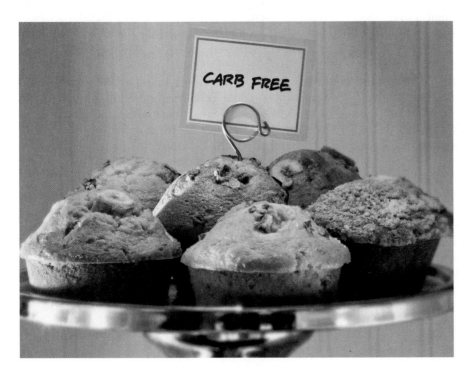

Fad diets, such as low-carbohydrate diets, often claim that if you limit certain types of foods, you'll lose weight. Which typical ingredients would need to be eliminated from muffins to make them "carb-free?" Do you think that "carb-free" muffins are a healthy choice?

programs, and others are commercial. Take Off Pounds Sensibly (TOPS), Weight Watchers, and Overeaters Anonymous are three well-known weight-management organizations. TOPS and Overeaters Anonymous are free and provide group support. TOPS focuses on teaching skills for healthy eating and exercising. Overeater's Anonymous meetings are based on the Alcoholics Anonymous 12-step program and may be more suitable for binge eaters or others with emotional issues related to weight.[28] Weight Watchers is a commercial program that provides social support and education about nutrition, exercise, and behavior management.

There are many other commercial diet organizations, some of which "guarantee" a weight loss of a certain number of pounds that will be kept off indefinitely. Many of these programs claim to be medically supervised, but medical supervision varies widely. You may see a physician for your initial screening and never again, or you may see one at each visit. Prescriptions for diet drugs (discussed in the next section) have also become popular in commercial centers. Remember to be skeptical of unrealistic promises and to use your critical thinking skills when considering weight-management programs. For some tips, see the box "Evaluating a Weight Loss Program."

The Medical Approach

Because obesity is a major risk factor for many health conditions, health centers have been involved in helping people find solutions. We consider three medical strategies used to treat obesity: very-low-calorie diets, diet drugs, and surgical procedures.

Very-Low-Calorie Diets (VLCDs)

An aggressive option for patients with high health risks because of obesity, VLCDs require a physician's supervision. These diets provide a daily intake of 800 calories or less and include at least 1 gram of high-quality protein per kilogram of body weight, little or no fat, and at least 50 grams of carbohydrate. Vitamin and mineral supplementation is provided to ensure sufficient nutrient intakes. Typical meals consist of a limited daily choice of foods (lean meat, fish, poultry), or a prescription powdered formula, or both.

VLCDs provide enough protein to fulfill a patient's daily protein requirements, but they provide little else as an energy source. Since the body needs energy all the time, it breaks down protein and fat stores to provide energy. The proteins release glucose and the fats release ketones, both of which can serve as a source of energy for the brain. Ketones can cause health problems if their levels become too high, so the process must be monitored closely.

VLCDs are used for moderately to severely obese patients (people with BMIs greater than 30) who are highly motivated but have not had success with more conservative

plans. Patients with BMIs of 27 to 30 with medical conditions that could improve with rapid weight loss are also candidates. Weight loss after a 26-week program averages 20 percent of the patient's initial weight. When patients are evaluated 5 years after the program, they seem to maintain a weight loss of only 5 percent.[28]

Prescription Drugs

No drug currently available can ensure permanent weight loss, and finding such a miracle drug is unlikely because of the complex factors that lead to obesity. Some products have been shown to affect weight loss, but the benefits must always be weighed against the potential side effects of any drug. Weight loss drugs are designed to work with lifestyle changes, such as increased physical activity and decreased food intake. Because of the expense, potential for side effects, and need for medical supervision, such drugs are intended for people who are at least 30 percent over their healthy body weight. There are three current categories of weight-loss drugs: appetite suppressants, thermogenic drugs, and fat-blocking drugs.

Appetite Suppressants   People take appetite suppressants to decrease their total caloric intake by decreasing their desire to eat. Amphetamines were once the most widely prescribed appetite suppressant. The continuous use of amphetamines curbs the appetite for about 3 months, but after that time, you must take higher and higher doses to maintain the effect. Before long, a dangerously high dose is needed for the desired effect of appetite suppression. Amphetamines also have addictive potential, so their prescription use in weight control has been discontinued.

Recently, certain appetite suppressants have been developed to take advantage of the fact that the levels of dopamine, serotonin, and norepinephrine in the brain are related to appetite. Drugs that increase the levels of these chemicals have been shown to have weight loss potential. Fenfluramine (part of the popular diet combination Phen-fen) was an effective medication in this category of drug. Fenfluramine was widely prescribed as an aid to weight loss in the 1990s, but when evidence linked it to an increased risk of heart valve abnormalities and primary pulmonary hypertension, the drug was removed from the market. The recall of fenfluramine has left dieters and health providers wary of prescription diet drugs. Phenteramine (the other component of the Phen-fen combination) is still used alone but is not as effective at producing weight loss without fenfluramine.

Sibutramine is an appetite suppressant that is currently approved for weight loss. It results in a weight loss of 3 percent to 8 percent when used as an adjunct to lifestyle modification. Side effects include mild increases in blood pressure, dry mouth, headache, and sleep difficulties.[29]

Consumer Clipboard

Evaluating a Weight Loss Program

If you're looking for a weight loss program, you'll have many choices—from programs that have been around for years to fad diets that come and go. Choosing an approach that is safe and effective starts with doing some research and taking a critical look at what each program offers. The American Heart Association recommends that you consider these points:

- **Diet and nutrition** A food plan that you can live with should take into account your current eating habits and food preferences. If you don't like the foods, chances are good you won't stay with the plan for long.

- **Realistic goals** The program should not promise more than a loss of 1 to 2 pounds per week. Women should eat at least 1,200 calories per day; men should eat at least 1,500 calories per day. Determining a healthy weight for you should be done in consultation with a medical professional.

- **Nutrition education** The focus of the program should be to encourage you to develop a lifetime of healthy eating habits. You should be working with a medical professional to individualize meal planning.

- **Physical activity** Promoting physical activitiy, such as walking, should be one of the highest priorities of the program. Participants without any health restrictions should be encouraged to get 30 to 60 minutes of moderate physical activity most days of the week.

- **Behavior modification** The approach to weight loss should be individualized, taking into account which of your habits need to be changed. Support group help should be offered.

Here are some red flags to watch out for:

- **Miracle foods that burn fat** Your body stores extra food as fat. Foods don't burn fat. You can burn fat by increasing your physical activity, decreasing the amount of food you eat, or doing both.

- **Bizarre quantities of only one food or food type** Eating only beef or tomatoes one day or unlimited amounts of grapefruit or cabbage soup doesn't make good nutritional sense. These foods are fine as part of an overall healthy diet, but eating them in large quantities or to the exclusion of other foods can lead to serious nutritional imbalances and unpleasant side effects.

- **Specific food combinations** There's no scientific evidence that eating foods in certain combinations or sequences aids in long-term weight loss.

- **No health warnings** If the weight loss program is a reputable one, it will issue warnings for people with diabetes or high blood pressure to consult with their physician before starting the program.

- **Easy access to prescription drugs** Prescription drugs for weight loss should be used only by individuals who are more than 20% over their ideal weight—and then only under close medical supervision. Many of these drugs can produce serious side effects.

- **Liquid diets** These diets don't teach you how to eat in a healthy way. Even though they may "work" in the short term, they're not a real solution to a weight problem.

If you're still wondering which way to go, discuss your situation with your health care professional. In fact, a good weight loss program will suggest that you do just that.

Source: AHA Guidelines for Selecting a Weight Loss and Maintenance Program, 2005, www.americanheart.org.

Thermogenic Drugs   Thermogenic drugs function as a stimulant to the body, increasing the BMR to produce the same effect as increased energy expenditure. Ephedrine and caffeine fall into this category. These drugs can cause shakiness, dizziness, and sleeping difficulties. Currently, no thermogenic drugs are approved for weight loss.

Fat-Blocking Drugs   This category of drugs reduces the absorption of dietary fat by the body. The breakthrough drug in this area is Orlistat, which works by inhibiting the action of *lipases,* enzymes that break down fat in the stomach and intestines. While you are taking Orlistat, digestion of the fat you eat is reduced by about 30 percent. The undigested fat passes through your body. The use of Orlistat leads to an average weight loss of 8 percent to 10 percent of initial body weight within 6 months. With continued use, the weight loss is maintained at 2 years. Orlistat also has a positive effect on blood cholesterol levels.

A drawback is that dietary fat is only part of the obesity equation; total caloric intake is also important. Fat-blocking drugs do little to promote changes in food serving size and food choice. In addition, Orlistat has some bothersome side effects, including stomach cramps, gas, and fecal incontinence (leaking stool). The reduction in fat absorption also leads to a loss of fat-soluble vitamins and beta carotene.[29]

Surgical Options

Because of the potential for complications, surgery is never a first-line approach to obesity. The National Institutes of Health has determined that surgical therapy should be considered for patients with a BMI of 40 or greater and a history of failed medical treatments for obesity, or for patients with a BMI of 35 or greater with other illnesses or risk factors.

Three surgical methods for treating obesity are available: gastric restriction, gastric bypass, and gastric banding. **Gastric restriction** is a procedure in which part of the stomach is stapled off, leaving the patient with a smaller stomach. In a **gastric bypass,** a large part of the stomach is stapled off, leaving a small pouch. The small intestine is surgically reconnected so that the pouch empties into the lower part of the small intestine, bypassing the upper part and reducing calorie absorption. Gastric banding is a surgical technique in which a band is placed around the upper part of the stomach, creating a smaller stomach pouch. Some of these surgeries can be performed laparoscopically (through a small instrument inserted into the abdomen). The advantages of the laparoscopic technique are that incisions can be much smaller and the risk of complications from surgery are lower.

The surgical procedures physically limit the amount of food the person can consume at one sitting. A large study evaluating patients undergoing weight loss surgery found that, on average, they lost 62 percent of excess weight. Most patients had significant improvement in or resolution of diabetes, hypertension, and other obesity-related conditions.[30] As with any surgical procedure, side effects can occur at the time of surgery or after surgery. The most serious risk is the development of a blood clot in a leg (due to bed rest at the time of surgery) or a tear in the gastrointestinal tract. Other risks that may develop after the surgery include wound problems (infection), vomiting, heartburn, anemia, and vitamin deficiency.

Nonprescription Diet Drugs and Dietary Supplements

Popular over-the-counter diet drugs and dietary supplements include diet teas, bulking products, starch blockers, diet candies, sugar blockers, and benzocaine. Herbal supplements have also become particularly popular, although data are limited on the effectiveness of these products. With the increased use, some safety concerns have arisen. One example is ephedra, a stimulant drug found in many over-the-counter weight loss supplements. Ephedra can cause cardiac arrhythmia (abnormal hearth rhythm) and even death by constricting blood vessels while increasing the heart rate and speeding up the nervous system. In February 2004, the FDA banned dietary supplements containing ephedra because of the association of this drug with heart attack, stroke, hypertension, and heat stroke. Again, consumers need to use their critical thinking skills when considering the use of any product, including herbal supplements, to help them lose weight.

THE SIZE ACCEPTANCE, NONDIET MOVEMENT

More than 80 million Americans go on diets each year. Their attempts to lose weight rarely succeed in the long run. Nearly 95 percent of people who lose weight while on diets regain the weight within 5 years. These failures in dieting have not kept health professionals from encouraging people to lose weight by dieting. A strong message has been that with the right diet and exercise program, anyone can lose weight.

The size acceptance, nondiet movement started in response to the frustration felt by many people in attempting to lose weight. The approach seeks to decrease negative body image and self-deprecating thoughts and to encourage self-acceptance and healthy eating patterns. The focus of the nondiet movement is on how people who are large can be healthy. The movement is based on six basic tenets.[31]

1. Good health is a state of physical, mental, and social well-being. All people can achieve good health through eating a variety of foods, being physically active, and appreciating their bodies as they are.

2. People come in a variety of shapes and sizes. This should be viewed as a positive characteristic of the human race.

3. There is no ideal body size, body shape, BMI, or body composition that everyone should strive to achieve.

4. Self-esteem and body image are strongly linked. Helping people feel good about their bodies and about who they are can help them achieve and maintain healthy behaviors.

5. Each person is responsible for taking care of his or her body.

6. Appearance stereotyping is wrong. No matter what the weight, all people deserve equal treatment in employment and the media and competent and respectful treatment by health professionals.

Perhaps in response to the nondiet movement, or perhaps in response to the increasing number of obese people, language is beginning to change in the direction of greater acceptance of overweight. Media and advertising describe large women as big-boned, generous-sized, or ample. Clothing manufacturers are downplaying the increasing girth of Americans by adjusting clothing sizes. The Institute of Standards Research in Philadelphia reports that a size 8 dress in 1942 had a 23-inch waist and a 34-inch hip. Today, a size 8 has a 27-inch waist and a 37-inch hip.[32] The movement has also had some political impact: Several states have passed laws against weight discrimination.

The size acceptance movement has made strides in changing health approaches from weight loss to weight management. A positive outcome would be a decrease in yo-yo weight loss and the use of unsustainable fad diets. However, the change in focus could have a negative effect if it does not include some of the important components associated with achieving a healthy body weight. Passionate pleas by the size acceptance movement should not obscure the fact that obesity is a serious medical problem. The goal is to find a balanced approach that combines personal acceptance with promotion of a healthy body composition.

ACHIEVING A HEALTHY BODY WEIGHT AND BODY COMPOSITION FOR LIFE

Obesity is a long-term problem, and it requires long-term solutions. If solutions are not found, we can expect to see not only more chronic health problems, at great personal and societal cost, but also a rise in such negative trends as eating disorders caused by cycles of weight loss followed by weight gain and discrimination toward overweight people that may discourage them from seeking health care and making lifestyle changes.[31] Both individuals and society have roles to play in reversing these trends.

Tasks for Individuals in Sustaining Healthy Body Weight

If your genetics and behavioral history predispose you to being overweight, you can still improve your overall health through moderate lifestyle changes. Weight reduction is not the sole indicator of improved health. The focus needs to be on a healthier lifestyle rather than on weight loss itself. A balanced plan of action includes six key components:

1. A goal of overall health improvement through targeted improvement in selected areas, such as blood pressure, cholesterol level, and blood sugar level.

2. A goal of 60 minutes of moderate-intensity physical activity five times a week. (This can be divided into smaller sections of time throughout the day.)

3. A diet emphasizing fruits and vegetables.

4. Inclusion of peer support groups.

5. Self-acceptance of body size.

6. Follow-up evaluation by a health care professional.

Set Realistic Goals

Research on behavioral management techniques, VLCDs, and drug therapy indicates that most people who lose weight by lifestyle intervention programs regain lost weight within 3 to 5 years. Most people regain weight lost through drug therapy within a single year. This failure to attain lasting weight loss has led the American Dietetic Association (ADA) to restructure the goal of obesity treatment from weight loss alone to weight management.[33] The ADA defines *weight management* as the adoption of sustainable eating and exercise behaviors associated with the reduction of risks for disease and improved feelings of vigor and well-being. The primary goal of weight management is to attain good health through a stable weight. A dieter should establish realistic goals; even small weight losses can significantly improve health status.

The American Health Foundation's Expert Panel on Healthy Weight concurs with the ADA's weight-management approach.[33] A healthy weight target of a BMI between 19 and 25 or a healthier weight goal for people above the target BMI of 25 should be used. A healthy weight goal for a person with a BMI greater than 25 could be to lower BMI by 1 to 2 points, the equivalent of about 10 pounds to 16 pounds below current weight. This amount of weight loss would reduce the obesity-associated risk of disease. The new BMI should remain stable for at least 6 months before any further attempts at weight loss occur. (See the box "Who Is Most Likely to Achieve and Maintain a Healthy Weight?")

Restrict Calories

The proportion of dietary energy from fat in the average American diet has increased during the past 25 years, and the total caloric intake for the average adult has increased by about 6 percent. For most people, some caloric restriction will be required for weight loss. Low-fat menus are generally suggested, because lowering fat also tends to decrease caloric intake. However, if you eat 10 fat-free

KEY TERMS

gastric restriction   Surgical procedure in which part of the stomach is stapled off to decrease its size.

gastric bypass   Surgical procedure in which a large part of the stomach is stapled off to create a small pouch. The small intestine is surgically reconnected to this pouch so that the stomach empties into the lower part of the small intestine, bypassing the upper part and reducing calorie absorption.

Beating the Odds

Who Is Most Likely to Achieve and Maintain a Healthy Weight?

Body mass index is a fairly reliable indication of healthy weight, but it can fluctuate with changes in phase and stage of life. People are often most vulnerable to weight gain during times of transition. Brief profiles of three people are presented here. Which of them do you think is most likely to achieve and maintain a healthy weight?

Eliana is a 30-year-old woman with a BMI of 32. Her diet consists of three meals a day with two small snacks. She follows a healthy diet, consuming lots of fruits and vegetables. She doesn't drink alcohol, smoke, or use drugs. She had her first child 6 months ago and is breast-feeding. She and her husband used to eat out about once a week, but now that they have the baby, they've been eating in more. Before pregnancy, she had a BMI of 25. She has been walking three times a week for 50 minutes with her husband. She feels she has a good support system and feels motivated to get back to her prepregnancy weight.

Austin is a 20-year-old college student with a BMI of 28. He eats two meals a day and tries to follow a high-protein diet, although he does like to snack during the day. He lives in the dorms and on weekends tends to drink up to 10 beers. Before starting college, he had a BMI of 25. He walks to class each day but does not exercise otherwise. Austin enjoys his group of friends; they tend to do a lot of partying together.

Peter is a 40-year-old man with a BMI of 35. He eats three meals a day with a snack late at night. He tries to follow a nutritious diet but tends to go heavy on the carbohydrates, including quite a lot of sugar. He does not drink alcohol or use drugs. Peter is recently divorced and is living alone, although he sees his teenage children on weekends. His BMI has fluctuated from 30 to 37 for the past 20 years. He does not exercise and feels he has a limited support network since his recent divorce.

OLC Web site Visit the **Online Learning Center** at www.mhhe.com/teague1e for comments by the authors.

cookies instead of 3 regular cookies, you have defeated the purpose of a low-fat diet. The real value lies in changing your eating patterns to include foods that are lower in both calories and fat, rather than just trying to limit serving sizes of higher fat and higher calorie foods. To establish healthful eating habits, you have to be aware of nutrition. Many resources are available for learning calorie-counting techniques, and at first you may need to watch labels on food closely to keep track of the total calories until you can trust your instincts.

Many people who want to reduce their calorie intake simply skip meals. Eating regular meals is as important as choosing the healthy contents of these meals. Your body requires a continuous source of energy. Skipping meals can initiate a starvation response when your body receives the signal that food is scarce. To lose weight, you need a slight energy deficit every day. A meal plan that decreases daily caloric intake by about 500 calories is generally advised. To prevent weight gain, a reduction of 50 calories to 100 calories a day may be all that is needed.[34] Start by reducing the empty calories in your diet, such as alcohol, sweets, and soft drinks, and then look at reducing the calories in your diet that come from fat. Your meals should meet the nutritional needs of your body for protein, carbohydrates, fats, vitamins, and minerals. Your meal plan must also be compatible with your lifestyle and financial needs; otherwise you will not be able to maintain it for the long term.

Manage Behavior

Many behavior management tools are available to help you learn new eating and activity patterns. Approaches may incorporate self-monitoring, stress management, and increased physical exercise. The following strategies may help you get started.

1. *Stimulus control.* Detect and respond to environmental cues associated with unhealthy eating habits and physical inactivity. Become conscious of when, where, and why you are eating. For example, if you live in a dorm and eat at night in your room when you study, you may be eating without paying attention to how much you are consuming.

2. *Self-supervision.* Keep a log of the foods you eat and the physical activity you do.

3. *Social support and positive reinforcement.* Recruit others to join you in your healthier eating and exercising habits. Exercise together, encourage each other, and plan nonfood rewards for reaching goals.

4. *Stress management.* Use relaxation techniques, exercise, and problem-solving strategies to handle the stresses in your life, instead of overeating.

5. *Cognitive restructuring.* Moderate your self-defeating thoughts and emotions, redefine your body image, and set realistic goals. Instead of resolving to start running 5 miles a day, set a realistic goal of walking 20 minutes a day.

Once you've achieved a healthy weight, keep up a regular program of physical activity to help maintain that weight level. Find an exercise that you enjoy and make it a part of your life.

Get Active

Physical activity helps in preventing chronic disease and weight gain, in treating obesity, and in maintaining a desirable weight after weight loss. Lean people are more active than obese people are, and regular exercise decreases the odds of weight gain. Physical activity enhances the weight loss achieved through dietary changes, although dietary changes appear to be more effective for initial weight loss. Physical activity is most important in maintaining weight loss. Even without weight loss, the addition of exercise to a daily routine confers health benefits for all people.[35]

As described in Chapter 8, the 2005 *Dietary Guidelines for Americans* recommend 60 minutes of moderate- to vigorous-intensity physical activity on most days of the week to manage body weight and prevent gradual weight gain in adulthood. To sustain weight loss in adulthood, the guidelines recommend 60 minutes to 90 minutes of daily moderate- to vigorous-intensity physical activity. Simple lifestyle changes that increase physical activity and that you can incorporate into your daily routine are the best way to guarantee long-term success, again as noted in Chapter 8. Take the stairs, walk to campus, bicycle to work, dance in the living room to your favorite music—just get up off the couch and move! Of course, more vigorous activity will help even more, but don't get discouraged by the false idea that a brutal exercise regimen is a necessity.

Tasks for Society in Sustaining Healthy Habits

So far we have focused on the individual's role in change, but society has also had an influence on the patterns of obesity in the United States. To change the patterns of the public at large, we need to construct new policies that benefit the health of our society without discriminating against individuals.

Define Obesity as a Chronic Degenerative Disease

A telephone survey conducted by the Centers for Disease Control and Prevention showed that nearly half of obese patients being treated for other conditions had *not* been told by their physicians to lose weight.[36] This was before the publication of the first National Guidelines on Obesity in 1998, which have brought obesity into the spotlight as a major preventable cause of death. Health officials hope that national recognition of the problem will trickle down to health providers and community activists.

Defining obesity as a chronic degenerative disease will help us move away from the "quick fix" mentality. As with any chronic disease, such as hypertension and diabetes, the focus must be on sustainable changes. Programs that combine nutritional education, exercise education, and lifestyle modification may help to promote healthier, more sustainable weight loss.

Extend Health Insurance Coverage to Prevention of Obesity

Medical insurers have been slow to cover all preventive health care, and prevention of obesity is no exception. Although conclusive evidence shows that obesity is associated with risks of multiple medical conditions, few insurance plans currently cover health visits for obesity education or treatment alone. With concern about health care and health care costs rising, we may see changes in the future. Employers and educational institutions can push legislators to make preventive medicine a priority for insurance companies. Individuals too can write to their representatives supporting insurance coverage for preventive medicine.

Healthy People 2010

OBJECTIVE AREA *Nutrition and Overweight*

- Increase the proportion of adults who are at a healthy weight.
- Reduce the proportion of adults who are obese.

"Between 1976 and 1994 the number of cases of obesity . . . increased more than 50 percent—from 14.5 percent of the adult population to 22.5 percent. . . . A concerted public effort will be needed to prevent further increases of overweight and obesity. Health care providers, health plans, and managed care organizations need to be alert to the development of overweight and obesity in their clients and should provide information concerning the associated risks. . . . To lose weight and keep it off, overweight persons will need long-term lifestyle changes in dietary and physical activity patterns that they can easily incorporate into their lives."

 For more information on Healthy People 2010 objectives, visit the Web site at www.healthypeople.gov.

For more information on Canadian health objectives, visit the Health Canada Web site at www.hc-sc.gc.ca/english.

Support Consumer Awareness

In a free society we avoid restricting the media and advertising, but consumers can become more conscious of their effects on eating patterns. Advertising is a supply-and-demand industry. If consumers don't buy the products depicted in ads, or if they complain about the content of ads, food manufacturers will eventually respond.

Parents can also limit children's exposure to media and advertising by limiting television viewing time. When children are encouraged to reduce TV time, they have a more positive attitude toward physical activity. Limiting TV time will also decrease the exposure to junk food advertising and decrease the amount of food consumed in front of the TV set.[20, 22]

Promote Healthy Foods

As noted in Chapter 7, markets in high-income neigborhoods sell more fruits and vegetables; markets in low-income neighborhoods sell more high-fat foods. Experiments have shown that price incentives can have a dramatic effect on food behavior. Lowering the price of low-fat, nutritious foods increases the rate at which people purchase fruits and vegetables.[17] Pricing strategies are a potentially broad-based intervention to alter eating patterns.

School-based programs can educate and promote healthy eating patterns among youth. The U.S. surgeon general has asked that all schools reduce junk food and promote healthy, balanced meals. In order for schools to meet this goal, they need to change the current trend of allowing fast-food options and candy and soda machines to be available in highly accessible locations on school campuses (see Chapter 7).

Support Active Lifestyles Through Community Planning

Continuing suburbanization and a focus on cars have given Americans great individual autonomy, but they have decreased our physical activity. As a society, we need to consider ways to encourage a more active lifestyle. As discussed in Chapter 8, observers have proposed many ideas, including attractive, easily visible stairways as an alternative to elevators; walking areas and parks in all communities; increased public transportation; and employee benefits for bicycling or walking to work.

Although the American girth has steadily grown in the recent past, this trend does not have to continue. People can successfully manage their weight by establishing careful eating habits and integrating physical activity and exercise into their daily routines. A healthy energy balance is the key to attaining lifelong weight control goals. Our communities and society need to support and encourage individuals in making these lifestyle changes.

You Make the Call

Should Schools Screen for Obesity?

In response to the rising tide of obesity among American youth, some elementary, middle, and high schools in the United States have begun screening students for obesity. If a student is identified as overweight or obese on the basis of height and weight, a message is sent home to his or her parents, along with educational information about the benefits of a healthy weight, the risks of obesity, and safe ways to manage weight. The goal is to combat obesity and to improve the health of students.

Proponents of this plan argue that many screening services are currently offered through public schools. Across the country, school-age children are routinely screened for hearing loss and visual impairment. Both of these are medical conditions that can significantly impair a student's ability to learn, and both have treatments that can improve the student's ability to learn. Schools also offer individualized education plans for children with physical or learning disabilities and chronic health conditions. The individualized plans are designed to help all children maximize their learning potential and health. Schools currently have federally funded programs to subsidize school breakfasts and lunches so that all children have adequate nutrition for learning. Each of these represents processes already in place to maximize the health and learning potential of all students.

Proponents also point out that obesity is associated with a number of serious health conditions. If healthy behaviors can be established in childhood, there is a higher likelihood of establishing and maintaining a healthy body weight in adulthood. They see screening as a way to reach this goal.

Opponents of school screening respond that there is no simple solution to overweight, as there is for impaired vision or hearing. Resources available to the child and his or her family for addressing obesity are limited. Currently, health insurance plans do not cover medical visits to prevent or treat overweight or obesity, and schools do not yet have programs designed to work with a child labeled as overweight or obese. Screening would simply stigmatize the overweight or obese child.

Opponents also argue that students would be better served by increasing access to activities that encourage healthy behaviors for all children, such as expanding physical education programs, role-modeling healthy nutrition by reducing access to soda and candy at school, and developing programs to promote healthy lifestyle choices.

Should public schools be involved in weighing and measuring students and notifying parents if their children are overweight or obese? What do you think?

Pros

- Obesity is a major health concern among youth.
- School screening is a way to reach most children and to identify those in need of weight loss.
- Attaining a healthy weight becomes more difficult if a child becomes overweight and stays overweight into adulthood.

Cons

- Obesity is not like other conditions screened for at school; there are no proven or readily available interventions for obesity.
- School screening for obesity may cause students to discriminate against overweight and obese children.
- School screening does little good if there is no follow-up with the family. Many overweight and obese children have parents who are also overweight. The issue is a complex one that needs to be addressed at the family, community, and societal levels, not just at the level of the child.
- Even if overweight or obesity is identified, most insurance plans currently do not pay for weight loss programs or healthier food choices.

OLC Web site For more information about this topic, visit the Online Learning Center at www.mhhe.com/teague1e.

SOURCES: "Pennsylvania to Require Schools to Record BMI of Students," www.eatrightpa.org; Arkansas School BMI Assessment Project, www.cbc.ca/consumers/market/files/health; The School Health Program, www.health.co.hernando.fl.us/school; Should MCPS Put BMI on Report Cards? Yes, Schools Should Fight Obesity, http://silverchips.mbhs.edu.

SUMMARY

- Overweight and obesity are major health concerns in the United States. More than half of all Americans are overweight, and one fifth are obese.

- Obesity is associated with increased risk for high blood pressure, diabetes, high cholesterol, heart disease, stroke, gallbladder disease, osteoarthritis, sleep apnea, lung problems, and some cancers.

- There is no ideal body weight, but there are ranges for healthy body weight.

- Body mass index (BMI) is a single number that represents height-to-weight ratio. A BMI of 18.5 to 25 without any medical conditions associated with a need for weight loss is considered healthy. Individuals with a BMI of 30 or higher are considered obese.

- Percentage of body fat is a measure of body composition, the proportion of body fat to fat-free mass (bones, muscles, and so on). Healthy body fat percentages are 12 percent to 20 percent for men and 20 percent to 30 percent for women.

- Body fat distribution is another important consideration, with "pear" shapes considered healthier than "apple" shapes.

- Genetics influences body weight and composition, but culture also plays a role. Other influences include gender and age, the food environments we inhabit, our sedentary lifestyles, repeated dieting, and stress.

- The key to weight management is energy balance, the relationship between caloric intake and caloric expenditure. A positive energy balance leads to weight loss; a negative balance leads to weight gain. Components of energy expenditure are physical activity, the thermic effect of food, adaptive thermogenesis, and basal metabolic rate, the rate at which energy is used for basic life functions.

- There are no quick fixes for overweight and obesity, but the diet industry and weight management organizations provide advice, support, and education for consumers seeking weight loss. Critical thinking skills are needed in evaluating commercial weight loss programs.

- Medical treatments for weight loss include very-low-calorie diets, surgery, and drugs that decrease appetite or block fat absorption. These options may be recommended for people with immediate health risks related to obesity. Nonprescription drugs and dietary supplements are popular for weight loss but carry some health risks.

- The size acceptance, nondiet movement promotes acceptance of people of all sizes, adoption of healthy behaviors, and rejection of discrimination based on weight.

- Reversing the trend toward obesity is the responsibility of both individuals and society. Individuals can choose healthier lifestyles, and society can adopt policies that benefit health without discriminating against individuals.

REVIEW QUESTIONS

1. What does body mass index measure? What factors are not taken into account by this measure?
2. What methods are used to evaluate body composition?
3. Why is it better to be pear shaped than apple shaped?
4. Why is it difficult to separate the effects of genetics from the effects of environment when investigating the causes of overweight?
5. Describe the differences between males and females in weight gain and weight distribution at different phases of life.
6. What additional meanings does food have in U.S. culture besides providing basic nutritional sustenance?
7. How does television viewing influence obesity patterns?
8. Explain the relationship of weight gain and weight loss to stress.
9. What three components are used to determine daily energy requirements?
10. Why does a higher fat intake result in a higher caloric intake?
11. What are the six key components of a balanced plan of action for weight loss?
12. List several steps society can take to help reverse the obesity trend.

WEB RESOURCES

American Diabetes Association: Highlighting diabetes prevention, this organization offers information about weight loss and exercise through its healthy recipes, tip sheets, and brochures. www.diabetes.org

American Heart Association: This site is a good resource for links to articles on weight loss and weight management, featuring topics such as fad diets. www.americanheart.org

Ask the Dietitian/Overweight: The Q&As on this site focus on real-life weight issues, offering tips on motivation, dealing with setbacks, and the challenges of lifetime weight management. www.dietitian.com

Calorie Control Council: This site offers an online calorie counter, an exercise calculator, and a BMI calculator. Healthy recipes and a guide to effective weight control are also offered. www.caloriecontrol.org

Centers for Disease Control and Prevention: The CDC information on overweight and obesity includes trends, contributing factors, health consequences, and economic consequences. Recommendations on weight management and various resources

are offered. To view height-weight tables, visit these sites: www.cdc.gov/growthcharts www.cdc.gov

Cyberdiet: This site features a free diet profile and takes you through a guided tour of Dietwatch, which focuses on a personal online plan for eating right, exercising smart, and feeling good. www.cyberdiet.com

U.S. Consumer Gateway/Health: Dieting and Weight Control: This site takes you to several government resources on weight loss and weight management, including dietary guidelines, how to lose weight safely, and finding a weight loss program that will work for you. www.consumer.gov

Weight-Control Information Network (WIN): An information service of the National Institute of Diabetes and Digestive and Kidney Diseases, WIN features government publications and other resources on weight control for adults, children, and pregnant women. http://win.niddk.nih.gov

REFERENCES

1. Centers for Disease Control and Prevention. (2005). U.S. obesity trends 1985–2003. www.cdc.gov.

2. National Center for Health Statistics. (2005). Prevalence of overweight among children and adolescents: United States 1999–2002. www.cdc.gov.

3. Hay, W., et al. (2003). Current pediatric diagnosis and treatment (16th ed.). New York: McGraw-Hill/Appleton & Lange.

4. Mokdad, A. H., Ford, E. S., Bowman, B. A., et al. (2003). Prevalence of obesity, diabetes, and obesity related health risk factors, 2001. *Journal of the American Medical Association, 289,* 76–79.

5. Must, A., Spadano, J., Coakley, E. H., Field, A. E., Colditz, G., & Dietz, W. H. (1999). The disease burden associated with overweight and obesity. *Journal of the American Medical Association, 282,* 1523–1529.

6. Mokdad, A. H., Marks, J. S., Stroup, D. F., & Gerberding, J. L. (2004). Actual causes of death in the United States, 2000. *Journal of the American Medical Association, 291,* 1238–1245.

7. Whitney, E. D., & Rolfes, S. R. (2002). *Understanding nutrition* (9th ed.). Belmont, CA: Wadsworth Publishing.

8. National Heart, Lung, and Blood Institute. (1998). Clinical guidelines on the identification, evaluation and treatment of overweight and obesity in adults: The evidence report. Rockville, MD: National Institutes of Health.

9. Flegal, K. M., Graubard, B. I., Williamson, D. F., & Gail, M. H. (2005). Excess deaths associated with underweight, overweight, and obesity. *Journal of the American Medical Association, 293* (15), 1861–1867.

10. Bray, G. A., Bouchard, C., & James, W. P. T. (Eds.). (1998). *Handbook of obesity.* New York: Marcel Dekker.

11. Gallagher, D., Heymsfield, S. B., Heo, M., Jebb, S. A., et al. (2000). Healthy percent body fat ranges: An approach for developing guidelines. *American Journal of Clinical Nutrition, 72,* 694–701.

12. Bray, G. A. (2003). *An atlas of obesity and weight control.* New York: The Parthenon Publishing Group.

13. Farooqi, I. S., & O'Rahilly, S. (2004). Monogenic human obesity syndromes. *Recent Progress in Hormone Research.* 59, 409–424.

14. Bray, G. (1997). Obesity. In A. S. Fauci, et al. (Eds.), *Harrison's principles of internal medicine,* 14th ed. (pp. 454–462). New York: McGraw-Hill.

15. Gordon-Larsen, P., Nelson, M. C., & Popkin, B. M. (2004). Longitudinal physical activity and sedentary behavior trends: Adolescence through adulthood. *American Journal of Preventive Medicine, 27* (4), 277–283.

16. Gunderson, E., & Abrams, B. (2000). Epidemiology of gestational weight gain and body weight changes after pregnancy. *Epidemiology Reviews, 22* (2), 261–274.

17. French, S. A., Strory, M., & Jeffery, R. W. (2001). Environmental influences on eating and physical activity. *Annual Reviews of Public Health, 22,* 309–335.

18. Drewnowski, A., & Specter, S. E. (2004). Poverty and obesity: The role of energy density and energy costs. *American Journal of Clinical Nutrition, 79* (1), 6–16.

19. Nielsen, S. J., & Popkin, B. M. (2003). Patterns and trends in food portion sizes 1977–1998. *Journal of the American Medical Association, 289,* 450–453.

20. Dietz, W. H., & Gortmaker, S. L. (2001). Preventing obesity in children and adolescents. *Annual Reviews of Public Health, 22,* 337–353.

21. Frank, L. D., Andresen, M. A., & Schmid, T. L. (2004). Obesity relationship with community design, physical activity and time spent in cars. *American Journal of Preventive Medicine, 27* (2), 87–96.

22. Hu, F. B., et al. (2003). Television watching and other sedentary behaviors in relation to risk of obesity and Type 2 diabetes mellitus in women. *Journal of the American Medical Association, 289* (14), 1729–1880.

23. Marshall, S. J., Biddle, S. H., Gorely, T., et al. Relationship between media use, body fatness and physical activity in children and youth: A meta analysis. *International Journal of Obesity and Related Metabolic Disorders, 28* (10), 1238–1246.

24. Carlos Poston, W., & Foreyt, J. P. (1999). Obesity is an environmental issue. *Atherosclerosis, 146,* 201–209.

25. Lambert, C. (2004, May-June). The way we eat now. *Harvard Magazine.*

26. Sherrid, P. (2003, June 16). Piling on the profit. Health and medicine. *US News & World Report.*

27. Astrup, A., Meinert Larsen, T., & Harper, A. (2004). Atkins and other low-carbohydrate diets: Hoax or an effective tool for weight loss? *Lancet, 364* (9437), 897–899.

28. Andersen, D. A., & Wadden, T. A. (1999). Treating the obese patient. *Archives of Family Medicine, 8,* 156–167.

29. Weigle, D. S. (2003). Pharmocological therapy of obesity: Past, present, and future. *Journal of Clinical Endocrinology and Metabolism, 88* (6), 2462–2469.

30. Buchwald, H., Andor, Y., Braunwald, E., et al. (2004). Bariatric surgery: A systematic review and meta-analysis. *Journal of the American Medical Association, 292* (14), 1724–1737.

31. Spark, A. (2001). Health at any size: The self-acceptance non-diet movement. *Journal of the American Medical Association, 56* (2), 69–72.

32. Fumento, M. (1998). *The fat of the land: Our health crisis and how overweight Americans can help themselves.* New York: Viking-Penguin.

33. Position of the American Dietetic Association: Weight Management. (1999). www.eatright.org.

34. U.S. Department of Agriculture. (2005). 2005 *Dietary guidelines for Americans.* www.health.gov/dietaryguidelines.

35. McInnis, K. J., Franklin, B. A., & Rippe, J. M. (2003, March 15). Counseling for physical activity in overweight and obese patients. *American Family Physician.*

36. Galuska, A., et al. (1999). Are health care professionals advising obese patients to lose weight? *Journal of the American Medical Association, 282* (1), 1576–1578.

Add It Up! WHAT ARE YOUR DAILY ENERGY NEEDS?

You can estimate your daily energy needs by (1) determining your BMR and (2) determining your energy expenditure above BMR from physical activity. Combining the two numbers gives you your total daily energy requirements.

1. First, estimate your BMR, the minimum energy required to maintain your body's functions at rest. Begin by converting your weight in pounds to weight in kilograms. Then multiply by the BMR factor, which is estimated at 1.0 calories/kg/hour for men and 0.9 for women. Then multiply by 24 hours to get your daily energy needs from BMR.

    Let's look at Gary, a 30-year-old, 180-pound man.

$$\frac{180 \text{ lb}}{2.2 \text{ lb/kg}} = 82 \text{ kg}$$

$$82 \text{ kg} \times 1 \text{ calories/kg/hour} = 82 \text{ calories/hour}$$

$$82 \text{ calories/hour} \times 24 \text{ hours/day} = 1{,}968 \text{ calories/day}$$

Gary's BMR—the energy he uses every day just to stay alive—is 1,968 calories.

Now let's look at Lisa, a 24-year-old 115-pound woman.

$$\frac{115 \text{ lb}}{2.2 \text{ lb/kg}} = 52 \text{ kg}$$

$$52 \text{ kg} \times 0.9 \text{ calories/kg/hour} = 47 \text{ calories/hour}$$

$$47 \text{ calories/hour} \times 24 \text{ hours/day} = 1{,}128 \text{ calories/day}$$

Lisa's BMR is 1,128 calories per day.
Now calculate your own BMR.

Your weight in lbs _____ /2.2 lb/ = _____ kg

_____ kg × 1 (men) = _____ calories/hour

_____ kg × 0.9 (women) = _____ calories/hour

_____ calories/hour × 24 = _____ calories/day

2. Next, estimate your voluntary muscle activity level. The following table gives approximations according to the amount of muscular work you typically perform in a day. To select the category appropriate for you, think in terms of muscle use, not just activity.

Lifestyle	BMR Factor
Sedentary (mostly sitting)	0.4–0.5
Lightly active lifestyles (such as a student)	0.55–0.65
Moderately active (such as a nurse)	0.65–0.7
Highly active (such as a bicycle messenger or an athlete)	0.75–1

A certain amount of honest guesswork is necessary. If you have a sedentary job but walk or bicycle to work every day, you could change your classification to lightly active (or even higher, depending on distance). If you have a moderately active job but spend all your leisure time on the couch, consider downgrading your classification to lightly active. Competitive athletes in training may actually need to increase the factor above 1.

Let's assume that Gary works in an office. He does walk around to talk to coworkers, go to the cafeteria for lunch, make photocopies, and do other everyday activities. We'll assess his lifestyle as sedentary but on the high side of activity for that category, say 0.5. To estimate Gary's energy expenditure above BMR, we multiply his BMR by this factor:

$$1{,}968 \text{ calories/day} \times 0.50 = 984 \text{ calories/day}$$

Let's assume that Lisa works as a stock clerk in a computer store. She spends a lot of time walking around and sometimes lifts fairly heavy merchandise. She doesn't own a car and rides her bike several miles to and from work each day and also for many errands, so she's at the high end of moderately active, say 0.7. To estimate Lisa's energy expenditure above BMR, we multiply her BMR by this factor:

$$1{,}128 \text{ calories/day} \times 0.70 = 790 \text{ calories/day}$$

Note that although Lisa is much more active than Gary, she uses less energy because of her lower body weight.

Now calculate your own estimated energy expenditure from physical activity.

_____ calories/day × BMR factor _____ =

_____ calories/day

3. To find your total daily energy needs, add your BMR and your estimated energy expenditure.

For Gary, this is
1,968 calories/day + 984 calories/day
= 2,952 calories/day

For Lisa, it is
1,128 calories/day + 790 calories/day
= 1,918 calories/day

Because several estimates are used in this method, total daily energy needs should be expressed as a 100-calorie range roughly centered on the final calculated value, which would be about 2,900–3,000 calories/day for Gary and about 1,870–1,970 calories/day for Lisa.

Now calculate your total daily energy needs.

BMR calories/day _____ + physical activity

calories/day _____ = _____ total calories/day

Finally, compare your daily energy needs with your daily calorie intake.

Your daily energy needs: _____

Your daily calorie intake: _____

Remember, if you want to lose weight, you need to take in less energy than you use up. You can shift the balance by increasing your activity level or decreasing your food intake. Moderate changes in both intake and activity level are the safest way to lose weight.

CHAPTER 10

Body Image: Viewing Yourself

DID YOU KNOW?

- As the ideal body image promoted for women becomes thinner, the rates of dieting and the incidence of eating disorders both increase. In the last 30 years, the number of diagnosed eating disorders in the United States has doubled. Eating disorders currently affect about 5 to 10 million women and 1 million men in the United States.

- If you have ever starved yourself to fit into a new pair of jeans or to make the cut on an athletic team, you are one of millions of people who have engaged in disordered eating behaviors at some point in their lives. In an unknown number of cases, disordered eating patterns escalate into full-blown eating disorders.

- An individual with anorexia may think she looks fat while she is actually starving herself to death. Anorexia has the highest death rate of any psychiatric disorder, about 10 percent.

OLC *Your Health Today*   www.mhhe.com/teague1e

Go to the Online Learning Center for *Your Health Today* for interactive activities, quizzes, flashcards, Web links, and more resources related to this chapter.

How do you evaluate how you look and decide whether it is acceptable? Your goal for appearance usually reflects the values of society and is shaped by family, peers, language, advertising, and the media, among other influences. In other words, it is a cultural ideal. Very often, such ideals are quite different from most people's natural appearance, and for some, the discrepancy can produce feelings of inadequacy, dissatisfaction, and self-criticism. For others, it can lead to a resolve to reach the ideal, no matter how unrealistic the goal or unhealthy the means. And for a few, it leads to a quest for perfection that results in psychological illness.

Chapter 9 focused on the current problem of overweight and obesity in U.S. society, and we explored ways to achieve and maintain a healthy body weight and body composition. This chapter considers the other side of the coin—society's obsession with thinness and dieting and the corresponding prevalence of eating disorders. The message about attaining a healthy body weight has to be balanced with a message about developing a healthy body image, setting realistic goals, and maintaining emotional well-being.

We begin this chapter with an exploration of the forces and influences that shape body image in our culture. We focus particularly on women's drive to be thin and men's drive to be muscular. We then look at the most common eating disorders—anorexia, bulimia, and binge-eating disorder—as well as other disorders related to body image, exploring how they are diagnosed, how they affect health, and how they can be treated. We close with an examination of various ways to raise awareness of these disorders and to prevent them.

WHAT SHAPES BODY IMAGE?

Like all ideas, values, attitudes, and beliefs, **body image**—the mental representation that a person has of his or her own body, including perceptions, attitudes, thoughts, and emotions—is strongly influenced by culture. U.S. culture places a premium on appearance, especially for women but increasingly for men. Every day we see hundreds of images and messages about how we should look, whether we are reading a magazine, seeing a movie, noticing ads in public places, or watching television in the privacy of our homes. The advertising industry and the media are relentless in selling the American consumer an image of the ideal body, and many of us buy into what they are selling. The message of the media is powerful.

Women and Body Image

For girls and women, beauty has long been held up as a desirable trait. Pioneering English feminist Mary Wollstonecraft pointed out back in 1792 that women would submit to anything to reach the ideal of beauty, even giving up the right to think for themselves. Repeated cycles of feminist thinking and activism over the last two centuries have attempted to change the message society sends to women and to free women from their obsession with the body.

Current Cultural Messages

Today, women have many more educational and occupational opportunities than ever before, and they fulfill a broad range of valued roles in society. Despite progress in many areas of women's rights, however, our culture still tells women that their most important job is to be beautiful. From infancy onward, when baby girls are described as "delicate," "soft," and "pretty," females are encouraged to define themselves in terms of their bodies. The female body continues to be portrayed by the media as an object of desire, and this objectification reinforces women's focus on their appearance. The media place a heavy emphasis on women's physical attributes rather than on their abilities, performance, or accomplishments.

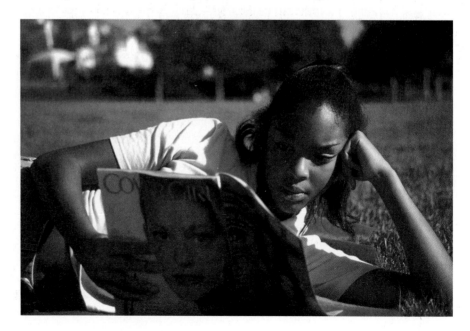

In their preteen years, girls are often influenced by the ideal of being model-thin. The "perfect body" shown in the media is perceived as the norm rather than the exception it actually is.

For the past 50 years, what is held to be the ideal female body in U.S. culture has been getting thinner. It is well known that actresses and beauty queens of the 1940s and 1950s had much more ample proportions than female movie stars and models do today. Marilyn Monroe wore a size 14 dress, for example, compared with the typical size 4 or 6 fashion model of today. Models and actresses now have about 10 percent less body fat than Monroe did and about 12 to 15 percent less than the average healthy woman. Many girls and women aspire to the weight and shape of the super-thin fashion model. Unfortunately, the average fashion model is thinner than 98 percent of all American women.[1] Models represent a tiny subset of the population but provide an unattainable goal for millions.

It is not surprising, then, that women experience high levels of dissatisfaction with their bodies. Women's magazines promote the ideal of thinness and provide advice on how to attain it. Magazines directed toward young women contain 10 times as many articles and advertisements that emphasize thinness as do magazines directed toward young men. These magazines can leave women feeling inadequate, preoccupied with a desire to be thin, unhappy with their own bodies, and afraid of becoming fat. Studies show that after women view media images of thin women, they are less satisfied with their own bodies than they are after viewing images of average-sized women.[2–4]

Striving for thinness often leads to a decision to diet, and dieting can sometimes lead to disordered eating behaviors, such as severely restricting calorie intake and getting rid of calories by purging. Disordered eating, in turn, can become compulsive and turn into an eating disorder. Eating disorders occur most often in cultures in which female attractiveness is linked with being thin.

About 90 percent of diagnosed eating disorders occur in women. Are men somehow protected from eating disorders? Are they less exposed to cultural reinforcements of thinness? Or is there a bias in our current medical system against the detection and diagnosis of eating disorders in men? Whatever the reason, women appear much more likely to take to heart the cultural goals of thinness and to have more of a body focus than do men.

Effects of Puberty

Eating disorders are most likely to develop during adolescence. As noted in Chapter 9, hormonal changes cause increases in body fat in girls, especially on the hips, buttocks, and thighs. The percentage of body fat in healthy girls increases from about 12 percent to about 25 percent during puberty. Given the cultural emphasis on thinness, many girls become concerned about their bodies at this time. However, many girls are concerned even before puberty. By sixth grade, twice as many girls as boys consider themselves fat, even though they are not overweight by objective standards. Sixth-grade girls are more likely to

want to lose weight to become thin, whereas boys are more likely to want to gain weight, especially in the upper body, to become more muscular.

Ethnicity and Body Image

Body satisfaction is also affected by one's ethnicity. Caucasian women are reported to have the most body dissatisfaction and the highest rates of eating disturbances. African American women report less body dissatisfaction, fewer weight concerns, and more positive self-image in comparison with Caucasian women.[5] Beauty ideals have been shown to differ between African American women and Caucasian women, with African Americans being more likely to base "looking good" on a certain self-image or style than on body shape or weight.[6] Their more weight-tolerant attitudes are considered a protective factor against eating disorders.

Levels of body dissatisfaction and disordered eating among Asian American women are about equal to those of Caucasian women. The data for Native Americans and Hispanics suggest that their rates are about the same as that of white women. However, Hispanic women report less concern about weight than do Caucasian women.[6] Research suggests that the more a person feels connected to mainstream, white middle-class society or strives to fit into it, the higher the levels of body dissatisfaction and disordered eating. More research is needed to help determine risk factors and protective factors for different ethnic groups. To test your sense of risk factors, see the box "Who Is Most Likely to Maintain a Healthy Body Image?"

Men and Body Image

Male body image has been less affected by cultural expectations and the media than female body image has. Historically, men have been judged by achievement and strength more than by looks. Media and advertising have promoted a masculine image that emphasizes power, performance, and choice for men, focusing on action and performance rather than on appearance. Correspondingly, men are more satisfied with their body size and appearance than women are.

However, men are not immune to body image concerns. Many studies show that males of all ages report body dissatisfaction.[7] Moreover, a new trend seems to be emerging, with men being increasingly drawn into the world of beauty and appearance. Hair, skin, and grooming

KEY TERMS

body image   Mental representation that a person has of his or her own body, including perceptions, attitudes, thoughts, and emotions.

Beating the Odds

Who Is Most Likely to Maintain a Healthy Body Image?

Factors that influence the likelihood of developing a distorted body image in U.S. culture include age, gender, ethnicity, personality characteristics, family characteristics, and genetic and biological factors. Brief profiles of three individuals are presented here. Which of them do you think is most likely to maintain a healthy body image?

Estella is a 16-year-old Caucasian teen who lives at home with her mom. Her parents recently divorced, and she spends weekends with her dad. She runs track and cross-country and gets straight As in school. Estella is 5 feet 6 inches tall, weighs 118 pounds, and has a BMI of 19. She started menstruating 2 years ago and has no health problems.

Lishondra is a 20-year-old African American woman who lives in the dormitory at her university. Her parents are happily married, and, although they live in a different state, she talks to them weekly by phone. She does well in school, maintaining a 3.25 grade point average. She runs daily for fun and fitness. Lishondra is 5 feet 6 inches tall, weighs 130 pounds, and has a BMI of 21. She started menstruating at age 11 and has no health problems.

Amelia is an 18-year-old Caucasian student who lives in the dormitory at her college. Her parents are married and live nearby. She has a sister at the same college. Amelia is on a scholarship for gymnastics and has had an ankle injury this year that has kept her from competition. She is 5 feet 2 inches tall, weighs 120 pounds, and has a BMI of 22. She started menstruating at age 13 and has a history of depression.

OLC Web site Visit the **Online Learning Center** at www.mhhe.com/teague1e for comments by the authors.

products directed toward men are making their use of beauty products acceptable, although they are pitched to a masculine image. Words like *musk, wood, spice,* and *surf* are used to describe scents, giving them a manly aura. Product names are chosen to suggest power ("Brut," "The Baron"). Men's fashion magazines have been around since the 1950s, but they are currently growing in popularity. Although their circulation does not approach that of *Playboy* or *Sports Illustrated,* the more fashion-oriented *GQ, Maxim, Young Black Male,* and *Esquire* all have significant male readership. In one survey of 6,000 men aged 18

to 55 asking how they would like to see themselves, three of the six top answers involved appearance: attractive to women, sexy, and good looking. The traditionally active male qualities of assertiveness and decisiveness trailed these responses.[8] The business of promoting body obsession among men has created a market with huge financial potential.

The marketing of the male body image has created an environment in which a man's physique is becoming as important as his possessions and accomplishments. As with women, the ideal male body shape has become more unrealistic, distorted, and extreme. The traditional V-shaped body is still admired, but today's male models have trimmer waists and bulkier biceps. The evolution of G.I. Joe action figures mirrors society's changing preferences. In 1964, G.I. Joe had the physique of an average man in reasonably good shape. By 1992, he had a build that most men could not attain without the use of anabolic steroids. Cartoons, video games, and other action heroes project the same image. Many professional athletes are also often highly muscled (in some cases, as a result of using steroids or other muscle-building and performance-enhancing drugs). Today, a man is expected to have large, well-defined muscles and a rippling abdomen complete with well-defined muscles, called a "six-pack." To attain this goal, many men not only undereat (to reduce body fat and create more muscle definition) but also overtrain and use steroids.

For some men, this unrealistic message about super-sized bodies can lead to a condition known as **muscle dysmorphia** (or muscle dysmorphic disorder; sometimes referred to as "bigorexia"). Men with this condition perceive themselves as being insufficiently massive or muscular in appearance, no matter how bulked up they really are. (Muscle dysmorphia is discussed in more detail in a later section of this chapter.) Some observers suggest that supermuscularity may be one way men believe they can distinguish themselves in a world of increasing gender equality.

About 10 percent of eating disorders are diagnosed in men.[2] There are many speculations about why eating disorders occur less among men. Perhaps the earlier societal focus on male accomplishments rather than physique is protective. As men buy into the cultural quest for physical perfection and pursue unrealistic goals, they may experience feelings of inadequacy, which in turn can lead to dieting and body-building. When asked why they diet, men give four answers that are rarely mentioned by women: (1) to avoid repetition of childhood teasing, (2) to improve sports performance, (3) to avoid weight-related medical problems that their fathers had, and (4) to improve gay relationships.[2]

Eating disorders among men may have been underdiagnosed, perhaps because they have been considered a female problem. For example, the diagnostic criteria for eating disorders include the cessation of menstrual periods.

Health care providers are beginning to take a closer look at the eating patterns of young men and are changing diagnostic criteria to include men and boys. Another factor in low diagnoses is that public discussion of men's anxiety about their bodies has remained a societal taboo. Thus, many men are secretive about their drive to bulk up. An increased rate of eating disorders among men is worrisome because average body fat in men is only about 15 percent of total body mass. Thus, men have less weight to lose before muscle mass starts to decrease.

Sports and Body Image

Participation in sports confers many health and fitness benefits, including higher levels of self-esteem in both boys and girls. Sports may provide protection against eating disorders by promoting a focus on performance rather than on appearance.[9] However, participation in sports also carries pressure, both from oneself and from coaches, teammates, and parents. High-level athletes often succeed because they have high expectations of themselves, accompanied by varying degrees of perfectionism and compulsiveness. Athletes often learn to disregard signals from their body, including pain, during training. Parents and coaches can directly and indirectly encourage disordered eating by commenting on appearance or performance when a young athlete has lost weight. They can also indirectly foster disordered eating by not recognizing patterns of rapid weight loss.

In some sports, such as wrestling, dance, gymnastics, swimming, cycling, distance running, and horse racing, a premium is placed on leanness. For some participants, the combination of the demands of the sport, pressure from parents and coaches, and their own individual traits can lead to an increased risk for an eating disorder. The risk appears to be greatest for athletes competing at elite levels, such as college teams. A large study evaluating the effects of sports on eating disorders found that women who competed in nonelite sports that do not emphasize leanness had the least risk of developing eating disorders.[7,10]

Body Art

Some people choose to use body art to express their public body image. Tattooing and body piercing, for example, are ways that individuals say something about themselves. The message might be "This is who I am" or "This is who I'd like to be." Like other forms of self-expression, body art is closely tied to an individual's sense of self, which may change over time. If you are thinking about having body art done, consider the health issues involved before making any permanent changes to your body (see the box "Tattooing and Body Piercing").

EATING DISORDERS

Eating disorders are chronic illnesses that jeopardize physical and mental health; they can be life threatening. The key characteristic of eating disorders is a severe disturbance in eating behavior. A second characteristic is a distorted body image. What begins as a diet takes on a life of its own, turning into self-induced starvation or repeated cycles of binging and purging. The most extreme forms of disturbed eating behavior are anorexia nervosa and bulimia nervosa, both of which are classified as psychiatric disorders in the American Psychiatric Association's *Diagnostic and Statistical Manual of Mental Disorders* (*DSM-IV-TR*). Binge eating is not officially classified as a psychiatric disorder, but it shares features with other eating disorders and is considered an area in which further research is needed.

Eating disorders occur primarily among people in Western industrialized countries. They occur in every ethnic, cultural, and socioeconomic group. They appear to become more prevalent when food is abundant and has taken on symbolic meanings, such as comfort, love,

In some sports, athletes must stay below a specified weight to compete in their category. In others, they are pressured by coaches or teammates to keep their weight low as a competitive advantage.

KEY TERMS

muscle dysmorphia Disorder in which a person perceives his body to be underdeveloped no matter how highly developed his muscles really are.

eating disorder Condition characterized by severely disturbed eating behaviors and distorted body image; eating disorders jeopardize physical and psychological health.

Consumer Clipboard

Tattooing and Body Piercing

The ankle tattoos and eyebrow rings you see on campus today may seem like a recent trend, but their roots go back to the Middle Ages, when Crusaders were tattooed with crosses so that they would be given a Christian burial, and to Ancient Egypt, where a pierced navel was a sign of royalty.

Like the clothes you choose to wear, a tattoo or piercing says something about you and becomes a part of your body image. If you're considering getting a tattoo or having a piercing done, review the facts before visiting your local "body art" shop.

Temporary, or decal-type, tattoos are commonly applied to the skin with a moistened piece of cotton and last several days. The color additives used for such tattoos, which should be approved by the FDA for cosmetic use on the skin, sometimes cause allergic reactions. Henna, a natural vegetable coloring, is FDA-approved for use as a hair dye only but not for direct application to the skin as done in tattooing.

Permanent tattooing involves making a puncture wound in the skin and injecting ink deep into the second layer of the skin, called the dermis, to make the tattoo long-lasting. This procedure is usually done with a handheld electric instrument that uses a tube and needle system. Some pain should be expected, and light bleeding may occur.

What are the risks associated with permanent tattooing? The most serious is the risk of infection, which usually results from using a nonsterile needle. Diseases such as hepatitis B or C, HIV/AIDS, and many other infectious diseases can be transmitted this way. Allergic reactions to the inks are rare, but they can be troublesome because it's difficult to remove the pigment that's causing the problem. If you decide that you want to have the tattoo removed later, the process can be painful and may involve several treatments and considerable expense. Removal is commonly done if the result is not satisfactory or the tattoo no longer seems appropriate.

Body piercing involves some of the same risks as tattooing. Certain body sites are more likely to result in problems than others. Piercings of the mouth and nose are often associated with infection because these areas harbor millions of bacteria, and tongue piercings can damage the teeth over time. If you change your mind about body piercing, the worn object can simply be removed. The piercing wound usually remains, and removal can cause scarring.

Both tattooing and body piercing should be approached with caution and careful consideration:

- Find out about the laws in your state related to permanent tattooing. If you're under 18, you may need your parent's consent.

- Get a recommendation from someone you trust. Find out about the experience and credentials of the person who will be performing the procedure.

- Visit the place where the procedure will be done. Is it clean and professional-looking? If possible, watch the procedure you plan to undergo and ask questions.

- Give yourself a 2-week waiting period before making a final decision to have a permanent body change.

Sources: Data from *Human Sexuality: Diversity in Contemporary America* (p. 449) by B. Strong, C. DeVault, B. W. Sayad, and W. Yarber, 2005, New York: McGraw-Hill; "Body Piercing" and "Tattoos" (fact sheets), www.kidshealth.org; "Tattoos and Permanent Makeup," 2004, and "Temporary Tattoos and Henna/Mehndi," 2001, U.S. Food and Drug Administration, www.cfsan.fda.gov.

belonging, fun, and control. They are also more common where being attractive is related to being thin. The frequency of eating disorders appears to be directly related to rates of dieting. In the last 30 years, the number of diagnosed cases in the United States has doubled. Of course, not all people who diet have eating disorders. In fact, using the strict diagnostic criteria proposed by the *DSM-IV-TR*, only about 1 percent of women in the United States have anorexia nervosa and about 3 percent have bulimia nervosa.[11] Rates are estimated to be about the same in Canada.

More common and widespread than eating disorders are **disordered eating behaviors,** such as restrictive dieting and binging and purging, which are not as severe or frequently practiced as those associated with diagnosed disorders. These behaviors may occur in response to emotional stress, an upcoming athletic event, concern about personal appearance, and so on. They may or may not develop into a full-blown eating disorder. The rates of disordered eating in the general population are not known but thought to be much higher than the rates of diagnosed eating disorders.

A person with anorexia nervosa may appear indifferent to food or may even seem repulsed by it. In reality that individual is obsessed by food and lives in fear of becoming fat.

Diagnosing Eating Disorders

As recently as the 1980s the terms *anorexia nervosa* and *bulimia nervosa* were virtually unknown to the general public. Today, disturbed eating patterns have become alarmingly common. In one study, 80 percent of eighth-grade girls thought that starving and purging are acceptable weight control methods.[8] Detecting when someone with disordered eating makes the transition to having an eating disorder is difficult. Guidelines for the diagnosis of eating disorders have been developed to standardize the determination of when abnormal eating and thinking patterns make the transition into disorders. In this section we review the most common eating disorders and their diagnostic criteria.

Anorexia Nervosa

The word *anorexia* is of Greek origin: *an,* which means "lack of," and *orexis,* which means "appetite." However, most people with **anorexia nervosa** do not have a lack of appetite; they are more likely to be obsessed with food. They have an intense fear of gaining weight and a disturbed perception of their body size or image, and they think they can stay in control of their lives by denying themselves food.

The diagnostic criteria for anorexia nervosa outlined in the *DSM-IV-TR* are as follows:[12]

- Refusal to maintain body weight at or above a minimally normal weight for age and height (usually less than 85 percent of expected body weight).

- Intense fear of gaining weight or becoming fat, even though underweight.

- Disturbance in the way in which one's body weight or shape is experienced, undue influence of body

weight or shape on self-evaluation, or denial of the seriousness of the current low body weight.

- Amenorrhea—the absence of at least three consecutive menstrual cycles.

Some people with anorexia control their weight just by severely restricting calories (*restricting type*), and others engage in binge-eating and purging behavior (for example, self-induced vomiting or the misuse of laxatives, diuretics, or enemas; *binge-eating/purging type*). To get a sense of how anorexia plays out in a person's life, see the box "Carmen: A Case of Anorexia Nervosa."

Bulimia Nervosa

The word *bulimia* is of Latin origin and means "hunger of an ox." People with **bulimia nervosa** consume a huge amount of food at one sitting and then use an inappropriate method to get rid of the calories they have

KEY TERMS

disordered eating behaviors Abnormal eating patterns (for example, vomiting, use of laxatives, extreme dieting) that may not fit the rigid diagnostic rules for anorexia or bulimia but affect quality of life.

anorexia nervosa Eating disorder marked by distortion of body image and refusal to maintain a minimally normal body weight.

bulimia nervosa Eating disorder marked by distortion of body image and repeated episodes of binge eating, usually followed by purging in the form of self-induced vomiting, misuse of diuretics or laxatives, excessive exercising, or fasting.

HIGHLIGHT ON HEALTH
Carmen: A Case of Anorexia Nervosa

Carmen had been an outstanding gymnast in high school and was recruited to be on her college gymnastics team. Although she had the small, compact body typical of the sport, she had always been conscious of her weight and how much she ate. At college, though, she started to become concerned about her body after her coach made some disparaging comments about another team member who had put on a few pounds. She very much wanted her coach's approval, so she started watching her weight more carefully and restricting what she ate.

By the middle of freshman year, Carmen seemed to have lost touch with what she really looked like. When she looked in the mirror, she saw a fat body that couldn't possibly belong to a successful gymnast. In reality, Carmen looked more like a walking skeleton. She wasn't taking in enough food to support her body functions, let alone her vigorous training routine. She had also developed some unrealistic thought patterns. She felt that nothing mattered as much as her coach's approval; in fact, she didn't feel worthy of anyone's respect without it. She felt she had to be perfect, and that included being thin. But somehow, she never felt satisfied that she was thin enough—or perfect enough—to stop dieting. She also saw things as black or white with no shades of gray; for example, if she wasn't thin, she was fat.

By spring semester, Carmen had lost a lot of weight and was showing signs of serious illness. She frequently felt dizzy when performing her gymnastic routines and had to stop. She had headaches and felt tired a lot of the time. She stayed home from classes more and more with minor illnesses; she just seemed to catch everything that was going around. She had not menstruated in months. The only symptom that really worried her, though, was that her abdomen seemed more prominent. This was partly because of constipation and bloating and partly because it was such a contrast to her sticklike arms and legs. When Carmen saw her protruding stomach in the mirror, she would become more determined to lose weight.

When Carmen went home for spring break, her parents were shocked by how thin she was. They called their family physician, who immediately told them to bring Carmen in for a physical exam. After talking to Carmen about her body image, her physical symptoms, and her eating patterns, the physician decided that Carmen was starving, despite Carmen's own continued insistence that she was fat. The physician told Carmen and her parents that she had anorexia nervosa and that without immediate hospitalization, her life was in danger. Carmen didn't want to go into the hospital, but her parents convinced her. Once she was there, the treatment team had to get Carmen to work with them in order to stabilize her condition. While the nurses provided her with the nutrition she needed, a psychologist began helping her see that starving herself was not a healthy way to achieve her goals, either in gymnastics or in life.

consumed. People with bulimia also have a disturbed perception of body size and image. Binge-eating and purging behaviors are usually socially isolating. The diagnostic criteria outlined for bulimia nervosa in the *DSM-IV-TR* are as follows:[12]

- Recurrent episodes of binge eating, characterized by both (1) eating, in a discrete period of time (for example, 2 hours), an amount of food that is definitely larger than most people would eat in that period of time, and (2) a sense of lack of control during the episode—a feeling that one cannot stop eating or control what or how much one is eating.
- Recurrent inappropriate compensatory behavior to prevent weight gain, such as self-induced vomiting; misuse of laxatives, diuretics, enemas, or other medications; fasting; or excessive exercise.
- The episodes occur, on average, at least twice a week for 3 months.

- Self-evaluation is unduly influenced by body shape and weight.

The *DSM-IV-TR* distinguishes between people who use purging behaviors to get rid of calories (*purging type*) and those who use fasting or excessive exercise (*nonpurging type*). To get a sense of bulimia, see the box "Lauren: A Case of Bulimia Nervosa."

Binge-Eating Disorder

Eating disorders are often thought of in association with underweight (anorexia) or normal weight (bulimia), but disordered eating patterns can also cause obesity. **Binge-eating disorder** has increasingly been recognized as a psychological disturbance that is associated with obesity.[13] This disorder involves binge-eating behaviors without vomiting or purging. About 10 percent of patients in weight loss clinics are believed to have binge-eating disorder. One quarter of patients seeking treatment are male, although the prevalence and gender distribution in the community are unclear.[14]

HIGHLIGHT ON HEALTH

Lauren: A Case of Bulimia Nervosa

Lauren was a 19-year-old sophomore in college with a healthy weight of 125 pounds. Her friends didn't know why she talked so much about not having any willpower around food, because they always saw her eat normal, or even small, amounts of food in public. But in fact, Lauren did eat a lot. No one saw it because she did it secretly. At night, she would frequently go out alone and buy a pint of ice cream or several hamburgers. On these evenings, it was not uncommon for her to consume 2,000 calories at one sitting. Afterwards, disgusted and panicked by how much she had eaten, Lauren would lock herself in her bathroom, stick her finger down her throat, and vomit everything she had just eaten. Sometimes she would use laxatives to help "get it all out of her system."

Lauren worried a lot about what other people thought of her. She felt that people were watching every bite she took in public and judging her for her lack of willpower. She forced herself to eat sparingly when she was with others and then binged when she was alone in her room. She also had a feeling that there was something missing in her life or in her, but she didn't know what it was. She didn't want to talk to her friends about this sense of inadequacy for fear she would lose their respect. She felt that if she wasn't perfect, she wasn't worthy of anyone's attention or love.

Lauren's teeth gave her a lot of problems. They had spots that were sensitive to heat and cold. She also frequently had heartburn, which she treated with antacids. When she took laxatives, she would often have diarrhea with cramps. She took this to mean that her attempts to clean out her system were working.

Lauren didn't know it, but she wasn't really hiding her problem from her family or friends. When she went home for break, her parents noticed that she seemed withdrawn and that she would get up from the table and go upstairs to the bathroom as soon as she finished a meal. Her roommate noticed that she went out alone at night a lot, and she sometimes found food that Lauren had hidden in their room. She also realized that Lauren was vomiting her food. She contacted Lauren's parents, and together they confronted Lauren with their concerns. Lauren agreed to seek treatment at the student health clinic.

At the clinic, Lauren was diagnosed with bulimia nervosa, but the physician determined that she was not in any immediate danger. As in many cases of bulimia, Lauren's weight was fairly normal, and she didn't have any severe chemical imbalances. Lauren agreed to see a psychotherapist twice a week to address and change her patterns of thinking and behavior.

People with binge-eating disorder have some differences from other obese people. They are more likely to have depression. They have more fluctuations in weight. Treatment for people with binge-eating disorder may need to be different from other obesity treatment programs. Emphasizing patterns of eating and putting less emphasis on dieting can be important.[8] As noted earlier, binge-eating disorder is not officially classified as a psychiatric disorder, but it is included in the *DSM-IV-TR* as an area in which further research is needed. The criteria for this disorder are as follows:[12]

- Recurrent episodes of binge eating, as defined for bulimia.

- The episodes are associated with (1) eating much more rapidly than usual, (2) eating to the point of feeling uncomfortably full, (3) eating large amounts of food when not feeling hungry, (4) eating alone because of being embarrassed by how much one is eating, (5) feeling disgusted with oneself, depressed, or guilty about overeating.

- Marked distress about binge eating.

- The binge eating occurs, on average, at least 2 days a week for 6 months.

- The binge eating is not associated with the regular use of inappropriate compensatory behaviors (purging, fasting, excessive exercise) and does not occur exclusively during the course of anorexia or bulimia.

To get a sense of binge-eating disorder, see the box "Zach: A Case of Binge-Eating Disorder."

Thought Patterns Associated With Eating Disorders

People with eating disorders share many psychological characteristics and patterns of thinking, including the following:[8]

- Low self-esteem
- Self-critical attitude

KEY TERMS

binge-eating disorder   Eating disorder marked by binge-eating behavior without the vomiting or purging of bulimia.

HIGHLIGHT ON HEALTH

Zach: A Case of Binge-Eating Disorder

Zach, a 21-year-old man who was working part-time and going to college, felt a lot of pressure to succeed. He was the first member of his family to attend college, and his parents bragged about him to everyone they knew. Sometimes, however, Zach felt depressed and unable to cope, and then he would find comfort by staying in his apartment and "pigging out." He might eat an entire large pizza in one sitting, followed by an entire box of cookies or a whole cake. Sometimes he wouldn't even bother to heat up his dinner in the microwave; he would just eat it cold. Zach frequently ate until he got so full it was unpleasant, even painful. He felt guilty and ashamed after these binges, but he couldn't seem to stop himself.

Zach had always been slightly overweight, but during his junior year in college he gained 25 pounds in 3 months. He began to feel disgusted with himself and his body and started avoiding people he knew. He noticed how much harder it was to move around and how fast his heart would beat after the slightest exertion. Zach wanted to lose weight but did not believe he had the ability to diet or to stop his food binges. He particularly worried about developing diabetes, which ran in his family, and it was this worry that finally brought him to a weight management program at his college wellness center. By working with experts to develop a sensible exercise and nutrition program, Zach began to take steps to bring his weight back under control.

- Belief in the importance of thinness
- Black-and-white thinking
- Feelings of emptiness
- Desire to be special or unique
- Need for power and control
- Desire for respect and admiration
- Difficulty in expressing feelings
- Need for escape or a safe place
- Lack of coping skills
- Lack of trust in self or others
- Being terrified of failure

Thoughts associated with anorexia and bulimia overlap, and not all of these patterns must be present for a person to have an eating disorder. Many of these patterns are also found in persons with anxiety disorders and mood disorders, such as depression.

The connection between eating disorders and depression and anxiety disorders is complicated. People with anorexia and bulimia frequently report symptoms of depression and anxiety. Family members of people with anorexia also have increased rates of depression and anxiety disorders. In the case of anorexia, diagnosing depression is difficult, because starvation produces some of the same symptoms produced by depression, including changes in sleep patterns, decreases in energy level, and decreases in interest in activities.[15] It is not clear why some people who diet go on to develop eating disorders and others do not, but the roles of depression and anxiety may be significant. Further research is needed in this area; more research is also needed to find new treatment options.

Health Consequences of Eating Disorders

Eating disorders have serious health implications; some short-term problems, such as heart rate abnormalities, can even lead to death. Long-term problems can cause significant disability. Although anorexia and bulimia often overlap, they are associated with slightly different medical problems.

Health Effects of Anorexia

Anorexia nervosa carries the highest death rate of all psychiatric diagnoses—10 percent, according to most studies.[16] The signs and symptoms of anorexia include severe weight loss and an imbalance in electrolytes—chemicals such as calcium and potassium that help conduct electricity in the body. When a person severely restricts calorie intake, the body becomes emaciated, enters starvation mode, and shuts down all unnecessary activity. Blood is directed toward the organs that are most vital in sustaining life, the brain and the heart, and away from all the other organs. The skin becomes dry, cold, and discolored. The kidneys are unable to clear excess fluid from the body, so the abdomen becomes bloated, the legs may become swollen, and constipation develops. In some individuals, a fine, downy hair called lanugo grows on the body. The bones become demineralized and depleted of calcium. Finally, even the brain and heart cannot be protected. Blood pressure decreases and heart rate slows as the body attempts to maintain heart function with minimal activity. With decreased blood flow to the brain and decreased energy stores, the person feels tired and lethargic and has a loss of coordination. The brain can actually decrease in size.

In women, the menstrual cycle becomes erratic or absent. In men, testosterone levels and testicle size decrease. In both men and women, the sex drive declines. Patients with anorexia have an increased risk of infection because of low white blood cell count and low body temperature, both of which interfere with the immune system's ability to fight off pathogens. Eventually, if the pattern of starvation continues, even the heart cannot continue. At this point, irregular heart rhythms can occur, and death may be imminent.

Most of these complications are reversible if the person receives enough calorie replacement. However, some complications do not appear to be reversible, most notably, bone loss. Decreased bone calcium (osteoporosis) is one of the most serious long-term effects of severe calorie restriction. Peak bone density is reached during the adolescent years. After that it remains relatively stable until the middle 30s, when it starts a slow decline. Thus, calorie restriction and low calcium intake in the teens and early 20s have a long-term effect on the bones. Studies of bone density in 20- to 25-year-old women with anorexia have shown them to have the bone strength of 70- to 80-year-old women.[8]

Health Effects of Bulimia

Bulimia is associated more with electrolyte imbalance than with starvation. The binge phase can cause the stomach to enlarge and in some rare cases even burst. Different methods of purging have different health effects. Vomiting causes electrolyte imbalances that can lead to irregular heart rhythms. It can cause inflammation of the esophagus, which manifests as heartburn. It can even cause the esophagus to tear, which results in severe bleeding and requires immediate medical attention. Tooth enamel erodes from frequent contact with stomach acid, and calluses can form on the hand used to induce vomiting.

Laxatives act mainly on the large intestine and can cause abnormalities in the normal function of the intestines, leading to bloating, diarrhea, and abdominal pain. Diuretics cause fluid loss and can affect blood pressure if dehydration occurs. Both methods cause electrolyte imbalance, which can lead to abnormalities in heart functioning.

Health Effects of Binge-Eating Disorder

The health consequences of binge-eating disorder are related primarily to obesity. As discussed in Chapters 8 and 9, obesity is a degenerative chronic health condition that often significantly shortens the life span. Diseases associated with overweight and obesity include cardiorespiratory disease, diabetes, high blood pressure, gallbladder disease, osteoarthritis, sleep apnea, and certain cancers.

Treating Eating Disorders

Aside from osteoporosis, most medical conditions associated with anorexia and bulimia are reversible. Keys to recovery appear to be early intervention, lower incidence of purging behavior, the support and participation of family members and loved ones, and lack of other diagnosed

---

Healthy People 2010

OBJECTIVE AREA *Mental Health Status Improvement*

- Reduce the relapse rates for persons with eating disorders, including anorexia nervosa and bulimia nervosa.

"Studies suggest that from 30 to 50 percent of patients treated successfully in the hospital [for anorexia nervosa] become ill again within 1 year of leaving the hospital. Efforts are underway to develop and test specific interventions that can prevent relapse in these patients. . . . Effective short-term treatments exist for [bulimia nervosa]. . . . Risk for relapse seems to drop after 4 years of being symptom-free."

For more information on the Healthy People 2010 objectives, visit the Web site at www.healthypeople.gov.

For more information on Canadian health objectives, visit the Health Canada Web site at www.hc-sc.gc.ca/english.

---

psychological problems. When patients with anorexia receive appropriate treatment, as many as 76 percent recover fully and 86 percent recover partially.[8] A person is considered to have recovered when weight is restored to within 15 percent of recommended weight. In women, recovery includes the return of regular menstruation and in men, the return to a normal testosterone level.

Recognizing the Problem

The first step toward treatment is the recognition that there is a problem. People with eating disorders often deny that they are ill and refuse treatment.[14] At the heart of many eating disorders is a desire to have a sense of control over one's life, and treatment involves both weight gain and a perceived loss of this control. Health care providers may face the dilemma of wanting to respect a patient's autonomy and wishes and at the same time wanting to provide effective treatment for a potentially life-threatening illness. Friends, roommates, parents, and others who are close to those with eating disorders may also deny that there is a problem or fail to recognize it, because dieting, exercise, and preoccupation with food are so much an accepted part of our culture. (See the boxes "Do You Know Someone With Anorexia?" and "Do You Know Someone With Bulimia?") Treatment is most effective when the patient and family members all recognize the problem and are involved in treatment decisions.

Challenges & Choices

Do You Know Someone With Anorexia?

A person with anorexia will usually deny that he or she is too thin. If you think someone you know has anorexia, you might want to ask someone at your school health center for advice on what to do. Signs of anorexia include the following:

Physiological Signs

- Large weight loss in a short period of time.
- Unusually pale skin.
- Cold body temperature.
- Dizziness or fainting spells.
- Cessation of menstrual periods without an obvious reason (such as pregnancy).

Behavioral Signs

- Fasting or severe dieting.
- Cutting food into tiny bites, counting bites of food, or preparing food for others but refusing to eat.
- Expressing an intense fear of becoming fat despite being painfully thin.
- Staying away from situations where food is available, such as parties.

- Maintaining a harsh, no-excuses exercise regimen.
- Dressing in layers to hide weight loss.
- Binging or purging (vomiting, using laxatives, enemas, or diuretics).

Psychological Signs and Attitude Shifts

- Mood swings.
- Perfectionism.
- Insecurity about abilities despite competence.
- Tendency to judge self-worth by what he or she eats or does not eat.
- Tendency to be withdrawn.

It's Not Just Personal . . .

Studies conducted by the National Association of Anorexia and Associated Eating Disorders indicate that 20 percent of people with anorexia will die prematurely as a result of the disorder. The death rate associated with anorexia is 12 times higher than the death rate from all causes for females aged 15–24.

Components of Treatment

Effective treatment of eating disorders usually involves a multidisciplinary or **multimodality team.** This group of health care providers with different expertise—physician, psychiatrist, psychologist, social worker, nutritionist, nurses—work together to address all areas of a patient's health. The process begins with a medical evaluation, ideally by a trusted health care provider who is familiar with eating disorders.

If severe weight loss or another medical abnormality has occurred, hospitalization may be required while adequate nutrition is restored. During the weight gain phase of treatment, the focus is simply on getting patients to gain enough weight so that the symptoms of starvation will improve. While patients are in a physical crisis, they may find it hard to work on long-term change. If patients do not appear to be in imminent danger, they can usually be treated while living at home.

Once weight is stabilized, the second phase of treatment—including psychotherapy, behavioral relearning and modification, and nutritional rehabilitation and education—can be initiated.[17] Because eating disorders are psychiatric illnesses, the most important part of treatment (aside from weight gain for severely anorexic patients) is psychotherapy. Once the patient has acknowl-

edged that there is a problem, therapy focuses on such issues as low self-esteem and overemphasis on body image and body weight. For bulimia, the use of cognitive behavioral therapy has been effective; this approach focuses on changing specific behaviors and the thought patterns that maintain the behaviors. Nutritional education includes information about healthy eating patterns, normal weight, and nutritional needs. Treatment for eating disorders often involves the entire family.

For individuals with anorexia, two treatment factors seem to be particularly effective. The first is hospitalizing the person long enough so that sufficient weight gain can occur; doing so appears to reduce the risk of readmission and perhaps improve long-term outcomes.[18] The second is maintaining outpatient treatment long enough so that risk of relapse is minimized. Because an eating disorder is a chronic illness, part of treatment is learning how to maintain self-esteem, a positive body image, and healthy eating patterns for life. A goal of treatment is to teach the person to recognize self-destructive patterns of behavior and to develop better coping skills. Some of the complex factors that influence eating disorder–related behaviors are shown in Figure 10.1.

In some cases, medication may be used as a component of treatment. As noted earlier, eating disorders have

Challenges & Choices

Do You Know Someone With Bulimia?

A person with bulimia is usually of normal weight. Signs of bulimia include the following:

Physiological Signs

- Swollen glands, puffy cheeks, or broken blood vessels under the eyes.
- Frequent sore throat without known causes.
- Fatigue and muscle aches without known causes.
- Unexplained tooth decay or erosion of tooth enamel.
- Yo-yo weight fluctuations within a 10- to 15-pound range.

Behavioral Signs

- Binging.
- Being secretive about food; stealing or hiding food.
- Talking constantly about food or weight.
- Avoiding restaurants, planned meals, or social events with food present.
- Putting oneself down for eating too much.

- Leaving the table and going to the bathroom right after a meal.
- Vomiting; using laxatives, enemas, or diuretics.
- Taking diet pills.
- Maintaining a harsh, no-excuses exercise regimen.
- Expressing an intense fear of becoming fat despite being of normal weight.

Psychological Signs and Attitude Shifts

- Mood swings that include depression, sadness, guilt, or self-loathing.
- Harsh self-criticism.
- Need for the approval of others.
- Self-worth based on weight.

It's Not Just Personal . . .

It is estimated that 10 percent of college-age women suffer from bulimia. About 10 percent of those with bulimia are men. An estimated 10 percent of individuals with bulimia will die from complications of the disorder, including cardiac arrest.

---

been linked to mood disorders, particularly depression, and individuals with eating disorders may manifest such symptoms as depressed mood, social withdrawal, and irritability. For this reason, antidepressants may be prescribed for eating disorders. During the weight gain phases of anorexia treatment, antidepressants do not appear to be beneficial, but they do seem to be somewhat helpful in reducing relapses during the weight maintenance phase. In the treatment of bulimia, the use of antidepressants leads to a rapid decrease in the binge-purge cycle.[14,19]

Treatment Settings

Treatment can occur either in or out of the hospital. Some programs have multiple treatment settings, and patients can move between settings depending on their needs. The options include inpatient treatment, day treatment, residential facilities, and halfway houses or recovery houses (Table 10.1). If possible, the patient should be actively involved in choosing the treatment option.

BODY DYSMORPHIC DISORDER

Many of us look at our bodies and see things we'd like to change. For some people, however, the pattern of seeing faults becomes an obsession that significantly interferes

with their lives. A key feature of **body dysmorphic disorder** is a preoccupation with a defect in appearance. The preoccupation can be about a wholly imagined defect or exaggerated concern about a slight defect. The diagnostic criteria outlined in the *DSM-IV-TR* for this body dysmorphic disorder are as follows:[12]

- Preoccupation with an imagined defect in appearance. If a slight physical anomaly is present, the person's concern is markedly excessive.
- The preoccupation causes significant distress or impairment in social, occupational, or other important areas of functioning.
- The preoccupation is not better accounted for by another mental disorder (such as anorexia).

KEY TERMS

multimodality team   Group of health care providers working together to ensure that all areas of a patient's health are addressed.

body dysmorphic disorder   Preoccupation with an imagined or exaggerated defect in appearance.

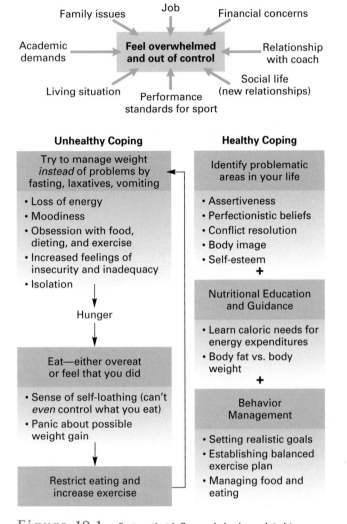

Figure 10.1 Factors that influence behaviors related to eating disorders. *Treatment requires that the therapy team identify and pay attention to a complex mix of influences.* Source: Reprinted from *Medical and Orthopedic Issues of Active and Athletic Women* (p. 149), by R. Agostini, 1994, with permission from Elsevier. (Courtesy of Priscilla Wright, PhD.)

Table 10.1	Treatment Settings for Patients With Eating Disorders
Setting	**Model**
Outpatient therapy	Visits to clinic or treatment center for family or individual counseling, nutritional counseling, and medical checkups at biweekly, weekly, or more frequent intervals as necessary.
Day treatment	Structured care in clinical setting for 4 to 8 hours a day; patient may return home at night.
Residential facility	Live-in facility providing 24-hour supervision; level of support and supervision varies.
Halfway house	Similar to residential facility, but programs are less structured and do not provide 24-hour supervision. These are usually transitional facilities to prepare patients for return home.
Inpatient setting	Twenty-four-hour hospital care focusing on immediate weight gain and medical problems.

The perceived fault can be in any part of the body. The person may worry about acne, wrinkles, skin color, baldness, facial or body asymmetry, or the size or shape of any body part, such as nose, eyebrows, ears, breasts, muscles, and so on. Concern about the perceived defect causes the person distress, and behaviors linked to the defect interfere with the normal activities of living. A person with body dysmorphic disorder may spend hours in front of the mirror (or may, alternatively, avoid mirrors). He or she may spend a good part of every day thinking about the defect and may avoid relationships or social situations out of embarrassment and self-consciousness.

Muscle Dysmorphia

Earlier in this chapter we mentioned muscle dysmorphia, a subcategory of body dysmorphic disorder. This condition, sometimes called bigorexia or reverse anorexia, oc-

curs in men who believe they appear thin and scrawny even though their muscles are actually quite large.[20] They are ashamed of their bodies and obsessed with working out with weights to develop muscular strength. They may avoid social contact because they believe other people are contemptuous of their bodies.

It is unclear why some people develop muscle dysmorphia. The condition may be related to obsessive-compulsive disorder, which is marked by recurring thoughts or compulsions that people can't get out of their heads. The disorder may originate in childhood experiences that undermine self-esteem, such as taunting by peers, and it may be aggravated by body-building magazines and media images that glorify bulging muscles and present them as a realistic goal. Still, many men are exposed to these experiences and images, and most do not develop muscle dysmorphia.

Cosmetic Surgery

Some people with body dysmorphic disorder turn to cosmetic surgery to correct their supposed flaw in appearance. However, not everyone who turns to cosmetic surgery has this disorder. In fact, cosmetic surgery and makeovers of every kind have become commonplace in U.S. society in the last decade. The increase is most likely related to the ever-growing emphasis on appearance. Between 2002 and 2003 there was a 20 percent

HIGHLIGHT ON HEALTH

Ron: A Case of Muscle Dysmorphia and Activity Disorder

Ron had been concerned about his muscular development ever since he was a kid. At the age of 18, he still felt he wasn't big enough, even though he was bigger and stronger than the average man and quite athletic. Ron didn't socialize or go out much, mostly because he was usually at the gym working out. He avoided talking to people while he was there, because he was sure that they were all secretly laughing at how scrawny he was. Ron couldn't really enjoy a meal at a restaurant or a friend's house, either. He kept to a strict diet of high-protein foods and dietary supplements. Ron lifted weights in competition and was actually quite strong, but his muscles didn't look bulky enough to him. He thought about trying steroids to further increase his muscle size.

Not only was Ron obsessed with his muscular development; he was also using exercise to control his moods. He never really felt in control except when he was lifting weights. On a few occasions he injured himself by lifting too much weight, yet he couldn't rest long enough to heal properly. When he felt too sore to lift, he would run or do calisthenics. All the extra activity actually kept his muscles from bulking up further, but he saw the lack of new bulk as a sign that he wasn't working hard enough. Ron wasn't able to see how his pattern of exercise was hurting his health. It took the intervention of a personal trainer at the gym to help him start to understand that he needed to seek psychological help.

---

increase in the number of cosmetic procedures performed in the United States, and between 1997 and 2003, there was a 293 percent increase.[21] Women had 87 percent of the total number of procedures. The most commonly performed surgical procedures were liposuction, breast augmentation, eyelid surgery, rhinoplasty (nose reshaping), and breast reduction. The most commonly performed nonsurgical procedures were Botox injections (for wrinkles), laser hair removal, skin resurfacing procedures, and collagen injections. In Canada, the statistics are similar, with liposuction, breast augmentation, and facelifts the most popular surgical procedures, and Botox treatments by far the most popular nonsurgical procedure.

By definition, cosmetic surgery is elective; it is not done to treat a medical condition. As with any surgery or medical procedure, there are risks. A key risk is psychological: If a person is unhappy with her appearance because she has a distorted body image or is comparing herself to an unrealistic ideal, it is unlikely that a single operation is going to make her significantly happier. There are also physical risks, both at the time of surgery (for example, reactions to anesthesia, blood loss, infection) and later (for example, reactions to the silicone in breast implants).

Cosmetic surgery can of course have psychological and physical benefits. Some people are happy with the results of cosmetic surgery. Some become more confident about their appearance and more successful socially or professionally. Surgeries such as otoplasty (cosmetic ear surgery) and rhinoplasty (nose reshaping) can change a physical characteristic that has caused a person emotional distress for years; breast reduction can enable a woman to feel less self-conscious about her appearance or engage in sports or activities that were previously uncomfortable.

EXERCISE DISORDERS

Like eating disorders, exercise disorders are on the rise, and researchers are beginning to look into exercise patterns that may be abnormal. Such patterns may exist in conjunction with eating disorders or by themselves. Here we look at one abnormal exercise pattern, known as activity disorder.[8]

People with **activity disorder** control their bodies or alter their moods by being overly involved in exercise or addicted to exercise. People who are addicted to exercise continue to exercise strenuously even when the activity causes such problems as illness, injury, or the breakdown of relationships. At the heart of activity disorder is the use of exercise to gain a sense of control and accomplishment, to maintain self-esteem, and to soothe emotions rather than to increase fitness, relaxation, or pleasure. The disorder is not about exercise itself but meeting psychological needs through exercise. The hallmark of activity disorder is a pattern of exercise that becomes detrimental to health rather than beneficial (see the box "Ron: A Case of Muscle Dysmorphia and Activity Disorder").

KEY TERMS

activity disorder Excessive or addictive exercising, undertaken to address psychological needs rather than to improve fitness.

The signs and symptoms of activity disorder often resemble those of anorexia and bulimia: There is a significant overlap among them. Physical symptoms of activity disorder include fatigue, reduction in performance, decreased focus, increased compulsion to exercise, decreased heart rate response to exercise, and muscle degeneration. Cycles of repetitive overuse injuries are common.

Activity disorder is more common among men than among women, a difference that may be related to childhood experiences and cultural values. Males tend to be more active than females are during childhood, and our culture continues to support male independence and physical achievement. The association between activity and achievement may influence active people with perfectionist tendencies to become addicted to exercise.

Treatment for activity disorder is similar to that for eating disorders, although most cases of pure activity disorder can be handled in an outpatient setting. Unfortunately, activity disorder often occurs in conjunction with an eating disorder; the combination can rapidly increase the physical problems of both disorders.

AWARENESS AND PREVENTION: PROMOTING A HEALTHY BODY IMAGE

In spite of a cultural obsession with the physical body, variations in size and shape are not accepted as the norm. Instead, ideal body images, one for women and one for men, are relentlessly promoted in advertising, art, entertainment, and fashion. Not only do these cultural ideals ignore normal physical differences; they also do not allow for the normal changes of healthy aging. Although we cannot escape or ignore these cultural messages, we can view them with critical awareness and make healthy choices about how we want to live. We can do this as individuals, and we can encourage and support programs and organizations that attempt to counter the prevailing cultural messages.

One step individuals can take in promoting healthy choices is to become more aware of their own attitudes about body image, body weight, and the roles of men and women in society. Many people are not aware of how they are conveying cultural messages or of the effect their comments can have on others. A dieting parent, for example, may comment on a healthy child's food choice, or a coach may reinforce weight loss for young athletes whose weight is normal. Even the casual comments people make to friends about other people's appearance or weight have an effect. Negative attitudes can be tempered by an increased acceptance of physical diversity and an emphasis on what people's bodies can do rather than on what they look like.

If you are a parent, you are a powerful role model for your son or daughter. You can communicate your own healthy body image, approach to weight management, and problem-solving skills to your children. You can emphasize the importance of a balance between inner and outer beauty, healthy eating patterns, healthy relationship patterns, and achievements. You can also help children interpret advertising and media and teach them to be smart consumers.

Many organizations and programs promote healthy body image and lifestyle patterns for young people. For example, the Girl Scouts' "Free to Be Me" program emphasizes inner strengths and healthy differences instead of outer appearances. It encourages girls to think about who they really are and what they like to do; to understand and resist peer pressure; to learn about eating disorders and substance abuse; and to celebrate their own diversity. The Boy Scouts' "Fit for Life" and "5-a-Day" badge programs, although not designed specifically to combat eating disorders, teach boys about healthy nutrition, fitness, and exercise.

Parents can foster healthy self-esteem in their children by paying attention to them, making time to do things together, and letting them know that they are loved for themselves rather than just for their appearance or accomplishments.

Challenges & Choices

Ten Tips for Dads of Daughters

1. Listen to your daughter, focusing on what is really important—what she thinks, feels, believes, dreams, and does—rather than how she looks.

2. Encourage her strengths and help her learn to recognize, resist, and overcome barriers.

3. Respect her uniqueness. Urge her to appreciate her body, and discourage dieting.

4. Participate in sports and physical activities with her, whether it's tag, catch, jump rope, basketball, Frisbee, hockey, soccer, or just taking a walk.

5. Get involved in her school—volunteer, chaperone, read to her class. Ask tough questions: Does the school have programs that raise awareness about body image and prevent eating disorders? Does it have zero tolerance of sexual harassment of boys or girls? Does it have ways to encourage girls to take advanced math and science classes? Does it have ways to help girls be leaders?

6. Get involved in her activities—coach, drive, direct a play, teach a class. Demand equal access to resources and facilities for girls.

7. Work with other parents to make the world better for girls. This includes working to end violence against women, media sexualization of girls, pornography, advertisements that play on girls' insecurities, and cultural messages that boys are more important than girls.

8. Take your daughter to work with you, and make sure your business participates in Take Our Daughters and Sons to Work Day every April. Show her how to pay bills and manage money.

9. Support positive alternative media for girls. Watch television programs that portray smart, strong girls; subscribe to healthy magazines edited by girls; and support Web sites run by girls.

10. Talk with other fathers, sharing experience, expertise, and encouragement. Together, fathers can exert a lot of influence; for example, they can stop negative ads.

It's Not Just Personal . . .

According to some surveys, more than 40 percent of girls in first through third grades in the United States want to be thinner, and more than 80 percent of 10-year-olds are afraid of being fat.

Source: Adapted from Ten Tips for Dads of Daughters: Things a Dad of Daughters Can Do Today, Dads and Daughters, www.dadsanddaughters.org. Copyright Dads and Daughters. Used with permission. (Contact info: Dads and Daughters, PO Box 3110, Duluth, MN 55803; phone 218-722-3942; fax 218-728-0314; e-mail info@dadsanddaughters.org.)

Girls, Inc., is a nationwide educational and advocacy organization that encourages girls to be "strong, smart, and bold." This organization's programs focus on building girls' interest and skills in math, science, and technology; on educating girls to prevent teen pregnancy; on developing media literacy, emotional literacy, strategies for self-defense, and leadership skills; and on helping girls participate in sports and take healthy risks in life.

Another organization, Dads and Daughters, is a national advocacy group that seeks to empower young women by helping fathers become more involved in their daughters' lives, in the community, and in their culture. One initiative, for example, encouraged people to write protest letters to the media company that produced a televised swimsuit model search. Dads and Daughters also provides tips for fathers of daughters on how to promote their healthy development. Although aimed specifically at fathers, these tips are equally valuable for any adults who are involved in the lives of girls or boys (see the box "Ten Tips for Dads of Daughters").

In addition to private efforts, the government sponsors a number of programs designed to promote healthy body image and healthy eating. For example, the Office of Women's Health, operating under the U.S. Department of Health and Human Services, sponsors "Body Wise," an educational campaign aimed at increasing knowledge about eating disorders, promoting healthy eating, and reducing preoccupation with body weight and size. This office publishes information sheets on boys and eating disorders as well. The U.S. government also sponsors Girl Power, a national educational campaign that encourages girls 9 to 13 to "make the most of their lives."

Finally, to counteract unhealthy attitudes, we can resist current cultural messages and become active in changing them. The advertising industry spends billions of dollars every year not just on selling products but also on finding out what consumers want. They conduct research on consumer attitudes and desires, hold focus groups, monitor sales, and pay attention to consumer reactions. By supporting healthy body images and buying products that reflect diversity, we can move our society in the direction of more realistic and accepting attitudes toward the body.

You Make the Call

Are the Media Responsible for Eating Disorders?

"What we want is a greater diversity of images of women," declared Tessa Jowell in front of fashion magazine editors, advertisers, clothes designers, and representatives of various women's groups at the UK Cabinet's Body Image Summit in June 2000. Jowell, the Minister for Women of the United Kingdom, organized and hosted the summit after the British Medical Association asserted that images of "abnormally thin" women were responsible for rising rates of eating disorders. The goal of the meeting was to address the increasingly unrealistic portrayal of women in the media and its effect on the female population.

Those at the summit emphasized that they did not want to tell women, the fashion industry, or the media what to do or how to do it. Rather, they wanted to raise awareness and stimulate debate. By the end of the meeting they had agreed on a number of recommendations. One of the most notable called for a media-led body that would develop a self-regulatory code for the industry designed to promote the use of more diverse images of women. This code would include such measures as banning anorexic-looking models from magazine pages and pressuring fashion houses to provide clothes in bigger sizes for photo shoots. Some people are skeptical that the media will abide by such self-monitoring, however; they think government regulation is required to force the media to present more diverse, realistic images.

Opponents of this view think it is absurd to suggest that eating disorders are caused by media images of women. They point out that there is no scientific evidence linking portrayals of women with the incidence of eating disorders. They argue that the media are actually very diverse, as are the images they present, and that the media have not been effective in influencing consumers in other ways. For example, although the media constantly promote diets and exercise plans, obesity continues to increase.

They also point out that different people respond to media images in different ways. Most readers and consumers of the media do not develop eating disorders; in fact, underlying psychological issues, such as low self-esteem, are at the heart of all eating disorders. They concede that for some vulnerable individuals—those, for example, who are going through a difficult emotional period—media images might have an undue influence on their thinking. However, they point out that the diet and weight loss industries also promote thinness as an ideal for women, yet they are not called to account the way the media are. Finally, they assert that responsibility for body weight and body image lies with individuals and their parents, families, schools, and communities. Consumers need to learn how to interpret media images and not be seduced into thinking they are attainable goals. In other words, the media don't need to change; individuals do.

Are the media and all their associated industries responsible for the growing incidence of eating disorders? Should they be regulated by the government and required to present more diverse images? What do you think?

Pros
- Eating disorders are serious, even life-threatening illnesses, and their incidence is increasing in U.S. society.
- As the body ideal presented for women becomes thinner, the rate of eating disorders increases.
- The media play an enormous role in shaping what a society defines as beautiful.
- By promoting an unattainable, unhealthy, and inhuman ideal, the media are preying on some of the most fragile and vulnerable members of society.
- By promoting an emphasis on appearance and the body, the media are perpetuating the oppression of women.

Cons
- Eating disorders are psychiatric illnesses; they are caused by a complex mix of factors. It's simplistic to blame the media.
- Advertising, fashion, entertainment, and the media are giving consumers what they want. If people don't like it, they don't have to buy into it.
- Regulation and censorship impinge on people's freedom of choice and their ability to make their own healthy or unhealthy decisions.
- It's up to individuals to take responsibility for their own behaviors and body image.

OLC Web site For more information on this topic, visit the Online Learning Center at www.mhhe.com/teague1e.

SOURCES: "UK Summit Condemns Unrealistic Media Image of Women," by Georgina Kenyon, June 21, 2000. Reuters Health, www.womenshealthchannel.com/WomensHealthWorld; "The Changing Shape of the Model," by Megan Lane, May 30, 2000, BBC News Online, http://news.bbc.co.uk; "Magazines Ban Anorexic Models," by Tara Womersley, June 22, 2000, Electronic Telegraph, www.caaws.ca/health.

SUMMARY

- The ideal female and male bodies portrayed by the media in U.S. culture do not represent realistic, healthy body images.

- American culture emphasizes appearance over achievement for women and currently places a premium on thinness. Striving for thinness leads to dieting and in some cases to eating disorders.

- Women account for about 90 percent of eating disorders, which are most likely to develop during adolescence and which appear to be most common in ethnic and cultural groups that are connected to mainstream, middle-class society or striving to fit into it.

- The ideal body image for men is becoming more muscular and oversized.

- Eating disorders are psychiatric conditions characterized by severely disturbed eating behaviors and distortions in body image. Disordered eating is a pattern of disturbed eating behaviors (such as fasting, vomiting) that falls short of meeting the criteria for a diagnosed eating disorder but affects quality of life.

- Anorexia nervosa is a disorder involving self-starvation and a seriously distorted body image. Bulimia nervosa is a disorder involving binge-purge cycles and a seriously distorted body image. Binge-eating disorder leads to obesity; it involves binges without the compensatory purging behaviors of bulimia.

- People with eating disorders have distorted patterns of thinking, including a self-critical attitude, black-and-white thinking, and a need for control. Many have symptoms of depression and anxiety disorders.

- Eating disorders have serious health consequences, including electrolyte imbalance, heart rhythm abnormalities, the cessation of menstruation in women, a decrease in testosterone levels in men, and osteoporosis, among others.

- Treatment of eating disorders is often complicated by the patient's denial of a problem. Individuals with severe emaciation usually have to be hospitalized to restore body weight. Thereafter, treatment includes psychotherapy focusing on self-esteem and body image, behavioral modification and relearning, and nutritional education and rehabilitation.

- Body dysmorphic disorder involves preoccupation with an imagined or exaggerated defect in appearance. Muscle dysmorphia is a subcategory of this disorder in which a person thinks his body and muscles are too small and underdeveloped. Many people, both with and without these disorders, are turning to cosmetic surgery to correct supposed flaws in appearance and reach for physical perfection.

- Activity disorder involves excessive exercising for the purpose of managing feelings rather than improving fitness.

- Prevention of eating disorders and other disorders characterized by distortions in body image requires that individuals become aware of cultural and media messages and replace them with healthy beliefs and attitudes. Organizations and programs, both private and governmental, exist to promote healthy eating and exercising behaviors.

REVIEW QUESTIONS

1. Give some examples of media and cultural influences on body image for women and for men.

2. What are some possible reasons for the greater incidence of eating disorders in women than in men?

3. What are some differences in body image and disordered eating among different ethnic groups?

4. What sports are especially associated with risks for disordered eating? Why?

5. What is the difference between an eating disorder and disordered eating?

6. What are the diagnostic criteria for anorexia nervosa? For bulimia nervosa? For binge-eating disorder?

7. What are some of the similarities between depression and the thought patterns associated with eating disorders?

8. Describe the differences between the health consequences of anorexia and those of bulimia.

9. What are the criteria for recovery from an eating disorder?

10. Why do you think the whole family is often involved in the treatment of an eating disorder?

11. How is body dysmorphic disorder different from normal concern about appearance?

12. What are some of the risks and some of the possible benefits of cosmetic surgery?

13. How is activity disorder different from normal exercising?

14. What steps can individuals take to prevent the occurrence of eating disorders and other body-image-related disorders?

WEB RESOURCES

Body Positive: This educational organization teaches critical thinking about our culture's focus on thinness. Its resources include BodyTalk, a video on body acceptance for teen girls and boys, and links to other organizations that offer information on body image. www.bodypositive.com

Dads & Daughters: Encouraging fathers to become actively involved in the lives of their daughters, this advocacy group works to counteract the cultural messages that devalue girls and women. www.dadsanddaughters.org

Girls, Inc.: Dedicated to inspiring all girls to be "strong, smart, and bold," Girls, Inc. offers educational programs throughout the United States, particularly to girls in high-risk, underserved areas. It teaches girls how to advocate for themselves and their communities and to promote positive change. www.girlsinc.org

National Association for Self-Esteem: The aim of this organization is to integrate self-esteem throughout U.S. society. Its Web site features a self-guided tour that lets you rate your self-esteem, as well as articles, a newsletter, FAQs, and links to other resources. www.self-esteem-nase.org

National Eating Disorders Association: Promoting public understanding of eating disorders, this organization offers programs and services related to treatment and support of families affected by these disorders. www.edap.org

TeensHealth: This site offers various topics of interest to teens, including body image and self-esteem, eating disorders, cutting, and emotional changes in adolesence. www.kidshealth.org/teen

Teen HealthFX: This site offers a wide range of online resources related to teen health, relationships, and sexuality. Its emotional health section addresses eating disorders, cutting, mood changes, and support groups. www.teenhealthfx.com

REFERENCES

1. National Eating Disorders Association. (2002). Statistics: Eating disorders and their precursors. www.nationaleatingdisorders.org.

2. Anderson, A. E., & Holman, J. (1997). Males with eating disorders: Challenges for treatment and research. *Psychopharmacology Bulletin 33* (3), 391–397.

3. Groesz, L. M., Levine, M. P., & Murnen, S. K. (2002). The effect of experimental presentation of thin media images on body satisfaction: A meta-analytic review. *International Journal of Eating Disorders 31*, 1–16.

4. Andrist, L. C. (2003). Media images, body dissatisfaction, and disordered eating in adolescent women. *Maternal Child Nursing-American Journal of Maternal/Child Nursing 28* (2), 119–223.

5. Johnson, C., Crosby, R., & Engel, S., et al. (2004). Gender, ethnicity, self-esteem and disordered eating among college athletes. *Eating Behaviors 5* (2), 147–156.

6. Wildes, J. E., Emery, R. E., & Simons, A.D. (2001). Roles of ethnicity and culture in the development of eating disturbance and body dissatisfaction. *Clinical Psychology Review 21* (4), 521–551.

7. Labre, M. P. (2002). Adolescent boys and the muscular male body ideal. *Journal of Adolescent Health 30* (4), 233–242.

8. Costin, C. (1999). *The eating disorder sourcebook: A comprehensive guide to causes, treatments and prevention of eating disorders.* Lincolnwood, IL: Lowell House.

9. Cafri, G., Thompson, J. K., Ricciardell, L., & McCabe, M. (2005). Pursuit of the muscular ideal: Physical and psychological consequences and putative risk factors. *Clinical Psychology Review 25* (2), 215–239.

10. Smolak, L., Murnen, S. K., & Ruble, A. E. (2000). Female athletes and eating problems: A meta-analysis. *International Journal of Eating Disorders 27* (4), 371–380.

11. Mehler, P. S., & Krantz, M. (2003). Anorexia nervosa medical issues. *Journal of Women's Health 12* (4), 331–340.

12. American Psychiatric Association. (2000). *Diagnostic and statistical manual of mental disorders* (4th ed., Text Revision). Washington, DC: American Psychiatric Association Press.

13. Haster, G., Pine, D. S., Gamma, A., & Milos, G., et al. (2004). The associations between psychopathology and being overweight: A 20-year prospective study. *Psychological Medicine 34* (6), 1047–1057.

14. Fairburn, C. G., & Harrison, P. J. (2003). Eating disorders. *Lancet 361* (9355), 407–416.

15. O'Brien, K. M., & Vincent, N. K. (2003). Psychiatric comorbidity in anorexia and bulimia nervosa: Nature, prevalence and causal relationships. *Clinical Psychology Review 23* (1), 57–74.

16. Zipfel, S., Lowe, B., Reas, D. L., Deter, H. C., & Herzog, W. (2000). Long-term prognosis in anorexia nervosa: Lessons from a 21-year follow up study. *Lancet 355*, 721.

17. Stewart, T. M., & Williamson, D. A. (2004). Multidisciplinary treatment of eating disorders. Part 2: Primary goals and content of treatment. *Behavior Modification 28* (6), 831–853.

18. Vandereycken, W. (2003). The place of inpatient care in the treatment of anorexia nervosa: Questions to be answered. *International Journal of Eating Disorders 34*, 409–422.

19. American Psychiatric Association Work Group on Eating Disorders. (2000). Practice guidelines for the treatment of patients with eating disorders (revision). *American Journal of Psychiatry, 157* (1 Suppl), 1–39.

20. Pope, H. G., Jr., Phillips, K. A., & Olivardia, R. (2000). *The Adonis complex: The secret crisis of male body obsession.* New York: Free Press.

21. 2003 Cosmetic Plastic Surgery Research. (2005). www.cosmeticplasticsurgerystatistics.com.

Add It Up!

DO YOU WORRY TOO MUCH ABOUT YOUR APPEARANCE?

This exercise is designed to help you think about your body image and eating patterns. It is not intended to diagnose an eating disorder. If you answer yes to any of the questions, you may benefit from talking to a counselor or health care provider. If you mark yes to several questions, you may have serious body image concerns and may have disordered eating. A professional consultation is recommended.

Check if any of the following statements are true or mostly true for you:

1. ☑ I feel more in control when I restrict the amount of food that I eat.
2. ☑ I consistently compare the way I look to others and perceive myself to be too heavy.
3. ☐ I would do almost anything to look more muscular and "ripped."
4. ☑ I make sure to exercise whenever I feel as though I have eaten too much.
5. ☑ I would agree to cosmetic surgery if it were free.
6. ☐ I am dissatisfied with my body size and shape.
7. ☐ I am anxious about how people perceive or judge me.
8. ☐ I have patterns or rituals around food and eating, and I follow them in order to improve my appearance.
9. ☐ I feel anxious about gaining weight.
10. ☑ I feel as though I am constantly on a diet.
11. ☐ I eat to make myself feel better when I am sad, upset, or lonely.
12. ☑ I feel good about myself only when I weigh a certain amount or look a certain way.
13. ☑ I believe that people would think less of me if I gained weight.
14. ☐ I often skip meals to lose weight.
15. ☑ If I work hard enough, I can look like a professional athlete.
16. ☑ I frequently feel anxious or depressed because of concerns about my appearance.
17. ☑ My preoccupation with food makes it hard to concentrate on my work or school.
18. ☐ I get excluded from social groups because of how I look.
19. ☑ I sometimes feel obsessed about food.
20. ☐ I often talk negatively about my body in a serious way to myself or others.

PART 3

Your Health at Risk

In Part 2 you learned about the importance of lifestyle choices in achieving good health. In Part 3 we address specific choices that can put your health at risk. First we consider alcohol consumption and how it affects your health and safety and that of others. Next we discuss drugs and addictive behavior as factors that can put your health at risk. Finally, we consider tobacco as a challenge to the health of smokers and nonsmokers alike. While studying these chapters, think about these issues in the context of your own life. Is your approach to any of these substances putting your health at risk?

THINK IT OVER

Is your social group made up of both drinkers and nondrinkers?

If all drugs were legal, would the drug problem be solved?

Do you see a pattern of smoking or nonsmoking in your family?

CHAPTER **11**

Alcohol: Responsible Approaches to Drinking

DID YOU KNOW?

- A woman who consumes the same amount of alcohol as a man will have a higher blood alcohol concentration than he does. Women metabolize alcohol less efficiently than men do and consequently absorb about 30 percent more alcohol into the bloodstream. Women also suffer more alcohol-related health effects than men do, and they experience them sooner.

- If you are a man who has ever consumed five drinks in a row or a woman who has consumed four, you meet the criteria for binge drinking. Nearly half of college students engage in binge drinking, a pattern of alcohol consumption associated with serious physical, academic, social, and legal consequences.

OLC *Your Health Today*   www.mhhe.com/teague1e

Go to the Online Learning Center for *Your Health Today* for interactive activities, quizzes, flashcards, Web links, and more resources related to this chapter.

The use of alcohol has been a part of American life since the nation's founding, but the tide of public opinion has periodically risen against it. In 1918, the Eighteenth Amendment to the U.S. Constitution was passed, inaugurating the era of Prohibition—a ban on the manufacture, sale, and transportation of intoxicating liquors in the United States. In 1933, the Twenty-First Amendment was passed, repealing the Eighteenth. Prohibition had been a miserable failure.

The nation's ambivalence reflects the two faces of alcohol. We use it to feel good, to celebrate, to toast one another and life, yet we also see the devastation it can cause when drinking gets out of control. Used responsibly, alcohol helps us enjoy life; used irresponsibly, it can destroy lives. U.S. society currently approves of the use of alcohol by adults, and alcohol advertising typically depicts drinkers as attractive, youthful members of a fun-loving circle of friends. We seldom if ever see images of drunks or alcoholics, nor do we see many images of drinkers vomiting, passing out, or being brought to hospital emergency rooms with alcohol poisoning.

Because alcohol is a **psychoactive drug**—it causes changes in brain chemistry and alters consciousness—it can have profound and wide-ranging effects on all aspects of our thinking, emotions, and behavior. It is in society's interest to regulate the use of such a powerful substance, but it is up to individuals to determine what role they want alcohol to play in their lives. The same is true of many other psychoactive drugs, including nicotine-containing tobacco products, over-the-counter drugs, and prescription medications—they are legal but regulated. Still other psychoactive drugs are currently illegal, including marijuana, cocaine, LSD, and heroin. We discuss the effects of such substances and the issues surrounding their use in Chapter 12. We discuss nicotine and tobacco use in Chapter 13.

In this chapter, we focus on the complex issues associated with alcohol. We begin by looking at who drinks alcohol and why—patterns of use and frameworks for understanding this use, especially when it becomes problematic. We then look at alcohol consumption on college campuses, with a special focus on binge drinking. Next, we explore the effects of alcohol on the body and brain, the health risks and possible benefits of alcohol use, the problems of alcohol abuse and dependence, and treatment options. Finally, we consider how you can evaluate your own use of alcohol and take steps to make sure your use is responsible.

WHO DRINKS: PATTERNS OF ALCOHOL USE

More than 60 percent of American adults drink, at least occasionally. About one third of the adult U.S. population label themselves **abstainers.** They do not drink at all, or less often than once a year. Of the two thirds who do drink, 10 percent are considered **heavy drinkers,** and the remainder are **light drinkers** and **moderate drinkers.**[1] (Moderate drinking is defined as two drinks a day for men and one drink a day for women; heavy drinking is defined as drinking more than this and light drinking as less.[2]) As many as 90 percent of American adults have had some experience with alcohol, and 60 percent of men and 30 percent of women have had a bad experience with alcohol, such as driving when intoxicated or missing work owing to a hangover.[3] **Intoxication** is an altered state of consciousness due to ingestion of alcohol or other substances.

There is tremendous variability in drinking patterns across individuals and groups, however. Demographic factors (age, gender, ethnicity, education, income, geography) influence who drinks and how much. In this section we consider some of these factors.

Patterns Across the Life Span

Drinking patterns for men and women in the United States, by age and ethnic group, are shown in Figures 11.1 and 11.2. As the tables indicate, the roots of drinking behavior are established by the adolescent years. Consumption of alcoholic beverages is highest between the ages of 18 to 25 for whites and then begins a steady descent. The peak period for heavy drinking among Hispanic and African American men occurs between the ages of 26 and 30, and the decline tends to be less marked than that for white men.[3] In general, people are more likely to drink at certain stages in the life span, such as adolescence and early adulthood, the threshold of middle age, and following retirement. (Later in this chapter we take a closer look at drinking in the college-age population.)

KEY TERMS

psychoactive drug   A substance that causes changes in brain chemistry and alters consciousness.

abstainer   A person who drinks no alcoholic beverages or drinks less often than once a year.

heavy drinker   A man who drinks more than two drinks a day or a woman who drinks more than one drink a day.

light drinker   A man who drinks less than two drinks a day or a woman who drinks less than one drink a day.

moderate drinker   A man who drinks no more than two drinks a day or a woman who drinks no more than one drink a day.

intoxication   Altered state of consciousness as a result of drinking alcohol or ingesting another substance.

Figure 11.1   *Percentage of males reporting having four or more drinks on any single day in the past 30 days, by age group and race/ethnicity.* Source: *Alcohol and Health* (p. 31), U.S. Department of Health and Human Services, National Institutes of Health, National Institute on Alcohol Abuse and Alcoholism, 2000.

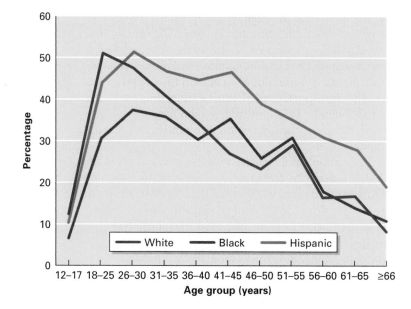

Older adults drink significantly less than younger adults do. A high percentage of older adults, particularly older women, abstain from alcohol.[4] Alcoholism is five times more prevalent in older adult men than in older adult women, and it is more common among whites than African Americans and Hispanic Americans.[5]

Women drink less than men do and start later. Sixty percent of American women drink alcohol on a regular basis, and about 5 percent have two or more drinks daily.[6] However, it takes less time for women to develop a drinking problem than it does for men. (Gender differences are also discussed later in the chapter.) Although the slope in drinking trajectories between men and women is different, recent research suggests that this gap is closing.

Ethnic Differences in Alcohol Use

As shown in Figures 11.1 and 11.2, alcohol consumption among whites is higher than among African Americans across most of the life span.[3] Alcohol consumption is high among Hispanic/Latino men, but it is very low among Hispanic/Latino women. Hispanic/Latino women are more likely to abstain from alcohol than are African American or white women. These differences may be the result of cultural norms and attitudes; in Hispanic culture, drinking tends to be encouraged for men but discouraged for women.[7]

Differences in alcohol consumption among ethnic groups are strongly influenced by sociocultural or environmental factors, including poverty, discrimination, feelings of powerlessness, immigration status, and degree

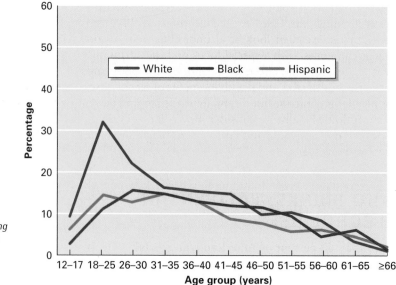

Figure 11.2   *Percentage of females reporting having four or more drinks on any single day in the past 30 days, by age group and race/ethnicity.* Source: *Alcohol and Health* (p. 32), U.S. Department of Health and Human Services, Public Health Services, National Institutes of Health, National Institute on Alcohol Abuse and Alcoholism, 2000.

of acculturation.[8] Economic factors, such as the heavy marketing of alcoholic beverages in minority neighborhoods, play a considerable role. For example, the number of liquor stories located in African American communities is proportionately much higher than the number in white communities.[3] Given these pressures, it is notable that alcohol consumption is generally lower among African Americans than among other groups.

Among Native Americans, alcoholism is recognized as the number one health problem.[3] The death rate from alcoholism for Native Americans is more than five times greater than that for other groups.[9] Four of the 10 leading causes of death for Native Americans are alcohol related. Numerous factors contribute to these disparities, most notably sociocultural factors such as poverty and discrimination. Scientists have also suggested that genetic factors may contribute to patterns of alcohol use by Native Americans. In addition, the cultural belief that alcoholism is a spiritual disorder rather than a physical disease makes it less likely that Native Americans will seek treatment. Treatment programs that reflect tribal values may be more effective, such as programs that incorporate traditional practices (sweat houses, prayers, dances) into the therapeutic process.[9]

Among Asian Americans, alcohol consumption overall is lower than among white Americans. Many Asian Americans tend to drink very little or abstain because of a genetically based biological reaction to alcohol (see Chapter 2). Approximately half of all Asian Americans have a gene that impairs the metabolism of alcohol, causing a set of unpleasant reactions (facial flushing, sweating, nausea) referred to as the flushing effect.[6]

WHY PEOPLE DRINK: FRAMEWORKS FOR UNDERSTANDING ALCOHOL USE

There are no simple explanations for why people drink or why some people develop drinking problems and others do not. One approach is to think of individuals as a host environment in which psychosocial and sociocultural factors interact to influence alcohol use and potential drinking problems. In this section we consider a variety of such factors.

Biological Factors in Alcohol Use

As discussed in Chapter 2, some people may be genetically susceptible to the influences of alcohol. Family, twin, and adoption studies have shown a family pattern of alcohol dependence, with the risk of alcoholism three to four times greater in close relatives of an alcoholic than in the general population.[3] Inborn temperament, too, may interact with poor parenting to make it more likely that a

child will grow up to have an alcohol problem, as discussed in the next section.

Psychosocial Factors in Alcohol Use

Psychosocial factors have a strong influence on why people drink and why some people are more likely to develop drinking problems. Experts have looked at these factors from a variety of perspectives.

The Motivational Perspective

Some researchers have looked at alcohol consumption from a motivational perspective, asking why people drink. Two broad underlying patterns identified by these researchers are compensatory drinking and drinking owing to external motivations.[3]

Compensatory drinking (drinking to cope) is the use of alcohol to soothe negative emotions, deal with stress, and reduce anxiety and tension. An example of compensatory drinking occurred after the terrorist attacks of September 11, 2001, when consumption of alcoholic beverages by New York City residents increased significantly. Under ordinary circumstances, people who tend to avoid life issues rather than confront them are more likely to drink for compensatory reasons.

People who use alcohol because of *external motivations* may drink to project a particular image or comply with social norms. For example, women who enter professions that have long been dominated by men (law enforcement, medicine, engineering, top corporate management) may be more vulnerable to drinking in excess as a way of fitting in. For them, drinking may be symbolic of status and equality.[10]

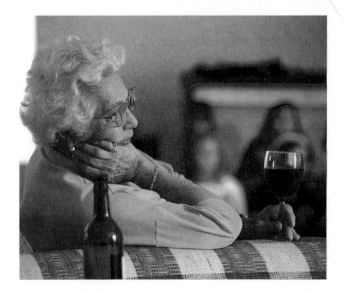

Once this woman didn't drink more than a glass of wine with dinner. Since her husband's recent death, she finds herself drinking regularly and to excess. Many people use drinking as a way of combating loneliness, job dissatisfaction, or financial troubles rather than taking positive steps to deal with these problems.

Parenting and the Family Environment

Other researchers have tried to understand alcohol use by looking at parenting and the family environment. A family history of alcoholism as a risk factor for the development of alcoholism is well established.[11] Children who grow up in families that include an alcoholic live in an environment of anxiety, tension, confusion, and denial. The risk for serious injury caused by child abuse and neglect is more than twice as high in children of mothers who drink as it is in those who don't.[3] This risk is higher when both parents drink.

Family dysfunction in general, even without an alcoholic parent, increases the likelihood that children will grow up to have alcohol problems. Physical or sexual abuse during childhood, for example, is frequently reported among women who are alcoholics.[12] Childhood traumas may predispose people to early alcohol use, which is associated with adult problem drinking.[3] Children in dysfunctional families are more likely to be exposed to high levels of stress and to experience negative emotions. Later, they may use drinking to soothe these negative feelings. Depression is associated with drinking at all stages of the life span for both men and women.

Note that most children who grow up in dysfunctional family environments do not develop problems with alcohol. Two key protective factors are believed to prevent these problems: (1) parent-child connectedness and (2) school connectedness. High parent-child connectedness exists when children feel close, loved, or wanted by one or both parents. School connectedness occurs when students feel close to other students, feel that they are recognized as part of the school community, and believe they are treated fairly by teachers.[3] Individuals are further protected in adulthood by having work and marriage responsibilities and a supportive social network.

The Developmental Effects Perspective

Some experts look at alcohol use from the perspective of developmental effects, focusing on how drinking patterns vary across the life span, with pressures to drink or not to drink concentrated at certain stages.[3] For example, alcohol use is high among adolescents and college students as individuals transition into adulthood and experiment with previously forbidden substances. Adults face new challenges in middle age; many people tend to drink more when they lose a valued social role, such as being a parent of young children or adolescents. In older adulthood, people may drink in response to stressors such as retirement, bereavement, social isolation, or loneliness.

Sociocultural/Environmental Factors in Alcohol Use

Because drinking occurs in a social and cultural context, sociocultural/environmental factors play an enormous role in how alcohol is used and misused. Some cultures

have higher acceptance of alcohol use, more tolerant attitudes toward drinking and drunkenness, and/or higher levels of alcohol consumption than others do. Economic factors, such as the availability and cost of alcohol and the ease of access, also play a role. Laws governing drinking age and the sale of alcoholic beverages affect who drinks. Stresses associated with minority status, including unemployment, discrimination, and poverty, are also associated with alcohol use. Again, the complex interaction of many factors—individual, psychological, social, cultural—determines who will drink and/or have a problem with alcohol and who will not.

DRINKING ON THE COLLEGE CAMPUS

If you take a walk on a college campus on a weekend morning, you may see broken liquor bottles, crushed beer cans, and flyers advertising specials at local bars littering the ground—the wreckage of the previous night's partying. Drinking rates at most colleges are very high; surveys indicate that up to 90 percent of college students drink alcoholic beverages.[13] Many students think of drinking as a recreational activity, part of having fun and letting off steam, but some engage in binge drinking, a particularly risky way to consume alcohol. In this section we consider how much students drink, why they drink, and what can be done to change these patterns.

Not long ago, binge drinking was viewed as a normal rite of passage on college campuses. With news reports of deaths that have resulted from this practice, this attitude is changing, and some student groups are taking action against binge drinking.

Binge Drinking

The problem of binge drinking was brought to the public's attention in 2000 by the Harvard School of Public Health College Alcohol Study (CAS).[13] **Binge drinking** is defined as the consumption of five or more drinks in a row for men and four or more drinks for women at least once in the previous 2-week period. (In North America, a **drink** is defined as 0.5 ounces, or 15 grams, of alcohol, the amount contained in about 12 ounces of beer, 5 ounces of wine, or 1.5 ounces of 80-proof distilled liquor.) In the Harvard study, students who binged three or more times in the previous 2 weeks or more than once a week on average were labeled *frequent binge drinkers*. Students who had binged one or two times in the 2-week period before the survey were labeled *occasional binge drinkers*. Students who had consumed alcohol in the past year but had not binged in the previous 2 weeks were labeled *non-binge drinkers*. *Abstainers* were students who had not consumed alcohol in the past year.[14]

The study found that most college students—84 percent—drank alcohol. About half of all students were binge drinkers (44 percent), and about one in five were frequent binge drinkers (23 percent).[14] About 10 percent of college students drank more than 15 alcoholic beverages per week. Levels of binge drinking were different among different segments of the student population, however. First-year college women were more likely to be frequent binge drinkers than sophomore, junior, or senior women were. A greater number of men were frequent binge drinkers (26 percent) than women (21 percent). Students living in fraternity and sorority houses reported the most frequent binge-drinking patterns (51 percent). Comparable levels of binge drinking occurred among dormitory residents (22 percent) and students living off campus (22 percent).[1]

Underage Drinking

Very often, binge drinking does not begin in college. Many students binge drink in high school and come to college expecting to continue drinking heavily.[15] The College Alcohol Study found that 15 percent of eighth graders and 30 percent of high school seniors binge drink.[1] This pattern suggests that colleges inherit the behavior of young people who binge drink. At the same time, college environments that promote drinking not only attract drinkers but also encourage drinking among people who were previously nondrinkers.

College students under the age of 21 consume 48 percent of all alcohol consumed by college students.[16] They drink less frequently than older students do, but they are more likely to binge during these episodes and to drink simply to get drunk.[17] They are also more likely to be injured or encounter trouble with law enforcement than are older students who binge drink. Underage drinking laws have not curbed this pattern.[3] Students can easily purchase alcohol without ID or with a false ID, and they have access to alcohol purchased by others. In states with tough drinking laws and in communities that strictly enforce these laws, underage drinking is less common.[18]

Consequences of Binge Drinking

Binge drinking can have profound physical, academic, social, and legal consequences. (To evaluate the importance of such consequences for you, see the Add It Up! feature at the end of the chapter.) Individuals who have been drinking heavily are more likely to be injured, to commit a crime or fall victim to violence, and to be involved with the law. Half to two thirds of campus homicides and serious assaults are believed to involve drinking by the offender, the

KEY TERMS

binge drinking Consumption of five or more drinks in a row by a man or four or more drinks in a row by a woman.

drink Beverage containing 0.5 ounces or 15 grams of alcohol, the amount contained in one 12-ounce beer, one 5-ounce glass of wine, or one 1.5-ounce shot of 80-proof distilled liquor.

HIGHLIGHT ON HEALTH

High-Risk College Drinking: A Snapshot of Consequences

Death: Each year, 1,400 college students between the ages of 18 and 24 die from alcohol-related unintentional injuries, including motor vehicle crashes.

Injury: Each year, 500,000 students between the ages of 18 and 24 are unintentionally injured under the influence of alcohol.

Assault: Each year, more than 600,000 students between the ages of 18 and 24 are assaulted by another student who has been drinking.

Sexual abuse: Each year, more than 70,000 students between the ages of 18 and 24 are victims of alcohol-related sexual assault or date rape.

Unsafe sex: In one year, 400,000 students between the ages of 18 and 24 had unprotected sex, and more than 100,000 students between the ages of 18 and 24 reported having been too intoxicated to know if they consented to having sex.

Academic problems: Each year, about 25 percent of college students report academic consequences of their drinking, including missing class, falling behind, doing poorly on exams or papers, and receiving lower grades overall.

Health problems/suicide attempts: More than 150,000 students develop an alcohol-related health problem every year, and between 1.2 and 1.5 percent of students indicate that they tried to commit suicide within the past year because of drinking or drug use.

Drunk driving: In one year, 2.1 million students between the ages of 18 and 24 drove under the influence of alcohol.

Vandalism: In one year, about 11 percent of college student drinkers reported that they damaged property while under the influence of alcohol.

Property damage: More than 25 percent of administrators from schools with relatively low drinking levels and over 50 percent from schools with high drinking levels say their campuses have a "moderate" or "major" problem with alcohol-related property damage.

Police involvement: Each year, about 5 percent of 4-year college students are involved with police or campus security as a result of their drinking, and an estimated 110,000 students between the ages of 18 and 24 are arrested for an alcohol-related violation, such as public drunkenness or driving under the influence.

Alcohol abuse and dependence: According to questionnaire-based self-reports about their drinking, 31 percent of college students met criteria for a diagnosis of alcohol abuse and 6 percent for a diagnosis of alcohol dependence in the previous 12 months.

Source: National Institute on Alcohol Abuse and Alcoholism, www.collegedrinkingprevention.gov.

---

victim, or both.[3] One study found that 74 percent of perpetrators of sexual assaults on college campuses had been drinking.[1] Women who binge drink are nearly 150 percent more likely to be victims of date rape, sexual battering, and unplanned sexual activity than are women who do not drink alcohol.[19] (See the box "High-Risk College Drinking: A Snapshot of Consequences.")

Binge drinkers also cause problems for other students. About 9 out of 10 students reported experiencing at least one adverse consequence of another student's drinking during the school year.[20] These "secondhand effects" of binge drinking include serious arguments, physical assault, damaged property, interrupted sleep or studying, unwanted sexual advances, sexual assault, and having to take care of a drunk student.

Why Do College Students Binge Drink?

Students binge drink for a variety of reasons. Some may drink simply because they can—they are away from

parental authority for the first time and see drinking as an assertion of autonomy and adult status. They may drink to ease social inhibitions, to fit in with peers, to imitate role models, or to celebrate. They also may drink to reduce stress, soothe negative emotions, self-medicate, or cope with academic pressure. Adapting to a new environment may influence some first-year students to binge drink. The mistaken belief that alcohol increases sexual arousal and performance (heavy drinking actually suppresses sexual arousal) may also account for some binge drinking.[1] Young people who are inexperienced with alcohol may not realize how binge drinking will affect them; as mentioned earlier, many people have had a negative experience with alcohol at some point in their lives, and most of them learn to moderate their drinking from these experiences.

Students who started drinking alcohol before age 16 are more likely to be binge drinkers, as are students with close friends or parents who binge drink. Binge drinking is also promoted by easy access to alcohol and cheap prices. Thus, social norms and the campus culture contribute to patterns of drinking. Students are more likely to binge drink on campuses where heavy drinking is the norm and less likely when drinking is discouraged.[21]

Changing the Campus Drinking Culture

Two broad approaches have been used to change the culture of drinking on college campuses. One is oriented toward restricting the use of alcohol, the other toward changing students' perceptions of social norms.

Restricting Alcohol Use

The restrictive approach focuses on reducing drinking and alcohol-related problems at the level of the individual student's behavior. Examples of strategies include identifying and treating high-risk students, punishing students who violate college alcohol policies or break the law, educating students to resist peer pressure to binge drink, and sponsoring alcohol-free social and cultural opportunities.

Some colleges have moved toward zero tolerance by implementing more restrictive policies, such as prohibiting alcohol at all college-sponsored events, maintaining alcohol-free residence halls and fraternity/sorority houses, and mandating participation in substance abuse programs for alcohol-related offenses. A controversial policy adopted by some schools is parental notification. When underage students are arrested for violations, the college sends a letter to their parents or guardians informing them of the incident. So far, such policies have not been found to violate students' privacy.

Colleges have also focused on restricting alcohol advertising and promotion on campus. In the 1980s, ads and promotions for beer dominated the campus landscape. Marketing research had established that most people develop brand loyalty between the ages of 18 and 24,[3] and college campuses provide an opportunity for the alcohol industry to reach entry-level drinkers before brand loyalty is entrenched. The Budweiser Clydesdale horses, for example, were a familiar sight at sports events.

In the 1990s, college administrators at many schools enacted policies to remove such ads and promotions from campus, and brewers and distillers moved their marketing efforts off campus. Many colleges now prohibit off-campus establishments from advertising alcoholic beverage promotions in college newspapers and on college radio stations. Restrictions at major sporting events have proved more troublesome, however, because the alcohol industry provides significant revenue to athletic programs.[1] Stadium signs, logos, and scoreboards are still adorned with beer and liquor ads. (This practice may be changing; see the box "College Sports and Alcohol.")

Consumer Clipboard

College Sports and Alcohol

Many colleges and universities struggle to reduce binge drinking among students—at the same time that their athletic programs receive financial support from makers of alcoholic beverages. Most of this support comes from breweries, which provide support in return for access to advertising space. Scoreboards, programs, radio broadcasts, and televised events all proclaim their sponsorship by brand-name alcoholic beverage companies.

Many people believe that this commercial practice undermines the educational mission of academic institutions and compromises their ability to implement credible and effective programs to curb binge drinking. Alcohol ads convey the impression that drinking is an important part of enjoying college sports, such as in tailgate parties at football games. The College Alcohol Study found that 53 percent of sports fans usually binge when drinking, compared to 41 percent of men and 37 percent of women who were not sports fans.

Efforts are under way to change this environment. In 1998 the U.S. Department of Health and Human Services called for the National Collegiate Athletic Association (NCAA) to sever the ties between college sports and alcoholic beverage sponsorship and advertising. By 2004, 210 NCAA schools had pledged to end alcohol advertising on college sports broadcasts. These pledges are part of a commitment to a nationwide effort promoted by the Campaign for Alcohol-Free Sports on TV. Another organization, the Center for Science in the Public Interest, has also initiated a major campaign called Time to End Alcohol Marketing in Sports (TEAMS). This campaign seeks to do the following:

- Eliminate alcoholic beverage sponsorship of college and Olympic sports.

- Prohibit alcohol advertising in sports broadcasting when 15 percent of the people in the viewing and listening audience, or 2 million persons (the lesser of the two), are under age 21.

- Eliminate alcohol sponsorship of youth sports events, athletic teams and leagues, and individual athletes.

If these efforts are successful, we may see an end to the mixed messages sent to the public, especially to young fans, about the role of alcohol in college and youth sports.

Source: Adapted from *Dying to Drink*, by H. Wechsler and B. Wuethrich, 2002, New York: Rodale Books.

Changing the Perceptions of Alcohol Use

The social norms approach focuses on changing students' perceptions about levels of drinking on their campus and attitudes toward alcohol use among their fellow students.[22] In other words, it attempts to bridge the gap between student-perceived levels of alcohol consumption and actual consumption of alcohol by most students. A common belief is that college students consume astronomical amounts of alcohol, but in fact, most students drink only at moderate levels.[1] In reality, binge drinking is not the norm on campus.[21,23] Positive, upbeat messages about drinking, in place of negative scare tactics, have been favorably received by most college students.

Critics of this approach claim that it is based on the assumptions that college students match their drinking to what they perceive to be the campus norm and that students drink more because they perceive this norm to be higher than it actually is.[24] Neither of these assumptions has been proven to be true. The approach has also been appropriated by the alcohol industry, which has used it to promote the notion that most people drink moderately and responsibly. This message would seem to relieve the industry of any responsibility for problem drinking and alcohol abuse.[25]

Combining Strategies to Combat Alcohol Use

To confront the frustrating problem of excessive drinking on college campuses, the National Institute on Alcohol Abuse and Alcoholism (NIAAA) created the Task Force on College Drinking, a distinguished panel of alcohol researchers, college administrators, and college students. In its 2002 report, the task force noted that although research on the prevention of college drinking is relatively new, the problem is clearly influenced by multiple factors and a comprehensive, integrated approach is needed. The report recommended interventions aimed at three constituencies: the student population as a whole, the college and its surrounding environment, and individual drinkers who are at risk for alcohol abuse or dependence.[25]

Addressing the problem at the level of the student population requires a direct focus on environmental contributors to high-risk drinking, such as widespread availability of alcohol, aggressive marketing and promotion of alcohol on the college campus, inconsistent enforcement of laws and policies that govern drinking, and student perceptions that high-risk drinking is the student norm.[25] Students are too often overlooked as essential agents of change. The 2001 CAS reported that the majority of students support tougher alcohol policies. For example, 67 percent want a crackdown on underage drinking, and 60 percent want kegs prohibited on the college campus.[1]

Interventions at the level of the college and its environment are more likely to occur when both the college and the community recognize high-risk drinking as a common problem. Examples of cooperative efforts include increased enforcement of minimum drinking age laws, "safe rides" programs, and limiting the density of alcohol outlets near campus. Intervention at the level of individual at-risk students requires effective screening programs. Campus student health services, for example, may conduct brief screening interviews with students during emergency room and health center visits. Screening tools that help students compare their drinking behavior with that of other students may also be useful.[25]

The task force emphasized the importance of visible leadership by college presidents to commit resources and support to programs that support these three levels of intervention. Active student participation in prevention policies and services is also essential.

EFFECTS OF ALCOHOL ON THE BODY

The body pays special attention to alcohol as soon as it enters the body. Alcohol is a very small molecule, and unlike food, which must be digested, it is quickly absorbed into the bloodstream through the walls of the stomach and the small intestine. Within minutes, alcohol is distributed to all the cells of the body, including the cells of the brain. In the brain, alcohol alters brain chemistry and changes neurotransmitter functions. It particularly affects the cerebellum—the center for balance and motor functions—and the prefrontal cortex—the center for executive functions, such as rational thinking and problem solving.

Alcohol is a **central nervous system depressant.** While alcohol levels in the blood and brain are rising, the person experiences feelings of relaxation and well-being, an expansive mood, and a lowering of social inhibitions. At higher levels, and especially when blood levels are falling, the drinker is more likely to feel depressed and withdrawn and to experience impairments in thinking, balance, and motor coordination. As alcohol concentrations in the brain increase, more functions are depressed and greater impairment occurs. These effects last until all the alcohol is metabolized (broken down into energy and wastes) and excreted from the body.

Alcohol Absorption

About 20 percent to 25 percent of the alcohol in a drink is absorbed into the bloodstream from the stomach, and 75 percent to 80 percent is absorbed through the upper part of the small intestine. A minimal amount of alcohol enters the bloodstream further along the gastrointestinal tract. Many factors affect alcohol absorption:

- *Food in the stomach.* The type of food has not been shown to have a meaningful influence on alcohol absorption.

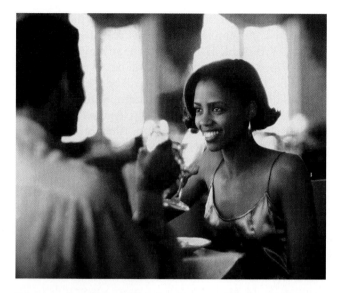

This man and woman may drink the same amount of wine with dinner, but they will metabolize the alcohol at different rates because of the difference in their body weights. In general, women feel the effects of drinking sooner than men do.

- *Gender.* Women absorb alcohol into the bloodstream more quickly than men do.
- *Age.* Older adults have a lower volume of water in the body; with less water to dilute alcohol, they are less tolerant of alcohol.
- *Drug interaction.* Interactions with many prescription and over-the-counter drugs can intensify a drinker's reaction to alcohol, leading to more rapid intoxication.
- *Cigarette smoke.* Nicotine extends the time alcohol stays in the stomach, increasing time for absorption into the bloodstream.
- *Mood and physical condition.* Fear and anger tend to speed up alcohol absorption. The stomach empties more rapidly than normal, allowing the alcohol to be absorbed more easily. People who are stressed, tired, or ill may also feel the effects sooner.
- *Alcohol concentration.* The more concentrated the drink, the more quickly the alcohol is absorbed. Hard liquor is absorbed faster than are beer and wine, which contain nonalcoholic substances that slow the absorption of alcohol.
- *Carbonation.* The carbon dioxide contained in champagne, cola, and ginger ale speeds the absorption of alcohol. Drinks that contain water, juice, or milk are absorbed more slowly.

Another factor that influences how alcohol affects a person is expectations. Studies using volunteers have found that people become more relaxed and talkative if they think they have been given alcoholic beverages, even when their drinks contained no alcohol.

Alcohol Metabolism

A small amount of alcohol is metabolized in the stomach, but 90 percent is metabolized in the liver. Between 2 and 10 percent is not metabolized at all; instead it is excreted unchanged in the breath, urine, and pores of the skin. This is why you can smell alcohol on the breath of someone who has been drinking.

In the liver, alcohol is converted to acetaldehyde by the enzyme *alcohol dehydrogenase (ADH).* Acetaldehyde is then quickly converted to acetic acid by the enzyme *acetaldehyde dehydrogenase.* Acetic acid is eventually broken down into carbon dioxide and water. The ability to metabolize alcohol is dependent on the amount and kind of ADH enzymes available in the liver. If more alcohol molecules arrive in the liver cells than the enzymes can process, the extra molecules circulate through the brain, liver, and other organs until enzymes are available to degrade them. Men make more ADH than women do, and alcoholics make less ADH than do nonalcoholics.

Blood Alcohol Concentration

Rates of alcohol absorption and metabolism affect how much alcohol is circulating in the blood at any given time. **Blood alcohol concentration (BAC)** is a measure of the amount of alcohol in grams in 100 milliliters of blood, expressed as a percentage. For example, for 100 milligrams of alcohol in 100 milliliters of blood, the BAC is .10 percent. BAC provides a good estimate of the alcohol concentration in the brain, which is why it is used as a measure of intoxication by state motor vehicle laws. The alcohol concentration in the brain corresponds well with alcohol concentration in the breath, so breath samples are accurate indicators of BAC. For this reason, breath analyzers are legal in most states for identifying and prosecuting drunk drivers.[3]

BAC is influenced by the amount of alcohol consumed and the rate at which the alcohol is metabolized by the body. Because alcohol is soluble in water and somewhat less soluble in fat, it does not distribute to all body tissues equally.[3] The more body water a person has, the more the alcohol is diluted and the lower the person's BAC will be. The more body fat a person has, the less alcohol is absorbed by body tissue and the more there is to circulate in the bloodstream and reach the brain. Thus, a

KEY TERMS

central nervous system depressant Chemical substance that slows down the activity of the brain and spinal cord.

blood alcohol concentration (BAC) The amount of alcohol in grams in 100 milliliters of blood, expressed as a percentage.

150-pound person with high body fat will have a higher BAC than will a 150-pound person with more lean body tissue who drinks the same amount. Body size alone influences BAC as well; a larger, heavier person has more body surface to diffuse the alcohol (as well as a higher body water content to dilute the alcohol).

Gender Differences in Alcohol Absorption and Metabolism

Women are generally more susceptible to the effects of alcohol and have a higher BAC than men do after drinking the same amount. Both of the factors just described—body size and body fat percentage—play a role in these gender differences. Women are generally smaller than men, and they have a higher body fat percentage. Another factor is that women absorb more of the alcohol they drink because they metabolize alcohol less efficiently than men do. Women produce less of the alcohol-metabolizing enzyme ADH than men do; consequently, they absorb about 30 percent more alcohol into the bloodstream than men do, even

if they consume the same number of drinks that the men consume. For example, if a 20-year-old, 200-pound man and a 20-year-old, 120-pound woman both have three beers in an hour, the man's BAC will be .06 percent at the end of the hour and the woman's will be .11 percent.

Besides body weight, body fat composition, and ADH differences, a woman's menstrual cycle may also influence alcohol absorption and excretion. Alcohol is absorbed more quickly in the premenstrual phase of a woman's cycle and possibly when she uses oral contraceptives.

These differences make women more vulnerable to the health consequences of alcohol, including alcohol-related liver disease, heart disease, and brain damage.[6] The risk for cirrhosis starts at 2½ drinks to 4 drinks a day for a man, but for a woman this risk starts to increase at less than 2 drinks.[26] The rate of atrophy (wasting) of the brain is almost twice as great for women who are chronic drinkers as for men. Women are more susceptible to illness and die at higher rates than men do for every cause of death associated with alcohol. The relationship between alcohol intake, BAC, and body weight for women and men is shown in Table 11.1.

Table 11.1 Relationships Among Gender, Weight, Alcohol Consumption, and Blood Alcohol Concentration

Absolute Alcohol (ounces)	Beverage Intake*	Blood Alcohol Concentrations (g/100 ml)					
		Female (100 lb)	Male (100 lb)	Female (150 lb)	Male (150 lb)	Female (200 lb)	Male (200 lb)
½	1 oz spirits** 1 glass wine 1 can beer	0.045	0.037	0.030	0.025	0.022	0.019
1	2 oz spirits** 2 glasses wine 2 cans beer	0.090	0.075	0.060	0.050	0.045	0.037
2	4 oz spirits** 4 glasses wine 4 cans beer	0.180	0.150	0.120	0.100	0.090	0.070
3	6 oz spirits** 6 glasses wine 6 cans beer	0.270	0.220	0.180	0.150	0.130	0.110
4	8 oz spirits** 8 glasses wine 8 cans beer	0.360	0.300	0.240	0.200	0.180	0.150
5	10 oz spirits** 10 glasses wine 10 cans beer	0.450	0.370	0.300	0.250	0.220	0.180

*in one hour
**100 proof

Source: *Drugs, Society, and Human Behavior,* 11th ed., by C. Ksir, C. L. Hart, and O. Ray, 2006, New York: The McGraw-Hill Companies.

Beating the Odds

Who Is Least Likely to Get Drunk?

Many factors influence how a person is affected by alcohol, including age, gender, physical and psychological condition, expectations, and many others. Brief profiles of three individuals are presented here. Which one do you think is least likely to get drunk?

Sondra is a 22-year-old woman with a large frame who weighs 150 pounds. She is studying for entrance exams to medical school and feels as if she is under a lot of pressure. She lets off steam by running every other day, which helps her stay in shape. On Saturday nights, she parties with friends and usually has three or four beers over the course of the evening. This week she felt overwhelmed by her work, and when her friends came over with a pizza, she quickly downed two beers. Within 2 hours she had had three slices of pizza and two more beers. She drank a bottle of water during the evening too, because she didn't want to get dehydrated.

Mike is a 60-year-old businessman contemplating retirement. His lifestyle is sedentary, and at 5 feet 10 inches and 190 pounds, he is overweight. He is divorced and lives alone with his cat and two dogs. He has been drinking moderately his whole life and is a frequent binge drinker. On this particular occasion, he ate dinner and sat down to enjoy a rented movie. Over the course of the evening he smoked five cigarettes and consumed half a bottle of bourbon, about 8 ounces of 80-proof liquor.

Francisco is a 21-year-old, 160-pound man in an apprenticeship program for roofers. He works hard and has been saving money to marry his high school sweetheart. He doesn't smoke and rarely drinks, even though some of his friends are heavy drinkers. Francisco was devastated this week when his girlfriend broke up with him. He could hardly get himself to work, and when the weekend came he went out drinking with his friends. Within 2 hours he had had three beers and four shots of tequila.

OLC Web site Visit the **Online Learning Center** at www.mhhe.com/teague1e for comments by the authors.

Rates of alcohol metabolism are affected not just by gender but also by ethnicity. As mentioned earlier in this chapter and as discussed in Chapter 2, some ethnic groups have genetically based differences in the enzymes that metabolize alcohol, causing concentrations of alcetaldehyde to build up in the brain and body tissues. This buildup causes the unpleasant reaction referred to as flushing syndrome or flushing effect.

Drinking behavior also influences alcohol metabolism. Chronic drinkers metabolize alcohol more rapidly than nondrinkers do and may become tolerant to alcohol, meaning they have to consume larger amounts to produce the same effects. Chronic users may have twice the tolerance for alcohol as the average person does.[27] (See the box "Who Is Least Likely to Get Drunk?")

Rates of Alcohol Metabolism

Alcohol is metabolized more slowly than it is absorbed. This means that the concentration of alcohol builds when additional drinks are consumed before previous drinks are metabolized. As a rule of thumb, people who have normal liver function metabolize about 0.5 ounce of alcohol (about one drink) per hour.[6] (Remember, rates of alcohol absorption and metabolism vary depending on gender, body weight, and numerous other factors.) For example, if you drink two drinks in 1 hour, you will still have 0.5 ounce of alcohol (one drink) in your system at the end of the hour. Let's say that a 200-pound man goes to a bar at 9:00 p.m. and consumes eight beers by 1:00 a.m. During the 4 hours he was at the bar, his liver would have metabolized 2 ounces of alcohol (four beers), leaving him with 2 ounces of alcohol (four beers) in his system. His BAC at 1:00 a.m. would be 0.11 (see Table 11.1).

You can use this rule of thumb and Table 11.1 to get a rough estimate of your BAC when you are drinking. Allow 1 hour for each drink you consume to be metabolized. Subtract the number of drinks metabolized from the total number of drinks you have consumed.

As noted, individuals differ in their sensitivity to alcohol, so people experience impairment at different BAC levels. Some people experience nausea, headache, and impaired motor skills at very low BAC levels. The National Highway Traffic Safety Administration reports that driving function can be impaired by BAC levels as low as .02 percent to .04 percent.[3] The behavioral effects of alcohol, based on studies of moderate drinkers, are summarized in Table 11.2. As you can see, alertness, ability to think clearly, and reaction time are disrupted even at very low BAC levels. As BAC levels increase, thinking and motor skills become increasingly impaired. A person with a BAC of .08 percent is considered legally drunk in many states; in other states, the cut-off is .10 percent.

Table 11.2 Blood Alcohol Concentration and Behavioral Effects

Percentage BAC	Stage	Behavioral Effects	Hours Required to Metabolize
0.01–0.05	Subclinical	Lowered alertness; bright, expansive mood; talkativeness; impaired judgment and memory; slowed reaction times; impaired motor function; reduced social inhibitions.	2–3
0.03–0.12	Euphoria	Large, consistent increases in reaction time; decrease in peripheral vision; unsteady balance; legally drunk at 0.08.	3–5
0.09–0.25	Excitement	Marked depression in sensory and motor function; loss of critical judgment; drowsiness; marked impairment of memory, comprehension, and perception.	7–10
0.18–0.30	Confusion	Severe motor disturbances; staggering; greatly impaired sensory perceptions; slurred speech; disorientation, increased pain threshold.	10–24
0.25–0.40	Stupor	No comprehension of surroundings although conscious; marked muscular incoordination; vomiting, incontinence.	More than 24
Above 0.35	Coma	Complete unconsciousness; incontinence; subnormal body temperature; death possible. Can result from rapid or binge drinking with few of the earlier effects.	More than 24
Above 0.50	Death	Death from respiratory arrest.	More than 24

Source: Alcohol and the Human Body, www.intox.com/physiology.asp.

Acute Alcohol Intoxication

People who drink heavily in a relatively short time are vulnerable to **acute alcohol intoxication** (also called acute alcohol shock or alcohol poisoning), a potentially life-threatening BAC level. Acute alcohol intoxication can produce collapse of vital body functions, notably respiration and heart function, leading to coma and/or death. A person in shock from acute alcohol intoxication usually has a rapid, weak pulse (100 beats per minute or more) and rapid, irregular breathing (one breath every 3–4 seconds). The skin is cool, damp, and pale or bluish in color, indicating a lower than normal level of oxygen in the blood. These color changes are most evident in the fingernails or membranes under the person's eyelids or inside the mouth.

Vomiting may occur during acute intoxication. The pyloric valve at the juncture of the stomach and small intestine tends to close when the liver is unable to effectively metabolize the amount of alcohol consumed. The additional alcohol remaining in the stomach irritates the lining of the stomach. This irritation causes involuntary muscle contractions that force stomach contents to flow back through the esophagus. If an unconscious drinker is lying in a position that allows the vomit to obstruct the airway passage, the person may die from asphyxiation (see the box "First Aid for Acute Alcohol Intoxication").

The vomiting reflex may be activated only if a BAC of .12 or higher is reached rapidly. Slow, steady drinking allows the vomiting reflex to be suppressed, and BAC can increase to dangerously high levels. At very high alcohol concentrations, .35 or greater, a person can become comatose, and death is possible.

Blackouts

A **blackout** is a period of time during which a drinker is conscious but has impaired memory function; later, he or she is not able to remember events that occurred during this time. The impairment is associated with changes in the hippocampus, a brain structure essential for memory and learning.[1] These changes may be temporary or permanent. Either way, a blackout is a warning sign that fundamental changes have occurred in the structure of the brain.

Researchers once assumed that blackouts were an indicator of alcoholism. Today, alcohol-induced blackouts are recognized as a common experience among nonalcoholics who binge drink. The 2001 College Alcohol Study reported that one in four binge drinkers experienced an alcohol-induced blackout during the school year. Two in four frequent binge drinkers experienced blackouts. Women black out at half the consumption levels of alcohol as reported by men; on average, women who reported blackouts consumed five drinks per occasion, whereas men consumed nine drinks per occasion.[1]

Hangovers

Less dangerous than blackouts but equally unpleasant, hangovers are a common reaction to alcohol toxicity.

Challenges & Choices

First Aid for Acute Alcohol Intoxication

People who have passed out from heavy drinking should be watched closely. All too often they are carried to bed and forgotten. For their safety, follow these measures:

- Know and recognize the symptoms of acute alcohol intoxication:
  — Lack of response when spoken to or shaken
  — Inability to wake up
  — Inability to stand up without help
  — Rapid or irregular pulse
  — Rapid, irregular respiration or difficulty breathing
  — Clammy, bluish skin
- Call 911. An intoxicated person who cannot be roused or wakened or has other symptoms listed above requires emergency medical treatment.
- Do not leave the person to "sleep it off." He or she may never awaken.

- Roll an unconscious drinker onto his or her side to minimize the chance of airway obstruction from vomit.
- If the person vomits, make certain his or her head is positioned lower than the rest of the body. You may need to reach into the person's mouth to clear the airway.
- Try to find out if the person has taken other drugs or medications that might interact with alcohol.
- Stay with the person until medical help arrives.

It's Not Just Personal . . .

Drinking games, hazing rituals, and other excessive drinking practices contribute to cases of acute alcohol intoxication among college students. Schools as diverse as MIT, Louisiana State University, and the University of Colorado have instituted measures to reduce drinking in response to student deaths and hospitalizations from alcohol poisoning.

They are characterized by headache, stomach upset, thirst, and fatigue. Despite the consistency of these symptoms, the biological reasons behind them are not well understood. Health experts speculate that alcohol disrupts the body's water balance, causing excessive urination and thirst the next day. The stomach lining may be irritated by increased production of hydrochloric acid, resulting in nausea. Alcohol also reduces the water content of brain cells. When the brain cells rehydrate and swell the next day, nerve pain occurs. Drinking more alcohol does not relieve these symptoms.[6] The only known remedy for a hangover is pain medication, rest, and time.

HEALTH RISKS OF ALCOHOL USE

Excessive alcohol consumption causes more than 100,000 deaths each year in the United States. Alcohol is toxic and has an effect on virtually all body organs and systems. The effects of alcohol are not restricted to the body, however; alcohol use can affect all aspects of a person's functioning. In this section we consider medical problems and social problems associated with the misuse of alcohol.

Medical Problems Associated With Alcohol Use

The major organs and systems damaged by alcohol use are the cardiovascular system, the liver, the brain, the immune system, and the reproductive system (Figure 11.3). Alcohol use is associated with certain cancers, and when pregnant women drink, it can cause a set of fetal birth defects known as **fetal alcohol syndrome (FAS)** (discussed in Chapter 16). Children born with FAS have permanent physical and mental impairments.

Heart Disease and Stroke

Chronic heavy drinking is a major cause of degenerative disease of the heart muscle, a condition called **cardiomyopathy,** and of heart arrhythmias (irregular heartbeat). Abnormal heart rhythm is one cause of sudden death in alcoholics, whether or not they already had heart disease. Heavy drinking also causes coronary heart disease (disease of the arteries serving the heart) and has been shown

KEY TERMS

acute alcohol intoxication   A life-threatening blood alcohol concentration.

blackout   Period of time during which a drinker is conscious but has impaired memory function as a result of changes in the hippocampus.

fetal alcohol syndrome (FAS)   Set of birth defects associated with use of alcohol during pregnancy.

cardiomyopathy   Disease of the heart muscle.

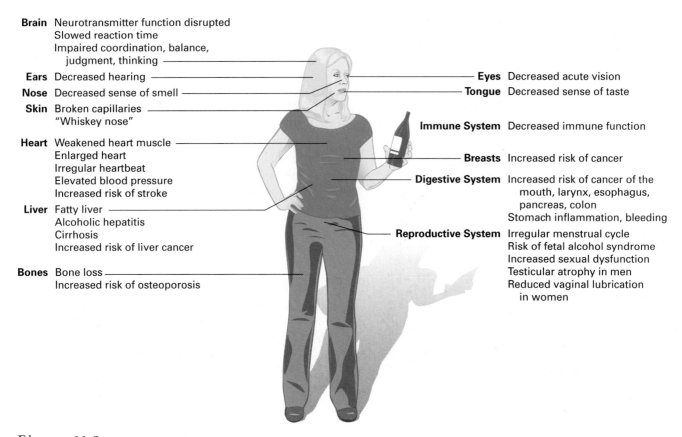

Figure 11.3   Effects of alcohol on the body.

to increase the risk for heart attacks owing to coronary heart disease. Some studies have reported that binge drinkers have six times the risk for fatal attacks than moderate drinkers do.[3]

In addition, long-term heavy drinking can elevate blood pressure and increase the severity of high blood pressure, which increases the risk for stroke (an interruption in the blood supply to the brain). Although some evidence indicates that moderate alcohol consumption has beneficial effects on blood pressure, it is generally held that consuming one drink a day can increase blood pressure in middle-aged adults and in older adults who already have high blood pressure.[3]

Liver Disease

The liver is a vital organ with many metabolic, digestive, and regulatory functions, including filtering toxins and pathogens from the blood. Alcohol-related liver disease occurs in three phases. The first, called **fatty liver,** occurs when the liver is flooded with more alcohol than it can metabolize, causing it to swell with fat globules. This condition can literally develop overnight as a result of binge drinking. In men, the alcohol capacity of the liver is about 70 grams to 80 grams, equivalent to about six drinks; in women it is three to four drinks. Drinking more than that at one sitting may cause fatty liver.

Fatty liver is not a serious problem for most drinkers, because with abstinence (usually about 30 days or so), stored fatty acids are used as fuel energy and the condition is completely reversed. Serious health problems may develop, however, when stored fatty-acid molecules increase in size and their cell membranes rupture, causing liver cells to die.[6]

The second phase of liver disease is called **alcoholic hepatitis,** which includes both liver inflammation and liver function impairment. This condition typically occurs in parts of the liver where cells are dead or dying. Alcoholic hepatitis can occur in the absence of a fatty liver, which suggests that direct toxic effects of alcohol may be the cause.[6]

The third phase of liver disease is **cirrhosis,** scarring of the liver tissue. Although other diseases can cause cirrhosis (such as viral hepatitis), between 40 and 90 percent of people with cirrhosis have a history of alcohol abuse.[3] The risk rises sharply with higher levels of consumption. It usually takes at least 10 years of steady, heavy drinking for cirrhosis to develop.[6]

As cirrhosis sets in, liver cells are replaced by fibrous tissue, called collagen, which changes the structure of the liver and decreases blood flow to the organ. Liver cells die and liver function is impaired, leading to fluid accumulation in the body, jaundice (yellowing of the skin), and an opportunity for infections or cancers to establish themselves. Jaundice is a sign that toxins are beginning to accumulate in the blood owing to liver failure. The prognosis for people with alcoholic hepatitis or cirrhosis is poor. The death rate exceeds 60 percent over a 4-year period, with most deaths occurring within the first year.[6]

Cancer

Alcohol is associated with several types of cancer, particularly cancers of the head and neck (mouth, pharynx, larynx, and esophagus); cancers of the digestive tract; and breast cancer.[3] Research suggests that cancers of the upper digestive tract are associated with both the consumption of alcoholic beverages and the number of drinks consumed.[6] There is insufficient evidence to conclude that alcohol causes an increased risk for stomach cancer. Alcohol causes inflammation of the pancreas, the gland that produces insulin, among other functions, but the link between this inflammation and pancreatic cancer remains unproven. There is a weak association between alcohol and colon and rectal cancers.[3] Tobacco is a suspected factor in these cancers when a person also drinks alcohol.

Substantial evidence from many countries suggests that the risk of breast cancer increases for women who consume more than three drinks per day compared with women who abstain.[3] The Nurses Health Study found that women who consumed two drinks a day have a 10 percent higher risk of breast cancer than do women who consumed one drink per day.[1] Scientists theorize that alcohol increases a woman's exposure to estrogen and androgens, hormones that may increase cancer risk. The risk is more pronounced at heavy intake levels.

Brain Damage

Heavy alcohol consumption causes anatomical changes in the brain and directly damages nerve cells. Alcohol can cause a loss of brain tissue, inflammation of the brain, and a widening of fissures in the cortex (covering) of the brain.[28] People who consume moderate amounts of alcohol do not experience changes in brain structure and function, according to most studies, but heavy drinking, especially binge drinking, has been shown to disrupt short-term memory and the ability to analyze complex problems.[3] In long-term alcohol abuse, loss of brain tissue is associated with a mental disorder called alcoholic-induced persisting dementia, an overall decline in intellect. Some of this loss may be reversible if the person abstains from alcohol use for a few months, but after age 40, there is little improvement even with abstinence.[28]

Because the brain continues to grow and mature until the early 20s (see Chapter 3), there is concern that heavy alcohol use during the teen years can be harmful to the developing brain. Studies have revealed that the hippocampus (a center for learning and memory) is 10 percent smaller in teenagers who drink heavily than in those who

don't.[28] Research has also found differences in the prefrontal cortex, the center for executive functions (rational thinking, planning). Teenagers who drink heavily score worse than nondrinkers do on tests, particularly tests involving verbal and nonverbal information recall, and they have an increased risk of school failure, social problems, depression, suicidal thoughts, and violence.[28,29]

Immune System Functioning

Heavy alcohol consumption can reduce the efficiency of the immune system, apparently by interfering with the production and secretion of immune cells. The overall effect is an impaired immune system that leaves the drinker vulnerable to infection. There is no evidence, however, that moderate alcohol consumption suppresses the immune system.[3,6]

Body Weight and Nutrition

There are 7 calories in each gram of alcohol and between 12 and 15 grams of alcohol in a standard drink. This means that between 84 and 105 calories are provided by the alcohol in one drink. Carbohydrates and other substances in alcoholic beverages provide additional calories: A regular beer has about 144 calories; a glass of wine, 100–105 calories, and a shot of gin or whiskey, 96 calories.[30] Mixers add more calories, as do *alcopops*—sugary, fizzy, fruit-flavored drinks popular among younger drinkers.

These calories are empty, providing almost no nutrients. According to the *Dietary Guidelines for Americans,* calories from alcohol have to come from the "discretionary calorie allowance," usually amounting to a few hundred calories a day, after nutrient requirements have been met (see Chapter 7). It's easy to see that consuming alcohol can lead to weight gain; these calories have a tendency to be deposited in the abdomen, giving drinkers the characteristic "beer belly."

On the other hand, long-term heavy drinkers who substitute the calories in alcohol for those in food are at risk for weight loss and malnutrition. They are also vulnerable to alcohol-induced persisting amnestic disorder, a mental disorder characterized by memory impairment and an inability to learn new information (a different disorder from alchohol-induced persisting dementia). This disorder is caused by thiamin deficiency (a B vitamin).

KEY TERMS

fatty liver   Condition in which the liver swells with fat globules as a result of alcohol consumption.

alcoholic hepatitis   Inflammation of the liver as a result of alcohol consumption.

cirrhosis   Scarring of the liver as a result of alcohol consumption.

Social drinking is a common way of loosening up at a party. As inhibitions fall, the result may be inappropriate social behavior, risky sexual behavior, or even violence.

Heavy drinkers are at risk for it not only because they fail to consume enough nutritious foods but also because alcohol interferes with thiamin absorption.

Social Problems Associated With Alcohol Use

Alcohol affects not just those who are drinking but also those around the drinkers. Social problems associated with alcohol use include high-risk sexual behavior, violence, injury, and suicide.

Sexual Behavior

Alcohol reduces social inhibitions, and reduced inhibition may lead to unplanned sexual activity and a lowered likelihood of practicing safe sex (such as using a condom). One study found that frequent binge drinkers were five times less likely to practice safe sex than were non-binge drinkers.[29] Heavy drinkers are more likely to have multiple sex partners and to engage in other high-risk sexual behaviors. These behaviors are associated with increased risk of sexually transmitted disease and unplanned pregnancy.[29]

Violence

The National Crime Victimization Survey (NCVS) has consistently found that alcohol is more likely than any other drug to be associated with violence. One study found that 15 percent of robberies, 28 percent of aggravated and simple assaults, and 37 percent of rapes and sexual assaults are committed by individuals who have been drinking. Alcohol is a factor in 67 percent of domestic violence cases and half of all homicides.[3] Women who binge drink or date men who binge drink are at increased risk for sexual exploitation (rape and other forms of non-consensual sex).[31]

Injury

The relationship between alcohol and risk of injury has been established for a wide variety of circumstances, including automobile crashes, falls, and fires. Reduced cognitive function, impaired physical coordination, and increased risk-taking behavior (impulsivity) are the alcohol-related factors that lead to injury. Alcohol has also been shown to increase the risk of serious injury and decrease the probability of survival because it impairs heart and circulatory system function. The risk of injury increases steadily with the amount of alcohol consumed.[3]

Suicide

Alcohol use is a factor in about one third of suicides, and it is second only to depression as a predictor of suicide attempts by youth.[6] The relationship between alcohol and depression is very strong. Estimates are that 20 percent to 36 percent of people who commit suicide were drinking shortly before their suicide or had a history of alcohol abuse.[3] Alcohol-associated suicides tend to be impulsive rather than premeditated acts.

Another View: Health Benefits

The Health Professional Study found that men and women who drink moderately on 5 to 7 days of the week have less risk of heart disease than do those who drink moderately on fewer days of the week.[32] Moderate drinkers also have less risk of heart disease than do either abstainers or heavy drinkers. The *Dietary Guidelines for Americans* note that the lowest rates of death occur among people who consume one to two drinks a day.

Scientists speculate that moderate alcohol consumption increases high-density lipoproteins (HDL) ("good cholesterol"), has an anticlotting effect on the blood, and reduces stress.[32] The beneficial effects of alcohol on HDL levels and blood clotting may be only temporary, lasting perhaps 24 hours, so that people who drink moderately every day maintain optimal protection against heart disease. It is apparently the pattern of drinking, not the type of alcoholic beverage, that confers benefits. People who drink wine, for example, tend to do so in small amounts every day rather than in large amounts. Binge drinking does not serve as a protective factor and can actually increase the risk for heart disease.[3] In women, the beneficial effects may be offset by an increased risk of breast cancer.

The *Dietary Guidelines for Americans* advise that moderate alcohol consumption—one drink a day for women and two drinks a day for men—can be beneficial for middle-aged and older adults, the age groups most susceptible to coronary heart disease. In younger adults, however, alcohol appears to have fewer, if any, health benefits, and it is associated with more deaths from injuries and accidents. Even light drinking can have adverse effects on certain people, such as individuals with liver disease or high blood pressure. It is not recommended that anyone begin drinking or drink more frequently because of anticipated health benefits.

ALCOHOL MISUSE, ABUSE, AND DEPENDENCE

Misusing alcohol can lead to a range of problems, from intoxication, to alcohol abuse, to alcohol dependence, to alcoholism. Between 20 and 25 percent of people who drink develop some alcohol-related problem(s) at some point.[6] About 4 percent to 5 percent develop alcohol dependence and are categorized as alcoholics.[33]

Problem drinking is a pattern of alcohol use that impairs the drinker's life, causing personal difficulties and difficulties for other people. For college students, such difficulties might be missed classes or poor academic performance. **Alcohol abuse** is a pattern of drinking that leads to distress or impairment and increases the risk of health problems and/or social problems.[11] It is the continued use of alcohol despite an awareness of these effects. According to the American Psychiatric Association's *Diagnostic and Statistical Manual of Mental Disorders (DSM-IV-TR)*, a diagnosis of alcohol abuse may be made if one or more of the following has occurred at any time in a 12-month period:

- Recurrent abuse of alcohol that impairs the drinker's ability to fulfill major obligations at home, work, or school (for example, work absenteeism).
- Recurrent alcohol abuse in situations that may be physically hazardous (for example, operating machine equipment).

- Recurrent alcohol abuse associated with legal problems (for example, drunk driving).
- Recurrent alcohol abuse despite frequent social problems associated with drinking (for example, fighting while drunk).[11]

Alcohol dependence is considered a separate disorder; it is characterized by a strong craving for alcohol.[18] People who are dependent on alcohol use it compulsively, and most will eventually experience physiological changes in brain and body chemistry as a result of alcohol use. One indicator of dependence is the development of **tolerance,** reduced sensitivity to the effects of a drug so that larger and larger amounts are needed to produce the same effects.[6] Another indicator is experiencing **withdrawal,** a state of acute physical and psychological discomfort, when alcohol consumption abruptly stops.

Alcohol dependence is also known as **alcoholism,** defined as a chronic disease with genetic, psychosocial, and environmental causes.[11] It is often progressive and fatal. The manifestations of alcoholism include lack of control over drinking, preoccupation with alcohol, use of alcohol despite adverse consequences, and distortions in thinking (most notably denial). This definition is similar to that of problem drinking, but there is a difference in degree. Alcohol becomes a problem when individuals are impaired by their drinking, but drinkers become alcoholics when they become dependent on alcohol. Alcoholics spend time anticipating their next drink (craving), planning when and where to get it, and hiding their alcohol use from others.

As mentioned in Chapter 2, evidence indicates that there may be two distinct types of alcoholism, both with a

KEY TERMS

problem drinking   Pattern of alcohol use that impairs the drinker's life, causing difficulties for the drinker and for others.

alcohol abuse   Pattern of alcohol use that leads to distress or impairment, increases the risk of health and/or social problems, and continues despite awareness of these effects.

alcohol dependence   Disorder characterized by a strong craving for alcohol, the development of tolerance for alcohol, and symptoms of withdrawal if alcohol consumption stops abruptly.

tolerance   Reduced sensitivity to the effects of a drug so that larger and larger amounts are needed to produce the same effects; a sign of dependence.

withdrawal   State of acute physical and psychological discomfort that occurs if use of a drug stops abruptly; a sign of dependence.

alcoholism   A primary chronic disease characterized by excessive, compulsive drinking.

genetic link.[6] Type I alcoholics often feel guilt, fear, or a loss of control about their drinking behavior. Their personality traits include shyness, rigidity, dependence, pessimism, high anxiety, and slowness to anger. They typically grew up in a home environment where heavy drinking was the norm and had at least one parent who was a problem drinker. Type I alcoholics usually start heavy drinking after age 25. This drinking pattern is typically triggered by environmental stressors, such as setbacks or losses. Alcohol reduces anxiety for Type I alcoholics.

Type II alcoholics become heavy drinkers before age 25; almost all are men. Their characteristics are the opposite of those of Type I alcoholics. They usually do not experience feelings of guilt, fear, or loss of control about their drinking behavior. They are impulsive, aggressive, adventurous, optimistic, independent, and quick to anger. Alcohol reinforces feelings of elation for Type II alcoholics. The genetic link is believed to be stronger in Type II alcoholism.

TREATMENT OPTIONS

Treatment options for alcohol-related disorders include brief interventions, inpatient treatment programs, outpatient treatment programs, and self-help approaches.

Brief Interventions

Some alcohol problems are discovered by primary care physicians through the use of screening surveys that identify individuals who have developed or may be at risk of developing health problems associated with drinking. If a drinking problem is discovered, steps can be implemented to help the patient avoid or minimize further problems. Advice and counseling are the principal intervention techniques used by the primary care physician. Research has shown that such brief interventions can be valuable in reducing a patient's problems with alcohol.[34] Brief interventions used with college students have also appeared to be effective for reducing alcohol use and long-term alcohol-related problems. It is not clear whether brief interventions are effective with patients who are already alcoholics.[3]

Inpatient Treatment

When alcohol-related problems are severe, individuals benefit from placement in a residential facility specializing in alcohol recovery. Studies suggest that inpatient treatments are highly successful: 70 percent of people who complete the program remain abstinent for at least five years.[3]

The first stage of treatment is detoxification, the gradual withdrawal of alcohol from the body. Withdrawal symptoms include profuse sweating, rapid heart rate, elevated blood pressure, nausea, headache, difficulty

sleeping, depression, and irritability.[33] People who have been heavy drinkers for a long time and/or who have an underlying medical condition may experience more severe withdrawal symptoms, such as seizures and, rarely, a disturbance called **delirium tremens (DTs).**[6] Symptoms of the DTs include delirium, disorientation, and hallucinations. An acute DT episode is a medical emergency requiring hospitalization.

The early phase of alcohol treatment may also include medications, such as anti-anxiety and antidepressant drugs, although such drugs are usually prescribed only when the person has an underlying medical or psychological disorder. Another drug that may be prescribed is disulfiram (Antabuse). This drug causes a person to become acutely nauseated if any alcohol is consumed, although it does not reduce alcohol cravings.[6] Researchers are exploring drugs that increase levels of the neurotransmitter serotonin as a way to reduce cravings and relapse.[3]

Counseling is an important component in any kind of alcohol treatment. Family members are often encouraged to participate in the recovery process. This participation helps them better understand how they are personally affected and how they can help their loved one recover from alcoholism.

Outpatient Treatment

Economic pressures have led to a reduction in the number of inpatient treatment days covered by health insurance companies, which in turn has led to greater use of outpatient programs. In these programs, patients participate in a treatment program during the day and return home in the evening. Treatment typically includes individual counseling, group counseling, and marital or family counseling. Research suggests that outpatient programs are as effective or more effective than inpatient programs are.[3]

Self-Help Programs

The best-known self-help program is Alcoholics Anonymous (AA). The goal of AA is total abstinence from alcohol. A basic premise of AA is that an alcoholic is biologically different from a nonalcoholic person and consequently can never safely drink any alcohol at all. Although alcoholics are not to blame for their problem, they still must take responsibility for their behavior. In the 12-step path to recovery, members recognize that they are "powerless over alcohol" and have to seek help from a "higher power." (For more on this aspect of AA, see the box "Spirituality and Alcohol Treatment Programs.") Other key components of AA are group support and the use of sponsors—members who are paired with new members and who provide support if the temptation to relapse becomes overwhelming.

Some people are uncomfortable with AA's focus on spirituality, and alternative programs have been developed

HIGHLIGHT ON HEALTH
Spirituality and Alcohol Treatment Programs

Because alcoholism is considered a disease of the body, mind, and spirit, AA and many other 12-step programs strongly emphasize the spiritual dimension of health and recovery. In AA, people are taught that they do not have the strength to maintain sobriety on their own; this strength can be acquired only through reliance on a higher power.

Such reliance can be a barrier to people who do not have a strong religious faith. Moderate management (MM) treatment programs are based on the premise that internal strength for sobriety can be derived from one's own power, from a higher power, or from a combination of the two. Personal responsibility is founded on self-control and self-discipline in MM programs.

The difference between AA and MM programs points up the different meanings people may attribute to the concept of spirituality. For some, it means belonging to an organized religion associated with a supreme being. For others, it means a more diffuse sense of belonging to something greater than oneself. Both views draw from a universal human need to understand the meaning of life. They share the beliefs that there is meaning and purpose to life, that life is worth living, and that each person has value and worth.

Source: Al-Anon Family Group Headquarters, Inc., www.al-anon.org.

that do not have this focus. One such group is Rational Recovery (RR), which focuses on self rather than spirituality. Members use reason instead of prayer, identify emotions that lead them to drink, and learn skills to control these emotional impulses. Like AA, RR stresses total abstinence.

Another objection to AA is its perceived masculine orientation, and alternative programs have been developed by and for women, such as Women for Sobriety (WFS). Like AA and RR, WFS is a mutual aid organization that encourages personal responsibility and aims for total abstinence. However, WFS pays more attention to some of the problems characteristic of female alcoholics. It focuses on building self-esteem, dealing with social disapproval, solving financial and child care issues, and addressing underlying psychological problems, such as anxiety, depression, and dependence on other substances. Although AA dominates self-help programs for alcoholism, it has not been shown to be more effective than some of these alternative programs.[3]

Self-help programs have also been developed for family members and friends of alcoholics. Al-Anon is a support program whereby individuals can explore how they may have enabled the alcoholic's behavior (for example, by covering up or rationalizing) and how they can change their behavior. Alateen is a support program for young people who have been affected by someone else's drinking. Adult Children of Alcoholics is a program that provides a supportive environment where people can confront the potentially lifelong emotional effects associated with growing up in an alcoholic household.

Relapse Prevention

Recovery from alcoholism is a lifelong process. The first two years after treatment are usually the hardest. The dif-

ficulty of recovery is thought to be due to the changes that alcohol has produced in the brain. The brain's circuitry has been reprogrammed such that pleasure has become associated primarily with alcohol. Craving can continue for years, even during sleep. MRI brain scans have shown that viewing a picture of an alcoholic drink activates a part of the frontal cortex in the brains of alcoholics but not in the brains of moderate drinkers. The mere thought of a drink can affect the brain of a recovering alcoholic.[35]

Some health experts estimate that more than 90 percent of people recovering from substance abuse use alcohol or other drugs within a 12-month period after treatment.[33] Still, about 70 percent of those who receive treatment stop drinking for prolonged periods. Relapse prevention focuses on social skills training (stress management, assertiveness, communication skills, self-control) and family and marital therapy. Despite a high relapse rate, those who participate in treatment programs clearly do better than those who do not.

The Harm Reduction Approach

Some health experts disagree with the disease model of alcoholism, in which it is viewed as a chronic disease that is either present or absent.[34] This view seems to rule out

KEY TERM

delirium tremens (DTs)   Severe condition characterized by delirium, disorientation, and hallucinations, associated with withdrawal from alcohol.

the possibility that there could be some middle ground or that some drinking by alcoholics might be acceptable. In contrast, the **harm reduction** approach focuses on reducing the harm associated with drinking, both to the individual and to society. An example of harm reduction is **controlled drinking,** which emphasizes moderation rather than abstinence.[18] Individuals are taught to practice responsible, controlled drinking through cognitive behavioral techniques, such as using a diary to chart drinking patterns, and consumption management techniques, such as limiting drinks to one per hour.

Controlled drinking programs have long been promoted in Great Britain and Canada.[18] These programs are controversial precisely because they do not require abstinence. Some experts fear that making controlled drinking an option for alcoholism treatment will cause a stampede of patients away from abstinence programs, although research has not shown that this happens.[36] Most mental health experts agree that total abstinence is the most effective approach for recovery from alcoholism.[3] Controlled drinking is considered appropriate for early-stage problem drinkers.[37]

Public Policies and Laws Aimed at Harm Reduction

A variety of public policies and laws are aimed at reducing the harm caused by alcohol consumption. These include the minimum drinking age, drunk driving laws, and various community ordinances.

Minimum Legal Drinking Age

Since 1984, all states have had laws prohibiting the purchase and public possession of alcohol by people under the age of 21. Despite inconsistent compliance with these laws, research suggests that they result in less underage drinking than occurred when the drinking age was 18.[38] Evidence also suggests that these laws result in less drinking after age 21.[3] Some people argue that the minimum drinking age laws are too restrictive and create a mystique about alcohol that fosters irresponsible drinking, but research does not support this argument.

Drunk Driving Laws and Sobriety Checkpoints

Studies show that tough drinking laws are effective in preventing drunk driving,[18] despite problems with enforcement and detection of intoxicated drivers. Still, many people continue to drink and drive. Education and treatment programs used in conjunction with punishments, such as mandatory suspension of drivers' licenses for first-time offenders, have not proven to be effective in preventing driving under the influence.[3] A practice that does substantially increase compliance with drunk driving laws is the use of sobriety checkpoints. Law enforcement agents

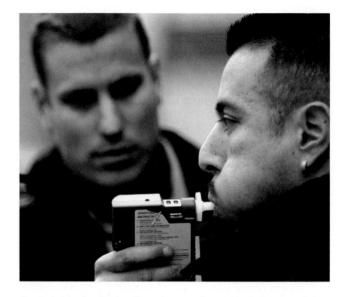

An alcohol sensor or a breath analyzer can be used to test a suspected drunk driver for intoxication. If this young man did not submit to such testing, what consequences might he face?

check drivers for intoxication with alcohol sensors and breath analyzer tests. Alcohol sensors are noninvasive tests that can detect the presence of alcohol on the breath when held in the vicinity of a driver. Breath analyzer tests measure the amount of alcohol exhaled in the breath.

Laboratory tests, such as urinalysis and blood tests, are sometimes used to confirm BAC level. Many states now require people suspected of driving under the influence of alcohol or illicit drugs to undergo blood testing. Refusal to submit to either a breath analyzer test or urinalysis when requested by law enforcement can result in immediate driver's license revocation.

Server Liability Laws

Server liability laws make licensed establishments liable for injuries or property damage caused by an intoxicated or underage customer who is served by the establishment. These laws also apply to private individuals who serve alcohol at social functions. Under server liability laws, a third party who has been injured by a drunk driver can file a civil suit against the server for damages. The jury is still out on whether server liability laws are effective.[3] Few cases have been prosecuted, and few licensed establishments have been cited for serving alcohol to intoxicated patrons.[3]

Restrictions on Liquor Sales and Outlets

Ease of access is a key factor in alcohol consumption. The more places there are to purchase alcohol within a certain geographical area, the higher the rates of alcohol consumption and alcohol-related harm.[3] Some communities have worked for a more even distribution of alcohol outlets throughout their area to curb this problem.

Studies show that alcohol is readily available to underage drinkers. Although parents and other adults are the most common source, underage drinkers also buy alcoholic beverages at convenience stores, liquor stores, and bars.[39] Recently, the Internet has become a source for underage purchase of alcoholic beverages. The National Academy of Sciences estimates that 10 percent of underage purchases of alcoholic beverages are ordered through the Internet or home delivery services. The amount of underage sales over the Internet is small, but health authorities are concerned that it could become a virtual vending machine for underage drinkers.[38]

Tax Increases

Another way to control alcohol consumption is by increasing taxation. Research suggests that an increase in price of alcohol is met by a corresponding decrease in consumption per capita. Higher prices appear to reduce consumption by underage and moderate drinkers but not by heavy drinkers. Raising prices too much might also create a black market for alcoholic beverages.[3,38,39]

Community Ordinances

Local communities have a variety of measures at their disposal for influencing alcohol consumption, including limiting drink specials at local bars, prohibiting out-of-sight sales (purchases made by one person for several others), and imposing a minimum drink price.[40] Communities can also enforce fines and revoke liquor licenses when bars serve underage drinkers. House parties can be controlled through public nuisance and noise laws. Research suggests that comprehensive community programs that unite city agencies and private citizens are effective in reducing drunk driving, related driving risks, and traffic deaths and injuries.[3]

TAKING ACTION

Is alcohol a problem in your life? Do you wonder what you can do to reduce or prevent harm from alcohol-related activities? In this section we provide some suggestions for individual actions.

Are You at Risk?

First, you need to determine whether you are at risk for alcohol-related problems. Physicians sometimes use the CAGE questionnaire to identify alcoholism. It consists of four questions:

- Have you ever tried to cut down on your drinking?
- Have you ever been annoyed by criticism of your drinking?
- Have you ever felt guilty about your drinking?
- Have you ever had a morning "eye-opener"?

A yes answer to one or more of these questions does not mean you are an alcoholic, but it does suggest that you may be at risk for alcohol dependence. To learn more about your risks, see the box "Assess Your Alcohol-Related Attitudes and Behavior."

Developing a Behavior Change Plan

If you decide you would like to change your behavior around alcohol, you can develop a behavior change plan following the steps described next.

Record Behavior Patterns

Recognize, review, and evaluate the role that alcohol plays in your life. Keeping a drinking diary can help you analyze your drinking patterns. A drinking diary is a record of when, where, and with whom you drink alcohol; how much you drink; antecedents (thoughts, moods, stressors, people, situations) that lead up to your drinking; your thoughts and feelings before, during, and after drinking; and any short- or long-term consequences of your drinking. Record your drinking behavior every day for 2 weeks.

Analyze Your Drinking Diary

To analyze your diary, look for patterns in your drinking. Do you drink only on weekends or only at parties? Do you drink when you are alone? Do you drink after a major exam or when you have completed an assignment? Or do you drink before a stressful event? Does a certain place, person, or emotion trigger your drinking? In short, analyze your diary to find out everything you can about your drinking behavior.

Establish Goals

If you decide you want to change your drinking behavior, set goals for yourself. Goals should be specific, motivating, achievable, and rewarding. "I'm going to drink less" is too vague a goal. "I'm going to drink only once a week and have no more than four drinks" is a more specific, measurable goal. Your goals should be modest and incremental.

KEY TERMS

harm reduction   Approach to alcohol treatment that focuses on a broader range of drinking behaviors and treatments than are associated with abstinence programs.

controlled drinking   Approach to drinking that emphasizes moderation rather than abstinence.

HIGHLIGHT ON HEALTH

Assess Your Alcohol-Related Attitudes and Behavior

Do you sometimes wonder if you have a problem with alcohol? This quick assessment will help you find out. Simply answer yes or no to the following questions.

1. Are you unable to stop drinking after a certain number of drinks?
2. Do you need a drink to get motivated?
3. Do you often forget what happened while you were partying (have blackouts)?
4. Do you drink or party alone?
5. Have others annoyed you by criticizing your alcohol use?
6. Have you been involved in fights with your friends or family while you were drunk or high?
7. Have you done or said anything while drinking that you later regretted?
8. Have you destroyed or damaged property while drinking?
9. Do you drive while high or drunk?
10. Have you been physically hurt while drinking?
11. Have you been in trouble with the school authorities or the campus police because of your drinking?
12. Have you dropped or chosen friends based on their drinking habits?
13. Do you think you are a normal drinker despite friends' comments that you drink too much?
14. Have you ever missed classes because you were too hungover to get up on time?
15. Have you ever done poorly on an exam or assignment because of drinking?
16. Do you think about drinking or getting high a lot?
17. Do you feel guilty or self-conscious about your drinking?

If you answered yes to three or more questions, you may be consuming alcoholic beverages in a harmful manner. Consider contacting your student health clinic or counseling center for information or help.

Source: From "Alcohol: Decisions on Tap," by permission of American College Health Association, P.O. Box 28937, Baltimore, MD 21240-8937.

Implement Your Plan

Develop specific strategies to attain your goals. For example, if you always have a drink when you get home from work or class and you want to eliminate that drink, don't keep alcohol in your house. If you drink in social situations or with certain people, learn to say no to some drinks. Tell people you feel better when you don't drink, and avoid people who can't accept that. Plan ahead what you will do when you're tempted to have a drink. Ask family and friends for their support. For more suggestions, see the box "Tips for Changing Your Alcohol-Related Behavior."

Evaluate Your Results

After a few weeks, evaluate the outcome of your behavior change plan. Did you achieve your goals? If not, what obstacles prevented you from succeeding? How can you overcome these obstacles? People who succeed at changing their behavior don't necessarily do so the first time they try. The key is to view each failure as an opportunity to learn more about yourself. Periodically assessing your progress allows you to devise alternative strategies for reaching your goals.

Be an Advocate

If you are interested in addressing the serious consequences of irresponsible alcohol consumption, you can join an advocacy organization or concerned citizens group on your campus or in your community. Mothers Against Drunk Driving (MADD) is a nationwide advocacy organization with hundreds of local chapters throughout North America. It was founded to educate citizens about the effects of alcohol on driving and to influence legislation on drunk driving. Recently, MADD has focused on the problem of binge drinking on college campuses and has created an honor roll of colleges that actively combat underage and binge drinking.

Students Against Destructive Decisions (SADD) initially focused on drunk driving by youth but has broadened its activities to include initiatives against underage drinking, illicit drug use, failure to use seat belts, and drugged driving. The central mission of SADD, however, remains a pact called "Contract for Life," an agreement parents and teenagers can make to provide safe transportation for one another, no questions asked, if any of them has become impaired by alcohol consumption.

Challenges & Choices

Tips for Changing Your Alcohol-Related Behavior

- Stock your refrigerator with healthy beverages—juice, bottled water, milk, sports drinks, diet soda.

- If you want to have alcoholic beverages on hand, buy small quantities—one or two bottles of beer rather than a six-pack, for example.

- If you drink when you're upset, lonely, or stressed out, learn how to handle these feelings in a healthier way, such as exercising, meditating, or talking with a friend or counselor.

- If you drink when you're with other people, learn how to socialize without alcohol; try hiking or playing sports with friends, or attend alcohol-free events.

- If others are pressuring you to drink, learn how to say no.

- When you are drinking, keep your BAC low by drinking slowly, drinking water and nonalcoholic beverages as well as alcoholic ones, eating food, and staying within your limits; avoid mixed or carbonated drinks.

- When you are the host, provide nonalcoholic beverages and food, and make sure no one who drives away from your house at the end of the party is drunk or impaired.

It's Not Just Personal . . .

Many people think that they can drink and still be capable of making rational decisions, that they can drive safely if they consume just a few drinks, that they can sober up quickly if they have to, and that drinking isn't dangerous. All are myths.

Boost Alcohol Consciousness Concerning the Health of University Students (BACCHUS) is an organization with hundreds of chapters across North America. It is run by student volunteers and promotes both abstinence and responsible drinking. Some BACCHUS chapters have joined with Greeks Advocating Mature Management of Alcohol (GAMMA) to provide a peer education network. This network program may be called BACCHUS or GAMMA on your college campus. The merging of BACCHUS and GAMMA has led to a broadening of approaches to health issues that affect college students.[1]

Many parents and students look into school alcohol policies as a factor in college selection. Some organizations publish rankings of the most notorious "party schools." Some colleges have signed on to national programs to combat binge drinking. These anti-alcohol actions have been fueled by the knowledge that a crackdown can play a key role in attracting applicants.

***

Whatever your attitudes toward alcohol, and whatever your alcohol-related behaviors have been thus far, remember that it is up to you to decide what role you want alcohol to play in your life. Many people do not drink at all, and many more drink only occasionally. Drinking is a serious problem for only about 5 percent to 10 percent of the population. You can make sure you are not among that group by making responsible decisions about alcohol use.

You Make the Call

Should Passive Alcohol Sensors Be Used by Law Enforcement?

The National Highway Safety and Traffic Administration estimates that about 40 percent of all traffic fatalities are alcohol related. One drunk driving death occurs every 30 minutes. To reduce alcohol-related crashes, law enforcement officials in many states now use passive alcohol sensors (PAS). PAS devices detect the presence of alcohol in the air surrounding the driver. They are often concealed in a flashlight or clipboard.

These devices are called passive because the driver being tested does not actually blow into the PAS. In fact, drivers are usually not aware that they are being tested for the presence of alcohol. The law enforcement officer holds the PAS 3 inches to 10 inches from the driver, and a light indicator displays an approximate level of alcohol in the air sample. The PAS reading is a simple pass or fail test; it does not measure BAC. If the driver fails, the officer may perform a breath analyzer test. Sensors have been used at sobriety checkpoints, during truck inspections, and during routine traffic stops.

A major legal issue is whether the use of PAS is a violation of an individual's rights under the Fourth Amendment, which provide protection from unreasonable search and seizure. Two exceptions to the Fourth Amendment may apply to this debate. One is the "plain view" doctrine—if something is in plain view, there cannot be a reasonable expectation of privacy. The argument is that a person's breath is openly displayed to the public. Law enforcement officers have long relied on sniffing the air for the presence of alcohol to determine whether the driver has been drinking. The other exception to the Fourth Amendment is the automobile exception doctrine, which holds that an individual should have less expectation of privacy in a vehicle than in his or her residence. In both cases, the law enforcement officer must be justified in making the stop. Sobriety checkpoints, truck stops, and stops for traffic violations have been found to meet this requirement.

Opponents of PAS object to their use as intrusive, sneaky, and a violation of civil rights. The American Civil Liberties Union (ACLU) has questioned their use because they allow law enforcement to check for alcohol without the knowledge or consent of the person being tested. According to the ACLU, such searches are conducted without probable cause.

Proponents point out that X-ray machines and dogs are used in airports to detect guns, explosives, drugs, and other dangerous or contraband items, often without probable cause. Drunk driving is a public health problem, and we should use advances in technology to protect the public. What do you think?

Pros

- PAS devices help officers identify a higher proportion of drivers who have been drinking, potentially reducing the number of injuries and deaths resulting from alcohol-related car crashes every year.

- Officers in routine traffic stops have only a short amount of time to evaluate drivers. The drivers' use of breath mints, cologne, and gum may interfere with the officer's ability to sniff alcohol. Car exhaust fumes can also interfere with this process. PAS devices provide a way around these problems.

- Arrests are not made on the basis of PAS results—a follow-up breath test is used to measure BAC—and PAS results cannot be used as evidence in court.

Cons

- Even if the use of PAS does not compromise an individual's civil liberties, it is intrusive and assumes guilt.

- PAS devices measure alcohol in the air and do not necessarily pinpoint its source. The alcohol they detect could be on the breath of passengers rather than on the breath of the driver.

- PAS devices detect alcohol at very low levels. Alcohol from mouthwash or liquid cold medications can cause a person to fail a PAS test.

- Environmental conditions—wind, dampness, and extreme temperatures—interfere with PAS readings, leading to errors.

- PAS devices are costly and have not yet proven to be cost effective for detecting drunk driving.

OLC Web site For more information about this topic, visit the Online Learning Center at www.mhhe.com/teague1e.

SOURCES: "Combating Hardcore Drunk Driving: A Source Book of Promising Strategies, Laws, and Programs: Enforcement," National Commission Against Drunk Driving, 1997, www.ncadd.com; "A Survey of Strategies for Reducing Alcohol-Impaired Driving and Underage Drinking," by K. Orlansky, S. Richards, and K. Baker-Hernandez, 2001, Office of Legislative Oversight, www.montgomerycountymd.gov; "Passive Alcohol Sensors and the Fourth Amendment—The Impaired Driving Update," Spring 2001, www.ndaa.org; "Using a Passive Alcohol Sensor to Detect Legally Intoxicated Drivers," National Commission Against Drunk Driving, 1993, *American Journal of Public Health*, 83 (4), 551–560; *Dying to Drink*, by H. Wechsler and B. Wuethrich, 2002, New York: Rodale Books.

SUMMARY

- Alcohol is a psychoactive drug that causes changes in brain chemistry that affect all aspects of a person's functioning. About one third of Americans are abstainers; of the remaining two thirds, 10 percent are heavy drinkers and the rest are light to moderate drinkers.

- The peak period of alcohol consumption is in adolescence and early adulthood, after which it declines. Older adults drink significantly less than younger adults do. Women drink less than men do and start later. Different cohorts of Americans have different drinking patterns.

- Generally speaking, Hispanic men drink at the highest levels across the life span, followed by white men and African American men. Hispanic women have low levels of alcohol consumption. Native Americans have high levels of alcoholism; Asian Americans have low levels.

- People drink and develop drinking problems for a variety of biological, psychosocial, and sociocultural reasons. There is a biological/genetic contribution to susceptibility to the effects of alcohol. Psychosocial factors include parenting and the family environment. A family history of alcoholism and other kinds of family dysfunction are strongly associated with alcohol problems, although most children who grow up in these families do not develop alcohol problems. Researchers also study alcohol use from the perspectives of motivation, developmental effects, cognitive effects, and sociocultural factors.

- Binge drinking is a serious problem among college students. Nearly half of all students who drink are binge drinkers. Underage drinkers consume about half of all alcohol consumed by students. Binge drinking can have physical, academic, social, and legal consequences. A comprehensive approach is needed to address this problem.

- Alcohol is a central nervous system depressant, at first causing feelings of relaxation and, later, feelings of depression, along with mental and physical impairment.

- Most alcohol is absorbed in the small intestine; speed of absorption is affected by food in the stomach, gender, age, other drugs, cigarette smoke, mood and physical condition, alcohol concentration in the drink, and carbonation. Expectations also play a role in intoxication.

- Most alcohol is metabolized in the liver by the enzymes alcohol dehydrogenase and acetaldehyde dehydrogenase. A small amount of alcohol is excreted in the breath, pores, and urine.

- Blood alcohol concentration (BAC) is a measure of the amount of alcohol, in grams, in 100 milliliters of blood, expressed as a percentage. BAC is influenced by the amount of alcohol consumed and the rate at which it is metabolized, which in turn is affected by body size, body fat, amount and type of enzymes in the liver, and other factors. Women metabolize alcohol less efficiently than men do and thus are more susceptible to both the intoxicating effects of alcohol and the long-term health consequences of alcohol abuse.

- Alcohol is metabolized more slowly than it is absorbed, so that BAC builds when additional drinks are consumed before previous drinks are metabolized. On average, it takes about 1 hour for the body to metabolize .5 ounces of alcohol, the amount in one drink. Although a person with a BAC of .08 to .10 is considered legally drunk, impairment can begin at much lower levels.

- Acute alcohol intoxication can occur when a person drinks a large amount of alcohol in a short period of time; it can result in death from cessation of breathing and heart function. A blackout is a period of time during which a drinker is conscious but has impaired memory function as a result of changes in the hippocampus. A hangover is a set of unpleasant symptoms that can follow alcohol consumption.

- Alcohol is a toxic substance and has far-reaching health effects. Major organs and systems damaged by alcohol include the cardiovascular system, the liver, the brain, the immune system, and the reproductive system. Alcohol is associated with cancers of the digestive system and with breast cancer, and it can cause fetal alcohol syndrome in children whose mothers drink during pregnancy. It has 7 calories per gram and can cause weight gain; with long-term use it can lead to malnutrition and vitamin deficiency.

- Social problems associated with alcohol include high-risk sexual behavior, violence, injury, and suicide.

- Moderate drinking is associated with cardiovascular benefits in middle-aged and older adults.

- The misuse of alcohol is associated with a range of serious problems. Problem drinking is a pattern of alcohol use that causes difficulties for the drinker and for others. Alcohol abuse is a pattern of drinking that causes distress and impairment and that continues despite awareness of these problems. Alcohol dependence is a disorder characterized by craving for alcohol, tolerance, and symptoms of withdrawal if consumption ends abruptly. Alcoholism is a chronic, progressive, often fatal disease characterized by alcohol dependence.

- Treatment options include brief interventions, inpatient treatment, outpatient treatment, and self-help programs like AA. Relapse prevention is difficult because alcohol causes changes in the brain. The harm reduction approach to treatment advocates moderation and controlled drinking rather than abstinence.

- Numerous laws and public policies, such as the minimum legal drinking age and drunk driving laws, are aimed at reducing the harm caused to the public by alcohol use.

- Responsible decisions about alcohol include controlling one's own consumption and advocating responsible uses of alcohol.

REVIEW QUESTIONS

1. Briefly explain the different drinking trajectories of white, black, and Hispanic men and women.

2. Why is alcohol consumption overall lower among Asian Americans than among white Americans?

3. What are three motivations for drinking identified by researchers, and how are they different?

4. Describe several ways that parenting and the family environment can lead to later problems with alcohol.

5. What phases of life are associated with greater alcohol use, and why?

6. What are some of the sociocultural or environmental factors associated with alcohol use?

7. Define the following terms: (a) binge drinking, (b) frequent binge drinking, (c) occasional binge drinking, and (d) abstinence.

8. List several reasons why college students tend to binge drink.

9. List several secondhand effects of binge drinking experienced by nondrinking students.

10. Describe the three approaches to changing the college drinking culture discussed in the chapter.

11. Explain blood alcohol concentration and list several factors that influence it.

12. Why are women more affected by alcohol than men are?

13. Describe the behavioral effects of alcohol at a BAC of .10 percent.

14. What are the physical symptoms of a person experiencing acute alcohol intoxication? What first aid steps should be taken?

15. What causes vomiting during intoxication?

16. Describe the progression of alcohol-induced liver disease.

17. Why does alcohol consumption lead to high-risk sexual behavior and other social problems?

18. Why is moderate alcohol use associated with lower risk of heart disease, according to scientists?

19. Distinguish problem drinking from alcohol abuse and alcohol dependence.

20. Explain tolerance and withdrawal. What do they indicate?

21. Describe the symptoms associated with detoxification.

22. Why is recovery from alcohol dependence so difficult?

23. Briefly explain the basic belief behind harm reduction, and list five harm reduction policies used to curb underage and excessive drinking.

24. Why is controlled drinking considered a controversial treatment approach?

25. List the steps in a behavior change plan for responsible drinking.

WEB RESOURCES

Al-Anon Family Group Headquarters: This Web site offers information about Al-Anon and Alateen groups in local communities. It provides resources to help you assess whether you are being affected by the drinking problem of someone close to you. www.al-anon.alateen.org

Alcoholics Anonymous (AA) World Services: This organization provides information on Alcoholics Anonymous, including the philosophy of its 12-step program. It features a preventive approach to alcohol abuse. www.alcoholics-anonymous.org

BACCHUS and GAMMA Peer Education Network: Made up of college and university students, this organization promotes peer education programs designed to prevent alcohol abuse. www.bacchusgamma.org

The College Alcohol Study, Harvard School of Public Health: To learn more about studies of binge drinking on college campuses, visit this site. www.hsph.harvard.edu/cas

College Drinking Prevention: This Web site features "A Call to Action: Changing the Culture of Drinking at U.S. Colleges," a Task Force Report by the National Institute on Alcoholism and Alcohol Abuse. www.collegedrinkingprevention.gov

HadEnough.org: This site features a self-quiz on binge drinking and other resources on this topic related to college life. www.hadenough.org

Mothers Against Drunk Driving (MADD): This organization is dedicated to the issues of underage drinking and drunk driving, providing information and literature on many related topics. www.madd.org

National Association for Children of Alcoholics (NACoA): Dedicated to addressing the special needs of children of alcoholics, this organization offers support and information. www.nacoa.net

National Clearinghouse for Alcohol and Drug Information/ Prevention Online: A good resource for information on alcohol abuse, this organization offers help to families and friends of individuals with alcohol problems. www.health.org

National Council on Alcoholism and Drug Dependence (NCADD): Besides offering counseling referrals, this council is a valuable resource for various types of information on alcoholism. www.ncadd.org

National Institute on Alcohol Abuse and Alcoholism (NIAAA): Visit this organization's Web site for authoritative information on alcohol abuse and alcoholism. NIAAA is dedicated to public education on these topics and offers various helpful publications. www.niaaa.nih.gov

Substance Abuse and Mental Health Services Administration: The U.S. Department of Health and Human Services sponsors this site, which features a wide range of resources on substance abuse and closely related issues, such as mental health, homelessness, and AIDS/HIV. www.samhsa.gov

REFERENCES

1. Wechsler, H., & Wuethrich, B. (2002). *Dying to drink: Confronting binge drinking on college campuses.* New York: Rodale Books.

2. American Pyschiatric Association. (2000). *Diagnostic and statistical manual of mental disorders* (4th ed., Text Revision [*DSM-IV-TR*]). Washington, DC: American Psychiatric Association Press.

3. National Institute on Alcohol Abuse and Alcoholism; National Institutes of Health. (2000). *Alcohol and health.* Washington, DC: U.S. Department of Health and Human Services.

4. Breslow, R. A., & Smothers, B. (2004). Drinking patterns of older Americans: National Health Interview Survey, 1997–2001. *Journal of Studies on Alcohol, 65* (2), 232–240.

5. Ferrini, A. F., & Ferreni, R. L. (2000). *Health in the later years.* (3rd ed.) New York: McGraw-Hill.

6. Ksir, C., Hart, C. L., & Ray, O. (2006). *Drugs, society, and human behavior* (11th ed.). New York: McGraw-Hill.

7. Suarez, L., & Ramirez, A. G. (1999). Hispanic/Latino health and disease. In R. M. Huff & M. V. Kline (Eds.), *Promoting health in multicultural populations.* Thousand Oaks, CA: Sage Publications.

8. Huff, R. M., & Kline, M. V. (1999). Health promotion in the context of culture. In R. M. Huff & M. V. Kline (Eds.), *Promoting health in multicultural populations.* Thousand Oaks, CA: Sage Publications.

9. Hodge, F. S., & Fredericks, L. (1999). American Indian and Alaska native populations in the United States: An overview. In R. M. Huff & M. V. Kline (Eds.), *Promoting health in multicultural populations.* Thousand Oaks, CA: Sage Publications.

10. Wild, T. C. (2002). Personal drinking and sociocultural drinking norms: A representative population study. *Journal of Studies on Alcohol, 63* (4), 469–475.

11. Morse, R. M., & Flavin, D. K. (1992). The definition of alcoholism: The Joint Committee of the National Council on Alcoholism and Drug Dependence, and the American Society of Addiction Medicine to Study the Definition and Criteria for the Diagnoses of Alcoholism. *Journal of the American Medical Association, 263,* 1012–1014.

12. Springer, K., & Kantrowitz, B. (2004, May 16). Alcohol's deadly triple threat. *Newsweek,* 90–102.

13. Wechsler, H., Lee, J. E., Kuo, M., & Lee, H. (2000). College binge drinking in the 1990s: A continuing problem. Results of the Harvard School of Public Health 1999 College Alcohol Study. www.hsph.harvard.edu.

14. Wechsler, H. (2000). College binge drinking in the 1990s: A continuing problem. Results of the Harvard School of Public Health 1999 College Alcohol Study. *Journal of American College Health, 48,* 199–210.

15. Wechsler, H., Lee, J. E., Nelson, T. F., and Kuo, M. (2002). Underage college students: Drinking behavior, access to alcohol, and the influence of deterrence policies. Findings from the Harvard School of Public Health College Study. *Journal of American College Health, 50* (5), 223–236.

16. Hill, D. S., Hawkins, J. B., Catalano, R. F., & Abbott, R. D. (2004). Adolescent heavy episodic drinking trajectories and health in young adulthood. *Journal of Studies on Alcohol, 65* (2), 204–212.

17. Okoro, C. A., Brewer, R. D., Darmi, T. S., Moriarity, D. G., Giles, W. H., & Mokdad, A. H. (2004). Binge drinking and health-related quality of life: Do popular perceptions match reality? *American Journal of Preventative Medicine, 26* (3), 230–233.

18. Larimer, M. E., Marlatt, G. L., Baer, J. S., et al. (1998). Harm reduction for alcohol problems. In G. A. Marlatt (Ed.), *Harm reduction: Pragmatic strategies for managing high risk behaviors.* New York: Guilford Press.

19. Hingson, R. (1998). College-age drinking problems. *Journal of American College Health, 47* (2).

20. Wechsler, H., Lee, J. E., Nelson, T. F., & Lee, H. (2001). Drinking levels, alcohol problems, and second-hand effects in substance-free college residences: Results of a national study. *Journal of Studies on Alcohol, 62* (1), 23–31.

21. Licciardone, J. C. (2003). Perceptions of drinking and related findings from the nationwide college survey. *Journal of Studies of American College Health, 51* (6), 247–256.

22. Trockel, M., Williams, J. R., & Reis, J. (2003). Considerations for more effective social norms based alcohol education on campus: An analysis of different theoretical conceptualizations in predicting drinking among fraternity men. *Journal of Studies on Alcohol, 64* (1), 43–49.

23. Borsoi, B., & Carey, K. B. (2002). Descriptive and injunctive norms in college drinking: A meta-analytic integration. *Journal of Studies on Alcohol, 64* (3), 331–341.

24. Wechsler, H., Nelson, T. F., Lee, J. E., et al. Perception and reality: A national evaluation of social norms marketing interventions to reduce college students' drinking study. *Journal of Studies on Alcohol, 62* (1), 23–31.

25. National Institute on Alcohol Abuse and Alcoholism. (2002). *A call to action: Changing the culture of drinking at U.S. colleges.* Washington, DC: U.S. Department of Health and Human Services.

26. Frezza, M., et al. (1990). High blood alcohol levels in women: The role of decreased gastric alcohol dehydrogenase activity and first-pass metabolism. *New England Journal of Medicine, 322* (4), 95–99.

27. Adolescents' binge drinking produces tolerance to alcohol. (2003). Health News. www.intelihealth.com.

28. American Medical Association. (n.d.). Brain damage risks. www.ama-assn.org.

29. Chesson, H. W., Harrison, P., & Stall, R. (2003). Changes in alcohol consumption and in sexually transmitted disease incidence rates in the United States: 1983–1998. *Journal of Studies on Alcohol, 64* (5), 623–630.

30. U.S. Department of Agriculture (2005). 2005 *Dietary guidelines for Americans.* www.health.gov/dietaryguidelines.

31. Giancola, P. R. (2002). Alcohol-related aggression during the college years: Theories, risk factors, and policy implications.

In National Institute on Alcohol Abuse and Alcoholism, *A call to action: Changing the culture of drinking at U.S. colleges.* Washington, DC: U.S. Department of Health and Human Services.

32. Simon, H. B. (2002). *The Harvard Medical School guide to men's health.* New York: The Free Press.

33. National Institute on Alcohol Abuse and Alcoholism. (2000). *10th special report to the U.S. Congress on alcohol and health.* Washington, DC: U.S. Department of Health and Human Services.

34. Helmkamp, J. C., Hungerford, D. W., Williams, J. M., et al. (2003). Screening and brief intervention for alcohol problems among college students in a university hospital emergency department. *Journal of American College Health, 52* (1), 7–10.

35. Brink, S. (2001, May 7). Your brain on alcohol. *U.S. News & World Report,* 50–57.

36. Peele, S. (2004, March/April). The new prohibitionists: Our attitudes toward alcoholism and doing more harm than good. *The Science News,* 14–19.

37. Oglivie, H. (2001). *Alternatives to abstinence: Controlled drinking and other approaches to managing alcoholism.* New York: Hatherleigh Press.

38. Wagenarr, A. C., & Toomey, T. L. (2000, March). Effects of minimum drinking age laws: Review and analyses of the literature from 1960 to 2000. *Journal of Studies of Alcohol.*

39. Williams, J., Chaloupka, F. J., & Wechsler, H. (2002). Are there differential effects of price and policy on college students' drinking intensity? *National Bureau of Economic Research I,* Working paper 8702.

40. Harwood, E. M., Erickson, D. J., Fabian L. E. A., et al. (2003). Effects of communities, neighborhoods and stores on retail pricing and promotion of beer. *Journal of Studies on Alcohol, 64* (5), 720–726.

Add It Up! CONSEQUENCES OF BINGE DRINKING

Compared with non-binge drinkers, binge drinkers are more likely to experience negative consequences from drinking. Primary consequences are alcohol-related problems experienced by the drinker. Secondary consequences are alcohol-related problems experienced by those around the drinker. For each of the items listed here, indicate on a scale of 1 to 5 whether this event would be very important to you (5), somewhat important (4), neither important nor unimportant (3), somewhat unimportant (2), or very unimportant (1).

	Important				Unimportant

Primary Consequences

Did something regrettable	5	4	3	2	1
Missed a class	5	4	3	2	1
Got behind in school work	5	4	3	2	1
Argued with friends	5	4	3	2	1
Drove after drinking alcohol	5	4	3	2	1
Engaged in unplanned sex	5	4	3	2	1
Had unprotected sex	5	4	3	2	1
Got hurt or injured	5	4	3	2	1
Got into trouble with police or college authorities	5	4	3	2	1
Damaged property	5	4	3	2	1
Had a poor performance on an exam	5	4	3	2	1
Engaged in pranks	5	4	3	2	1
Made unwanted sexual advances	5	4	3	2	1

Secondary Consequences

Experienced unwanted sexual advances	5	4	3	2	1
Had studying disrupted	5	4	3	2	1
Had sleep disrupted	5	4	3	2	1
Had to take care of a drunk fellow student	5	4	3	2	1
Been insulted or humiliated	5	4	3	2	1
Had my property damaged	5	4	3	2	1
Was physically assaulted	5	4	3	2	1

Scoring

Add up your points for Primary Consequences: _____
Add up your points for Secondary Consequences: _____

Interpreting Your Scores

Primary Consequences

59–65	Consequences of binge drinking are very important to you.
46–58	Consequences of binge drinking are somewhat important to you.
33–45	Consequences of binge drinking are neither important nor unimportant to you; you are neutral toward them.
13–32	Consequences of binge drinking are of little or no importance to you.

Secondary Consequences

32–35	The secondhand effects of binge drinking are very important to you.
25–31	The secondhand effects of binge drinking are somewhat important to you.
18–24	The secondhand effects of binge drinking are neither important nor unimportant to you; you are neutral toward them.
7–17	The secondhand effects of binge drinking are of little or no importance to you.

If the consequences of binge drinking are important to you, now is the time to take action to change your behavior or to influence those around you to change their behavior.

SOURCE: Adapted from "Trends in College Binge Drinking During a Period of Increased Prevention Efforts: Findings from the Harvard School of Public Health College Study Surveys: 1993–2001," by H. Wechsler et.al., 2002, *Journal of American College Health, 50,* p. 207.

CHAPTER 12

Drugs and Addictive Behavior: Use, Abuse, and Control

DID YOU KNOW?

- If you smoked marijuana in high school, you have something in common with the nearly 20 percent of Americans between the ages of 12 and 17 who have tried the drug at least once. The psychoactive effects of marijuana can be relatively mild, but its effects on the lungs are not. Marijuana smoke contains more carcinogens than tobacco smoke does; habitual use is associated with damage to the airways and acute and chronic bronchitis.

- You can be addicted not just to drugs but to patterns of behavior, such as gambling, shopping, exercising, or using the Internet. The defining characteristic of addictive behaviors is that they are compulsive and out of control. Scientists speculate that something about these behaviors may trigger the same pleasure and reward pathway in the brain that is activated by addictive drugs like cocaine and heroin.

OLC *Your Health Today*   www.mhhe.com/teague1e

Go to the Online Learning Center for *Your Health Today* for interactive activities, quizzes, flashcards, Web links, and more resources related to this chapter.

Like alcohol, drugs have a pervasive presence in American life. We use them for headaches, insomnia, anxiety, stress—and some of us use them for fun. According to a nationwide survey in 2003, an estimated 19.5 million Americans aged 12 and older were current users of illicit (illegal) drugs, representing more than 8 percent of the population.[1] An estimated 110 million Americans aged 12 and older—more than 46 percent of the population—have used an illicit drug in their lifetime. The most commonly used drug is marijuana, followed by cocaine and hallucinogens (Table 12.1). In 2003 an estimated 6.3 million Americans were current users of medical drugs taken nonmedically, including pain relievers, tranquilizers, stimulants, and sedatives.[1]

Drugs are used by different people for different reasons. Many people take drugs as a recreational activity—to alter their state of consciousness, to relax and feel more sociable, to experience euphoria, to "get high." Some people take drugs to rebel—to experiment, take risks, seek new and exciting sensations. Others take drugs to conform—to fit in with a peer group or to avoid having to say no. For some people, drug use is a way to cope with stress, pain, or adversity, whether the adversity comes in the form of an unexpected life event, such as loss of a job, or in the form of oppressive social conditions experienced daily, such as poverty and discrimination. And for some people, drug use is a way of life, a behavior they can no longer control.

In Chapter 11 we discussed the use of alcohol in U.S. society; in this chapter we discuss the use of psychoactive drugs other than alcohol. We begin with a look at the context of drug use in the United States, a brief history of how drugs were alternately introduced and banned over the years. We continue with an examination of terms related to drugs, types of drugs, and the use, misuse, and abuse of drugs. We then consider the effects of drugs on the body and the brain, and we explore addiction and addictive behaviors other than drug use. Next, we look at the characteristics and effects of specific drugs in six different categories. We end with a discussion of approaches to the drug problem in our society.

Table 12.1   Illicit Drug Use in Lifetime, Past Year, and Past Month Among Persons Aged 12 or Older: Percentages, 2003

Drug	Time Period		
	Lifetime	Past Year	Past Month
Any illicit drug	46.4	14.7	8.2
Marijuana and hashish	40.6	10.6	6.2
Cocaine	14.7	2.5	1.0
Crack	3.3	0.6	0.3
Heroin	1.6	0.1	0.1
Hallucinogens	14.5	1.7	0.4
LSD	10.3	0.2	0.1
PCP	3.0	0.1	0.0
Ecstasy	4.0	0.9	0.2
Inhalants	9.7	0.9	0.2
Nonmedical use of any psychotherapeutic*	20.1	6.3	2.7
Pain relievers	13.1	4.9	2.0
Tranquilizers	8.5	2.1	0.8
Stimulants	8.8	1.2	0.5
Methamphetamine	5.2	0.6	0.3
Sedatives	4.0	0.3	0.1
Any illicit drug other than marijuana	29.9	8.5	3.7

*Prescription medications; does not include over-the-counter drugs.

Source: *National Survey on Drug Use and Health, 2003,* Substance Abuse and Mental Health Services Administration, 2003, Rockville, MD: Office of Applied Studies.

THE CONTEXT OF DRUG USE

In Chapter 11 we commented on Prohibition, a 15-year period when the government tried (and failed) to restrict the manufacture, sale, and transport of alcoholic beverages within the United States. Similar efforts have been made to restrict other drugs as well. Two major "epidemics" of drug use and abuse have occurred, with corresponding legislative attempts to control use through prohibition and punishment.

The first of these epidemics began in the mid-19th century and lasted four or five decades, during which access to drugs was easy and legal. As drugs were discovered, refined, and introduced to the public, they were hailed for their beneficial effects; only later did their harmful effects, including their addictive properties, become apparent. Cocaine, for example, was made readily available as an "ideal tonic" by Parke-Davis and other drug manufacturers starting in 1884. The result was widespread popular consumption of the drug in several easy-to-use applications, including injection, sniffing, smoking, and as a salve. Even Coca-Cola contained cocaine until 1900. In 1910 President William Howard Taft described cocaine use as "the most threatening of the drug habits that has ever appeared in this country."

Opium and its active ingredient, morphine, enjoyed a similar popularity. By 1895, there were an estimated 250,000 opium and morphine addicts in the United States. In 1898, heroin, a derivative of morphine, entered the commercial market as a cough suppressant marketed by the Bayer Company. At a time when vast numbers of people were dying from illnesses marked by coughing, a powerful cough medicine that gave symptom relief was warmly welcomed. By 1915, heroin had overtaken morphine as the leading cause of opiate-related admissions

to New York City's Bellevue Hospital, prompting the city's health commissioner to call teenage heroin use "an American disease."

This period of American history ended in 1914 with the passage of the Harrison Narcotics Act, which required physicians, pharmacists, and other vendors to submit paperwork on all drug transactions. Initially designed as a tax law, the act was used to put many physicians and pharmacies out of business. This law was the seed of all subsequent federal controlled-substance regulations. The war on drugs had begun.

The second major drug epidemic in the United States was propelled by the counterculture of the 1960s and 1970s. Drug use represented rejection of traditional family and societal values, lifestyles, and politics, as well as membership in a special group. It was commonplace for drug enthusiasts to claim that regular drug use would change the nature of society for the better. Harvard psychologist Timothy Leary advocated use of LSD and urged young people to "turn on, tune in, drop out." Social and legal changes were proposed—such as legalizing marijuana and other drugs—but ultimately none of them was adopted. By 1980 public opinion had shifted again, and legislation was moving in the direction of stiffer penalties for drug-related crimes (Figure 12.1). The Reagan administration initiated an aggressive war on drugs that is currently still in place.

Today, drug use in our society continues to be high, despite efforts to curtail it. In addition to the human costs, illicit drug use causes considerable economic damage. An estimated $160 billion was drained from the U.S. economy by drug use in 2000, largely in lost productivity owing to drug-related illness and death and in health care costs.[2] In 2002 more than 670,000 drug-related hospital

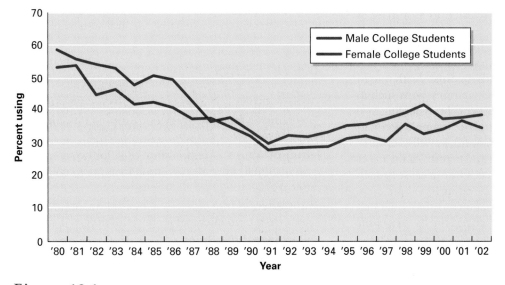

Figure 12.1   Annual trends in illicit drug use by male and female college students, 1980–2002.

Source: University of Michigan, Institute for Social Research, Monitoring the Future study, 2003, www.monitoringthefuture.org.

emergency room visits were reported in the United States.[3] The most common reason for these visits was consumption of alcohol in combination with other drugs, followed by use of cocaine, marijuana or hashish, and heroin. Other economic costs of illicit drug use include social welfare costs, workplace accidents, property damage, incarceration of otherwise productive individuals, goods and services lost to crime, work hours missed by victims of drug-related crime, costs of law enforcement, and costs of the criminal justice system. A large part of these costs—about $20 billion annually—is incurred by the war on drugs, especially the operation of the prison system. Clearly, drug use is a problem both for individuals and for society.

WHAT IS A DRUG?

The dictionary defines **drug** as a substance other than food that affects the structure or the function of the body through its chemical action. Alcohol, caffeine, aspirin, and nicotine are all drugs, as are amphetamines, cocaine, hallucinogens, sedatives, and inhalants. Penicillin is an example of a drug used to treat physical illness. The drugs discussed here are *psychoactive drugs*—substances that cause changes in brain chemistry and alter consciousness, perception, mood, and thought. This state is known as *intoxication.*

Psychoactive drugs are used for both medical and nonmedical (recreational) purposes. For example, Ritalin, a central nervous system (CNS) stimulant with effects similar to amphetamine, is prescribed to treat hyperactivity in children—a medical use. Cocaine, another CNS stimulant, is used recreationally to cause a burst of pleasurable sensations and to increase energy and endurance—a nonmedical use. When a medical drug is used for nonmedical (recreational) purposes, or when a drug has no medical uses, it is referred to as a **drug of abuse.**

All drugs have the potential to be toxic, that is, poisonous, dangerous, or deadly. We saw in Chapter 11 that alcohol damages body organs and can cause death if used in sufficient amounts to suppress vital functions such as respiration. The same is true of other central nervous system depressants such as barbiturates (for example, Seconal) and tranquilizers (for example, Valium), as well as opium-derived drugs such as morphine and heroin. At the other extreme, CNS stimulants such as cocaine can cause sudden death by speeding up heart rate, elevating blood pressure, and accelerating other body functions to the point that systems are overwhelmed and collapse. In its *Diagnostic and Statistical Manual of Mental Disorders (DSM-IV-TR)*, the American Psychiatric Association (APA) uses the term **substance** to refer to a drug of abuse, a medication, or a toxin.[4] In this chapter we use the terms *drug* and *substance* interchangeably.

Types of Drugs

Drugs are classified in several different ways. A basic distinction is often made between legal drugs and illicit (illegal) drugs. *Legal drugs* include medications prescribed by physicians, over-the-counter (OTC) medications, and herbal remedies. Drugs developed for medical purposes, whether OTC or prescription, are referred to as **pharmaceutical drugs.**

OTC medications can be purchased easily by consumers without a prescription. They include common remedies for headache, pain, colds, coughs, allergies, stomach upset, and other mild symptoms and complaints. Herbal remedies are usually botanical in origin; there are more than 700 substances in this group. At this time, the federal government's Food and Drug Administration (FDA) does not regulate herbal remedies before they are brought to market the way it regulates the development and approval of pharmaceutical drugs. The FDA does have the power to remove an herbal remedy from the market if it has proven harmful. This was the case with the dietary supplement ephedra, a stimulant used for weight loss and body building, which the FDA banned after it was linked with more than 100 deaths from heart attack and stroke. See the box on "Taking a Smart Approach to Self-Medication."

Prescription drugs can be ordered only by a licensed medical doctor (MD). They must undergo a rigorous testing and approval process by the FDA. Today the legal pharmaceutical industry is one of the largest and most profitable industries in the United States, with sales well over $100 billion a year. Despite these astronomical sales, however, more than half of all prescriptions are filled with only 200 drugs.

Illicit drugs are generally viewed as harmful, and it is unlawful to possess, manufacture, sell, or use them. Many drugs that are available by prescription are legal when obtained through a physician but illicit when manufactured or sold outside of the regulated medical system. Tobacco

(KEY) TERMS

drug Substance other than food that affects the structure or function of the body through its chemical action.

drug of abuse Medical drug used for nonmedical (recreational) purposes or a drug that has no medical uses.

substance Drug of abuse, a medication, or a toxin; the term is used interchangeably with *drug.*

pharmaceutical drugs Drugs developed for medical purposes, whether over the counter or prescription.

illicit drugs Drugs that are unlawful to possess, manufacture, sell, or use.

Consumer Clipboard

Taking a Smart Approach to Self-Medication

More than 700 products sold over the counter today include ingredients or dosage strengths that were available only by prescription just 30 years ago. With this wide range of products to choose from, self-medication—whether it's for relief from a cold or an approach to boosting the immune system—has become common.

Helpful as these products may be, like all medicines, they need to be approached with caution and common sense. When choosing to use over-the-counter (OTC) drugs, keep these points in mind:

- Inform yourself about OTC drugs by reading and understanding the label information. Read and follow the directions carefully (how much to take, how to take it, and how long to take it). Also note the active ingredients (therapeutic substances), purpose (product category), uses (symptoms or diseases to be treated or prevented), warnings (when not to use the product, when to stop taking it, when to see a doctor, and possible side effects), and other product information.

- Read the label each time you purchase an OTC product. Products from the same brand family are not always used to treat the same conditions, and they don't necessarily contain the same ingredients. Also, the ingredients may change.

- If you're planning to take an OTC drug for a recurring condition, such as migraine headaches or minor pain of arthritis, consult with your physician first.

- When it comes to medicine, more does not necessarily mean better. Don't misuse OTC medicines by taking them longer or in higher doses than the label recommends. If your symptoms persist, you need to see a physician.

- Be alert for possible interactions between drugs. These are just a few cautions involving some common OTC ingredients:

  — Avoid alcohol if you're taking antihistamines, cough or cold products that contain dextromethorphan, or drugs used to treat sleeplessness.

  — Don't use drugs for sleeplessness if you're taking prescription sedatives or tranquilizers.

  — If you're taking a prescription blood thinner, or if you have diabetes or gout, check with your physician before taking any product that contains aspirin.

  — Unless your physician has instructed you to do so, don't use a nasal decongestant if you're taking a prescription drug for high blood pressure or depression, or if you have thyroid disease, diabetes, or prostate problems.

- Dietary supplements are not regulated by the Food and Drug Administration, so the ingredient amounts listed on the label are not always accurate. In addition, the manufacturer's claims about their safety and effectiveness are not always backed up by solid research.

- When you're asked at the physician's office to list the medications you take, include everything—prescription drugs and all OTC drugs, including daily multivitamins and aspirin.

Confused about taking OTC medications? Talk to your physician or pharmacist about any questions or concerns you may have.

Source: Data from "Over-the-Counter Medicines: What's Right for You?" 2005, U.S. Food and Drug Administration, www.fda.gov.

---

and alcohol are illegal drugs in the hands of minors, but they are usually not considered illicit because of their widespread availability to adults.

In an effort to reduce the use of illegal drugs and the nonmedical use of certain prescription drugs, Congress passed the Comprehensive Drug Abuse Prevention and Control Act, usually referred to as the Controlled Substance Act, in 1970. This act categorized drugs into five groups according to their addictive quality and medical uses. Schedule I drugs have a high potential for abuse and have no currently accepted medical purpose. Heroin and LSD are Schedule I drugs. Schedule II drugs have a high potential for abuse but have a medical purpose; examples are morphine and cocaine. Schedule III, IV, and V drugs have accepted medical uses and a moderate to limited potential for abuse. Substances that are not controlled include over-the-counter medications and herbal remedies. These drugs appear to be nonaddictive and have few harmful side effects. Table 12.2 summarizes the controlled substance schedules and gives examples for each group.

Table 12.2   Summary of Controlled Substance Schedules

Schedule	Criteria	Examples
Schedule I	a. High potential for abuse b. No currently acceptable medical use in treatment in the United States c. Lack of accepted safety for use under medical supervision	Heroin Marijuana LSD
Schedule II	a. High potential for abuse b. Currently accepted medical use c. Abuse may lead to severe psychological or physical dependence	Morphine Cocaine Methamphetamines
Schedule III	a. Potential for abuse less than I and II b. Currently accepted medical use c. Abuse may lead to moderate physical dependence or high psychological dependence	Anabolic steroids Most barbiturates Dronabinol
Schedule IV	a. Low potential for abuse relative to III b. Currently accepted medical use c. Abuse may lead to limited physical or psychological dependence relative to III	Alprazolam (Xanax) Barbital Chloral hydrate Fenfluramine
Schedule V	a. Low potential for abuse relative to IV b. Currently accepted medical use c. Abuse may lead to limited physical or psychological dependence	Mixtures having small amounts of codeine or opium relative to IV

Source: *Drugs, Society, and Human Behavior* (11th ed.), by C. Ksir, C. L. Hart, and O. Ray, 2006, New York: The McGraw-Hill Companies.

The Controlled Substance Act schedules govern the legal distribution and use of most substances with a significant potential for abuse. The primary federal agency charged with enforcing these regulations and with coordinating national and international efforts to reduce the illicit drug supply is the Drug Enforcement Administration (DEA). Hence, this classification scheme is often referred to as the DEA Schedules.

Drug Use, Misuse, and Abuse

As we saw in the use of the term *illicit,* terms used in discussing drugs and drug problems are often used in different ways. The term *drug use* can refer to taking two aspirins for a headache, but we usually don't think of that as a problem, either for ourselves or for society. We do think of drug use as a problem if it involves the use of particular drugs (for example, cocaine) by particular people (for example, middle school students), and we expect our society to address it in some way.

The term **drug misuse** generally refers to the use of prescription drugs for purposes other than those for which they were prescribed or in greater amounts than prescribed. The term can also refer to the use of nonprescription drugs or chemicals such as glues, paints, or solvents for any purpose other than that intended by the manufacturer.

The term **drug abuse** generally means the use of a substance in amounts, situations, or a manner such that it causes problems, or greatly increases the risk of prob-

lems, for the user or for others. The *DSM-IV-TR* definition of substance abuse refers to both alcohol abuse and drug abuse (see Chapter 11). It defines *substance abuse* as a maladaptive pattern of use leading to impairment or distress that continues despite serious adverse consequences. These consequences may be failure to fulfill major role obligations at work, school, or home (for example, being fired from a job, being expelled from school); experiencing social or interpersonal problems (for example, getting into arguments or fights); experiencing legal problems (for example, being arrested); or exposing oneself to physically dangerous situations (for example, driving or operating a machine while using the drug).[4]

Drug abuse is not the same as drug dependence; a person can abuse a drug—for example, by binge drinking or taking Ecstasy on weekends—without being dependent on it. We discuss drug dependence later in the chapter.

EFFECTS OF DRUGS ON THE BODY

All psychoactive drugs have an effect on the brain, and they reach the brain by way of the bloodstream. In Chapter 11 we saw that when alcohol is consumed, most of it is absorbed through the walls of the small intestine and travels quickly to the brain. Like alcohol, some psychoactive drugs are consumed by mouth, but other routes of administration are used as well.

Routes of Administration

Psychoactive drugs are taken by one of four methods: orally (by mouth), injection, inhalation, or application to the skin or mucous membranes. The speed and efficiency with which the drug acts are strongly influenced by the route of administration.

Most drugs are taken orally. Although this is the simplest way for a person to take a drug, it is the most complicated way for the drug to enter the bloodstream. A drug in the digestive tract must be able to withstand the actions of stomach acid and digestive enzymes and not be deactivated by food before it is absorbed.

The injection route involves using a hypodermic syringe to deliver the drug directly into the bloodstream (intravenous injection), to deposit it in a muscle mass (intramuscular injection), or to deposit it under the upper layer of skin (subcutaneous injection). With an intravenous (IV) injection ("mainlining"), the drug enters the bloodstream directly; onset of action is more rapid than with oral administration or other means of injection. IV injection carries the danger of introducing pathogens into the blood, either from the skin or from contaminated needles and syringes. Intramuscular (IM) injection affords less rapid absorption than does IV injection but more rapid absorption than subcutaneous (SC) injection ("skin popping"). Muscles have a better blood supply than the underlying layers of the skin do and thus provide more capillary area through which the drug can be absorbed.

The inhalation route is used for smoking tobacco, marijuana, and crack cocaine; for snorting cocaine; and for "huffing" gasoline, paints, and other inhalants. It is also used medically to administer various anesthetics (for example, during surgery). An inhaled drug enters the bloodstream quickly because capillary walls are very accessible in the lungs. For psychoactive drugs, inhalation can produce even more rapid effects than IV injection.

Application to the skin or mucous membranes is a less common method of drug administration. Most drugs are not well absorbed through the skin. *Dermal absorption* occurs when an oil or ointment is rubbed on the skin, producing a topical, or local, effect. *Transdermal absorption* occurs when a longer lasting application produces a systemic effect, such as when a patch delivers estrogen or nicotine. The advantage of the transdermal route is that it affords slow, steady absorption over many hours, producing stable levels of the drug in the blood.

Application of a drug to the mucous membranes results in more rapid absorption than application to the skin, because the mucous membranes are moist and have a rich blood supply. When people snort cocaine powder into the nose, they experience a rapid effect because the drug quickly dissolves and is absorbed through the mucous membranes. People who chew tobacco absorb nicotine directly into the bloodstream through the mucous

Some inhalants, such as spray paint, glue, and cleaning fluids, are readily accessible to young teens looking for a cheap way to get high. Depending on the chemical involved, the effects can range from intoxication lasting a few minutes to loss of consciousness or even sudden death.

membranes lining the mouth. Rectal and vaginal suppositories are also absorbed quickly, although these methods are less commonly used.

Factors Influencing the Effects of Drugs

The effect a drug has on a person depends on a number of variables, including the characteristics of the drug, the characteristics of the person, and the characteristics of the situation. The first of these categories includes the chemical properties of the drug and its actions. Depending on the drug's chemical composition, it may speed up body processes or slow them down, produce a mild high or

KEY TERMS

drug misuse Use of prescription drugs for purposes other than those for which they were prescribed or in greater amounts than prescribed, or the use of nonprescription drugs or chemicals for purposes other than those intended by the manufacturer.

drug abuse Use of a substance in amounts, situations, or a manner such that it causes problems, or greatly increases the risk of problems, for the user or for others.

Beating the Odds

Who Is Most Likely to Remain Drug Free?

Both protective factors and risk factors come into play in determining whether a particular person will become dependent on drugs or remain drug free. Someone with multiple risk factors—a chaotic home environment, for example, or parents who abuse drugs—may nevertheless have enough protective factors—resilience, social skills, a strong adult role model—to overcome obstacles and stay drug free. Brief profiles of three people are presented here. Which person do you think has the best chances of remaining drug free?

Jason is a 17-year-old high school senior living in a white, upper-middle-class community in the Midwest. His parents are both professionals with no history of addiction. They are very busy with their careers, and family time together is not a high priority for them. They give Jason a lot of freedom and seldom ask him where he is going. He is not close to his younger sister, who also seems to lead her own separate life. Jason gets good grades in high school, plays on the basketball team, and writes for the school newspaper. It is very important to his self-esteem to be well liked and popular. He started dating at 13 and became sexually active at 15. Next year he is planning to attend a state university that is known as a party school. It is located several hundred miles from his home.

Victor is a 16-year-old Latino living in Los Angeles. His father was arrested for heroin use when Victor was in elementary school and has been in prison ever since. His mother works as a nurse's aide in a local hospital. She keeps a close eye on her family and makes sure they eat dinner together every night. All the kids help out with shopping, cleaning, and chores around the house. They spend a lot of time with their extended family, which includes grandparents, aunts and uncles, and cousins on both sides of the family. Victor occasionally hangs out with kids in the neighborhood, some of whom are getting involved in selling drugs, but his grandfather tells him to stay away from them. Victor is a good student, and his school counselor says he can get a scholarship to attend college. He would be the first one in his family to go beyond high school, and he feels uneasy about doing something so different.

Janis is a 14-year-old girl living on a farm in rural New England. Both of her parents work the family farm and have difficulty making ends meet. Janis considers her family loving, but she often feels alone. On her mother's side, there is a history of alcoholism and depression, although neither of her parents drinks. Janis is an average student and spends a lot of her free time listening to heavy metal music and surfing the Web. On weekends she goes to the mall and hangs out with her friends at the video game arcade. She and her friends all think the town is dead and would like their lives to be more exciting. They hang out with older kids when they can. At this point, Janis is unsure what she wants to do after she graduates from high school.

OLC Web site Visit the **Online Learning Center** at www.mhhe.com/teague1e for comments by the authors.

---

acute anxiety, or cause disorientation or hallucinations. These effects also depend on how much of the drug is taken, how often it is taken, and how recently it was taken.

Characteristics of the person include age, gender, body weight and mass, physical condition, mood, experience with the drug, and expectations, as we saw in the case of alcohol. Generally speaking, the same amount of a drug has less effect on a 180-pound man than on a 120-pound woman. If a person has taken other drugs, the interactions of the chemicals can influence outcomes, as when one CNS depressant intensifies the effect of another. The effects of drugs are also influenced by the characteristics of the situation or the environment. Taking a drug at home while relaxing with a group of friends may produce a different experience than will taking the same drug at a crowded, noisy bar or club, surrounded by strangers.

Drug Dependence

As we saw in the case of alcohol, continued use of a drug can lead to *dependence,* a condition characterized by a strong craving for a drug and by compulsive use of the drug despite serious negative consequences. (Drug dependence is commonly known as **drug addiction,** but the APA uses the more precise term *dependence.*) Dependence usually means that physiological changes have taken place in brain and body chemistry as a result of using the drug. One indicator of physiological dependence is the development of *tolerance,* reduced sensitivity to the effects of the drug. Tolerance means that the user has to keep increasing the drug dose to get the same high. For example, a heroin user may have to take 10 times the amount initially taken to achieve the desired effect. Tolerance usually occurs because the body seeks to compensate for the chemical imbalance caused by the drug and achieves a "new normal." More of the drug is needed to move the body from that level.

Another sign of physiological dependence is that stopping drug use leads to the unpleasant and uncomfortable set of symptoms known as *withdrawal*. Withdrawal symptoms are different for different drugs. For example, withdrawal from amphetamines is marked by intense feelings of fatigue and depression, increased appetite and weight gain, and sometimes suicidal thinking. Withdrawal from heroin causes nausea, vomiting, sweating, diarrhea, yawning, and insomnia.

Drug dependence is considered a mental disorder by the American Psychiatric Association, and risk factors are the same as for other mental disorders. They include inadequate parenting, excessive shyness or aggressiveness, lack of coping skills, identification with a deviant peer group, neighborhood disorganization, poverty, and many others. See Table 3.2 in Chapter 3 (p. 62) for a more detailed list. There are also factors that protect people from developing drug dependence, such as good communication skills, family cohesion, and employment opportunities. See Table 3.1 in Chapter 3 (p. 61). To check your ability to recognize such factors, see the box "Who Is Most Likely to Remain Drug Free?"

Drug users can experience **psychological dependence** as well as physical dependence. Even without physiological dependence, people who are dependent on a drug may spend a great deal of time trying to obtain the substance, give up important parts of their lives to pursue and use the substance, and make repeated, unsuccessful attempts to cut down or control their use of the drug. They may withdraw from family activities, school, work, or hobbies in order to use the substance or to spend more time with substance-using friends. They continue using the drug even though they know it is causing them severe problems. These behaviors are usually present when there is physiological dependence, but they may also be present in the absence of physiological dependence, that is, when dependence is psychological. To assess whether you are at risk for developing dependence on a drug, see the Add It Up! feature at the end of the chapter.

Effects of Drugs on the Brain

What accounts for the phenomenon of dependence? Scientists studying the effects of drugs on the brain have found that many addictive drugs, including cocaine, marijuana, opioids, alcohol, and nicotine, act on neurons in three brain structures—the ventral tegmental area (VTA) in the midbrain, the nucleus accumbens, and the prefrontal cortex.[5] Neurons in these three structures form a pathway referred to as the **pleasure and reward circuit** (Figure 12.2).

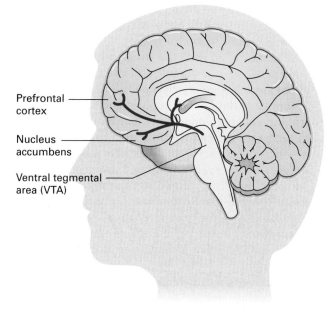

Figure 12.2   **The pleasure and reward circuit in the brain.** *The drug reward system includes neurons using dopamine in the ventral tegmental area, which connect to neurons in the nucleus accumbens and the prefrontal cortex. All psychoactive drugs operate via this pathway, but some drugs also act on other neurotransmitters and structures.* Source: "The Brain's Drug Reward System," NIDA Notes, September/October 1996, www.drugabuse.gov.

When molecules of an addictive drug reach neurons in the VTA, these neurons increase production of dopamine, a neurotransmitter associated with feelings of pleasure. The VTA neurons pass messages to clusters of neurons in the nucleus accumbens, where the release of dopamine produces intense pleasure, and to the prefrontal cortex, where thinking, motivation, and behavior are affected. Addictive drugs also increase the sensitivity and the

KEY TERMS

drug addiction   Drug dependence, characterized by physiological changes that cause tolerance to develop and that lead to withdrawal symptoms if use is stopped abruptly.

psychological dependence   Dependence on a substance or behavior in the absence of physiological dependence, as evidenced by such signs as spending a great deal of time trying to obtain the substance and continuing to use the substance despite adverse consequences.

pleasure and reward circuit   Pathway in the brain involving three structures—the ventral tegmental area, the nucleus accumbens, and the prefrontal cortex—associated with drug dependence.

responsiveness of the dopamine-producing neurons in the VTA, a condition associated with craving. Nonaddictive drugs do not cause these changes.

All or nearly all addictive drugs, whether "uppers" or "downers," operate via this pleasure and reward circuit, but some also operate via additional mechanisms. An example is the opioids (opium and its derivatives, morphine, codeine, and heroin). The brain has neurons with receptors for **endorphins,** its own "natural opiates"—brain chemicals that block pain when the body undergoes stress, such as during extreme exercise or childbirth. The structure of drugs in the opium family is similar to the structure of endorphins, so opioids readily bind to endorphin receptors, reducing pain and increasing pleasure. These effects occur in addition to the dopamine-related changes in the pleasure and reward circuit.

Researchers have found that stress causes changes in the brain that are identical to those caused by some addictive drugs, such as cocaine. Stress is one of the most powerful triggers for relapse in people with addictions, even after long periods of abstinence. Stress may activate the hypersensitive neurons in the VTA, increasing craving for the addictive drug. Even a simple reminder of the drug may be stressful enough to cause craving, such as an ad for cigarettes or the sight of someone smoking, for someone who has recently quit a tobacco habit.

ADDICTION AND ADDICTIVE BEHAVIORS

Human beings have always experimented with plants and their products and have long been aware of their diverse effects, from euphoria, to sleepiness, to hallucinations, to craving. The affliction of drug dependence is as old as human history. Until the 20th century the most common view of individuals addicted to drugs was that they were weak-willed, self-indulgent, immoral malingerers. As a result of research on the brain and neurotransmitters like that described earlier, addiction is now seen not as evidence of a character flaw but as an illness with a clear biological basis.

No one starts using drugs believing that he or she will become addicted. Most people believe they are smart enough or strong enough not to get hooked. Typically, a person begins by using a substance to reduce pain or anxiety or to produce feelings of pleasure, excitement, confidence, or connection with others. With repeated use, users can come to depend on being in this altered state, and without the drug, they may feel worse than they did before they ever took it. Besides such symptoms as nausea and anxiety, users in withdrawal may feel that life is not worth living without the drug. Many people need help in tolerating the short-term discomfort of withdrawal and

directing their attention to the long-term benefits of being drug free.

Addictive Behaviors

Although addiction is usually associated with drug use, many experts now extend the concept of addiction to other areas in which behavior can become compulsive and out of control, such as gambling, exercise, and sex. Except for gambling, most research does not indicate clearly that compulsive behaviors in other areas should be considered mental disorders. However, some scientists speculate that they may follow the same pleasure pathway as drugs do in the brain. The behaviors themselves produce the high, and the brain adjusts in such a way that the person experiences a strong desire to repeat the behavior as well as a craving for the behavior when it stops.

Compulsive Gambling

Gambling can produce intense excitement and rapidly shifting emotions, from elation to despair; these compelling feelings give it its potential for addiction. The *DSM-IV-TR* includes **pathological gambling** as an impulse-control disorder, characterized by a preoccupation with the activity (reliving past wins, thinking about how to get money for bets); desire for the action and excitement even more than the money; and the need to bet increasingly large amounts of money to achieve the same excitement. Compulsive gamblers lie to family members about their gambling, commit crimes to get money, and jeopardize their careers, relationships, and well-being in many other ways to pursue their habit.

For some people, gambling starts out as a form of entertainment but turns into an addiction. It is as real and powerful as addiction to a drug like heroin.

Cultural factors affect the particular type of gambling a person engages in, whether horse racing, cock fighting, college sports, the stock market, casino betting, or some other kind of risk-taking activity. A compulsive gambler is always looking for something to bet on and will bet on anything. The prevalence of pathological gambling in a society is directly related to the availability of legalized gambling.[4]

Pathological gambling is more common in men than in women. Some individuals are hooked from their first bet, but for others, the habit gradually takes over their lives, often with an escalation in gambling in response to a stressful event. Men who have been diagnosed with pathological gambling have been found to have abnormalities in neurotransmitter systems, including serotonin, dopamine, and norepinephrine systems.[4] As with other mental disorders, experts do not know whether these changes occur before or after the onset of the disorder.

Estimates are that 3 percent to 4 percent of those who gamble do so compulsively. Gamblers Anonymous was founded in 1957 for people who could not control their gambling behavior. Based on the Alcoholics Anonymous model, this organization asserts that gambling is a progressive illness that can be arrested but not cured. It provides a 12-step program with meetings and group support.

Other Compulsive Behaviors

Some people use the Internet compulsively, spending endless hours shopping, chatting, developing virtual relationships, playing games, viewing pornography, or simply searching for and downloading information. Others are "addicted" to sex: They have frequent sexual encounters, often with different partners; spend a great deal of time thinking about their next sexual encounter; engage in behaviors that put them at risk for disease or arrest; and avoid sex with a spouse but pursue it with someone they do not know. Still other people exercise, eat, or shop compulsively, with such predictable consequences as underweight, overweight, or credit card debt, respectively.

The key component in all these addictions is that the person feels out of control and powerless over the behavior. As with drug dependence, the pattern of behavior has several other telling characteristics: The person uses the activity to self-medicate or escape from negative feelings; is preoccupied with the activity when not engaged in it; pursues the activity despite the problems it causes; and feels shame and distress about the behavior. Both psychotherapy and self-help groups are available to assist individuals struggling with these troubling behavior patterns.

DRUGS OF ABUSE

Now that we have considered the general characteristics and effects of drugs (and behaviors) that produce changes in the brain, we turn to a discussion of specific drugs, organized into categories according to their chemical effects: stimulants, depressants, opioids, hallucinogens, inhalants, and marijuana.

Central Nervous System Stimulants

Drugs that speed up activity in the brain and sympathetic nervous system are known as **stimulants.** Their effects are similar to the response evoked during the fight-or-flight reaction (see Chapter 5). Heart rate accelerates, breathing deepens, muscle tension increases, the senses are heightened, and attention and alertness increase. These drugs can keep people going, mentally and physically, when they would otherwise be fatigued. The drugs may stimulate movement, fidgeting, and talking, and they may produce intense feelings of euphoria and create a sense of energy and well-being.

Caffeine

The mild stimulant caffeine is probably the most popular psychoactive drug. Common sources of caffeine include coffee, tea, soft drinks, headache and pain remedies like Excedrin, stay-awake products like NoDoz, and weight loss aids. Chocolate contains caffeine but at much lower levels than these sources. Average caffeine intake among Americans is about 200 milligrams a day (about 2 cups of coffee or 4–5 cups of tea).

At low doses, caffeine increases alertness; at higher doses it can cause restlessness, nervousness, excitement, frequent urination, and gastrointestinal distress. At very high levels of consumption (1 gram a day, or 8–10 cups of coffee), symptoms of intoxication can include muscle twitching, irregular heartbeat, insomnia, flushed face, excessive sweating, rambling thoughts or speech, or excessive pacing or movement. People can develop tolerance to caffeine and experience withdrawal symptoms (usually irritability, headache, and fatigue) when cutting back or eliminating it. If you think you might be consuming too much caffeine, see the box "Tips for Cutting Back on Caffeine." (Another commonly used mild stimulant, nicotine, is discussed in Chapter 13.)

KEY TERMS

endorphins Natural chemicals in the brain that block pain during stressful or painful experiences.

pathological gambling Compulsive, out-of-control gambling, characterized by signs of psychological dependence; classified as an impulse-control disorder.

stimulants Drugs that speed up activity in the brain and the sympathetic nervous system.

Challenges & Choices

Tips for Cutting Back on Caffeine

Student life often includes hours of sedentary, stressful work and a need to concentrate despite fatigue. If you are like many students, you may count on coffee or caffeinated soda to keep you going when you're studying for exams or trying to meet a term paper deadline. Usually, however, caffeine doesn't help unless you are actually sleepy, and you will be sleepier when it wears off. If you consume more than 250 milligrams of caffeine a day, you may feel nervous or jittery, have sleep problems, or experience other symptoms of caffeine intoxication. Here on some tips on how to cut back.

- Keep track of how much caffeine you consume. See the table for caffeine content of common products.

- Set a daily limit for caffeine intake, and restrict your consumption to that amount. You may want to limit consumption to a specific time of day—a cup of coffee in the morning, for example—so you won't have to make a decision at any other time. For some people, abstinence is easier than moderation. If you experience withdrawal symptoms, cut back gradually.

- Find other ways to keep your energy up. If you are fatigued, make sure you are getting enough sleep and exercise and eating properly.

- Keep noncaffeinated drinks on hand—water, juice, herbal tea.

It's Not Just Personal . . .

Caffeine consumption is associated with bone loss and osteoporosis in women, but drinking milk throughout adult life helps to prevent caffeine-related bone loss.

Caffeine Content of Common Products (in milligrams)	
Gourmet coffee, 16 oz	550
Gourmet coffee, 12 oz	375
Gourmet coffee, 8 oz	250
Regular coffee, 8 oz	135
Cappuccino, 8 or 12 oz	35
Caffe latte, 8 or 12 oz	35
Espresso, 1 oz	35
Hot chocolate, 8 oz	5
Tea, 8 oz	50
Green tea, 8 oz	30
Dark chocolate, 1 oz	20
Maximum Strength No-Doz	200
Vivarin	200
Regular No-Doz	100

Source of table data: *Nutrition Action Health Letter,* December 1996.

Amphetamines

For centuries, practitioners of Chinese medicine have made a medicinal tea from herbs called Ma-huang. In the 1920s a chemist working for the Eli Lilly Company identified the active ingredient in Ma-huang as the compound ephedrine. The actions of this compound include opening the nasal and bronchial passages, allowing people to breathe more easily. The drug quickly became an important treatment for asthma, allergies, and stuffy noses. Researchers worked to develop synthetic forms of this botanical product, and a few years later, amphetamine was synthesized. Nasal amphetamine inhalers quickly grew in popularity; consumers found that they not only cleared the bronchioles but produced elation.

In the 1930s amphetamines were put to additional uses: helping patients with narcolepsy stay awake, suppressing appetite in people who wanted to lose weight, and treating depression. Students began to take amphetamines to cram for exams, and truck drivers took them to drive long hauls without stopping for sleep. In the 1940s soldiers fighting in World War II took amphetamines to stay alert and combat drowsiness. By the 1960s amphetamines were so widely available that they were quickly swept up into the drug culture of that period.

Amphetamines, Schedule II substances, are still used to treat narcolepsy, but they are no longer recommended for depression or weight control. Particularly in the case of depression, a host of newer, more effective drugs is available. Amphetamines are still used to treat attention deficit/hyperactivity disorder (ADHD) in children and adults. Although they are stimulants, they have a paradoxical effect in individuals with ADHD, helping them gain control of their behavior. More than 1 million children in the United States now take Ritalin and other amphetamines to control hyperactivity. It is not clear whether the increase in use of these drugs is due to a greater incidence of the disorder or greater awareness. Some people believe it is just a way to exert social control over very active children, especially boys, in school settings. More research and better screening tools are needed before these questions can be answered.

HIGHLIGHT ON HEALTH

Signs of Cocaine Use

- Dilated pupils (when large amounts are taken)
- Dry mouth, frequent lip licking
- Excessive activity, difficulty sitting still, lack of interest in food or sleep
- Irritable, argumentative, nervous
- Talkative but unfocused; conversation jumps around

- Runny nose, chronic sinus/nasal problems, nose bleeds
- Use or possession of drug paraphernalia, such as small spoons, razor blades, or plastic, glass, or metal straws

Amphetamines are usually taken orally or intravenously. Concerns about their use involve their effects on the heart, lungs, and many other organs. At low levels they may cause loss of appetite, rapid breathing, high blood pressure, and dilated pupils. Decision making can be impaired even at moderate dosage levels. At higher levels, amphetamines can cause paranoia, panic, fever, sweating, headaches, blurred vision, dizziness, and sometimes aggressiveness and violence. Very high doses may cause flushing, rapid or irregular heartbeat, tremors, and even collapse. Deaths due to heart failure and burst blood vessels in the brain have also been reported. Withdrawal symptoms after continued amphetamine use include a drop in energy, feelings of helplessness, and thoughts of suicide or death, as mentioned earlier. The person may "crash" into depression or sleep for 24 hours. Some symptoms can continue for days or weeks.

Methamphetamine ("speed") has a chemical structure similar to that of amphetamine and produces similar but more intense effects. It is manufactured easily in laboratories with relatively inexpensive over-the-counter ingredients. It is usually snorted. A very pure form of methamphetamine, called "ice" or "crystal meth," can be smoked, producing an intense rush of pleasure lasting a few minutes. Snorting or smoking produces the same euphoric high within about 3 to 5 minutes, and oral ingestion produces it within about 20 minutes.[6]

Like amphetamine, methamphetamine is a Schedule II substance, legally available only with a prescription. It is used medically to treat narcolepsy, ADHD, and sometimes obesity. Its effects include increased wakefulness and physical activity and decreased appetite. High doses can elevate body temperature to dangerous, sometimes lethal, levels and cause convulsions. Dependence is a possible outcome of use, as it is with amphetamines.

Cocaine

A powerful CNS stimulant, cocaine heightens alertness, inhibits appetite and the need for sleep, and provides intense feelings of pleasure. The use of cocaine has been traced back hundreds of years to the Inca Empire in Peru. Natives of the Andes Mountains still chew the leaves of the coca plant, both to produce pleasure and to increase endurance. Pure cocaine was first extracted from coca leaves in Europe in the mid-19th century; it was introduced as a remedy for a number of ailments and used medically as an anesthetic.[7] Today cocaine is classified as a Schedule II drug, meaning that it has high potential for abuse.

Cocaine can be consumed in various ways. Coca leaves can be chewed or sucked, allowing the cocaine to be absorbed slowly into the system, or they can be mixed with other compounds to form coca paste, which is smoked. Both of these practices are limited largely to cocaine-producing areas in Central and South America. The most common form of pure cocaine is cocaine hydrochloride powder, made from coca paste. It can be snorted or mixed with water and injected intravenously. Snorting produces a relatively quick effect that lasts from 15 to 30 minutes; IV injection produces a rapid, powerful, and brief effect.

Two other methods of use are freebasing and smoking crack cocaine. Freebasing involves heating cocaine hydrochloride with a volatile solvent such as ether or ammonia and smoking it. This practice is dangerous because the solvent can ignite and burn the user. Crack is a form of cocaine that appeared in the mid-1980s and led to an epidemic of cocaine use in the United States. When crack is smoked in a pipe, its effects are extremely rapid and intense. This method of use also produces the highest rate of dependence. Cocaine mixed with heroin produces a drug called a "speedball."

Cocaine is still used as a local anesthetic, often for surgeries in the areas of the nose and throat. Most uses, however, are recreational. Like other CNS stimulants, cocaine causes an acceleration of heart rate, elevated blood pressure, dilation of the pupils, and an increase in alertness, muscle tension, and motor activity. It produces feelings of euphoria, often accompanied by talkativeness, sociability, and a sense of grandiosity (see the box "Signs of Cocaine Use"). These effects appear almost immediately after a single dose and usually last for 15 minutes to an hour. When the effects wear off, the user typically wants to repeat the experience. Dependence can occur after only a few uses. Withdrawal after prolonged use is characterized by a depressed mood, fatigue, sleep disturbances, unpleasant dreams, and increased appetite.

At higher doses, cocaine use can lead to cardiac arrhythmias, respiratory distress, bizarre or violent behavior, psychosis, convulsions, seizures, coma, and even death. Regular snorting can irritate the nasal passage and result in a chronic runny nose. Some users may become malnourished because the drug suppresses appetite. Chronic users with cocaine dependence may spend huge amounts of money on the drug in a short period of time, neglecting work, school, and family responsibilities in pursuit of the drug.

MDMA

Also known as Ecstasy or XTC, MDMA has chemical similarities both to stimulants (such as methamphetamine) and hallucinogens (such as mescaline).[8] Thus, it produces both types of effects. MDMA appears to elevate levels of the neurotransmitter serotonin, the body's primary regulator of mood, perhaps in a manner similar to the action of antidepressants. Users experience increased energy, feelings of euphoria, and a heightened sense of empathy and closeness to those around them. Some users report enhanced hearing, vision, and sense of touch, but only a few report actual visual hallucinations.

In addition to the drug's euphoric effects, MDMA can cause increased heart rate, elevated body temperature (sometimes to dangerous levels), profuse sweating, dry mouth, muscle tension, blurred vision, and involuntary teeth clenching. Serious risks include dehydration, hypertension, and heart or kidney failure. MDMA use can apparently lead to psychological problems, such as depression, anxiety, confusion, paranoia, and sleep disturbances. Findings from several studies show that long-term users of MDMA can suffer cognitive defects, including problems with memory. However, more research on the long-term effects of this drug is needed.

Central Nervous System Depressants

Central nervous system **depressants** slow down activity in the brain and sympathetic nervous system. This category of drugs includes sedatives (for example, barbiturates), hypnotics (sleeping medications), and most anti-anxiety drugs. They can be deadly if misused, especially when mixed with one another or with alcohol (another CNS depressant). They are available both by prescription and from illicit sources. CNS depressants carry a high risk for dependence.

Barbiturates and Hypnotics

Barbiturates ("downers") are powerful sedatives that produce pleasant feelings of relaxation when first ingested, usually followed by lethargy, drowsiness, and sleep. Users experience impairments in judgment, decision making, and problem solving, as well as slow, slurred speech and lack of coordination. Dependence is common among middle-aged and older adults who use barbiturates as sleep aids. Withdrawal is difficult, and symptoms, including insomnia, anxiety, tremors, and nausea, can last for weeks; they can be mitigated by gradually tapering off the drug.

Hypnotics are prescribed for people with insomnia and other sleep disorders. People working on the night shift or traveling through multiple time zones may use them to get to sleep quickly and at odd hours. Hypnotics are also used to control epilepsy and to calm people before surgery or dental procedures.

Anti-Anxiety Drugs

The most widely prescribed CNS depressant is the group of anti-anxiety drugs known as the benzodiazepines; examples are Xanax, Valium, and Ativan. Also known as tranquilizers, the benzodiazepines are used to control panic attacks and anxiety disorders. Users are at risk for dependence and for increasing dose levels as they become tolerant. Another concern is the **rebound effect,** which occurs when a person stops using a drug and experiences symptoms that are worse than those experienced before taking the drug. A person who stops taking Xanax, for example, may experience high anxiety for a few days, followed by a return to more typical anxiety levels. The rebound effect can make it difficult to stop taking a particular medication.

Rohypnol

A relatively new CNS depressant is Rophynol (flunitrazepam). This powerful sedative, also called "roofies," has depressive effects and causes confusion, loss of memory, and sometimes loss of consciousness. It is especially dangerous when mixed with alcohol. Rohypnol is known as a "date rape drug" because men have slipped it into women's drinks in order to sexually assault them later. As of this time the drug's manufacturer has changed the formulation of this drug so it will not remain colorless when dissolving in a drink. In addition, a Florida-based company is developing a coaster that reacts when drops from a contaminated drink splash onto its surface.

GHB

Another so-called date rape drug is Gamma hydroxybutyrate (GHB). This CNS depressant produces feelings of pleasure along with sedation and is a drug of choice among young people at bars, clubs, and parties. It can be produced in several forms, including a clear, tasteless, odorless liquid and a powder that readily dissolves in liquid. Like Rohypnol, it has been slipped into the drinks of women who later did not remember being sexually assaulted. It usually takes effect within 15 to 30 minutes and lasts from

Clubs that offer all-night dancing, alcoholic beverages, and drugs are designed to attract a young crowd. In this kind of atmosphere, risky behavior is often viewed as part of the excitement.

3 to 6 hours. Besides sedation and amnesia, GHB can cause nausea, hallucinations, respiratory distress, slowed heart rate, loss of consciousness, and coma. Users are at risk for dependence with sustained use. GHB is sometimes used to counteract the effects of stimulants (cocaine, methamphetamine) or hallucinogens (LSD, mescaline).

GHB, Rohypnol, and MDMA are sometimes referred to as "club drugs" because of their widespread use at clubs and parties. Their use is particularly dangerous because of the unpredictable setting in which they are usually taken. When GHB and Rohypnol are consumed with alcohol, the combined sedative effects can lead to life-threatening conditions. Additionally, all of these drugs are typically produced in basement labs, so dose and purity are uncertain.

Opioids

Natural and synthetic derivatives of opium, a product harvested from a gummy substance in the seed pod of the opium poppy (*Papaver somniferum*), are known as **opioids.** Opium originated in the Middle East and has a long history of medical use for pain relief and treatment of diarrhea and dehydration. Currently, opioids are prescribed as pain relievers, anesthetics, antidiarrheal agents, and cough suppressants.

Drugs in this category include morphine, heroin, codeine, and oxycodone. Also known as narcotics, opioids are commonly misused and abused. They produce a pleasant, drowsy state in which cares are forgotten, the senses are dulled, and pain is reduced. They act by altering the neurotransmitters that control movement, moods, and a number of body functions, including body temperature, digestion, and breathing. They produce feelings of pleasure and block sensations of pain.

With low doses, opioid users experience euphoria, followed by drowsiness, constriction of the pupils, slurred speech, and impaired attention and memory. With higher doses, users can experience depressed respiration, loss of consciousness, coma, and death. When first used, opioids often cause nausea, vomiting, and a negative mood rather than euphoria. Chronic users usually experience dry mouth, constipation, and vision problems.

Opioids can be smoked, snorted, injected, or taken orally. They have a high potential for dependence. Withdrawal symptoms include anxiety, restlessness, craving, irritability, nausea, muscle aches, negative mood, runny nose, insomnia, and diarrhea.

Morphine

The primary active chemical in opium, morphine is a powerful pain reliever. Its first widespread use, facilitated by the development of the hypodermic syringe in the 1850s, was during the Civil War. So many soldiers became addicted that after the war, morphine addiction was called "the soldier's disease."[9] Because of the high risk of dependence, physicians prescribing morphine today do so conservatively.

KEY TERMS

depressants   Drugs that slow down activity in the brain and sympathetic nervous system.

rebound effect   Phenomenon that occurs when a person stops using a drug and experiences symptoms that are worse than those experienced before taking the drug.

opioids   Natural and synthetic derivatives of opium.

HIGHLIGHT ON HEALTH

Signs of Oxycodone Use

- Energetic and talkative initially, becoming relaxed and content
- Slightly slurred speech
- Impaired coordination

- Drowsiness
- Constricted pupils, unresponsive to light
- Use or possession of drug paraphernalia, such as syringes and needles

Heroin

Heroin is three times more potent than morphine. It was developed in the late 19th century as a supposedly nonaddictive substitute for codeine (another derivative of morphine, useful for suppressing coughs). Just as Civil War veterans suffered from morphine addiction, many soldiers came home from the war in Vietnam addicted to heroin.

Whereas morphine has medical uses, heroin is almost exclusively a drug of abuse. Its use is associated with unemployment, divorce, and drug-related crimes. Users are at risk for such diseases as hepatitis, tuberculosis, and HIV infection from contaminated needles. Heroin dependence is also associated with a high rate of death, primarily from overdoses, accidents, injuries, AIDS, and incidents involving violence.[4] Babies born to women who used heroin during pregnancy are often drug dependent at birth. Heroin itself does not appear to cause any long-term damage to the body aside from collapsed veins. When heroin addicts are seen scratching their bodies in a frantic way, it usually indicates the drug was mixed with additives or contaminants prior to sale and is causing an allergic reaction.

Synthetic Opioids

Some of the most widely prescribed drugs in the United States are synthetic opioids, made from oxycodone hydrochloride. Brand names include OxyContin, Vicodin, Demerol, Percocet, and Percodan. Some people who start using these drugs for pain become addicted and misuse or abuse them (see the box "Signs of Oxycodone Use"). OxyContin, for example, provides long-lasting, timed-release relief for moderate to severe chronic pain when taken in tablet form. If the tablets are chewed, crushed and snorted, or dissolved in water and injected, they provide an immediate, intense rush similar to that of heroin. One group particularly susceptible to opioid misuse is medical personnel with access to controlled substances.

Hallucinogens

LSD, psilocybin, and mescaline are a few of the so-called **hallucinogens** (also called psychedelics). They differ chemically, but their effects are similar: They alter perceptions and thinking in characteristic ways. They produce intensification and distortion of visual and auditory perceptions as well as hallucinations. Some hallucinogens are synthetic (for example, LSD), and others are derived from plants (for example, mescaline, from peyote, and psilocybin, from psilocybin mushrooms). They are Schedule I drugs with no current medical uses.[10]

LSD

Lysergic acid diethylamide (LSD) is a synthetic hallucinogen that alters perceptual processes and enhances emotionality. It was first synthesized in 1938 by chemist Albert Hofmann, working for the Swiss pharmaceutical company Sandoz, from ergot, a fungus that grows on rye and other grains. Hofmann accidentally absorbed a bit of LSD through the skin and experienced dizziness, visual distortions, and a vivid stream of fantastic images. He and other researchers continued to study LSD, hoping to discover some therapeutic properties, but their research proved unproductive.

In the 1960s the recreational use of hallucinogens, particularly LSD, became a hallmark of the counterculture. Enthusiasts promised that an LSD trip would change consciousness, provide deep insights, and inspire feelings of love, spirituality, and community. Psychedelic artwork reflected the brilliant colors and flowing, exotic imagery users experienced in their minds. Use of LSD peaked in the late 1960s and then declined, as reports circulated of "bad trips," prolonged psychotic reactions, "flashbacks," self-injurious behavior, and possible chromosomal damage.

LSD is one of the most potent psychoactive drugs known. It is odorless, colorless, and tasteless, and a dose as small as a single grain of salt (about .01 mg) can produce mild effects. At higher doses (.05 mg to .10 mg), hallucinogenic effects are produced. Most users take LSD orally; absorption is rapid. Effects last for several hours and vary depending on the user's mood and expectations, the setting, and the dose and potency of the drug. It usually takes hours or days to recover from an LSD trip. Although LSD is thought to stimulate serotonin receptors in the brain, its exact neural pathway is not completely understood.

Besides visual distortion, LSD can produce auditory changes, a distorted sense of time, changes in the perception of one's own body, and *synesthesia,* a "mixing of senses," in which sounds may appear as visual images or a visual image changes in rhythm to music. Feelings of euphoria may alternate with waves of anxiety. In a bad trip, the user may experience acute anxiety or panic.

Tolerance to the effects of LSD develops quickly for some users, and they must increase their intake of LSD to get the same effects. Repeated daily doses become ineffective in 3 to 4 days. LSD does not produce compulsive drug-seeking behaviors, and physiological withdrawal symptoms do not occur when use is stopped.

Phencyclidine (PCP)

First developed in the 1950s as an anesthetic, PCP was found to produce such serious side effects—agitation, delusions, irrational behavior—that its use was discontinued. Since the 1960s it has been manufactured illegally and sold on the street, often under the name "angel dust." It has fewer hallucinogenic effects than LSD and more disturbances in body perception. A drug with similar effects is ketamine.

PCP is a white crystalline powder that is readily soluble in water or alcohol. It can be smoked, snorted, or injected intravenously. At low doses, it produces euphoria, dizziness, nausea, slurred speech, rapid heartbeat, high blood pressure, numbness, and slowed reaction time. At higher doses it causes disorganized thinking and feelings of unreality, and at very high doses it can cause amnesia, seizures, and coma. A person who has taken PCP is anesthetized enough to undergo surgery. The drug is particularly associated with aggressive behavior, probably as a result of impaired judgment and disorganized thinking. Combined with insensitivity to pain, these effects can produce dangerous or deadly results. PCP is involved in about 3 percent of drug-related emergency room visits and about 3 percent of drug-related deaths.[4]

PCP use does not lead to physical dependence, but users often develop a profound psychological dependence, despite the unpredictability of the drug and the behavioral impairment it causes. Users may spend a significant amount of time on the drug, leading to problems in social and occupational functioning, and their lives may become chaotic. Some users have attributed their continued use to the feelings of strength, power, and invulnerability it gives them, along with its numbing effect on the mind.

Inhalants

The drugs called **inhalants** are breathable chemical vapors that alter consciousness, typically producing a state of intoxication that resembles drunkenness. The vapors come from substances like paint thinners, gasoline, glue, and spray can propellant. The active ingredients in these products are chemicals like toluene, benzene, acetone, and tetrachlorethylene—all powerful toxins and carcinogens.

Inhalants are commonly classified into four categories: volatile solvents (liquids that vaporize at room temperature: paint thinners, dry cleaning fluids, gasoline, glues, correction fluids); aerosols (spray paints, hair sprays, deodorants); gases (medical anesthetics like nitrous oxide, ether, and chloroform); and nitrates (sexual enhancers like amyl and butyl nitrate, sometimes called "poppers"). Many compounds that are inhaled contain multiple intoxicating substances.[11]

Vapors can be inhaled using different methods. A user can inhale the fumes from a rag that has been soaked in the substance and placed over the mouth and nose ("huffing") or breathe into a bag containing the substance ("bagging"). Users also inhale fumes directly from containers and even spray aerosols into the nose and mouth. Vapors reach the lungs and enter the bloodstream very quickly.

At low doses, inhalants cause light-headedness, dizziness, blurred vision, slurred speech, lack of coordination, and feelings of euphoria. At higher doses, they can cause lethargy, muscle weakness, and stupor. An overdose of an inhalant can result in a loss of consciousness, coma, or death. Inhalants can also cause behavioral and psychological changes, including belligerence, confusion, apathy, and impaired social and occupational functioning. Perhaps the most significant negative effect for chronic users is widespread and long-lasting brain damage.

Marijuana

The most widely used illicit drug in the United States is marijuana. In 2003, there were an estimated 14.6 million users among Americans aged 12 and older (6.2 percent of the population), and nearly 20 percent of young people aged 12 to 17 had used marijuana at least once.[1]

Marijuana is derived from the hemp plant, *Cannabis sativa.* The leaves of the plant are usually dried and smoked, but they can also be mixed in tea or food. Hashish is a resin that seeps from the leaves; it is usually smoked. The active ingredient in marijuana is delta-9-tetrahydrocannabinol (THC). The potency of the drug is determined

KEY TERMS

hallucinogens Drugs that alter perceptions and thinking, intensifying and distorting visual and auditory perceptions and producing hallucinations; also called psychedelics.

inhalants Breathable chemical vapors that alter consciousness, producing a state resembling drunkenness.

HIGHLIGHT ON HEALTH
Signs of Marijuana Use

- Rapid, loud talking and bursts of laughter in early stages of intoxication
- Drowsiness or stupor in later stages of intoxication
- Dry mouth
- Increased appetite
- Bloodshot eyes, dilated pupils

- Forgetfulness while conversing
- Tendency to drive slowly (below speed limit)
- Distorted sense of time passage (tendency to overestimate time intervals)
- Use or possession of drug paraphernalia, such as cigarette papers or pipes

by the amount of THC in the plant, which in turn is affected by the growing conditions. Since the 1960s, the amount of THC in marijuana sold on the street has increased from 1–5 percent to as much as 10–15 percent.

Marijuana use produces mild euphoria, sedation, lethargy, short-term memory impairment, distorted sensory perceptions, a distorted sense of time, impaired motor coordination, and an increase in heart rate (see the box "Signs of Marijuana Use"). Effects typically begin within a few minutes and last from 3 to 4 hours. Sometimes the drug causes anxiety or a negative mood. At high doses, marijuana can have hallucinogenic effects, accompanied by acute anxiety and paranoid thinking. Chronic, heavy users of marijuana may develop tolerance to its effects and experience some withdrawal symptoms if they stop using it, but most dependence seems to be psychological.

Researchers have found that THC has a variety of effects on the brain. One effect is the suppression of activity in the information processing system of the hippocampus, perhaps accounting for some impairments in problem solving and decision making associated with being high on marijuana. Marijuana smoke has negative effects on the respiratory system; it contains more carcinogens than tobacco smoke does and is highly irritating to the lining of the bronchioles and lungs. In addition to coughs and chest colds, users may experience more frequent episodes of acute bronchitis and may be more likely to develop chronic bronchitis.[4]

Cannabis has been known from ancient times and used as a medical treatment for conditions ranging from rheumatism to absent-mindedness. Since 1970, marijuana has been a Schedule I controlled substance, with no accepted medical uses. Many people claim that marijuana does have medical uses, especially as a treatment for glaucoma, for the pain and nausea associated with cancer and chemotherapy, and for the weight loss associated with AIDS. Research suggests that smoking marijuana is no more effective than taking THC in pill form for these purposes,

but the use of marijuana for medical uses has become a matter of political debate. Proponents of its use assert that it makes life livable for many people with painful and debilitating medical conditions and that there is no reason not to legalize it. Opponents argue that legalizing marijuana would imply approval of its use for recreational purposes and open the floodgates to abuse of all drugs.

Like alcohol, marijuana affects the skills required to drive a car safely, including concentration, attention, coordination, reaction time, and the ability to judge distance. Because it also impairs judgment, people who are high may not realize their driving skills are impaired. It also appears that marijuana use during pregnancy affects both the likelihood of miscarriage and the health of the fetus.[12] Babies born to mothers who use marijuana may be smaller and more likely to develop health problems once they are born. During infancy and early childhood, these children may have more behavioral problems and cognitive deficits, and in school, they have more difficulty with tasks requiring memory, attention, and decision making.[13]

APPROACHES TO THE DRUG PROBLEM

As mentioned, drug use and dependence are problems both for individuals and for society. The U.S. government continues to wage a war on drugs, with mixed results. Government approaches to the drug problem have traditionally fallen into two broad categories: supply reduction and demand reduction. A newer approach to the drug problem is harm reduction, an approach used in alcohol treatment programs as well (see Chapter 11).

Supply Reduction Strategies

Strategies to reduce the supply of drugs are aimed at controlling the quantity of illicit substances that enter or are produced in the United States. An example is **interdiction,** the interception of drugs before they enter the country, as when customs officials use dogs to sniff out drugs at airports or when the Coast Guard boards ships to search for drugs as they enter U.S. waters.

The U.S. government also puts pressure on governments in other countries to suppress the production and exportation of drugs. Unfortunately, the plants that yield drugs are important and profitable cash crops for peasant farmers in many countries, and the drug smuggling business is controlled by criminal interests that are often beyond the control of the government. The profits from illegal drugs are so high that a drug-trafficking organization can lose 90 percent of its product and still make money. Efforts to reduce the drug supply at the international level have led to human rights abuses, an expansion of oppressive regimes, and increased corruption among police, government, and military personnel.

The government also attempts to prevent domestic production of drugs by raiding suspected underground drug labs or stamping out enterprises that grow marijuana on a large scale. Another domestic supply side strategy is to obstruct the distribution of drugs, such as when a massive police presence is used in an area where drugs are sold or when legal means are used to disrupt money laundering and other practices that underlie the financial structures of the drug business. Federal statutes now authorize the seizure of any property used in connection with the sale or possession of illegal drugs, including cars, boats, planes, and homes.

Despite the money spent on these efforts and impressive seizures of drugs every year, foreign drugs are cheaper and more available today than they were 2 decades ago, and domestic production has been increasing.

Demand Reduction Strategies

Demand-side strategies include penalizing users through incarceration; preventing drug use, primarily through education; and treating individuals once they have become dependent on drugs.

Incarceration for Drug-Related Crimes

Penalizing users means enforcing the laws against drug possession, arresting offenders, and putting people in prison. The assumptions behind this approach are that incarceration will reduce drug-related crime by getting users off the streets and that the threat of punishment will deter others from using drugs. Most states mandate harsh prison terms for the possession or sale of relatively small quantities of drugs, regardless of whether the person is a first-time or repeat offender. As a result, U.S. prisons are crowded with people convicted of drug-related crimes; in

fact, more than half of the people in U.S. prisons are serving time for such offenses. The United States imprisons a larger percentage of its population than does any other nation. Elsewhere, low-level crimes like drug possession do not draw a prison sentence.

Since prisoners are a captive audience, it would make sense to provide treatment while they are in jail, but only a small percentage of prisoners who need drug treatment receive it. Instead, prison time serves mainly to disrupt people's lives and turn young people who may have been experimenting with drugs into criminals. Incarceration does little to address the larger problem of drug use in our society.

Prevention Strategies

A second demand-side strategy is prevention through education. Prevention strategies focus on reducing the demand for drugs by increasing an individual's ability to decline drug use when confronted with an opportunity to experiment. Programs involve primary, secondary, or tertiary prevention, depending on their targeted audience. Primary, or universal, prevention programs are designed to reach the entire population without regard to individual risk factors. Public service commercials on television asking us to imagine a world without cigarettes or billboards referring to crystal meth as "crystal mess" are examples of primary prevention strategies. Secondary, or selective, strategies focus on those subgroups that are at greatest risk for use or abuse, with the aim of increasing protective factors and decreasing potential risk factors. An example is a class that teaches problem-solving skills to adolescents. Tertiary, or indicated, strategies target at-risk individuals rather than groups, again focusing on protective factors such as academic, interpersonal, social, or job skills. An example is a program that tutors individual students in ways to manage emotions and maintain self-esteem without drugs.

A prevention strategy used in the workplace is drug testing, usually random urine screening. The goal of drug testing is not to catch drug users and fire them but to create an environment in which it is clear that drug use is not condoned. Companies also want to limit their liability by reducing the likelihood that an employee will make a mistake that causes someone harm. Federal law requires that people in jobs involving transportation, such as air traffic controllers, train engineers, and truck drivers, undergo regular testing to ensure public

KEY TERMS

interdiction   Interception of drugs before they enter the country.

Healthy People 2010

OBJECTIVE AREA *Substance-Free Youth*

- Increase the age and proportion of adolescents who remain alcohol and drug free.

"Strengthening the ability of children and teenagers to reject [illicit drugs] is an important and critical element in prevention activities, because the required skills and attitudes can carry over into adulthood, long after family constraints and other influences have lost their effectiveness. . . . Comprehensive, community-based programs include interventions that influence individual behavior and attitudes through education and interventions that change environments through controls on the availability of substances."

For more information on Healthy People 2010 objectives, visit the Web site at www.healthypeople.gov.

For more information on Canadian health objectives, visit the Health Canada Web site at www.hc-sc.gc.ca/english.

safety. U.S. military personnel also undergo regular drug testing. Although some see the practice as an infringement on privacy, so far it has withstood judicial challenges.

Drug Treatment Programs

The third type of demand-side strategy is helping people to stop using drugs after they have started, that is, providing treatment. Evidence indicates that treatment is a more effective strategy for reducing drug use than locking up dealers or cutting off supplies at our borders.[14,15] As with alcohol, treatment is available in a variety of formats, from hospital-based inpatient programs, to community-based outpatient programs, to self-help/mutual-help groups such as Narcotics Anonymous (NA).

Most experts agree that treatment for addiction is a lifelong process requiring vigilance and hard work. The first step is acknowledging that there is a problem and getting into a treatment program. Treatment is more successful when the program lasts at least 3 months, includes individual counseling, and has components that address all aspects of the individual's life, including medical treatment, family therapy, living skills, and occupational skills. Many programs have had success with cognitive and behavioral approaches to therapy. Individuals do better when they have a support system of family and friends, are employed, and do not have coexisting psychiatric

problems. At the completion of the treatment program, they need to continue with follow-up care and possibly join a self-help program. Some treatment programs are covered by insurance but usually less comprehensively than are treatments for physical illnesses such as cancer or heart disease.

Harm Reduction Strategies

Both of the approaches discussed so far—supply reduction and demand reduction—assume that drug use should be prevented and that government intervention is necessary to protect both individuals and society from their threat. As we saw in Chapter 11, harm reduction strategies are based on a different idea—that attempting to completely eliminate drugs is futile and that efforts should be focused on helping addicts reduce the harm associated with their drug use.[16,17,18]

Advocates of the harm reduction approach assert that the decision to use drugs is not immoral and that drug users are in need of treatment rather than punishment. Examples of harm reduction strategies are needle exchange programs, in which addicts are provided with sterile needles in exchange for their used ones, and drug substitute programs, in which individuals are maintained on addictive but less debilitating drugs, such as methadone for heroin addicts. Other harm reduction strategies include controlled availability (certain drugs are available through a government monopoly), medicalization (drugs are available by prescription but only to individuals who are already addicted to them), and decriminalization (the penalty for possession of certain drugs is reduced or eliminated if the quantity held is below a certain limit).

Proponents of harm reduction strategies claim that they represent a more realistic approach to the drug problem and would allow resources to be directed away from punishment, which is ineffective, and toward treatment, which is effective. Opponents of harm reduction strategies argue that they are thinly disguised forms of drug legalization and that any softening of a zero tolerance position would result in an epidemic of drug use. As noted in Chapter 11, effective harm reduction programs have been in place in England and Canada for years, and numerous programs exist in the United States. However, harm reduction is rejected as an official policy by the U.S. government.

***

The use of drugs in our society is widespread. If you have not already had a personal encounter with recreational drugs, you are likely to have one at some point in your life. As with other aspects of health-related behavior, making responsible decisions about drug use depends on information, self-knowledge, and behavioral strategies and skills. Use the material in this chapter as the basis for making the right decision for yourself.

You Make the Call

Is Law Enforcement the Best Way to Fight the War on Drugs?

Imagine that your child is about to start attending a high school where drug use has been increasing and a star athlete recently overdosed on cocaine. You and other parents meet with teachers, school and district administrators, and local and state government officials to discuss solutions to the growing drug problem. To your surprise, the range of opinions is broad and the debate is heated. Some people want to build up the police force, use drug-sniffing dogs to patrol the school, and impose mandatory drug testing for school athletes. Others want to implement drug awareness and education programs and set up more after-school clubs and activities. At the end of the evening, the advocates of increased law enforcement have prevailed.

A local debate such as this mirrors the national debate over solutions to the drug problem. The ratio of government spending on prevention, education, and treatment to spending on law enforcement (including spending on military interdiction by the Department of Defense, court costs incurred by the Justice Department, and maintenance of the prison system by the Bureau of Prisons) is roughly 30:70, despite abundant evidence that law enforcement is not solving the problem. Although billions of dollars are spent every year on the war on drugs, illicit substances are readily available in high schools, on college campuses, and in communities across the country.

Proponents of the law enforcement approach point out that possession of drugs, even in small quantities, is illegal and that to have an orderly and safe society the law must be upheld. Arresting individuals who use drugs and sentencing them to jail discourages dealers and sellers and serves as a deterrent to those considering drug use. Because adolescents often have poor judgment, lack impulse control, and take risks without thinking about consequences, efforts to get through to them have to be tough and harsh.

Opponents of this approach point out that research supports prevention and treatment as far more effective responses to the drug problem than enforcement. They argue that drugs will always be available and that families, schools, and communities need to help young people acquire problem-solving and decision-making skills. Relying on the police and drug testing can lead to civil rights abuses and violations of privacy rights. In the war on drugs, one side lines up with a "law and order" approach, and the other emphasizes prevention and treatment. What do you think?

Pros

- Criminal activity calls for criminal punishment.
- Drug dealers and sellers need to be driven from the community.
- Harsh punishments deter young people from trying drugs.
- Public safety and security are of the highest importance and override concerns about civil liberty abuses.

Cons

- Most young people are experimenting with drugs; they are not criminals. Arrests and jail time can permanently derail the lives of promising young citizens.
- Imprisonment and long sentences have not been shown to reduce the number of subsequent drug arrests; the deterrent argument is faulty.
- We always need to be vigilant about our civil liberties, especially when the public is vulnerable to fears about safety and security.
- Drug users are in need of treatment and rehabilitation, not punishment and incarceration.

OLC Web site For more information about this topic, visit the Online Learning Center at www.mhhe.com/teaguele.

SUMMARY

- There have been two major "epidemics" of drug use in the United States, one in the second half of the 19th century, the other in the 1960s and 1970s. About 8 percent of the American population currently use an illicit drug.

- A drug is a substance other than food that affects the structure or function of the body through its chemical action. A psychoactive drug is a substance that causes changes in brain chemistry and alters consciousness, perception, mood, and thought.

- A drug of abuse is a medical drug used for nonmedical (recreational) purposes or a drug with no medical purposes.

- Legal drugs include prescription medications, over-the-counter medications, and herbal remedies. Illicit drugs are illegal.

- Drugs with potential for abuse are regulated by the Controlled Substances Act of 1970.

- Drug abuse is the use of a substance in amounts, situations, or a manner such that it causes problems, or greatly increases the risk of problems, for the user or for others.

- Psychoactive drugs can be taken orally, by injection, by inhalation, or by application to the skin or mucous membranes.

- The effect of a drug depends on the characteristics of the drug, the characteristics of the person, and the characteristics of the situation.

- Drug dependence, or drug addiction, is characterized by a strong craving for a drug and by compulsive use of the drug despite serious negative consequences, usually because physiological changes have occurred; tolerance and withdrawal are signs of dependence. Dependence can also be psychological.

- Addictive drugs produce their effects and produce dependence by acting on the pleasure and reward circuit in the brain.

- Behaviors can also be addictive; pathological gambling is classified as an impulse-control disorder characterized by loss of control over gambling behavior.

- Drugs of abuse are classified as CNS stimulants, CNS depressants, opioids, hallucinogens, inhalants, and marijuana.

- CNS stimulants speed up the activity of the sympathetic nervous system; they include caffeine, amphetamines, methamphetamine, and cocaine. MDMA has both stimulant and hallucinogenic effects.

- CNS depressants slow down the activity of the sympathetic nervous system; they include barbiturates and hypnotics, anti-anxiety drugs, Rohypnol, and GHB.

- Opioids are natural and synthetic derivatives of the opium poppy that act on natural receptors in the brain for endorphins. Also known as narcotics, they block pain and produce drowsiness and feelings of pleasure; they include opium, morphine, heroin, and synthetic opioids.

- Hallucinogens alter perceptions and thinking and produce visual and auditory distortions and hallucinations. They include natural substances such as peyote and mescaline and synthetic substances such as LSD and PCP.

- Inhalants are breathable chemical vapors that alter consciousness and produce a state resembling drunkenness. They come from highly toxic and carcinogenic substances.

- Marijuana comes from the hemp plant; it produces mild euphoria and sedation, among other effects. It is the most widely used illicit drug in the United States.

- Government's attempts to control drugs fall mainly into two categories: supply reduction and demand reduction.

- Supply reduction strategies include stopping drugs at the borders, pressuring other countries to control drug production, and obstructing domestic production and distribution.

- Demand reduction strategies include arresting and imprisoning users, preventing use through education and drug testing, and treating users.

- Harm reduction strategies focus on helping addicts reduce the harm associated with their drug use. Examples are needle exchange and methadone programs.

REVIEW QUESTIONS

1. What addictive drugs were commonly available in the 19th century? Why was it not known that they were addictive?

2. What are some of the costs to society of drug abuse and the war on drugs?

3. What is a psychoactive drug? What is a drug of abuse?

4. How are pharmaceutical drugs and herbal remedies treated differently by the FDA?

5. What are the five categories of controlled substances?

6. What is the difference between drug misuse and drug abuse?

7. Describe the differences in speed of effect between the four methods of drug administration.

8. What factors contribute to the effects of a drug?

9. Explain how tolerance and withdrawal are related to dependence. How can dependence be psychological?

10. Describe the pleasure and reward pathway in the brain. What additional mechanism accounts for the effects of opioids?

11. What are the characteristics of addictive behavior?

12. Describe the effects of CNS stimulants. How are they like the fight-or-flight response?

13. What are the medical uses of amphetamines? Of cocaine?

14. What are the medical uses of barbiturates, hypnotics, and anti-anxiety drugs?

15. What are some of the dangers associated with club drugs?

16. How are synthetic opioids abused?

17. Why is the use of PCP dangerous? What dangers are associated with the use of inhalants?

18. What are some negative effects of marijuana use on the body?

19. Describe three supply reduction strategies and three demand reduction strategies for drug control.

20. What features make a treatment program effective?

21. Why is harm reduction controversial as an approach to drug control?

WEB RESOURCES

ClubDrugs.Org: This Web site offers information on club drugs such as Ecstasy, GHB, and LSD, including trends and statistics for these and other drugs of abuse.
www.clubdrugs.org

Gamblers Anonymous: This organization answers questions about compulsive gambling through its Web site, describing the characteristics of people who become addicted to gambling. The site features a self-assessment for determining whether you have a gambling problem.
www.gamblersanonymous.org

Habitsmart: Habit endurance and habit change are the focus of this site. In addition to addiction, this site addresses topics such as depression, anger management, harm reduction, and cognitive therapy.
www.habitsmart.com

Higher Education Center for Alcohol and Other Drug Abuse and Violence Prevention: This government organization looks at problems of drug abuse and violence in context, emphasizing the importance of managing the environment, using educational campaigns, and promoting early intervention treatment and recovery strategies.
www.edc.org/hec

Narcotics Anonymous (NA): NA resources include drug information, helplines, contact information, news features, publications, and links.
www.na.org

National Clearinghouse for Alcohol and Drug Information: This site features a RADAR network—Regional Alcohol and Drug Awareness Resource—consisting of more than 700 active centers for substance abuse prevention and treatment.
www.health.org

National Council on Problem Gambling: With an online directory of National Certified Gambling Counselors, this organization offers help to compulsive gamblers through its literature, links, and treatment information.
www.ncpgambling.org

National Institute on Drug Abuse: This site features in-depth information on various drugs of abuse, offering research reports and drug information facts along with many other helpful resources.
www.nida.nih.gov

Substance Abuse and Mental Health Services Administration (SAMHSA): SAMHSA offers information and resources on mental health, drug abuse prevention and treatment, and workplace issues.
www.samhsa.gov

U.S. Drug Enforcement Administration: Drugs of Abuse: This comprehensive resource includes fact sheets on drugs of abuse and briefs and background information on topics such as drug trafficking and abuse, law enforcement, and drug policy.
www.dea.gov

REFERENCES

1. Substance Abuse and Mental Health Services Administration. (2004). *Overview of findings from the 2003 National Survey on Drug Use and Health.* Rockville, MD: Office of Applied Studies.

2. Executive Office of the President. (2001). *The economic costs of drug abuse in the United States: 1992–1998.* Washington, DC: Office of National Drug Control Policy.

3. Substance Abuse and Mental Health Services Administration. (2003). *Emergency department trends from the drug abuse warning network, final estimates 1995–2002.* Rockville, MD: Office of Applied Studies.

4. American Psychiatric Association. (2000). *Diagnostic and statistical manual of mental disorders* (4th ed., Text Revision [*DSM-IV-TR*]). Washington, DC: American Psychiatric Association Press.

5. Saal, D., Dong, Y., Bonci, A., & Malenka, R. C. (2003). Drugs of abuse and stress trigger a common synaptic adaptation in dopamine neurons. *Neuron, 37* (4), 577–582.

6. Methamphetamine abuse and addiction. (2002, January). NIDA Research Report. www.nida.nih.gov.

7. Cocaine abuse and addiction. (2004, November). NIDA Research Report. www.nida.nih.gov.

8. MDMA (Ecstasy) abuse. (2004, April). NIDA Research Report. www.nida.nih.gov.

9. Ksir, C., Hart, C. L., & Ray, O. (2006). *Drugs, society, and human behavior* (11th ed.). New York: McGraw-Hill.

10. NIDA Research Report. (2001, March). Hallucinogens and dissociative drugs. www.nida.nih.gov.

11. NIDA Research Report. (2005). Inhalant abuse. www.nida.nih.gov.

12. NIDA. (2005, February). Marijuana: facts for teens. www.nida.nih.gov.

13. Marijuana. (2005). NIDA Info Facts. www.drugabuse.gov.

14. Glaze, S. (1995). Treating addiction. *Congressional Quarterly Researcher, 5* (1), 1–24.

15. Califano, J. (1998). Crime and punishment—and treatment too. National Center on Addiction and Substance Abuse at Columbia University. www.casacolumbia.org.

16. Marlatt, G. A. (Ed.). (1998). *Harm reduction: Pragmatic strategies for managing high-risk behaviors.* New York: Guilford Press.

17. Drug Policy Alliance. (2004). Reducing harm: Treatment and beyond. www.drugpolicy.org.

18. NIDA InfoFacts. (2005). Drug addiction treatment methods. www.nida.nih.gov.

Add It Up!   ARE YOU AT RISK FOR DRUG DEPENDENCE?

If you wonder whether you are becoming dependent on a drug, ask yourself the following questions. Answer yes (Y) or no (N).

_____ 1. Do you take the drug regularly?

_____ 2. Have you been taking the drug for a long time?

_____ 3. Do you always take the drug in certain situations or when you're with certain people?

_____ 4. Do you find it difficult to stop using the drug? Do you feel powerless to quit?

_____ 5. Have you tried repeatedly to cut down or control your use of the drug?

_____ 6. Do you need to take a larger dose of the drug in order to get the same high you're used to?

_____ 7. Do you feel specific symptoms if you cut back or stop using the drug?

_____ 8. Do you frequently take another psychoactive substance to relieve withdrawal symptoms?

_____ 9. Do you take the drug to feel "normal"?

_____ 10. Do you go to extreme lengths or put yourself in dangerous situations to get the drug?

_____ 11. Do you hide your drug use from others? Have you ever lied about what you're using or how much you use?

_____ 12. Do people close to you ask you about your drug use?

_____ 13. Are you spending more and more time with people who use the same drug as you?

_____ 14. Do you think about the drug when you're not high, figuring out ways to get it?

_____ 15. If you stop taking the drug, do you feel bad until you can take it again?

_____ 16. Does the drug interfere with your ability to study, work, or socialize?

_____ 17. Do you skip important school, work, social, or recreational activities in order to obtain or use the drug?

_____ 18. Do you continue to use the drug despite a physical or mental disorder or despite a significant problem that you know is worsened by drug use?

_____ 19. Have you developed a mental or physical condition or disorder because of prolonged drug use?

_____ 20. Have you done something dangerous or that you regret while under the influence of the drug?

The more questions you answered yes, the more likely it is that you are becoming dependent on a drug. If the problem is still in its early stages, try the behavior change strategies suggested for alcohol-related behaviors at the end of Chapter 11 (p. 299). If the problem is more serious, talk to your physician or to a health care provider at your student health center before it gets worse.

If you think a friend or family member is developing a drug problem, you may want to talk to the person about your concerns. Be prepared for the person to deny that there is a problem or to get angry at you. Provide the person with information about treatment resources in the community or on your campus. The less judgmental and more supportive you can be, the more likely you will be able to help.

SOURCE: Wellness Worksheet #47 for *Core Concepts in Health* (10th ed.), by P. M. Insel and W. T. Roth, 2006, New York: The McGraw-Hill Companies.

CHAPTER 13

Tobacco: The Smoking Challenge

DID YOU KNOW?

- If you smoke, but only occasionally—for example, in social situations where people are talking and drinking—you may belong to the 30 percent of current smokers who consider themselves social smokers. Individuals in this group use tobacco regularly but not daily and don't consider themselves hooked. Historical behavior patterns suggest that many of these individuals may eventually become heavy smokers.

- Cigars may seem safer than cigarettes because they take longer to smoke, and many cigar smokers don't inhale. However, cigar smokers have higher rates of oral cancer than cigarette smokers do, and the secondhand smoke from cigars is more toxic than that from cigarettes. The air quality in some cigar lounges has been found to be comparable to that in a poorly ventilated garage with a car engine running or a major metropolitan freeway at rush hour.

OLC *Your Health Today*   www.mhhe.com/teague1e

Go to the Online Learning Center for *Your Health Today* for interactive activities, quizzes, flashcards, Web links, and more resources related to this chapter.

Like alcohol, tobacco poses a problem for society. Adults are free to use it, but such use causes a vast array of health problems, both for those who smoke and for those around them. Tobacco use is the leading preventable cause of death in the United States, implicated in a host of diseases and debilitating conditions. The health hazards of tobacco are well known, yet one in five Americans continues to smoke, and nearly 6,000 teenagers and children under the age of 18 start smoking every day.[1]

The use of tobacco, a plant native to the Americas, can be traced back thousands of years. In more recent history, the Spanish explorers brought tobacco back to Europe in the 16th century, where its use quickly caught on and was just as quickly condemned as foul smelling and harmful to the brain and lungs. John Quincy Adams, sixth president of the United States, took up smoking and chewing tobacco as a young man. He eventually freed himself from his dependence and wrote, "I have often wished that every individual . . . afflicted with this artificial passion could force it upon himself to try but for three months the experiment which I made, sure that it would turn every acre of tobacco land into a wheat field, and add five years to the average of human life."[2] The question is, If the harmful and addictive qualities of tobacco have been known for hundreds of years, why do millions of Americans continue to embrace this "artificial passion"?

In this chapter, we explore the complex issues associated with tobacco use. We begin by looking at patterns of tobacco use in the population, and we consider the nature of tobacco and tobacco products. We then examine the health hazards associated with tobacco use and the factors that lead people to start and continue smoking. Next, we explore various approaches to quitting and treatment. Finally, we consider how the challenge posed by tobacco use in our society can be addressed.

WHO SMOKES: PATTERNS OF TOBACCO USE

More than 22 percent of the adult population of the United States 18 years old and over are smokers—about one in five Americans (Table 13.1). In Canada, rates are similar—about 20 percent of all Canadians 15 years old and over are smokers.[3] The percentage of Americans who smoke is down from a high of nearly 42 percent in 1965. In that year, more than half of all men smoked (51.2 percent), and a third of all women smoked (33.7 percent).[4] The decline in the last 40 years has occurred largely as a result of public health campaigns about the hazards of smoking, beginning with the 1964 Surgeon General's Report on Smoking and Health. Although the prevalence of smoking in the United States continues to decline, the rate of decline has slowed since 1990. Rates of smoking vary across states, with the highest rates in Kentucky, Alaska, West Virginia, Tennessee, and Indiana and the lowest rates in Utah, California, Massachusetts, New Jersey, and Connecticut.[5]

Gender and Age Group Differences

The rates of smoking are higher among men than women. In the United States, 24.8 percent of men and 20.1 percent of women smoke, and in Canada, 23 percent of men and 17 percent of women smoke.[3,6] More than 20 percent of Americans are former smokers, and about 60 percent have never smoked.[1] By far the most popular tobacco product is cigarettes, followed by cigars and smokeless tobacco (chewing tobacco). Sixteen percent of men and 4 percent of women smoke cigars, and 9 percent of men and 1 percent of women use smokeless tobacco.[5]

Rates of smoking are higher among young people than among older people. Among adults aged 18–44, the rate is more than 25 percent; among those aged 45–64, it is about 22 percent; and among those aged 65 and higher, it is about 9 percent. In 2003, 22 percent of high school students reported smoking cigarettes, a decline from the 36 percent who reported smoking in 1997. Still, 20 percent of high school seniors, 12 percent of 10th graders, and 5.5 percent of 8th graders smoke cigarettes daily. Most smokers get hooked in adolescence—more than 90 percent of smokers begin smoking before the age of 21.[1] Many young smokers think they can easily quit at any time, but adolescents who smoke regularly have just as hard a time quitting as older smokers do.

Currently, college students are more likely to smoke than is the general population. About 26 percent of college students smoke. Women are more likely to smoke in college; 26.5 percent of women smoke, compared with 24.6 percent of men.[7] Overall, cigarette smoking is strongly correlated with educational attainment. Adults with less than a high school education are three times as likely to smoke as those who graduate from college.[4] Other psychosocial factors that increase the likelihood that a person will smoke include having a parent or sibling who smokes, associating with peers who smoke, being from a lower socioeconomic status family, doing poorly in school, and having positive attitudes about tobacco.

Smoking and Ethnicity

Smoking is more prevalent among the white population (25 percent) than among African Americans (23 percent) or Hispanics (20 percent).[6,8] The highest rates of smoking—34 percent—occur among American Indians and Alaska natives. The lowest rates occur among Asian Americans and Pacific Islanders (17 percent). Women smoke less than men do in all ethnic groups. African American women smoke less than white women. The lowest rates of smoking occur among Hispanic, Pacific Islander, and Asian American women.[8,9]

Smoking rates can vary tremendously among groups within broad ethnic categories. For example, despite low

Table 13.1	Cigarette Smoking by Persons 18 Years of Age and Over, United States, Selected Years 1965–2002				
	Percentage of Persons Who Are Current Cigarette Smokers				
	1965	**1985**	**1995**	**2000**	**2002**
All persons	41.9	29.9	24.6	23.1	22.4
Male	51.2	32.2	26.5	25.2	24.8
Female	33.7	27.9	22.7	21.1	20.1

Source: *Health, United States, 2004.* National Center for Health Statistics, 2004, Hyattville, MD.

rates of smoking overall among Asian Americans and Pacific Islanders, rates are very high among some of the 50 distinct ethnic groups that fall under this umbrella label. Among Tongan American men, the smoking rate is 65 percent; among Cambodian American men, 71 percent; and among Laotian American men, 72 percent.[9] Clearly, behaviors like smoking are influenced by socio-cultural factors, including acculturation and access to health information and health care.

Types of Smokers

People who smoke more than 10 cigarettes a day are considered **heavy smokers.** Those who smoke fewer than 10 cigarettes a day are referred to as **chippers.** A relatively new phenomenon seen among college students and other young people is **social smoking,** smoking regularly but not daily, primarily in social situations or as an accessory to social drinking. This pattern of smoking may be a response to strict antismoking laws, particularly smoke-free workplaces and public spaces. Many people under the age of 25 have grown up in smoke-free environments. Although the effects have been beneficial, health experts speculate that their experience has led them to consider cigarettes a strictly social, and therefore mostly harmless, pleasure. Social smokers still exercise considerable control over their smoking; they tend to buy cigarettes by the pack rather than by the carton, and when the price of cigarettes goes up, their consumption goes down.[10]

An estimated 30 percent of today's smokers are social smokers.[10] Health experts are not sure whether they will continue smoking at a low level, stop smoking, or become heavy smokers at a later time. Historical behavior patterns of smoking suggest that many social smokers and chippers are likely to become heavy smokers, although tobacco

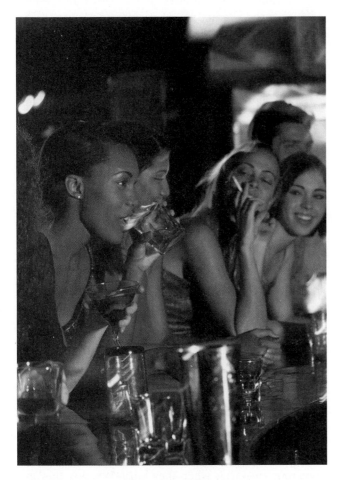

Social smokers may not smoke at all when they're alone, but at a party they often reach for a cigarette automatically. Although such individuals usually show control over their smoking, they may go on to become regular, or even heavy, smokers.

KEY TERMS

heavy smoker Person who smokes more than 10 cigarettes a day.

chipper Person who smokes fewer than 10 cigarettes a day.

social smoking Practice of smoking regularly but not daily, primarily in social situations.

control laws creating smoke-free environments may change this progression.

TOBACCO PRODUCTS

Tobacco is a broad-leafed plant that grows in tropical and temperate climates. Tobacco leaves are harvested, dried, and processed in different ways for the variety of tobacco products—rolled into cigars, shredded for cigarettes, ground into a fine powder for inhalation as snuff, or ground into a chewable form and used as smokeless tobacco.

Substances in Tobacco

When tobacco leaves are burned, more than 4,800 distinct substances are produced. So far, nearly 70 of these substances have been identified as carcinogenic, and many more are harmful in other ways. The most harmful substances are tar, carbon monoxide, and nicotine.

Tar

Tar is a thick, sticky residue that consists of hundreds of different chemical compounds and contains many of the carcinogenic substances in tobacco smoke. Tar coats the smoker's lungs and creates an environment conducive to the growth of cancerous cells. Tar is responsible for many of the changes in the respiratory system that cause the hacking "smoker's cough."

Carbon Monoxide

When tobacco is lit, many gaseous compounds are created. One of the most hazardous is carbon monoxide, the same toxic gas emitted from the exhaust pipe of a car. Carbon monoxide interferes with the ability of red blood cells to carry oxygen, so that vital body organs, such as the heart, are deprived of oxygen. Many of the other gases produced when tobacco burns are carcinogens, irritants, and toxic chemicals that damage the lungs. For example, tobacco smoke contains nitrous oxide and hydrogen cyanide,[11] two gases that cause lung cancer; toluene, an industrial solvent; and acetone, otherwise known as nail polish remover.

Nicotine

Nicotine is the primary addictive ingredient in tobacco. It is carried into the body in the form of thousands of droplets suspended in solid particles of partially burned tobacco. These droplets are so tiny that they penetrate the alveoli (small air sacs in the lungs) and enter the bloodstream, reaching body cells within seconds.

Nicotine is both a poison (it is used as a pesticide) and a powerful psychoactive drug. The first time it is used, it usually produces dizziness, light-headedness, and

nausea, signs of mild nicotine poisoning. These effects diminish as tolerance grows. Nicotine causes a cascade of stimulant effects throughout the body by triggering the release of adrenaline.[2] As we saw in Chapter 5, adrenaline is a body chemical involved in the stress response; it increases arousal, alertness, and concentration. Nicotine also stimulates the release of endorphins, the body's "natural opiates" that block pain and produce a mild rush of pleasure. (We discuss the effects of nicotine in greater detail later in the chapter.)

Cigarettes

Cigarettes account for nearly 95 percent of the tobacco market in the United States.[5] Nicotine from a cigarette reaches peak concentration in the blood in about 10 minutes and is reduced by half within about 20 minutes, as the drug is distributed to body tissues. Rapid absorption and distribution of nicotine enable the smoker to control the peaks and valleys of nicotine absorption and effect. This process of control—absorption, distribution, elimination—makes cigarettes an effective drug-delivery system for nicotine.[2]

The unfiltered cigarettes of the 1940s and 1950s, laden with high amounts of nicotine and tar, are no longer popular, nor are the king-size filtered cigarettes of the 1960s.[12] They have been replaced by low-nicotine, low-tar cigarettes and ultra-low nicotine, ultra-low tar cigarettes. All tobacco products, however, are hazardous to your health.[13]

Clove Cigarettes

Clove cigarettes, which consist of about 60 percent tobacco and 40 percent cloves (an aromatic spice), are promoted as safer cigarettes. However, they actually contain higher levels of tar and carbon monoxide than regular cigarettes. The active ingredient in cloves causes a numbing effect that allows smokers to inhale the smoke more deeply and to hold the smoke in their lungs for a longer time, giving the smoke more time to do damage.

Herbal Cigarettes

Herbal cigarettes contain herbs such as ginseng rather than tobacco. They come in flavors like cherry and mint and are packaged to look like candy cigarettes. Since they contain no tobacco or nicotine, they are billed as healthier alternatives to tobacco or as aids to quitting.[14] They are not subject to FDA regulation or to the laws that prevent sale to minors. Between 1997 and 1999, herbal cigarettes increased in sales by over 300 percent.[15]

Despite their popularity, herbal cigarettes are harmful to health. Like tobacco, herbs produce an assortment of dangerous chemicals when they burn. Whether they are more or less harmful than tobacco is not known at this time. Smoking herbal cigarettes also ingrains the behaviors associated with smoking tobacco cigarettes and may make it more likely that a young person will move on to cigarettes.

Bidis

Bidis are cigarettes made in India from unprocessed, sun-dried tobacco. They are smaller than cigarettes, contain less tobacco, and come in flavors like chocolate and strawberry. No chemicals or additives are used in their manufacture.[16] They are less expensive than cigarettes and can be sold to minors in some states.

Because they contain only natural ingredients, their manufacturers claim they are safer than regular cigarettes. Health experts disagree and call them "cigarettes with training wheels."[17] The unprocessed tobacco in bidis actually produces smoke three times higher in nicotine, three times higher in carbon monoxide, and four times higher in tar than that from cigarettes. Because the tobacco is wrapped in a nonporous leaf rather than cigarette paper, bidis do not burn well, forcing smokers to inhale more deeply to keep the cigarette lit. Studies from India suggest that bidis pose a greater risk for cancers of the oral cavity, throat, lung, esophagus, stomach, and liver, as well as for coronary artery disease, than regular cigarettes do.[17]

Most bidi smokers are Latino and African American teens and adults in their twenties.[17] Bidis account for less than 1 percent of all cigarette sales in the United States, but health experts are concerned about their appeal to youth and their marketing on the Internet. At the request of the U.S. government, some importers are voluntarily putting health warning labels on bidis.

Cigars

Cigars have more tobacco and nicotine per unit than cigarettes do, take longer to smoke, and generate more smoke and more harmful combustion products than cigarettes. The tobacco mix used in cigars has a different pH (relative acidity) than does the tobacco mix used in cigarettes, making it easier for cigar smoke to be absorbed through the mucous membranes of the oral cavity than is the case with cigarettes. Nicotine absorbed via this route takes longer to reach the brain than nicotine absorbed in the lungs and has a less intense but longer lasting effect.

Cigar smokers typically do not inhale; those who do are usually former cigarette smokers. Cigar smokers who do not inhale have lower mortality rates than cigar smokers who do.[18] Inhalation substantially increases the cigar smoker's exposure to carcinogenic chemicals and increases the risk for lung cancer and chronic respiratory disease.[19] Whether or not smoke is inhaled, cigar smoking exposes the oral mucosa to large amounts of carcinogenic chemicals; consequently, cigar smokers have a higher risk for oral cancers than cigarette smokers. When compared with people who don't smoke at all, cigar smokers have

8 times the risk for oral cancers, 7 times the risk for throat cancer, 4.5 times the risk for obstructive lung disease, and twice the risk for lung cancer.[18]

Pipes

Pipe smoke has more toxins than cigarette smoke does and is more irritating to the respiratory system. Pipe smokers who do not inhale are at less risk for lung cancer and heart disease than cigarette smokers are. Like cigar smokers, however, pipe smokers who are former cigarette smokers tend to inhale and consequently are exposed to more toxins than they were when they smoked cigarettes. Pipe smokers are just as likely as cigarette smokers to develop cancer of the mouth, larynx, throat, and esophagus.[20]

Smokeless Tobacco

There are two types of smokeless tobacco, snuff and chewing tobacco. **Snuff** is a powdered form of tobacco that can be inhaled through the nose or placed between the bottom teeth and lower lip. **Chewing tobacco** is used by lodging a cud or pinch of smokeless tobacco between the cheek and gum. It is available as loose leaf or as a plug (a compressed, flavored bar of processed tobacco). Smokeless tobacco is sometimes called *spit tobacco* because users spit out the tobacco juices and saliva that accumulate in the mouth. Spittoons were a common sight in public places well into the 20th century, until spitting was recognized as a public health hazard because it spread diseases like tuberculosis.[2]

Because users do not inhale toxic gases, manufacturers of smokeless tobacco have promoted their product as a safe alternative to cigarettes. This is not the case. Tobacco does not have to burn to cause health hazards. Spit tobacco contains at least 28 carcinogens, and using spit tobacco is believed to cause about 10 percent to 15 percent of oral cancers, leading to about 6,000 deaths each year. When spit

KEY TERMS

tar Thick, sticky residue formed when tobacco leaves burn, containing hundreds of chemical compounds and carcinogenic substances.

nicotine Primary addictive ingredient in tobacco; a poison and a psychoactive drug.

snuff Powdered form of tobacco, usually inhaled through the nose or placed in the mouth between the bottom teeth and lower lip and absorbed through the mucous membranes of the oral cavity.

chewing tobacco Form of tobacco placed in the mouth and absorbed through the mucous membranes of the oral cavity; also called spit tobacco.

tobacco is kept in contact with the oral mucosa, it can cause *dysplasia,* an abnormal change in cells, and *oral lesions,* whitish patches on the tongue or mouth that may become cancerous. Spit tobacco also causes gum disease, tooth decay and discoloration, and bad breath.[21-24]

EFFECTS OF TOBACCO USE ON HEALTH

By the 18th century, scientists suspected that tobacco smoke caused cancer. By the mid-20th century, research showed that it was also a causal factor in heart disease, respiratory diseases, and numerous other debilitating conditions. Today, overwhelming evidence indicates that smoking is the single greatest preventable cause of illness and premature death in North America.[25]

Short-Term Effects of Tobacco Use

When a smoker lights up, nicotine reaches the brain within 7 to 10 seconds, producing both sedating and stimulating effects. As noted earlier, nicotine increases levels of both endorphins and adrenaline; it also affects levels of dopamine and other neurotransmitters. Adrenaline causes heart rate to increase by 10 to 20 beats per minute, blood pressure to rise by 5 to 10 points,[12] and body temperature in the fingertips to decrease by a few degrees.[2] It also suppresses hunger sensations, inhibits urine production, and signals the liver to convert glycogen to glucose, raising blood sugar levels.

The tar and toxins in tobacco smoke damage olfactory cells and taste buds, dulling the senses of smell and taste. Tobacco smoke damages cilia, the hairlike structures in the bronchial passages that prevent toxins and debris from reaching delicate lung tissue. It also blocks the function of mucus, which normally traps foreign materials, so these irritants remain in contact with lung tissue longer. Researchers believe that chemicals in tar, such as benzopyrene, switch on a gene in lung cells that causes cell mutations that can lead to cancerous growth.[26] These chemicals may also damage a gene with a role in killing cancer cells.

Carbon monoxide in tobacco smoke affects the way smokers process the air they breathe. Normally, oxygen is carried through the bloodstream by hemoglobin, a protein in red blood cells. When carbon monoxide is present, hemoglobin binds with carbon instead of oxygen. Since there is only so much hemoglobin in the body at any given time, oxygen delivery to the cells is impaired. Smoker's bodies try to compensate by creating more red blood cells, but such compensation is insufficient. Heavy smokers quickly become winded during physical activity because the cardiovascular system cannot effectively deliver oxygen to muscle cells.[2]

During waking hours, carbon monoxide remains in a smoker's blood for 2 hours to 4 hours; during sleep, however, carbon monoxide will remain in the blood up to 8 hours.[11] Chain smokers are particularly at risk for the buildup of carbon monoxide in the blood. The highest concentration of carbon monoxide exits the blood within a few minutes of lighting up. Chain smokers do not provide the blood even a brief respite from carbon monoxide buildup. An overview of the short-term effects of smoking on the body is presented in Figure 13.1.

Long-Term Effects of Tobacco Use

Smoking accounts for 15 percent of all adult deaths in a given year—more than AIDS, car crashes, alcohol, homicides, illegal drugs, suicides, fires, poor diet, and physical inactivity combined.[27] The greatest health concerns associated with smoking are heart disease, cancer, and chronic lower respiratory diseases.

Cardiovascular Disease

The short-term effects of nicotine on the heart have long-term effects in regular smokers. Increased heart rate, increased tension in the heart muscle, and constricted blood vessels lead to hypertension (high blood pressure), which is both a disease in itself and a risk factor for other forms of heart disease, including coronary artery disease, heart attack, stroke, and peripheral vascular disease. Nicotine also makes blood platelets stickier, increasing the tendency of blood clots to form. It raises blood levels of low-density lipoproteins ("bad cholesterol") and decreases levels of high-density lipoproteins ("good cholesterol").[28] People who smoke more than one pack of cigarettes per day have three times the risk for heart disease and congestive heart failure as nonsmokers.[25]

Cancer

Smoking is implicated in about 30 percent of all cancer deaths. It is the cause of 87 percent of deaths from lung cancer, and it is associated with cancers of the pancreas, kidney, bladder, breast, and cervix. Smoking and using smokeless tobacco play a major role in cancers of the mouth, throat, and esophagus. Among men, oral cancers are the seventh most frequently occurring cancer. Oral cancers caused by smokeless tobacco tend to occur early in adulthood. About 50 percent of smokeless tobacco users also smoke cigarettes, thus increasing their risk of developing cancer. The use of alcohol in combination with tobacco increases the risk of oral cancers. Cancer of the esophagus is of particular concern, because its survival rates are very low.[22,23,25,29]

Smoking also increases the cancer-causing potential of occupational and environmental pollutants, such as asbestos and radon. The lung cancer risk associated with exposure to radon, for example, is 6 to 11 times higher in smokers than nonsmokers.[25]

Brain Nicotine reaches the brain within 7 to 10 seconds, triggering release of chemicals that affect mood; effects are both sedating and stimulating. Effects peak in about 10 minutes and are reduced by half within about 20 minutes.

Nose Tar and toxins irritate membranes in nose, dull sense of smell.

Mouth and throat Tar and toxins irritate membranes in mouth, dull taste buds, stain teeth, cause raspy voice.

Lungs Smoke increases mucus production and damages cilia in airway, preventing them from filtering out particles. Tar collects in lungs, creating conditions conducive to cancer. Tobacco smoke is absorbed into bloodstream and travels throughout body.

Heart and blood Nicotine causes heart rate to increase, blood pressure to rise, blood vessels to constrict. The heart must work harder to deliver oxygen to cells. Tobacco smoke makes blood stickier and adversely affects cholesterol levels.

Liver Liver converts glycogen to glucose, causing an increase in blood sugar.

Digestive system Nicotine is secreted from the bloodstream into saliva, swallowed, and reabsorbed in the stomach, increasing risk for cancers of the digestive tract.

Adrenal glands Adrenal glands increase production of adrenaline, causing stimulating effects throughout body.

Kidneys Nicotine inhibits production of urine.

Skin Nicotine causes constriction of blood vessels and decreased blood flow to skin; smoke contains chemicals that damage collagen and elastin, causing excess wrinkling.

Reproductive system Toxins in tobacco smoke are secreted into cervical mucus and increase risk of cervical cancer. In pregnant women, nicotine and tobacco chemicals are passed to fetus.

Figure 13.1   Short-term effects of smoking on the body.

The association between smoking and cancer varies greatly according to the number of cigarettes smoked per day, the degree of inhalation, the age of smoking initiation, and, if the person no longer smokes, the number of years since he or she quit.[26] The likelihood of dying from lung cancer increases with the number of cigarettes smoked, deeper inhalation, and earlier initiation age.

Chronic Obstructive Pulmonary Disease

Smoking is a key factor in causing the diseases encompassed by the category *chronic obstructive pulmonary disease* (COPD, also called chronic lower respiratory disease). These are emphysema, chronic bronchitis, and asthma. **Emphysema** is an abnormal condition of the lungs in which the alveoli (air sacs) become enlarged and their walls lose their elasticity. Late in the disease, it becomes increasingly difficult to breathe. Although there may be a hereditary component, people with emphysema almost always have a history of smoking. Bronchitis is irritation and inflammation of the bronchi, the airway passages leading to the lungs. **Chronic bronchitis** is characterized by mucus secretion, cough, and increasing difficulty in breathing. **Asthma** is a respiratory disorder characterized by

recurrent episodes of difficulty in breathing, wheezing, coughing, and thick mucus production. Almost as many people die from COPD today as from lung cancer.[25] Thousands more people live with COPD complications and discomfort that seriously compromise their quality of life.

Other Health Effects of Tobacco Use

Tobacco is associated with a variety of health conditions other than cardiovascular disease, cancer, and respiratory

KEY TERMS

emphysema   Abnormal condition of the lungs characterized by decreased respiratory function and increased shortness of breath.

chronic bronchitis   Respiratory disorder characterized by mucus secretion, cough, and increasing difficulty in breathing.

asthma   Respiratory disorder characterized by recurrent episodes of difficulty in breathing, wheezing, coughing, and thick mucus production.

diseases. These conditions include changes in the skin (wrinkling), increased risk during surgery, infertility and sexual dysfunction, periodontal disease, duodenal ulcers, and osteoporosis. Smoking causes oxidative stress in the eyes that contributes to the development of cataracts (thickening and clouding of the lens). Smoking also reduces the effectiveness of some medications, particularly anti-anxiety drugs and penicillin. Nicotine and other substances in tobacco may interfere with drug metabolism by speeding up the body's use of the drug and its elimination. This means a smoker may have to take a higher drug dosage to produce the desired effect.

Special Health Risks for Women

Formerly, men had much higher rates of lung cancer, heart disease, and respiratory disease than women did in part because of their higher rates of smoking. Increased smoking among women over the last 35 years has led to an increase in rates of all these diseases in women; deaths from lung cancer in women, for example, have increased by 400 percent.[30,31]

In addition, smoking is associated with fertility problems in women, menstrual disorders, early menopause, and problems in pregnancy. Women who smoke during pregnancy are at increased risk for miscarriage, stillbirths, preterm delivery, low birth weight in their infants, and perinatal death (infant death a few months before or after birth). Research indicates that infants are at higher risk for sudden infant death syndrome (SIDS) if their mothers smoked during pregnancy. Their risk continues to be higher after birth if they are exposed to environmental tobacco smoke.[32]

Special Health Risks for Men

The overall drop in smoking rates by men in the past three decades has led to a reduction of lung cancer

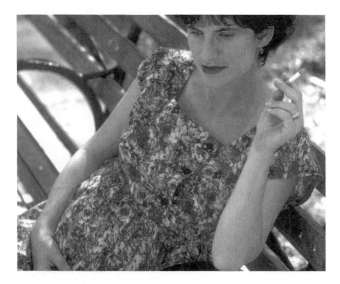

Despite the surgeon general's health warning label on cigarettes, some women continue to smoke during pregnancy, increasing the risk for miscarriage, stillbirth, preterm delivery, low birth weight in their infants, newborn death, and sudden infant death syndrome.

deaths in men, but the greater use of other forms of tobacco by men—cigars, pipes, and smokeless tobacco—places them at higher risk for cancers of the mouth, throat, esophagus, and stomach. Like women, men who smoke experience problems with sexual function and fertility. Smoking adversely affects blood flow to the erectile tissue, leading to a higher incidence of erectile dysfunction (impotence); it also alters sperm shape, reduces sperm motility, and decreases the overall number of viable sperm.[33]

Special Health Risks for Ethnic Minority Groups

Mortality rates from several diseases associated with tobacco use, including cardiovascular disease, cancer, and SIDS, are higher for ethnic minority groups than for whites.[8] For example, African American men and women are more likely to die from lung cancer, heart disease, and stroke than are members of other ethnic groups, despite lower rates of tobacco use. Reductions in smoking among African Americans over the past two decades have led to a decline in lung cancer for African American men and a leveling off in African American women. Reduced smoking rates have also led to a decrease in lung cancer deaths in Hispanic men.[9]

Dependence on tobacco and desire to quit appear to be prevalent across all ethnic groups, but groups vary in rates of smoking, smoking patterns, quitting behavior, and awareness of the health effects of smoking. Health experts stress the need to deliver effective and appropriate tobacco intervention programs to various ethnic groups, and a broad aim of Healthy People 2010 is to reduce disparities among segments of the population.

Benefits of Quitting

Smokers greatly reduce their risk of many health problems when they quit. Health benefits begin immediately and become more significant the longer the individual stays smoke free (see the box "When You Quit Smoking: Health Benefits Timeline"). Respiratory symptoms associated with COPD, such as smoker's cough and excess mucus production, decrease quickly after quitting. Infection rates for bronchitis and pneumonia drop significantly, and recovery from illnesses like colds and flu is more rapid. Taste and smell return and circulation improves, raising body temperature in the hands and feet and improving brain, heart, and lung function.

Within 1 year, the risk of heart attack and coronary artery disease is reduced by half, and within 5 years, risk approaches that of nonsmokers, as does the risk of stroke.[26] Within 5 years, the risk of oral and esophageal cancer is cut by half,[34] and within 10 years, the risk of lung cancer is cut by 30 percent to 50 percent. Ex-smokers also have a lower risk of cervical and bladder cancer compared to continuing smokers.

HIGHLIGHT ON HEALTH
When You Quit Smoking: Health Benefits Timeline

Immediately	You stop polluting the air with secondhand smoke; the air around you is no longer dangerous to children and adults.
20 minutes	Blood pressure decreases; pulse rate decreases; temperature of hands and feet increases.
12 hours	Carbon monoxide level in blood drops; oxygen level in the blood increases to normal.
24 hours	Chance of heart attack decreases.
48 hours	Nerve endings start to regrow; exercise gets easier; senses of smell and taste improve.
72 hours	Bronchial tubes relax, making breathing easier; lung capacity increases.
2–12 weeks	Circulation improves; lung functioning increases up to 30 percent.
1–9 months	Fewer coughs, colds, and flu episodes; fatigue and shortness of breath decrease; lung function continues to improve.
1 year	Risk of smoking-related heart attack is cut by half.
5 years	Risk of dying from heart disease and stroke approaches that of a nonsmoker; risk of oral and esophageal cancers is cut by half.
10 years	Risk of dying from lung cancer is cut by half.
10–15 years	Life expectancy reaches that of person who never smoked.

Source: Health Canada: On the Road to Quitting, www.hc-sc.gc-ca.

Quitting also increases longevity. Individuals who quit before the age of 50 cut their risk of dying within the next 15 years in half. Men who quit between ages 35 and 39 add an average of 5 years to their life span, and women add 3 years. People who quit between the ages of 65 and 69 increase their life expectancy by 1 year or more.[34] Even quitting after the age of 70 substantially lowers the risk of dying and improves the quality of life.

Effects of Environmental Tobacco Smoke

You don't have to be a smoker to experience adverse health effects from tobacco smoke. Abundant evidence indicates that inhaling the smoke from other people's tobacco products—called **environmental tobacco smoke (ETS),** secondhand smoke, or passive smoking—has serious health consequences (see the box "Health Effects of Environmental Tobacco Smoke"). In 1993 the Environmental Protection Agency designated ETS a Class A carcinogen—an agent known to cause cancer in humans—and in 2000 the U.S. Department of Health and Human Services added it to their list of known human carcinogens.

The effects of ETS vary depending on whether the smoke is coming from the burning end of a cigarette or cigar or the burning tobacco in a pipe (**sidestream smoke**) or has been inhaled and exhaled by the smoker (**mainstream smoke**). Because sidestream smoke is not filtered by the tobacco, the cigarette filter, or the body of the smoker, it contains more tar, nicotine, carbon monoxide, and other toxic and carcinogenic compounds than mainstream smoke does.[35] About 85 percent of ETS is sidestream smoke, and 15 percent is mainstream smoke.

The tobacco used in cigars generates much more hazardous ETS than does the tobacco in cigarettes. The air in some cigar lounges has been found to have pollutant levels 60 times higher than federal standards for clean air.[18] This level is comparable to that found in a poorly ventilated garage with a car engine running or a major metropolitan freeway at rush hour.

Nearly 30 percent of the American population is exposed to ETS on a regular basis. Scientists estimate that for every pack of cigarettes smoked by a smoker, the nonsmoker sharing a common air supply will have involuntarily inhaled the equivalent of three to five cigarettes. Scientific evidence supports a significant relationship between long-term exposure to ETS and both heart disease and cancer. ETS is responsible for about 48,000 deaths from heart disease every year in the United States and about 3,000 deaths from lung cancer. Nonsmokers exposed to regular smoke for long periods can suffer impaired lung function equivalent to that of smokers who

KEY TERMS

environmental tobacco smoke (ETS) Smoke from other people's tobacco products; also called secondhand smoke or passive smoking.

sidestream smoke Smoke coming from the burning end of a cigarette or cigar or the burning tobacco in a pipe.

mainstream smoke Smoke that has been inhaled and exhaled by the smoker.

HIGHLIGHT (ON) HEALTH

Health Effects of Environmental Tobacco Smoke

Area	Known Causal Effects	Possible Causal Effects
Developmental effects	Babies born with low birth weight or small for gestational age	Spontaneous abortion (miscarriage)
	Sudden infant death syndrome (SIDS)	Adverse impact on child's cognition and behavior
Respiratory effects	Acute lower respiratory tract infections in children (bronchitis, pneumonia)	Exacerbation of cystic fibrosis
	Asthma induction and exacerbation in children	Decreased lung function
	Chronic respiratory symptoms in children	
	Middle ear infections in children	
	Eye and nasal irritation in adults	
Cardiovascular effects	Acute and chronic coronary heart disease	
	Higher death rate from heart disease	
Carcinogenic effects	Lung cancer	Cervical cancer
	Nasal sinus cancer	Breast cancer

Source: "Health Effects of Exposure to Environmental Tobacco Smoke," 1999, Monograph 10, p. ES-2, Washington, DC: National Cancer Institute.

smoke 10 cigarettes daily. ETS may also increase the risk of breast cancer, especially if exposure to the smoke occurs during a period when the breasts are growing rapidly, such as puberty or first pregnancy.[35]

ETS can also cause allergic reactions, with symptoms such as eye irritation, headache, cough, nasal congestion, and asthma. About 15 percent of ETS allergies are severe enough to cause disability and qualify people with allergies for occupational disability insurance.[35] This is one reason that employers have implemented smoke-free workplaces.

Even short-term exposure to ETS can be hazardous. Breathing ETS for 5 minutes can cause stiffening of the aorta, which makes the heart work harder to pump blood. Twenty minutes' exposure causes changes in blood platelets, increasing the risk of blood clots forming in the bloodstream. Thirty minutes' exposure impairs coronary arteries and the ability of the blood to manage low-density lipoproteins. Two hours' exposure can cause heart arrhythmias (irregular heartbeats), which increase the risk of a heart attack.[36]

Because of their smaller body size, infants and children are especially vulnerable to the effects of ETS. Children exposed to ETS experience 10 percent more colds, flu, and other acute respiratory infections than do those not exposed. ETS aggravates asthma symptoms and increases the risk of SIDS.[35] For some ideas on how to protect yourself and your loved ones from ETS, see the box "What You Can Do About Environmental Tobacco Smoke."

WHY DO PEOPLE SMOKE?

If smoking is so bad for your health, why do people smoke? And if quitting is so beneficial, why don't more people quit? Tobacco use and its relationship to health are complex issues that involve nicotine addiction, behavioral dependence, weight control, and aggressive marketing by tobacco companies, among other factors.[37]

Nicotine Addiction

Nicotine is a highly addictive psychoactive drug—some health experts believe it is the most addictive of all the psychoactive drugs—and tobacco products are very efficient delivery devices for this drug. Once in the brain, nicotine follows the same pleasure and reward pathway—involving the ventral tegmental area (VTA), the nucleus accumbens, and the prefrontal cortex—as other psychoactive drugs follow (see Chapter 12 and Figure 12.2). Increases in release of the neurotransmitter dopamine produce feelings of pleasure and a desire to repeat the experience. Nicotine also affects alertness, energy, and mood by increasing levels of endorphins and other neurotransmitters, including serotonin and norepinephrine.

With continued smoking, neurons in the VTA become more sensitive and responsive to nicotine, causing *addiction,* or dependence on a steady supply of the drug; *tolerance,* or reduced responsiveness to its effects; and *withdrawal* symptoms if it is not present (see Chapters 11

Challenges & Choices

What You Can Do About Environmental Tobacco Smoke

In Your Home

- Post a polite sign on your front door telling visitors that your house is a smoke-free zone.
- If visitors miss the sign and begin to light up, be ready to politely request that they smoke outside.
- Remove all ashtrays.
- Encourage family members who smoke to quit. Until they do, ask them not to smoke inside the home. Teach your children how to discreetly remove themselves from ETS that they encounter in other people's homes (moving to another room, playing outside).

In Your Workplace

- Work with your employer to make your workplace a smoke-free zone.

In Public Places

- When making reservations with hotels, rental car agencies, restaurants, and tour companies, ask for the no-smoking option. If one isn't available, take your business elsewhere, and let the company know the reason for your choice.
- If you are exposed to ETS, politely ask the smoker to put out his or her cigarette or to move. If you encounter resistance or hostility, ask the management to intervene, or, if you are outdoors, find a healthier location.
- Write letters or e-mail supporting clean air policies to your elected officials and to newspapers.
- Support organizations in your area that are working to restrict smoking and promote nonsmokers' rights.

It's Not Just Personal . . .

According to the World Health Organization, more than 50 percent of children worldwide are exposed to environmental tobacco smoke in their homes. These children have an increased risk of respiratory tract infections, ear infections, asthma, and sudden infant death syndrome.

---

and 12 for more on these concepts). Nicotine withdrawal symptoms include irritability, anxiety, depressed mood, difficulty concentrating, restlessness, hostility, decreased heart rate, increased appetite, and increased craving for nicotine.

More than two thirds of cigarette smokers who attempt to quit relapse within 2 days, unable to tolerate the period when withdrawal symptoms are at their peak. It takes about 2 weeks for a person's brain chemistry to return to normal. Withdrawal symptoms decrease and become more subtle with prolonged abstinence, but some smokers continue to experience intermittent cravings for years. Smoking tobacco may cause permanent changes in the nervous system, which may explain why some people who haven't smoked in years can become addicted again after smoking a single cigarette.[37-39]

Tobacco manufacturers long argued that nicotine use is a habit and not an addiction, but in 1988, the surgeon general issued a report stating that nicotine meets all the criteria for classification as an addictive drug. According to this report, cigarettes and other forms of tobacco are addictive, nicotine is the drug in tobacco that causes this addiction, and pharmacological and behavioral processes that determine tobacco addiction are similar to those that determine addiction to other drugs such as cocaine and heroin.[39] The American Psychiatric Association's *Diagnostic and Statistical Manual of Mental Disorders* (*DSM-IV-TR*) includes nicotine dependence as a disorder with the same characteristics as other substance dependence disorders. (See the box "Who Is Most Likely to Quit Smoking?")

Behavioral Dependence

People who smoke are not just physiologically dependent on a substance; they also become psychologically dependent on the habit of smoking. Through repeated paired associations, the effects of nicotine on the brain are linked to places, people, and events. Individuals may associate smoking with drinking a cup of coffee in the morning, drinking alcohol in the evening, studying or writing papers, using the computer, socializing with friends, driving, or other daily activities. Any of these sensory or environmental stimuli may trigger the urge for a cigarette. Tobacco companies design their advertising to take advantage of these associations, picturing attractive, healthy people smoking cigarettes while drinking alcohol and relaxing with friends.

Many smokers have a harder time imagining their future life without cigarettes than they do dealing with the physiological symptoms of withdrawal. Simply holding a cigarette may have a tranquilizing effect on some smokers.

Beating the Odds

Who Is Most Likely to Quit Smoking?

Many factors go into the decision to quit smoking, including information and knowledge about the health effects, skills and strategies to manage withdrawal, social support, environmental factors, and personal health history, among others. Brief profiles of three people are presented here. Which one do you think is most likely to quit smoking?

Rachel is 24 years old and is starting medical school in a few months. She grew up in a household with smokers and has been smoking since she was 16. Her mother has quit, but her father still smokes. Currently, Rachel smokes about half a pack a day. She has tried to quit twice before; on her second try she made it to the 3-month mark but relapsed while studying for the medical school entrance exams. She is well aware of the negative effects of smoking on her health and would like to quit. However, she was discouraged by her failure the last time, and she worries that medical school will be so stressful that she'll relapse again. She's also afraid of gaining weight. Her current boyfriend doesn't smoke and strongly urges her to quit. He exercises daily and encourages her to join him.

Matthew is 38 and works as a stockbroker on Wall Street. He started smoking in college and currently smokes a pack a day. On Fridays he usually goes to a cigar bar with his colleagues after work and smokes a cigar while drinking scotch or bourbon. Matthew recently moved into an apartment after breaking up with his wife, to whom he was married for 10 years. The last time he had a medical appointment, his physician suggested he see a psychiatrist for depression, and he also advised Matthew to quit smoking. He said he would prescribe a nicotine replacement drug for him and gave him a referral to a treatment program. Matthew has tried to quit smoking three times in the past; he is worried that this might not be the right time, but he's also worried that he has been smoking for almost 20 years. The fact that his grandfather died of lung cancer is a source of additional pressure.

Antonio is 18 and a college freshman. A lot of the men in his family smoke, so it seemed natural for him to start smoking in high school. He smoked only a few cigarettes a day when he was living at home, but now that he's on his own, he's been smoking more. Some of his friends have joined the cross-country team, and he's thinking about doing the same, but he worries about his stamina. He's noticed that he gets out of breath quickly, just going up the stairs to his apartment. He's thought about quitting, but every time he goes for a day without a cigarette, he gets such a strong craving that he buys a pack. One of his friends told him he can get a nicotine patch at the student health center, but he thinks he ought to be able to quit on his own.

OLC Web site Visit the **Online Learning Center** at www.mhhe.com/teague1e for comments by the authors.

A pack-a-day smoker holds a cigarette 20 times a day, 140 times a week. It can take a long time for these associations to dissipate and be replaced by new, nonsmoking associations. Some ex-smokers remain vulnerable to sensory and environmental stimuli—smelling tobacco smoke, seeing a cigarette ad, drinking alcohol, being around a friend who smokes—for years after quitting.[2] Stress is a common cause of relapse.

Weight Control

Nicotine suppresses appetite and slightly increases basal metabolic rate (rate of metabolic activity at rest). People who start smoking often lose weight, and continuing smokers gain weight less rapidly than nonsmokers. Weight control is one of the major reasons young women give for smoking, and weight gain can be a deterrent to quitting.[40] When individuals stop smoking, their appetite returns, along with craving for sweet foods, which nico-tine also suppresses. In addition, many people eat more while they are quitting just to have something in their mouths. Gaining 7 pounds to 10 pounds is typical before the body adjusts to the absence of nicotine.[26] Once a person has successfully quit, this weight can be lost through exercise and sensible eating.

Tobacco Marketing and Advertising

Every day, the tobacco industry loses 4,600 smokers, either to quitting or to death.[39] These users have to be replaced if tobacco companies are to stay in business. Because most smokers get hooked in adolescence, prime targets of tobacco advertising are children and teenagers. Tobacco advertising aimed at children associates smoking with characters like Joe Camel, a highly successful advertising image that was discontinued in 1997 because of intense criticism. Advertising aimed at teenagers associates smoking with alcohol, sex, and independence and presents it as an illicit pleasure that can initiate a young person into the adult world. Tobacco ads play to the vulnerabilities of teenagers, most of whom are striving for status, dealing with stress, and trying to establish their identities. Judging by the number of new smokers who take up tobacco use every year, tobacco advertising and marketing are extremely effective. Although the industry continues to claim that it does not market its products to children, research suggests otherwise.[39,41]

QUITTING AND TREATMENT OPTIONS

Once a person becomes an established smoker, quitting is exceptionally difficult. Nearly four of every five smokers want to quit smoking. Many daily smokers believe they will not be smoking in 5 years, but 75 percent are still smoking 5 years to 6 years later. In 2002, 52 percent of current smokers had tried to quit in the previous year, and 72 percent had been advised by their physicians to quit. However, only about 7 percent of smokers who quit successfully abstain a year later. Even among smokers who have lost a lung or undergone major heart surgery, only about 50 percent stop smoking for more than a few weeks.[5,26,42]

The good news is that smokers who quit for a year have an 85 percent chance of maintaining their abstinence. Those who make it 5 years have a 97 percent chance of continued success. Most people don't succeed the first time they try to quit—in fact, the average number of attempts required for successful smoking cessation is seven—but many succeed on subsequent attempts.[34]

Treatment Programs to Quit Smoking

Treatment programs can be quite effective. Twenty to forty percent of smokers who enter good treatment programs are able to quit smoking for at least a year.[42] Some programs are provided by hospitals. At the Mayo Hospital Nicotine Dependence Center, for example, smokers participate in an intensive residential smoking cessation program. Smokers are tested for blood levels of nicotine so that treatment can be individually adjusted to alleviate withdrawal symptoms and cravings. Other program components include daily group and individual therapy, stress reduction techniques, nutrition and diet information, supervised exercise, and a 12-step program similar to Alcoholics Anonymous.

Many programs encourage smokers to limit or eliminate their consumption of alcohol while they are quitting, because alcohol interacts with nicotine in complex ways and can make quitting more difficult. Dieting is not recommended while trying to quit, despite the potential for weight gain. Research suggests that individuals who diet while also trying to stop smoking are vulnerable to relapse. A more effective strategy is to tolerate the weight gain for the time being and address it after successfully quitting. Combining exercise with smoking cessation appears to be the most effective approach to managing the potential for weight gain. Another element is social support and encouragement by important people in the smoker's life. Some programs also use aversive techniques, such as rapid puffing, to foster an intense dislike of smoke and a desire to avoid tobacco.

Medications to Quit Smoking

In **nicotine replacement therapy (NRT),** a controlled amount of nicotine is administered, which gradually reduces daily nicotine use with minimal withdrawal symptoms. The transdermal patch and nicotine gum are the most common delivery systems. Although nicotine is addictive no matter how it is administered, and people do become addicted to nicotine gum, NRT products contain none of the carcinogens or toxic gases found in cigarette smoke, so they are a safer form of nicotine delivery.[43]

Using one or more of the NRT products doubles a person's chances of success in quitting and boosts smoking cessation rates to about 25 percent. NRT is beneficial when used as part of a comprehensive physician-promoted cessation program. It can help control withdrawal symptoms and craving while the individual is learning new behavioral patterns.[26,44,45] For a description of various forms of NRT, see the box "Comparing Nicotine Replacement Products."

Bupropion is a prescription drug approved in 2001 by the FDA as an aid to smoking cessation and marketed under the trade name Zyban. Bupropion and newer, similar drugs do not provide nicotine in substitute forms; rather, they act on the neurotransmitters affected by nicotine, though not at comparable levels. They are started a week before a person's quit date and continued for 7 weeks to 12 weeks after quitting. According to one review, a combination of medication and professional and/or social support consistently pushed smoking cessation rates to about 30 percent. This review also found that nicotine gum and bupropion seemed to help prevent weight gain.[44]

Quitting on Your Own: Developing a Behavior Change Plan

Physiological, psychological, and social forces affect your smoking behavior, but the decision to smoke, not to

KEY TERMS

nicotine replacement therapy (NRT)   Treatment for nicotine addiction in which a controlled amount of nicotine is administered to gradually reduce daily nicotine use with minimal withdrawal symptoms.

Consumer Clipboard

Comparing Nicotine Replacement Products

Different nicotine replacement products may appeal to different kinds of smokers. Smokers who experience severe cravings, for example, may do better with nicotine inhalers or sprays, which require frequent use but provide rapid, on-demand nicotine delivery. Other smokers may prefer the nicotine patch, which supplies a steady level of nicotine in the bloodstream and is applied only once a day. Here is a comparison of the features, benefits, and costs of several nicotine replacement products.

Nicotine gum is available over the counter and delivers nicotine on demand. It can be used for 12 weeks (or longer with a physician's approval), usually at a rate of 9 to 24 pieces a day and a cost of $4 to $18 a day. The advantages are that it is fast and easy to use, can be matched to need, and may limit weight gain. A major disadvantage is that many kinds have an unpleasant taste (though improved flavors are becoming available) and can cause nausea. Nicotine gum requires frequent use throughout the day and many not be adequate for heavy smokers. It reduces craving for a cigarette but does not help with some of the other symptoms of withdrawal.

The *nicotine patch,* also available without a prescription, is a self-adhesive, nicotine-containing circle that sticks to the skin like a Band-Aid. It is worn all day and slowly releases a steady supply of nicotine into the outer layer of skin. It takes up to three hours for the nicotine from the patch to enter the bloodstream, and nicotine continues to enter the bloodstream for several hours after the patch is removed. The delayed entry allows the wearer to achieve a near-constant level of nicotine in the body. The patch is applied once a day, is used for 6 to 12 weeks, and costs about $3 per day.

The advantages of the patch are that it is easy to use and helps with withdrawal symptoms. The disadvantages are that it doesn't work equally well for everyone, doesn't help with sudden cravings or eliminate withdrawal symptoms entirely, and can cause a skin rash. The FDA warns against smoking while wearing the patch or for 12 hours after removal, because doing so can produce very high nicotine levels. The 24-hour patch almost always causes vivid, colorful dreams and sleeping difficulties. The 16-hour patch may not produce the sleep side effects but may leave the person craving a cigarette upon waking in the morning.

The *nicotine inhaler,* nicknamed "the puffer," is a thin plastic cartridge that contains a nicotine plug in its base. When the person puffs on the cartridge, a nicotine vapor is extracted and absorbed through the membranes lining the mouth. Each cartridge delivers up to 400 puffs of nicotine vapor (the nicotine in one cigarette is about the same as 80 puffs on a cartridge.) The inhaler is used for about 6 months, with 6 to 16 uses a day. The cost averages out to about $6 a day.

The advantages of the inhaler are that it is fast, easy, and convenient. Some people prefer the inhaler because handling the cartridge and inhaling mimic the behavioral aspects of smoking. It also provides the kind of rapid spike in nicotine that smoking delivers. The disadvantages are that it requires frequent use and usually causes mouth and throat irritation, coughing, runny nose, and upset stomach. These side effects are usually mild and disappear after regular use of the inhaler.

The *nicotine spray* is a pump containing a gaseous suspension of nicotine. When it is sprayed into the nostrils, nicotine is quickly absorbed by the mucous membranes lining the nose. Like the inhaler, the spray provides a quick "hit" of nicotine, making it attractive to some highly dependent smokers. It is used for 3 to 6 months, 8 to 40 times a day, at a cost of about $6 a day. The advantages are that it is fast, easy to use, and convenient. The disadvantages are that it requires frequent use and causes nose and throat irritation, watering eyes, sneezing, and coughing. After a week of use, these side effects usually disappear. The nicotine spray has a greater potential for dependency than other NRT products do and should be used only under the direction of a physician.

Source: Adapted from *Treating Tobacco Use and Dependence: Clinical Practice Guideline,* by M. C. Fiore, W. C. Bailey, S. S. Cohen, et al., 2000, Rockville, MD: U.S. Department of Health and Human Services, Public Health Service.

smoke, or to quit is ultimately your own. Health-related behaviors consist mainly of habits, and changing these behaviors can disrupt your life. In the case of smoking, quitting means going through withdrawal, feeling stressed, probably gaining a little weight, and having to avoid situations that increase craving. Despite these hardships, quitting is worth it, and the majority of people who quit do so on their own.

One approach is to develop a behavior change plan similar to the one we described for cutting back on

Challenges & Choices

Enhancing Motivation to Quit Smoking

A person who smokes and does not want to quit may lack information about the harmful health effects of tobacco, may have fears or concerns about quitting, or may be demoralized by previous failures to quit. If someone you know smokes, you can help him or her move to a different stage of change by using an approach sometimes used by physicians to enhance motivation to quit. You can also use this approach to enhance your own motivation to quit. The approach relies on five Rs—relevance, risks, rewards, roadblocks, and repetition.

- **Relevance**   Make quitting as personally relevant and specific as possible. Information that is relevant to a smoker, such as age, family situation, or family health history, is likely to have the greatest motivational impact. The effect of smoking on children in the home is an example of relevant information.

- **Risks**   Help the smoker identify the negative consequences of smoking. Risks can be divided into three categories: (1) acute risks: shortness of breath, sexual dysfunction, infertility, harm to fetus in pregnancy, exacerbated asthma; (2) long-term risks: heart attacks, strokes, cancer, chronic respiratory diseases, long-term disability and need for extended care; and (3) the effects of secondhand smoke on those around the smoker: increased risk of lung cancer and heart disease in partners; higher prevalence of smoking by children of tobacco users; increased risks for SIDS, low birth weight, asthma, middle ear disease, and respiratory infections in children of smokers.

- **Rewards**   Help the smoker identify potential benefits of quitting. The benefits most relevant to the smoker need to be highlighted. Examples of rewards include feeling better physically, having a better sense of smell, rediscovering the taste of food, enjoying better health, saving money, breathing more easily, having healthier children, performing better in physical activities, reducing wrinkling/aging of skin, and not worrying about exposing others to secondhand smoke.

- **Roadblocks**   Help the smoker identify barriers to quitting. Examples include withdrawal symptoms, fear of failure, fear of weight gain, lack of social support, depression, and enjoyment of tobacco. Various kinds of treatment interventions can help with these roadblocks.

- **Repetition**   Most people make repeated attempts to quit. In this part of the approach to quitting, reinforce the smoker's decision to quit, review the benefits of quitting, and assist the smoker in overcoming impediments to quitting.

It's Not Just Personal . . .

Studies suggest that African Americans who smoke are highly motivated to quit, yet the number of African Americans who have succeeded in quitting smoking is lower than that of whites. According to the U.S. surgeon general, African Americans tend to smoke fewer cigarettes per day than whites do. They also begin smoking later in life than whites do. Yet death from smoking-related diseases is significantly higher among African Americans than among whites. More research is needed to determine the factors involved in these apparent contradictions.

Source: Adapted from *Treating Tobacco Use and Dependence: Clinical Practice Guideline,* by M. C. Fiore, W. C. Bailey, S. S. Cohen, et al., 2000, Rockville, MD: U.S. Department of Health and Human Services, Public Health Service.

alcohol consumption in Chapter 11. A first step is determining your readiness to quit. As discussed in Chapter 1, trying to change a behavior when you are not ready to change is pointless and counterproductive. It will only lead to failure and discouragement. Refer to the box "Assesssing Your Stage of Change" in Chapter 1 (p. 11) for a quick evaluation of your own stage of change in regard to quitting smoking. You can also refer to the box "Enhancing Motivation to Quit Smoking" for tips on increasing your motivation. If you are in the contemplation or action stage, you can develop a behavior change plan by following the steps described next.

Record Your Smoking Behavior Patterns

Use a health diary to record your tobacco-related behaviors for 2 weeks. Include when, where, and with whom you smoke; the triggers for smoking; and your thoughts and feelings before, during, and after smoking.

Analyze Your Smoking Patterns

What patterns do you see in your smoking behavior? Do you always smoke in certain situations? With certain people? The Add It Up! activity at the end of the chapter can help you analyze your patterns of smoking and identify your reasons for smoking.

Challenges & Choices

Preparing to Quit Smoking

When you have decided to quit and set a quit date, you can make adjustments in your environment and lifestyle that will improve your chances of success. Here are some tips:

- Make your home a smoke-free zone; post signs and do not allow anyone to smoke in your home. If feasible, ask your friends not to smoke around you.
- Throw away all your cigarettes and ashtrays.
- Get your clothes cleaned so they don't smell of cigarette smoke. Air out your car and house.
- Make an appointment with your dentist to get your teeth cleaned.
- If you want to use nicotine replacement therapy, consult with your physician about what product may work best for you.
- Stock up on low-calorie munchies to help you handle cravings with minimal weight gain.
- Make sure your social support system is established. Let your family and friends know your quit date.

- Try to make your last few days of smoking inconvenient, such as smoking only outdoors when it is very cold.
- Write a good-bye letter to cigarettes as a symbolic way of letting go.

It's Not Just Personal . . .

The decision to quit smoking is a personal one. Yet experts say that "going public" with this decision is usually best. You'll need the support of those closest to you—family and friends—to help you create an environment for success and to keep you going when you want to give up.

Sources: *Dying to Quit: Why We Smoke and How to Stop*, by J. Brigham, 1998, Washington, DC: National Academy Press; *Treating Tobacco Use and Dependence: Clinical Practice Guideline*, by M. C. Fiore, W. C. Bailey, S. S. Cohen, et al., 2000, Rockville, MD: U.S. Department of Health and Human Services, Public Health Service.

Establish Goals

Set a specific date to quit. Choose a time when you will be relatively stress free—not during exams, for example—so you will have the needed energy, attention, and focus. Experts recommend aiming for some time within 2 weeks of when you begin to plan. Plan to quit completely on that date; tapering off rarely works because it only prolongs withdrawal.

Prepare to Quit

Your most important asset in quitting is your firm commitment to do so. At the same time, you can take specific, concrete steps to increase your chances of success. Consider these questions:

- Why do you want to quit? Make a list of your reasons and post them on your refrigerator or in another prominent place in your home. Examples are better health, cleaner clothes, more spending money, and a sense of achievement.
- If you tried to quit in the past, what helped and what didn't? Learn from your mistakes. Don't be discouraged—as noted earlier, many people try several times before they finally succeed in quitting.
- What situations are going to be the most difficult? How can you plan ahead to handle them? To the

extent you can, reorganize your life to avoid situations in which you were accustomed to smoking and to include situations that are smoke free.

- What pleasures do you get from smoking? How can you get those pleasures from life-enhancing activities instead of smoking?
- Who can help you? Tell your family and friends you are planning to quit and ask for their support. Find a phone friend or an Internet buddy who will help you resist relapse. See the box "Preparing to Quit Smoking" for more tips.

Implement Your Plan

Make sure you no longer have any tobacco products when your quit day arrives. Be prepared to experience symptoms of withdrawal and have a plan for handling them, even if it's just "toughing it out." Exercise will help ease cravings for nicotine and elevate your mood, so make sure you exercise daily. About one in five smokers may experience mild depression after quitting. Exercise will also improve sleep and help you limit weight gain. Drink plenty of fluids; they help flush nicotine from your body. Don't drink as much caffeine as you are used to, though; the effects of caffeine become more pronounced when you stop smoking and can lead to nervousness or jitters.

Table 13.2   What to Expect When You Quit

Symptom	Reason	Duration	Relief
Irritability	Body craves nicotine.	2–4 weeks	Take walks, hot baths; use relaxation techniques.
Fatigue	Nicotine is a stimulant.	2–4 weeks	Take naps; don't push yourself.
Insomnia	Nicotine affects brain waves.	2–4 weeks	Avoid caffeine after 6:00 p.m.; use relaxation techniques.
Coughing, dry throat, nasal drip	Body is getting rid of excess mucus.	A few days	Drink fluids; try cough drops.
Dizziness	Brain is getting more oxygen.	1–2 days	Be cautious moving; change positions slowly.
Poor concentration	Nicotine is a stimulant, boosts concentration.	1–2 weeks	Get enough sleep; exercise; eat well.
Tightness in chest	Muscles are tense from nicotine craving or sore from coughing.	A few days	Use relaxation techniques, especially deep breathing; take hot baths.
Constipation, gas, stomach pain	Intestinal movement decreases for brief time.	1–2 weeks	Drink fluids; add fiber to diet (fruits, vegetables, whole grains).
Hunger	Nicotine craving can feel like hunger.	Up to several weeks	Drink water or low-calorie drinks; have low-calorie snacks on hand.
Headaches	Brain is getting more oxygen.	1–2 weeks	Drink water; use relaxation techniques.
Craving for a cigarette	Withdrawal from nicotine.	Most acute first few days; can recur for months	Wait it out; distract yourself; exercise; use relaxation techniques.

Source: www.quitnet.com.

Prevent Relapse

Symptoms of nicotine withdrawal last from 2 to 3 weeks, although the most acute symptoms may last only a few days. See Table 13.2 for a summary of symptoms, their causes, and suggested relief strategies.

Abstinence becomes easier with time, although it can still be difficult. Most relapses occur within the first 3 months.[26] There are two main lines of defense for maintaining prolonged abstinence. First, avoid high-risk situations. Relapse episodes are much more likely to occur if you are near someone else who smokes or you are in a smoky environment. Seek out smoke-free restaurants and bars and make your home smoke free.[46]

Second, develop coping mechanisms. Relapses are prompted by stress, anger, frustration and depression.[44] Make sure you have strategies to deal with these feelings, whether relaxation techniques, exercise, social support, or cognitive techniques. Examples of cognitive techniques are reminding yourself of why you quit, thinking about the people you know who have quit, adjusting your self-image so that you think of yourself as an ex-smoker or a nonsmoker rather than a smoker, reminding yourself that withdrawal symptoms mean your body is flushing out toxic nicotine residue, and congratulating yourself every time you beat an urge to smoke. Remember, you are overcoming an addiction to an extremely harmful drug; your discomfort and effort will be repaid with better health and longer life.

CONFRONTING THE TOBACCO CHALLENGE

The cost of tobacco use to individuals and society is enormous. An estimated 440,000 Americans die every year from smoking-related causes. Health care costs attributable to smoking-related diseases are estimated at nearly $160 billion. When the value of lost earnings and productivity from illness, disability, and premature death are added, the total cost nearly doubles. Given this devastation, why are the manufacture and sale of tobacco products legal in this country?

The answer to this question is complex. Tobacco has been part of the agricultural economy of the country since colonial times, and today it is a multibillion-dollar industry with tremendous lobbying power and a huge impact on the nation's economic health. Many state economies depend on tobacco, and elected representatives from those states make sure tobacco interests are protected at the federal level. Because we are a free society and smoking is viewed as a personal decision, there are many constraints on the government's ability to protect citizens and consumers from the hazards of tobacco use. Still, significant inroads have been made in confronting the challenge posed by tobacco, and the tobacco industry is facing tremendous pressure on many fronts.

The Nonsmokers' Rights Movement and Legislative Battles

In the 1970s and 1980s, a nonsmokers' rights movement took shape as a result of growing public awareness and outrage at the damage inflicted by tobacco. The movement was reinforced by three important studies:

- 1986 surgeon general's report identifying ETS as a cause of disease, including lung cancer, in healthy nonsmokers and a factor in the increased frequency of respiratory infections in children of parents who smoke
- 1993 Environmental Protection Agency report classifying ETS as a Class A carcinogen—an agent known to cause cancer in humans
- 1999 National Cancer Institute report attributing about 53,000 premature deaths each year to ETS

Smoking came to be seen as both a public health problem and an antisocial behavior.[47]

Although some antismoking actions took place at the state level, nonsmoking advocates realized their best chances of success were at the local level. Local municipalities are farther from the reach of tobacco industry lobbying and political contributions, and local laws are easier to pass and enforce and more likely to receive citizen support. By 2003, thousands of local laws and ordinances were in place across the country, creating smoke-free workplaces, restaurants, bars, and public places.

The tobacco industry responded to the nonsmokers' rights movement with public relations campaigns, efforts to influence local politics, and underwriting for smokers' rights groups. The industry also lobbied for preemptive legislation at both the state and the federal levels—legislation that prevents local jurisdictions from passing laws to regulate tobacco use. Preemptive legislation has been successful in curtailing the passage of local tobacco control laws, particularly in restaurants and bars. In Iowa, for example, the state supreme court in 2004 overturned the smoke-free restaurant law passed by the city of Ames as a violation of the state's preemptive legislation. Tobacco control advocates are pushing for the removal of preemptive legislation that prevents local governments from initiating smoke-free laws.

Some tobacco control laws have been passed at the state level. In 1975, Minnesota became the first state to enact a clean indoor air act requiring nonsmoking areas in public places. California has had a ban on smoking in workplaces since 1994 and on smoking in bars since 1998. Other states have a variety of regulations on smoking in public places. The federal government also has tobacco control measures in place, such as the ban on smoking on domestic airline flights.

Lawsuits and Court Settlements

Tobacco companies spent much of the 20th century denying that nicotine was addictive and that smoking was dangerous to one's health. With their vast resources, they were able to defend themselves against lawsuits brought by

With its powerful advertising campaigns and vast resources, the tobacco industry was successful in fighting lawsuits brought by individuals for many years. In the 1990s this situation changed when individual smokers joined together and mounted class action lawsuits claiming health injury from smoking.

individual claimants, but in the 1990s they began to face class action suits, cases representing claims of injury by hundreds or thousands of smokers. In addition, states began suing tobacco companies for losses incurred by state health insurance funds used to pay for tobacco-related diseases.

These pressures led to the 1998 Multi Settlement Agreement (MSA), in which the tobacco industry agreed to pay $206 billion to 46 states over a 25-year period in exchange for protection from future lawsuits by the states and other public entities. Other provisions of the MSA included a ban on billboard advertising and restrictions on advertising aimed at children. The settlement money from the MSA was to be used by the states primarily to fund tobacco education and prevention programs.

Some of the money went to the American Legacy Foundation's "Truth" campaign, a nationwide effort to tell the truth about tobacco products to youth. Studies indicate that this campaign was successful in deterring children and teenagers from taking up smoking.[48] Still, the campaign's $59 million annual spending pales in comparison with the $12.5 billion spent by tobacco companies on advertising and promoting tobacco products in 2002 in the United States alone. Furthermore, money from the settlement may dry up as a result of loopholes in the agreement.[49]

Regulation and Taxation: Harm Reduction Strategies

Since 1964 the surgeon general has released volumes of reports documenting the harmful effects of tobacco use. Use has declined since that time, but the decline has not been as great as one might expect, given the extremely negative effects of smoking on health. The government cannot prohibit tobacco use by adults or force individuals to stop smoking, but it can take actions aimed at reducing the harm associated with the use of tobacco products by those who continue to smoke.

The relationship between smoking and disease is dose related: The more you smoke, the higher your risk.[50] A harm reduction approach focuses on reducing a smoker's exposure to nicotine, tar, and carbon monoxide. One way to achieve this is by limiting access to tobacco products, such as by increasing the price through taxes. Another way, one promoted by tobacco companies, is the use of "light" cigarettes. The latter approach has proved to be just another way to dupe consumers.

Limiting Access to Tobacco

Access to tobacco can be limited by increasing cost, reducing physical availability, and regulating tobacco marketing campaigns. When taxes on tobacco products are increased, raising their price, sales and use decline. For example, tax increases of 10 percent in Canada resulted in a

14 percent decline in the prevalence of smoking among 15- to 19-year-olds.[51] Cigarette tax increases have been particularly effective in discouraging people from starting smoking.[51]

Physical availability of tobacco products is reduced when the laws restricting sales to minors are enforced. States are required to conduct random, unannounced inspections of places where tobacco is sold, and reports detailing results of these inspections must be submitted to the federal government each year. Physical availability is also reduced when smoking is prohibited in workplaces and public spaces.

Restrictions on tobacco advertising may affect access to tobacco as well.[52] Tobacco companies argue that their advertising efforts are aimed solely at creating brand loyalty, not at attracting new smokers. Antitobacco activists draw from extensive research to refute this claim. Tobacco marketing campaigns appear to be specifically directed at children, women, and minorities. Children as young as age 6, for example, have reported familiarity with cigarette ads using cartoon characters.[39]

The Scam of "Light" Cigarettes

"Light" cigarettes with lower levels of tar and nicotine have been promoted by the tobacco industry as safer than regular cigarettes. This marketing campaign has been successful: Lower tar cigarettes have become the best selling cigarettes in North America.[26] They are popular with college students and other young people, and they are likely to be the first tobacco product adopted by children and adolescents.

Lower tar cigarettes are not safer than regular cigarettes. Smokers who switch to these cigarettes compensate for reduced yields of tobacco and nicotine by taking more puffs per cigarette, inhaling more deeply, and smoking more cigarettes per day.[26] Large studies of mortality risks have found no evidence that lower tar cigarettes reduce health risks.[53] Public health experts strongly argue that the tobacco industry should not be allowed to market cigarettes using the terms *mild, light,* or *ultra-light,* and the World Health Framework Convention on Tobacco Control specifically outlaws these terms. The truth is that there is no such thing as a safe cigarette.

Education and Prevention: Changing the Cultural Climate

Fifty years ago, cigarette smoking was an accepted part of everyday life. People smoked in restaurants, movie theaters, concert halls, college classrooms, offices, and airplanes. On television, quiz show panelists, newshour anchormen, and sitcom characters smoked on the air. In movies, smoking was associated with the elegant, sophisticated lifestyle of characters played by actors such as Katherine Hepburn and Humphrey Bogart.

Healthy People 2010

OBJECTIVE AREA *Tobacco-Free Youth*

- Reduce the initiation of tobacco use among children and adolescents.

"School-based tobacco prevention programs identify the social influences that promote tobacco use among youth and teach skills to resist these influences. Such programs have demonstrated consistent and significant reductions or delays in adolescent smoking. The effects dissipate over time if they are not followed by additional education interventions or linkages to community programs."

For more information on Healthy People 2010 objectives, visit the Web site at www.healthypeople.gov.

For more information on Canadian health objectives, visit the Health Canada Web site at www.hc-sc.gc.ca/english.

Those days are gone, along with the social norms that made smoking a socially acceptable behavior. (Also gone are many of the stars who smoked, including Humphrey Bogart, Louis Armstrong, Lucille Ball, Sammy Davis, Jr., Nat King Cole, and Walt Disney—all the victims of smoking-related diseases.) Awareness of the health hazards of smoking and ETS, greater skepticism toward tobacco advertising and promotion, and increased willingness on the part of nonsmokers to assert their rights have all contributed to changes in the cultural climate surrounding tobacco use.

Clearly, however, there is more to do. Movies still depict attractive characters smoking, cigarette ads still lead young people to associate smoking with popularity and relaxation, and teenagers still try cigarettes every day. Antismoking campaigns that focus on the risks of smoking fail to counter the positive images that are conveyed by movies, media, and advertising and that motivate young people to take up smoking.[54] Research indicates that perception of risk is not a deterrent when teenagers are thinking about experimenting with tobacco.

One recommendation by health experts is that antismoking campaigns use some of the same strategies that have worked for the tobacco companies.[54] For example, they should target specific market segments, focusing on young people and their attitudes, values, and lifestyles. Messages should be delivered repeatedly over long periods of time in a multitude of formats, and they should be varied to appeal to the age and ethnic/cultural identity of the intended audience. As many forms of media as possible should be used, including public service announcements, paid advertising during prime time, and celebrity endorsement and support.

Community interventions are also recommended, working through schools, local government, civic organizations, and health agencies. Many colleges and universities are now smoke-free environments, as are many fast-food restaurant chains and a majority of the country's shopping malls. All of these efforts have the potential to create a fundamental change in social norms and in public attitudes toward tobacco use. Such a change, in turn, has the potential to close the pipeline of new smokers and motivate current smokers to quit.

You Make the Call

Smoking Restrictions in Public Places

There is no longer any doubt that environmental tobacco smoke (ETS) significantly increases the risk of smoking-related diseases in individuals who do not smoke. For example, the rate of lung cancer among spouses of smokers is higher than among spouses of nonsmokers, and rates of respiratory infections in children are higher in families with smokers than in families without smokers. In such cases, smoking or not smoking is a personal issue with ethical dimensions.

ETS becomes a public policy issue when smoking affects people in public accommodations, where access is open to everyone. There are two types of public accommodations: those operated by the government on behalf of taxpayers and those operated by private business owners on their own behalf. Most people agree that facilities operated with taxpayer support, such as public universities, courthouses, and libraries, have the right to ban smoking, since most taxpayers—75–80 percent of the population—are nonsmokers. (Some people do argue that public facilities should take into consideration the rights of smokers as well, since they are also taxpayers.)

More controversial are efforts to ban smoking in facilities operated by private owners, such as restaurants, bars, movie theaters, and stores. Technically, any place that allows a person to walk in off the street can be defined as a public accommodation, and many cities include such small businesses in their laws and ordinances restricting smoking. In some local jurisdictions, nonsmoking restrictions are extended to outdoor areas like beaches, parks, pedestrian malls, and areas within a certain distance—for example, 30 feet—of doors and entries to buildings. Proponents of smoking restrictions argue that government has not only the right but the duty to protect the public from known health hazards. They cite rates of disease and death from ETS and point out that even brief exposure causes respiratory irritation. People who work in bars and restaurants are particularly at risk from ETS when patrons are allowed to smoke. Proponents argue that the right of nonsmokers to breathe clean air supersedes the rights of smokers to light up.

Opponents of smoking restrictions argue that the government does not have the right to intrude on small businesses. They view such restrictions as an oppressive crusade by nonsmokers to impose their tastes and preferences on smokers, and they suggest government controls may next extend into private residences. They point out that businesses like bars and restaurants depend on customer satisfaction, and when smoking is prohibited, revenues may go down. Evidence to date has not been conclusive on this possible effect.

Laws are changing, but restrictions on smoking in public places are still controversial. What do you think?

Pros

○ Since the 1986 surgeon general's report, ETS has been identified as a cause of cancer, including lung cancer, in healthy nonsmokers and has been associated with an increased frequency of respiratory infections in the children of smokers.

○ Even brief exposure to ETS can cause headaches, coughing, dizziness, nausea, and irritation to the eyes, nose, and throat.

○ Nonsmoking employees and patrons are exposed to ETS when patrons are allowed to smoke.

○ Loss of revenue by restaurants and bars who adopt smoke-free accommodations has not been proven by objective studies.

○ Any greater revenue taken in by bars and restaurants that allow smoking is offset by higher costs in other areas—maintenance expenses (cleaning of carpets, drapes, clothes), insurance premiums (fire, health, worker compensation), and labor costs (absenteeism, productivity).

○ The right to smoke should not interfere with the nonsmoker's right to breathe smoke-free air.

Cons

○ Restaurant owners are entrepreneurs and have the right to operate their businesses without undue local government interference.

○ Bans on smoking may reduce revenue at restaurants and bars and put them out of business.

○ Many restaurants and bars have implemented self-imposed bans; government action is not needed.

○ If people don't like smoke, they can go to another restaurant.

○ If local government can control the actions of private citizens in restaurants, what is to stop it from extending its reach into private residences?

OLC Web site For more information about this topic, visit the Online Learning Center at www.mhhe.com/teaguele.

SOURCE: "Reducing Tobacco Use: A Report of the Surgeon General," U.S. Department of Health and Human Services, 2000, Atlanta, GA: Centers for Disease Control and Prevention.

SUMMARY

- About 22 percent of Americans and about 20 percent of Canadians smoke. The prevalence of smoking has declined substantially in the last 40 years, but the rate of decline has slowed since 1990. Smoking rates are higher among men than women, among younger people than older people, and among whites than members of ethnic minority groups.

- Social smoking is a relatively new phenomenon; research has not determined whether social smokers will quit, continue smoking at a low level, or become heavy smokers. People who smoke more than 10 cigarettes a day are considered heavy smokers; people who smoke fewer than 10 cigarettes a day are called chippers.

- Tobacco contains hundreds of toxic and carcinogenic substances; the most harmful are tar, carbon monoxide, and nicotine. Cigarettes are by far the most popular tobacco product; other products include cigars, pipes, and smokeless tobacco. All forms of tobacco—including clove cigarettes, herbal cigarettes, and bidis—carry health hazards.

- Smoking causes cardiovascular disease, cancer, respiratory diseases, and many other debilitating conditions. It is the leading preventable cause of death in the United States. Tar and toxins dull the senses of smell and taste, damage the lungs, and lead to conditions conducive to cancer throughout the body. Carbon monoxide impairs the delivery of oxygen to body cells. In the brain, nicotine produces both sedating and stimulating effects.

- Smoking is associated with fertility problems and sexual dysfunctions in both men and women. Tobacco use during pregnancy increases the risk of miscarriage, low birth weight in infants, and other reproductive problems, as well as SIDS. Members of ethnic minority groups have higher mortality rates from tobacco-related diseases even when their rates of smoking are lower.

- Quitting smoking has health benefits both immediately and in the long term. Within 5 years, the risk of heart disease and stroke approaches that of nonsmokers, and within 10 years, the risk of lung cancer is cut by half.

- Environmental tobacco smoke (ETS) has been found to cause cardiovascular disease, lung cancer and other cancers, respiratory diseases, and other negative health effects in healthy nonsmokers. Sidestream smoke—the smoke coming from the burning end of a cigarette or cigar—is more dangerous than mainstream smoke—the smoke exhaled by the smoker. Cigars generate much more hazardous ETS than cigarettes.

- People smoke because they are addicted to nicotine, because they have become psychologically and behaviorally dependent on smoking, because they hope to lose weight, and because they are influenced by the sophisticated advertising and marketing campaigns of tobacco companies.

- Quitting smoking is exceptionally difficult. Options include formal treatment programs, medications such as nicotine patches and nicotine gum, and quitting on your own.

- Tobacco companies powerfully influence public policy on tobacco use through lobbying and political contributions. Challenges to the tobacco industry include the nonsmokers' rights movement, local laws restricting smoking in public places, lawsuits and monetary settlements, and such harm reduction strategies as taxes on tobacco products, enforcement of laws restricting sales to minors, and restrictions on tobacco advertising.

- "Light" cigarettes and low-tar, low-nicotine tobacco products are not any safer than regular ones.

- As smoking becomes less socially acceptable, tobacco use should decline further. However, the tobacco industry continues to recruit young smokers, and nicotine addiction prevents many current smokers from quitting.

REVIEW QUESTIONS

1. What trends have occurred in the last 40 years in tobacco use? What accounts for these trends?

2. What demographic and psychosocial factors predict tobacco use in young people?

3. What is social smoking? What is probably behind this phenomenon? How are chippers and heavy smokers defined?

4. What are the most harmful substances in tobacco?

5. Explain why cigarettes are effective delivery systems for nicotine.

6. Describe the dangers of clove cigarettes, herbal cigarettes, and bidis.

7. What is the difference in how nicotine from cigarettes and cigars is absorbed?

8. What are the health hazards of spit tobacco?

9. Describe the effects of nicotine, tar, and carbon monoxide on the brain and body.

10. How does smoking contribute to cardiovascular disease?

11. What cancers are particularly associated with smoking?

12. What special risks of tobacco use apply to women? To men?

13. Describe some of the benefits of quitting.

14. What are some of the risks associated with environmental tobacco smoke?

15. Describe the addictive effects of nicotine. Why is it so hard to quit smoking?

16. What associations are promoted in tobacco advertising aimed at children? At adolescents?

17. What components make a smoking cessation treatment program effective?

18. How does nicotine replacement therapy work? How does bupropion work?

19. Describe the steps of a behavior change plan to quit smoking. What are two strategies to prevent relapse?

20. What reports propelled the nonsmokers' rights movement in the 1970s and 1980s?

21. What is preemptive legislation at the state level?

22. What is the Multi Settlement Agreement?

23. What are three harm reduction strategies used by the government to limit the damage associated with tobacco use?

24. What factors have contributed to the reduced social acceptability of tobacco use?

WEB RESOURCES

Action on Smoking and Health (ASH): This site covers a wide range of information on smoking, including nonsmokers' rights, guidelines on quitting smoking, smoking risks, and statistics on smoking.
www.ash.org

American Cancer Society: Look for the Detailed Guides for information on lung cancer: risk factors, cancer terminology, treatment options, and talking with your doctor.
www.cancer.org

American Council on Science and Health: At this organization's Web site, go to the tobacco section, which includes news and publications on health issues related to smoking. www.acsh.org

American Lung Association: See the Quit Smoking feature of the association's Web site for news articles, resources for support, information on legislation, and fact sheets. www.lungusa.org

Americans for Nonsmokers' Rights: This organization offers information on environmental smoke; how to protect yourself from smoke at home, at work, and in the community; legal issues related to smoking; and special concerns for youth. www.no-smoke.org

CDC's Tobacco Information and Prevention Sources (TIPS): The tips offered on this site are directed at kids, teens, and adults. Everything from the surgeon general's reports to Celebrities Against Smoking and community action programs can be found here. www.cdc.gov/tobacco

Center for Tobacco Cessation: Look for the Resources section of this site for a varied list of links offering information on smoking cessation, including special groups such as women and young girls, useful information for smokers, and vital information on nicotine addiction. www.ctcinfo.org

National Heart, Lung, and Blood Institute: This organization's Web site offers health information and publications on diseases and conditions of the heart and the lungs related to smoking. www.nhlbi.nih.gov

Quitnet: This online support group offers general information for the public and members-only features, including self-assessment tools and a directory of local support groups. www.quitnet.com

Smokefree.Gov: The online guide to quitting smoking offered at this site includes practical steps for preparing to quit, quitting, and "staying quit." You can also instant-message an expert or get telephone support. www.smokefree.gov

Tobacco.Org: This Web site features tobacco news, advertising information, contacts in tobacco control and the tobacco industry, an activism guide, and links to other resources. www.tobacco.org

World Health Organization Tobacco Free Initiative: The WHO considers tobacco use a public health priority and sponsors the World No Tobacco Day. Its Web site includes press releases and news articles on tobacco use and health. www.who.int/toh

REFERENCES

1. American Lung Association. (2003). Adolescent smoking statistics. www.lungusa.org.

2. Krogh, D. (1999). *Smoking: The artificial passion.* New York: W. H. Freeman and Company.

3. Health Canada. (2004). Canadian tobacco use monitoring survey. www.hc-sc.gc.ca.

4. National Center for Health Statistics. (2004). *Health, United States, 2004.* Hyattsville, MD: Author.

5. Centers for Disease Control and Prevention. (2002). State-specific prevalence of current cigarette smoking among adults, United States. *Morbidity and Mortality Weekly Report,* Atlanta, GA: Author.

6. Tomar, S. L. (2003). Trends and patterns of tobacco use in the United States. *American Journal of the Medical Sciences, 326* (4), 248–254.

7. Johnston, L. D., O'Malley, P. M., & Bachman, J. G. (2002). *Monitoring the future: National survey results on drug use, 1975–2001.* Volume II: *College students and adults ages 19–40.* (NIH Publication No. 02-5107). Bethesda, MD: National Institute on Drug Abuse.

8. Centers for Disease Control and Prevention. (1998). *Tobacco use among U.S. racial/ethnic minority groups: A report of the surgeon general.* Atlanta, GA: Author.

9. Centers for Disease Control and Prevention. (2000). *Tobacco use among U.S. racial/ethnic minority groups—African Americans, American Indians and Alaska Natives, Asian Americans and Pacific Islanders, and Hispanics: A report of the surgeon general.* Atlanta, GA: Author.

10. Baer, J. S., & Murch, H. B. (1998). Harm reduction, nicotine, and smoking. In A. Marlatt (Ed.), *Harm reduction.* New York: The Guilford Press.

11. Das, S. K. (2003). Harmful health effects of cigarette smoking. *Molecular and Cellular Biochemistry, 253* (1–2), 159–165.

12. Fairchild, A., & Cosgrove, J. (2004). Out of the ashes: The life, death and rebirth of the "safer" cigarette in the United States. *American Journal of Public Health, 94* (2), 192–204.

13. Hyand, A., Hughes, J. R., Farrell, M., & Cummings, K. (2003). Switching to lower tar cigarettes does not increase or decrease the likelihood of future quit attempts. *Nicotine & Tobacco Research, 5* (5), 665–671.

14. Hoffman, D., Hoffman, I., & El-Bayoumy, K. (2001). The less harmful cigarette: A controversial issue. *Chemical Research in Toxicology, 14* (7), 767–790.

15. Koch, W. (1999, August 5). The rage: Flavored cigarettes. *USA Today,* pp. 1A–2A.

16. Watson, C. H., Polzin, G. M., Calafat, A. M., & Ashley, D. L. (2003). Determination of tar, nicotine, and carbon monoxide yields in the smoke of bidi cigarettes. *Nicotine & Tobacco Research, 5* (5), 747–753.

17. Rahman, M., & Fukij, T. (2000). Bidi smoking and health. *Public Health, 114* (2), 123–127.

18. National Cancer Institute. (1998). *Cigars: Health effects and trends.* Monograph No. 9. Washington, DC: Author.

19. Baker, F., Ainsworth, S. R., Dye, J. T., et al. (2000). Health risks associated with cigar smoking. *Journal of the American Medical Association, 284,* 735–740.

20. Shaper, A. G., Wannamethee, S. G., & Walker, M. (2003). Pipe and cigar smoking and major cardiovascular events, cancer incidence and all-cause mortality in middle-aged British men. *International Journal of Epidemiology, 32* (5), 802–808.

21. Cancer Net from the National Cancer Institute. Questions and answers about smokeless tobacco and cancer. www.meb.uni-bonn.de/cancer.gov.

22. Severson, H. H. (2003). What have we learned from 20 years of research on smokeless tobacco cessation? *American Journal of the Medical Sciences, 326* (4), 206–211.

23. U.S. Department of Health and Human Services. (1986). *The health consequences of using smokeless tobacco: A report of the advisory committee to the surgeon general.* Washington, DC: Author.

24. Hatsukami, D. K., & Severson, H. H. (1999). Oral spit tobacco: Addiction, prevention, and treatment. *Journal of Nicotine and Tobacco Research, 1,* 21–44.

25. U.S. Department of Health and Human Services. (2004). *The health consequences of smoking: A report of the surgeon general.* Atlanta, GA: Author.

26. Kozlowski, L. T., Henningfield, J. E., & Brigham, J. (2001). *Cigarettes, nicotine, and health: A biobehavioral approach.* Thousand Oaks, CA: Sage Publications.

27. Glantz, S. A. (1996). *The cigarette papers.* Berkeley, CA: University of California Press.

28. Levington, S. (2003). The importance of cholesterol, blood pressure, and smoking for coronary heart disease. *European Heart Journal, 24* (19), 1703–1704.

29. Flanders, W. D., Lally, G. A., Zhu, B. P., Henley, S. J., & Thun, M. J. (2003). Lung cancer mortality in relation to age, duration of smoking, and daily cigarette consumption: Results from Cancer Prevention Study II. *Cancer Research, 63* (19), 6556–6562.

30. U.S. Department of Health and Human Services. (2001). *Women and smoking: A report of the surgeon general.* Washington, DC: Author.

31. New evidence links smoking and lung cancer in women. (2003, January 9). *Women's Health Weekly,* p. 18.

32. Venners, S. A., Wang, X., Chen, C., et al. (2004). Paternal smoking and pregnancy loss: A prospective study using a biomarker of pregnancy. *American Journal of Epidemiology, 159* (10), 993–1001.

33. Ronald Y., & McVory K. (2003). Smoking and erectile dysfunction: How strong a link? *Contemporary Urology, 15* (3), 34.

34. U.S. Department of Health and Human Services. (1990). *The health benefits of smoking cessation: A report of the surgeon general.* Rockville, MD: Author.

35. National Cancer Institute. (1999). *Health effects of exposure to environmental tobacco smoke.* National Cancer Institute, Monograph 10. Washington, DC: Author.

36. Regents of the University of California. (2004). A little is dangerous. Tobacco scam. www.tobaccoscam.ucsf.edu.

37. Henningfield, J. E. (2000). Tobacco dependence treatment: Scientific challenges, public health opportunities. *Tobacco Control, 9* (suppl. 1), 13–110.

38. Davies, G. M., Willner, P., James, D. L., & Morgan, M. J. (2004). Influence of nicotine gum on acute cravings for cigarettes. *Journal of Psychopharmacology, 18* (1), 83–87.

39. Glantz, S. A. (2003). *Tobacco biology and politics.* Waco, TX: HEALTH EDCO.

40. Saarni, S. E., Silvertoinen, K., Rissanen, A., et al. (2004). Intentional weight loss and smoking in young adults. *International Journal of Obesity, 28* (6), 796–802.

41. Choi, W. S., Ahluwalia, J. S., Harris, K. J., & Okuyemi, K. (2002). Progression to established smoking: The influence of tobacco marketing. *American Journal of Preventive Medicine, 22* (4), 137–145.

42. Brigham, J. (1998). *Dying to quit: Why we smoke and how to stop.* Washington, DC: National Academy Press.

43. Bussian, B. (2002). Strategies for nicotine replacement therapy. *Drug Discovery Today, 8* (17), 778–779.

44. Fiore, M. C., Bailey, W. C., Cohen, S. S., et al. (2000). *Treating tobacco use and dependence: Clinical practice guideline.* Rockville, MD: U.S. Department of Health and Human Services, Public Health Service.

45. Schuurmans, M. M., Diacon, A. H., Van Biljon, X., & Bolliger, C. T. (2004). Effect of pre-treatment with nicotine patch on withdrawal symptoms and abstinence rates in smokers subsequently quitting with the nicotine patch: A randomized controlled trial. *Addiction, 99* (5), 634–640.

46. Brandon, T. H., Herzog, T. A., & Webb, M. S. (2003). It ain't over until it's over: The case for offering relapse-prevention interventions to former smokers. *American Journal of the Medical Sciences, 326* (4), 197–200.

47. Americans for Nonsmokers' Rights. (2003). Recipe for a smoke free society. www.no-smoke.org.

48. Kessler, D. (2001). *A question of intent: The great American battle with a deadly industry.* New York: Public Affairs.

49. Givel, M., & Glanz, S. A. (2004). The global settlement with the tobacco industry 6 years later. *American Journal of Public Health, 94* (2), 218–224.

50. Farrelly, M. C., Davis, K. C., Haviland, M. L., Messeri, P., & Healton, C. G. (2005). Evidence of a dose-response relationship between "truth" antismoking ads and youth smoking prevalence. *American Journal of Public Health, 95,* 425–431.

51. Gruber, J., Sen, A., & Stabile, M. (2003). Estimating price elasticities when there is smuggling: The sensitivity of smoking to price in Canada. *Journal of Health Economics, 22* (5), 821–842.

52. Federal Trade Commission. (1997). *Report to Congress: Pursuant to the Federal Cigarette Labeling and Advertising Act.* Washington, DC: Author.

53. Burns, D., Shanks, T., Major, J., & Thun, M. (2002). *Evidence on disease risk in public health consequences of low yield cigarettes,* Smoking and Tobacco Control Monograph, 13. Washington, DC: National Cancer Institute.

54. Mecklenburg, R. E. (2003). Public health issues in treating tobacco use. *American Journal of the Medical Sciences, 326* (4), 255–261.

Add It Up!   WHY DO YOU SMOKE?

People smoke for different reasons—for example, to enhance mood, to relieve tension, or to have something in their hands. If you are a smoker, knowing why you smoke will give you tools to help you quit. For each of the following statements, circle one number indicating how often the statement is true for you.

	Never	Seldom	Sometimes	Often	Always
A. I smoke cigarettes in order to keep from slowing down.	1	2	3	4	5
B. Handling a cigarette is part of my enjoyment in smoking.	1	2	3	4	5
C. Smoking cigarettes is pleasant and relaxing.	1	2	3	4	5
D. I light up a cigarette when I feel angry about something.	1	2	3	4	5
E. When I run out of cigarettes, I find it unbearable until I can get them.	1	2	3	4	5
F. I smoke cigarettes automatically, without even being aware of it.	1	2	3	4	5
G. I smoke cigarettes to stimulate myself, to perk myself up.	1	2	3	4	5
H. Part of my enjoyment in smoking a cigarette comes from the steps I take to light up.	1	2	3	4	5
I. I find cigarettes pleasurable.	1	2	3	4	5
J. When I feel uncomfortable or upset about something, I light up a cigarette.	1	2	3	4	5
K. When I am not smoking a cigarette, I am very much aware of it.	1	2	3	4	5
L. I light up a cigarette without realizing I still have one burning in the ashtray.	1	2	3	4	5
M. I smoke cigarettes to give me a lift.	1	2	3	4	5
N. When I smoke a cigarette, part of my enjoyment is watching the smoke as I exhale it.	1	2	3	4	5
O. I want a cigarette most when I am comfortable and relaxed.	1	2	3	4	5
P. When I feel blue or want to take my mind off cares and worries, I smoke a cigarette.	1	2	3	4	5
Q. I get a real gnawing hunger for a cigarette when I haven't smoked for a while.	1	2	3	4	5
R. I've found a cigarette in my mouth and not remembered putting it there.	1	2	3	4	5

Scoring

Enter the number you have circled for each question in the spaces on the next page. Add the three scores on each line to get your totals. Most people smoke for one or more of six broad reasons: (1) stimulation, a sense of increased energy; (2) handling, the satisfaction of manipulating things; (3) pleasurable feelings, a state of enhanced well-being; (4) a decrease in negative feelings and tension; (5) psychological addiction, a complex pattern of craving for tobacco; (6) habit, an automatic response to environmental stimuli or internal craving.

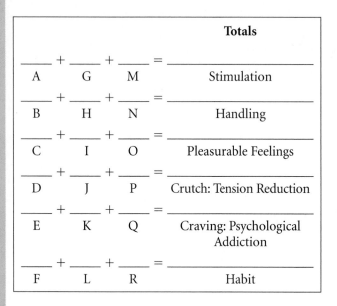

			Totals
____ + ____ + ____ =			_____
A	G	M	Stimulation
____ + ____ + ____ =			_____
B	H	N	Handling
____ + ____ + ____ =			_____
C	I	O	Pleasurable Feelings
____ + ____ + ____ =			_____
D	J	P	Crutch: Tension Reduction
____ + ____ + ____ =			_____
E	K	Q	Craving: Psychological Addiction
____ + ____ + ____ =			_____
F	L	R	Habit

Interpreting Your Score

The highest score possible in a category is 15. A score of 11 or above on any factor suggests that this factor is an important source of satisfaction for you. The higher your score, the more important a particular factor is in your smoking. Your smoking cessation efforts should include strategies that help you address each of the dimensions that strongly influence your smoking. Here are some suggestions:

Stimulation: Try substituting a brisk walk or some other form of exercise.

Handling: Try playing with a pen or pencil, a smooth stone, or a coin. If you want to have something in your mouth, try sugarless gum.

Pleasurable feelings: Try exercising, socializing, or eating or drinking low-calorie foods or drinks.

Tension reduction: Same as pleasurable feelings.

Craving: Quitting may be especially hard for you. However, many smokers with this primary motivation have a low risk of relapse because once they quit, they never want to have to go through it again. Nicotine replacement therapy can help.

Habit: Quitting may be relatively easy for you. Ask yourself, Do I really want this cigarette?

SOURCE: "Why Do You Smoke?" NIH Publication No. 93-1822, Reprinted October 1992, U.S. Department of Health and Human Services.

Your Relationships and Sexuality

In Part 4 we consider the role that relationships and sexuality play in your health. We see how a strong social network offers connection and meaning and a solid foundation for personal growth. Next we discuss your sexuality, as an expression of you as an individual and a reflection of the influences of society and culture. Interconnected with your relationships and your sexual health are the reproductive choices that you will need to consider. All three elements—relationships, sexuality, and reproductive choices—will have a strong impact on your life and your health.

THINK IT OVER

Are family ties, friendships, or intimate relationships most important to you at this time in your life?

What does being sexually responsible mean to you?

What factors influence your opinions about reproductive choices?

CHAPTER **14**

Relationships: Connection and Communication

DID YOU KNOW?

- Friendships are important relationships that increase your sense of belonging, purpose, and self-worth. People with friendships and other kinds of social support have better mental and physical health, cope with stress more successfully, and may even live longer than those without such support.

- If you are between the ages of 20 and 24 and have never been married, you are part of the rapidly growing segment of people in U.S. society who are delaying marriage or choosing singlehood. Between 1970 and 2003, the percentage of single men in this age group increased from 55 percent to 86 percent, and the percentage of single women more than doubled, from 36 percent to 75 percent.

OLC *Your Health Today*   www.mhhe.com/teague1e

Go to the Online Learning Center for *Your Health Today* for interactive activities, quizzes, flashcards, Web links, and more resources related to this chapter.

Relationships are at the heart of human experience. We are born into a family; grow up in a community; have classmates, teammates, and colleagues; find a partner from among our acquaintances and friends; and establish our own family. Yet for all their importance in our lives, relationships are fraught with difficulties and challenges. More than half of all marriages in the United States end in divorce, and many children grow up in a single-parent or blended family of one kind or another. Many people also live alone in the United States, either by choice or by chance.

We sometimes take relationships for granted, but they deserve as much attention and effort as other aspects of our lives. They are a vital part of wellness. People with a strong social support system have better mental and physical health, are more capable of dealing with stress and adverse life events, and may even live longer than those without such support.[1] Social isolation contributes to depression and feelings of helplessness and hopelessness; being isolated undermines a person's self-esteem and sense of purpose in life.

In this chapter we consider some of the many dimensions of relationships. We begin by exploring the characteristics and behaviors that contribute to healthy relationships and the processes by which we find a partner and fall in love. We then take a look at communication, the key to successful relationships, and we continue with a brief examination of the relational aspects of sex and gender. Finally, we explore the major institutions in our society, both formal and informal, that provide the norms and structures by which we form, maintain, and end our most significant relationships.

HEALTHY RELATIONSHIPS

Three kinds of important relationships are the one you have with yourself, the ones you have with friends, and the ones you have with intimate partners. In each, certain qualities serve to enhance the relationship's positive effects.

A Healthy Sense of Self

All your relationships begin with who you are as an individual. A healthy sense of self, reasonably high self-esteem, a capacity for empathy, and the ability both to be alone and to be with others are examples of such individual attributes. Many people develop these assets growing up in their families, but if you experience deficits in childhood, you can still make up for them later in life.

In Chapter 3 we discussed the characteristics of mentally healthy people. They include optimism, resilience, a sense of self-efficacy, and emotional intelligence. We also discussed ways of enhancing your mental health, such as cultivating a supportive social network, developing good communication skills, and maintaining a healthy lifestyle. The attributes and skills that enhance the mental health of individuals are also the building blocks of healthy relationships.

Friendships and Other Kinds of Relationships

If you think about the people you consider your friends, you may come up with a range of relationships. One

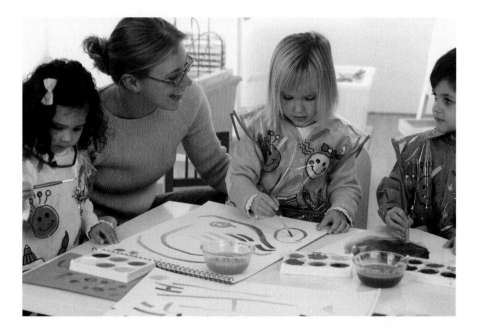

Individuals with a healthy sense of self "feel good in their skin." They like themselves, feel confident in their abilities, are open to new ideas, and enjoy other people. Generally optimistic, they cope well with life's challenges.

Challenges & Choices

Expanding Your Circle of Friends

Some people prefer a small circle of friends, and others enjoy having a large and diverse social support system. If you want to expand your circle of friends, here are some tips:

- *Get out with your pet.* Take your dog to a beach or dog park. Conversation happens naturally between pet owners.

- *Work out.* Join a class at the gym or community center, get a group of people to take yoga at lunchtime, or start a walk group.

- *Do lunch.* Invite someone to join you for lunch, or for breakfast or dinner.

- *Volunteer.* Many organizations need volunteers, including museums, concert halls, churches, hospitals, community centers, and campus programs. Common interests are a positive basis for relationships.

- *Join an organization in support of an issue or cause you believe in.* People working toward common goals often form strong bonds, whether it's cleaning up the environment, working in a political campaign, or rescuing abandoned animals.

- *Join a hobby group.* Find a group with similar interests, such as gardening, hiking, cycling, books, crafts, or singing.

- *Go back to school.* Take a college course or adult education class in something you've been meaning to pursue but never had time for before, such as painting, interior design, or auto mechanics.

It's Not Just Personal . . .

According to the U.S. Bureau of Labor Statistics, about 64.5 million Americans, or 28.8 percent of the population over 16 years of age, volunteer through organizations every year. About one fourth of all men and one third of all women do some kind of volunteer work.

Source: "Social Support: A Buffer Against Life's Ills," Mayo Clinic, 2005, www.mayoclinic.com.

---

researcher has identified several different "degrees of friendship": [2]

- *"Familiar strangers."* These are acquaintances and people we have just met. We exchange hellos and stop to talk to them on the street, but our relationships with them are superficial.

- *Neighbors.* We see and hear a great deal about their lives and we help one another out, but we might not otherwise have much in common with them.

- *Confederates.* These are people with whom we share a common activity or goal, such as serving together on a school committee or belonging to a babysitting co-op.

- *Pals.* We share an activity with pals, such as a weekly game of basketball or poker; we are fairly equal in ability and stature with our pals. Without the activity, these relationships might not survive.

- *Family members, or kin.* Family relationships can develop into friendships, such as sometimes happens between parents and their adult children.

- *Coworkers.* We often spend more time with coworkers than with anyone else in our lives, and we share many life events with them.

- *Friends.* Defined by feelings rather than by proximity or shared goals, friends are some of the most important people in our lives.

Friendship is a reciprocal relationship based on mutual liking and caring, respect and trust, interest and companionship. We often share a big part of our personal history with our friends. Compared with romantic partnerships, friendships are usually more stable and longer lasting; in fact, some last a lifetime. Many people have hundreds of acquaintances but only three to seven people they would really call friends.

Research shows that friendships, along with family ties and involvement in social activities, offer a psychological and emotional buffer against stress, anxiety, and depression. They help protect you against illness, and they help you cope with problems if you do become ill. Friendships and other kinds of social support increase your sense of belonging, purpose, and self-worth.[1] For tips on cultivating friendships, see the box "Expanding Your Circle of Friends."

Strengths of Successful Partnerships

An intimate relationship with a partner has many similarities with friendships, but it has other qualities as well. Compared with friendships, partnerships are more

HIGHLIGHT ON HEALTH
Seeking: Someone Just Like Me

Most people are seeking a partner who is similar to them in qualities such as income, beauty, and desire to have children. In one study, participants were asked to rate themselves on a scale from 1 to 9 on the following attributes: financial resources, physical attractiveness, faithfulness, parenting qualities, social status, health, desire for children, ambition, and strength of family bonds. They were then asked to rate the importance of

each of these attributes in their choice of a long-term partner on the same 1–9 scale. The biggest predictor of the importance of any attribute in a partner was where the participant placed him- or herself on the scale.

Source: "Cognitive Processes Underlying Human Mate Choice: The Relationship Between Self-Perception and Mate Preference in Western Society," by P. M. Buston and S. T. Emlen, 2003, *Proceedings of the National Academy of Sciences, 100* (15), 8805–8810.

exclusive, involve deeper levels of connection and caring, and have a sexual component. The divorce rate tells us that many intimate partnerships are not successful. What makes them succeed? The following are some characteristics of successful partnerships:

- The more mature and independent individuals are, the more likely they are to establish intimacy in their relationship. Independence and maturity often increase with age; in fact, the best predictor of a successful marriage is the age of the partners.
- The partners have both self-esteem and mutual respect.
- The partners understand the importance of good communication and are willing to work at their communication skills.
- The partners have a good sexual relationship, one that includes the open expression of affection and respect for the other's needs and boundaries.
- The partners enjoy spending time together in leisure activities, but they also value the time they spend alone pursuing their own interests.
- The partners are able to acknowledge their strengths and failings and take responsibility for both.
- The partners are assertive about what they want and need in the relationship and flexible about accommodating the other's wants and needs. They can maintain a sense of self in the face of pressure to agree or conform.
- The partners are friends as well as lovers, able to focus unselfish caring on each other.
- The couple has good relationships with family and friends, including in-laws, members of their extended family, and other couples.
- The partners have shared spiritual values.

Developing and maintaining a successful intimate relationship takes time and effort, but it is a challenge worth pursuing.

LOVE AND INTIMACY

How do we go about finding the right person for a successful partnership, and what is involved when we fall in love? Is it all about magic and chemistry, or is there something more deliberate and purposeful about it?

Attraction

People appear to use a systematic screening process when deciding whether someone could be a potential partner. According to one scholar, love is not blind, and we do not fall in love accidentally.[3] Some of the conscious and unconscious factors that affect this process include proximity, physical attractiveness, similarity, and perhaps even a bit of biological instinct.

Proximity is an often overlooked but significant factor in how we find our romantic partners.[4,5] Simply being physically close to people makes it more likely that we will establish a relationship with them. College students develop relationships with other students in their dorms and classes, and workers develop relationships with those who work near them. Sometimes attraction is a function of familiarity, and proximity determines how often we are exposed to another person.

Of the people in proximity to us, we are most interested in those we find physically attractive. Only if we find a person attractive are we willing to consider his or her other traits. In general, people who are perceived as attractive in our society have an advantage. They are evaluated more positively by parents, teachers, and potential employers; make more money; and report having better sex with more attractive partners.

We are also drawn to people who are similar to ourselves, usually in characteristics such as age; physical traits such as height, weight, and attractiveness; educational attainment; family, ethnic, and cultural background; religion; political views; and values, beliefs, and interests. (See the box "Seeking: Someone Just Like Me.") We are attracted to people who agree with us, validate our opinions, and share our attitudes. Even though opposites may initially attract, partners who are like each other tend to have more successful relationships. The more differences partners have, the more important communication skills become.

Some theorists propose that our attractions to potential mates have a biological, evolutionary basis. They suggest that on some level, women seek mates who have or can obtain necessary resources and can provide a safe and comfortable home for them and their children. They are less interested in a man's physical attractiveness and more interested in his social and economic status, his ambition and power, and his character and intelligence.[3] Women are willing to marry less attractive older men if they earn more money and have more education than the women do.

Men, according to this view, seek mates who can give them strong and healthy children, and consequently they pursue women who are physically attractive (which can be an indicator of good health). Men are willing to marry women who are younger than them, who have less education, who are not likely to hold a steady job, and who are likely to earn less money than they do, all because such women are thought (on some level) to be better procreators. This evolutionary view has incited controversy and debate, with opponents insisting such differences in attraction are the result of socialization and learning.

The Process of Finding a Partner: Dating and More

How do people actually find a suitable mate? A generation or two ago, dating fulfilled this function. Dating relationships followed a somewhat predictable course. People met through their friends or daily activities, and the man took the initiative in asking the woman for a date. After a period of formal and informal dating, the two might make a commitment to "go steady" or get engaged. After months or even years in a committed relationship, the couple might decide to get married, usually after the man proposed.

Does this model of mate selection still apply in the 21st century? For some couples, it does. Others prefer a different approach. According to a survey of more than 1,000 college women, the newer trends of "hanging out" and "hooking up" are popular alternatives to traditional dating.[6] Singles might hang out with a group of 5 or 10 friends rather than pairing off with a partner and doing only couple's activities. Hooking up (sex without commitment) was reported to be widespread on many campuses and had many levels, from kissing, to oral sex, to intercourse. The survey found it was rare for college men to ask women out on dates or to acknowledge they had become a

couple. Still, the study reported that marriage remains a major life goal for the majority of college women; most would like to meet a spouse while at college.

Both in and out of college, many people prefer a more flexible approach to finding a life partner than traditional dating. For example, women often take the lead in asking men out and playing a more assertive role in the development of the relationship. Many people place personal ads in newspapers, search for partners on the Internet, or use dating services to find a suitable mate. Others participate in "speed dating" events, in which they spend a designated period of time talking with each of several other participants over the course of the evening, often over dinner.

It makes sense to cast a wide net in the search for a partner. Even participating in such activities as social groups, volunteering, sports, and church may not bring you in contact with a broad range of people. Furthermore, most people lead busy lives, and these approaches to dating enhance your ability to be selective. For example, Internet dating services provide detailed personal profiles of potential partners so you can eliminate those who will not be a good match for you. Still, you need to be cautious in pursuing a relationship with someone you meet over the Internet. For some guidelines, see the box "Tips for Internet Dating."

No matter how you approach the process of finding a suitable partner, it should be a time for fun and mutual enjoyment and a way to get to know another person. The following are some suggestions for making this experience rewarding:

- Take things slowly. Reveal information about yourself gradually; otherwise, it can be overwhelming to the other person.
- Do not feel the need to become physically involved right away; becoming friends first is better for a relationship.
- Get to know the person's friends and family members if you can. You can learn a great deal about someone from the other people in his or her life. Also notice how the person treats other people. Look for someone who is respectful to everyone.
- Keep in mind that the traits you dislike in the beginning will probably bother you even more as time goes by.
- Be honest about who you are.

Theories of Love

Of all the people we are attracted to and all the potential mates we screen, what makes us fall in love with one or two or a few in a lifetime? The beginning stages of falling in love can feel like a roller-coaster ride, taking the lovers from the heights of euphoria to the depths of despair. They may actually become "love sick" and find themselves

Consumer Clipboard

Tips for Internet Dating

Know how to guard your safety, privacy, and emotional energy when dating through the Internet. Here are some tips.

- Allow for the "cyber exaggeration" factor. Most people lie a little about their age, looks, job, salary, or marital status. Some people lie a lot.

- Use your instincts. If you feel uncomfortable, discontinue the conversation and do not meet the person. Advise the dating service or bulletin board if you feel your experience with the person was threatening or dangerous.

- If you decide to meet someone in person, choose a public place and make it a coffee date. A person who insists on meeting for dinner or at a bar might be overeager or need to drink to feel comfortable.

- Tell a friend you are meeting someone you met on the Internet and say where and when. Print the profile of the person you are meeting and give it to your friend. Ask your friend to call you on your cell phone during the meeting to check in with you.

- Be aware that communication on the Internet can become intimate quickly and you may find yourself writing things you would never say to someone in person at an early stage of a relationship. When meeting in person, do not skip the usual steps in getting to know someone. Act in a manner appropriate to meeting a person for the first time, regardless of previous conversations or perceived closeness.

- Schedule a half-hour meeting at most. If it's not working out, be ready with a simple statement, such as "I've really appreciated meeting you, but I think I'm looking for a different match and I don't want to take more of your time. Thank you and good luck." Don't invent ridiculous excuses. Be polite and decisive.

- Limit your search to people who live within 30 or 40 miles of you. Otherwise, you may end up having a long-distance relationship, or the relationship will suffer from time and distance strains.

- Don't get discouraged. Ask your friends for their support and encouragement in your search.

---

unable to eat, sleep, or think of anything but the object of their desire. These early stages of a love relationship are typically romantic, idealistic, and passionate. The lovers are absorbed in each other and want to spend all their time together, sometimes to the exclusion of other people and everyday responsibilities.

Researchers think this experience of love involves increased levels of the neurotransmitter dopamine in the brain.[4] As we have seen in the context of psychoactive drugs (Chapter 12), dopamine is associated with the experience of pleasure. Love also causes arousal of the sympathetic nervous system, as evidenced by such physiological signs as increased heart rate, respiration, and perspiration.

These responses gradually decrease as the relationship develops and progresses. Intense passion may subside as lovers become habituated to each other. In some cases, passion continues at a more bearable level and intimacy deepens; the relationship becomes more fulfilling and comes to include affection, empathy, tolerance, caring, and attachment. The partners are able to become involved in the world again, while maintaining their connection

with each other. In other cases, the lessening of passion signals the ending of the relationship; the lovers drift apart, seeking newer, more satisfying partnerships.

Similarity Theories

Some theories of love propose that these experiences of passion and fascination occur because people have found partners with whom they share many important similarities. In other words, according to **similarity theories,** not only are individuals attracted to people similar to them, but they also fall in love with them and choose them as partners. Many people prefer a partner

KEY TERMS

similarity theories Theories of attraction and mate selection stating that people fall in love with people who are similar to themselves.

with similar personality traits. Having a partner with a similar personality validates and reinforces our perceptions of ourselves. The **theory of narcissism** proposes that we tend to love in other people what we love in ourselves.

Research has supported the idea that similarity underlies romantic love and perhaps even the ability to reproduce. Differences can be exciting in a relationship, but couples with great similarity seem to have higher fertility rates, greater marital harmony, and greater overall life satisfaction than do couples with more differences.

Social Exchange Theory

A rather unromantic view of love is offered by **social exchange theory.** This theory suggests that falling in love and choosing a partner are based on the exchange of "commodities." These commodities include love, represented by warmth, affection, care, and comfort; status, an increase or decrease in self-worth; information, attained by advice and knowledge; property and money; goods; and services, such as mechanical skills or cooking.[7]

Most of our interactions involve some type of exchange; for example, we return love when we receive love. The social exchange theory of love proposes that we are looking for someone who can meet not just our emotional and sexual needs but also our needs for security, status, money, goods, and more. Studies report that partners seldom cite "filling of needs" when asked what they seek in a romantic relationship,[8,9] but psychologists suggest that "filling needs" may not be a socially acceptable answer.

Sternberg's Love Triangle

Psychologist Robert Sternberg has proposed a view of love that can give us insight into its various aspects. In this view, love has three dimensions: intimacy, passion, and commitment. **Intimacy** is the emotional component of love and includes feelings of closeness, warmth, openness, and affection. **Passion** is the sexual component of love; it includes attraction, romance, excitement, and physical intensity. **Commitment** is the decision aspect of a relationship, the pledge that you will stay with your partner through good times and bad, despite the possibility of disappointment and disillusionment.[10]

Different combinations of these three components produce different kinds of love. When there is only intimacy, the relationship is likely to be a friendship. Passion alone is infatuation, the high-intensity early stage of a love relationship. Commitment alone is characteristic of a dutiful, obligatory relationship, one that many people would consider empty. When there is both intimacy and passion, the relationship is a romantic one; commitment may develop in time. When there is passion and commitment, the relationship has probably developed rapidly, without

the partners' getting to know each other very well; when passion fades, there may not be much substance to this type of relationship. When there is intimacy and commitment but no passion, the relationship may have evolved into more of a long-term friendship; Sternberg calls this relationship **companionate love.** Finally, when all three components are present, the couple has **consummate love.**[10] This type of relationship is what we all dream of, but it's difficult to find and even harder to sustain. To evaluate your relationship, see the Add It Up! feature at the end of this chapter.

Some researchers have found that life satisfaction is more strongly predicted by companionate love (high levels of commitment and intimacy, low level of passion) than by passionate love (high level of passion).[11] Companionate love is more characteristic of couples who have been married for years. Passionate love includes more intense emotions, both positive and negative. However love is conceptualized, it is something that enhances happiness and satisfaction in life.

COMMUNICATION

We establish, maintain, and nourish our relationships—or, alternatively, damage and destroy them—through communication. Clear, positive communication is a key to successful intimate relationships. This doesn't mean you should "tell all" at the beginning of a relationship or deliver the "brutal truth" in the middle of a heated argument. It does mean that you are honest and open and communicate in a caring, respectful way. It also means learning to listen when your partner has the floor.

Nonverbal Behavior and Metamessages

A good deal of communication takes place as **nonverbal communication,** through facial expressions, eye contact, gestures, body position and movement, and spatial behavior (how far apart people sit or stand). People tend to monitor their verbal behavior—what they say—much more carefully than their nonverbal behavior, yet nonverbal communication may convey their real message. Researchers studying nonverbal communication in married couples have found correlations between the quality of a relationship and nonverbal behavior. Couples with less disagreement in their relationship sit closer to each other, touch each other more during discussion, make eye contact more frequently, and display more open body postures than do couples with more disagreement.

Nonverbal behavior is part of the **metamessage,** the unspoken message you send or get when you are communicating. The metamessage encompasses all the conscious and unconscious aspects of a message, including the way something is said, who says it, when and where it is said,

Healthy People 2010

OBJECTIVE AREA *Health Communication*

- Use communication strategically to improve health.

"Studies indicate that patients find communicating with their health care providers difficult . . . and report that providers do not give them enough information, even though they highly value the information and want to know more. . . . Clear, candid, accurate, culturally and linguistically competent provider-patient communication is essential for the prevention, diagnosis, treatment, and management of health concerns . . ."

 For more information on the Healthy People 2010 objectives, visit the Web site at www.healthypeople.gov.

For more information on Canadian health objectives, visit the Health Canada Web site at www.hc-sc.gc.ca/english.

or even that it is said at all. It includes the meaning and intent behind a message. Often, the metamessage is what triggers an emotional response rather than just the words someone says. When you find yourself in an escalating argument, stop and "metacommunicate," or talk about the way you are talking. What you are perceiving as condescending or insulting, for example, may not be meant that way; if you seek clarification, you may discover this. On the other hand, a gut reaction can be an accurate reading of intent, and metacommunicating is a way to explore feelings and meanings that may be hidden or unconscious.

Building Communication Skills

People who are good communicators have many personal attributes that contribute to their success, such as empathy, interest in others, a sense of humor, and a history of positive interactions with others. There are also some specific skills that people can learn and practice in order to be better communicators, both when they speak and when they listen.

One aspect of being an effective communicator when you speak is knowing what you want to say. Examine your own feelings, motives, and intentions before you speak. When you do speak, use "I" statements to state what you feel or want in a clear, direct way without blaming or accusing the other person. Using "I" statements helps you take responsibility for your own emotions and reactions rather than trying to place responsibility on someone else. For example, it is more productive to say, "I

feel . . . when you . . ." than to say, "You make me feel . . ." Saying what you would like to have happen is also more productive than complaining about what isn't happening. Other keys to positive, effective communication are avoiding generalizations, making specific requests, and remaining calm. If you feel yourself starting to get angry, take a time-out and come back to the conversation after you cool off.

When you are the listener, do just that—listen. Don't interrupt, give advice, explain, judge, analyze, defend yourself, or offer solutions. Give the other person the floor, along with the time and space to say fully what is on his or her mind, just as you would like when you are speaking. Show with your body language that you are paying attention and are present. If you don't understand something, seek clarification at an appropriate point. Attentive listening shows that you respect the other person and care about him or her. It is the cornerstone of good communication.

KEY TERMS

theory of narcissism   The view that people love in other people what they love in themselves.

social exchange theory   Theory stating that people fall in love and choose a mate based on the exchange of commodities, such as love, status, money, and services.

intimacy   Emotional component of love, including feelings of closeness, warmth, openness, and affection; one of the three dimensions of love in Sternberg's love triangle.

passion   Sexual component of love, including attraction, romance, excitement, and physical intensity; one of the three dimensions of love in Sternberg's love triangle.

commitment   The decision aspect of a relationship, the pledge to stay with a partner through good times and bad; one of the three dimensions of love in Sternberg's love triangle.

companionate love   In Sternberg's theory, love with intimacy and commitment but no passion.

consummate love   In Sternberg's theory, love with intimacy, passion, and commitment.

nonverbal communication   Communication that takes place without words, mainly through body language.

metamessage   The unspoken message in a communication; the meaning behind the message, conveyed by nonverbal behavior and by situational factors such as how, when, and where the message is delivered.

HIGHLIGHT ON HEALTH

A Caring Approach to Conflict Resolution

Research indicates that all couples fight and that most fights are never resolved. The difference between unhappy and happy couples is *how* they fight. Although effective listening contributes to the overall health of a relationship, it appears that being a good listener requires too much of partners when the argument gets heated. Instead, partners in successful marriages seem to be able to moderate their responses during conflict to avoid inflicting permanent damage on the relationship. Here are some characteristics of this approach to conflict:

- Gentleness and compassion are key ingredients in successful relationships. Partners who couch their criticisms and complaints in a gentle, soothing, and even humorous approach are more likely to have a happy relationship than those who are belligerent.

- Successful relationships are strongly correlated with men yielding to the influences of their partners. When partners share power, conflicts are more readily resolved.

- Anger itself is not destructive in a relationship, but criticism, defensiveness, contempt, and stonewalling are counterproductive and damaging during conflict. They can lead to escalation, withdrawal, and distancing, all of which are associated with lower relationship satisfaction.

- When the focus is more on having a good discussion than on finding a solution to a problem, the outcome is more satisfactory. Discussion and problem solving can be treated as two separate parts of conflict resolution.

- Couples who report being happy have come to terms with their irresolvable differences and have learned to work around them while continuing to love each other. They don't let the differences poison the wonderful things in their relationship.

Sources: "Predicting Marital Happiness and Stability from Newlywed Interactions," by J. Gottman, et al., 1998, *Journal of Marriage and Family, 60,* pp. 5–22 © 1998 by the National Council on Family Relations, 3989 Central Ave. NE, Suite 550, Minneapolis, MN 55421, reprinted by permission; "Married with Problems? Therapy May Not Help," by Susan Gilbert, April 19, 2005, *The New York Times.*

If you and your partner are experiencing conflict, good communication skills can help you resolve it constructively. Conflict is a normal part of healthy relationships. Often, it is a sign that partners are maintaining their right to be different people and to have different points of view; it can also indicate that the relationship is changing or growing. See the box "A Caring Approach to Conflict Resolution" for some insights on how partners in successful relationships approach conflict.

When you are trying to resolve a conflict with your partner, keep the topic narrow. Try not to generalize to other topics, incidents, or issues. You might want to set a specific time and place to have your conversation, making sure it's quiet and private. You might also want to set a time limit on your discussion. Avoid being either passive or aggressive; **assertiveness** means speaking up for yourself without violating someone else's rights. Don't exaggerate or use sarcasm, and don't be afraid to admit you are wrong or sorry. Be prepared to negotiate and compromise, but don't give up something that is really important to you (for example, time to keep up your other friendships). If you feel that demands are being made on you that you cannot or do not want to meet, this may not be the right relationship for you. Communicating clearly about that is important, too.

Gender Differences in Communication Styles

Like other aspects of behavior, patterns of communication are learned and therefore subject to social and cultural influences, including gender expectations. According to linguistics scholar Deborah Tannen, gender differences in communication patterns have a significant impact on relationships. Tannen suggests that men are more likely to use communication to compete and women are more likely to use communication to connect. Men want to establish their dominance, competence, and knowledge in a conversation, and women are interested in finding commonalities, sharing experiences, and giving and receiving support.[12]

Consider this example: A woman comes home from work and tells her partner about an upsetting incident that occurred that day. He responds by giving her advice on what she should have done and said. A few days later, she tells him about another, similar incident at work. He responds by saying, "I already told you how to handle this situation." The woman feels unsupported and disappointed by this response, and her partner doesn't understand why. In this example, the woman wants to talk about the incident and have her partner show his understanding and caring by listening to her. The man wants to fix the problem; he shows his understanding and caring by giving her advice.

Although these patterns are broad and general, they are sometimes at the root of misunderstandings between men and women. If you find yourself experiencing confusion or conflict in your communications with the other sex, consider whether gender differences may be involved. Neither style is right or wrong, better or worse—they are just different.

SEX AND GENDER

Most adult partnerships and intimate relationships include a sexual component. Sexuality encompasses not just sexual behavior but also a broad set of values, beliefs, attitudes, and social behaviors. It includes biological, psychological, sociological, and cultural dimensions. We consider many of these aspects of sexuality in Chapters 15 and 16. In this section, we consider just two such dimensions—gender roles and sexual orientation.

Gender Roles

Although they are often used interchangeably, the terms *sex* and *gender* have different meanings. **Sex** refers to a person's biological status as male or female; it is usually established at birth by the appearance of the external genitals. A person with female genitals usually has XX chromosomes, and a person with male genitals usually has XY chromosomes. Sex is not always clear-cut, however. As discussed in Chapter 2, chromosomes are sometimes added, lost, or rearranged during the production of sperm and ova, causing such conditions as Klinefelter syndrome (XXY) and Turner syndrome (XO). Sometimes, as a result of genetic factors or prenatal hormonal influences, a baby is born with ambiguous genitals—a condition referred to as **intersex.** In such cases, parents and physicians are faced with the difficult task of deciding which sex to "assign" the child to. Other times, a person experiences a sense of inappropriateness about his or her sex and identifies psychologically or emotionally with the other sex.

Gender refers to the behaviors and characteristics considered appropriate for a male or female in a particular culture. "Masculine" and "feminine" traits are largely learned via the process of socialization during childhood. **Gender role** is the set of behaviors and activities a person engages in to conform to society's expectations. In our culture, for example, the traditional male gender role has been that of breadwinner and provider, and the traditional female gender role has been homemaker, wife, and mother. Gender role stereotypes suggest that a masculine man is competitive, aggressive,

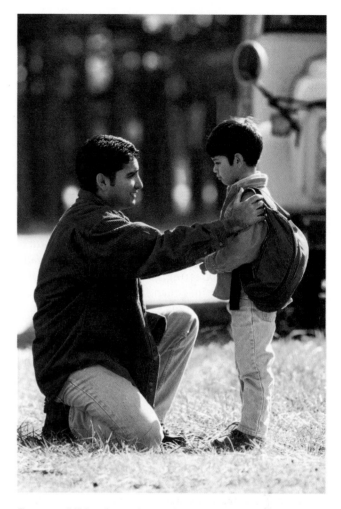

The responsibilities of parenting are often shared, with both fathers and mothers taking an active part in caring for their children. As work patterns change, gender stereotypes are being replaced by flexible parental roles.

KEY TERMS

assertiveness The ability to stand up for oneself without violating other people's rights.

sex A person's biological status as a male or a female, usually established at birth by the appearance of the external genitals.

intersex Condition in which the genitals are ambiguous at birth as a result of genetic factors or prenatal hormonal influences.

gender Masculine or feminine behaviors and characteristics considered appropriate for a male or a female in a particular culture.

gender role Set of behaviors and activities a person engages in to conform to society's expectations of his or her sex.

ambitious, power-oriented, and logical and that a feminine woman is cooperative, passive, nurturing, supportive, and emotional.

Today, we commonly assume that both genders are
capable and can be successful in a variety of roles at
home and at work. However, gender roles and gender
stereotypes are learned in childhood and become part of
who we are. They are ingrained and hard to change, even
when we are aware of them. For example, both men and
women have been shown to play the stereotyped role assigned to their gender in order to appear romantically
attractive to the other sex, and both men and women
may be initially attracted to romantic partners because
they fit the gender role stereotype.[13] After the initial attraction phase of a relationship, however, many partners
are irritated by the stereotypical traits they originally
found exciting or endearing, such as talkativeness in a
woman or reticence in a man. In long-term relationships, both sexes value traits such as honesty, empathy,
responsibility, open-mindedness, and humor, and both
tend to prefer a partner who integrates so-called masculine and feminine traits. Still, different socialization
processes are at the root of much misunderstanding and
conflict in relationships.

Sexual Orientation

Sexual orientation refers to a person's emotional, romantic, and sexual attraction to a member of the same sex, the
other sex, or both. It exists along a continuum that ranges
from exclusive heterosexuality (attraction to individuals
of the other sex) through bisexuality (attraction to individuals of both sexes) to exclusive homosexuality (attraction to individuals of one's own sex). Although the role of
genes in sexual orientation is not clearly understood (see
Chapter 2), sexual orientation is known to be influenced
by a complex interaction of biological, psychological, and
societal factors, and these factors may be different for
different people.

Sexual orientation involves a person's sense of identity. Most experts believe that it is not a choice and does
not change. It is not the result of how a person was raised
or of experiences the person had as a child. A person's sexual orientation may or may not be evidenced in his or her
appearance or behavior, and the person may choose not
to act on his or her sexual orientation. For example, a bisexual may have a committed relationship with a person
of one sex and therefore decide not to act on an attraction
to the other sex. Some people who are homosexual or bisexual may choose to hide their sexual orientation or live
as heterosexuals to avoid prejudice or, if their sexual orientation is incompatible with their personal beliefs, to
avoid their own internal dilemmas.

Heterosexuality is defined as emotional and sexual
attraction to members of the other sex. Heterosexuals are
often referred to as *straight*. Throughout the world, laws

related to marriage, child rearing, health benefits, financial matters, sexual behavior, and inheritance generally
support heterosexual relationships. **Homosexuality** is defined as emotional and sexual attraction to members of
the same sex. In today's usage, homosexual men are typically referred to as *gay,* and homosexual women are referred to either as gay or as *lesbians.*

Homosexuality occurs in all cultures, but researchers
have generally had difficulty determining exactly what
proportions of the population are straight and gay. Sex researcher Alfred Kinsey estimated that about 4 percent of
American males and 2 percent of American females were
exclusively homosexual.[14,15] The popular media tend to
place the combined figure for gay men and lesbians at
about 10 percent of the population.

People who are emotionally and sexually attracted to
both sexes are referred to as **bisexuals.** They may date
members of both sexes, or they may have a relationship
with a member of one sex for a period of time and then a
relationship with a member of the other sex for a period
of time. After having relationships with members of both
sexes, a bisexual may move toward a more exclusive orientation, either heterosexual or homosexual.

Individuals who experience discomfort or a sense of
inappropriateness about their sex (called *gender dysphoria*) and who identify strongly with the other sex are
referred to as cross-gender identified, transsexual, or
transgendered. Such individuals have a sense of identity
as male or female that conflicts with their biological sex.
Many dress in the clothes of the other sex (*cross-dressing*)
and live in society as the other sex. Some undergo surgery
and hormone treatments to experience a more complete
transformation into the other sex. Transgendered individuals have typically experienced gender dysphoria since
earliest childhood, but most children who do not fit the
cultural stereotype of masculinity or femininity do not
grow up to be transgendered. A very small percentage of
the population is transgendered.

Whether straight, gay, bisexual, or transgendered, human beings seek the same things in relationships, whether
conceptualized as intimacy, passion, and commitment or
some other combination of qualities and experiences. We
all want to be affirmed, to be wanted, to love someone and
be loved in return, to belong. These (and many others) are
basic human needs and desires that are fulfilled only in relationships with other human beings.

COMMITTED RELATIONSHIPS AND LIFESTYLE CHOICES

Society has an interest in how we form and formalize
our committed relationships, especially when child
rearing will be involved. In this section we consider
marriage, one of the most important social and legal institutions in societies throughout the world, along with

other relationship and lifestyle choices that many people make today.

Marriage

Marriage is not only the legal union of two people but also a contract between the couple and the state. In the United States, each state specifies the rights and responsibilities of the partners in a marriage. Although marriage has traditionally meant the union of a man and a woman, many same-sex couples are interested in marriage, and some states now issue marriage licenses to same-sex couples.

Marriage is by far the most popular living arrangement for adults (Table 14.1). Despite high divorce rates, 72 percent of Americans have been married by the age of 34, and 96 percent of Americans have been married by age 65. Among Americans aged 25 to 34, 48 percent of the men and 55 percent of the women are married and living with their spouse.[16]

Marriage is an opportunity to develop a physically and emotionally intimate and supportive relationship with another person. Marriage partners typically merge their social networks and their financial resources as well as their lives. Most married couples expect to become parents and view raising children as a purpose of the marriage.

Marriage confers benefits in many domains. Partnerships and family relationships provide emotional connection for individuals and stability for society. Married people live longer than single or divorced people, partly because they lead a healthier lifestyle. Married people report greater happiness than do single, widowed, or cohabiting people. Married couples have sex more frequently and consider their sexual relationship more satisfying emotionally and physically than single people. Married people are more successful in their careers, earn more, and have more wealth. Children brought up by married couples tend to be more academically successful and emotionally stable.

Characteristics of a Successful Marriage

One predictor of a successful marriage is positive reasons for getting married. Positive motivations include companionship, love and intimacy, supportive partnership, sexual compatibility, and interest in sharing parenthood. Poorer reasons for getting married, those associated with less chance of having a successful marriage, include premarital pregnancy, rebellion against parents, seeking independence, seeking economic security, family or social pressure, and rebounding from another relationship.

Love alone is not enough to make a marriage successful. Research has found that the best predictors of a happy marriage are realistic attitudes about the relationship and the challenges of marriage; satisfaction with the personal-

ity of the partner; enjoyment of communicating with the partner; ability to resolve conflicts together; agreement on religious and ethical values; egalitarian roles; and a balance of individual and joint leisure activities. (To test your ideas about strengths in marriage, see the box "Who Is Most Likely to Stay Married?") The characteristics associated with successful and unsuccessful marriages are typically present in a couple's relationship before they are married.[17]

Premarital Counseling

Because of the high divorce rate, many couples now participate in premarital counseling programs. Such programs had their origin in religious organizations in the 1950s, but today a wide variety of premarital programs is available. In 2000, between one fourth and one third of all those getting married in the United States, Australia, and Great Britain were participating in some form of relationship education.[18]

Premarital programs focus on communication skills, problem solving, conflict resolution, and positive ways of enhancing relationships. Practicing these skills before making a formal commitment allows people to find out if their partner responds in ways that will increase the relationship's chance of success. Most marriages have periods of happiness, productivity, and mutual admiration alternating with periods of unhappiness, frustration, and disillusionment. Premarital counseling programs teach couples that marriage has ups and downs and that struggles, challenges, and differences often provide opportunities for growth, both personally and in the relationship. Couples who invest some time and effort in counseling before marriage often find they can later avoid many problems and especially the trauma of divorce.

KEY TERMS

sexual orientation A person's emotional, romantic, and sexual attraction to a member of the same sex, the other sex, or both.

heterosexuality Emotional and sexual attraction to members of the other sex.

homosexuality Emotional and sexual attraction to members of the same sex.

bisexuality Emotional and sexual attraction to members of both sexes.

transgendered Having a sense of identity as a male or female that conflicts with one's biological sex; transgendered individuals experience a sense of inappropriateness about their sex and identify strongly with the other sex.

Table 14.1   U.S. Households by Type and Selected Characteristics, 2003 (In thousands, except average size)

Characteristic	Family Households				Nonfamily Households		
			Other Families				
	Total	Married Couple	Male House-holder	Female House-holder	Total	Male House-holder	Female House-holder
All households	75,596	57,320	4,656	13,620	35,682	16,020	19,662
Age of householder							
15 to 24 years	3,551	1,379	789	1,383	3,060	1,507	1,552
25 to 34 years	13,438	9,536	1,011	2,892	5,617	3,343	2,274
35 to 44 years	18,741	14,001	1,087	3,652	5,328	3,278	2,051
45 to 54 years	16,863	13,297	922	2,644	5,760	2,971	2,789
55 to 64 years	11,261	9,543	413	1,305	4,999	2,023	2,976
65 years and over	11,741	9,565	434	1,743	10,918	2,898	8,020
Race and ethnicity of householder							
White only	62,297	49,915	3,500	8,881	29,349	13,070	16,278
Non-Hispanic	53,845	44,101	2,674	7,070	27,321	11,968	15,353
Black only	8,928	4,165	762	4,000	4,538	2,043	2,495
Asian only	2,845	2,286	223	337	1,073	526	547
Hispanic (of any race)	9,090	6,189	872	2,029	2,249	1,228	1,021
Size of households							
1 person	(X)	(X)	(X)	(X)	29,431	12,511	16,919
2 people	32,047	24,310	1,992	5,745	5,031	2,660	2,371
3 people	17,076	11,526	1,403	4,147	813	556	257
4 people	15,672	12,754	733	2,185	295	212	83
5 people	6,969	5,719	296	955	60	42	17
6 people	2,489	2,004	142	344	31	19	12
7 or more people	1,343	1,007	90	246	22	19	2
Average size	3.19	3.22	3.11	3.12	1.24	1.32	1.17
Number of related children under 18							
No related children	36,685	30,261	2,240	4,183	35,682	16,020	19,662
With related children	38,911	27,059	2,416	9,437	(X)	(X)	(X)
1 child	16,511	10,378	1,429	4,704	(X)	(X)	(X)
2 children	14,333	10,800	683	2,850	(X)	(X)	(X)
3 children	5,771	4,235	220	1,317	(X)	(X)	(X)
4 or more children	2,296	1,646	84	566	(X)	(X)	(X)

Source: *Current Population Survey*, Annual Social and Economic Supplement, 2003, U.S. Census Bureau.

Note: A *household* contains one or more people; everyone living in a housing unit makes up a household.

A *family household* has at least two members related by birth, marriage, or adoption. Family households are maintained by married couples or by a man or woman living with other relatives; children may or may not be present.

A *nonfamily household* can be either a person living alone or a person who shares the housing unit only with people who are not his or her relatives, such as roommates or boarders.

Gay and Lesbian Partnerships

Like heterosexual couples, same-sex couples desire intimacy, companionship, passion, and commitment in their relationships. Because they often have to struggle with "coming out" and issues with their families, gay men and lesbians frequently have communication skills and strengths that are valuable in relationships. These qualities include flexible role relationships, the ability to adapt to a partner, the ability to negotiate and share decision-making power, and effective parenting skills among those who choose to become parents.[19,20] Unfortunately, gay men and lesbians often have to deal with **homophobia**

Beating the Odds

Who Is Most Likely to Stay Married?

Predictors of a successful marriage include emotional maturity, motivation for getting married, similarities in background and beliefs, willingness to work at the relationship, communication skills, level of commitment, and many more. Brief profiles of three couples are presented here. Which couple do you think has the best chances of staying married?

Jeff and Jolene Spencer are newlyweds. She is 24 and he is 27. They were engaged for almost 3 years before getting married. For part of that time, Jeffrey was away on a religious mission. Jolene does not have the same religious background, but she respects Jeffrey's beliefs and commitment to his faith. She has agreed to raise their children in his church. Jolene's parents were divorced when she was 12, and she is determined to make her marriage work. Jeffrey's parents wish he had chosen someone from his own religion. They feel they have nothing in common with Jolene or her parents.

Marcus Tucker and Tanya Anderson have been going together since they were sophomores in high school. They were married in their senior year, after Tanya got pregnant. They live with Marcus's parents while trying to save enough money to get their own apartment. Tanya's mother takes care of the baby during the day while they are at work, and both families help out with babysitting and financial assistance when they can. Tanya and Marcus have participated in couples workshops at the local community college and are committed to providing a secure home for their child.

Eric and Jenny Lee are both physicians in their 40s. They met in medical school, and although they weren't attracted to each other at first, they gradually came to know and respect each other. They own their own home and are financially secure, but their family members are scattered around the country. Two years ago, they lost their only child, Julie, to leukemia at the age of 6. They do not seem to have recovered from this trauma yet. Eric feels that he is going through the motions of living and drifting without purpose; Jenny has buried herself in her work. They no longer eat dinner together or sleep in the same bed.

OLC Web site Visit the **Online Learning Center** at www.mhhe.com/teague1e for comments by the authors.

(irrational fear of homosexuality and homosexuals) and discrimination as well. Same-sex relationships do not receive the same level of societal support and acceptance that heterosexual relationships do.

Researchers looking at relationship satisfaction among comparable samples of gay, lesbian, and heterosexual couples found that all three groups reported similar levels of relationship quality and satisfaction.[21] The options of domestic partnership, civil union, and marriage have become available for same-sex partners in some states. For a discussion of the debate surrounding the issue of same-sex marriage, see You Make the Call at the end of the chapter.

Cohabitation

The U.S. government defines **cohabitation** as two people of the opposite sex living together as unmarried partners. Since the 1960s, cohabitation has become one of the most rapidly growing social phenomena in the history of our society. The rate of cohabitation has increased tenfold since the 1960s, when about half a million people were living together. In 2003 approximately 4.6 million couples, or 9.2 million men and women, were identified as cohabiting. The proportion of all households identified as cohabiting couples increased from 2.9 percent in 1996 to 4.2 percent in 2003.[16]

Cohabitation seems to have become an accepted part of the process of finding a mate. Most couples today believe it is a good idea to live together in order to decide if they should get married, and more than 50 percent do live together before getting married. Yet an estimated 40 percent of these arrangements do not result in marriage.[22]

Currently, cohabitation is more common among individuals of lower socioeconomic levels. Recent data show that among women between 19 and 44 years of age, 60 percent of high school dropouts have cohabited, while

KEY TERMS

homophobia   Irrational fear of homosexuality and homosexuals.

cohabitation   Living arrangement in which two people of the opposite sex live together as unmarried partners.

Same-sex couples are gaining greater acceptance in society, but their relationship often involves stresses that heterosexual couples don't experience. If same-sex couples have children, the parents and the children both face special challenges.

37 percent of college graduates have done so. Cohabitation is also more common among individuals who have been divorced or have experienced the divorce of their parents. Individuals who are less religious than their peers, have been fatherless, or grew up in families with serious marital conflict are also more likely to cohabit.[22]

Some studies have shown that cohabitation actually decreases the likelihood of success in marriage and increases the likelihood of divorce. Such findings are controversial, however, because of the difficulty in determining whether this effect results from the characteristics of those who choose to cohabit before marriage or from the experience itself of living together before marriage.[22,23]

Divorce

For a large percentage of couples, the demands of marriage prove too difficult, and the couple chooses to divorce. The divorce rate rose rapidly in the 1970s and 1980s in the Untied States and leveled off in the 1990s. About 52 percent of marriages in the United States currently end in divorce.[24] Between 30 and 40 percent of marriages end in divorce in Canada.[25]

Most people who divorce in the United States are younger than 45 years old. Couples who marry when they are 20 or younger are more likely to split up than couples who are older when they marry. Overall, people with lower incomes and less education tend to have higher rates of divorce. Two thirds of all divorces are initiated by women, probably because it gives them a better chance of retaining custody of their children in most states. Women may also be less satisfied with their marriages than men.

Why do so many couples divorce in our society? Many couples simply cannot handle the challenges of married life. They may not have the problem-solving skills, or they may not be sufficiently committed to the relationship. Many people enter marriage with unrealistic expectations, and some people choose an unsuitable mate. Although most people marry again, at least 50 percent of those who remarry get divorced a second time.

Although divorce may seem to be a single event in a person's life, the termination of a marriage is almost always a traumatic process lasting months or years. Divorce is a leading cause of poverty, leaving many children in impoverished homes headed by a single parent, often the parent with the lower income. The number of single-mother families in the United States rose from 3 million in 1970 to 10 million in 2003, and the number of single-father families rose from under half a million to 2 million in the same period. In all, there were 12 million single-parent families in 2003.[16] Most single-parent families cannot maintain the same lifestyle that they had before the divorce.

Divorce also appears to damage physical health. Gastrointestinal and respiratory problems increase after divorce, as does the incidence of hypertension. Divorce is one of the most stressful life events a person can experience. It is especially hard on children, leading to different kinds of problems for children of different ages. Counseling can help both children and adults deal with the stress of divorce and adjust to a new life. Children are best served by continuing to have contact with both parents as long as the adults can get along.

Blended Families

Many divorced people eventually remarry, and **blended families,** in which one or both partners bring children from a previous marriage, are becoming a common form of family. Some observers suggest that blended families will be the most prevalent type of family in the United States by 2010.

Just as it takes time for a family to reorganize and stabilize itself after a divorce, it also takes time for a blended family to achieve some measure of cohesion after parents remarry. It can take 2 or more years for stepparents and stepchildren to build relationships. Adults should allow time for trust and attachment to develop before they take on a parenting role with their stepchildren. When children regularly see their noncustodial parent, they are better able to adjust to their new family. Children also adjust better if the parents in the blended family have a low-intensity relationship and if the relationships between ex-spouses are civil.

Singlehood

Although marriage continues to be a popular institution, a growing number of people in our society are unmarried. In 2003, 25 percent of women and 32 percent of men over the age of 15 had never been married. For the age group 30 to 34, 33 percent of men and 23 percent of women had never been married.[16] The biggest change in the profile of U.S. families between 1970 and 2003 was the increase in the percentage of households that were one-person households, from 17 percent to 26 percent (Figure 14.1). In other words, one in four Americans lived alone in 2003.

Part of the reason for this shift is that young people have been staying single longer and getting married later. Between 1970 and 2003, age at first marriage in the United States rose from 20.8 to 25.3 for women and from 23.2 to 27.2 for men.[16] A similar trend has occurred in Canada. Between 1980 and 2000, age at first marriage among Canadians rose from 25.9 to 31.7 for women and from 28.5 to 34.3 for men.[26]

As the age of first marriage rises, the number of single people in the population increases. Many of these young adults are delaying marriage to pursue educational and career goals, but an increasing number of people view singlehood as a legitimate, healthy, and satisfying alternative to marriage. Some people, including some highly educated professionals and career-oriented individuals, prefer to remain unmarried. In singlehood they find the freedom to pursue their own interests, spend their money as they wish, invest time in their careers, develop a broad network of friends, have a variety of sexual relationships, and enjoy opportunities for solitude. For them, being single is a positive choice.

The ranks of the single also include those who are involuntarily single, however. These include people who are divorced, separated, and widowed; they may or may not be satisfied with their unmarried state. People who enjoy being single are those who feel socially and psychologically independent, are able to handle loneliness, are able

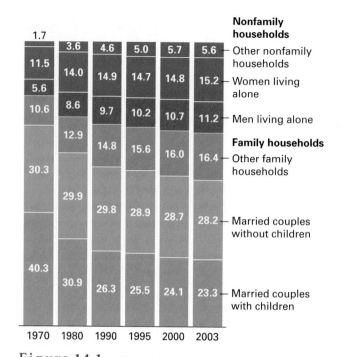

Figure 14.1   U.S. households by type, 1970–2003 (Percentage Distribution). Source: *Current Population Survey*, March and Annual Social and Economic Supplements: 1970–2003, U.S. Census Bureau.

Note: A *household* contains one or more people; everyone living in a housing unit makes up a household. A *family household* has at least two members related by birth, marriage, or adoption. Family households are maintained by married couples or by a man or woman living with other relatives; children may or may not be present. A *nonfamily household* can be either a person living alone or a person who shares the housing unit only with people who are not his or her relatives, such as roommates or boarders.

to make it on their own financially, and are proactive about creating an interesting life.

Keeping Your Relationships Strong and Vital

A characteristic of relationships—both partnerships and families—is that they change over time. Many researchers and clinicians have studied how individuals deal with roles and developmental tasks within a relationship or family unit as they move through the life cycle. No matter what specific challenges come up, three basic qualities seem to make partnerships and families strong: cohesion, flexibility, and communication.[27]

Cohesion is the dynamic balance between separateness and togetherness in both couple and family relationships. Relationships are strongest when there is a balance

KEY TERMS

blended families   Families in which one or both partners bring a child or children from a previous marriage.

HIGHLIGHT ON HEALTH
Keeping Your Relationship Vital

- Compliment your partner once or twice each day.
- Set aside 15 minutes each week to discuss one or two issues and one or two strengths of your relationship.
- Do something nice unexpectedly. Plan surprises to spice up your relationship.
- Be assertive. Ask for what you want, so your partner does not have to guess.

- Listen to your partner with care.
- Make a date with each other at least once a week, just as you did at the beginning of your relationship.
- Resolve issues as soon as possible, before they become serious.
- At least once a year, enjoy a romantic weekend away together or attend a workshop to enrich your relationship.

between intimacy and autonomy. There are times when partners and family members spend more time together and other times when they spend more time apart, but they come back to a comfortably cohesive point. *Flexibility* is the dynamic balance between stability and change. Again, relationships are strongest when there is a balance. Too much stability can cause rigidity; too much change can cause chaos. Communication is the tool that partners and families use to adjust levels of cohesion or flexibility when change is needed. (For other strengths of healthy families, see the box "Factors That Make Families Resilient" in Chapter 5, p. 122.)

How can you translate these concepts into specifics to keep your relationship strong and vital? For one thing, bringing new experiences to the relationship can help to keep it fresh and alive. This might mean trying a new restaurant or vacation site or leaving your partner a love note in the morning. For more ideas, see the box "Keeping Your Relationship Vital."

When a relationship seems to need more than revitalizing, professional counseling can be helpful. If the problem persists for 2 or 3 months and you are not able to resolve it, you should probably seek help. Couples who receive help with difficulties before they become too severe have a better chance of overcoming the problems and developing a stronger relationship than do those who delay. Marriage and family therapists are specifically trained to help couples and families with relationship problems. Look for a therapist who is licensed by your state or who is a certified member of the American Association for Marriage and Family Therapists (AAMFT). Your physician or clergy person may be able to recommend a qualified professional. A couples therapist can help you develop the strengths and resources you need to nourish and enhance this vital part of your life.

You Make the Call

Should Same-Sex Marriage Be Legal?

Although marriage has traditionally been defined as a religious and legal commitment between a man and a woman, many committed same-sex partners are challenging this definition and demanding the right to marry. In a few states, they have won some rights. In Vermont and Connecticut, same-sex civil unions offer couples many of the rights of marriage, and Hawaii's Reciprocal Beneficiaries law offers some marriagelike benefits. Maine, New Jersey, and California offer domestic partnerships, with a range of rights and benefits. In Massachusetts, same-sex couples are entitled to full marriage rights as a result of a 2003 Supreme Court ruling in that state. Changes in state laws and court rulings are ongoing.

Other states have passed "defense of marriage" acts, stating that marriage is a union between one man and one woman. They have done so because the "full faith and credit" clause of the U.S. Constitution requires that any law passed in one state be honored in all other states. To further circumvent this clause, President Clinton signed the Defense of Marriage Act (DOMA) in 1996, making the same claim law at the federal level. The passage of these laws creates a conflict with laws allowing same-sex unions. The debate continues.

What is at stake in this issue? Proponents of same-sex marriage point out that the Fourteenth Amendment to the U.S. Constitution prohibits the states from denying any citizen the equal protection of the laws, and many state constitutions protect equal rights for all. Proponents claim that same-sex couples are being discriminated against and denied equal rights by not being allowed to marry. Marriage gives heterosexual couples hundreds of legal, economic, and social benefits and rights, in areas such as child custody, joint ownership of property, taxation, health insurance, Social Security and pensions, medical decision making, inheritance, legal protection, and many others. Proponents argue that gay people are unfairly denied access to the same benefits that are available to heterosexual people.

Opponents of same-sex marriage argue that the Bible condemns homosexuality and that virtually all major religions consider gay relationships sinful or immoral. They further argue that a nation's laws should reflect the moral values on which it is founded and that many U.S. laws have their origin in religious teachings, such as the injunction against murder. Because laws imply moral approval of a behavior and shape the attitudes of society, legalizing same-sex unions condones behavior that the majority of people find unacceptable. Some but not all opponents with a religious orientation also argue that the purpose of marriage is procreation and because same-sex couples do not produce children, they are not entitled to be married.

Supporters of same-sex marriage respond to the religious argument by citing the U.S. Constitution. The First Amendment prohibits the establishment of a state religion, which is the basis for the separation of church and state in the United States. Laws based on religious views are not constitutional, nor is discrimination against an individual or a group on the basis of religious views. Even if certain churches do not want to perform same-sex marriages, marriage as a secular institution should be available to all.

Another argument against legalizing same-sex marriage is that doing so threatens the sanctity of marriage, one of society's most revered institutions. Marriage is the basis of the family, and one of the family's most important functions is raising and socializing children. Marriage is already in a precarious state in the United States, and legalizing gay marriage would further weaken it and cause it to lose respect, according to this view. Some opponents argue that if marriage is opened up to same-sex couples, it would lead down the "slippery slope" to marriage between multiple persons, marriage between friends for tax purposes, or even marriage to an animal. We need a firm definition of marriage to discourage such an explosion of possibilities, in the opinion of these opponents.

Supporters of same-sex marriage respond that society is changing and that sometimes the law has to take the lead in securing social justice for all. They point out that civil rights laws had to be passed to back up principles on which the United States was founded, such as that all people have equal rights. They note that interracial marriage was illegal in the United States until the Supreme Court ruled otherwise in 1967. Prohibiting marriage between same-sex partners is a form of minority discrimination, as it would be if African American or Hispanic partners were not allowed to marry. Like interracial marriage, gay marriage is an idea whose time has come.

Proponents also say that allowing gay people to marry would only strengthen the institution of marriage, creating more families and environments for child rearing and promoting family values. They note that no research has ever shown that being raised by same-sex parents results in psychological or emotional harm or causes children to become gay or lesbian. They assert that the institution of marriage is far less threatened by gay marriage than by the social forces that have been eroding it for the past 50 years.

Some opponents say that same-sex partners who want to publicly declare their commitment to each other should be satisfied with the options of civil union or domestic partnership where available, leaving the institution of marriage to heterosexual couples. Proponents respond that these are second-class options, analogous to the "separate but equal" schools and facilities provided for African Americans until they were declared unconstitutional by the Supreme Court in 1954.

Should marriage be an option for everyone, or should it be limited to heterosexual couples? What do you think?

Pros

- All citizens are entitled to equal rights and equal protection under the law. When same-sex partners are prohibited from marrying, they are denied access to the many rights and benefits available to their fellow citizens who are heterosexual and thus allowed to marry. Prohibiting same-sex marriage is a form of discrimination.

- Prohibiting gay marriage on religious grounds is unconstitutional, as is discrimination based on religious views.

- Society is changing, and sometimes law and society have to lead the way in areas of social justice, setting a standard that encourages people to reconsider their prejudices. This was the case with many civil rights laws. Gay marriage is an idea whose time has come.

- Gay people form the same kind of loving, committed relationships as heterosexual people and have the same right to formalize their relationships in the eyes of society and the law.

- Gay marriage increases the number of committed relationships and families in society and promotes family values.

- Domestic partnerships and civil unions provide couples some rights at the state level, but many of the rights and benefits of marriage are conferred at the federal level, as, for example, in tax laws. Thus, these options are not the same as marriage.

Cons

- Virtually all major religions consider homosexuality sinful or immoral; this value should be reflected in the nation's laws. Legalizing gay marriage would

- condone behavior that the majority of people consider immoral or unacceptable.
- Legalizing gay marriage weakens the institution of marriage and threatens its sanctity. Opening up marriage to same-sex partners would lead to new definitions of marriage and family, contributing to a further devaluation of marriage and a decline in family values.

- The purpose of marriage is procreation. Since same-sex couples do not procreate, they do need the protection or validation of marriage.
- Marriage is one of the most important traditional social institutions, and in nearly all societies it is considered to be a union between one man and one woman.

OLC Web site For more information about this topic, visit the Online Learning Center at www.mhhe.com/teaguele.

SUMMARY

- Relationships and social support are a vital part of wellness. Healthy relationships start with a healthy sense of self.
- Friendships are important relationships based on mutual liking and caring, respect and trust, interest and companionship. They increase a person's sense of belonging, self-worth, and purpose.
- Partnerships have many similarities with friendships but are more exclusive, involve deeper levels of caring and connection, and include a sexual component.
- Individuals employ a systematic screening process to identify potential mates. Attraction is influenced by proximity, physical attractiveness, similarity, and perhaps biological instincts. Methods of finding a partner range from traditional dating to searching for a match on the Internet.
- Falling in love is an intense experience of fascination with and absorption in another person, accompanied by high levels of desire and passion. Theories propose that people fall in love with people who are like them or with whom they can have an equitable exchange of so-called commodities, such as love, status, money, or services. Sternberg's love triangle identifies intimacy, passion, and commitment as the three main components of love.
- Communication is the key to successful relationships. A large proportion of communication is nonverbal.
- Communication skills include clearly and honestly stating your feelings, thoughts, and needs and attentively and respectfully listening to your partner's statements. Good communication skills can help couples resolve conflict.

- Gender differences in communication styles can make it difficult for partners to understand each other's meanings and intentions.
- Gender roles are the behaviors and activities that people adopt to conform to their society's expectations for people of their sex. Most people prefer partners who can be successful in a variety of roles and who integrate both masculine and feminine traits in their personalities.
- Sexual orientation is a person's emotional and sexual attraction to members of the same sex (homosexuality), the other sex (heterosexuality), or both sexes (bisexuality). No matter what their sexual orientation, all human beings seek love, affirmation, and other positive experiences in relationships.
- Marriage, the legal union of two people, is the most popular living arrangement for adults. Cohabitation is a rapidly growing social phenomenon that seems to have become an accepted part of the mate selection process.
- More than half of all marriages in the United States end in divorce, leading to an increasing prevalence of blended families made up of previously married adults and their children. Singlehood is another rapidly growing choice in relationship status and lifestyle.
- Three basic qualities that make relationships and partnerships strong are cohesion, flexibility, and communication. Most people find that relationships are worth the attention, time, and energy they require.

REVIEW QUESTIONS

1. Why are friendships and other kinds of social support important?
2. How is an intimate relationship different from a friendship? What are some qualities that contribute to the success of an intimate relationship?
3. Why are people attracted to partners who are similar to them?
4. Describe some differences in what women and men may be looking for in a mate. Explain the possible evolutionary basis for these differences.

5. What is the social exchange theory of attraction and mate selection?

6. Describe how the three components of the love triangle might be combined to result in different kinds of relationships.

7. What are some components of nonverbal communication? Why is it important?

8. What are some qualities of good communication when you are the speaker? When you are the listener? What are some guidelines for effective conflict resolution?

9. Explain how gender differences might affect the ability of couples to communicate.

10. What is the difference between sex and gender?

11. Describe the three kinds of sexual orientation. What does it mean to be transgendered?

12. What are some features of a successful marriage? What are some predictors of marital dissatisfaction?

13. Why do some couples choose to live together as unmarried partners rather than get married?

14. What are some of the negative effects of divorce?

15. What are some of the reasons people choose to be single?

16. What are cohesion and flexibility in the context of strong relationships and families?

WEB RESOURCES

American Association for Marriage and Family Therapy: At this Web site, you can view FAQs about marriage and family therapy, read updates on family problems, locate a family therapist in your area, and find listings of books, articles, and other resources related to family problems. www.aamft.org

American Psychological Association Help Center: The Families and Relationships section of this site features a wide variety of information, such as communication tips, psychological tasks for a good marriage, stepfamily issues, and social life problems. www.apahelpcenter.org

E-Mail Communication and Relationships: Featured on the Rider University Web site, this article addresses the topic of how e-mail affects communication and relationships. With a light-hearted look at how this medium affects the message, it addresses such issues as e-mail stress and cross-cultural e-mail. www.rider.edu/~suler/psycyber/emailrel.html

Family Pride Coalition: This organization promotes equality for lesbian, gay, bisexual, and transgendered parents and their children. The site offers educational information on parenting and diversity issues, legal rights, adoption, school environment, and other related topics. www.familypride.org

National Council on Family Relations: This professional organization offers information on families and family relationships.

Go to its Families section for family tips, expert information on family life, and links to other resources on family issues. www.ncfr.org

Parents Without Partners: This international organization addresses the special issues of rearing children alone for adults who are divorced, widowed, or never married. In addition to study groups, publications, and social activities for families and adults, it offers a parenting e-mail newsletter and links to many other parenting resources. www.parentswithoutpartners.org

Prepare-Enrich / Life Innovations: This site offers a stronger-marriage inventory, a quiz for couples, information on finding a marriage counselor, and other resources for couples. www.prepare-enrich.com

Psychology Today: This journal's Web site offers a relationships section that addresses topics such as how to make marriage work and conflict resolution. It also features self-assessments on communication skills, argument styles, and relationship pitfalls. www.psychologytoday.com

Whole Family Center: This site has resources for the whole family, teens, married couples, parents, and seniors. Its interactive features let you observe counseling in action and follow real-life family dramas in dialogue and video format. www.wholefamily.com

REFERENCES

1. Social support: A buffer against life's ills. (2005). www.mayoclinic.com.

2. Pogrebin, L. C. (1988). *Among friends: Who we like, why we like them, and what we do with them.* New York: McGraw-Hill.

3. Pines, A. M. (1999). *Falling in love: Why we choose the lovers we choose.* New York: Routledge Press.

4. Fisher, H. (2004). *Why we love: The nature and chemistry of romantic love.* New York: Henry Holt.

5. Moreland, R. L., & Beach, S. (1992). Exposure effects in the classroom: The development of affinity among students. *Journal of Experimental Social Psychology, 28,* 255–276.

6. Glenn, N., & Marquardt, E. (2001). Hanging out, hooking up, and hoping for Mr. Right. Institute for American Values. www.americanvalues.org.

7. Gangestad, S. W., & Simpson, J. A. (2000). The evolution of human mating: Tradeoffs and strategic pluralism. *Behavioral and Brain Sciences, 23,* 573–644.

8. Kendrick, D. T., Grot, G. E., Trose, M. R., & Sadalla, E. (1993). Integrating evolutionary and social exchange perspectives on relationships: Effects of gender, self-appraisal and involvement level on mate selection criteria. *Journal of Personality and Social Psychology, 64,* 951–969.

9. Pines, A. M. (2001). The role of gender and culture in romantic attraction. *European Psychologist, 6* (2), 96–102.

10. Sternberg, R. J. (1988). *The triangle of love.* New York: Basic Books.

11. Jungsik, K., & Hatfield, E. (2004). Love types and subjective well-being: A cross-cultural study. *Social Behavior and Personality: An International Journal, 32,* 173–182.

12. Tannen, D. (2001). *I only say this because I love you.* New York: Random House.

13. Gallup Organization. (2000, December). Gallup poll: Traits of males and females.

14. Kinsey, A. C., Pomeroy, W. B., & Martin, C. E. (1948). *Sexual behavior in the human male.* Reprint edition, 1998. Bloomington, IN: Indiana University Press.

15. Kinsey, A. C., Pomeroy, W. B., Martin, C. E., & Gebhard, P. H. (1953). *Sexual behavior in the human female.* Reprint edition, 1998. Bloomington, IN: Indiana University Press.

16. Fields, J. (2004, November). America's families and living arrangements. 2003. *Current Population Reports,* 1–25. Washington, DC: U.S. Census Bureau.

17. Olson, D. H., & Olson, A. K. (2000). *Empowering couples: Building on your strengths.* Minneapolis, MN: Life Innovations.

18. Halford, W. K., et al. (2002). Relationship enhancement. In D. H. Sprenkle (Ed.), *Effectiveness research in marriage and family therapy.* Alexandria, VA: American Association of Marriage and Family Therapy.

19. Bepko, C., & Johnson, T. (2000). Gay and lesbian couples in therapy: Perspectives for the contemporary family therapist. *Journal of Marital and Family Therapy, 26* (4), 409–419.

20. van Wormer, K., Wells, U., & Boes, M. (2000). *Social work with lesbians, gays, and bisexuals: A strengths perspective.* Boston: Allyn & Bacon.

21. Gottman, J., & Levenson, R. L. (2004). 12-year study of gay and lesbian couples. Gottman Institute. www.gottman.com.

22. Popenoe, D., & Whitehead, B. D. (2004). *The state of our unions: The social health of marriage in America.* The National Marriage Project. Rutgers, The State University of New Jersey. http://marriage.rutgers.edu.

23. Cohan, C., & Kleinbaum, S. (2000). Toward a greater understanding of the cohabitation effect: Premarital cohabitation and marital communication. *Journal of Marriage and Family, 64,*180–192.

24. *Statistics.* (2001). Washington, DC: U.S. Census Bureau.

25. Canadian statistics. (2003). www.rainbows.ca/statistics.html.

26. Child and Family Canada. (2005). Divorce: Facts, figures and consequences. www.cfc-ef.ca.

27. Olson, D. H., & Defrain, J. (2003). *Marriage and families: Intimacy, diversity, and strength* (4th ed.). New York: McGraw-Hill.

Add It Up!

STERNBERG'S TRIANGULAR LOVE SCALE

How does Sternberg's triangular love model relate to your relationships? Consider an important love relationship you have had with someone in the last few years. Read the following statements and rate your agreement with each one, on a scale of 1 to 9, with 1 indicating you don't agree at all, 5 indicating you agree moderately, and 9 indicating you agree strongly. After rating all the items, consult the scoring key at the end of the scale.

1	2	3		4	5	6		7	8	9
Not at all				Moderately				Strongly		

Intimacy Component

_____ 1. I actively support my partner's well-being.

_____ 2. I have a warm relationship with my partner.

_____ 3. I can count on my partner in times of need.

_____ 4. My partner can count on me in times of need.

_____ 5. I am willing to share my possessions and myself with my partner.

_____ 6. I receive considerable emotional support from my partner.

_____ 7. I give considerable emotional support to my partner.

_____ 8. I communicate well with my partner.

_____ 9. I value my partner greatly in my life.

_____ 10. I feel close to my partner.

_____ 11. I have a comfortable relationship with my partner.

_____ 12. I feel that I really understand my partner.

_____ 13. I feel that my partner really understands me.

_____ 14. I feel that I can really trust my partner.

_____ 15. I share deeply personal information about myself with my partner.

Passion Component

_____ 16. Just seeing my partner excites me.

_____ 17. I find myself thinking about my partner frequently during the day.

_____ 18. My relationship with my partner is very romantic.

_____ 19. I find my partner very attractive.

_____ 20. I idealize my partner.

_____ 21. I cannot imagine another person making me as happy as my partner does.

_____ 22. I would rather be with my partner than with anyone else.

_____ 23. Nothing is more important to me than my relationship with my partner.

_____ 24. I especially like physical contact with my partner.

_____ 25. There is something almost "magical" about my relationship with my partner.

_____ 26. I adore my partner.

_____ 27. I cannot imagine life without my partner.

_____ 28. My relationship with my partner is passionate.

_____ 29. When I see romantic movies and read romantic books, I think of my partner.

_____ 30. I fantasize about my partner.

Decision/Commitment Component

_____ 31. I know that I care about my partner.

_____ 32. I am committed to maintaining my relationship with my partner.

_____ 33. Because of my commitment to my partner, I would not let other people come between us.

_____ 34. I have confidence in the stability of my relationship with my partner.

_____ **35.** I could not let anything get in the way of my commitment to my partner.

_____ **36.** I expect my love for my partner to last for the rest of my life.

_____ **37.** I will always feel a strong responsibility for my partner.

_____ **38.** I view my commitment to my partner as a solid one.

_____ **39.** I cannot imagine ending my relationship with my partner.

_____ **40.** I am certain of my love for my partner.

_____ **41.** I view my relationship with my partner as permanent.

_____ **42.** I view my relationship with my partner as a good decision.

_____ **43.** I feel a sense of responsibility toward my partner.

_____ **44.** I plan to continue my relationship with my partner.

_____ **45.** Even when my partner is hard to deal with, I remain committed to our relationship.

Scoring Key

Add your ratings for each of the three sections—intimacy, passion, and decision/commitment—and write the totals

in the blanks below. Divide the score from each section by 15 to get an average score for each section.

_____ ÷ 15 = _____
Intimacy score   Intimacy average

_____ ÷ 15 = _____
Passion score   Passion average

_____ ÷ 15 = _____
Decision/   Decision/
commitment score   commitment average

Each average score can range from 1 (low agreement) to 9 (strong agreement). If your average score on any component is 7 to 9, that component is a very strong part of your relationship. If your average score on any component is 1 to 3, that component is not a very strong part of your relationship. If your average score on any component is 4 to 6, that component is a moderately strong part of your relationship. Refer to the chapter discussion for an overall characterization of your relationship based on your scores. Remember, though, that relationships change over time—intimacy can deepen, commitment can grow, and even passion can be renewed. Remember, too, that a relationship does not have to fit a model to be a satisfying and important part of your life.

SOURCE: Sternberg's _Triangular Love Scale_ (adapted) from _The Triangle of Love_, by Robert J. Sternberg. Reprinted by permission of Robert J. Sternberg.

CHAPTER 15

Sexual Health: Biology, Society, and Culture

DID YOU KNOW?

- If you are sexually active and use condoms, you are in the majority of people who practice safer sex. Sixty-one percent of young adults aged 18 to 24 report using condoms, and 73 percent report using them if they have three or more sexual partners.

- Many women experience difficulty having an orgasm at some point in their lives, and many men experience difficulty achieving or maintaining an erection. Common causes include anxiety about sexual performance, lack of appropriate stimulation, alcohol or drug use, and relationship issues. Most of these problems are transient.

OLC *Your Health Today*   www.mhhe.com/teague1e

Go to the Online Learning Center for *Your Health Today* for interactive activities, quizzes, flashcards, Web links, and more resources related to this chapter.

Sexuality is a vital aspect of physical and psychological wellness. In the context of intimate relationships, sexuality plays a role in some of life's most meaningful experiences. Sexual activity is a source of pleasure, excitement, and connection with other people, and it is even good for your health. Studies show that an active sex life reduces the risk of heart disease, decreases risk of depression, provides temporary relief from chronic pain, boosts the immune system, and lowers the risk of death.[1] But sexuality is a complex human behavior, and it can be associated with negative experiences, such as worries and anxieties, relationship discord, health issues, and social problems.

Like health in general, sexual health is not limited to the absence of symptoms of disease. It includes healthy sexual functioning across the life span, satisfying intimate relationships based on mutual respect and trust, and the ability and resources to procreate if so desired. It involves acceptance of one's own sexual feelings and tolerance for those of others. It also includes knowledge about sexuality and access to the information needed to make responsible decisions about your sexual health.

In this chapter we explore some of the biological, psychological, sociological, and cultural aspects of sexual health. We begin with a brief consideration of sexual pleasure, and then we take a closer look at sexual anatomy, functioning, and response. We also consider sexual development and health in different stages of life. We continue with some of the varieties of sexual behavior and expression and some of the common sexual dysfunctions. We discuss personal issues in protecting your sexual health, and we conclude with a look at some of the cultural issues society faces in the 21st century.

Ads for drugs that enhance sexual performance suggest changing attitudes toward sex. Having sex for personal pleasure, rather than for procreation, is widely accepted in today's society.

BIOLOGY, CULTURE, AND SEXUAL PLEASURE

Although sexual anatomy and physiology are similar in all human beings, sexual behavior and expression vary tremendously across societies, cultures, and eras. There are even differences in what is considered sexually pleasurable, a phenomenon that highlights the role of the brain in sexuality. **Sexual pleasure** has been defined as positively valued feelings induced by sexual stimuli.[2] Sensory signals arriving in the brain are not inherently pleasurable; rather, the brain interprets them as pleasurable. This interpretation and evaluation of stimuli by the brain as sexually pleasurable is influenced by everything the individual has learned about sex in his or her society and culture, including expectations, attitudes, and values. Thus, the experience of sexual pleasure is profoundly affected by context and culture.

American culture projects mixed attitudes about sex and sexual pleasure. Our Puritan forebears believed

that the sole purpose of sexuality was procreation and that sexual expression for any other purpose was sinful. Partly as a result of these attitudes, sexuality was shrouded in mystery and silence for generations, and this puritan legacy continues to influence our cultural character today. On the other hand, the 20th century, especially the second half of the 20th century, was characterized by a drive for greater openness and freedom of expression, including sexual expression. The "sexual revolution" of the 1960s and 1970s made sexuality something to be talked about, studied, and celebrated.

Sexual attitudes in U.S. society are marked by an ongoing tension between the two poles of sexual restrictiveness and sexual freedom. As with all issues, attitudes toward sex shift over time (see the box "Contemporary Trends in Sexual Behavior"). The sexual revolution gave way to a more conservative climate in the 1980s and 1990s. Prevailing attitudes toward sex and sexual pleasure in the early 21st century will be determined, in part, by college students and other young adults.

HIGHLIGHT ON HEALTH

Contemporary Trends in Sexual Behavior

Popular American culture is saturated with sexual imagery and content, suggesting that sexuality pervades every aspect of life. Is the media view accurate? Two recent studies have provided insight into current sexual practices among Americans. Here is a brief snapshot.

- **Premarital Sexual Activity**   Average age of first sexual experience is about 17 for women and about 16 for men. Average age of first marriage is 25 for women and 27 for men. The implication is that women have about 8 years of premarital sexual activity and men have about 11 years.

- **Committed Relationships**   Most people are engaged in committed, monogamous relationships. Among college students aged 18 to 24, 60 percent of women and 38 percent of men report being in a committed relationship. College students between the ages of 18 and 24 average about one partner per year.

- **Extramarital Affairs**   Extramarital affairs are fairly uncommon. The best estimate is that 3 percent to 4 percent of currently married couples have an affair in a given year, with lifetime prevalence of 15 percent to 18 percent. Affairs are more common among young adults and twice as common among men as women.

- **Frequency of Sexual Intercourse**   On average, adults engage in sexual intercourse 62 times a year, or about once a week. Frequency varies with age and relationship status. Frequency is 85 times a year for young adults, 63 times a year for middle-aged adults, and 10.5 times a year for older adults.

- **Sexual Inactivity**   Between 15 and 28 percent of nonmarried adults aged 18 to 49 are sexually inactive, whereas only 1 percent to 2.4 percent of married adults are sexually inactive. About 32 percent of college men and 18 percent of college women aged 18 to 24 were sexually inactive over the past year. Abstinence and very low frequency of sexual intercourse are most prevalent in youth and older adulthood.

- **Use of Condoms**   Since 1970, condom use has gradually increased for both men and women, although usage leveled off in the 1990s. Overall, 61 percent of young adults aged 18 to 24 use condoms, and 73 percent use them if they have three or more sexual partners. Frequency of condom use is higher among young adults, those who have never been married, and those with low incomes; it is not associated with level of education.

- **Knowledge of Safer Sex**   In response to the AIDS epidemic, high-risk groups reported increased use of safe sex practices, including reduced number of sexual partners, decreased frequency of sex, condom usage, abstinence, and restriction of sex to partners they knew well. Since 1993, however, safe sex practices have not increased by either high-risk or low-risk groups. Most adults know the basics of safe sex, but many are unaware of important details. For example, 62 percent of college men and women aged 18 to 24 believed they could tell if a partner had a sexually transmitted disease (STD) from the appearance of the person's genitals. (Some STDs do not have any visible signs.) Although 74 percent of college students said that contraception should be discussed before the first sexual experience with a partner, 32 percent of men and 24 percent of women said they did not have this discussion.

Sources: "American Sexual Behavior: Trends, Socio-Demographic Differences, and Risk Behavior," by T. W. Smith, April 2003, GSS Topical Report No. 25, National Opinion Research Center, University of Chicago; "What's Really Going on Behind Closed Doors," Smarter Sex Organization, March 30, 2005, www.smartersex.org.

SEXUAL ANATOMY AND FUNCTIONING

Although sexuality serves many purposes in human experience, the biological purpose of sexuality is reproduction. In this section we explore some of the biological aspects of sexuality.

Sexual Anatomy

The male and female sex organs arise from the same undifferentiated tissue during the prenatal period, becoming male or female under the influence of hormones (discussed later in this section). In this sense, the sexual organs of males and females are very similar, although their purpose and functions are complementary. The female sex organs are responsible for the production of ova and,

KEY TERMS

sexual pleasure   Positively valued feelings induced by sexual stimuli.

if pregnancy occurs, the development of the fetus. The male sex organs are responsible for producing sperm and delivering them into the female reproductive system to fertilize the ovum.

Female Sex Organs and Reproductive Anatomy

In both sexes, there are external and internal sex organs. The external genitalia of the female are called the vulva and include the mons pubis, the labia majora and labia minora, the clitoris, and the vaginal and urethral openings (Figure 15.1). The mons pubis is a mound or layer of fatty tissue that pads and protects the pubic bone. The labia majora (major lips) and labia minora (minor lips) are folds of tissue that wrap around the entrance to the vagina. Pubic hair typically covers the mons pubis and the outer surface of the labia majora. The inner surfaces of the labia majora are smooth and contain several oil and sweat glands. The labia minora form a protective hood, or prepuce, over the clitoris. The clitoris is a highly sensitive,

cylindrical body about 3 centimeters in length that fills with blood during sexual excitement. Consisting of a glans, corpus, and crura, the clitoris is located at the top of the vulva between the lips of the labia minora.

The urethral opening, the passageway for urine from the urinary bladder, is located immediately below the clitoris. The hymen is a thin membranous fold, highly variable in appearance, which may partially cover the opening of the vagina. The hymen has no known biological function and is frequently absent. The perineum is the area between the bottom of the vulva and the anus. It contains many nerve endings. The anus is the lower opening of the digestive tract.

The internal sex organs of the female include the vagina, cervix, uterus, fallopian tubes, and ovaries. The vagina is a hollow, muscular tube extending from the external vaginal opening to the cervix. It serves as both the organ for heterosexual intercourse and the birth canal. In most women, it is 3 to 4 inches long. The walls of the

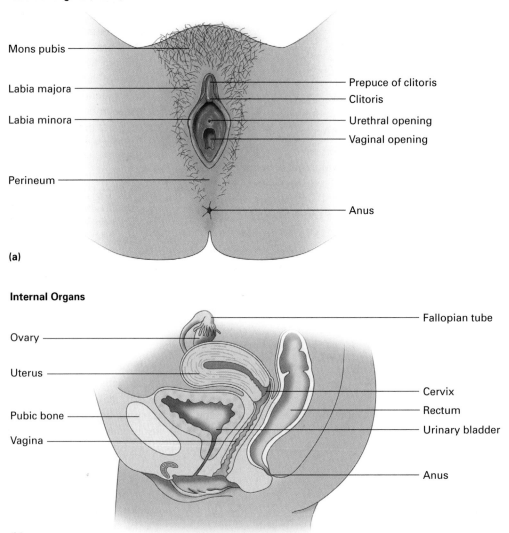

External Organs (Vulva)

Mons pubis

Labia majora

Labia minora

Perineum

Prepuce of clitoris

Clitoris

Urethral opening

Vaginal opening

Anus

(a)

Internal Organs

Ovary

Uterus

Pubic bone

Vagina

Fallopian tube

Cervix

Rectum

Urinary bladder

Anus

(b)

Figure 15.1
Female sexual and reproductive anatomy.
(a) External structures;
(b) internal structures.

vagina are soft and flexible and have several layers. The existence of an area called the G-spot on the lower front wall of the vagina is a subject of debate; if it is present, it may feel like an elevated bump. Located on either side of the vagina under the labia are the crura, extensions of the clitoris.

The cervix is the lower part of the uterus; it extends into the vagina and contains the opening to the uterus. The cervix produces a mucus that changes with different stages of the menstrual cycle. The uterus is the organ in which a fertilized egg develops into an embryo and then a fetus. Approximately the size of a pear (3 inches long), the uterus is made up of several layers of muscle and tissue. The endometrium is the layer that is shed during menstruation.

The ovaries are the female reproductive glands that store and release the ova (eggs) every month, usually one at a time—the process of ovulation. They also produce the female sex hormones estrogen and progesterone. The ovaries are about 1½ inches long and are located on either side of the uterus. Extending from the upper sides of the uterus are the fallopian tubes (or oviducts), the passageways through which ova move from the ovaries into the uterus. They are about 4 inches long. Their openings are lined with fimbria, appendages with beating cilia that sweep the surface of the ovaries during ovulation and guide the ovum down into the tubes.

The mammary glands, or breasts, are also part of female sexual and reproductive anatomy. They consist of 15 to 25 lobes that are padded by connective tissue and fat. Within the lobes are glands that produce milk when the woman is lactating following the birth of a baby. At the center of each breast is a nipple, surrounded by a ring of darker colored skin called the areola. The nipple becomes erect when stimulated by cold, touch, or sexual stimuli.

Male Sex Organs and Reproductive Anatomy

The external genitalia of the male include the penis and the scrotum, which contains the testes (Figure 15.2). The penis, when erect, is designed to deliver sperm into the female reproductive tract. The shaft of the penis is formed of three columns of spongelike erectile tissue that fill with blood during sexual excitement. The glans, or head of the penis, is an expansion of the corpus spongiosum (one of the three columns of erectile tissue in the penis shaft). The glans contains a higher concentration of nerve endings than the shaft and is highly sensitive.

The corona is a crownlike structure that protrudes slightly and forms a border between the glans and the shaft; it is also highly sensitive. The frenulum is a fold of skin extending from the corona to the foreskin. The foreskin, or prepuce, covers the glans, more or less completely. **Circumcision** involves removing this skin and leaving the head of the penis permanently exposed. The urethral opening, through which both urine and semen

pass (at different times), is located at the tip of the penis in the glans. The urethra runs the length of the penis from the urinary bladder to the exterior of the body.

The scrotum, a thin sac composed of skin and muscle fibers, contains the testes. The scrotum is separated from the body to keep the testes at the lower temperature that is needed for sperm production. The area between the scrotum and the anus is the perineum; as in females, it contains many nerve endings. The anus is the lower opening of the digestive tract.

The male internal reproductive organs include the testes; a series of ducts that transport sperm (the epididymis, vas deferens, ejaculatory ducts, and urethra); and a set of glands that produce semen and other fluids (the seminal vesicles, prostate gland, and Cowper's glands). The two testes, located in the scrotum, are the male reproductive glands; they produce both sperm and male sex hormones such as testosterone. Once sperm are produced in the testes, they enter the epididymis, a highly coiled duct lying on the surface of each testis. As they move along the length of the epididymis (which, if uncoiled, would measure about 20 feet in length), immature sperm mature and develop the ability to swim.

When the male ejaculates, sperm are propelled from the epididymis into the vas deferens, another duct, which joins with ducts from the seminal vesicles to form the short ejaculatory ducts. The two seminal vesicles, located at the back of the bladder, produce about 60 percent of the volume of semen, the milky fluid that carries sperm and contains nutrients to fuel them. The sperm and semen travel through the ejaculatory ducts to the prostate gland, a doughnut-shaped structure that encircles the urethra and contributes the remaining volume of semen. The semen is then ejaculated through the urethra. The two Cowper's glands, located below the prostate gland, produce a clear mucus that is secreted into the urethra just before ejaculation. The volume of semen in one ejaculation is about 2 milliliters to 5 milliliters, containing between 100 and 600 million sperm.

Sexual Response

In order for reproduction to occur, ova and sperm have to be brought into close association with each other. The psychological and motivational mechanism for this is the human sexual response, which includes sex drive, sexual arousal, and orgasm.

KEY TERMS

circumcision   Removal of the foreskin of the penis; a procedure often routinely performed on newborn male infants in the United States.

External Organs

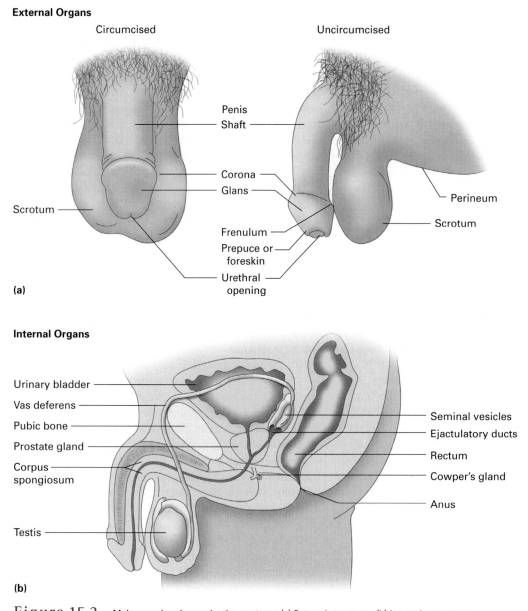

(a)

Internal Organs

(b)

Figure 15.2   **Male sexual and reproductive anatomy.** (a) External structures; (b) internal structures.

Sex Drive

Sex drive—sexual desire, or libido—is defined as a biological urge for sexual activity. The principal hormone responsible for the sex drive in both males and females is testosterone, produced by the testes in males and by the adrenal glands in both sexes. Testosterone stimulates increased release of the neurotransmitters dopamine and serotonin in the brain; they are thought to be involved in making external stimuli arousing. Levels of these two neurotransmitters peak at orgasm and then decline.[3] Serotonin is thought to have an effect on feelings of sexual satisfaction after orgasm. The hormones epinephrine (adrenaline) and norepinephrine (noradrenaline), released by the adrenal glands, are involved in arousal,

increasing heart rate, blood pressure, respiration, and other autonomic nervous system functions.

People usually seek to satisfy the sex drive through physical stimulation and release, either with a partner or through self-stimulation. Although the biological mechanisms of the sex drive and sexual arousal are essentially universal, the stimuli that create arousal are largely determined by one's culture, as noted earlier. Besides hormones, sex drive is also influenced by sexual imagery and sexual fantasies. It can be stimulated by sights, sounds, smells, tastes, and myriad other external stimuli, as well as by one's own thoughts and fantasies. The ultimate goal of arousal also varies by culture. Western cultures typically focus on attaining orgasm. Some cultures encourage the suppression or sublimation of the sex drive; other cultures emphasize spiritual and sensual outcomes as the goals of sexual activity.[4]

Sexual Arousal

Sexual arousal on the physiological level usually begins with physical stimulation of the **erogenous zones**—parts of the body that are particularly sensitive to sexual stimulation, such as the penis, clitoris, and nipples. Men and women both experience the physiological responses of vasocongestion and myotonia during arousal.

Vasocongestion is the inflow of blood to tissues in erogenenous areas. In men, the arterioles supplying blood to the erectile tissue of the penis are normally constricted. Sexual arousal causes nerves in the penis to release nitric oxide, which in turn activates an enzyme that relaxes the arterioles and allows the penis to fill with blood. Engorgement compresses the veins in the penis and prevents blood from flowing out. In women, a similar process causes engorgement of the clitoris, labia, vagina, and nipples; vaginal lubrication also increases. **Myotonia** is a voluntary or involuntary muscle tension occurring in response to sexual stimuli. Both vasocongestion and myotonia build up during sexual excitement and decrease afterward.[4]

The Human Sexual Response Model

In the 1960s, sex researchers William Masters and Virginia Johnson conducted detailed studies of sexual activity and developed a four-phase model of the human sexual response (Figure 15.3) The four phases are excitement, plateau, orgasm, and resolution.[4]

The excitement stage begins with stimulation that initiates vasocongestion and myotonia. The first sign of excitement in men is penis erection. In women, signs include vaginal lubrication and, frequently, nipple and clitoral erection. Heart rate and respiratory rate generally increase in both men and women. The excitement phase can last less than a minute or continue for up to several hours.

The plateau phase is a leveling-off period just before orgasm. Like the excitement phase, it can last for a few seconds or an hour or more. Increased muscle tension continues during the plateau phase. The heart rate remains elevated and breathing is deep. Both men and women may experience a "sex flush," a flushing effect caused by increased circulation of the blood to the skin. The penis increases in size and length, and the upper two thirds of the vagina widens and expands.

Orgasm is a physiological reflex in which a massive discharge of nerve impulses occurs in the nerves serving the genitals, usually in response to tactile stimulation, causing rhythmic muscle contractions in the genital area and a sensation of intense pleasure. In men, contractions occur in the penis, ducts, glands, and muscles in the pelvic and anal region; orgasm is accompanied by the ejaculation of semen. In women, contractions occur in the uterus, vagina, and pelvic and anal region.

Resolution is the return to an unexcited, relaxed state. The sex flush fades, if it was present, and heart and respiratory rates return to normal. Men enter a **refractory period,** lasting from minutes to hours, during which vasoconstriction of the arterioles supplying the erectile tissue causes the penis to become flaccid again. During the refractory period, the man is not able to have another orgasm. Most young men can have one to three orgasms in an hour, as can some older men.

In women, orgasm is not followed by a refractory period, so women can experience multiple orgasms during a single sexual experience. Multiple orgasms may be experienced as part of the general climactic wave or as a series of orgasms as much as 5 minutes apart.

An Alternative Model of the Sexual Response

An alternative model suggests that many women, especially those in long-term relationships, may not experience sexual desire (conscious sexual urges) moving to sexual arousal. Instead, sexual arousal more commonly precedes sexual desire. Sexual desire occurs only after a sufficient period of sexual arousal and is more of a responsive event than a spontaneous event.[5] The choice to initiate sexual arousal is often more dependent on intimacy needs (needs for emotional closeness, bonding, love, affection) than a need for physical sexual arousal or release. Intimacy benefits and appreciation for the sexual well-being of the partner serve as the motivational factors to move from sexual neutrality to sexual arousal.[5] This model may also apply to some men in long-term relationships.

KEY TERMS

sex drive   Biological urge for sexual activity; also called sexual desire or libido.

erogenous zones   Parts of the body that are particularly sensitive to sexual stimulation, such as the penis, clitoris, and nipples.

vasocongestion   Inflow of blood to tissues in erogenous areas.

myotonia   Voluntary or involuntary muscle tension occurring in response to sexual stimuli.

orgasm   Physiological reflex characterized by rhythmic muscle contractions in the genital area and a sensation of intense pleasure.

refractory period   Time following orgasm when a man cannot have another orgasm.

Female

Excitement

Uterus rises

Vaginal lubrication occurs
Clitoris enlarges
Labia minora swell
Labia majora swell

Plateau

Uterus rises further

Upper part of vagina
expands
Vaginal walls expand

Color of labia darkens

Orgasm

Contractions in uterus

Rhythmic contractions
in vagina
Rectal sphincter
contracts

Resolution

Uterus lowers

Vagina returns to
normal state
Clitoris returns to
unaroused position
Labia return to normal
size and color

Male

Excitement

Vasocongestion of
penis leads to erection

Partial erection

Unstimulated state
Testes rise
Skin of scrotum tenses,
thickens, and rises

Plateau

Cowper's gland
secretion
Color of penile glans
darkens
Prostate gland enlarges

Testes enlarge and
are fully elevated
Scrotum thickens and tenses

Orgasm

Contractions of penis
Sperm and semen expelled
by rhythmic contractions
of urethra
Vas deferens contracts
Internal sphincter of
bladder contracts
Prostate gland contracts
Seminal vesicles contract
Rectal sphincter contracts

Resolution

Erection subsides
Unstimulated state

Scrotum thins, folds return
Testes lower to normal position

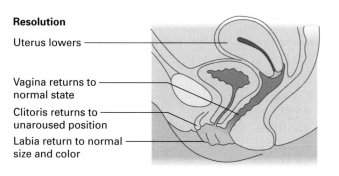

Figure 15.3   The human sexual response model.

Challenges & Choices

Discussing a Sexual Problem With Your Partner

Conversations about sex are part of virtually all successful intimate relationships. Sexual desires are personal, and partners can't read each other's minds. At some point you may need to speak up about a sexual problem. Here are some guidelines:

- Be assertive about your needs, but be tactful and considerate. Sex is a sensitive topic for most people.

- Admit frustration but avoid anger. Anger is a roadblock to effective communication.

- Avoid blame. Take responsibility for whatever part of the problem you may have control over.

- Avoid words like *should, ought,* and *must.* They sound like demands and imply that there is some standard your partner has to meet. Improving a sexual relationship means working together for your mutual pleasure and satisfaction.

- If your partner approaches you with a problem, try not to be defensive. When people want to solve sexual problems, it means they care about the relationship.

It's Not Just Personal . . .

If you and your partner are having a sexual problem, keep in mind that this is more common than you might think. For example, 8% of women say that they rarely achieve orgasm. For men, premature ejaculation is common, with 28% reporting that they experience this problem often.

Sources: *The Sexual Male: Problems and Solutions,* by R. Milstein and J. Slowinsky, 1999, New York: W. W. Norton and Company; Sexuality Information and Education Council of the United States, www.siecus.org.

Regardless of whether sexual desire precedes or follows sexual arousal, sufficient time spent in creating a pleasurable physical experience, through both genital and nongenital stimulation, helps ensure that the arousal phase operates efficiently. If excitement is not ignited, motivation to continue with sexual activity can quickly fade.

The Experience of Orgasm

Although orgasm is physically experienced in the genitals, it is also a cerebral event. The subjective experience of orgasm can be influenced by an infinite variety of physical, emotional, psychological, interpersonal, and environmental factors. Examples include the time of day, the setting, your physical condition, your prior experience with your partner, and the quality of the relationship. Some people claim that every orgasm is different. Still, there are some universals.

Most people experience a feeling of deep warmth or pressure when orgasm is imminent or inevitable. Orgasm is usually felt as waves of intense pleasure accompanied by contractions in the penis, vagina, or uterus. The sensations may be localized to the genitals, or they may be generalized over the whole body.

About a third of women reach orgasm from the sensations produced in the vagina by the thrusting of the penis, but many women need direct stimulation of the clitoris to reach orgasm.[6] Since most intercourse positions do not include such direct pressure or stimulation, intercourse alone may not be completely satisfying for a

woman. Active stimulation of the clitoris with fingers or a vibrator can help women reach an orgasm. When a woman is unable to reach an orgasm, it is usually due to inhibition or lack of needed stimulation. Some women may be tempted to fake an orgasm, perhaps out of fear of being perceived as sexually deficient, but doing so can undermine a relationship. A satisfying relationship includes having honest discussions about what helps both partners respond orgasmically (see the box "Discussing a Sexual Problem With Your Partner").

As noted earlier, the existence of a sensitive spot on the front wall of the vagina, called the G-spot, is a matter of debate. Some women report that a steady pressure on this spot produces a different kind of orgasm. However, research has failed to show that the G-spot plays a significant role in sexual satisfaction.[7]

Sexual Development and Health Across the Life Span

The biology of sexual and reproductive development is directed by hormones, beginning in the womb. Male sex hormones, called **androgens,** are secreted primarily by

KEY TERMS

androgens   Male sex hormones, secreted primarily by the testes.

the testes, and female sex hormones, called **estrogens** and **progestins,** are secreted by the ovaries. The adrenal glands also secrete androgens in both males and females. The pituitary gland and the hypothalamus in the brain both have roles in regulating levels and functions of the sex hormones.

Prenatal Development

During prenatal development, the presence of a Y chromosome causes the reproductive glands to develop into testes; the testes produce testosterone, which causes the undifferentiated reproductive structures to become male sex organs. If there is no Y chromosome, the glands develop into ovaries and the reproductive structures become female sex organs. At birth, the appearance of the external sex organs signals the biological sex of the baby to the world.

Puberty

Hormones come into play again at puberty, when the secondary sex characteristics appear and the reproductive system matures. There is a growth spurt in both sexes (about 2 years earlier in girls than in boys), the sex organs become larger, and pubic and underarm hair appears. In boys, the voice deepens, facial hair begins to grow, and the onset of **ejaculation** occurs. Boys begin to experience **nocturnal emissions** (orgasm and ejaculation during sleep), and the testes start to produce sperm. In girls, breasts develop, body fat increases, and **menarche,** the onset of menstruation, occurs.

Menstruation

Every month between the ages of about 12 and about 50, except during pregnancy, women experience monthly menstrual periods. During the first half of the cycle, the lining of the uterus thickens with blood vessels in preparation for the possibility of pregnancy, and an ovum matures in one of the ovaries. About halfway through the cycle, the ovum is released (ovulation) and is carried into the uterus. If sperm are present, the ovum may be fertilized and begin to develop into an embryo. If sperm are not present, the uterine lining is shed, causing **menses,** and the cycle begins again.

Some girls and women experience uncomfortable physical symptoms during their periods, such as cramps and backache, and some experience physical and emotional symptoms before their periods, such as headache, irritability, and mood swings, referred to as premenstrual tension or premenstrual syndrome (PMS). If symptoms are severe and interfere with usual work, family, or social activities, the woman may be diagnosed with premenstrual dysphoric disorder (PMDD). The exact causes of PMS and PMDD are not known, but lifestyle changes, such as exercising, eating well, and avoiding alcohol, may help relieve symptoms. A physician may prescribe medications for more severe symptoms.

Menopause

In middle age, hormonal changes cause a gradual reduction in ovarian functioning that culminates in **menopause,** the cessation of menstruation. Although the average age of menopause in the United States is 52, a small percentage of women experience premature menopause before age 40.[3]

During the time leading up to menopause, a period of 3 years to 7 years called *perimenopause,* many women experience symptoms caused by hormonal fluctuations, such as hot flashes, night sweats, irritability, and insomnia.

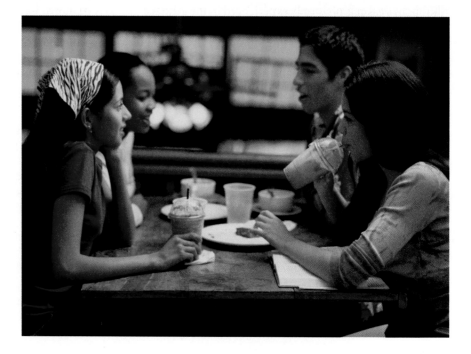

As body changes appear, preteens become more aware of themselves as sexual beings. Besides paying greater attention to their physical appearance, they may engage in flirting behavior, group dating, and, sometimes, early sexual exploration.

A decrease in estrogen production can cause less visible symptoms as well, such as a reduction in bone density and changes in blood levels of cholesterol. These changes contribute to women's increased risk of osteoporosis and heart disease later in life.

Loss of estrogen also causes changes in the genitals, which can lead to changes in sexual functioning. These changes may be minimal for some women but very dramatic for others. The vaginal walls become thinner and lubrication may decrease, making intercourse less comfortable. Vaginal lubrication during the excitement phase may take from 1 to 5 minutes to occur, whereas in a young woman it takes only 15 seconds to 20 seconds. It may take longer to reach orgasm, and orgasm may be less intense. In some women, sex drive may decrease. Because sexuality has so many emotional, psychological, and interpersonal dimensions, however, the physical changes associated with menopause do not necessarily have a major impact on a woman's sex life.

Hormone replacement therapy (HRT) has been a popular treatment for the symptoms of menopause. At first, estrogen was used alone, but evidence surfaced that estrogen replacement therapy (ERT) increased the risk of endometrial cancer. Then, estrogen and progesterone were used together in HRT, not only to treat the symptoms of menopause but also to lower the risk of heart disease and osteoporosis in menopausal women. In 1991 the National Institutes of Health began a research project called the Women's Health Initiative Study to provide definitive conclusions on the relationship between HRT and osteoporosis, breast cancer, heart disease, stroke, blood clots, and colon cancer. Results were due in 2005, but in 2002, the portion of the study involving women taking a combination of estrogen and progestin was abruptly stopped when researchers concluded that the risks of HRT far outweighed their benefits.[8] The risk of breast cancer rose more quickly for women on HRT after 4 years, and the risk of heart disease and blood clots increased each year for women on HRT. Women are advised to consult with their physicians to determine whether the benefits of taking HRT outweigh their personal risks.

"Viropause"

Men do not experience a dramatic change in reproductive capacity in midlife as women do; the testes continue to produce sperm throughout life. Some researchers believe, however, that middle-aged men experience a 5-to-12-year period during which their testosterone levels fluctuate.[9] The term **viropause** (pronounced "VEER-o-pause") has been coined to refer to changes in virility or sexual desire in middle-aged men, analogous to menopause in women. The condition is also referred to as Androgen Decline in Aging Males. Common symptoms include irritability, sluggishness, mild to moderate mood swings, and a sense of declining vitality. A sudden loss of self-respect may

reduce testosterone levels, which can in turn reduce a man's sex drive.[9]

As testosterone levels decline in later life, men experience some changes in sexual functioning. It may take up to several minutes to achieve an erection during stimulation, whereas in younger men it takes from 3 to 5 seconds. It may also take longer to reach orgasm, and orgasm may be less intense. The refractory period usually becomes longer as men get older.

For both men and women, biological changes in the sexual response phases have only a marginal effect on sexual interest and activity. There does tend to be a slow, steady decline in sexual activity over the course of life, caused by lower levels of sex hormones and physiological changes in the body. The more sexually active a person is, the less effect these biological changes have.

VARIETIES OF SEXUAL BEHAVIOR AND EXPRESSION

What is "normal" sexual behavior? By now it should be clear that what is defined as normal depends on social and cultural context. For example, individuals with a disability will have special issues related to having a sexual life (see the box "Sexuality and Disability"). Rather than thinking in terms of normalcy, social scientists think in terms of behavior that is typical and behavior that is less typical. In this section we consider both types of sexual behavior.

Typical and Common Forms of Sexual Expression

Typical forms of sexual behavior and expression in U.S. society include celibacy, kissing, erotic touch, self-stimulation, oral-genital stimulation, and intercourse.

KEY TERMS

estrogens   Female sex hormones; secreted by the ovaries.

progestins   Female sex hormones; secreted by the ovaries.

ejaculation   Emission of semen during orgasm.

nocturnal emission   Orgasm and ejaculation during sleep.

menarche   Onset of menstruation.

menses   Flow of menstrual blood; the menstrual period.

menopause   Cessation of menstruation.

viropause   Changes in virility or sexual desire in middle-aged men.

HIGHLIGHT ON HEALTH
Sexuality and Disability

A wide range of disabling conditions can affect a person's sexuality, from Down syndrome to spinal cord injury. Although individuals with disabilities may experience limitations on their sexuality or may have to develop new or alternative forms of sexual activity, most people with disabilities can have a rewarding sex life. Information and education can help individuals with disabilities, as can counseling that focuses on building self-esteem; overcoming shame, guilt, fear, anger, and unrealistic expectations; and developing a holistic approach to sexuality that includes all activities that offer pleasure and intimacy. Information and education are also important for members of the general public, who too often fail to acknowledge the full humanity of individuals with disabilities, including their sexuality.

For people with physical limitations, a major challenge can be finding a sexual partner. Individuals may not want to risk rejection and may hide their feelings behind a mask of anger or indifference. Potential partners may need to be open-minded, patient, persistent, and willing to experiment to find out what works. Depending on the type of condition or injury, different forms of sexual expression may be possible. A person with a spinal cord injury may or may not be able to have an orgasm, but he or she may be able to have intercourse, may experience sensuous feelings in other parts of the body, and may be able to have a child. As in any relationship, the key is discovering who the other person is and nurturing emotional as well as sexual intimacy. When a partner in an established relationship is facing a disability, the couple may want to seek information and counseling on how the disability will affect their sexual functioning.

Changes in sexual functioning and desire can also be caused by chronic diseases, such as diabetes, arthritis, and cardiovascular disease, as well as by the medications used to treat them. Diabetes can cause nerve damage and circulatory problems that affect erectile functioning in men; arthritis causes pain that can make sexual activity uncomfortable; cardiovascular disease can lead to depression or to fear that sexual activity will cause another heart attack or stroke. Individuals and couples may have to make significant adjustments in their forms of sexual expression to accommodate such disabling conditions.

Individuals with mental or developmental disabilities also face challenges in sexual expression. Depending on the degree of disability, some such individuals may be unable to learn the basics of reproduction or how to behave appropriately in public, while others are able to marry and raise children. Sex education is important for all people with developmental disabilities, especially adolescents. Children and young teens need to know about puberty and the hormonal and physical changes they will experience, and they especially need to know that these changes are normal. Boys have to learn about erections and nocturnal emissions, and girls have to learn about menstruation. Both boys and girls need to learn about masturbation and that, if done, it should be done in private.

For more severely disabled people, education may be limited to teaching them not to undress or touch their genitals in public. For those with milder disabilities, learning about companionship, safe sex practices, and sexual relationships is appropriate. In general, the best approach is to tailor sex education to the needs of the individual.

Sources: *Human Sexuality*, 5th ed. by B. Strong, C. DeVault, B. Sayad, and W. Yarber, 2005, New York: McGraw-Hill; *The Sexual Male: Problems and Solutions*, by R. Milsten and J. Slowinski, 1999, New York: W. W. Norton and Company.

Celibacy

Continuous abstention from sexual activities with others is called **celibacy.** People may be completely celibate (do not engage in masturbation) or partially celibate (engage in masturbation). Moral and religious beliefs lead some people to choose celibacy. Lack of a suitable sexual partner or sexual relationship may be another reason for celibacy.[6]

Some people use the term *abstinence* interchangeably with *celibacy,* but **abstinence** usually means abstention only from sexual intercourse. As such, abstinence is promoted as a way to avoid sexually transmitted diseases and unintended pregnancy. It is discussed further later in this chapter and in Chapter 16.

Kissing

Kissing is usually the first sexual experience with another person. The act of kissing stimulates all of the body senses simultaneously. The lips physically respond to a kiss by swelling, darkening in color, and congesting with blood. These physical changes make nerve endings in the lips more sensitive, heightening the pleasurable sensation.

Erotic Touch

Touch is a sensual form of communication that can elicit feelings of tenderness and affection as well as sexual feelings. It is an important part of **foreplay,** touching that increases sexual arousal and leads to sexual intercourse. Some areas of the body are more sensitive to touch than others. Skin in the nonspecific erogenous zones of the body (the inner thighs, armpits, shoulders, feet, ears, and sides of the back and neck) contains more nerve endings than do many other areas; these areas are capable of being aroused by touch. Skin in the specific erogenous zones (penis, clitoris, vulva, perineum, lips, breasts, and buttocks) has an even higher density of nerve endings, and nerve endings are closer to the skin surface.[6] These erogenous zones are more sensitive to sexual arousal by touch. The landscape of erotic touch includes holding hands, stroking, caressing, squeezing, tickling, scratching, and massaging.

Self-Stimulation

The two most common self-stimulation sexual activities, called **autoerotic behaviors,** are sexual fantasies and masturbation. Sexual fantasies are mental images, scenarios, and daydreams imagined to initiate sexual arousal. They range from simple images to complicated erotic stories.[10] The fact that the body can become aroused when a person thinks about sex highlights the fact that the brain is a major player in sexual functioning. Many people feel guilty about their sexual fantasies,[6] but fantasies are actually effective and harmless ways of exploring sexual fulfillment. People often fantasize about situations and behaviors they would never engage in in real life.

Masturbation is self-stimulation of the genitals for sexual pleasure. It is usually done manually or with a vibrator or other sex toy. The stigma attached to masturbation is left over from a previous era, when it was considered sinful and dangerous to one's health, probably because its purpose was pleasure rather than procreation. Today, masturbation is better understood and more widely accepted as a natural and healthful sexual behavior. Masturbation is a part of sex therapy programs designed to help people overcome sexual problems, and mutual masturbation is promoted as a way to practice safer sex. Still, about half of all men and women feel guilty about masturbating.[11]

Oral-Genital Stimulation

Cunnilingus is the oral stimulation of the female genitals with the tongue and lips; it includes licking, kissing, and gently sucking the clitoris, labia, or vaginal area. **Fellatio** is the oral stimulation of the male genitals with the tongue, lips, and mouth. Oral stimulation can be part of foreplay, or it can be a sexual activity leading to orgasm. Some people find oral-genital stimulation very pleasurable; others refrain because of religious or moral beliefs. Oral sex is not an entirely safe form of sex, because infections can be transmitted via the mouth. Using some form of protection during oral sex is recommended, as discussed later in this chapter.

Anal Intercourse

A small percentage of heterosexual couples and a larger percentage of gay male couples practice anal intercourse, the penetration of the rectum with the penis. The anal area has a high density of nerve endings and is sensitive to stimulation. Because the skin and tissue of the anus and rectum are delicate and can be easily torn, anal intercourse is one of the riskiest sexual behaviors for the transmission of infections. Condom use is strongly recommended during anal intercourse.

Sexual Intercourse

Sexual intercourse, also known as coitus or making love, is by far the most common form of adult sexual expression. (If you are thinking about starting a relationship that will include sexual intercourse, see the box "Are You Ready for Sex?") It is a source of sexual pleasure for most couples, as well as the primary way that human reproduction occurs. In sexual intercourse, a man typically inserts his erect penis into a woman's vagina and thrusts with his hips and pelvis until he ejaculates. A woman who is aroused responds with matching hip and pelvic thrusts, but she may or may not reach orgasm solely from penetration and thrusting, as mentioned earlier.

Sexual intercourse can be performed in a variety of positions. The most common is the so-called missionary position, in which the man lies on top of the woman. In this position, the penis can penetrate deeply into the vagina. When the woman lies on top of the man, penetration may not be as deep, but the woman has more control,

KEY TERMS

celibacy Continuous abstention from sexual activities with others.

abstinence Abstention from sexual intercourse, usually as a way to avoid conception or STDs.

foreplay Touching that increases sexual arousal before sexual intercourse.

autoerotic behaviors Self-stimulating sexual activities, primarily sexual fantasies and masturbation.

masturbation Self-stimulation of the genitals for sexual pleasure.

cunnilingus Oral stimulation of the female genitals with the tongue and lips.

fellatio Oral stimulation of the male genitals with the tongue, lips, and mouth.

HIGHLIGHT ON HEALTH

Are You Ready for Sex?

If you are an adult and are trying to decide whether you're ready to have sex with a partner, consider the following guidelines. You may be ready for sex if these guidelines seem to apply to your situation.

- You feel comfortable in the relationship.
- Neither you nor your partner is pressuring the other for sex.
- You are not trying to
  - Prove your love for your partner
  - Increase your sense of self-worth
  - Prove that you are mature
  - Show that you can attract a sexual partner
  - Get attention, affection, or love
  - Rebel against parents or society

- Sex will be an expression of your current feelings, not an attempt to solve problems in a struggling relationship or ignite a relationship that is growing cold.
- You and your partner can discuss your sexual histories and sexual health issues.
- You and your partner can discuss and agree on an effective method of birth control and share the details, responsibilities, and costs.
- You and your partner can discuss and agree on what both of you will do if conception occurs.
- Being in a sexual relationship is consistent with your moral values and beliefs.

Adapted with permission from SIECUS Report 13.6. Copyright 1985 by the Sex Information Council of the United States, Inc., 120 W. 42nd St., Suite 2500, New York, NY 10036.

---

an important psychological factor for some women. When the woman sits or kneels on top of the man, penetration is deeper and the woman can increase clitoral stimulation by rocking back and forth.[6]

In the rear-entry position, the woman lies face down and the man lies on top of her, or both lie on their sides. Although penetration is not as deep in this position, there is more opportunity for clitoral stimulation by either the woman or the man. Side-by-side positions may be popular for sexual partners with significant weight differences, pregnant women, partners with chronic pain disorders like arthritis, and partners who do not enjoy deep thrusting.[6]

Atypical Sexual Behaviors and Paraphilias

Some sexual practices are much less common statistically in our society than those already described. If they are practiced between consenting adults and no physical or psychological harm is done to anyone, they are simply considered atypical. Examples are sex games in which partners enact sexual fantasies, use sex toys (vibrators, dildos), or engage in phone sex (talk about sex, describe erotic scenarios). Another kind of sex game is bondage and discipline, in which restriction of movement (using handcuffs or ropes, for example) or sensory deprivation (using blindfolds or masks) is employed for sexual enjoyment. Most sex games are safe and harmless, but partners need to openly discuss and agree beforehand on what they are comfortable doing.

Atypical sexual practices that do not meet the criteria described above (being consensual and causing no harm) are called paraphilias; they are classified as mental disorders, and many are illegal. According to the American Psychiatric Association's *Diagnostic and Statistical Manual of Mental Disorders* (*DSM-IV-TR*), a **paraphilia** is a mental disorder characterized by recurrent, intense sexual urges, fantasies, or behaviors generally involving (1) nonhuman objects, (2) the suffering and humiliation of oneself or one's sexual partner, or (3) children or other nonconsenting adults.[12] The urges occur over a period of at least 6 months and cause significant distress or impairment. Examples of paraphilias are exhibitionism (exposing one's genitals to strangers), voyeurism (observing others' sexual activity without their knowledge), and pedophilia (sexual attraction to and activity with children). A person with a paraphilia usually seeks treatment only when forced to by the law. Treatment focuses initially on reducing the danger to the patient and potential victims and then on strategies to suppress the behavior. Relapse prevention is essential since these behaviors are usually long-standing.[6]

SEXUAL DYSFUNCTIONS

At some point in their lives, many people experience some kind of **sexual dysfunction**—a disturbance in sexual drive, performance, or satisfaction—at some point in their lives. Up to 50 percent of couples report having experienced sexual dissatisfaction or dysfunction.[9] Sexual difficulties may occur at any point in the sexual response, although

Couples who have jobs and children to care for may not always have the time or energy to enjoy a satisfying sex life. Scheduling "date" nights or weekends away together can help foster the intimacy needed for a rewarding sexual relationship.

lack of sexual desire is cited as the most frequent problem in marriage and long-term relationships.[13] Fortunately, most forms of sexual dysfunction are treatable.

Female Sexual Dysfunctions

Common sexual dysfunctions in women include pain during intercourse, sexual desire disorder, female sexual arousal disorder, and orgasmic dysfunction.

Pain During Intercourse

Some women experience pain during intercourse as a result of **vaginismus,** intense involuntary contractions of the outer third of the muscles of the vagina that tighten the vaginal opening when penetration is attempted. The muscle spasm may range from mild, causing discomfort during intercourse, to severe, preventing intercourse altogether. Vaginismus may be caused by the physiological effects of a medical condition, such as a pelvic or vaginal infection, or it may be caused by psychological factors, such as fear of intercourse. A woman who has experienced sexual trauma, such as abuse or rape, may develop vaginismus. In treating this condition, a physician should first rule out medical problems. He or she may then recommend **Kegel exercises,** the alternating contraction and relaxation of pelvic floor muscles, which can help relieve vaginismus. Referral to psychotherapy or sex therapy may be needed if the condition persists.

Pain during intercourse can result from factors other than vaginismus. A common cause is lack of vaginal lubrication due to insufficient arousal or to hormone fluctuation. If greater attention to foreplay does not help resolve the problem, commercial products are available that provide lubrication.

Sexual Desire Disorder

Sexual desire disorder is characterized by lack of sexual fantasies and desire for sexual activity. Because individuals have different normal levels of sexual desire, a problem is considered to exist only if a person is dissatisfied with her own or her partner's level of sexual desire. Low sexual desire can have physical causes. Medications and drugs, hormonal changes, alcohol, nicotine, recreational drugs, some antidepressants, birth control pills, and medical problems such as chronic pain may affect sexual desire.[14]

Low sexual desire can also be caused by psychological, emotional, and relationship problems. A person experiencing a decline in sexual desire should consider what

KEY TERMS

paraphilia Mental disorder characterized by recurrent, intense sexual urges, fantasies, or behaviors generally involving (1) nonhuman objects, (2) the suffering and humiliation of oneself or one's sexual partner, or (3) children or other nonconsenting adults.

sexual dysfunction Disturbance in sexual drive, performance, or satisfaction.

vaginismus Intense involuntary contractions of the outer third of the muscles of the vagina that prevent penetration or make it uncomfortable.

Kegel exercises Alternating contraction and relaxation of pelvic floor muscles, performed to help relieve vaginismus, among other effects.

HIGHLIGHT ON HEALTH
A Double Standard

Throughout much of the 20th century, sex education was presented from a male point of view. Boys received extensive warnings about hormonal impulses that would trigger sexual desire, while girls were taught about the menstrual cycle. If girls were told anything at all about sex, it was to avoid getting boys too excited. The message was that only boys wanted to have sex; female sexual pleasure was rarely if ever mentioned.

Women who were interested in their own sexuality risked disapproval and worse if they did not conform to society's norms. If they were sexually active outside marriage, they were likely to be labeled *promiscuous*, a word that might also be applied to gay men but not to heterosexual men. Even if women were willing to pursue their own pleasure, little information on female sexuality was available.

In the 1970s, feminists rebelled against this situation. In books like *Our Bodies, Ourselves,* they edu-cated women about their bodies and especially about the role of the clitoris in sexual pleasure. According to some feminists, most American women were ignorant of the role of the clitoris in sexual pleasure until the 1960s. Some misinformation can be traced back to Freud's theories of sexuality, which held that mature women derived sexual satisfaction from vaginal penetration rather than clitoral stimulation. However, much of the ignorance surrounding women's sexuality can be attributed to our society's reluctance to acknowledge the important role of sexuality in women's lives.

Sources: *Women,* by N. Angier, 1999, Boston: Houghlin Mifflin; *With Pleasure: Thoughts on the Nature of Human Sexuality,* by P. R. Abramson and S. D. Pinkerton, 1995, New York: Oxford Press; *Our Bodies, Ourselves: A New Edition for a New Era,* Boston Women's Health Book Collective, 2005, New York: Touchstone Books.

else is occurring in her life, such as financial worries, anxiety about work, or problems communicating with her partner. When people are tired, overworked, or stressed, they may give sex a low priority. To have a satisfying sex life, partners have to at least take the time to have sex. Setting aside a particular time may be a solution. Adding variety to sex, such as by trying different positions, sharing sex fantasies, or playing sex games, can also help.

Female Sexual Arousal Disorder

This disorder is characterized by an inability to attain or maintain the lubrication-swelling response of sexual arousal to the completion of sexual activity. The symptoms do not occur because of insufficient or misplaced sexual stimulation. Like sexual desire disorder, this disorder is considered a problem only if the individual experiencing it considers it a problem.

Orgasmic Dysfunction

Orgasmic dysfunction is defined as the persistent inability to have an orgasm following normal sexual arousal. Between 25 and 35 percent of women report having had difficulty with orgasm on one or more occasions, and 10 percent to 15 percent of women report that they have never had an orgasm.[15] Some women can achieve orgasm through masturbation or oral sex but not with penile penetration. Although orgasm is not necessary for conception or enjoyment of sex, difficulty achieving orgasm can become a frustrating and distressing experience.

Orgasmic dysfunction may be influenced by psychological and emotional factors, by lack of knowledge and experience, or by the person's beliefs and attitudes about sex.[16] Certain medications, including some antidepressants, also reduce the ability to reach orgasm. Orgasmic dysfunction may be more common in younger women; as they gain experience, learn more about their bodies, and are exposed to a wider variety of stimulation, they may be less likely to have difficulties reaching orgasm. Therapy for orgasmic dysfunction focuses on encouraging women to experiment with their own bodies to discover what stimulates them to orgasm. They are then encouraged to transfer this learning to their sexual relationships.

Treatment of Female Sexual Dysfunctions

For most of the 20th century, understanding of female sexuality was grounded in ignorance (see the box "A Double Standard"). Even today, sexuality and sexual pleasure are defined primarily in male terms.[17] What is known about the neurophysiology of sexual arousal, desire, and orgasm has come mainly from research on men and has been extrapolated to women. But women's sexuality is different from men's and much more complex than previously thought. Currently, there is a new interest in female sexuality on the part of scientists, sex therapists, and pharmaceutical companies, partly as a result of the success of Viagra in relieving men's sexual problems.

In the past, the sexual problems sometimes associated with menopause were treated with hormones, but health risks have reduced this practice. Another approach is testosterone replacement therapy. As noted earlier, testosterone is responsible for sex drive in both men and women. Women typically experience a 15 percent drop in testosterone levels during their 30s and 40s.[3] Women with deficient testosterone levels may experience decreased sexual arousal, less sexual fantasizing, and less sensitivity to the stimulation of their nipples, vagina, or clitoris. Sensibly prescribed, medically necessary testosterone can increase a woman's sex drive without serious side effects. Scientists are experimenting with both oral supplements and patches that deliver the drug through the skin. Benefits have included increased feelings of vitality and sexual desire, but possible side effects include increased risk of heart disease and liver damage. A higher-than-normal testosterone level exposes women to the same health risks as those experienced by men.[3]

Viagra has been tried in women to treat low sexual desire, but results have been disappointing. Viagra has the same effect on the clitoris as it has on the penis, allowing tissue to swell with blood during sexual arousal. However, physiological arousal does not lead to sexual desire as easily in women as it does in men. Although the ability to become aroused may be enhanced, the desire to have sex may not. Despite setbacks, the drug market for treating female sexual dysfunction is likely to reach $2 billion by 2008.[14]

Male Sexual Dysfunctions

Male sexual dysfunctions include pain during intercourse, sexual desire disorder, erectile dysfunction, and ejaculation dysfunction.

Pain During Intercourse

Pain during intercourse or after intercourse is rarely cited as a sexual dysfunction in men, but it can reduce sexual pleasure and satisfaction. Penile pain usually results from infections from sexually transmitted diseases. Herpes can cause painful lesions on the penis, and gonorrhea and chlamydia cause a penile discharge and pain with urination or ejaculation for most men. Peyronie's disease, an abnormal curvature of the penis, can also make intercourse painful. Infections of the prostate and epididymis also cause pain and should be treated.

Sexual Desire Disorder

Like women, men sometimes experience reduced interest in sex. Sexual desire disorders are frequently caused by emotional problems, including relationship difficulties, depression, guilt over infidelity, worry, stress, and overwork. Reduced sexual desire also can have some physical causes, such as changes in testosterone level. Some health conditions can reduce the production of testosterone by the testes.

Erectile Dysfunction

As noted earlier, erection occurs when arterioles supplying blood to the penis relax, allowing the spongy chambers of the penis to fill with blood. In men with **erectile dysfunction (ED),** smooth-muscle cells constrict the local arteries and reduce blood flow to a trickle, preventing a buildup of blood. The penis remains flaccid (soft) if the smooth-muscle cells are contracted.

The causes of erectile dysfunction (formerly called impotence) can be psychological or physical or both. The best way to determine the cause is to observe overnight erection patterns. Starting in early childhood, males experience erections during normal sleep. If the cause of ED is emotional, erections will continue to occur during sleep. Less than 20 percent of ED cases have emotional causes.[18] Examples of such causes are anxiety about sexual performance and problems in the relationship with the partner. Some of the physical causes of ED are low testosterone levels, medications (some antidepressants, blood pressure medications), drugs (alcohol, tobacco), injury, vascular disease, blood flow problems in the genitals, and nerve damage, such as from diabetes, injury, or prostate surgery (see the box "Who Is Least Likely to Experience Erectile Dysfunction?").

Long-term excessive pressure from riding a bicycle also may cause erectile dysfunction. Blood vessels that supply the penis are located in the area between the base of the scrotum and the anus, and excessive pressure in this area can reduce blood flow to the penis. Numbness in the penis and scrotum is a warning sign of excessive pressure. If you experience this problem, try adjusting the bicycle seat so your legs don't extend as far while pedaling, or buy a wider bicycle seat. Personnel in most bicycle shops can help you adjust your seat properly.[9]

Ejaculation Dysfunction

Premature ejaculation, defined as a tendency to ejaculate before or shortly after the beginning of intercourse, is

KEY TERMS

erectile dysfunction (ED)   Condition in which the penis does not become erect before sex or stay erect during sex.

Beating the Odds

Who Is Least Likely to Experience Erectile Dysfunction?

A variety of factors can contribute to erectile dysfunction, including medical conditions, lifestyle habits, psychological issues, and age. Brief profiles of three men are presented here. Which one do you think is least likely to experience ED?

Jason is a 26-year-old paramedic. He is not currently in a relationship. He is 30 pounds overweight and doesn't get a lot of exercise, though his job is physically active. He spends most of his free time trying to meet women over the Internet, but so far he has not been successful in finding a good match. Jason has a high-fat diet and takes medication for high blood pressure, which runs in his family. He typically drinks two or three beers every evening; he is a light smoker.

Ramiro is a 35-year-old computer technician. He was diagnosed with diabetes when he was 10 years old, and since then he has taken medication daily. Because he knows that exercise is important for people with diabetes, he has become an avid bicyclist and regularly participates in competitive cycling events. He consumes a low-fat, high-fiber diet and doesn't drink or smoke. He is single and has an active sex life.

Aidan is a 42-year-old investment banker. He finds his work highly stressful, and he unwinds at the end of the day at a local cigar bar, drinking and smoking. He is not overweight, but he doesn't exercise or pay attention to his diet. Aidan recently broke up with his girlfriend after a 5-year relationship because she wanted to get married and start a family. He would like to get married, but he doesn't want to have children. He takes antidepressants and occasionally uses cocaine and marijuana recreationally.

OLC Web site Visit the **Online Learning Center** at www.mhhe.com/teague1e for comments by the authors.

---

probably the most common type of ejaculation dysfunction.[19] Like ED, premature ejaculation often results from anxiety about sexual performance or unreasonable expectations. For example, a man might be worried about maintaining an erection and rush to a climax.[9]

Treatment of Male Sexual Dysfunction

Treatment of sexual dysfunction in men often relies on testosterone. Men with a low testosterone level may benefit from testosterone replacement therapy. It can be injected, administered through a patch, or applied to the skin as an ointment. It is not prescribed for men with normal testosterone levels because it can increase blood pressure, affect blood cholesterol levels, and possibly increase risk for prostate cancer.[9]

Treatments for erectile problems include drugs taken orally and by injection, mechanical devices (penile implants), and surgery to repair arteries supplying blood to the penis. Today, Viagra (sildenafil) is the treatment of choice for ED. Viagra was introduced in 1998 and has become the most frequently prescribed drug in the United States. Taken an hour before sex, Viagra works by increasing the concentration of the chemical that allows smooth-muscle cells in the erectile tissue to stay relaxed so the spongy chambers of the penis can remain filled with blood. Its effects last about 4 hours. Studies suggest that about 80 percent of men with varying degrees of ED have benefited from Viagra.[9]

Common side effects of Viagra include flushing, indigestion, nasal congestion, nausea, and headaches. Overuse can cause a dangerous condition called priapism, a state of continuous erection that can permanently damage the penis. Use of Viagra is dangerous for men with preexisting health conditions such as heart disease, high blood pressure, and diabetes, and fatalities have been reported in connection with its use.

Viagra is just one of several new drugs developed to treat erectile problems. Levitra (Vardenafil) and Cialis (Tadolifil) are chemically similar to Viagra but more potent and efficient. Levitra takes about 16 minutes to work and may last 2 hours longer than Viagra. Cialis also takes about 16 minutes to work but may last up to 36 hours. Both have side effects similar to those of Viagra.

Sex therapy for male sexual dysfunctions focuses on modifying counterproductive behaviors, improving communication between partners, and teaching specific techniques to enhance sexual performance. Drug approaches to sexual dysfunctions do not take into account the importance of relationships. They may offer a temporary confidence-builder, but they do not provide a long-term solution to issues that may lie behind sexual problems. Correcting unhealthy lifestyles, working on relationships, and cultivating a more realistic expectation of aging can improve mid- and late-life sexuality. Exercise, good nutrition, and emotional intimacy with one's partner are as important as Viagra.

Healthy People 2010

OBJECTIVE AREA *STDs and HIV*

- Increase the proportion of sexually active persons who use condoms.

"Unintended pregnancies and sexually transmitted diseases (STDs), including infection with the human immunodeficiency virus that causes AIDS, can result from unprotected sexual behaviors. Abstinence is the only method of complete protection. Condoms, if used correctly and consistently, can help prevent both unintended pregnancy and STDs...."

"About one-half of all new HIV infections in the United States are among people under age 25 years, and the majority are infected through sexual behavior. HIV infection is the leading cause of death for African American men aged 25 to 44 years. Compelling worldwide evidence indicates that the presence of other STDs increases the likelihood of both transmitting and acquiring HIV infection."

For more information on Healthy People 2010 objectives, visit the Web site at www.healthypeople.gov.

For more information on Canadian health objectives, visit the Health Canada Web site at www.hc-sc.gc.ca/english.

PROTECTING YOUR SEXUAL HEALTH

One of the biggest threats to your sexual health is infection with a sexually transmitted disease (STD). These infections range from annoyances like pubic lice to life-threatening diseases like AIDS. We discuss STDs in detail in Chapter 20; here, we discuss **safer sex** practices, which prevent the exchange of body fluids during sex. Two safer sex practices are using condoms and having sex that does not involve genital contact or penetration. A third practice is abstinence, considered the only way to completely guarantee protection against STDs. (These practices are also discussed in Chapter 16 as ways to prevent conception.) Another key to safeguarding your sexual health is communicating about sex.

Using Condoms

Condoms (or *male condoms*) are thin sheaths, usually made of latex, that fit over the erect penis during sexual intercourse. They provide a barrier against penile, vaginal, or anal discharges and genital lesions or sores. Although condoms do not provide complete protection against all STDs, they greatly reduce the risk of infection when used correctly (see Figure 16.2 in the next chapter). Latex condoms should not be used with any oil-based lubricants (such as Vaseline or hand lotion) because such products cause latex to deteriorate. Plastic (polyurethane) condoms are also available and can be used by people who are allergic to latex. They are thinner, stronger, and less constricting than latex, and they are not eroded by oil-based lubricants. However, they are more expensive than latex condoms and have not been as fully tested for effectiveness.

Protection against STDs is also offered by the **female condom,** a soft pouch of thin polyurethane that is inserted into the vagina before intercourse. The female condom has a soft flexible ring at both ends. The ring at the closed end is fitted against the cervix, and the ring at the open end remains outside the body (see Figure 16.3 in the next chapter). Both male and female condoms can be purchased at drug stores and grocery stores. The female condom covers more of the genital area, so it may provide more protection against an STD lesion or sore than the male condom does. Spermicidal foam can be used with both kinds of condoms to kill some bacteria.

Condoms and **dental dams** (a small latex square placed over the vulva) should be used during oral sex because bacteria and viruses can be transmitted in semen and vaginal fluids. Plastic wrap placed over the vulva, or a piece of latex cut from a latex glove, is an alternative to a dental dam. Protection is especially important if there are any cuts or sores in the mouth; even bleeding gums can increase the risk of getting an infection.

Sexual activities that do not involve genital or skin contact are safer than those that do. Many people find enjoyment in such activities as hugging, massage, and erotic touching, stroking, and caressing with the clothes on.

KEY TERMS

safer sex   Sexual activities that do not include exchange of body fluids during sex.

condom   Thin sheath, usually made of latex, that fits over the erect penis during sexual intercourse to prevent conception and protect against STDs.

female condom   Soft pouch of thin polyurethane that is inserted into the vagina before intercourse to prevent conception and protect against STDs.

dental dam   Small latex square placed over the vulva during oral sex.

Consumer Clipboard

Ten Questions to Ask Your Partner Before Beginning a Sexual Relationship

"There's something I need to tell you." It's far better to hear these words before you have sex with a partner than after. Partners need to discuss their sexual histories and health before beginning a sexual relationship. They also need to be realistic about the risks they're taking and assertive about their right to be safe. Both partners should be willing to ask and answer the following 10 questions:

1. Are you having sex with anyone else?
2. How many sexual partners have you had?
3. Have you ever had an STD?
4. Have you ever had a sexual partner who had HIV or another STD?
5. Have you been tested for HIV or another STD?
6. If so, how many sexual partners have you had since then?
7. Have you ever had genital warts or other sores or lesions on your genitals?
8. Do you have any STD symptoms—sores, warts, pain, vaginal or penile discharge?
9. Do you know how to tell if you are infected with an STD?
10. Are you willing to get tested for HIV and other STDs and then have a monogamous relationship? If not, are you willing to use condoms every time we have sex?

Source: Harvard Medical School's Consumer Health Information, www.intelihealth.com.

Practicing Abstinence

People practice abstinence for a variety of reasons. Some are abstinent for moral or religious reasons; they believe that sexual activity should be reserved for marriage. Abstinence is often promoted as a positive choice for young people; when this is the case, however, individuals should be provided with information and education about both contraception and STDs. Some unmarried couples choose to be abstinent until they are married, and some married couples use periodic abstinence as a contraceptive method. As noted earlier, abstinence is the only way that people can be completely certain they are not at risk for STDs and unintended pregnancy.

Avoiding Alcohol

Whether you plan to use a condom, limit your sexual activities, or not have sex at all, it's a good idea to avoid drinking alcohol when you are in a situation where sex might occur. Alcohol lowers sexual inhibitions and impairs judgment, decision making, effective listening, rational thinking, and the ability to accurately assess risky behaviors and potentially dangerous situations. Honesty, respect, trust, and communication are all likely to be compromised under the influence of too much alcohol. Decreased neurological function can even make it difficult to use a condom properly. In addition, alcohol impairs sexual performance and reduces sexual satisfaction. Psychoactive drugs like marijuana and Ecstasy also increase your risk of engaging in behavior you might regret later.

Communicating About Sex

Conversations about sexual topics can be awkward and difficult, but they are important to your health, your partners' health, and the success of your relationship. If you are about to begin a sexual relationship, take the time to tell your partner your sexual health history and find out about his or hers. See the boxes "Ten Questions to Ask Your Partner Before Beginning a Sexual Relationship" and "Tips for Telling a Partner You Have an STD" for guidelines on how to approach these discussions.

Also take the time to clarify your values, attitudes, and standards about your own sexuality. Is your behavior consistent with your values? Are you influenced by media images and peer pressure, or are your decisions about sexual activity intentional and voluntary? Along with all the sexual information, knowledge, and freedom available to individuals in our society comes the responsibility to make informed, healthy choices.

SEX AND CULTURE: ISSUES FOR THE 21ST CENTURY

Woody Allen's 1973 movie *Sleeper* may have captured some of the sexual realities of our current cultural scene. In this movie, set in the future, all of a person's

Challenges & Choices

Tips for Telling a Partner You Have an STD

Telling a partner you have an STD is not easy. Being candid and honest at the outset of the relationship is highly recommended. Here are some tips:

- If you are currently undergoing treatment for the STD, tell your partner; do not have sex until treatment is complete.

- Be open about how you contracted the STD and share the information you have about the disease. Do not share any medication you are taking. Most antibiotics are effective only if you take the entire course prescribed for you.

- Encourage your partner to be tested if it is possible that he or she has become infected. This might happen if you realize you have an STD after you and your partner begin a sexual relationship. Symptoms of some STDs don't appear for some time; other STDs don't have any visible symptoms at all.

- If your partner resists getting tested, emphasize that consequences can be very serious if an STD is left untreated.

- You can be reinfected with an STD after you have been treated if your partner isn't treated as well. Some STDs are passed back and forth between partners several times, sometimes becoming more resistant to treatment. Make sure you are both free of infection before you start or resume sexual activity.

It's Not Just Personal...

According to the CDC National Prevention Information Network (www.cdcnpin.org), the United States has the highest rates of STDs in the industrialized world. In fact, those rates are 50 to 100 times higher than those of other industrialized countries. An estimated 15.3 million new cases of STDs are reported each year in the United States.

Source: *Sex Q & A*, by A. Hooper, 2001, New York: DK Publishing.

---

sexual needs can be taken care of by a sophisticated mechanical masturbator called an "orgasmatron." People no longer have to deal with the difficulties and hang-ups associated with relationships to get sexual satisfaction.

Like the orgasmatron, the Internet offers people immediate, anonymous, and solitary sex without the complexities of relationships. The same can be said for pornography and prostitution, two other commonplace features of contemporary culture. In this section, we take a brief look at these three phenomena.

Cybersex

Sex is ubiquitous on the Internet, whether you're looking for it or not. Sexual images, invitations, and products can pop up on your computer screen or in your e-mail in-box at almost any time. If you are seeking sexual topics, you can easily find pornography, sexually explicit Web sites, erotic chat rooms, interactive games, and sex toys for sale. Some Web sites offer instant partners for mutual sexual fantasies, and some provide live video of performers who can respond to suggestions made by the viewer.

People access this explicit but virtual sex for many reasons—to obtain sexual gratification, to search for

romance, to relieve boredom, to satisfy their curiosity. Issues arise over whether the availability of **cybersex** has harmful consequences, for adults, for children, for society. An exploration of the issues associated with cybersex is provided in You Make the Call at the end of the chapter.

Pornography

The definition of **pornography** has been a matter of debate for generations, but it is widely held to include materials created, distributed, or sold for the sole purpose of sexual arousal. Pornography has long been part of human culture, but every society and era has its own versions. An issue for our time is whether pornography

KEY TERMS

cybersex   Sexual material and activity available on the Internet, including pornography, sexual chatting, and interactive sex with a virtual partner.

pornography   Materials created, distributed, or sold for the sole purpose of sexual arousal.

promotes violence against women and sexual abuse of children. Some social scientists have suggested that exposure to depictions of sexual violence and exploitation can increase criminal behavior, especially on the part of men with psychological problems or other vulnerabilities. Some feminists have argued that pornography contributes to the sexual subordination of women and ongoing social inequalities for women.[20] The distribution of child pornography on the Internet has vastly increased its availability and emboldened its practitioners. For reasons such as these, some people want government to do more to suppress X-rated materials and punish those who promote them.

Defenders of pornography respond that the use of explicit sexual materials by adults is protected by the right to free speech. They argue that pornography—both "hard core" and "soft core" (erotic material aimed more at couples)—provides harmless pleasure and has educational and therapeutic benefits. They also point out that research has yet to establish a relationship between pornography and sexual violence.[20] With the Internet becoming ever more pervasive in our society, the debate is likely to continue.

Prostitution

Like pornography, **prostitution**—the exchange of sex for money—has been around since the beginning of recorded history and probably before. An issue in our era is the spread of HIV infection and AIDS by prostitutes throughout the world. Commercial sex is associated with very high rates of HIV infection worldwide. In some developing countries, prostitution is forced on young girls and adolescents, and condom use by men is rare. In some places, these "sex workers" are organizing to protect their health and human rights.

In the United States, many prostitutes use injection drugs, one of the principal sources of HIV infection, or have customers who use them. In some parts of the country, up to 50 percent of the prostitutes are estimated to be infected with HIV.[9] Some public health experts have argued that prostitution should be decriminalized so that prostitutes can be licensed and required to have regular health exams. They point to the counties in Nevada where prostitution is legal and prostitutes are required by law to use condoms and be tested monthly for HIV. No legal working prostitute in these counties is HIV positive. Decriminalizing prostitution on a national level is unlikely at this time, however; at most, it will remain a major cultural issue in the 21st century.

KEY TERMS

prostitution   Exchange of sex for money; prostitutes are sometimes called sex workers.

You Make the Call

Cybersex: Harmless Fun or Moral Black Hole?

Cybersex, cyber porn, virtual sex—whatever you call it, it's available on the Internet. A major objection to the widespread availability of this material is that children can easily access it. Although owners of adult Web sites say they are not interested in attracting children, there is no foolproof way to prevent sexually curious children from gaining access to many of these sites. Some children use their parents' credit cards to pay for access and simply click on the "I am over 18" button. Other children come across the sites by accident when researching innocent topics.

In 1995, Congress passed the Communications Decency Act (CDA), imposing fines and possible prison sentences on anyone who knowingly made sexually explicit material on the Internet available to children. The Supreme Court struck down the CDA in 1997 as a violation of the right to free speech guaranteed by the First Amendment. In 1998, President Clinton signed the 1998 Child Online Protection Act, but this act has also been challenged under the First Amendment.

Another objection is that the Internet has vastly expanded the range over which pornographic material, including child pornography, can be distributed. It has emboldened pedophiles and enhanced their ability to pursue their activities, and it has led people to explore a world of atypical sexual behaviors and sexual subcultures in ways that were not feasible in the past.

Opponents also question the effect of cybersex on mental health; they argue that engaging in sex with virtual partners impairs real relationships and robs people of the ability to experience sexual pleasure through interpersonal connections and intimacy. Laboratory studies have found that men are less enthusiastic about the attractiveness of their real-life partner after viewing attractive women in pornographic videos. Some people become addicted to Internet sex and devote large portions of their lives and financial resources to it, at the expense of their relationships, families, and jobs. Finally, opponents argue that the proliferation of sexual material on the Internet represents a degradation of society's morals and standards of decency.

Defenders of cybersex point out that it is intended for adults, who have the right to choose what they want to view on the Internet. Parents are responsible for keeping their children from accessing explicit sexual materials. Censoring or suppressing this material would be a violation of First Amendment rights, as the courts have already ruled. Defenders also argue that all forms of sexual expression are natural and that it is puritanical to condemn the behaviors depicted in pornography as immoral or abnormal. Defenders argue in addition that the kind of sexually explicit material available on the Internet can be used to educate and treat people with sexual dysfunctions by exposing them to a broad range of sexual activity without negative judgments.

Some people see cybersex as harmless entertainment that provides a needed outlet for responsible adults. Others view it as a threat to the moral development of children and the moral fiber of society. What do you think?

Pros

- Cybersex is a healthy outlet for sexual expression that fulfills sexual fantasies and needs for both men and women.

- Cybersex is not harmful. A 1970 review of scientific evidence by the Commission on Obscenity and Pornography concluded that pornography is not harmful. Cybersex would fall into the same category.

- Cybersex is an educational tool that can be used to teach sexual anatomy and functioning to people as

they become sexually mature. It reinforces acceptance of a wide range of behaviors and enhances people's ability to enjoy their full sexuality.

- Cybersex is a useful therapeutic treatment for some sexual problems and dysfunctions, especially for sexually inhibited individuals.

- Adults have the right to view sexually explicit materials if they wish. Cybersex is protected by the First Amendment right to free speech.

- There is no practical way to regulate and police sexual material on the Internet.

- Children are much more likely to be exposed to sexual images and references in movies, television shows, and song lyrics than on the Internet.

Cons

- Like pornography, cybersex objectifies and exploits women. Much of the sexually explicit material on the Internet depicts women in dehumanizing ways.

- Cybersex endangers children by facilitating the widespread distribution of child pornography and promoting pedophilia.

- The findings of the 1970 review of obscenity and pornography are not relevant today. Sexually explicit material today is much more violent and exploitative than in 1970.

- Pornography is illegal for children under age 18, but the Internet does not have any effective ways to block children from accessing sexually explicit sites. Operators of adult sites know they are going to break the law.

- Cybersex has a negative effect on people's real lives and relationships.

- Cybersex is degrading and has an emotionally and morally damaging effect on people.

OLC Web site For more information about this topic, visit the Online Learning Center at www.mhhe.com/teaguele.

SOURCES: *Pornography: The Production and Consumption of Inequality,* by G. Dines, R. Jensen, and A. Russo, 1998, New York: Routledge; *Growing Up Digital: The Rise of the Net Generation,* by D. Tapscott, 1998, New York: McGraw-Hill; *Tangled in the Web: Understanding Cybersex from Fantasy to Addiction,* by K. S. Young, 2001, Austin, TX: 1st Book Library; *The Psychology of the Internet,* by P. Wallace, 1999, New York: Columbia University Press.

SUMMARY

- Sexual health has biological, psychological, sociological, and cultural aspects. It includes healthy sexual functioning across the life span, satisfying intimate relationships, and the ability and resources to procreate if so desired.

- Sexual pleasure is strongly influenced by cultural attitudes and values. American society is characterized by

an ongoing tension between its puritan heritage and an affinity for freedom and open expression.

- The external female sex organs include the mons pubis, the labia majora and labia minora, the clitoris, and the vaginal and urethral openings, collectively referred to as the vulva. The internal female sex organs include the vagina, cervix, uterus, fallopian tubes, and ovaries. The mammary glands are also part of female sexual anatomy.

- The external male sex organs include the penis and the scrotum, which contains the testes. The internal male sex organs include the testes; a series of ducts that transport sperm (the epididymis, vas deferens, ejaculatory ducts, and urethra); and a set of glands that produce semen and other fluids (the seminal vesicles, prostate gland, and Cowper's glands).

- Sex drive is the biological urge for sexual activity; it is regulated by hormones and other body chemicals. Sexual arousal is marked by increased blood flow and muscle tension in the genitals and other erogenous zones of the body.

- The human sexual response model includes four stages: excitement, plateau, orgasm, and resolution. Orgasm is a physiological reflex characterized by rhythmic muscle contractions in the genital area and a sensation of intense pleasure. The subjective experience of orgasm can vary depending on a wide array of factors and circumstances.

- The biology of sexual and reproductive development is directed by hormones. During prenatal development, the presence of a Y chromosome stimulates the development of testes, which produce testosterone and cause the reproductive structures to become male sex organs. Without the Y chromosome, ovaries and female sex organs develop. At puberty, secondary sex characteristics appear and both sexes become sexually mature.

- The menstrual cycle is the monthly cycle of changes in the uterus that culminate in menstruation, the shedding of the uterine lining, if conception does not occur. Ovulation, the release of an ovum, occurs about halfway through the cycle. Menopause is the cessation of menstruation, usually occurring around age 50.

- Men do not experience a dramatic change in reproductive capacity in midlife as women do, but they do experience a gradual decline in sexual activity in mid- to later life.

- "Normal" sexual expression is defined by societal and cultural expectations. Typical sexual behaviors and forms of sexual expression in U.S. society include celibacy, kissing, erotic touch, self-stimulation (sexual fantasies and masturbation), oral-genital stimulation, and intercourse.

- Atypical sexual behaviors include activities that are less statistically common but that are consensual and do not cause harm, such as the use of sex toys. Paraphilias are sexual practices that are considered mental disorders and may be illegal.

- A sexual dysfunction is a disturbance in sexual drive, performance, or satisfaction. It may be temporary or long lasting. Common sexual dysfunctions in women include pain during intercourse, sexual desire disorder, female sexual arousal disorder, and orgasmic dysfunction. Male sexual dysfunctions include pain during intercourse, sexual desire disorder, erectile dysfunction, and ejaculation dysfunction. Sexual dysfunctions can have both physical and psychological causes; treatments include hormones, drugs, psychotherapy, and sex therapy.

- Safer sex practices are those that prevent the exchange of body fluids during sex. They include using male condoms, female condoms, and dental dams; having sex that does not include genital contact or penetration; and practicing abstinence. Communicating about sex is an important part of intimate relationships and sexual health.

- Cybersex, pornography, and prostitution are three areas of sexual behavior that present problems for society.

REVIEW QUESTIONS

1. What are some of the components of sexual health?

2. What accounts for the complementarity of the male and female sex organs?

3. Describe the external and internal female sexual organs. What is the dual function of the vagina? What are the functions of the ovaries?

4. Describe the external and internal male sexual organs. Describe the process by which sperm move from the testes to the urethra. What are the functions of the seminal vesicles, prostate gland, and Cowper's glands?

5. What are some of the problems associated with hormone replacement therapy?

6. What hormones and neurotransmitters are involved in regulating sex drive?

7. Describe the process by which the penis becomes erect.

8. What are the four phases of the human sexual response model? What happens in each phase? What is the refractory period?

9. Why do many women not reach orgasm from penile thrusting alone?

10. What glands and organs are involved in producing sex hormones?

11. Describe the effects of puberty for males and for females.

12. What are the physical and emotional changes associated with menopause? With viropause?

13. What are some reasons that people choose celibacy or abstinence?

14. What is foreplay? Why is it important? What are the most common sexual behaviors and forms of expression?

15. What makes a sexual behavior atypical? What are the basic criteria that distinguish atypical behaviors from paraphilias?

16. What is the definition of a paraphilia? What are some examples?

17. What is the most frequently cited sexual problem in long-term relationships?

18. What are two causes of pain during intercourse for women? What are some causes of orgasmic dysfunction in women? Why is Viagra not very effective in women?

19. What are some of the emotional and physical causes of erectile dysfunction? What are three approaches to the treatment of male sexual dysfunction?

20. Why should you not use an oil-based product with a latex condom?

21. What are some sexual and sensual activities that do not include genital or skin contact?

22. How does alcohol affect sexual decision making?

23. What questions should you ask your partner and be prepared to answer before starting a sexual relationship?

24. What are some of the problems and issues associated with sexual material available on the Internet? With pornography? With prostitution?

WEB RESOURCES

Go Ask Alice: This Columbia University site features questions and answers of interest to young adults. The section on sexuality addresses a wide range of topics—from kissing to achieving orgasm. The sexual health section offers information on issues such as reproduction, contraception, and STDs.
www.goaskalice.columbia.edu

National Men's Health Network: In addition to offering basic information related to men's health, this site includes a resource center with links to articles, books, government sites, health organizations, and other health resources of special interest to men.
www.menshealthnetwork.org

National Sexuality Resource Center: This organization addresses issues in contemporary sexuality. Its sexual literacy campaign is designed to counteract negative messages about sexuality and promote healthy attitudes toward sexuality.
http://nsrc.sfsu.edu

National Women's Health Network: Organized to promote women's involvement in the health care system, this group offers news updates, fact sheets, and health information packets. It encourages critical analysis of health issues related specifically to women.
www.womenshealthnetwork.org

Planned Parenthood: The Sexual Health section of this Web site offers a guide to sexuality for young women and another for young men. It also features topics such as safer sex, condom use, and STDs, with questions and answers on a variety of sexuality issues.
www.plannedparenthood.org

Sexuality Information and Education Council of the United States: This organization's Web site includes FAQs, information updates, fact sheets on sexuality at different life stages, gay and lesbian issues, and approaches to sex education.
www.siecus.org

Talking with Kids: This site features a series of "tough topics" that parents face with their children. It offers 10 tips on how to approach discussions on sex, including the importance of initiating such conversations, giving age-appropriate information, and creating an atmosphere for openness.
www.talkingwithkids.org

REFERENCES

1. Hutcherson, H. (2002). *What your mother never told you about sex.* New York: G. P. Putnam's Sons.

2. Abramson, P. R., & Pinkerton, S. D. (1995). *With pleasure: Thoughts on the nature of human sexuality.* New York: Oxford University Press.

3. Crenshaw, T. L. (1996). *The alchemy of love and lust.* New York: Pocket Books.

4. Masters, W., & Johnson, L. (1966). *Human sexual response.* Boston: Little, Brown.

5. Basson, R. (2000). The female sexual response: A different model. *Journal of Sex and Marital Therapy, 26,* 51–65.

6. Godson, S. (2002). *The sex book.* London: Cassell Illustrated.

7. Hooper, A. (2001). *Sex Q & A.* New York: DK Publishing.

8. Writing Group for the Women's Health Initiative Investigators. (2002). Risks and benefits of estrogen plus progestin in healthy premenopausal women. *Journal of American Medical Association, 28* (3), 324–333.

9. Milsten, R., Slowinski, J. (1999). *The sexual male: Problems and solutions.* New York: W. W. Norton and Company.

10. Bader, M. (2002). *Arousal: The secret logic of sexual fantasies.* New York: St. Martin's Press.

11. *Masturbation—From stigma to sexual health.* (2002). New York: Planned Parenthood Federation of America.

12. American Psychiatric Association. (2000). *Diagnostic and statistical manual of mental disorders* (4th ed., Text Revision *[DSM-IV-TR]*). Washington, DC: American Psychiatric Association Press.

13. Surgeon general. (2004). The surgeon general's call to action to promote sexual health and responsible sexual behavior. U.S. Department of Health and Human Services. www.ejhs.org/volume4/calltoaction.htm.

14. Leland, J. (2000, May 29). The science of women and sex. *Newsweek*, 48–54.

15. Heiman, J. R. (2000). Orgasmic disorders in women. In S. R. Leiblum & R. C. Rosen (Eds.), *Principles and practice of sex therapy.* New York: Guilford Press.

16. Barlik, B., & Goldberg, J. (2000). Female sexual arousal disorders. In S. R. Leiblum & R. C. Rosen (Eds.), *Principles and practice of sex therapy.* New York: Guilford Press.

17. Crawford, M., & Popp, D. (2003). Sexual double standards: A review and methodological critique of two decades of research. *The Journal of Sex Research, 40* (1), 13–26.

18. Marieb, E. N. (2001). *Human anatomy and physiology* (5th ed.). San Francisco: Benjamin Cummings.

19. Symond, T., Roblin, D., & Hart, K. (2003). How does premature ejaculation impact a man's life? *Journal of Sex & Marital Therapy, 29,* 361–370.

20. Dines, G., Jensen, R., & Russo, A. (1998). *Pornography: The production and consumption of inequality.* New York: Routledge.

Add It Up! SEXUAL PROBLEM QUESTIONNAIRE

Sexual problems in a relationship can often be traced to the emotional dimension of the relationship, to general sexual misinformation, or to inadequate communication between partners. Many people prefer not to think about sexual problems, but self-reflection is the vital first step in addressing them. If you think you might be experiencing a sexual problem in your relationship, consider the following five questions and answer them as honestly as you can. Use a scale of 1 to 5, with 1 representing "not at all," 3 representing "somewhat," and 5 representing "very much." Then read the discussion that follows the questions.

1. Do you think about the   1 2 3 4 5
    problem often?

2. Has the problem affected   1 2 3 4 5
    your self-image?

3. Do you fear discussing the   1 2 3 4 5
    problem with your partner?

4. Does the problem affect   1 2 3 4 5
    your daily life?

5. Have you sought advice or   1 2 3 4 5
    thought about seeking advice
    about the problem from a friend?

Scoring

1.   Determining whether there is a sexual problem in your relationship is the critical first step. The amount of time you spend worrying or thinking about the problem is an indicator of its seriousness. A high score here indicates greater seriousness and a greater need to address the problem. For example, if you feel anxious much of the day as you visualize what may happen later that evening, you need to address the problem.

2.   Does the problem affect how you feel about your body? Does it damage your ability to develop relationships? For example, do you avoid intimate relationships out of fear that a sexual encounter will embarrass you? A high score on this question indicates that this problem may be damaging your self-esteem and your ability to develop healthy relationships.

3.   People often complain that their partner does not understand the depth of their frustration or anxiety about a sexual problem. A high score here indicates a fear or reluctance to discuss the issue with your partner. Sexual problems affect both partners and have to be addressed by both. Fear and withdrawal isolate you and increase the distance in the relationship.

4.   A high score on this question is a warning that the problem is affecting areas of your life other than your sexual relationship. For example, a preoccupation with feelings of sexual inadequacy may interfere with your ability to concentrate at work or make you feel depressed or short-tempered at home. These feelings can snowball into overall dissatisfaction with the relationship and eventually destroy it. Sexual dissatisfaction is a primary cause of divorce in the United States and Canada.

5.   Seeking advice about a sexual problem from a friend is probably not a good idea. Many partners would consider it a betrayal of trust. Discussion of sexual problems is best kept within the relationship. If you cannot resolve the problem by yourselves, first rule out physical or medical causes and then seek help from a counselor or sex therapist. A valuable source for referrals is the American Association of Sex Educators, Counselors, and Therapists.

SOURCE: Adapted from *The Sexual Male: Problems and Solutions,* by R. Milstein and J. Slowinski, 1999, New York: W. W. Norton & Company.

CHAPTER 16

Reproductive Choices: Contraception, Pregnancy, and Childbirth

DID YOU KNOW?

• If you or your partner takes birth control pills, you are using the most popular form of contraception used by unmarried women in the United States. The advantages of birth control pills include their effectiveness, safety, convenience, ease of use, and reversibility. Their main disadvantage—and it is a big one—is that they provide no protection against sexually transmitted diseases (STDs).

• If you are a woman of childbearing age who might become pregnant, make sure your diet includes at least 400 micrograms of folic acid a day. This nutrient plays a role in preventing neural tube defects (defects in the brain and spinal cord) in a developing fetus. It is recommended that women have high levels of folic acid in their bodies at least 3 months *before* they become pregnant.

OLC *Your Health Today*   www.mhhe.com/teague1e

Go to the Online Learning Center for *Your Health Today* for interactive activities, quizzes, flashcards, Web links, and more resources related to this chapter.

Are you ready to be a parent? If your answer is no, many safe and effective methods of contraception are available that you and your partner can use to avoid an unintended pregnancy. If your answer is yes, a wealth of knowledge is available that you can use to increase the likelihood that your pregnancy is a positive experience and that your baby is healthy. If you want to have children some time in the future, planning for it now—by using contraception and choosing healthy lifestyle behaviors—can give you peace of mind and the knowledge that you are doing everything you can to protect the health of your future family.

In Chapters 14 and 15 we explored intimate relationships and sexuality. In this chapter we build on those topics to discuss reproductive choices and issues in creating a family. We begin by looking at the different contraceptive methods that are available to sexually active couples, from abstinence to sterilization, and then we consider the options open to people who do have unintended pregnancies. We continue with a look at infertility and the technologies developed to treat it. We then explore the many dimensions of pregnancy, prenatal care, and fetal development. We conclude the chapter with a discussion of labor, delivery, and the postpartum period.

CHOOSING A CONTRACEPTIVE METHOD

Choosing and using a contraceptive method that is right for you is important for one very significant reason: It lowers your risk of unintended pregnancy. More than half of all pregnancies are unintended, and many are unwanted, either because the couple doesn't want a child at this time or because they don't want a child at all. Unintended pregnancies occur among women of all ages and ethnic groups, and they nearly always cause stress and life disruption. They also have poorer health outcomes. Compared with women having planned pregnancies, women with unintended pregnancies are less likely in general to receive adequate prenatal care, are more likely to drink alcohol and smoke, and are more likely to have babies with **low birth weight** (less than 5.5 pounds).[1]

The most worrisome unintended pregnancies are those that occur among teenagers. Nearly 80 percent of teen pregnancies are unintended. Compared with nonteenage mothers, teenage mothers are less likely to marry or stay married, less likely to finish high school or attend college, and more likely to require public assistance.[1]

Throughout history, people have used their ingenuity to prevent unwanted pregnancies, devising vaginal barriers, spermicidal agents, and condoms from a variety of natural materials. Greater understanding of when and how pregnancy occurs, along with advances in reproductive technology, have led to the development of more acceptable and reliable contraceptive methods. In this section, we take a look at several of these methods.

Healthy People 2010

OBJECTIVE AREA *Family Planning*

- Increase the proportion of females at risk of unintended pregnancy (and their partners) who use contraception.

"Poor or nonexistent contraceptive use is one of the main causes of unintended pregnancy, with unintended pregnancy occurring among two groups: females using no contraception and females whose contraceptives fail or are used improperly. . . . Reducing the proportion of sexually active persons using no birth control method and increasing the effectiveness (correct and consistent use) with which persons use contraceptive methods would do much to lower the unintended pregnancy rate. Just reducing the proportion of females not using contraception by half could prevent as many as one-third of all unintended pregnancies and 500,000 abortions per year."

For more information on Healthy People 2010 objectives, visit the Web site at www.healthypeople.gov.

For more information on Canadian health objectives, visit the Health Canada Web site at www.hc-sc.gc.ca/english.

Abstinence

The only guaranteed method of preventing pregnancy is **abstinence.** As noted in Chapter 15, abstinence is usually defined as abstention from sexual intercourse; that is, there is no penile penetration of the vagina. In heterosexual couples who have vaginal intercourse and use no contraceptive method, 85 percent of the women will become pregnant in one year.[2] Abstinence is the only contraceptive method that is effective all the time and has no side effects or risks.

The Fertility Awareness Method

Women can usually become pregnant in a window of time around ovulation (release of an ovum). The **fertility awareness method** of birth control, sometimes called the **rhythm method,** is based on abstaining from sex during the time that conception might take place. Ovulation usually occurs 14 days before the menstrual period begins (Figure 16.1). For a woman with a 28-day cycle, ovulation usually occurs on day 14. The ovum is most likely to become fertilized within 24 hours after release from the ovary if it is to happen at all; however, the ovum can remain viable for 4 days. Sperm can survive up to 7 days in

Figure 16.1   *The fertility awareness, or rhythm, method uses the menstrual cycle to determine when fertilization is likely to occur and when unprotected sexual intercourse should be avoided.*

cervical mucus. Thus, any sperm deposited in the vagina after day 8 of the menstrual cycle could still be around on day 14, when the woman ovulates. To avoid pregnancy, the couple would need to avoid intercourse or use another method of contraception between day 8 and day 19.

The fertility awareness method requires that the woman have a regular cycle, because abstinence or barrier methods must be used for 7 days before ovulation. Although it's normal to have either a consistent cycle with the same number of days between periods or a cycle with variations in the number of days, the fertility awareness method is appropriate only for women with a consistent cycle.

Ovulation is accompanied by certain signs that a woman can recognize in order to learn her own patterns before she starts using this method. Couples also use these signs to pinpoint the time of ovulation when they are trying to conceive. One sign is that cervical mucus becomes thinner and stretchier, resembling egg white, and increases in quantity before ovulation, so the vagina feels wetter. Another sign is that, because of hormone activity, basal body temperature rises by about half a degree when

ovulation occurs and remains higher until the end of the cycle. A woman can take her temperature each morning with a basal temperature thermometer to see when this increase occurs.

Some couples who use the fertility awareness method rely on withdrawal when they have intercourse during the fertile period; that is, the man removes his penis from the woman's vagina before he ejaculates. With perfect use, withdrawal may be an effective form of contraception; however, for typical users, this is not an effective or reliable way to prevent conception, for several reasons. One is that sperm are frequently released before ejaculation; another is that sperm ejaculated near the entrance to the vagina can sometimes find their way inside; a third is that the man may not be able to withdraw quickly enough.

Barrier Methods

Contraceptive methods known as **barrier methods** physically separate the sperm from the female reproductive tract. These methods include the male condom, the female condom, the diaphragm, the cervical cap, and the contraceptive sponge. To increase their effectiveness, the diaphragm and cervical cap should be used with **spermicide,** chemical agents that kill sperm. Spermicide usually comes in a foam or jelly and can be purchased at a grocery or drug store at a cost of $10–$15 per tube.

The chance of becoming pregnant while using a barrier method is low if the method is used consistently and correctly. Correct use of a barrier method means that the barrier is used 100 percent of the time in which there is contact between the penis and the vagina and that spermicide is correctly applied with the diaphragm and cervical cap. Unfortunately, this is often not the case. The typical pregnancy rates are 15 percent with the male condom and 16 percent with the diaphragm. With correct use during every act of intercourse, however, the pregnancy rates drop to 2 percent for condoms and 6 percent for diaphragms.

KEY TERMS

low birth weight   Birth weight of less than 5.5 pounds, often as a result of preterm delivery.

abstinence   Abstention from sexual intercourse.

fertility awareness method (rhythm method)   Contraceptive method based on abstinence during the window of time around ovulation when a woman is most likely to conceive.

barrier methods   Contraceptive methods based on physically separating sperm from the female reproductive tract.

spermicide   Chemical agent that kills sperm.

Challenges & Choices

Buying and Using Condoms

The advantages of condoms are that they are available over the counter, relatively low in cost, fairly convenient to use, effective in protecting against STDs, and moderately effective in protecting against unintended pregnancy. Here are some tips to ensure the lowest risk of an unwanted outcome:

- Buy latex condoms if you are not allergic to them. Latex is the best material for preventing the spread of STDs.

- Check the expiration date before buying or using condoms. Outdated condoms are more likely to break during use.

- Condoms are available with or without spermicide. The most commonly used spermicide is nonoxynol-9. Because of recent evidence that this product can cause skin irritation, it is currently recommended that condoms without spermicide be purchased.

- Don't remove the condom from its wrapper until you are ready to use it.

- Don't leave condoms in the glove compartment of your car. Temperature extremes weaken the condom and make it more likely to break. Don't store them in your wallet either.

- Use only water-based lubricants. Oil-based products quickly cause latex to deteriorate, leading it to leak or break.

- If you are buying a female condom, check the expiration date and make sure it includes directions. Practice inserting the condom before you actually use it. During use, make sure the man's penis is inserted inside the condom.

- Correct use of condoms means not only that they are placed on the penis correctly before intercourse and removed correctly afterward (see Figure 16.2) but also that they are used for every occasion of sexual intercourse and do not leak or break. Most failures occur because of incorrect or inconsistent use.

It's Not Just Personal . . .

In many developing nations, such as Ivory Coast, Togo, and Ghana in West Africa, condoms are widely used for contraception because of their availability and their low cost in comparison with oral contraceptives. Even when not used specifically to prevent the spread of HIV/AIDS and other STDs, condoms have this added benefit in countries where such diseases are often present at epidemic levels.

Condoms

The only form of contraception proven to decrease the risk of contracting a sexually transmitted disease is the male condom. As described in Chapter 15, the *male condom* is a thin sheath, usually made of latex, that is rolled down over the erect penis before any contact occurs between the penis and the woman's genitals. The correct application of a condom is illustrated in Figure 16.2. Male condoms come with or without spermicide. There is no evidence that spermicide is necessary to reduce the risk of pregnancy, and spermicide can cause irritation for some users. Condoms can be purchased in grocery and drug stores and do not require a prescription from a physician (see the box "Buying and Using Condoms"). They cost between 27 cents and 1 dollar each, but they are often given out free at clinics.

Also as described in Chapter 15, the *female condom* is a pouch of thin polyurethane that is inserted into the vagina before intercourse (Figure 16.3). Like male condoms, female condoms can be purchased at grocery stores or drug stores for about $2.

In addition to helping prevent unwanted pregnancy, male and female condoms protect against sexually transmitted diseases. Condoms can be purchased at drugstores and grocery stores without a prescription.

Figure 16.2   Use of the male condom. *(a) Place the rolled condom over the head of the erect penis. Hold the top one-half inch of the condom with one hand, and squeeze the air out to allow space for semen. (b) With the other hand, unroll the condom downward, smoothing out any air bubbles. (c) Continue unrolling the condom down to the base of the penis. (d) After ejaculation, hold the condom around the base of the penis until the penis has been withdrawn completely to avoid any leakage of semen.*

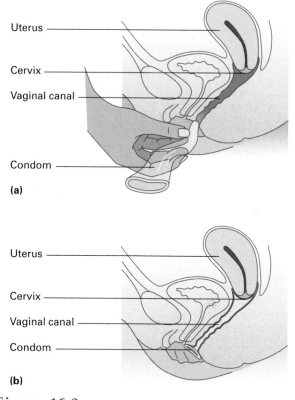

Figure 16.3   Use of the female condom. *(a) Take the smaller ring of the condom and flex it gently to fit into the vaginal canal. Follow the manufacturer's detailed instructions for insertion. (b) When the condom is in place, the smaller ring covers the cervix and the larger ring remains outside the vagina.*

Diaphragm

The vaginal **diaphragm** is a circular rubber dome that is inserted in the vagina before intercourse; correct placement is shown in Figure 16.4. It fits between the pubic bone and the back of the vagina and covers the cervix. Spermicidal jelly or foam is placed in the dome, or cup, of the diaphragm before it is inserted; thus, the spermicide covers the cervix, where it provides the best protection. Spermicide must be reapplied into the vagina if a second act of sex occurs. The diaphragm is removed 6 to 12 hours after sex. A woman has to be fitted with the correctly sized diaphragm by a health care provider and shown how to insert and remove it. The cost of this method includes the physician visit (between $50 and $150), the diaphragm (usually $30–$50), and spermicide. A diaphragm can be used for 2 years with correct care.[2]

Cervical Cap

The **cervical cap** is a small, cuplike rubber device that covers only the cervix; correct placement is shown in Figure 16.5. The cervical cap is kept in place on the cervix by natural suction. A small amount of spermicidal jelly or foam is placed in the center of the cap before it is inserted. The cervical cap can be left in place for up to 48 hours or removed 6 hours after intercourse. As with the diaphragm, a

woman has to be fitted with a cervical cap and shown how to insert and remove it. The cost of this method includes the physician visit (between $50 and $150), the cervical cap ($30–$50), and spermicide. A cervical cap may be used for 2 years with correct care.[2]

Contraceptive Sponge

The Today **contraceptive sponge** recently became available in the United States again after being absent from the market since 1994, when the manufacturer stopped

KEY TERMS

diaphragm   Circular rubber dome that is inserted in the vagina before intercourse to prevent conception.

cervical cap   Small, cuplike rubber device that covers only the cervix and is inserted in the vagina before intercourse to prevent conception.

contraceptive sponge   Small polyurethane foam device presaturated with spermicide that is inserted in the vagina before intercourse to prevent pregnancy.

(a)

(a)

(b)

(b)

(c)

(c)

Figure 16.4   Use of the diaphragm. *(a) With clean hands, place about 1 tablespoon of spermicide (jelly or cream) in the diaphragm, spreading it around the diaphragm and its rim. (b) Using the thumb and forefinger, compress the diaphragm. Insert it into the vagina, guiding it toward the back wall and up into the vagina as far as possible. (c) With your index finger, check the position of the diaphragm to make sure that the cervix is covered completely and the front of the rim is behind the pubic bone.*

Figure 16.5   Placement of cervical cap. *(a) With clean hands, fill one third of the cap with spermicide. (b) Separate the labia with one hand while squeezing the rim of the cap together with the other hand. Holding the cap with the dome side down, insert it into the vagina, and push it up and onto the cervix. (c) Press the rim around the cervix, and pinch the rounded end to create suction. Sweep your finger around the cap to make sure that the cervix is covered completely. Check for a dimple in the dome of the cap, which means there is enough suction.*

making it because of production problems. The Today sponge is a small polyurethane foam device that is presaturated with 1 gram of the spermicide nonoxynol-9. It is inserted into the vagina and fits snugly over the cervix (Figure 16.6). It is available over the counter and dispos-

able; one size fits all. The Today sponge remains effective for 24 hours without requiring any additional application of spermicide. For women who have not had a previous pregnancy, effectiveness is about the same as that of a male condom.

The diaphragm (left) and the cervical cap (right) must be used with a spermicide. Correct placement and care of these contraceptive devices are important for effectiveness.

The IUD

The **intrauterine device (IUD)** has a complex history in the United States. Because of a design flaw, IUDs in the 1960s and 1970s were associated with a high rate of pelvic inflammatory disease, an infection of the ovaries and fallopian tubes. The design of IUDs has been made safer, and they are currently regaining popularity. Two types are used, the copper IUD and the progesterone IUD. Both are small, T-shaped devices that a health care provider inserts through the cervix into the uterus. A correctly placed IUD is shown in Figure 16.7.

The IUD is believed to work by altering the uterine and cervical fluids to reduce the chance that sperm will move up into the fallopian tubes where they can fertilize an ovum. In addition, some women using the progesterone-containing IUD do not ovulate, and so fertilization is not possible.

IUDs are highly effective and require little maintenance after they are in place, but several problems are associated with their use. Women can experience irregular bleeding. The IUD can move or fall out of the uterus, so the woman must learn how to check to make sure the device is still properly located each month. Currently, the role that IUDs play in the spread of sexually transmitted infection and pelvic inflammatory disease is unclear. Any woman at risk for sexually transmitted infection should use condoms.

The cost of an intrauterine device is about $200 to $300, including the physician fee and the cost of the device. The copper IUD can remain in place for up to 10 years; the progesterone IUD can remain in place for 5 years.

Hormonal Contraceptive Methods

Hormonal methods come in a variety of forms—pills, injections, patches, and vaginal rings—and work by preventing ovulation. They also alter cervical mucus, making it

(a)

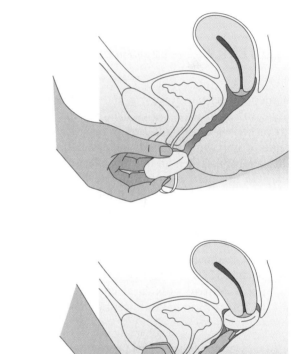

(b)

(c)

Figure 16.6   Placement of Today sponge. *With clean hands, remove the sponge from the package. (a) Hold it in one hand with the dimple side facing up and the loop hanging down. Wet the sponge thoroughly with clean tap water. Squeeze the sponge gently to produce suds and activate the spermicide. (b) With the dimple side facing up, fold the sponge in half and insert it deep into the vagina, along the back wall, to cover the cervix. (c) With your finger, check the position of the sponge. The dimple should be facing the cervix, and the loop should be facing away from it.*

KEY TERMS

intrauterine device (IUD)   Small T-shaped device that when inserted in the uterus prevents conception.

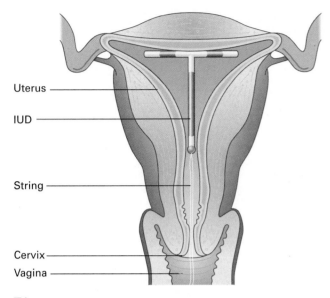

Figure 16.7   T-shaped IUD correctly positioned in the uterus.

harder for sperm to reach ova, and they affect the uterine lining so a fertilized egg is less likely to be implanted. They are prescribed or administered by a physician. The advantages of hormonal methods include their effectiveness, their ease of use, their limited side effects, and the fact that they do not permanently affect fertility. They do not require any action at the time of intercourse. In addition, they offer some general health benefits. They reduce menstrual cramping and blood loss, premenstrual symptoms, and the risk of endometrial and ovarian cancer. Their main disadvantage is that they do not provide any protection against STDs.

Birth control pills (oral contraception) are the most popular form of contraception among unmarried

Birth control pills are highly effective and easy to use, making them the most popular form of birth control among unmarried women in the United States. Although they offer protection against some diseases, such as ovarian cancer, possible side effects range from bloating and weight gain to more serious ones such as increased risk of stroke and heart attack.

women in the United States. They are easy to use and highly effective if taken as directed. Some types are taken every day of the month, and others are taken 3 weeks out of 4. During the 4th week, the woman has a light period. Some women have difficulty remembering to take the pill every day; missing even 1 day can increase the risk of pregnancy.

Birth control pills contain either a combination of estrogen and progesterone or progesterone only. They can cause a variety of minor side effects, including symptoms of early pregnancy (nausea, bloating, weight gain, tender breasts), depression, and headaches. More serious side effects include increased risk of stroke, blood clots, high blood pressure, and heart attack, especially in older women and in women who smoke (see the box "Side Effects of Birth Control Pills"). Serious side effects are rare and are primarily associated with the estrogen component of hormonal contraceptives. Many types of pills are available; if one doesn't seem to work well for you, consult with your physician to find one that does. The cost of birth control pills is usually $15 to $50 per month.[2]

Injectables, patches, and vaginal rings are newer methods of administering hormonal contraceptives. They combine the effectiveness of birth control pills with ease of use. Injectable contraceptives are longer lasting. An injection of Depo-Provera, which contains progesterone, lasts about 3 months, and an injection of Lunelle (not currently available in the United States), which contains estrogen and progesterone, lasts about 1 month. Injections are highly effective and require little action on the part of the woman or couple except for regular visits to the health care provider.

The contraceptive skin patch works by slowly releasing hormones transdermally (through the skin) into the bloodstream. The woman places a new patch on her skin every week for 3 weeks; during the 4th week, she has a light period. The patch is very effective and has few side effects. These side effects are similar to those of combination birth control pills; an additional possible side effect is a skin reaction at the patch site.

The vaginal contraceptive ring is a soft, flexible plastic ring containing estrogen and progesterone. The ring is placed in the vagina every 28 days. It is left in place for 21 days and then removed for 7 days. The ring slowly releases hormones. Women and their partners report that they rarely feel the ring during intercourse. The side effects are similar to those of combination birth control pills.

Contraceptive implants are small capsules filled with synthetic progesterone that are placed under the skin by a physician. They slowly release hormones for several years. The best known implant, Norplant, is not currently available in the United States because of lawsuits, but it is widely used in other parts of the world,

HIGHLIGHT ON HEALTH

Side Effects of Birth Control Pills

Although hormonal birth control options have become remarkably safe, there are some rare but potentially serious side effects. If you are taking birth control pills, you should know the warning signs; you can remember them from the acronym ACHES. If you develop one or more of these symptoms, it may or may not be related to your contraceptive method. See your health care provider for an assessment of the symptom and a determination of whether it is safe for you to continue using birth control pills.

A Abdominal pain (Possible causes: blood clot in pelvic veins or liver, benign tumor in liver, gall stones)

C Chest pain (Possible causes: blood clot in lungs, heart attack, breast mass)

H Headaches (Possible causes: migraine, hypertension, stroke)

E Eye problems (blurry vision or loss of vision) (Possible causes: migraine, blood clot behind eye, change in shape of cornea so contact lenses don't fit)

S Severe leg pain (Possible cause: blood clot in leg)

Source: *Managing Contraception,* by R. A. Hatcher, A. L. Nelson, M. Zieman, et al., 2003, Tiger, GA: Bridging the Gap Foundation.

---

including in many European countries. Implanon is another progesterone implant that is currently undergoing FDA review.

Post-Sex Contraception

The so-called **morning-after pill,** or **emergency contraception,** contains either a combination of estrogen and progesterone or progesterone alone in concentrations that are higher than those in birth control pills. One pill is taken as soon as possible after unprotected sex. A second pill is taken 12 hours later. This pill should be taken within 48 to 72 hours of unprotected sex to prevent conception, but it may be effective up to 5 days after sex. In the United States, emergency contraception is sold under the trade name Preven or Plan B. It costs between $15 and $40 per use.

Emergency contraception reduces the chance of pregnancy after unprotected intercourse by 85 percent by preventing fertilization or implantation. It does not cause an abortion. Emergency contraception is useful when a barrier method fails, such as when a condom breaks, and in cases of rape or incest. Many physicians are starting to routinely prescribe the morning-after pill for women who use barrier methods of contraception so they can have it on hand if their barrier method fails. In 33 countries, emergency contraception is available from a pharmacist without a prescription. The FDA recently rejected a proposal for over-the-counter sale of such contraception in the United States.[3]

The morning-after pill is not considered an **abortogenic agent** (an agent that causes the termination of an established pregnancy), for two reasons. One reason is

that pregnancy requires a fertilized ovum. Because the morning-after pill works by altering hormones to prevent fertilization, pregnancy is not considered to have occurred. The other reason is that, according to some definitions, including that of the World Health Organization, pregnancy does not start until the fertilized ovum is implanted in the wall of the uterus. Because the morning-after pill prevents implantation if an ovum is fertilized, pregnancy, again, is not considered to have occurred.

Sterilization

Sterilization is a surgical procedure that permanently prevents any future pregnancies. It is the most commonly chosen form of contraception and is especially popular

KEY TERMS

birth control pills (oral contraception) Combinations of hormones (estrogens and progestins) that provide contraception by preventing ovulation.

morning-after pill (emergency contraception) Pill containing hormones that can be taken within 48 to 72 hours of unprotected sex to prevent pregnancy.

abortogenic agent Agent that causes the termination of an established pregnancy.

sterilization Surgical procedure that permanently prevents any future pregnancies.

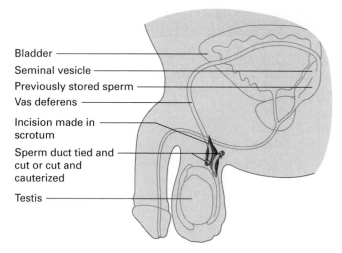

Figure 16.8   Vasectomy. *With only local anesthesia needed, this surgical procedure offers permanent sterilization.*

Figure 16.9   Tubal ligation. *This surgical procedure is often performed via laparoscopy, which involves creating two small incisions, one for the scope device and the other for the surgical instruments. It usually requires only local anesthesia.*

with married couples who do not want to have any more children. Besides condoms, sterilization is currently the only form of contraception available to men.

The male sterilization procedure is **vasectomy.** In this procedure, a health care professional makes a small incision or puncture in the scrotum, then ties off and severs the vas deferens, the duct that carries sperm from the testes to the seminal vesicle, where sperm would mix with semen (Figure 16.8). This is done on both sides of the scrotum because each testicle has a vas deferens. Vasectomy is usually a relatively quick procedure performed with a local anesthetic. Most men return to their usual activities within 2 to 3 days. Vasectomy does not interfere with sexual function or alter the level of male hormones. Semen is still produced and does not change in appearance. The cost of a vasectomy can range from $350 to $755, and the sterilization effect lasts for life.

The most common female sterilization procedure is **tubal ligation.** In this procedure, a physician makes an incision in the abdomen, then severs and ties or seals the fallopian tubes, the ducts through which ova pass from the ovaries to the uterus (Figure 16.9). The procedure can be done via a surgical method called *laparoscopy.* A laparoscope, a tube that the surgeon can look through with a tiny light on the end, is inserted through a small incision, and the surgical instruments are inserted through another small incision. The procedure can be done with a spinal anesthetic, although a general anesthetic can also be used. Recovery usually takes somewhat longer than recovery from a vasectomy. When a cesarean section is performed to deliver a baby, a tubal ligation can be done at the same time.

Tubal ligation does not alter a woman's menstrual cycle or hormone levels. The ovaries continue to function,

but ova are prevented from traveling through the fallopian tubes to the uterus and thus cannot be fertilized. A tubal ligation costs between $1,200 and $2,500 and lasts for life.[2] Although in rare cases pregnancy does occur after a vasectomy or tubal ligation, these procedures should be considered permanent.

Another effective technique for permanent sterilization in women, called Essure, was approved by the FDA in 2003. It involves the placement of a micro-rod in each of the fallopian tubes. Tissue begins to develop around the micro-rods, and after 3 months this tissue barrier prevents sperm from reaching the egg. During this 3-month period another form of birth control should be used. This sterilization procedure can be performed on an outpatient basis and does not require general anesthesia.

Which Contraceptive Method Is Right for You?

Given all the options available for contraception and the number of variables that have to be taken into account in choosing a method—effectiveness, cost, convenience, permanence, safety, protection against STDs, and consistency with personal values—deciding which method is the best one for you can be difficult. Here are some questions to consider:

• Is your main concern preventing pregnancy? Or do you also need to worry about sexually transmitted diseases? If you are concerned about STDs, you need to use condoms. If you are in a mutually faithful, monogamous relationship and neither

Table 16.1   Effectiveness of Selected Contraceptive Methods

Contraceptive Method	Women Who Become Pregnant Within 1 Year with Typical Use of Method (%)	Women Who Become Pregnant Within 1 Year with Perfect Use of Method (%)
No method	85	85
Spermicide alone	29	18
FAM (rhythm)	25	1–9
Withdrawal	27	4
Cervical cap		
Women with prior birth	32	26
Women with no prior births	16	9
Diaphragm	16	6
Condom		
Female condom	21	5
Male condom	15	2
Birth control pill	8	0.3
Contraceptive sponge (Today sponge)		
Women with prior birth	32	20
Women with no prior births	16	9
Birth control patch (Evra patch)	8	0.3
Vaginal ring (Nuva ring)	8	0.3
IUD		
Copper	0.8	0.6
Progesterone (Mirena)	0.1	0.1
Depo-Provera	3	0.3
Norplant	0.05	0.05
Sterilization		
Female sterilization	0.5	0.5
Male sterilization	0.15	0.10

Source: Adapted from *Contraceptive Technology*, 18th ed. (p. 792), by R. A. Hatcher, J. Trussell, F. Stewart, et al., 2004, New York: Ardent Media.

you nor your partner has an STD, then a barrier method may not be necessary. You may want to consider birth control pills, an injectable contraceptive, or an IUD. Table 16.1 shows the effectiveness of various contraceptive methods.

- Are you planning to have children with this partner at some time in the future? If so, are you comfortable with a form of contraception that may be slightly less reliable but that has other advantages? The male and female condoms, the diaphragm, the cervical cap, and the contraceptive sponge are all safe, nonpermanent methods.

- Do you already have children and know that you do not want any more? Surgical sterilization is a highly effective method with no hassles after the initial procedure.

- How much can you afford to pay for contraception? There are several factors to consider here. For example, how often do you need contraception? If you have sex daily, the cost of buying condoms for every time can quickly add up,

KEY TERMS

vasectomy   Male sterilization procedure, involving tying off and severing the vas deferens to prevent sperm from reaching the semen.

tubal ligation   Female sterilization procedure involving severing and tying off or sealing the fallopian tubes to prevent ova from reaching the uterus.

whereas the one-time cost of an IUD or sterilization may be less. If you have sex once a month or less, the opposite may be true. If you need to use two forms of contraception, one to prevent STDs and one to increase your chances of avoiding pregnancy, again, the costs can add up. Don't forget to take into account the cost if you or your partner gets pregnant with the form of contraception you select. It might be the cost of having an abortion, or it might be the cost of raising a child.

- Are you worried about the safety and health consequences of contraception? These concerns are important considerations for anyone choosing a contraceptive method. Frequently, however, people are surprised to learn how safe all the contraceptive options available today have become. To put the risks associated with contraception in perspective, see Table 16.2.

- Is your choice influenced by your religious, spiritual, or ethical beliefs? Some people are not

Table 16.2	Risks of Contraception in Perspective
Activity	**Risk of Death in a Year**
Risk to men and women all ages participating in:	
Motorcycling	1 in 1,000
Automobile driving	1 in 5,900
Risk to women aged 15 to 44 participating in:	
Tampon use	1 in 350,000
Pregnancy prevention:	
Birth control pills	
Smoker (>25 cig per day)	1 in 1,700
Nonsmoker	1 in 66,700
IUD	1 in 10,000,000
Diaphragm, condom	None (potential of allergic reaction)
Sterilization	
Tubal ligation	1 in 38,500
Vasectomy	1 in 1,000,000
Pregnancy carried past 20 weeks	1 in 10,000
Termination of pregnancy by legal abortion:	
Before 9 weeks	1 in 262,800
Between 9 and 12 weeks	1 in 100,100
Between 12 and 15 weeks	1 in 34,400
After 15 weeks	1 in 10,200

Source: Adapted from *Contraceptive Technology*, 18th ed. (p. 236), by R. A. Hatcher, J. Trussell, F. Stewart, et al., 2004, New York: Ardent Media.

comfortable with any method that interferes with natural processes. Periodic abstinence or the fertility awareness method may be the right choice.

UNINTENDED PREGNANCY

If you or your partner becomes pregnant unexpectedly, you have to make a monumental decision in a very short period of time. You will probably feel a range of emotions, from frightened to excited to angry to awed, and your feelings may fluctuate from one extreme to another. You may feel isolated, but millions of men and women have been in your position before. The important thing is to see your physician or health care provider as soon as possible to discuss your options. They are to (1) carry the pregnancy to term and raise the child, (2) carry the pregnancy to term and place the child in an adoptive family, or (3) terminate the pregnancy.

If you are a teenager, most states allow you to seek **prenatal care** (or care related to pregnancy) on your own, without permission of a parent or guardian.[4] If you are afraid to discuss your pregnancy with family members, a health care provider can help you determine the best way to share the news with them. Alternatively, if you believe it would be unwise to involve your family, a health care provider can help you find the resources you need.

The decision to raise a child is one of the biggest decisions you will ever make (see the box "Who Is Most Likely to Have an Unintended Pregnancy?"). Although there is little regulation covering who can become a parent, the effects of parenting are pervasive and long lasting, both for individuals and for society. A life is literally in your hands. Parenthood is one of life's great joys, but it is also a tremendous responsibility. Estimates are that one third to one half of all babies born in the United States every year are the result of unintended pregnancies, either mistimed or unwanted.[5]

Are you ready to become a parent? Here are some questions you need to consider:

- What are your long-term educational, career, and life plans? How would having a child at this time fit in with those plans?

- What is the status of your relationship with your partner? Is he or she someone you want to commit to and share parenthood with? If you are the mother, the greater part of the pregnancy experience will fall on you, but parenting will involve making decisions with your partner about child rearing. Do you have similar goals for a child? Can you communicate well with each other?

- Do you feel emotionally mature enough to take on the responsibility of raising a child? Parenthood can be demanding, bewildering, and frustrating, and it requires patience, sacrifice, and the ability to

Beating the Odds

Who Is Most Likely to Have an Unintended Pregnancy?

There are many reasons for postponing pregnancy or not wanting a child at all, and there are also many ways to make sure an unintended pregnancy doesn't occur. Brief profiles of three couples are presented here. Which couple do you think is most likely to experience an unintended pregnancy?

Maggie and Zach are college juniors, both 20 years old. They have been dating for a year and have been sexually involved for the past 6 months. Maggie was taking birth control pills, but she stopped because of the weight gain she experienced. Now they use condoms most of the time, usually the kind that come with a spermicide. Sometimes they have to search Zach's apartment to find a condom, and if they can't, they take a chance. Both Maggie and Zach are healthy and active; neither of them smokes or takes any medications. They both want to have children someday, but they want to finish college and get launched in careers first. They haven't thought too much about how committed they are to each other for the future.

Julia and Kirk have been married for 4 years and have a 1-year-old daughter. They are both 27. Kirk is the floor manager at a local auto plant and experiences a lot of job-related stress. He struggles with an alcohol problem and occasionally binges on weekends. He is thinking about joining AA. Julia is an interior designer and has been able to continue working part-time since having a child. She is breast-feeding their daughter and has not been getting her period since the birth. When they have sex, Kirk withdraws before ejaculating. They would like to have another child in 3 to 4 years.

Vicki and Justin are 35 and 40 years old, respectively. They have been married for 10 years and have two children, aged 4 and 7. Vicki is a research associate at the local university and Justin is a real estate lawyer. They are both healthy, exercise regularly, and drink moderately. They do not want to have any more children. Vicki has an IUD, but they have been talking about the possibility of Justin getting a vasectomy.

OLC Web site Visit the **Online Learning Center** at www.mhhe.com/teague1e for comments by the authors.

---

put aside your own needs to meet the needs of another person.

- What are your financial resources at this point? Having a child is expensive. Short-term costs include the medical costs of pregnancy, prenatal care, and delivery and the cost of supplies for the baby. Long-term costs are all the costs of raising a child to age 18 or beyond. If you are the father, even if you do not want to be emotionally or physically involved, you will probably be legally required to remain financially involved.

- How large is your social support system? Do you have family members and friends who will help you? Does your community have resources and support services? Social support has been found to be one of the most important factors in helping couples make a successful adjustment to parenthood.

- What is your health status and age? Do you smoke, drink, or use recreational drugs? Do you have an STD or other medical condition that needs to be treated? Are you under 18 or over 35? Babies born to teenagers and women over 35 have a higher incidence of health problems (see the box "When Is the Best Time to Have a Baby?").

Adoption

Adoption can be a positive solution for an unintended pregnancy if you and your partner are not able or willing to become parents at this time in your lives. Adoption provides a permanent family for a child in need. Many couples are unable to conceive or choose not to have a biological child and want to adopt. If you are considering adoption, either as a solution to an unplanned pregnancy or as an adoptive parent, you can choose either an open adoption or a closed adoption. For couples seeking to adopt, international adoptions are another alternative. All forms of adoption require that both biological parents relinquish their parental rights.

Open Adoption

In an open adoption, the biological parents help to choose the adoptive parents and maintain a relationship with

KEY TERMS

prenatal care   Regular medical care during pregnancy, designed to promote the health of the mother and the fetus.

Successful parenthood requires emotional maturity on the part of both partners. Other factors that contribute to effective parenthood include a stable relationship between the partners, adequate financial resources, and a strong social support system.

them and the child. The degree of involvement can range from the exchange of information through a third party to a close and continuous relationship among all parties throughout the child's life. This choice can make it easier for parents to give up a baby, and it allows the child to know his or her biological parents, siblings, and relatives. Many adoption agencies offer this option.

Closed Adoption

In a closed adoption, the more traditional form of adoption, the biological parents do not help choose the adoptive parents, and the adoption records are sealed. This type of adoption provides more privacy and confidentiality than open adoption does. In some states, the child may access the sealed records at the age of 18, and many states are in the process of passing legislation that would open previously sealed records, even for adoptions that occurred decades ago. This change could affect many men and women who thought their adoption decisions would remain confidential forever. One of the reasons for the proposed change is the realization that knowledge about one's biological parents can be important for both psychological and health reasons.

International Adoption

International adoptions have become increasingly common, with children being adopted from Central America, South America, Eastern Europe, and Asia. For many couples, the decision to adopt a child from another country is based on a desire to help a child who is already alive and in need of care. A major legislative change now allows children in international adoptions to automatically be granted U.S. citizenship at the time of their adoption.

Elective Abortion

Terminating the pregnancy through **elective abortion** is the third option for a woman with an unintended pregnancy. (This type of abortion is called *elective* to distinguish it from **spontaneous abortion,** or miscarriage.) Since 1973 elective abortion has been legal in the United States. In the case of *Roe v. Wade,* the U.S. Supreme Court ruled that the decision to terminate a pregnancy must be left up to the woman, with some restrictions applying as the pregnancy advances through three trimesters (divisions of the pregnancy into parts, each about three months long). In the second trimester, states can apply restrictions to protect the mother's health, and in the third trimester, when the fetus could survive outside the womb, some states even ban abortion.

Since the passage of *Roe v. Wade,* many attempts have been made at state and national levels to limit access to legal abortion. The debate over abortion between pro-life and pro-choice activists is one of the most highly charged political issues of our time. In November 2003 Congress passed a ban on a particular type of abortion. A similar ban had previously been found unconstitutional by the U.S. Supreme Court, and the current ban is being challenged. At this time, a woman can legally elect to end a pregnancy without the agreement of the father. In many states, a teenager is protected in her right to end a pregnancy without the notification of her parents.

If you are pregnant and considering abortion, seek health care counseling to discuss all your options, the risks associated with the procedure, and the technique to be used. Your health care provider will confirm the stage of your pregnancy with a physical exam and possibly with

HIGHLIGHT ON HEALTH

When Is the Best Time to Have a Baby?

How old do you want to be when you have a child? Although this is a highly personal decision influenced by many factors—educational and career plans, relationship status, health issues, and others—there is information that you can use to make the best decision from a health perspective.

Studies suggest that both the woman and the child experience the least health risk if the woman has her pregnancy after the age of 18 and before the age of 35. Before the age of 18, a woman's body is still growing and developing. The additional demands of pregnancy and nursing can impair a woman's health, and the baby is more likely to be born early and have a low birth weight.

After the age of 35, a woman is more likely to have difficulty getting pregnant, because fertility declines as a woman gets older. Many women who have delayed childbearing until their late 30s or early 40s have been disappointed to find that it takes much longer to become pregnant or that they have to turn to reproductive

technology to conceive. After 35, women are also at increased risk for medical problems during pregnancy, including miscarriage, and for having a baby who is born prematurely, has low birth weight, or has a genetic abnormality like Down syndrome.

Once there is a child in the family, many parents plan to have a second or third. For health reasons, it appears that waiting until the first child is 2 years old before getting pregnant again may be best. A woman's body can take up to 2 years to fully recover from pregnancy and nursing. If a pregnancy occurs too quickly after the birth of a child, the mother is at increased risk for anemia (low blood iron) and decreased energy and strength. The new child is at increased risk for early birth and low birth weight, and the older child may suffer from a decrease in attention and sometimes the sudden cessation of nursing.

Source: United Nations Children's Fund, www.unicef.org.

---

ultrasound. Most abortions are performed during the first trimester, and before the 16th week of gestation. The most common technique currently in use is surgical abortion, but the use of medical abortion is increasing.

Surgical Abortion

In **surgical abortion,** the embryo or fetus and other contents of the uterus are removed through a surgical procedure. (Between 2 and 8 weeks of gestation, the term *embryo* is used; after the 8th week, the term *fetus* is used.) The most common method of surgical abortion performed between the 6th and 12th weeks is vacuum aspiration; it is used for about 90 percent of all abortions performed in the United States.[6] A licensed physician performs this procedure in a clinical setting, such as a medical office or hospital. The cervix is numbed with a local anesthetic and opened with an instrument called a dilator. After the cervix has been opened, a catheter, a tubelike instrument, is inserted into the uterus. The catheter is attached to a suction machine, and the contents of the uterus are removed.

The procedure takes about 10 minutes and requires a few hours' recovery before the woman can return home. A follow-up appointment is needed about 2 weeks after the procedure to ensure that the body is healing. When performed in a legal and safe setting, elective abortion does not increase the risk of infertility or of complications in future pregnancies.

Medical Abortion

An alternative to surgical abortion is **medical abortion,** in which a pharmaceutical agent is used to induce an abortion. The drug mifepristone (formerly known as RU 486) has been approved by the FDA as a medication to induce abortion. Mifepristone acts by blocking progesterone receptors on the surface of the body's cells. Progesterone is needed by the cells of the uterine lining to support a pregnancy; without it, the lining sloughs off, along with any fertilized egg that has been implanted in it.

Mifepristone can be used only during the first 7 weeks of gestation (or 9 weeks of pregnancy, dated from day 1 of the last menstrual period). It is taken in the form of a pill and followed 2 or 3 days later with another drug,

KEY TERMS

elective abortion Voluntary termination of a pregnancy.

spontaneous abortion Involuntary termination of a pregnancy, or miscarriage.

surgical abortion Surgical removal of the contents of the uterus to terminate a pregnancy.

medical abortion Use of a pharmaceutical agent to terminate a pregnancy.

misoprostol, which induces contractions. Most women have cramping and bleeding and abort the pregnancy within 2 weeks, although in some cases this may occur within a few hours or days. The success rate is nearly 90 percent, and serious complications are rare. If abortion does not occur, a surgical abortion is recommended, because the drugs can harm the developing embryo.[7]

WHEN CONCEPTION IS DIFFICULT

For a small percentage of couples, becoming pregnant is difficult. About 7 percent of married couples experience **infertility,**[8] the inability to become pregnant after not using any form of contraception during sexual intercourse for 12 months. Many couples think they will become pregnant immediately once they make the decision to stop using contraception. Older couples who have delayed childbearing can be especially surprised and distressed when conception does not occur quickly. The longer childbearing is delayed, the higher the chances that conception will be difficult and that pregnancy will be complicated.

Causes of Infertility

Identifying the cause of infertility determines what treatment to use. In about one third of cases, infertility stems from male factors, such as low sperm count or lack of sperm motility. In another one third of cases, infertility results from blockage in the woman's fallopian tubes, often scarring that has occurred as a result of pelvic inflammatory disease or another complication of an STD. Blockage can also be caused by an unsterile abortion or by endometriosis, a condition in which uterine tissue grows outside the uterus. In the remaining one third of cases, the problem is lack of ovulation, abnormalities in the cervical mucus or in anatomy, or unknown causes.

Treatment Options for Infertility

The decision to seek treatment for infertility can be difficult. The couple will be asked to discuss their sex life in detail. The evaluation and treatment can strain a relationship, with sex becoming scheduled and goal oriented rather than spontaneous and pleasure oriented. Infertility treatment can also be expensive and may not be covered by insurance.

In many cases, the cause of the infertility can be determined. Treatments include surgery to open blocked tubes or correct anatomical problems; fertility drugs to promote ovulation and regulate hormones; and more advanced reproductive techniques, as described in the box "Treatment Options for Infertility." Most treatments increase the likelihood of multiple births.

PREGNANCY AND PRENATAL CARE

Many women do not realize they are pregnant until they are beyond the crucial early phase of development. During this time they may have inadvertently caused harm to their developing child by drinking, smoking, taking medications or recreational drugs, or being exposed to hazardous substances. Research is now indicating that events and conditions during pregnancy can not only cause **congenital abnormalities** (birth defects) but also influence the individual's development throughout life, affecting cognitive development in childhood and health risks, including mental health risks, in adulthood. The best approach to ensuring good health is to give every child the best possible start in life.

Prepregnancy Counseling

With increased control over when to have children, couples also have the opportunity to improve their health before conception. Couples who practice family planning can take advantage of **prepregnancy counseling,** which may include an evaluation of current health behaviors and health status, recommendations for improving health, and treatment of any existing conditions that might increase risk. Couples with increased risk of having a child with a genetic disease, because of their ethnic background, for example, or because of the presence of someone with a genetic disease in the family health tree, may be referred for genetic counseling (see Chapter 2). Because so many women become pregnant unintentionally, however, every sexually active woman who might become pregnant should be aware of the importance of healthy lifestyle factors.

Nutrition and Exercise

A balanced, nutritious diet before and during pregnancy helps ensure that both you and your child get required nutrients. Total calorie intake needs increase by about 300 calories a day during the second and third trimester, equivalent to an extra apple and glass of milk each day. The goal for weight gain during pregnancy is 20 to 30 pounds, most of it during the second half of pregnancy.[9]

A baby needs calcium for its growing bones, and this is linked to the mother's calcium intake. A pregnant teenager needs to consume more calcium than an older woman does because she needs more calcium for her own bones. Getting folic acid in food or in a folate supplement is also recommended to reduce the risk of neural tube defects (problems in the development of the brain and spinal cord). Women should increase their folic acid intake during the 3 months *before* getting pregnant so they have a high level of folic acid in their bodies at the time of conception. The 2005 *Dietary Guidelines for Americans* recommend that all women of childbearing age who may become pregnant consume at

HIGHLIGHT ON HEALTH

Treatment Options for Infertility

Method	How It Works
Hormonal treatments	Drugs induce ovulation; used when infertility is caused by lack of ovulation or irregular ovulation.
Intrauterine (artificial) insemination	Sperm are collected and placed in the woman's uterus by syringe or catheter; used when infertility results from low sperm count, low sperm motility, or thick cervical mucus. Donor sperm can be used if the partner's sperm have a genetic abnormality or if the partners are a lesbian couple.
Gamete intrafallopian transfer (GIFT)	The ovaries are stimulated to produce multiple eggs, the eggs are collected, and eggs and sperm are surgically placed in the fallopian tube for fertilization.
Zygote intrafallopian transfer (ZIFT)	The ovaries are stimulated to produce multiple eggs, the eggs are collected and fertilized, and fertilized eggs are placed in the fallopian tube.
In vitro fertilization (IVF)	The ovaries are stimulated to produce multiple eggs, the eggs are collected and fertilized, and fertilized eggs are transferred to the woman's uterus.

least 400 micrograms of folic acid a day and that pregnant women consume 600 micrograms a day.[10] You can reach this intake by eating several servings of dark green, leafy vegetables a day, by taking vitamin supplements, or by eating grain products and cereals fortified with folic acid.

Pregnant women, women who might become pregnant, nursing mothers, and young children are advised to monitor their fish and shellfish intake because of contamination with mercury. They can eat up to 12 ounces of fish (two average servings) that is low in mercury, such as canned light tuna, salmon, pollock, or catfish, per week. They should not eat swordfish, shark, tilefish, or king mackerel. For information about the safety of locally caught fish, check local advisories.[11] Foodborne infections can have more serious effects in pregnant women than in the general population, and the FDA advises pregnant women to avoid unpasteurized foods, soft cheese (for instance, brie, camembert, and feta), and raw or smoked seafood.

Regular exercise during pregnancy is recommended to help maintain muscle strength, circulation, and general well-being. Pregnancy is not the time to train for a marathon, but women can maintain their prepregnancy level of activity. In the second and third trimesters, women should be cautious about exercise that might cause injury or trauma, such as team sports, skiing, or horseback riding. Instead, they should choose safer forms of cardiorespiratory endurance exercise, such as walking, swimming, or stationary cycling. Women with difficult pregnancies may be advised to avoid exercise altogether.

Maternal Immunizations

Women should be vaccinated for two infectious diseases before pregnancy, rubella (German measles) and hepatitis

B. Rubella can cause a spontaneous abortion or serious birth defects, including deafness and blindness. Hepatitis B is a highly infectious disease that causes liver damage. It can be transmitted sexually, through nonsexual contact, and from mother to child during pregnancy and delivery (called **vertical transmission**). If you become pregnant and have not had these immunizations, do not get them during pregnancy but plan to get them after the birth of your baby. Try to avoid exposure to these infections while you are pregnant.

Medications, Drugs, and Toxic Substances

The uterus is a highly protected place, but most substances that the mother ingests or that otherwise enter

KEY TERMS

infertility Inability to become pregnant after not using any form of contraception during sexual intercourse for 12 months.

congenital abnormality Birth defect.

prepregnancy counseling Counseling before conception that may include an evaluation of current health behaviors and health status, recommendations for improving health, and treatment of any existing conditions that might increase risk.

vertical transmission Transmission of an infection or disease from mother to child during pregnancy and delivery.

her bloodstream eventually reach the fetus. These include prescription medications the mother may be taking for a health condition as well as other drugs and toxic substances. Some substances, called **teratogens,** can cause physical damage or defects in the fetus, especially if they are present during the first trimester, when rapid development of body organs is occurring. Tobacco and alcohol are the most commonly used drugs during pregnancy, with 22 percent of pregnant women using tobacco and 20 percent using alcohol. Women report lower rates of illegal drug use with pregnancy, with 7 percent using marijuana and 2 percent using cocaine, heroin, or methamphetamine. Almost 50 percent of women will stop using these drugs once they learn they are pregnant.[12]

If you have a condition for which you take prescription medication, such as diabetes, epilepsy, high blood pressure, acne, or asthma, consult with your physician to make sure the medication does not cause harm to a fetus. You may need to change medications or consider making lifestyle changes to maintain your health during pregnancy while also protecting the health of your fetus. If you suffer from depression or anxiety, your symptoms may worsen during pregnancy and the **postpartum period** (the 3-month period following childbirth) as a result of hormonal and emotional fluctuations. Your physician may be able to help you find natural ways to deal with these changes or recommend starting or continuing medication.

Tobacco Use During Pregnancy

Risk of spontaneous abortion, low birth weight, early separation of the placenta from the uterine wall, and infant death increases with the use of tobacco during pregnancy. The risk increases with the number of cigarettes smoked. If you smoke, try to quit before you get pregnant or abstain during pregnancy and after the baby is born. Avoid places where you and your child will be exposed to environmental tobacco smoke. Babies living in homes where adults smoke have a higher incidence of respiratory infections and **sudden infant death syndrome (SIDS).** Smoking cessation programs and treatments, including the nicotine patch, can help you quit.

Alcohol and Pregnancy

Consuming three or more ounces of alcohol daily (about six drinks) during pregnancy is associated with **fetal alcohol syndrome (FAS).** This condition is characterized by abnormal facial appearance, slow growth, mental retardation, and social, emotional, and behavior problems in the child. A safe level of alcohol consumption during pregnancy has not been established, and even occasional binge drinking may carry significant risk. If you are pregnant or may become pregnant, avoid drinking alcohol.

Illicit Drugs and Pregnancy

Illicit drugs have a variety of effects on a fetus, depending on the chemical action of the drug. Cocaine causes blood vessels to constrict in the placenta and fetus, increasing the risk of early separation of the placenta from the uterine wall, low birth weight, and possible birth defects. Heroin can cause retarded growth or fetal death as well as behavior problems in a child exposed to it in the womb. A baby whose mother used heroin during pregnancy is born addicted and experiences withdrawal symptoms, which can include seizures, irritability, vomiting, and diarrhea. Illicit drugs are also dangerous because they are often contaminated with other agents, such as glass, poisons, and other drugs.

Work Environment During Pregnancy

The U.S. Pregnancy Discrimination Act makes it illegal to exclude a woman from a job because she is or may become pregnant, and half of women in their reproductive years work outside the home. Most women can maintain their usual activity level during pregnancy and continue

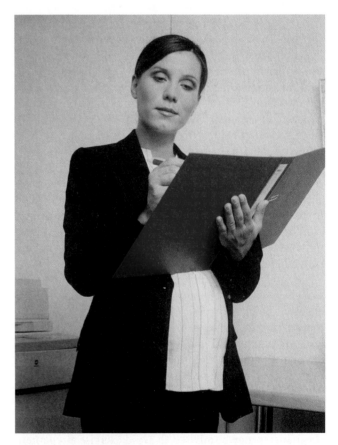

Women who work throughout their pregnancy need to attend to work demands that could adversely affect their pregnancy. During pregnancy, such women need to avoid occupational chemical exposure, which could cause a birth defect. In the later stages, they may find long periods of standing difficult to tolerate and may need to alternate between tasks that require standing and those that can be done while sitting.

working until delivery. They may need to adjust their activities if their work involves prolonged periods of standing, heavy lifting, or work with dangerous machines or hazardous materials. If you work with any chemicals, paints, or cleaning agents, check with your health care provider to make sure exposure is safe during pregnancy.

Abusive Relationships

Approximately 4 million women are assaulted by their male partners each year in the United States. Unfortunately, many women mistakenly believe that becoming pregnant and having a child will improve an abusive relationship. The fact is that abuse is a pattern of behavior that continues during pregnancy. Approximately 2 percent to 6 percent of women report abuse from their husband or intimate partner during pregnancy.[13] Abused women are less likely to seek prenatal care and are more likely to go into labor early and have a low-birth-weight baby. Abused women and their babies are more likely to die during pregnancy and the following year than are women who are not abused.[14] Women who are hit, kicked, or pushed by their partners need to seek help; they should not assume the abuse will stop when they become pregnant.

Regular Health Care Provider Visits

Every pregnant woman should visit her health care provider once a month until the 30th week, once every 2 weeks from the 31st to the 36th week, and once a week from the 37th to the 40th week (see the box "Choosing a Health Care Provider for Labor and Delivery"). Week of pregnancy is calculated from the date of the last menstrual period, which is 2 weeks before ovulation and conception occurred. A full-term baby has a gestational period of 38 weeks and is considered to have reached its due date 40 weeks after the woman's last menstrual period.

If the woman has not had prepregnancy counseling, the first prenatal visit will include a physical exam, a health history, and blood work to screen for illness, infections, and chronic disease and to ensure that the embryo or fetus is properly located in the uterus. The father's health history is also reviewed to determine whether the embryo or fetus has an increased risk for any condition or disease. After this first visit, the health care provider uses the subsequent visits to monitor the fetus for normal growth and development and the woman for complications of pregnancy.

Complications of Pregnancy

Although it is shocking to hear that a woman has died in childbirth in the 21st century, such deaths do occur. Mortality is higher in ethnic and racial minority groups, pointing to the role of socioeconomic factors, such as lack of prenatal care, lack of access to health information, and dietary differences.[15]

Early complications of pregnancy include the diagnosis of STDs. Experts recommend that all women be screened at the first pregnancy visit for gonorrhea, chlamydia, syphilis, hepatitis B, and human immunodeficiency virus (HIV) infection. Gonorrhea, chlamydia, and syphilis are treated and cured with antibiotics. The viral sexually transmitted diseases (hepatitis B, genital herpes, and HIV) cannot be cured, but the risk of passing these infections to the infant can be reduced. For hepatitis B, the infant receives hepatitis B vaccination and immunoglobulin immediately after birth. For genital herpes, the mother can take antiviral medication near the time of delivery to reduce the risk of a herpes outbreak at delivery. If a woman has a genital lesion at the time of labor, a cesarean section can further reduce risk of infection for the infant. For HIV, antiviral medication during pregnancy, labor, and delivery substantially reduces the risk of transmission to the infant. Current rates for vertical transmission of HIV in the United States are less than 2 percent. HIV-infected women with access to clean water and formula are advised not to breast-feed.[16]

Complications of pregnancy occur more frequently near the end of pregnancy. An especially dangerous condition is **preeclampsia,** characterized by high blood pressure, fluid retention, possible kidney and liver damage, and potential fetal death. The woman may notice swelling in her face or experience a severe headache or blurred vision. If not treated, the condition can develop into **eclampsia,** a potentially life-threatening disease

KEY TERMS

teratogens Substances that can cause physical damage or defects in the fetus, especially if they are present during the first trimester, when rapid development of body organs is occurring.

postpartum period Three-month period following childbirth.

sudden infant death syndrome (SIDS) Unexpected death of a healthy baby during sleep.

fetal alcohol syndrome (FAS) Combination of birth defects caused by prenatal exposure to alcohol, characterized by abnormal facial appearance, slow growth, mental retardation, and social, emotional, and behavior problems.

preeclampsia Dangerous condition that can occur during pregnancy, characterized by high blood pressure, fluid retention, possible kidney and liver damage, and potential fetal death.

eclampsia Potentially life-threatening disease that can develop during pregnancy, marked by seizures and coma.

Consumer Clipboard

Choosing a Health Care Provider for Labor and Delivery

When you are thinking about prenatal care and delivery, you have a number of options. Factors influencing your choice include your personal preferences, your medical and health history, and the likelihood of complications during your pregnancy. Here is a general description of the kinds of providers who may be available.

Midwives can be certified nurse-midwives or licensed midwives. A certified nurse-midwife has graduated from a school of nursing, passed a nursing certification exam, and received additional training in midwifery. A licensed midwife has completed a training program in midwifery similar to that of a certified nurse-midwife but may or may not have a prior background in nursing. Licensing laws for midwives vary from state to state. Depending on the state, midwives may be allowed to deliver babies at home, in birthing centers, or in hospitals. Midwives usually take patients who are at low risk for medical or pregnancy complications. If complications develop during prenatal care or delivery, a midwife will refer the case to a family physician or an obstetrician. Midwives tend to view pregnancy and birth as a family event. They are usually trained in support techniques (such as breathing and relaxation techniques) so the woman can have a delivery without anesthetic medications, and they usually stay with the woman throughout labor.

Family physicians have completed 4 years of medical school and 3 years in a residency training program. Some family physicians provide pregnancy-related care only for low-risk pregnancies; others receive extra training so they can manage complicated pregnancies and perform caesarean sections if necessary. Family physicians may deliver babies in birthing centers or hospitals but rarely perform home births. Like midwives, many family physicians view pregnancy and birth as a family event, and some use the same kind of support techniques.

Obstetricians have completed 4 years of medical school and an additional 4 years in a residency training program in obstetrics and gynecology. They are trained to handle all kinds of pregnancies, from low risk to high risk. Obstetricians tend to spend limited time at the bedside of a laboring patient; instead, they monitor labor for signs of problems and are present for delivery. Obstetricians usually have a medical orientation to labor management and delivery.

Perinatologists are obstetricians with additional training in the management of high-risk pregnancy. These specialists consult with and accept referrals from obstetricians. They are usually found at major medical centers. Most women see a perinatologist only if serious complications arise in the pregnancy.

---

marked by seizures and coma. A woman with pre-eclampsia may have to deliver her baby early to protect her own and the baby's health. The cause of this condition is not known.

Complications of Pregnancy for the Child

The most serious risk for the child during pregnancy is infant death, or **stillbirth.** About 1.2 percent of all pregnancies result in infant deaths. Half of these deaths occur before the fetus is born, and 80 percent occur before the 28th week of pregnancy. After birth, the leading causes of infant death are preterm birth, low birth weight, and SIDS. Before 1980, an infant born early and weighing less than 750 grams (about 1.65 pounds) would not have survived. Now it is standard practice to treat any infant weighing at least 500 grams (about 1.1 pounds).[15] Rates of both low birth weight and infant mortality are significantly higher for African Americans in the United States than for members of other groups. Reducing such disparities

through improved access to health information and prenatal care is a national health goal.

Diagnosing Problems in a Fetus

About 5 percent of babies born in the United States have a birth defect.[8] Several tests have been developed to detect abnormalities in a fetus before birth. The most frequently performed tests are alpha-fetoprotein (AFP) measurement, ultrasound, and chromosomal analysis through chorionic villus sampling or amniocentesis.

Alpha-Fetoprotein Measurement

Alpha-fetoprotein (AFP) is a protein produced by the infant and released into the amniotic fluid. It then crosses into the mother's blood, where it can be measured and compared with normal ranges. Abnormally high levels have been associated with problems in brain and spinal cord development, and abnormally low levels have been associated with chromosomal abnormalities in the fetus, especially Down syndrome. AFP testing is often done as part of triple screening or quadruple screening (screening for certain hormone levels) at 16 to 18 weeks of pregnancy. If an increased risk of problems or abnormalities is identified, more precise testing is performed.

Ultrasound

Commonly used to determine the size and gestational age of the fetus, its location in the uterus, and any major anatomical abnormalities, **ultrasound** is the use of high-frequency sound waves to produce a visual image of the fetus in the womb. It can also reveal the sex of the fetus. Health care professionals are debating whether all pregnant women should have an ultrasound or whether it makes sense only for women at risk for particular problems. Because it is usually not medically necessary, many insurance plans no longer cover routine ultrasound screening.

Chromosomal Analysis

Many chromosomal abnormalities are fatal and cause spontaneous abortion, but some are not fatal. Chromosomal abnormalities cause from 20 to 25 percent of all birth defects. The most common is Down syndrome (see Chapter 2 for more on this syndrome). Chromosomal abnormalities occur with greater frequency as maternal age increases. For example, the risk of Down syndrome in a 20-year-old woman is 1 in 1,400, but the risk in a 40-year-old woman is 1 in 100.[15] The most common reasons for chromosomal testing are advanced maternal age (35 years or older) and an abnormal AFP finding. Other reasons are a previous pregnancy with a chromosomal or genetic abnormality, a family history of children with chromosomal or genetic abnormalities, or an abnormal ultrasound finding.

In both **chorionic villus sampling (CVS)** and **amniocentesis,** a needle is passed through the abdomen of a pregnant woman into the uterus. (CVS can also be done by passing a thin catheter through the vagina and cervix.) In CVS, a sample is taken from the chorionic villus, part of the placenta or fetal support system in the uterus. In amniocentesis, a sample of amniotic fluid, the fluid that fills the pouch enclosing the fetus in the uterus, is taken. In both cases, fetal cells from the samples are grown in the lab and then subjected to chromosomal analysis. CVS can be performed between weeks 10 and 12, and amniocentesis can be performed between weeks 14 and 18. If a chromosomal problem is detected, the parents are faced with the difficult choice of continuing or terminating the pregnancy (see Chapter 2).

Fetal Development

Within 30 minutes of fertilization in the fallopian tube, the single-celled fertilized ovum, called a *zygote,* starts to divide. By the end of 5 days, the cluster of cells has made its way down the tube into the uterus. By the end of a week, it attaches to the uterus and starts to send small rootlike attachments into the uterine wall to draw nourishment. By the end of the second week, it is fully embedded in the lining of the uterus.

The period from week 2 to week 8, called the embryonic period, is a time of rapid growth and differentiation. By 4 weeks, the cluster of cells has divided into cells of different types, forming an embryo, a **placenta,** and an **amniotic sac.** By 8 weeks, all body systems and organs are present in rudimentary form, and some, including the heart, brain, liver, and sex organs, have started to function.

The period from the end of the 8th week after conception to birth is called the fetal period. By 12 weeks bones have formed and blood cells are beginning to be produced in the bone marrow. By 16 weeks, the sex of the fetus can be readily determined, and the mother can feel fetal movements. By 24 weeks, the fetus makes sucking movements with its mouth. It typically weighs about 640 grams and is starting to assume a fetal position because of space restrictions in the uterus. If a fetus is born between about 24 and 25 weeks of gestation, it can survive with aggressive medical intervention.

By week 26 the eyes are open, and by week 30, a layer of fat is forming under the skin. At 36 weeks, the fetus weighs about 2,500 grams and has an excellent chance of survival. The lungs are usually mature at this point. As noted earlier, a baby is considered to be full term at

KEY TERMS

stillbirth Infant death before or at the time of expected birth.

alpha-fetoprotein (AFP) Protein produced by the infant and released into the amniotic fluid; AFP measurement is used to screen for some fetal abnormalities.

ultrasound Technique for producing a visual image of the fetus using high-frequency sound waves.

chorionic villus sampling (CVS) Technique for testing fetal cells for chromosomal abnormalities by removing cells from the chorionic villus, part of the placenta in the uterus.

amniocentesis Technique for testing fetal cells for chromosomal abnormalities by removing a sample of amniotic fluid from the amniotic sac.

placenta Structure that develops in the uterus during pregnancy and links the circulatory system of the fetus with that of the mother.

amniotic sac Membrane that surrounds the fetus in the uterus and contains amniotic fluid.

Time	Changes/milestones
8 weeks (end of embryonic period)	*By week 8, pregnancy is detectable by physical examination.* Head is nearly as large as body First brain waves can be detected Limbs are present Ossification (bone growth) begins Cardiovascular system is fully functional All body systems are present in at least basic form Crown-to-rump length: 30 mm (1.2 inches) Weight: 2 grams (0.06 ounces)
9–12 weeks (third month)	*By week 10, fetus responds to stimulation.* Head is still large, but body is lengthening Brain is enlarging Spinal cord shows definition Facial features begin to appear Internal organs are developing Blood cells are first formed in bone marrow Skin is apparent Limbs are well molded Sex can be recognized from genitals Crown-to-rump length: 90 mm
13–16 weeks (fourth month)	*By week 14, skeleton is visible on X-ray.* Cerebellum becomes prominent Sensory organs are defined Blinking of eyes and sucking motions of lips occur Face has human appearance Head and body come into greater balance Most bones are distinct Crown-to-rump length: 140 mm
17–20 weeks (fifth month)	*By week 17, mother can feel movement of fetus.* Fatty secretions (vernix caseosa) cover body Lanugo (silky hair) covers skin Fetal position is assumed Limbs are reaching final proportions Mother feels "quickening" (movement of fetus) Crown-to-rump length: 190 mm
21–30 weeks (sixth and seventh month)	*By weeks 25–27, survival outside the womb is possible.* Substantial weight gain occurs Myelination (formation of sheath around nerve fibers) of spinal cord begins Eyes are open Bones of distal limbs ossify Skin is wrinkled and red Fingernails and toenails are present Tooth enamel is forming Body is lean and well proportioned Blood cells are formed in bone marrow only In males, testes reach scrotum at seventh month Crown-to-rump length: 280 mm
30–40 weeks (eighth and ninth month)	*Between weeks 32 and 34, survival outside the womb is probable.* Skin is whitish pink Fat is present in subcutaneous tissue Crown-to-rump length: 360–400 mm Weight: 2.7–4.1 kg (6–10 pounds)

Figure 16.10 Fetal development. *By the end of the first trimester, the anatomy of the fetus is almost completely formed. In the second trimester, the fetal heartbeat can be heard. During the last trimester, the greatest weight gain occurs.* Sources: Data from *Human Anatomy and Physiology* (6th ed.), by E. N. Marieb, 2004, San Francisco: Benjamin-Cummings; *Understanding Children and Adolescents* (4th ed.), by J. A. Schickedanz et al., 2001, Boston: Allyn & Bacon.

38 weeks of gestation, 40 weeks after the mother's last menstrual period. Full-term babies usually weight about 7½ pounds and are about 20 inches long. An overview of fetal development is shown in Figure 16.10.

CHILDBIRTH

By the ninth month, the pregnant woman is usually uncomfortably large and eager to have the baby, despite any apprehension she may harbor about the process of giving birth. Most parents find childbirth exciting, exhilarating, and even astounding. They finally get to meet the human being they have created.

Labor and Delivery

Labor begins when hormonal changes in both the fetus and the mother cause strong uterine contractions to begin. The pattern of labor and delivery can be different for every woman, and some women wonder how they will know it is time to call the midwife or go to the hospital. There are many subtle signs that labor is about to begin. In the days preceding labor, a woman may have diarrhea and a vaginal discharge containing mucus and sometimes a small amount of blood. The uterus may start to contract irregularly. In early labor or when the uterus is practicing in the weeks leading up to labor, the contractions may feel like a tightening of the stomach, mild menstrual cramps, or a dull backache that lasts from 30 to 60 seconds.

When labor begins in earnest, the contractions will become regularly spaced and begin to get stronger and more painful. The contractions cause the cervix to gradually pull back and open (dilate), and they put pressure on the fetus, forcing it down into the mother's pelvis. This first stage of labor can last from a few to many hours. When the cervix is completely open, the second stage of labor begins. The baby slowly moves into the birth canal, which stretches open to allow passage. The soft bones of the baby's head move together and overlap as it squeezes through the pelvis. When the top of the head appears at the opening of the birth canal, the baby is said to be *crowning*. After the head emerges, the rest of the body usually slips out easily. The third stage of labor is the delivery of the placenta, which usually takes another 10 minutes to 30 minutes. An overview of the process of labor and delivery is shown in Figure 16.11.

Many techniques have been developed to help women with the discomfort of the labor and delivery process. Many women and their partners take childbirth preparation classes to learn breathing and relaxation techniques to use during contractions. Several medication options are available in hospitals to further help with the discomfort. A woman may choose to have a pain medication given through an IV in the arm, or she may choose to have an *epidural,* a small catheter placed in the spine, through which pain medication can be administered.

Occasionally, the birthing process does not go smoothly. Sometimes the infant is too big to pass through the mother's pelvis. Sometimes an infant is in the wrong position, either sideways, buttocks first, or face first. Occasionally, the placenta covers the cervix so the baby cannot move into the birth canal. And sometimes the infant just does not tolerate the stress of the process well. In these situations, the health care provider usually recommends **cesarean section,** or **C-section,** the surgical delivery of the infant through the abdominal wall. Although most women are not enthusiastic about this option, it has saved many infants' and mothers' lives. Most hospitals now allow a woman to have her support person with her during the surgery. She can be awake and see her infant as it is born.

Newborn Screening

Babies are evaluated at birth to determine whether they require any medical attention or will need developmental support later. The Apgar scale is used as a quick measure of the baby's physical condition: a score of 0 to 2 is given for heart rate, respiratory effort, muscle tone, reflex irritability, and color. The scores are added for a total score of 0 to 10. The baby's neurological condition may also be assessed, and various screening tests may be given, such as tests for hearing and for phenylketonuria (see Chapter 2). Most babies are pronounced healthy and taken home within 24 to 48 hours of birth.

The Postpartum Period

Many expectant parents spend the 9 months of pregnancy focusing on the upcoming birth and thinking about the baby's sex, possible names, **circumcision** (whether or not to remove the foreskin of the penis), and breast-feeding versus bottle feeding. They may have spent little time thinking about exactly what it is like to be responsible for a baby. The first few weeks or months of parenthood are a period of profound adjustment, as parents learn how to care for their newborn (or **neonate**) and the newborn takes his or her place in the family. A few issues that deserve attention are growth and nutrition, illness and vaccinations, and attachment.

KEY TERMS

labor   Physiological process by which the mother's body expels the baby during birth.

cesarean section (C-section)   Surgical delivery of the infant through the abdominal wall.

circumcision   Removal of the foreskin of the penis; a procedure often performed routinely on baby boys in the United States.

neonate   Newborn.

Early first stage

The cervix thins (*effacement*) and begins to open (*dilation*). Short contractions (30 seconds) occur in 15- to 20-minute cycles. If the mucous plug that blocked the opening of the cervix during pregnancy gives way, light bleeding may occur (*bloody show*). The amniotic sac may also rupture (*water breaking*).

Late first stage

In the transition phase contractions become stronger and more frequent. These contractions may last from 60 to 90 seconds and occur every 1 to 3 minutes. When the cervix is completely open, with a diameter of about 10 centimeters, it is ready for passage of the baby's head.

Second stage

With strong and frequent contractions, the baby moves downward through the pelvic area, past the cervix, and into the vagina. The mother is instructed to "bear down" with the contractions to aid in the baby's passage through the birth canal. The baby's head emerges first, followed by the shoulders and rest of the body.

Third stage

Contractions of the uterus continue, and the placenta (*afterbirth*) is expelled. If the placenta is not expelled naturally, the health care provider puts pressure on the mother's abdomen to make this happen. The entire placenta must be expelled from the uterus or bleeding and infection may result.

Figure 16.11   Labor and delivery. *(a) In the first stage of labor the cervix thins and dilates, ending with the transition phase (b). (c) Delivery of the baby occurs in the second stage. (d) In the third stage the placenta is expelled.*

Growth and Nutrition

Babies have very high calorie requirements. One reason for this is their rapid rate of growth—they triple their birth weight by their first birthday—and another reason is the great relative mass of the infant's organs, especially the brain and liver, compared with muscle. Organs have much higher metabolic and energy requirements than muscle does.

The American Academy of Pediatrics and the American Academy of Family Physicians agree that breastfeeding is the best way to feed babies. Breast milk is perfectly suited to babies' nutritional needs and digestion; it also contains antibodies that reduce the risk of infections, allergies, asthma, and SIDS. For mothers, breast-feeding enhances bonding with the baby, contributes to weight loss after pregnancy, and may decrease the risk of ovarian cancer and breast cancer after menopause.[17] Breast-feeding is also more convenient and less expensive than bottle feeding. New mothers who have difficulty with breast-feeding can get advice and support from a lactation consultant, their health care provider, or support groups like LaLeche League. When a woman is breast-feeding, she may not get her menstrual period for up to 6 months after giving birth; however, ovulation can still occur, so breast-feeding is not a reliable form of birth control.

Because of illness, breast infection, or other reasons, about 10 percent of women are unable to breast-feed, and they bottle feed their infants instead. Bottle feeding provides adequate nutrition and enables parents to know how much food the baby is consuming. It also allows the mother more freedom and gives other family members the opportunity to feed and bond with the baby.

Illness and Vaccinations

Childbirth and the neonatal period are times of increased risk of infection for an infant. An infant under 2 months of age who develops a fever should be taken to see a health care provider immediately. Starting at 2 months, children receive vaccinations against several childhood diseases that, in the past, caused serious illness and death. They include diphtheria, pertussis (whooping cough), tetanus, measles, rubella (German measles), mumps, and polio, among others. The vaccinations are inexpensive and safe, especially when compared with the physical, emotional, and social costs of childhood diseases. Most states require that children be vaccinated before they are allowed to start public school. The National Immunization Survey reports that current childhood vaccination levels are at their highest ever, with 90 percent of children receiving the primary recommended vaccines. However, rates vary among racial and ethnic groups; again, reducing such disparities is a goal of national health policies.

Adjustment and Attachment

Although babies are tiny, they quickly become the center of attention in the household. They spend their time in recurring states of crying, alertness, drowsiness, and sleep. Parents spend much of their time feeding their newborn (at first, every 2 hours or so), changing diapers, and trying to soothe the crying infant. The strong emotional bond between parents and infant known as **attachment** develops during this period, and the infant begins to have feelings of trust and confidence as a result of a comforting, satisfying relationship with parental figures. This sense of trust is crucial for future interpersonal relationships and social and emotional development. Thus, a healthy infancy lays the foundation for a healthy life.

KEY TERMS

attachment   Deep emotional bond that develops between an infant and its primary caregivers.

You Make the Call

Surrogate Motherhood

Imagine this scenario: You and your spouse postponed having a family in order to develop your careers. Now you are both 42 and have been trying unsuccessfully to conceive a child for 4 years. For the past 2 years, you have been working with a fertility clinic, trying hormone treatments, intrauterine fertilization, and in vitro fertilization, all to no avail. Your physician has not been able to pinpoint the reason for your infertility. You are afraid that adoption would add more years to your wait, and you feel that time is slipping away. You have started thinking about surrogate motherhood.

Surrogate motherhood—hiring a woman to bear a child for you—has a long history dating back to biblical times. However, new reproductive technologies have created previously unforeseen options for surrogacy. The most common form is artificial insemination of the surrogate mother with sperm from the man in the infertile couple (the man and woman in the couple are referred to as the *intended parents* or *social parents*). The child is genetically related to the surrogate mother, who provides the egg, and to the intended father, who provides the sperm; the intended mother has to adopt the child when it is born. In another form of surrogacy, an egg from the intended mother is fertilized with sperm from the intended father, and the fertilized egg is implanted in the surrogate mother. The child is genetically related to both intended parents and unrelated to the surrogate mother. This option is usually chosen when pregnancy would be medically dangerous or impossible for the intended mother, as might be the case if she has a medical condition that would be worsened by pregnancy or if she is taking medication that would harm a fetus.

Typically, the couple pays the costs of the surrogate mother's prenatal and medical care during the pregnancy. In some cases they also pay the surrogate mother a fee, with some fees ranging up to $20,000 or more. When no fee is involved, the surrogate mother is usually a relative or friend of the couple who is carrying the pregnancy for altruistic reasons. The law varies from state to state, but some states ban surrogacy in exchange for money.

People considering surrogacy are advised to have legal agreements drawn up documenting the preconditions and contingency plans for the pregnancy and birth. These agreements need to cover such issues as the surrogate mother's health-related behaviors during the pregnancy (for example, smoking and drinking), any prenatal diagnoses indicating that the child may have a genetic abnormality, the death of one of the intended parents or divorce by the couple, the birth of a baby with a disability, and the decision by the surrogate mother to break the agreement and attempt to retain custody of the child. About 1 percent of surrogate mothers change their mind about giving up the child (compared to 75 percent of mothers with unplanned pregnancies who plan to give their baby up for adoption).

In cases where there is a custody dispute, the courts take several factors into account, including what is best for the child, the rights of the birth mother, and the genetic links of the child to the parents. In many cases, these factors conflict. The first case to bring surrogate motherhood into the public spotlight was the 1987–1988 case of "Baby M." When the birth mother in this case refused to give up her daughter and turned down the agreed-upon fee of $10,000, the genetic father sued for custody of the child. The New Jersey courts awarded custody of the baby to the father, allowed his wife to adopt the baby, and terminated the rights of the birth mother. The New Jersey Supreme Court then reversed the decision on appeal, calling it a dispute between two genetic parents with equal rights. They gave custody to the father, annulled the adoption by his wife, and granted visitation rights to the birth mother.

Surrogacy also raises ethical issues. Opponents warn that the practice trivializes reproduction and treats a child as a commodity to be bought and sold. The practice is depersonalizing for the surrogate woman, whose body is used as a vehicle for the genetic perpetuation of others. Because the couple seeking a child are often more affluent, better educated, and of higher socioeconomic status than the surrogate mother, there is a potential for exploitation. On the other hand, a woman who repeatedly bears children from others may be perceived as selling babies for profit. Some surrogate mothers, however, may be motivated by altruism; studies suggest that women who seek to become surrogates are slightly more altruistic, accept a higher degree of risk-taking behavior, and have easier pregnancies than their peers.

Surrogate motherhood always creates an extremely complex and intense situation and set of relationships. Supporters argue that the practice benefits both a couple who want a child and a woman who wants to bear a child for them, either for altruistic reasons or for a fee. Opponents argue that it involves buying and selling babies and is morally and ethically questionable. What to you think?

Pros

- Surrogate motherhood allows an infertile couple to have a child who is genetically related to them; often, adoption is not a viable option.

- Surrogate motherhood is an opportunity for a person to give the gift of a child to a couple who desperately wants one; the surrogate mother may derive satisfaction from her act.

- The freedom to conceive and bear a child is a protected right in U.S. society. Prohibiting surrogacy limits people's autonomy.

- Surrogacy is a contract between consenting adults; there is nothing illegal or unethical about it.

- Surrogacy provides women in financial need with the opportunity to earn money.

Cons

- It is wrong for a woman to loan her body to someone else for money.

- Women in financial need may be exploited by couples with the means to pay them to carry a child.

- Women may agree to surrogacy to earn a living; this amounts to buying and selling children.

- The child may suffer psychological harm; for example, there may be an acrimonious custody battle, or the child may be rejected by all parties because of a disability.

- The surrogate mother may suffer physical or psychological harm, and if she has other children or a spouse, they may be subject to social disapproval.

- Because of changing emotions and attitudes, a woman cannot give truly informed consent to surrender her baby until she actually gives birth.

- Surrogacy redefines motherhood in a way that threatens traditional concepts of parenting and family.

- All technological means of creating children, including artificial insemination, in vitro fertilization, and surrogacy, interfere and are at odds with the natural origins of life.

OLC Web site For more information on this topic, visit the Online Learning Center at www.mhhe.com/teague1e.

SOURCE: *Ethics in Obstetrics and Gynecology* (2nd ed.), American College of Obstetricians and Gynecologists, 2004, Washington, DC: Author.

SUMMARY

- Choosing the right contraceptive method lowers the risk of unintended pregnancy. More than half of all pregnancies, and 80 percent of teen pregnancies, are unintended.

- Abstinence is the only guaranteed method of preventing pregnancy.

- The fertility awareness method, or rhythm method, is based on abstaining from intercourse during the window of time around ovulation when a woman is most likely to conceive.

- Barrier methods of contraception use a physical barrier to prevent sperm from reaching ova. Spermicidal products should be used with some barrier methods (diaphragm and cervical cap) to increase their effectiveness. Barrier methods include the male condom, the female condom, and the Today contraceptive sponge, all of which are available over the counter, and the diaphragm and the cervical cap, both of which need to be fitted by a health care provider.

- The IUD is a small T-shaped device that is inserted in the uterus by a physician; it is believed to prevent conception by changing the cervical mucus and uterine secretions so sperm are less likely to reach the fallopian tubes and by changing the uterine lining so a fertilized egg is less likely to be implanted.

- Hormonal contraceptive methods—combinations of female hormones—work by preventing ovulation and also by altering the cervical mucus and the lining of the uterus. Birth control pills are taken every day or 3 weeks out of 4; during the 4th week, the woman has a light menstrual period. Injectable contraceptives (for example, Depo-Provera) are administered every month or every 3 months. The contraceptive skin patch is applied every week for 3 weeks; during the 4th week the woman has a period. The vaginal ring is placed in the vagina every 28 days; it is removed after 21 days to allow 7 days without the ring. Contraceptive implants (for example, Norplant) are placed under the skin by a physician and slowly release hormones for several years. They are not currently available in the United States.

- Emergency contraception is a hormonal method that can be taken within 48 to 72 hours after unprotected sex to prevent conception.

- Sterilization is a surgical procedure that permanently prevents conception. Male sterilization, called vasectomy, involves tying off and severing the vas deferens, preventing sperm from getting from the testes to the semen. Female sterilization, called tubal ligation, involves tying off and severing or sealing the fallopian tubes, preventing ova from getting from the ovaries to the uterus.

- Factors to consider when choosing a contraceptive method include effectiveness, cost, convenience, permanence, safety, protection against STDs, and consistency with personal values.

- In the case of an unintended pregnancy, three options are available: parenthood, adoption, and abortion. Adoptions can be open or closed; some couples are choosing international adoptions.

- In a surgical abortion, the contents of the uterus are removed by vacuum aspiration. In a medical abortion, the woman takes a drug, most often mifepristone, that causes the lining of the uterus to be shed, followed by another drug (misoprostol) that causes uterine contractions.

- Infertility is the inability to become pregnant after having unprotected intercourse for 12 months. Several methods are available to treat infertility, depending on whether it is caused by male factors, female factors, or both. They include surgery, hormone treatments, and advanced technology such as in vitro fertilization.

- Prenatal care is important for improving the chance for a successful pregnancy and lifelong good health for the child.

- A serious complication of pregnancy for the mother is preeclampsia, a condition of unknown cause characterized by high blood pressure and fluid retention. If not treated, it can lead to eclampsia, a life-threatening condition for the mother.

- The most serious complication of pregnancy for the child is infant death, or stillbirth. After birth, complications include preterm birth, low birth weight, and sudden infant death syndrome (SIDS).

- Fetal problems can be screened for by alpha-fetoprotein measurement and ultrasound. Fetal chromosomes can be analyzed through chorionic villus sampling (CVS) and amniocentesis.

- When conception occurs, the ovum is fertilized in the fallopian tubes, and the fertilized egg starts to divide and makes its way to the uterus. The period of the embryo, from week 2 to week 8, is a period of rapid growth and differentiation, at the end of which all body organs and systems are formed. The period of the fetus, from the end of the 8th week to birth, is a period of continued development and growth.

- A full-term baby is born after 38 weeks of gestation; it typically weights 7½ pounds and is about 20 inches long.

- The first stage of labor is the long period of uterine contractions during which the cervix is pulling back and opening and the baby is being pushed down into the mother's pelvis. The second stage of labor is the passage of the baby through the birth canal to the outside world. The third stage of labor is the delivery of the placenta.

- Some women prepare for childbirth by learning relaxation and breathing techniques so they can have unmedicated births. Pain medications are also available. Sometimes a cesarean section is necessary to save the mother's or baby's life.

- Newborns have very high nutritional requirements. Breast-feeding is recommended, but both breast-feeding and bottle feeding can meet the baby's nutritional and emotional needs.

- Illness during the neonatal period can be serious and should be treated. Starting at 2 months, infants receive vaccinations for many childhood diseases.

- The neonatal period is also the time when attachment develops and when the infant develops a sense of trust, the foundation for future healthy social and emotional development.

REVIEW QUESTIONS

1. What are some of the negative consequences of unintended pregnancies?
2. What is the only contraceptive method that is 100 percent effective?
3. What are the limitations of the fertility awareness method?
4. What physical signs accompany ovulation? How can they be used in family planning?
5. Why is withdrawal a less effective method of contraception than other types?
6. What is the single greatest advantage of condoms? What are their disadvantages?
7. How does the IUD work? What are the disadvantages of this method?
8. What are the potentially dangerous side effects of birth control pills?
9. Describe the procedures involved in vasectomy and tubal ligation. What are the advantages and disadvantages of these methods?
10. What factors should be considered when choosing a contraceptive method?
11. What factors should be considered when deciding on whether to become a parent?
12. Describe the procedures involved in surgical abortion and medical abortion.
13. What are some possible causes of infertility?
14. What are some benefits of prepregnancy counseling?
15. What are some dietary recommendations for pregnant women?
16. Explain how weeks of pregnancy are calculated.
17. What are the most serious complications of pregnancy for the mother and for the infant?
18. Describe four techniques used in diagnosing fetal abnormalities.
19. Why is the first trimester a time of great vulnerability for the developing fetus?
20. Describe the three stages of labor. What is a cesarean section?
21. What are the advantages of breast milk and breast-feeding?
22. What is attachment? Why is the period of infancy important for subsequent social and emotional development?

WEB RESOURCES

Alan Guttmacher Institute: This organization publishes journals and special reports related to sexual and reproductive health. Its online articles include topics such as abortion, pregnancy and childbirth, contraception, and STDs.
www.agi-usa.org

American Academy of Family Physicians: This site offers information on many issues for men and women, including contraceptive options, pregnancy and childbirth, reproductive health, and STDs.
http://familydoctor.org

American Society for Reproductive Medicine: Offering publications on sexual and reproductive health, this organization also provides fact sheets, FAQs, and information booklets.
www.asrm.org

Association of Reproductive Health Professionals: The Contraception Resources Center on this Web site features a glossary of terms, patient education brochures and guides, interactive tools, and information on emergency contraception.
www.arhp.org

Managing Contraception: This site offers a Q&A page with helpful information about sexual and reproductive health issues. It also features links related to abortion, contraception, counseling, and emergency contraception.
www.managingcontraception.com

Planned Parenthood Federation of America: This organization provides health information on birth control, emergency contraception, abortion, adoption, and pregnancy. Its resources include fact sheets, reports, and links.
www.plannedparenthood.org

Reproductive Health Online: This site offers sections on family planning and maternal and neonatal health. The family planning section highlights contraceptive methods, including emergency contraception. The maternal and neonatal health section includes information on complications related to pregnancy and to the newborn.
www.reproline.jhu.edu

National Abortion and Reproductive Rights Action League: This pro-choice organization works for better access to effective contraceptive options and to reproductive and other health care services. Featuring reproductive rights, the site offers educational and legislative information.
www.naral.org

National Adoption Information Clearinghouse: This organization offers a national directory search for adoption agencies according to state. Its publications address legal issues, access to family information, and collection of information about adopted persons, birth parents, and adoptive parents.
www.naic.acf.hhs.gov

National Right to Life Committee: This group works for legislative reform related to abortion and promotes alternatives to abortion. Its Web site features fact sheets and links to other resources.
www.nrlc.org

REFERENCES

1. Prevalence of selected maternal behaviors and experiences, Pregnancy Risk Assessment Monitoring System (PRAMS) 1999. (2002). *Morbidity and Mortality Weekly Review Surveillance Summaries, 51* (SS02), 1–26. www.cdc.gov/mmwr.

2. Hatcher, R. A., Trussell, J., Stewart, F., et al. (2004). *Contraceptive Technology* (18th ed.). New York: Ardent Media.

3. Tanne, J. H. (2004). FDA rejects over-the-counter status for emergency contraceptive. *British Medical Journal, 328* (7450), 1219.

4. English, A., & Kenney, K. E. (2003). *State minor consent laws: A summary* (2nd ed.). Chapel Hill, NC: Center for Adolescent Health and the Law.

5. PRAMS 1999 surveillance report. (2003). Atlanta, GA: Centers for Disease Control and Prevention.

6. Elam-Evans, L. D., et al. (2002). Abortion surveillance—United States, 1999. *Morbidity and Mortality Weekly Report Surveillance Summaries, 51* (9), 1–28. www.cdc.gov/mmwr.

7. Hausknecht, R. (2003). Mifepristone and misoprostol for early medical abortion: 18-month experience in the United States. *Contraception, 67,* 463–465.

8. Fertility, family planning, and women's health. (2000). www.cdc.gov/NCHS.

9. Gunderson, E., & Abrams, B. (2000). Epidemiology of gestational weight gain and body weight changes after pregnancy. *Epidemiology Reviews, 22* (2), 261–274.

10. U.S. Department of Agriculture (2005). 2005 *Dietary guidelines for Americans.* www.health.gov/dietaryguidelines.

11. What you need to know about mercury in fish and shellfish. EPA and FDA advice for: women who might become pregnant, women who are pregnant, nursing mothers and young children. (2004). www.epa.gov/waterscience.

12. Chasnoff, I. J., et al. (2005). The 4P's Plus screen for substance use in pregnancy: Clinical application and outcomes. *Journal of Perinatology,* online publication no. 10, www.nature.com/jp.

13. Beck, L. F., et al. (2002). Prevalence of selected maternal behaviors and experiences, Pregnancy Risk Assessment Monitoring System (PRAMS), 1999. *Morbidity and Mortality Weekly Report Surveillance Summaries, 51* (2), 1–27.

14. Boy, A., & Salihu, H. M. (2004). Intimate partner violence and birth outcomes: A systematic review. *International Journal of Fertility and Women's Medicine, 49* (4), 159–164.

15. Cunningham, F. G., et al. (2001). *Williams obstetrics* (21st ed.). New York: McGraw-Hill.

16. Allen, D., et al. (2001). Revised recommendations for HIV screening of pregnant women. *Morbidity and Mortality Weekly Report, 50* (RR19), 59–86. www.cdc.gov/mmwr.

17. Moreland, J., & Coombs, J. (2000). Promoting and supporting breast-feeding. *American Family Physician, 61* (7), 2093–2100, 2103–2104.

Add It Up!

RISKS FOR UNINTENDED PREGNANCY AND KNOWLEDGE OF POSSIBLE OUTCOMES

If you are sexually active, are you at risk for an unintended pregnancy? If you do become pregnant, are you at risk for difficulties during pregnancy or health problems in your child? And have you thought about your options if you should become pregnant? Answer the following questions to assess your risks.

1. Have you ever felt pressured in a relationship to have sex when you did not want to do so?   Yes   No

2. In your relationships, do you feel you can express your views with a partner and have him or her respect your opinion?   Yes   No

3. Do you always avoid having sex while under the influence of drugs or alcohol?   Yes   No

4. Do you discuss your partner's and your own history of sexually transmitted diseases before initiating sexual contact?   Yes   No

5. If you have had an STD in the past, has it been completely treated?   Yes   No

6. Do you discuss your partner's and your own thoughts and feelings about unintended pregnancy before initiating sexual contact?   Yes   No

7. Do you know your partner's thoughts about having children in the future?   Yes   No

8. Do you use an effective method of contraception every time you have sexual intercourse?   Yes   No

9. Do you use a method of contraception that protects you against STDs?   Yes   No

10. If you are a woman, do you get the recommended amount of folic acid in your diet or with supplements?   Yes   No

11. If you are a woman, do you avoid smoking, drinking, and using recreational drugs?   Yes   No

12. Are you between the ages of 18 and 35?   Yes   No

13. Do you know if you are at risk for sickle cell disease, Tay-Sachs disease, or cystic fibrosis?   Yes   No

14. Do you know your family health history for congenital birth defects, including Down syndrome?   Yes   No

15. If you become pregnant, do you know that parenthood, abortion, and adoption are your three choices?   Yes   No

16. If you are considering parenthood, do you feel ready—in terms of your financial resources, educational goals, relationship status, and emotional maturity—to have a baby at this point in your life?   Yes   No

17. Is either abortion or adoption an acceptable choice for you?   Yes   No

If you answered yes to 12 or more questions, you are well educated about communicating with your partners and knowing your risks for unintended pregnancy and the possible outcomes. If you answered yes to 9–11 questions, you are probably taking some risks; it would be a good idea to learn more about your own health and communication with partners. If you answered yes to fewer than 9 questions, you are taking significant risks and may be on your way to an unintended pregnancy.

PART 5

Challenges to Your Health

Part 5 highlights broad issues presenting challenges to your health and that of society as a whole—violence, unintentional injury, and environmental problems. Can you as an individual make a positive impact in an increasingly violent world? Is safety a personal issue or everyone's responsibility? When you think of environmental issues, do you focus on what's going on in your own backyard or around the world? These are important questions to consider as you study these chapters. Take the time to discuss these topics with your friends, balancing your ideas with other points of view.

THINK IT OVER

How would you communicate the idea of nonviolence to a violent person?

Have your ideas about safety changed since Hurricane Katrina in 2005?

Do you think it's possible to improve the environment for future generations?

CHAPTER 17

Violence: Prevention and Protection

DID YOU KNOW?

- If you have ever used alcohol in a sexual situation, you know that being intoxicated can make it harder to assess potentially dangerous situations, to assert yourself, to defend yourself, to listen, to make responsible decisions, and to inhibit aggressive impulses. Of those involved in college campus rapes, 75 percent of men and 50 percent of women had been drinking when the sexual assault occurred.

- If you are young and male, you have a much higher risk of being involved in a violent incident than does any other group. Homicide is the second leading cause of death for people aged 10 to 24 in the United States. Of those killed in this age group, about 85 percent are male. Of those arrested for violent crimes, 44 percent are under 25 years of age, and 82 percent are male.

- Although many women fear violence at the hands of a stranger, violence against women is far more likely to be inflicted by people they know. Of women raped in the United States, more than 60 percent know their assailant. Of women killed in the United States, a third are killed by their husbands or partners.

OLC *Your Health Today*   www.mhhe.com/teague1e

Go to the Online Learning Center for *Your Health Today* for interactive activities, quizzes, flashcards, Web links, and more resources related to this chapter.

Most of us see media images of violence nearly every day—school shootings on the nightly news, suicide bombings on the front page of the newspaper, murders and rapes on television police dramas, gun battles in action movies. For some Americans, violence is also part of daily life, whether experienced as neighborhood drug wars, domestic violence, gang violence, or robbery at the corner store. For others, violence is something remote and unreal; violent incidents occur rarely in their lives. Still others experience a single violent event—a rape or an assault, for example—that haunts them for the rest of their lives. As the terrorist attacks of September 11, 2001, demonstrated, however, no one is immune to the threat of violence or exempt from its effects. Violence affects everyone.

More than many of the other health topics discussed in this text, violence is a societal issue. Although violent acts are committed by individuals, the causes of violence are rooted in social and cultural conditions. This does not mean that people who commit violent crimes are not held accountable for their actions—they are. In fact, the United States incarcerates a larger proportion of its population than any other nation.[1] It does mean that taking action individually to reduce violence is difficult for people, unlike deciding to improve their diet or get more exercise. What you as an individual can do about violence falls into two categories: knowing how to reduce your own risk of encountering violence and working to create safer communities and to prevent violence in society.

In this chapter we look first at violent crime in the United States, factors that contribute to violence, and the recent decline in crime rates. We turn next to violence among youth, especially school violence and youth gangs, and we examine violence on the college campus, in particular, hazing and hate speech. We then consider sexual violence, including rape and sexual harassment, and we explore family and intimate partner violence. We touch briefly on violence in the workplace, hate crime, and terrorism, and we conclude with a discussion of some issues related to violence prevention. Throughout the chapter, the focus is on how individuals can change their behavior to keep themselves safe.

VIOLENCE IN THE UNITED STATES

Violence is defined as the use of force or the threat of force to inflict intentional injury, physical or psychological, on oneself or another person. Murder, robbery, and **assault** are all violent crimes, but violence also occurs in association with child abuse, sexual harassment, suicide, and several other kinds of conduct.

Crime Rates and Violence Facts

The United States is commonly believed to be one of the most violent nations in the industrialized word. Actually,

Compared with other nations, the United States has the highest number of homicides involving firearms. In contrast to the United Kingdom, where the use of firearms is strictly controlled, guns are readily available in the United States.

rates of violent crime in the United States are lower than those in many other developed countries, except in one area—homicide, especially homicide committed with a firearm. The number of firearm homicides in the United States is higher than in any other country; it is almost 15 times higher than in Canada.[2,3] Most experts attribute this difference to the ready availability of firearms in the United States.

The U.S. Justice Department and the Federal Bureau of Investigation (FBI) count cases of homicide, assault, robbery, and rape as violent crimes. According to these agencies, a total of 1.38 million violent crimes were committed in the United States in 2003, with aggravated assault accounting for 62 percent of them; robbery, 30 percent; rape, 7 percent; and homicide, 1.2 percent.[4] This amounts to 858,000 aggravated assaults, 413,400 robberies, 92,400 rapes, and 16,500 homicides (see the box "The FBI's 'Crime Clock'").

In 2003, firearms were involved in 30 percent of all violent crimes and 71 percent of all homicides.[4] Of the firearms used in homicides, 80 percent were handguns and the remainder were rifles, shotguns, and other kinds

KEY TERMS

violence   Use of force or the threat of force to inflict intentional injury, physical or psychological, on oneself or another person.

assault   Attack by one person on another using force or the threat of force to intentionally inflict injury. *Aggravated assault* is an attack that causes bodily injury, usually with a weapon or other means capable of producing grave bodily harm or death. *Simple assault* is an attack without a weapon that causes less serious physical harm.

HIGHLIGHT ON HEALTH
The FBI's "Crime Clock"

According to the FBI, one violent crime occurs every 22.8 seconds in the United States, and one property crime occurs every 3 seconds. Here is the breakdown:

Violent Crime		Property Crime	
Every 31.8 minutes	1 murder	Every 25 seconds	1 motor vehicle theft
Every 5.6 minutes	1 rape	Every 14.6 seconds	1 burglary
Every 1.3 minutes	1 robbery	Every 4.5 seconds	1 larceny-theft
Every 36 seconds	1 aggravated assault		

Source: *Crime in the United States—2003*, Federal Bureau of Investigation, Uniform Crime Reports, www.fbi.gov.

of firearms. About 78 percent of homicide victims knew their assailant; in about 22 percent of cases, the assailant was a stranger. In aggravated assault, equal numbers of attackers are known and unknown to their victims. Of women killed in 2003, a third were killed by their husbands or boyfriends. Of men, 2.5 percent were killed by their wives or girlfriends.[4] One in five child homicide victims was killed by a family member.[5]

What Accounts for Violence?

How can we understand violent crime? Although the causes are complex, some risk factors can be identified. Risk factors are not causes; rather, they are factors that increase the likelihood that a person will engage in a behavior or suffer harm. Age and sex are among the most reliable risk factors for violence.[6] The typical offender is a young male between the ages of 15 and 24. Forty-four percent of those arrested for violent crimes are under 25 years of age. Men are much more likely to commit a violent act than women are; 82 percent of those arrested for violent crimes are men.[4] Women do commit violent acts, but it is often in self-defense; for example, when women kill their husbands, it is typically after they have endured years of physical abuse and believe their lives are in danger.

Being a member of a minority group is a significant risk factor for violence. Although African Americans make up 12 percent of the population, they make up nearly half (48 percent) of all homicide victims (Figure 17.1).[7] The probability of being murdered before the age of 45 is 2.21 percent for African American men, compared with 0.29 for white men.[8] Similarly, African Americans account for 46 percent of homicide offenders. Thirty-seven percent of those arrested for violent crimes are African American; 60.5 percent are white, and the remainder are Native American, Asian, or Pacific Islander. (People of Hispanic ethnic origin are included in the racial categories "black" and "white" in these statistics.)

Where a person lives also influences the risk of being affected by violence. Violence is more prevalent in large cities—90 percent of violent crimes occur in metropolitan areas—and the larger the city, the higher the crime rate. Rates of violent crime in the United States are higher in the South and West than in the Northeast and Midwest.[4]

Like risk factors for mental illness, risk factors for violence occur at many levels. Risk factors at the societal and cultural levels include poverty, poor schools, disorganized neighborhoods, use of alcohol and drugs, availability of guns, exposure to media violence, and lack of economic, educational, and employment opportunities. Violence is also more common on college campuses than in the general population, perhaps because of the transient nature of the community.

Risk factors at the family level include child abuse, substance abuse or criminal activity by family members, lack of positive role models, and chaotic family organization. There is a higher risk of violence when parents are not involved in children's lives, do not supervise their

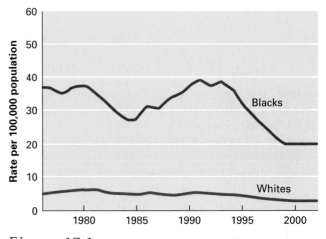

Figure 17.1   Homicide rates by race of victim, United States, 1976–2002. *Blacks were six times more likely than whites to be murdered in 2002.* Source: Bureau of Justice Statistics, www.ojp.usdoj.gov/bjs.

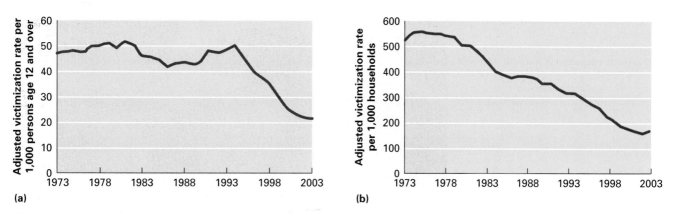

Figure 17.2   Crime rates in the United States, 1973–2003. (*a*) *Violent crime rates have declined since 1994, reaching the lowest level ever recorded in 2003.* (*b*) *Property crime rates declined through 2002 and stabilized in 2003.* Source: Bureau of Justice Statistics, www.ojp.usdoj.gov/bjs.

activities, and use harsh, lax, or inconsistent discipline. Risk factors at the individual level include such biological factors as genetics, brain structure, brain chemistry, and medical disorders; low intelligence; certain personality traits, such as aggressiveness and poor impulse control; and a history of previous criminal or antisocial behavior.[6] Other individual risk factors include attention deficit disorder and hyperactivity in children; deficits in cognitive and social cognitive functioning; poor impulse and behavior control; and early antisocial and aggressive behaviors. Problems are exacerbated for children who do poorly in school, are rejected by classmates, associate with deviant peers, and become involved with gangs. Conversely, protective factors, which buffer young people from the effects of risk factors, include high IQ, a positive social orientation, and involvement in school activities.[9] No single factor is sufficient to explain why violence occurs or why levels of violent crime rise or decline in different time periods.

Trends in Violent Crime

Rates of violent crime in the United States rose in the 1950s and 1960s, held steady in the 1970s and 1980s, and then declined precipitously in the 1990s. Between 1994 and 2003, the rate of violent crime (homicide, rape, robbery, and assault) fell by 33.4 percent, and the rate of property crime (burglary, theft, and motor vehicle theft) fell by 23 percent (Figure 17.2).[10] Experts have proposed a variety of explanations for this trend:[1]

- *Demographics.* Rates of violence fall when the segment of the population responsible for most occurrences of violent crime—young men aged 14–24—decreases in size. This commonly offered explanation is inadequate in this case, because the size of this group changed very little between 1994 and 2003.
- *Crack cocaine.* The boom in crack cocaine in the 1980s, accompanied by drug wars and gun violence, was followed by a steep decline in demand for crack in the early 1990s. Marijuana replaced crack as the drug of choice among younger drug

users; the marijuana trade is associated with less violence than is the trade in crack.
- *Economic expansion.* The economy improved in the 1990s, creating more opportunities for people to earn a living in legitimate ways.
- *Law enforcement and incarceration.* Mandatory sentencing policies, as exemplified by "three strikes" laws (automatic maximum sentences for people convicted of a third felony, even a nonviolent one), and the sharp increase in incarceration rates in the 1980s and 1990s removed many criminals from the streets. The prison population in the United States quadrupled between 1980 and 2000.
- *Expansion of resources for victims.* Resources for those affected by domestic violence increased in the 1980s and 1990s, including hotlines, shelters, legal advocates, and increased availability of judicial protections (such as restraining orders).

None of these explanations is sufficient by itself to explain the drop in crime; some combination of these factors and others is probably responsible for the overall trend. More research is needed to determine what policies and programs are effective and actually result in a reduction in violent crime. Areas for study include, among others, responses to drug offenses other than imprisonment, effective interventions in domestic violence, and approaches to gangs and gun use by young people.

Despite improvement in crime rates, the rate of violent crime is still unacceptably high in the United States, especially among minority populations. With crime rates leveling off and perhaps starting to creep upward again, it is imperative that the issue of violence be addressed in a rational and methodical way.

YOUTH VIOLENCE

Among people aged 10 to 24, homicide is the second leading cause of death in the United States (unintentional injuries, or accidents, are the first). In 2001 nearly

The school shooting at the Red Lake Indian Reservation in Minnesota in 2005 was a tragic reminder that violence can erupt in a normally peaceful setting. Is this a case of troubled individuals being out of control? Or does it reflect broader societal issues?

5,500 people in this age group were murdered, 85 percent of them male. In 2002 more than 877,000 people aged 10 to 24 were injured in violent acts, and 1 in 13 was hospitalized.[10]

School Violence

School shootings like those at Columbine High School in Littleton, Colorado, in 1999 and on the Red Lake Indian Reservation in Minnesota in 2005 highlight not just youth violence but issues such as depression and mental disorders in teenagers, bullying and social isolation, and access to weapons. Such mass shootings are shocking but rare in U.S. schools. Like violence in general, school violence has decreased in recent years, as evidenced, for example, by a decline in the percentage of high school students who were involved in a physical fight in 2003 (42 percent in 1991, 33 percent in 2003) and by the percentage of high school students who carried a weapon in 2003 (26 percent in 1991, 17 percent in 2003).[11]

Still, about 50 murders or suicides occur each year near schools, according to U.S. Education Department statistics.[12] A National Institute of Education study estimates that 23 percent of students and 11 percent of teachers are physically attacked on or near school grounds every month. About 9 percent of high school students in the United States were threatened or injured with a weapon in 2003, and 5.4 percent did not go to school one or more days because of concerns for their safety.[11]

Schools have responded to violence primarily by tightening security and strengthening punitive measures. Two federal laws, the Gun-Free Schools Act and the Safe and Drug-Free Schools Act, both passed by Congress in 1994, created a **zero-tolerance policy** that calls for expelling any student who brings weapons or drugs to school. The teachers' union, the American Federation of Teachers, strongly supports zero-tolerance policies, claiming that principals need to be able to respond quickly, decisively, and fairly to acts or threats of violence and drug abuse.[13]

Healthy People 2010

OBJECTIVE AREA *Injury and Violence Prevention*

- Reduce weapon carrying by adolescents on school property.

"Violence prevention programs for youth need to focus on strategies that reduce involvement in physical fighting and discourage weapon carrying on school property. [Such] strategies should begin early in life and must be tailored to youth of widely varying social, economic, cultural, and ethnic backgrounds. . . . Physicians and other health professionals are in a position to provide effective primary prevention messages to youth and their families."

 For more information on Healthy People 2010 objectives, visit the Web site at www.healthypeople.gov.

 For more information on Canadian health objectives, visit the Health Canada Web site at www.hc-sc.gc.ca/english.

On the other hand, some child advocates, educators, parents, and citizens consider zero-tolerance initiatives too inflexible. Children have been expelled from school for wearing Halloween costumes with paper swords and bringing plastic knives in lunch bags. These experts recommend such measures as providing mental health services for students, social support for families, classes in anger management, and more extracurricular activities that will get students involved in school and positive peer relationships. They also endorse measures that would reduce access to guns by children and adolescents.

Youth Gangs

Youth gangs are associations of adolescents and young adults aged 12 to 24 organized to control a territory, usually in an inner city, and to conduct illegal activities like drug trafficking. Gangs are associated with violence not just because of their illegal activities but because violence is part of members' lives, in their families and communities, before they ever join a gang. Many gang members derive a sense of belonging, purpose, and self-esteem not otherwise available in their lives, as well as security, protection, and a source of income, from gang membership.[14]

Efforts to reduce gang violence focus on preventing adolescents from joining gangs by keeping them in school and providing opportunities for legitimate success, such as meaningful employment opportunities. Community social controls can be increased by strengthening social institutions, such as schools and churches, and encouraging parents and community leaders to play a role in supervising adolescents' activities. Programs are needed in prisons, such as job training and drug treatment programs, that prevent the recycling of adult gang members back into the community crime scene. Finally, efforts to remove guns from the streets need to be enhanced.[15] Several cities have model programs in place, aimed at reducing gang violence through these strategies and others.

VIOLENCE ON THE COLLEGE CAMPUS

Would you think a community was safe that, in the past year, had 1 murder, 2 rapes, 13 robberies, 20 aggravated assaults, 190 burglaries, 66 car thefts, 160 arrests for alcohol violations, 158 arrests for drug violations, and 32 arrests for weapon violations? Would it surprise you to learn that this community is a university campus, a place traditionally viewed as a tranquil environment for intellectual pursuits?[16] In fact, there were a total of 77 murders on U.S. college and university campuses in 2002, according to U.S. Department of Education statistics, as well as thousands of other violent crimes, including 7,600 robberies, 3,600 forcible sex offenses, and 7,846 cases of aggravated assault.[17] Like other crime statistics, these numbers represent a decline from previous years. Still, violent crime represents a significant threat to students (see the box "Who Is Least Likely to Be Assaulted?").

Most colleges have responded to campus violence by raising the visibility of campus security officers, tightening security controls, and implementing stringent discipline programs.[18] Two federal laws regulate how campus crime is treated. The 1990 Campus Security Act (CSA) requires colleges and universities receiving federal funding to report annually all campus felony statistics to the U.S. Secretary of Education; to students, faculty, and staff of their respective institutions; and, on request, to prospective students and their parents. The 1992 Assault Victim's Bill of Rights Act (AVBRA) requires college administrators to provide justice, medical treatment, and psychological counseling for crime victims and survivors. Amendments to AVBRA passed in 1998 require colleges to promote educational awareness programs on sexual assault, facilitate the reporting of sexual assault, and help survivors who want to change their academic and living situation, among other requirements. Schools that fail to comply may lose federal funds, including student loan funding.

Hazing

A controversial practice on many campuses, associated especially with fraternities, sororities, and athletic teams, is hazing. According to the Fraternities Executive Association, **hazing** is "any action taken or situation created intentionally, whether on or off fraternity premises, to produce mental or physical discomfort, embarrassment, or ridicule."[19] Hazing is typically imposed as an initiation rite or a requirement for joining an organization.

Hazing activities have included kidnapping, alcohol chugging, forced swallowing of food and nonfood items, sleep deprivation, beatings, and calisthenics to the point of exhaustion. Deaths have occurred as a result of hazing, most often fraternity hazing. A common cause is alcohol

KEY TERMS

zero-tolerance policy Policy stating that any student who brings weapons or drugs to school will be expelled.

youth gangs Associations of adolescents and young adults aged 12 to 24 organized to control a territory and conduct illegal activities.

hazing Actions taken to cause mental or physical discomfort, embarrassment, or ridicule in individuals seeking to join an organization.

Beating the Odds

Who Is Least Likely to Be Assaulted?

Protecting yourself from assault, sexual or otherwise, requires common sense and vigilance. Sometimes individuals are naïve about risks, and other times they are in the wrong place at the wrong time. Brief profiles of three women are presented here. Which one do you think is least likely to be assaulted?

Candice attends a university located in a major metropolitan area. She often studies in the library until closing time and then walks to her dorm. Her college security department offers an escort service for students on campus after 10:00 p.m., but she doesn't think she needs to use it. Candice runs nearly every day in a 1,500-acre city park with extensive exercise trails and heavy shrubbery. She usually runs at the end of the day and is sometimes out until dark. Candice knows that some women have been accosted on her campus, so she is very alert while running. She took a course in self-defense when she was in high school and considers herself in excellent physical condition.

Kelly grew up in a small town in the Midwest and is now a freshman at a large university several hundred miles from home. She has been to several fraternity parties and is still learning to limit her alcohol consumption. Several older students have asked her out; she enjoys their attention but doesn't want to get involved with anyone yet. Kelly jogs by herself several afternoons a week; she always follows the same route, one that takes her into remote areas. She carries a cell phone with her, and for company, she listens to music on headphones. She always tells her roommate where she's going and when she expects to be back.

Abigail is a senior at a small college in the Northeast, 70 miles from a large city. She lives off campus with several housemates. They often neglect to lock the doors and occasionally find someone they don't know sleeping in their living room. On weekends, Abigail likes to go clubbing in the city with a few friends. They drink a fair amount of alcohol, smoke marijuana, and sometimes take other drugs. They have an agreement that they will never leave anyone alone at a club and that they will always go home together. One time they were followed by three men from a club, but they managed to get to their car before the men could approach them.

OLC Web site Visit the **Online Learning Center** at www.mhhe.com/teague1e for comments by the authors.

---

poisoning, but death can also occur from such practices as forcing pledges to drink huge quantities of water, which causes "water intoxication" and death from swelling of the brain stem. The number of deaths is difficult to determine accurately, because causes of death may be listed as accidents, alcohol overdoses, suicides, stabbings, shootings, and fires without indicating that the deaths occurred during a hazing acitivity.[19]

Although sorority hazing has caused fewer injuries and deaths than fraternity hazing, a significant number of sorority women have died of alcohol poisoning and alcohol-related falls and car crashes. Campus hazing is also practiced by clubs, bands, and athletic teams. At one university, 80 percent of responding college athletes reported that they had faced questionable or unacceptable initiation activities, including kidnapping and beating.

Hazing is illegal in many states and may be either a misdemeanor or a felony, depending on the state and the severity of the offense. Parents whose children have died in these senseless incidents have filed wrongful death suits against both colleges and fraternities. Hazing has also been reported as an initiation rite among firefighters, police officers, and employee groups.

Free Speech vs. Hate Speech

College and university campuses are places where debate and free expression are encouraged in the service of learning and intellectual freedom. Because of this commitment, institutions of higher education often find themselves at the center of free speech controversies. Maintaining an atmosphere of civility that allows respect for different opinions while protecting people from the violence that may be incited by offensive speech has become a major challenge.[20]

Hate speech—defined as verbal, written, or symbolic acts that convey a grossly negative view of particular persons or groups based on their gender, ethnicity, race, religion, sexual orientation, or disability[20]—is particularly troublesome. Its intent is to humiliate or harm rather than to convey ideas or information, and it has the potential to incite violence. Epithets, slurs, taunts, insults, and intimidation are common modes of hate speech; posters, flyers, letters, phone calls, e-mail, Web sites, and even T-shirts are media by which the message is distributed.

Some schools have adopted speech codes that require civility in discourse for all campus community members.[20] Some of these codes have been struck down by the courts as a violation of First Amendment rights. According to the rulings, hate speech must be proven to inflict real, not trivial, harm before it can be regulated. The U.S. Supreme Court has made it clear that colleges and universities cannot suppress speech simply because it is offensive. For this reason, many colleges and universities have adopted conduct codes that regulate certain actions associated with hate speech but not the speech itself.[20]

SEXUAL VIOLENCE

Sexual violence includes not just rape but sexual harassment, stalking, and other forms of forcible or coercive sexual activity.

Sexual Assault

In most states, the term *rape* has been replaced by the more comprehensive term *sexual assault,* which includes different kinds of attacks and varying degrees of severity. **Sexual assault** is any sexual behavior that is forced on someone without his or her consent. At the least, the victim is made to feel uncomfortable and intimidated; at the worst, he or she is physically and emotionally harmed.[21] Sexual assault includes forced sexual intercourse (rape), forced sodomy (oral or anal sexual acts), child molestation, incest, fondling, and attempts to commit any of these acts. Sexual assaults may be classified as misdemeanors or felonies. Another category of victimization is called **sexual coercion,** defined as imposing sexual activity on someone through the threat of nonphysical punishment, promise of reward, or verbal pressure rather than through force or threat of force.

According to studies, 25 percent to 60 percent of men have engaged in sexual assault and coercive sexual behavior.[22] The causes of this behavior are complex. Perpetrators may have been socialized in a way that promotes male power and encourages controlling behavior by males; they may not have the same understanding of sexual situations that women and other men do. They may accept stereotypes about gender roles and relationships. They may have had early sexual experiences, or they may have predisposing personality traits, such as irresponsibility or lack of social conscience. Also involved are situational factors, including time and place of assault, use of alcohol and other drugs, and the relationship between victim and perpetrator. No matter what their characteristics, only about 2 percent of men who rape ever go to prison.[23] Rape prevention efforts need to focus on changing the environment that promotes violence against women.

Rape

A study called the Sexual Victimization of College Women Survey found that about 35 women per 1,000 female students were victims of completed or attempted rape in any given academic year (fall and spring semesters). Rape was defined as unwanted vaginal, anal, or oral penetration by penis, finger, or object by force or threat of force.[22] Thus, a college with 10,000 female students could experience more than 350 rapes a year. These researchers estimated that 20 percent to 25 percent of college women experience completed or attempted rape during their college years.

According to findings of the National Violence Against Women Survey, about 18 percent of women in the United States survived a completed or attempted rape in 2000.[24] More than half of rape and sexual assault victims are under the age of 18, and one in five are under the age of 12. When a victim is younger than the "age of consent," usually 18, the perpetrator can be charged with **statutory rape** whether there was consent or not. Only 25 percent to 50 percent of all rapes are reported to the police, for a variety of reasons.[22] Victims may be embarrassed or traumatized, may not be sure that what happened to them qualifies as rape, may think they won't be believed, may blame themselves or feel guilty, or may not want to identify someone they know as a rapist.

Relatively few rapes are **stranger rapes,** that is, rapes committed by someone unknown to the victim. In 62 percent of rapes and sexual assaults, the victim knows the perpetrator.[23] In 40 percent of cases, the perpetrator is a friend or an acquaintance; **acquaintance rape** can be committed by a classmate, coworker, or someone else casually known to the victim. Unfortunately, only about 16 percent of acquaintance rapes are reported to the police.[25] **Date rape,** sexual assault by a boyfriend or someone with

KEY TERMS

hate speech Verbal, written, or symbolic acts that convey a grossly negative view of particular persons or groups based on their gender, ethnicity, race, religion, sexual orientation, or disability.

sexual assault Any sexual behavior that is forced on someone without his or her consent.

sexual coercion The imposition of sexual activity on someone through the threat of nonphysical punishment, promise of reward, or verbal pressure rather than through force or threat of force.

statutory rape Sexual intercourse with someone under the "age of consent," usually 18, whether consent is given or not.

stranger rape Rape committed by someone unknown to the victim.

acquaintance rape Rape committed by someone known to the victim.

date rape Rape committed by someone with whom the victim has a dating relationship.

HIGHLIGHT ON HEALTH
Alcohol, Rape, and Responsibility

Alcohol can increase your risk of being involved in rape, whether as a victim or as a perpetrator. Keep the following points in mind when deciding whether and how much to drink:

- Being intoxicated impairs your ability to communicate clearly, making it harder for you to state your expectations and limits regarding sexual activity.

- Being intoxicated impairs your ability to assess a situation that makes you vulnerable to assault and reduces your ability to defend yourself.

- Being intoxicated impairs your ability to make responsible decisions. Alcohol can diminish normal inhibitions against behaving aggressively.

- Being intoxicated makes it harder for you to listen carefully to your companion. A person who is drunk is not necessarily willing to have sexual intercourse. Having sex with someone who is too intoxicated to give informed consent is legally considered rape.

- Criminal law does not distinguish between acquaintance rape and stranger rape. Forced sexual intercourse of any kind is rape.

- Even if someone uses poor judgment by engaging in unwise behavior, such as drinking to excess or walking alone in an isolated area, the responsibility for sexual assault lies entirely with the person who uses force.

- Being drunk is not an excuse for using threats, intimidation, or physical force to coerce another person, and it does not reduce your responsibility for such behavior in either a criminal court or a college disciplinary hearing.

- If you do not pay attention to a refusal of sexual advances, you may commit an act punishable by permanent expulsion from school or imprisonment.

Source: Judith Scott, University Sexual Harassment Officer, University of North Carolina at Chapel Hill, 104 Vance Hall, CB 1040, Chapel Hill, NC 27599; 919-962-3026, 1991, rev. 8/97.

whom the victim has a dating relationship, is a type of acquaintance rape. In about 18 percent of rapes and sexual assaults, the perpetrator is the victim's intimate partner or husband.[23] Many states now allow rape charges to be brought by a woman against her husband.

Acquaintance rape survivors are more likely to have consumed alcohol or drugs before the assault, possibly reducing their awareness of signs of aggression in the rapist or their ability to respond to violence. (For more reasons to monitor alcohol consumption, see the box "Alcohol, Rape, and Responsibility.") One study found that 75 percent of men and 50 percent of women involved in campus acquaintance rapes had been drinking before the sexual assault.[26]

Sexual predators also use so-called date rape drugs, including rohypnol, gamma hydroxybutyrate (GHB), ketamine, and Ecstasy, to incapacitate their victims. To avoid this risk, drink bottled beverages, watch bartenders mix your drink, and do not ever leave drinks unattended. For more on date rape drugs, see Chapter 12.

Male Rape

In about 5 percent of completed and attempted rapes in the United States, the victim is male. About 1 in 33 men reports being a victim of a completed or attempted rape in his lifetime.[27] Like women, men are reluctant to report that they have been raped. They may feel embarrassed or ashamed, or they may not want to believe they have been raped. Law enforcement personnel, medical personnel, and social service agencies may be less supportive of male rape victims than of female rape victims because of similar misperceptions and misinformation.[27] The law is clear, however, on defining forced penetration as rape or sodomy. Male rape victims require the same level of medical treatment, counseling, and support as female victims.

Effects of Rape

Rape is a crime about dominance, power, and control, not about sex. Victims are intimidated and made to feel helpless. For many victims, the effects of rape can be profoundly traumatic and long lasting. Physical injuries usually heal quickly, but psychological pain can endure. Victims often experience fear, anxiety, phobias, guilt, nightmares, depression, substance abuse, sleep disorders, sexual dysfunctions, and social withdrawal. They may develop rape-related post-traumatic stress disorder, experiencing flashbacks and impaired functioning. Between 4 and 30 percent of victims contract an STD from the rape, and many worry that they may have been infected with HIV.[28] Some state laws now mandate HIV testing of an alleged rapist if the victim requests it.

Many victims blame themselves for the rape, and our society tends to foster self-blame. Myths about rape include the false beliefs that women or men who are raped did something to provoke it, put themselves in dangerous situations and so deserved it, or could have fought off their attacker. The fact is that no matter what a person does, nobody ever has the right to rape.

What to Do if You Are Raped

If you are raped, you may or may not be able to fight back. There is not a way to respond that works in all cases, and authorities recommend that you do whatever you need to do and can do to survive. It may be yelling, screaming, kicking, and fighting; it may be threatening to call the police; or it may be appeasing the perpetrator by going along. No matter how you respond, remember that your attacker is violating your rights and committing a crime; rape is not your fault.

After the rape, seek help as soon as you can. If you choose to call the police, there is a better chance that the perpetrator will be brought to justice and will be prevented from raping others. To preserve evidence, do not shower, change your clothes, or clean or straighten the crime scene.[28] You may want to write down everything you can remember about the attack, because memory is diminished during and after traumatic events. Include what the assailant looked like, what he said, his language and use of slang, the kind of sexual activities he wanted, and any threats or weapons he used. Writing this down can help you regain your sense of control, in addition to helping the police find and arrest the attacker.[28]

When the police arrive, tell them exactly what happened, being straightforward and truthful. Most likely they will take you to the hospital, where you will be given a rape exam. A physician may prescribe antibiotics and antiviral medications to decrease your chance of contracting an STD and hormonal medications to prevent pregnancy. In some communities, police departments have sexual assault response teams consisting of law enforcement officers, legal advocates, and medical personnel to help you.

Rape counseling is critical to your recovery from the attack. Talking about the rape, either one-on-one with a rape counselor or in a rape survivors' support group, can help you come to terms with your reactions and feelings. Rape crisis hotlines are available when you need immediate help. One such hotline is the Rape, Abuse, Incest National Network hotline at (800) 656-HOPE. It takes time to recover from rape, so be patient and take care of yourself.

Obtaining immediate attention from a health care professional and reporting the crime are the first steps to take after a rape. For many victims the process of recovery, which may take years, is aided by professional counseling.

Child Sexual Abuse

Any interaction between a child and an adult or an older child for the sexual gratification of the perpetrator is defined as **child sexual abuse.** This definition includes intercourse, fondling, and viewing or taking pornographic pictures. Rates of child sexual abuse are difficult to verify because many cases go unreported. The most frequently abused children are age 9 to 11.[29] Girls are sexually abused three times as often as boys.[5] The abuse is usually committed by a family member or other person known to the family. **Incest,** sexual activity between family members, is a particularly traumatic form of child sexual abuse because of the profound betrayal of trust involved.

Victims of sexual abuse usually suffer long-term effects, including anxiety, depression, post-traumatic stress disorder, and sexual dysfunctions. The seriousness of these problems is influenced by the frequency of abuse, the kind of sexual abuse, the child's age when the abuse began, the child's relationship with the abuser, the number of perpetrators, the victim's sex, and the perpetrator's sex. The most common form of child sexual abuse is abuse of a girl by her father, stepfather, brother, or uncle. Abuse of a boy by his mother is rare.[29]

Child sexual abusers may or may not be pedophiles. A pedophile is a person who is sexually attracted to and

KEY TERMS

child sexual abuse Any interaction between a child and an adult or an older child for the sexual gratification of the perpetrator.

incest Sexual activity between family members.

Challenges & Choices

Protecting Your Children From Online Predators

The following recommendations for parents may protect children from online pornography and sexual predators.

- Tell children they should never give their real name, phone number, address, or e-mail address to anyone on the Internet without a parent's permission.

- Keep computers with Internet access in a central area of the house where you can monitor what children are viewing. Find out who the children's online buddies are and check the computer's bookmarks to find out what Web sites children are accessing.

- Use the control functions provided by Internet services that allow parents to block content.

- Notify the police, FBI, or local customs service office if you believe your child is being exploited.

- Keep your credit cards away from your children. To enter pornography sites, a person must usually key in a valid card number.

- For more information, visit the Web site of the Center for Missing and Exploited Children, www.missingkids.org.

It's Not Just Personal . . .

In its *Highlights of the Youth Internet Safety Survey,* the U.S. Department of Justice reports that one in five children aged 10 to 17 receive unwanted sexual solicitations while they are online.

Source: Adapted from *Family Violence: Legal, Medical, and Social Perspective,* by H. Wallace, 2002, Boston: Allyn & Bacon.

aroused by children. Pedophiles often claim to "love" children and seek opportunities to be around them. Individuals who abuse or molest children who are not pedophiles are more likely to be opportunists with psychological problems and poor impulse control. Many such individuals spend little time around children, interact with them only sexually, and often dislike them.[30] They are commonly described as predatory, antisocial, and exploitative.

As described in Chapter 15, pedophiles have found a community on the Internet, where they share stories in chat rooms and clubs and buy and sell child pornography (see the box "Protecting Your Children From Online Predators"). A 2000 federal law requires Internet Service Providers such as AOL and Yahoo to report violations of child pornography laws to federal law enforcement authorities. The National Center for Missing and Exploited Children (NCMEC) acts as a clearinghouse for tips about sexual exploitation, which it distributes to law enforcement agencies. The FBI has also created the Innocent Images Task Force to hunt down online sex offenders. Such measures may slow down pedophiles and sex offenders but do little to deter the child abuser in the family.

If you know of a situation that may involve child sexual abuse, do not ignore it. Seek advice from someone you trust at your student health center or mental health clinic. Most abusers were abused themselves as children, although most children who are abused do not grow up to be abusers. The cycle of abuse can be broken. If you were sexually abused as a child and have not told anyone, getting counseling as soon as possible is imperative. Dealing with abuse is the only way to overcome the past and move on with your life.

Sexual Harassment

Sexual harassment includes two broad types of behavior or situations:

- A person in a position of authority, such as an employer or a teacher, offers benefits for sexual favors or threatens retaliation for the withholding of sex.

- Suggestive language or intimidating conduct creates a hostile atmosphere that interferes with a person's work or academic performance.

For example, a manager may seek sexual favors from an employee under the threat of job loss or demotion, or a professor may give a lower grade to a student who rejects his advances. A hostile environment can be created by visual images (for example, sexually explicit photos); language (for example, jokes, derogatory comments, obscene e-mails); or behavior (for example, inappropriate touching). Of all sexual harassment claims, 95 percent result from actions that create a hostile environment.[31]

Educational institutions that receive federal money are required to establish policies and grievance procedures for sexual harassment to ensure that complaints are properly investigated and corrective measures taken. If they fail to comply, they can lose their federal funds and be sued by the harassed person. Under federal regulations, colleges and universities are liable for sexual harassment perpetrated by their faculty or staff, regardless of whether the advance is accepted or rejected.

If you have experienced sexual harassment, keep a written record of all incidents of harassment, including the date, time, place, people involved, words or actions, and any witnesses. If you can, speak up and tell your harasser that the behavior is unacceptable to you. If you do not feel comfortable confronting the harasser in person, consider doing so by letter. If confrontation does not change the harasser's behavior, complain to a manager or supervisor. If that person does not respond properly to your complaint, consider using your organization's internal grievance procedures. Legal remedies are also available to you through your state Human Rights Commission and the federal Equal Employment Opportunity Commission. The threat of a lawsuit may end the harassment, but if it doesn't, don't give up. People who sexually harass others are sexual predators who will continue their unacceptable behavior until stopped.

Stalking and Cyberstalking

Another form of potentially dangerous conduct is **stalking,** in which a person repeatedly and maliciously follows, harasses, or threatens another person. Women are four times as likely as men to be victims of stalking; it is estimated that 1 in 12 women and 1 in 8 college women have been stalked. Four out of five victims know their stalker, who is often a former partner or boyfriend who wants to control or intimidate the victim.[32] In some cases, however, the stalker is a stranger or an acquaintance who has become obsessed with the victim and may have delusional beliefs about their relationship.[33]

The harassment typically includes surveillance at work, school, or home; frequent disturbing telephone calls; vandalism of the target's property; physical encounters; and attempts to get the victim's family and friends to aid the stalker. Targets of stalkers live in constant fear. They may be forced to change their lives significantly to avoid the stalker. If someone is stalking you, tell your family, friends, and coworkers so they do not unwittingly divulge information about you.

Many states have passed laws to protect individuals who are being stalked, but in some cases it is difficult to arrest and prosecute stalkers without violating their rights, such as the right to be present in a public place. If you plan to report a stalker to the police, keep a written record of all stalking incidents. Include dates, times, locations, witnesses, and types of incidents (personal encounters, telephone calls, e-mails). Some law enforcement departments and social service agencies provide forms for recording this information.

A variation on stalking is **cyberstalking,** the use of electronic media to pursue, harass, or contact another person who has not solicited the contact.[34] Online stalkers may send threatening, harassing, sexually provocative, or other unwanted e-mails to the target, or attack or impersonate the person on bulletin boards or in chat rooms. Laws against cyberstalking are in place in some states, but prosecution is hampered by Internet

protocols that preserve anonymity as well as by constitutional protection of free speech rights. If you are experiencing this kind of harassment, you can contact the stalker's Internet Service Provider (ISP) and complain about their client; they will often take action to try to stop the conduct. For more details on how to protect yourself from stalking and cyberstalking, see the box "Tips on Handling a Stalker."

FAMILY AND INTIMATE PARTNER VIOLENCE

All of us want to have loved ones we can count on to protect us from harm and a home where we feel safe. Unfortunately, this is not the case for millions of people in the United States. Violence in families can be directed at any family member, but women, children, and older adults are the most vulnerable. A *family* is defined by the U.S. Census Bureau as a group consisting of two or more persons related by marriage, birth, or adoption and living together in a household.[5] Because this usage excludes dating or cohabiting partners, gay and lesbian partners, and divorced partners, the Census Bureau also uses the term *intimate partners,* which includes all these relationships as well as married partners. Violence between intimate partners is called **intimate partner violence** or **domestic violence.**

Family Violence

Family violence is a broad term that includes several forms of violence and abuse. In this section we consider child abuse, elder abuse, and abuse of persons with disabilities.

KEY TERMS

sexual harassment   Behavior in which a person in authority offers benefits for sexual favors or threatens retaliation if sexual favors are withheld, or sexually oriented behavior that creates an intimidating or hostile environment that interferes with a person's work or academic performance.

stalking   Malicious following, harassing, or threatening of one person by another.

cyberstalking   Use of electronic media to pursue, harass, or contact another person who has not solicited the contact.

intimate partner violence or **domestic violence** Violence between two partners in an intimate relationship.

Challenges & Choices

Tips on Handling a Stalker

The National Center for Victims of Crime provides the following practical tips for dealing with a stalker.

- If you feel you are in imminent danger, go immediately to a safe place such as a police station, the home of a friend, or a domestic violence shelter; at a minimum, go to a public place where you will be near other people.

- If you know your stalker, consider getting a restraining order.

- Ask the local prosecutor's office whether your state or municipality has stalking laws that apply to your situation.

- Notify police if the stalker commits illegal acts such as entering your residence without permission or destroying your property.

- Document all evidence of stalking. Take photos of any injuries or vandalized property, save answering machine tapes with stalking messages, and keep a detailed written log.

- Develop a plan for escape from your home.

- Improve your home security (for example, install solid doors with dead bolts; trim bushes around windows).

- Consider getting assistance from domestic violence shelters, rape crisis counselors or programs, and victim-assistance coordinators in the prosecutor's office.

To protect yourself from cyberstalking, follow these guidelines:

- Create a gender-neutral, unprovocative e-mail address. This address should not reveal your general geographic area or your whole name.

- Use the software offered by chat rooms or similar forums to remove any personal information from your profile.

- Avoid attaching an e-mail signature to all your outgoing mail; you may be providing information you do not want revealed to some people.

- Use your e-mail software to turn off the header on your e-mail, since it may contain identifying features such as your name and e-mail address.

- When posting information to newsgroups, use a third-party e-mail site such as Yahoo or Hotmail or an anonymous e-mail service that strips out the identity information of the original sender.

It's Not Just Personal . . .

Australia, India, the United Kingdom, and at least 45 states in the United States have laws against cyberstalking. In many other countries, cyberstalking can be prosecuted under laws against stalking and criminal harassment.

Sources: National Center for Victims of Crime, www.ncvc.org; Cyberstalking: Risk Management, www.crimelibrary.com.

Child Abuse

Maltreatment of a child, or **child abuse,** includes physical abuse, sexual abuse, emotional abuse, and neglect. It occurs in all cultural, ethnic, and socioeconomic groups, with the highest rates of abuse occurring among the poorest children and among those who are disabled.[29] In 2002 an estimated 1,500 children died from injuries caused by abuse or neglect.[35] The highest number of victims are among newborns and infants, who are the most fragile, followed by teenagers.

Abusive parents often lack the emotional resources to cope with the stress of child rearing; they may not be knowledgeable about normal child development and have unrealistic expectations of their children. Some may have been abused themselves as children. Social conditions like unemployment, poverty, and isolation can be contributing factors, as well as alcohol or drug abuse. When a case of child abuse comes to light, the abusive parent or guardian is usually removed from the home to keep the child safe. Therapy typically focuses on the abuser but includes all family members.

Elder Abuse

Maltreatment of an older adult, or **elder abuse,** can include physical abuse (slapping, bruising); sexual abuse; emotional abuse (humiliating, threatening, intimidating); financial abuse (illegal or improper exploitation of funds); and neglect (abandonment, denial of food or health-related services). The legal determination of whether these actions constitute abuse varies from state to state and depends on their frequency, duration, and intensity. Inconsistent definitions have made it difficult to obtain accurate incidence data,[29] but estimates are that 4 percent to 10 percent of people age 65 and older are abused in the United States.[5]

The abuser is usually a family member, often an adult child, who is taking care of an aging parent or other elderly

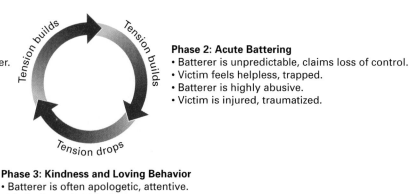

Phase 1: Tension Building
• Victim is compliant, tries to please batterer.
• Batterer experiences increased tension.
• Victim denies anger, minimizes threats.
• Batterer takes more control.
• Victim withdraws.
• Tension becomes unbearable.

Phase 2: Acute Battering
• Batterer is unpredictable, claims loss of control.
• Victim feels helpless, trapped.
• Batterer is highly abusive.
• Victim is injured, traumatized.

Phase 3: Kindness and Loving Behavior
• Batterer is often apologetic, attentive.
• Victim has mixed feelings.
• Batterer is manipulative.
• Victim feels guilty and responsible.
• Batterer promises change.
• Victim considers reconciliation.

Figure 17.3   Cycle of domestic violence. Source: Adapted from Understanding Abuse, Gay Partner Abuse Project, www.gaypartnerabuseproject.org.

relative. Abuse is more likely when the older person is frail, disabled, or impaired, such as by Alzheimer's disease or a physical ailment. It is also more likely when the abuser has substance abuse problems, has a mental illness, or is financially dependent on the older person.[5] Social isolation of the family and lack of community resources also contribute. Research suggests that daughters are more likely to be abusive through neglect than through physical abuse; they are also more likely than sons to be caring for parents who have severe health problems.[29]

Interventions for elder abuse include counseling and support groups for caregivers; battered women's services tailored to the needs of older women; family counseling that attempts to improve relationships within the family; and community services such as Meals-on-Wheels, home health programs, and elder day care.

Violence Against Persons With Disabilities

Children and adults with disabilities are especially vulnerable to abuse by family members; research indicates that they are abused five times more often than those who are not disabled.[29] Because disabled persons often depend on others to report abuse, their abusers are less likely than others to be prosecuted and convicted. One intervention strategy to prevent this form of abuse is to include personal safety training in programs for disabled individuals. When this approach is not feasible, strategies focus on making reporting laws more stringent, improving services to families with a disabled family member, and, where abuse occurs in institutional settings, improving the screening and hiring of staff.[29]

Intimate Partner Violence

Intimate partner violence, or domestic violence, is defined as abuse by a person against his or her partner in an intimate relationship. This definition includes the inten-

tional use of fear and humiliation to control another person. The vast majority of domestic violence victims—95 percent to 98 percent—are women. In 2000, half a million women were victims of nonfatal violence by their intimate partners, and 1,247 women were killed by their intimate partner in 2001.[36] The American Medical Association has stated that the home is more dangerous to women than city streets.[37]

Cycle of Abuse

Domestic violence is usually characterized by a cycle of abuse, a recurring pattern of escalating violence in an intimate relationship. This pattern can occur in any relationship, including gay male and lesbian partnerships. If the couple is heterosexual, it is sometimes referred to as **battered woman syndrome.** Typically, tension builds up in the relationship until there is a violent outburst, followed by a "honeymoon" period in which the abuser is contrite, ashamed, apologetic, and nonviolent.[29] Often he begs his partner to forgive him and promises it will never happen again. Unless the abuser gets help, however, the violence does recur and the cycle repeats itself, almost always becoming more severe (Figure 17.3). Research

KEY TERMS

child abuse   Maltreatment of a child; can be physical, sexual, or emotional abuse or neglect.

elder abuse   Maltreatment of an older adult; can be physical, sexual, emotional, or financial abuse or neglect.

battered woman syndrome   Cycle of abuse in an intimate relationship, characterized by escalating tension, a violent episode, and a period of lowered tension and nonviolence.

indicates that men who batter are more likely to abuse drugs and alcohol, suffer from mental illness, and have financial problems. They need help in dealing with the problems that cause them to act violently.

Most women who are battered eventually leave their abusive relationships, but they may make several attempts before they succeed. Battered women's shelters provide a safe haven where the woman and her children cannot be found by the abuser. They provide housing, food, and resources to help the woman start a new life. When shelters aren't available, private homes are sometimes available as safe houses, and churches, community centers, and YWCAs may also offer temporary facilities.[29]

A variety of factors can make it more difficult for some women to receive protection from domestic violence. In rural areas, women often have little or no access to shelters, safe homes, or social service agencies. Older women may be less able to access help, either because of physical impairment or generational attitudes; they may also be subjected to both partner battering and elder abuse. Cultural factors, ethnic traditions, and racism may hinder a woman's ability to obtain help. Women who are not citizens may fear being turned over to the Immigration and Naturalization Service and deported. Men in abusive relationships may also have difficulty finding support, because fewer services are available for men. Lesbians and gay men, similarly, may have limited access to appropriate support.[29]

Dating Violence

Dating violence is widespread. Researchers estimate that 1 in 10 high school students and 2 in 10 college students have been physically abused in dating relationships.[38] The Centers for Disease Control and Prevention (CDC) reported that almost 9 percent of high school students said they were hit, slapped, or hurt on purpose by their boyfriend or girlfriend in 2003, and 9 percent were physically forced to have sexual intercourse against their will.[11]

Some studies suggest that males and females inflict and receive dating violence in equal proportion, but women inflicting violence are usually defending themselves. Other studies find that twice as many women as men are victims of dating violence and that women are more likely to be physically injured. Studies show that individuals at risk for dating violence are more likely than others to have been sexually assaulted, to have peers who have been sexually victimized, and to accept dating violence. Perpetrators are more likely than others to abuse alcohol or drugs, to have adversarial attitudes toward others, to have sexually aggressive peers, and to accept dating violence.[39]

The FBI reports that 20 percent of female homicide victims are 14 to 18 years old.[23] Most killings occur in dating relationships dominated by control and physical abuse. Despite the seriousness of dating violence, young girls face more barriers in finding help than adult women

do. Many states require a parent's or guardian's permission before granting a protective order to a minor, and community shelters and counseling programs often require an adult's permission before admitting a minor. Families, schools, and communities need to work together to educate young people about what behavior is acceptable and unacceptable in a relationship.

Unhealthy relationships with the potential for abuse often involve power and control issues. One partner may make all the significant decisions, set numerous rules, restrict his or her partner's visits to friends and family, monitor phone calls and e-mails, control the couple's money, and be obsessed with what the partner is doing at all times. The abusive person may embarrass his or her partner in front of others and use derogatory names for the partner. Other signs of an unhealthy relationship are excessive jealousy, intimidation, and explosive anger. If you recognize any of these signs in your relationships, you may want to consider getting help to deal with these issues or ending the relationship.[29]

Resources for Survivors of Intimate Partner Violence

If you are concerned that someone you know may be in an abusive relationship, try talking to the person about the nature of the relationship and giving him or her information about resources available in your community. Encourage the person to maintain contact with friends and family members while getting support to leave the relationship and begin building a new life.[29]

Women who decide to leave abusive relationships may be overwhelmed by the prospect of finding another place to live, supporting themselves and their children, and changing their lifestyle. They need to assess their options for financial support, employment, health care, housing, and education. Help is available from social service agencies, educational programs, hotlines, shelters, advocacy organizations, and informational books and packets provided by national, state, and local organizations.

WORKPLACE VIOLENCE, HATE CRIME, AND TERRORISM

Violence can occur where there are high levels of stress, where there is bias, and where there is perceived injustice. In most cases, however, multiple risk factors are present; very often, the perpetrator of violence is psychologically disturbed.

Violence in the Workplace

Workplace violence is defined as violent acts, including physical assault and threats of assault, directed toward persons at work or on duty. It can include threatening or aggressive behavior, verbal abuse, intimidation, or harassment. It can be committed by strangers, customers or clients, coworkers, or people with personal relationships with workers. People in some occupations are at higher risk of experiencing workplace violence. Workers with the most dangerous jobs are police officers, followed by security guards, taxi drivers, prison guards, bartenders, mental health professionals, convenience and liquor store clerks, and schoolteachers.[40]

The National Institute for Occupational Safety and Health estimates that about 20 workers are murdered and 18,000 are assaulted each week while at work.[23] Employers can take measures to lower the risk of workplace violence, such as careful pre-employment screening, appropriate security measures in the workplace, the establishment of procedures for resolving disputes, awareness training for employees and management, and employee assistance programs that provide counseling for employees experiencing psychological problems or high levels of stress. Individuals can also be alert to warning signs of possible violence by others in the workplace, such as extreme changes in behavior, outbursts, conflicts with others, or bringing a weapon to work.

Hate Crime

A **hate crime** is defined as a crime motivated by bias against the victim's ethnicity, race, religion, sexual orientation, or disability.[4] Hate crimes tend to be excessively brutal, are frequently inflicted at random on people the perpetrators do not know, and are often committed by multiple perpetrators.[41]

In 2003 nearly 7,500 hate crimes were reported in the United States, involving 9,100 victims and 6,900 offenders. More than half of these crimes were committed because of the offender's racial bias (primarily anti-black);

Hate crimes are prohibited on many college campuses, in many states, and by the federal government. Characterized by bias against a particular group, this type of violence is often brutal and random.

18 percent were committed because of the offender's religious bias (primarily anti-Jewish); 16 percent because of the offender's sexual orientation bias (primarily anti-gay men); 14 percent because of the offender's ethnic or national origin bias (primarily anti-Hispanic); and less than 0.5 percent because of the offender's bias against persons with physical or mental disabilities.[4]

Most states have hate crime laws in place, as does the federal government. Many colleges and universities have policies prohibiting hate crimes and harassment of individuals in targeted groups, as well as programs that promote cultural knowledge and diversity.[42] Because hate crimes against lesbian, gay, bisexual, and transgendered (LGBT) persons have increased on campuses in recent years,[43,44] many colleges and universities have specific policies forbidding violence directed toward LGBT students. Many colleges have hotlines for reporting hate crimes; there are also local, state, and federal hotlines for getting information about and reporting hate crimes.

Terrorism

Terrorism is a form of violence directed against persons or property, including civilian populations, for the purpose of instilling fear and engendering a sense of helplessness. Often, terrorist acts are committed in supposed furtherance of political or social aims. Internationally, terrorist acts include kidnappings, murders, and bombings of churches, mosques, nightclubs, buses, and city streets. In the United States, such acts have included the 1993 bombing of the World Trade Center in New York City, the 1995 bombing of the Federal Building in Oklahoma City, and the September 11, 2001, attacks on the World Trade Center and the Pentagon in Washington, D.C.

Since the September 11, 2001, attacks, psychologists have established that people's deepest fears involve uncontrollable catastrophic events that are likely to affect future generations. Americans most fear the use of weapons of mass destruction—nuclear, chemical, and biological weapons—that could cause massive casualties.[45] In response to the September 11 attacks, the U.S. government created the Department of Homeland Security to prevent and guard against future attacks and the Homeland

KEY TERMS

hate crime Crime motivated by bias against the victim's ethnicity, race, religion, sexual orientation, or disability.

terrorism Violence directed against persons or property, including civilian populations, for the purpose of instilling fear and engendering a sense of helplessness.

Challenges & Choices

Protecting Yourself From Violence

In Your House or Apartment

- Keep doors and windows locked, even when you are at home.
- Before you open your door, make sure the caller is legitimate. If you are expecting a repairman, insist on proper identification. If the person wants to use your phone, offer to make the call for him or her but do not let the person inside. If your door does not have a peephole, consider getting one installed.
- If you have children, tell them not to open the door to strangers.
- If you are a woman living alone, use only your initials on your mailbox and in telephone directories.
- If you live in an apartment building, avoid being alone in the laundry room or garage, especially late at night.

On Campus and in Public Places

- Be aware of your surroundings; avoid walking through secluded areas and high-crime neighborhoods.
- Avoid listening to music on headphones; it reduces your attention to warning signs that may be occurring around you.
- Stay with others when possible; groups of three or more are rarely attacked.
- Act and walk in a confident manner. Most assaults occur because the assailant perceives an opportunity to attack someone who appears vulnerable.
- Walk close to the curb, facing oncoming traffic. You will be less vulnerable to attacks from people in cars or hiding in doorways, alleys, or bushes.

- When carrying packages or luggage, try to keep one arm free.
- Hold your purse firmly under your arm with the carrying strap over your opposite shoulder. Avoid carrying a wallet in a hip pocket, or transfer money and credit cards to a front pocket.
- When you are in any public place, do not display large amounts of cash. Be alert when using an ATM.
- Rely on your instincts. If you think you are being followed, walk quickly to a lighted area. If you feel that you are in immediate danger, scream and run.
- Encourage older and disabled persons to use community transportation services.
- If you jog, do so with a partner. Vary your route and the time you run; and if you run at night, be sure the area is well lighted. Don't wear headphones while jogging.
- Consider taking a class in self-defense.

It's Not Just Personal . . .

Whereas young people are most likely to be victims of violent crime, people over 65 are most likely to be victims of property crime (burglary, auto theft, property theft). Ninety percent of crimes committed against older adults are property crimes, compared with 40 percent of crimes committed against people aged 12 to 24.

Source: Adapted from *Safety: A Personal Focus* (pp. 178–180), by D. L. Bever, 1996, New York: McGraw-Hill.

Security Advisory System, a color-coded warning system, to alert citizens of the likelihood of attack.

In addition, the Federal Emergency Management Agency (FEMA) published a booklet called *Are You Ready? An In-Depth Guide to Citizen Preparedness* that provides guidelines in the event of any kind of disaster, including terrorist attack. The booklet explains how people can become informed about local emergency plans, how they can develop an emergency communication plan, and what they should do before, during, and after a disaster. The publication also describes what to include in a disaster supplies kit, including water, food, tools, and first-aid supplies. Instructions for obtaining free copies of the booklet are available at the FEMA Web site (www.fema.gov).

PREVENTING VIOLENCE

Although protecting yourself from terrorism is difficult, there are ways you can limit your risks in life; for strategies and tips, see the boxes "Protecting Yourself From Violence" and "Preventing Identity Theft." At the same time, self-protection measures must be part of a more comprehensive approach that addresses violence at the societal level.

Consumer Clipboard

Preventing Identity Theft

Have you ever been a victim of identity theft? If someone has possessed or used your name, address, Social Security number (SSN), bank or credit card account number, or other identifying information without your knowledge with the intent to commit fraud or other crimes, the answer is *yes*.

How does identity theft occur? Thieves obtain information from businesses or institutions by stealing records, conning or bribing employees, or hacking into computers. They can use "skimming" devices to steal credit and debit account numbers as your card is being processed. Low-tech approaches include rummaging through your trash, stealing wallets and purses, stealing mail, or stealing personal information from your home. In some cases identity thieves obtain the information directly from you—by luring you into a scam or by posing as a legitimate business person or government official.

What are some of the results of identity theft? Someone who steals your account numbers can buy big-ticket items, such as computers, and quickly resell them. They can take out an auto loan or establish phone or wireless service in your name. They can drain your current bank account or open a new one in your name. They can file for bankruptcy under your name or give your name to the police during an arrest.

How can you protect yourself against identity theft? Here are some tips to minimize your chance of being a victim of identity theft:

- Don't give out personal information on the phone, via mail, or over the Internet unless you've initiated the contact or know for sure who you're dealing with.
- Don't carry your SSN number with you; instead, keep it in a secure place. Give your SSN only when absolutely necessary.
- Protect all personal information in your home and at work.

- Deposit all mail in post office boxes or at your local post office.
- Guard your trash by shredding all billing, medical, and business documents.
- Carry only the ID information and credit and debit cards that you really need.
- Choose passwords for your credit card, bank, and phone accounts with care. Don't use your mother's maiden name, your birth date, the last 4 digits of your SSN, your phone number, or a series of consecutive numbers.
- Pay attention to your billing cycles. A missing bill could mean that someone has taken over your account.
- Watch out for promotional scams in the form of phony offers.
- Keep your computer secure with a firewall, virus-protection software, and password protection for key files. Before disposing of a computer, remove all data with a "wipe" utility program.

What are the first steps to take if you're a victim of identity theft?

- For financial account information, such as credit card or bank accounts, close those accounts immediately.
- For SSNs, call the toll-free fraud number of any of the three major credit bureaus, and place an initial fraud alert on your credit reports. Review those credit reports.
- For driver's license or other ID documents, contact the issuing agency about placing fraud flags.
- File a report with your local police. Get a copy of the police report.
- File a complaint with the Federal Trade Commission so that this information can be added to its database.

Source: Data from Federal Trade Commission. www.consumer.gov/idtheft.

Current efforts to curb violence focus primarily on arresting and imprisoning offenders. Strategies are also needed that prevent violence before it occurs—that is, interventions that change the social conditions underlying violence. In this section we briefly consider three areas in which measures might be taken to reduce or prevent violence.

The Role of Guns: Facilitating Violence

As noted earlier, firearms, especially handguns, play a large role in the high death rate associated with crime in the United States. Guns contribute to the lethality of any incident involving violence.

Gun control is a controversial issue in the United States. The Second Amendment to the U.S. Constitution protects the right of citizens to "keep and bear arms," a right that was important in colonial times but that may not be as important today. The gun industry, along with its powerful lobby and many clubs, organizations, and individual enthusiasts, defends the right of Americans to own guns with minimal restrictions. Some laws are in place regulating gun sales, such as computerized background checks on persons seeking to buy guns, aimed at screening out convicted felons and certain other groups. Proponents of gun control support these and other measures, including waiting periods for gun purchases, licensing of guns, and restrictions on access to guns by young people.[46] Proponents of gun control also support the design of safer guns, such as guns with trigger locks, but gun manufacturers point out that gun owners frequently do not use the locks, and the U.S. Congress concluded that locks were effective only with children younger than 6.[47]

The gun industry has come under fire in recent years for its marketing practices, which include targeting women, children, and minorities. The marketing campaign aimed at women focuses on three themes—empowerment, protection, and participation in shooting sports.[48] Playing on women's fears of rape, gun-wielding assailants, and terrorist acts, these campaigns encourage women to buy guns despite statistics showing that guns in the home are much more likely to kill a family member than a stranger.[49]

The gun industry has also used a variety of strategies to cultivate children as gun enthusiasts, including advertising in youth magazines, financing shooting ranges, providing gun training programs for schools, and manufacturing smaller firearms for children. The huge number of video games that involve shooting also stimulate children's interest in guns. The gun industry can be expected to increase its marketing to ethnic minorities as well. Rates of gun ownership by African Americans and Hispanics is considerably lower than that by whites, even though death rates from firearms are higher.[48] The complex issues surrounding the manufacture, sale, and ownership of guns are likely to be part of our national debate for some time to come.

The Role of Media and Entertainment: Glorifying Violence

Killing, maiming, torture, and rape are all part of the fare served up by the media and entertainment industries in U.S. society. Violent acts occur much more frequently in movies and television shows than they do in real life.[50] Exposure to such images may lead to increased fearfulness, depression, and pessimism, particularly in children.[51] Repeated exposure to violence may also lead to habituation and **desensitization,** a raised threshold for

reaction to violence and a loss of compassion. Repeated exposure to graphic images of violence also feed the appetite for more intense violence.[51]

The American Academy of Pediatrics (AAP) and five other prominent medical groups concluded in 2000 that there is a connection between violence in mass media and increases in both acceptance of aggressive attitudes and aggressive behavior in children.[52] Reports from the National Academy of Sciences and the CDC have supported these conclusions.[53] The entertainment industry maintains that these studies demonstrate only possible associations between media violence and aggression. Media defenders warn that attempts at regulation would border on censorship.

In response to this information, communities have organized boycotts of products of companies that sponsor violent and sexually explicit programs. Parents are using blocking technologies to keep their children from seeing selected television programs and Internet sites. The entertainment industry has started to regulate itself, primarily to avoid government regulation.[54] The video rental industry, for example, has introduced a "Pledge to Parents," promising that movies rated R (restricted) and video games rated M (mature) will not be rented to children under age 17, and the National Association of Theater Owners has promised to enforce the movie ratings system vigorously.

Supporting Families and Communities

In a healthy society, families carry out a vital function: teaching children self-control. Individuals with high levels of self-control are less likely to engage in criminal acts than are those with less self-control. Families can also teach children constructive ways to deal with anger, frustration, and destructive impulses. When children show signs of delinquency, schools and communities can provide parental education and support. Positive family interventions emphasize consistent parenting, clear rules and appropriate consequences, supervision of children's activities, and constructive management of family conflicts. There is no evidence that nontraditional families with young or single parents are any less effective at instilling values in children than are traditional families.[55]

The health of individuals and families is supported by healthy communities. Common sense suggests that safe physical environments—those with well-lit streets, for example—are less conducive to criminal activity than run-down environments. Communities where neighbors

KEY TERMS

desensitization   Raised threshold of reaction to violence and a loss of compassion.

look out for one another, as with neighborhood watch programs, are less inviting to criminals. Communities also have to support social changes that enhance economic and social stability.[56] To bring about change, communities have used strategies such as the following:[57,58]

- Cleaning up trash and graffiti and fixing broken windows
- Providing organized leisure activities and mentoring programs for youth
- Encouraging parent involvement in school activities
- Supporting low-income housing to curb an exodus of middle-income residents of all races
- Maintaining municipal services

- Curtailing street-corner loitering, panhandling, prostitution, and public drinking
- Increasing police presence in high-risk areas

Individuals who want to take action against violence have a variety of options, from volunteering at women's shelters to supporting public policies that address the root causes of violence in our society. Keeping a sense of perspective about violence is important, however. Some observes have suggested that Americans live in a media-driven "culture of fear," frightened by overblown accounts of crime, drugs, and violence.[59] The key is to take media portrayals of violence with a grain of salt while using your common sense to keep yourself safe.

You Make the Call

Is Profiling Justified?

Profiling (or *racial profiling*) is the practice of targeting people by their race, ethnicity, or religion for questioning in police, immigration, airport security, or other types of security procedures. In the United States, African Americans, Hispanics, Asians, middle Europeans, Middle Easterners, and people of many other backgrounds are subjected to profiling in a variety of situations.[61] They may be stopped on the highway, followed by salespeople in stores, pulled out of line at airports, or asked for multiple sources of identification when making credit card purchases. In a typical scenario, a young African American male driver is pulled over by a police officer and asked for his driver's license and registration; sometimes he is asked to step out of the vehicle, or the vehicle is searched.

Since the terrorist attacks of September 11, 2001, airlines and airports have increased their profiling of people who appear to be of Middle Eastern descent or followers of the Muslim faith, a practice sometimes called *airline profiling*. Once targeted, such individuals are typically taken to secluded waiting areas where they are searched and subjected to intense interrogation. Numerous complaints have been filed by Americans who felt harassed and humiliated by such treatment, claiming that it violated their Fourth Amendment rights to protection against unreasonable search and seizure and their Fourteenth Amendment rights to due process and equal protection under the law. According to Amnesty International USA, approximately 32 million Americans have been victims of racial profiling; the practice affects men, women, and children of all age groups and socioeconomic backgrounds.

Profiling is generally considered a violation of human rights. In 2001 President Bush said that "racial profiling is

wrong," and in 2003 the U.S. Justice Department issued guidelines forbidding racial profiling by federal law enforcement officials. Some law enforcement agencies are providing training in multicultural competence and are recording interactions between officers and citizens to ensure that police treat those they stop in a professional manner.[64] Many states have laws banning racial profiling, but most do not ban profiling based on religion or religious appearance. A federal law called the End Racial Profiling Act of 2004 is pending in Congress; if enacted and funded, it would afford broad protection against profiling.

At the same time, however, the political climate, as represented by the passage of the USA Patriot Act without debate a few weeks after 9/11, is favorable to increased caution and surveillance. Supporters of such measures argue that the need for better intelligence about terrorist activities and protection against future attacks justifies activities that might be construed as infringing on civil liberties. They claim that airline profiling is a reasonable approach to improving security in an area that has been shown to be vulnerable. Justified security or violation of rights—what do you think?

Pros

- Airline profiling is a sensible, statistically based tool that focuses resources efficiently on crime and terrorism prevention. The main perpetrators of violent terrorist acts involving airplanes have been Islamic extremists, mostly young Arab men. It makes sense to target individuals who seem to fit this profile.

- Immigration, law enforcement, and airline security systems would be seriously remiss if they didn't use any and every means possible to prevent another 9/11.

- Insurance companies use risk profiles (age, accident history, sex, marital status) to determine insurance rates. The same principles can be used to predict the likelihood of terrorist acts by certain individuals.

Cons

- Profiling is a violation of human rights, civil rights, and U.S. constitutional rights. It also promotes prejudice against certain groups.

- Racial profiling fosters anger and undermines confidence in the criminal justice system, potentially reducing its effectiveness.[62] If citizens mistrust police testimony in criminal cases, undeserved acquittals and hung juries may result.[63]

- Profiling distracts law enforcement officers from paying attention to suspicious behavior, which is the key indicator of a potential terrorist. After the 1995 bombing of the federal building in Oklahoma City, for example, bomber Timothy McVeigh was able to flee the scene because officers were looking for "Arab terrorists." It is more effective to focus on when and how passengers bought their tickets, how they are acting, and where their luggage is located.

- "Smart profiling" is more effective than racial profiling. Airlines can run names through their databases to identify high-risk passengers and screen them thoroughly.

OLC Web site For more information about this topic, visit the Online Learning Center at www.mhhe.com/teague1e.

SOURCES: Report on Racial Profiling, Amnesty International USA, www.amnestyusa.org/racial_profiling/report; *Driving While Black*, by K. Meeks, 2000, New York: Broadway Books; *Profiles in Justice*, by D. A. Harris, 2002, New York: The New Press; *A Resource Guide on Racial Profiling Data Collection Systems: Promises and Practices Learned*, U.S. Department of Justice, 2000, NCJ 184768; "Blind Spot," by R. Kennedy, 2002, *Atlantic Monthly, 289* (4), p. 24.

SUMMARY

- Violence is the use of force or the threat of force to inflict intentional injury, physical or psychological, on oneself or another person. Violent crimes include homicide, assault, rape, and robbery, among others.

- Rates of violent crime in the United States are comparable to those in other countries except homicide rates, which are much higher. Experts attribute this difference to the ready availability of firearms in the United States.

- The typical offender in violent crime is a male aged 15–24. Members of minority groups are more likely to be victims of violent crime as well as offenders. Living in a large city and living in the South or West also increase the likelihood of experiencing violence. Violence is more common on college campuses than in the general population.

- Risk factors for violence, besides age, sex, minority status, and geographic location, can be thought of as occurring at the level of society and culture (for example, poverty, media violence), the family (for example, substance abuse), and the individual (for example, poor impulse control).

- Rates of both violent crime and property crime declined dramatically in the United States in the 1990s. A variety of explanations has been proposed, but more research is needed to determine exact causes.

- Homicide is the second leading cause of death among people aged 10–24 in the United States.

- School violence includes not just shootings by an angry or depressed student but physical fights, murders, suicides, and attacks on students and teachers. Many schools have responded with zero-tolerance policies regarding guns and weapons.

- Youth gangs are associations of adolescents and young adults organized to control a territory and conduct illegal activities. Many cities have model programs in place designed to deter young people from joining gangs and to prevent adult gang members from returning to criminal activity in the community when they are released from prison.

- Crime is prevalent on college campuses and has been addressed by increased security precautions, among other responses. Hazing by fraternities, sororities, athletic teams, and other organizations results in injuries and deaths every year. Colleges have been constrained in their restrictions of hate speech by First Amendment protections of free speech.

- Sexual assault includes forced sexual intercourse (rape), forced sodomy (oral or anal sexual acts), child molestation, incest, fondling, and attempts to commit any of these acts. Causes of sexual assault may include socialization of males to be controlling and to accept gender stereotypes, personality traits like irresponsibility, and situational factors.

- An estimated 20 percent to 25 percent of women are raped during their college years. In most rapes, the perpetrator is known to the victim. In most rapes, both the perpetrator and the victim have been consuming alcohol.

- Male rape is less common than female rape but equally traumatizing.

- Rape is a crime about dominance and control. The psychological effects can be severe and long lasting. There is no single right way to respond to a rape attempt. Medical treatment and counseling are needed after a rape.

- Child sexual abuse may be committed by a pedophile or by an opportunistic person with psychological problems. The effects of sexual abuse can be long lasting; survivors should receive counseling.

- Sexual harassment includes unwanted sexual advances by a person with authority over another or the creation of a hostile or intimidating environment through the use of sexual images, language, or behavior.

- Stalking includes surveillance at home or work, telephone calls, trespassing, and intimidating physical encounters by a person who is following or harassing another. Cyberstalking is the use of electronic media to harass, attack, or impersonate another.

- Women, children, and older adults are the most common targets of family violence. Child abuse includes physical, sexual, and emotional maltreatment, as well as neglect. Elder abuse includes physical, sexual, emotional, and financial maltreatment, as well as neglect. Children and adults with disabilities are especially vulnerable to abuse.

- Intimate partner violence, or domestic violence, includes physical violence as well as threats and humiliation. Ninety-five percent of victims are women. Abuse is often marked by a cycle of escalating tension and violence, followed by a period of remorse by the abuser. This pattern can occur in any intimate relationship.

Violence also occurs in 10 percent to 20 percent of dating relationships. Many organizations offer help for victims and survivors of domestic violence.

- Workplace violence can be perpetrated by strangers, clients or customers, coworkers, or individuals with personal relationships with workers. Employers need to take measures to create secure workplaces for their employees.

- Hate crimes are motivated by bias against a victim's race, ethnicity, religion, sexual orientation, or disability. They tend to be excessively brutal and inflicted on strangers by multiple perpetrators.

- Terrorism is a form of violence directed against persons or property for the purpose of instilling fear and engendering a sense of helplessness. People's deepest fears involve uncontrollable catastrophic events that are likely to affect future generations, such as the use of weapons of mass destruction.

- Individuals can take many steps to protect themselves against violence, including being aware of their surroundings and avoiding alcohol and drugs when they are in certain situations.

- Current societal efforts to curb violence focus mainly on arresting and imprisoning offenders. Prevention efforts also need to focus on changing the social conditions that underlie violence. Restricting access to guns and reducing the depiction of violence in the media are two controversial areas for future consideration. In the meantime, families and communities need to be supported in their efforts to prevent and reduce violence.

REVIEW QUESTIONS

1. What is the relationship between media depictions of violence and the occurrence of violent crime in U.S. society?

2. What is believed to account for the high rates of homicide in the United States?

3. Of the crimes considered violent crimes by the Justice Department and FBI, which occur most frequently? Which occur least frequently?

4. What proportion of victims know their assailants in homicides? In aggravated assaults?

5. What are the two most reliable risk factors for violence? What are several other risk factors?

6. What explanations have been offered for the decline in violent crime in the United States since 1994? How well does each explanation fit the facts?

7. What evidence is there that school violence has declined in recent years? Describe the measures that lawmakers and schools have taken to reduce violence. What other measures have been recommended?

8. Describe efforts that have been taken to reduce youth gang violence.

9. Describe legislative measures to reduce violent crime on college campuses.

10. What is the challenge posed to colleges by individuals distributing messages of hate?

11. What acts are included in the definition of sexual assault? What is the difference between sexual assault and sexual coercion?

12. What are some possible factors that lead men to commit sexual assault? Why are many rapes not reported to police?

13. What proportion of rapes are committed by strangers versus someone known to the victim?

14. What are some of the effects of rape?

15. What factors influence the effect child sexual abuse has on the victim?

16. What are some differences between pedophiles and opportunists who molest children?

17. What actions can a person take who is experiencing sexual harassment?

18. What steps can you take to protect yourself from a stalker? From a cyberstalker?

19. What is the difference between family violence and intimate partner violence? What factors contribute to child abuse? To elder abuse?

20. Describe the cycle of abuse. Why do you think individuals remain in abusive relationships once abuse has begun? What are some signs of unhealthy relationships?

21. What measures can employers take to reduce the likelihood of workplace violence?

22. What groups are most likely to be targeted in hate crimes?

23. What form of terrorism do people most fear?

24. Describe the controversies over gun control and media violence.

25. What are some strategies used by communities to reduce crime?

WEB RESOURCES

The Chronicle of Higher Education: This journal publishes annual statistics for crime on college campuses, such as which schools report the highest rates for alcohol, drug, and weapons arrests.
www.chron.com/stats/crime

Crisis Prevention Institute: This organization offers a program in nonviolent crisis intervention, teaching professionals how to deal with disruptive and violent behavior through behavior management.
www.crisisprevention.com

CyberAngels: This organization acts as a neighborhood watch for online safety. Its Web site features information on child pornography, cyberstalking, identity theft, and fraud.
www.cyberangels.org

National Center for Victims of Crime: This Web site offers information on the cycle of abuse, child abuse, rape, domestic violence, stalking, dating violence, and violence against women.
www.ncvc.org

National Coalition Against Domestic Violence: This organization offers information packets and guides about violence, including teen dating violence. It features a directory of domestic violence programs throughout the United States.
www.ncadv.org

National Organization for Victim Assistance: Online publications of this organization cover topics such as crisis intervention, the psychological trauma of crime, supportive counseling, victim rights and services, and the Victims Movement.
www.trynova.org

National Sexual Violence Resource Center: This site operates as a collection and distribution center for information, statistics, and resources on sexual violence. Its publications include newsletters, a directory of projects working toward the end of sexual violence, and news releases.
www.nsvrc.org

Prevent Child Abuse America: This organization is dedicated to building awareness of child abuse and providing education on the abuse and neglect of children. Its publications include tips for parents, information for kids, newsletters, and fact sheets.
www.preventchildabuse.org

Rape, Abuse, and Incest National Network (RAINN): This site provides information about what to do if you or a friend is sexually assaulted, how to reduce your risk of sexual assault, and how to protect your child from sexual abuse. RAINN also offers A Parent's Guide to Internet Safety (FBI publication) and operates the free, confidential National Sexual Assault Hotline (1-800-656-HOPE).
www.rainn.org

REFERENCES

1. Rosenfeld, R. (2004, February). The case of the unsolved crime decline. *Scientific American.*

2. Bureau of Justice Statistics. (2004). Cross-national studies in crime and justice. NCJ 200988. www.ojp.usdoj.gov/bjs.

3. Lynch, J. (2002). Crime in international perspective. In J. Q. Wilson & J. Petersilia (Eds.), *Crime: Public policies for crime control* (pp. 5–42). San Francisco: ICS Press.

4. Federal Bureau of Investigation. (2003). Uniform Crime Reports, *Crime in the United States, 2003.* www.fbi.gov.

5. Barnett, O. W., Miller-Perrin, C. L., & Perrin, R. D. (2004). *Family violence across the lifespan: An introduction* (2nd ed.). Thousand Oaks, CA: Sage Publications.

6. Scott, B. G., & McLaughlin, K. (2002, January/February). Violence prevention—who's responsible? In "Closing the

Gap," *Newsletter of the Office of the Surgeon General.* Washington, DC: U.S. Department of Health and Human Services.

7. National Center for Victims of Crime. (2004). Crime & victimization in America: Statistical overview. www.ncvc.org.

8. Davis, G. G., & Muhlhausen, D. B. (2000). Young African-American males: Continuing victims of high homicide rates in urban communities. The Heritage Foundation. www.heritage.org/research/crime.

9. Greenwood, P. W. (2002). Juvenile crime and juvenile justice. In J. Q. Wilson & J. Petersilia (Eds.), *Crime: Public policies for crime control* (pp. 75–108). San Francisco: ICS Press.

10. Bureau of Justice Statistics, Crime and Victims Statistics. www.ojp.usdoj.gov/bjs.

11. Grunbaum, J., et al. (2004). Youth risk behavior surveillance—United States, 2003. *Morbidity Mortality Weekly Report 2004, 53* (No. SS-2). www.cdc.gov/mmwr/preview.

12. Nims, D. R. (2000). Violence in our schools: A national crisis. In D. S. Sandhu & C. B. Aspy (Eds.), *Violence in American schools*. Alexandria, VA: American Counseling Association.

13. Cauchan, D. (1999, July 13). Schools struggling to balance "zero tolerance," common sense. *USA Today,* 1A–2A.

14. Klein, M. W. (2002). Street gang cycles. In J. Q. Wilson & J. Petersilia (Eds.), *Crime: Public policies for crime control.* San Francisco: ICS Press.

15. Howell, J. C., & Decker, S. H. (1999). The youth gangs, drugs, and violence connection. Office of Juvenile Justice and Delinquency Prevention, *Juvenile Justice Bulletin.* www.ncjrs.org.

16. Smith, M. C., & Fossey, R. (1995). *Crime on campus.* Westport, CT: Oryx Press.

17. U.S. Department of Education. (2005). Summary, campus crime and security statistics. www.ed.gov.

18. Schuh, J. H. (1998). Campus vulnerability. In A. M. Hoffman, J. H. Schuh, & R. H. Fenske (Eds.), *Violence on campus: Defining the problems, strategies for action.* Gaithersburg, MD: Aspen Publishers.

19. Nuwer, H. (1999). *Wrongs of passage: Fraternities, sororities, hazing, and binge drinking.* Bloomington, IN: Indiana University Press.

20. Schuh, J. H. (1998). Matters of civility on campus. In A. M. Hoffman, J. H. Schuh, & R. H. Fenske (Eds.), *Violence on campus: Defining the problems, strategies for action.* Gaithersburg, MD: Aspen Publishers.

21. Interassociation Task Force of the Association for Student Judicial Affairs. (2003, December). National baseline study on campus sexual assault: Adjudicating sexual assault cases. http://asja.tamu.edu.

22. Fisher, B. S., Cullen, F. T., & Turner, M. G. (2000, December). The sexual victimization of college women. *National Institute of Justice Research Report.* Rockville, MD: National Criminal Justice Reference Center.

23. Bureau of Justice Statistics. National Crime Victimization Survey, 2003. Department of Justice. www.ojp.usdoj.gov/bjs.

24. Tjaden, P., & Thoennes, N. (2000). Full report of the prevalence, incidence, and consequences of violence against women: Findings from the National Violence Against Women Survey. Report NCJ 183781. Washington, DC: National Institute of Justice.

25. Acquaintance rape: A program of the National Center for Victims of Crime. www.ncvc.org.

26. Mohler-Kuo, M., Dowdall, G. W., Koss, M. P., & Wechsler, H. (2004). Correlates of rape while intoxicated in a national sample of college women. *Journal of Studies on Alcohol, 65* (1), 37–46.

27. Jacobson, N. (1997). *Male on male rape.* New York: Plenum Press.

28. Sexual assault. InfoLink. National Center for Victims of Crime. www.ncvc.org.

29. McGoldrick, M., Broken Nose, M. A., & Potenza, M. (1999). Violence and the family life cycle. In B. Carter & M. McGoldrick, *The expanded family life cycle: Individual, family, and social perspectives* (3rd ed.). Boston: Allyn & Bacon.

30. Wallace, H. (2002). *Family violence: Legal, medical, and social perspectives* (3rd ed.). Boston: Allyn & Bacon.

31. Keller, E. A. (2000). Consensual amorous relationships between faculty and students: The constitutional right to privacy. In E. Wall (Ed.), *Sexual harassment: Confrontations and decisions* (Rev. ed.). Amherst, NY: Prometheus Books.

32. Stalking. Fact Sheet. National Center for Victims of Crime. www.ncvc.org.

33. Morewitz, S. J. (2003). *Stalking and violence: New patterns of trauma and obsession.* New York: Kluwer Academic.

34. Cyberstalking: Risk management. www.crimelibrary.com.

35. Centers for Disease Control and Prevention, National Center for Injury Prevention and Control. (2004). Child maltreatment: Fact sheet. www.cdc.gov.

36. Intimate partner violence 1993–2001. (2003, February). Bureau of Justice Statistics Crime Data Brief (Publication No. NCJ 197838).

37. Berry, D. B. (2000). *The domestic violence sourcebook* (3rd ed.). New York: McGraw-Hill.

38. Bateman, P. (1998). The context of date rape. In B. Levy (Ed.), *Dating violence: Young women in danger.* Seattle, WA: Seal Press.

39. Gamache, D. (1998). Domination and control: The social context of dating violence. In B. Levy (Ed.), *Dating violence: Young women in danger.* Seattle, WA: Seal Press.

40. Occupational Safety and Health Administration. Workplace violence: Awareness and prevention. www.osha.gov.

41. Perry, B. (2001). *In the name of hate: Understanding hate crimes.* New York: Routledge.

42. Fenske, R. H., & Gordon, L. (1998). Reducing race and ethnic hate crimes on campus: The need for community. In A. M. Hoffman, J. H. Schuh, & R. H. Fenske (Eds.), *Violence on campus: Defining the problems, strategies for action.* Gaithersburg, MD: Aspen Publishers.

43. Gerstenfeld, P. B. (2003). *Hate crimes: Causes, controls, and controversies.* Thousand Oaks, CA: Sage Publications.

44. Evans, N. J., & Rankin, S. (1998). Heterosexism and campus violence: Assessment and intervention strategies. In A. M. Hoffman, J. H. Schuh, & R. H. Fenske (Eds.), *Violence on campus: Defining the problems, strategies for action.* Gaithersburg, MD: Aspen Publishers.

45. Stern, J. (2002). *The ultimate terrorists.* Cambridge, MA: Harvard University Press.

46. Smith, T. W. (2000). Public perspectives: Public opinion about gun policies. *The Future of Children, 12,* 155–163.

47. Teret, S. P., & Culross, P. L. (2000). Product-oriented approaches to reducing youth gun violence. *The Future of Children, 12* (2), 119.

48. Diaz, T. (2000). *Making a killing: The business of guns in America.* New York: The New Press.

49. A deadly myth: Women, handguns, and self-defense. (2001, January). Washington, DC: Violence Policy Center.

50. *Some things you should know about media violence and media literacy.* (2004). Elk Grove Village, IL: American Academy of Pediatrics.

51. Bok, S. (1999). *Mayhem: Violence as public entertainment.* New York: Basic Books.

52. Joint statement on the impact of media violence on children. (2000, July 26). Washington, DC: Congressional Public Health Summit.

53. Carlson, C., & Felitzen, C. L. (Eds.). (1998). *Children and media violence: Yearbook from the UNESCO clearinghouse on children and violence on the screen.* Nordicom, Goteborg University, Goteborg, Sweden.

54. Bork, R. (1996). *Slouching towards Gomorrah: Modern liberalism and American decline.* New York: HarperCollins.

55. Farrington, D. P. (2002). Families and crime. In J. Q. Wilson & J. Petersilia (Eds.), *Crime: Public policies for crime control* (pp. 129–148). San Francisco: ICS Press.

56. Taylor, R. B. (2002). Physical environment, crime, fear and resident-based control. In J. Q. Wilson & J. Petersilia (Eds.), *Crime: Public policies for crime control* (pp. 413–434). San Francisco: ICS Press.

57. Samson, R. J. (2002). The community. In J. Q. Wilson & J. Petersilia (Eds.), *Crime: Public policies for crime control* (pp. 225–252). San Francisco: ICS Press.

58. Murray, C. (2002). The physical environment. In J. Q. Wilson & J. Petersilia (Eds.), *Crime: Public policies for crime control* (pp. 349–361). San Francisco: ICS Press.

59. Glassner, B. (1999). *The culture of fear.* New York: Basic Books.

Add It Up! HOW SAFE ARE YOU?

Violence does not have to be part of your everyday life. To see how well you are protecting yourself from unsafe situations, consider the following statements and decide whether each one is always, sometimes, or never true for you.

General Safety Considerations	Always	Sometimes	Never
I am aware of my surroundings.			
I tell someone where I'm going whenever I leave home.			
I'm careful about giving personal information or my daily schedule to people I don't know.			
I vary my daily routine and walking patterns.			
If I walk at night, I walk with others.			
Auto Safety	**Always**	**Sometimes**	**Never**
I look in the back seat before I get in my car.			
I look around before parking, stopping, or getting into or out of my car.			
I keep my car doors locked at all times.			
I have a plan of action in case my car breaks down.			
I scan ahead of me and behind me, with my mirrors, for potential dangers.			
I avoid dangerous, high-risk places whenever possible.			
If hit from behind, I drive to the nearest police station or well-lighted, populated area, motioning for the person who hit me to follow.			
If I notice anyone loitering near my car, I go straight to a safe place and call the police.			
I never hitchhike.			
ATM Safety	**Always**	**Sometimes**	**Never**
I avoid using ATMs at night.			
I try to take someone with me when I use an ATM.			
I look for suspicious people or activity before entering or driving into an ATM area.			
I do not write my personal identification number on any paper I carry with me.			
I take all my ATM and credit card receipts with me to avoid leaving behind personal information.			

(continued)

Violence, Rape, and Homicide	Always	Sometimes	Never
I carefully limit my alcohol intake at parties.			
I do not drink alcohol on a first date.			
I refuse to be with anyone who seems violent.			
I do not allow anyone to strike me.			
I don't stay around anyone who has a gun and is drinking alcohol or using other drugs.			
I break off any relationship that is verbally or physically abusive.			
Ramps and Parking Lots	**Always**	**Sometimes**	**Never**
I park in well-lighted areas.			
I avoid walking down ramps in parking lots if there are other options.			
I keep my arms as free as possible when walking to my car.			
I check the back seat of my car before getting in.			
Public Transportation	**Always**	**Sometimes**	**Never**
While waiting for transportation, I am aware of my immediate surroundings.			
While waiting for transportation, I place myself so that I am protected from behind.			
I hold items under my arm so that they will be difficult to grab.			
While riding on buses or trains, I look aware and alert.			

Scoring

Give yourself 3 points for each Always answer, 2 points for each Sometimes, and 0 points for each Never.

Your Score	Your Risk
90–99	You are probably safe as long as you continue to follow these precautions.
80–89	You may need to reexamine some of your habits and make changes to improve your safety.
79 or less	You may need to make significant changes in your habits to improve your safety.

SOURCE: Adapted from *Wellness: Concepts and Applications*, 5th ed. (pp. 335–336), by D. J. Anspaugh, M. H. Hamrick, and F. D. Rosato, 2005, New York: The McGraw-Hill Companies.

CHAPTER **18**

Injury: Creating Safe Environments

DID YOU KNOW?

- If you are a male, your risk of dying from an unintentional injury is much higher than that of females. The greatest number of injury deaths in males occurs at age 21, and the total remains high until about age 50. The greatest number of injury deaths in females occurs after age 75.

- If you are ever distracted while driving because you are talking on your cell phone or changing a CD, you are at an increased risk of injury or death in a motor vehicle crash. Driver inattention is believed to be involved in at least 25 percent of all highway crashes. Such crashes account for nearly half of all unintentional injury deaths.

- Millions of people visit emergency rooms every year for injuries suffered while playing a sport or engaging in a recreational activity. ER physicians treat more than 500,000 bicyclists and 250,000 in-line skaters a year. In the 5-year period from 1997 to 2001, nearly 12,000 people were treated for injuries incurred while playing paintball.

OLC *Your Health Today*   www.mhhe.com/teague1e

Go to the Online Learning Center for *Your Health Today* for interactive activities, quizzes, flashcards, Web links, and more resources related to this chapter.

Unintentional injuries are the leading cause of death for children and adults between the ages of 1 and 39 and the fifth leading cause of death for Americans of all ages. Millions of people also suffer nonfatal injuries every year. These injuries and deaths occur as a result of car crashes, falls, fires, and scores of other incidents that could be prevented. Public health experts now avoid the term *accident* in referring to these incidents, because it implies that injury is a chance occurrence or unpreventable mishap over which individuals have no control.[1] These experts emphasize that injuries are preventable if people adopt behaviors that promote safety and if society does its part in reducing environmental hazards. Examples of safety-promoting behaviors are wearing safety belts in cars, keeping medications in locked cabinets out of the reach of children, and having working smoke detectors in the home.

Unintentional injuries are injuries that are not purposefully inflicted,[1] in contrast to intentional injuries like homicides, assaults, or rapes. The leading cause of unintentional injury death for Americans of all ages is motor vehicle crashes, followed by falls, poisoning, choking, and drowning. Common causes of injury death are different for different age groups. For example, for infants under 1 year of age, the leading cause of injury death is suffocation; for children aged 1 to 14, the second leading cause (after motor vehicle crashes) is drowning, and the third is fire and flames. For individuals aged 15 to 54, the second leading cause (after motor vehicle crashes) is poisoning, typically from drugs. For those over 75 years of age, the leading cause of injury death is falls.[2]

Leading causes of injury death also vary by ethnicity and race. For African Americans and people of Hispanic background, the second leading cause of death is poisoning, whereas for non-Hispanic whites and all other groups, it is falls. African Americans and Hispanics are also more likely to die from drownings and fires than from suffocation, while the opposite is true for whites and other groups. Across all groups, however, more males than females die from unintentional injuries from birth to age 80, and males have a higher rate of death per 100,000 people than females throughout the life span (Figure 18.1). For males, the greatest number of deaths occurs at age 21, and totals remain high until the early 50s; for females, the greatest number of deaths occurs after age 75.[2]

In this chapter we take a look at several different types of unintentional injury, along with measures that can be taken to avoid and prevent them. We begin with motor vehicle injuries, focusing on auto safety, motorcycle safety, and pedestrian safety. We then turn to recreational activities and consider bicycling, in-line skating, swimming and other water activities, and hunting. We then examine safety in the home, looking at falls, poisoning, fire, and choking, among other causes of injury, and safety in the workplace, focusing on back injury and computer use. We conclude with a brief look at natural disasters. Throughout the chapter we include guidelines and tips that will help you avoid unintentional injuries.

MOTOR VEHICLE SAFETY

Motor vehicle crashes account for 44 percent of all unintentional injury deaths. The highest number of motor vehicle deaths occur in the young and the old—those aged 16–19 and those aged 75 and older. Men are more likely than women to be killed in car crashes, although the ratio of male to female deaths dropped from 5 to 1 in 1975 to 3 to 1 in 2000. The change is attributed to an increase in the number of women who drive and the number of miles women drive. Women are more likely to be involved in car crashes, fatal and nonfatal combined, than men. [2-4]

What Factors Contribute to Motor Vehicle Crashes?

About 85 percent of motor vehicle crashes are believed to be caused by **improper driving,** defined as speeding, failing to yield the right of way, disregarding signals and stop signs, making improper turns, and following too closely,

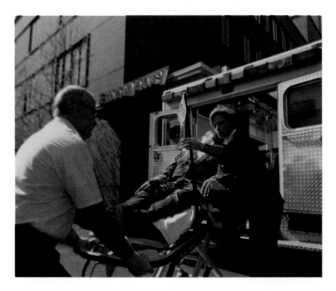

Motor vehicle crashes account for the greatest number of unintentional injury deaths. Many such deaths, including those from falls, poisoning, choking, and drowning, could be prevented through standard safety measures.

KEY TERMS

unintentional injury Injury that is not purposefully inflicted.

improper driving The cause of most motor vehicle crashes, including speeding, failing to yield right of way, following too closely, and passing on a yellow line.

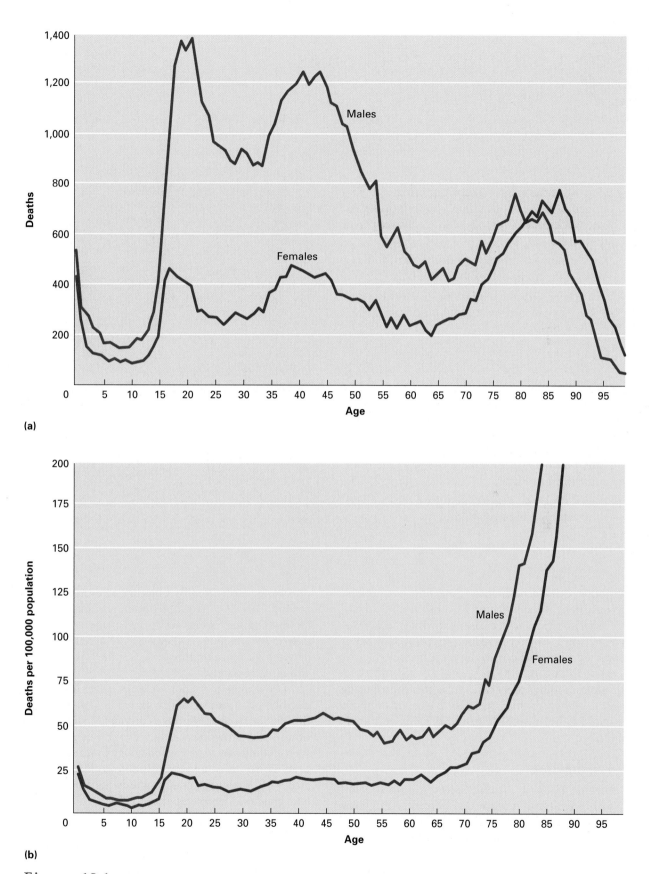

(a)

(b)

Figure 18.1   Unintentional injury deaths, United States, 2001—total number of deaths (a) and rates of death per 100,000 population (b). *(a) Unintentional injury deaths by sex and age. More males than females die from unintentional injuries at all ages from birth to age 80. (b) Unintentional injury death rates by sex and age. As people become older, their rates of death from unintentional injury soar.* Source: *Injury Facts*, 2004, National Safety Council.

Challenges & Choices

Defensive Driving

Defensive driving means anticipating potential hazards by keeping your eyes on other drivers and monitoring changing environmental conditions. The National Safety Council stresses nine defensive driving guidelines:

- Don't start the engine without securing each passenger in the car, including children and pets. Safety belts save thousands of lives each year. Lock all doors.
- Remember that driving too fast or too slow can increase the likelihood of collisions.
- If you plan to drink, designate a driver who won't drink. Alcohol is a factor in almost half of all fatal motor vehicle crashes.
- Be alert. If you notice that a car is straddling the center line, weaving, making wide turns, stopping abruptly, or responding slowly to traffic signals, the driver may be impaired.
- Avoid an impaired driver by turning right at the nearest corner or exiting at the nearest exit. If it appears that an oncoming car is crossing into your lane, pull over to the roadside, sound the horn, and flash your lights.
- Notify the police immediately after seeing a motorist who is driving suspiciously.

- Follow the rules of the road. Don't contest the "right of way" or try to race another car during a merge. Respect other motorists.
- Don't follow too closely. You can determine an appropriate following distance by using the "three-second rule." Select a fixed object on the road ahead, such as a sign or an overpass. When the car in front of you passes it, count "one one thousand, two one thousand, three one thousand." If you pass the object before you complete the count, you are following too closely. In poor driving conditions, double or triple your distance (to 6 or 9 seconds).
- While driving, be cautious, aware, and responsible.

It's Not Just Personal . . .

According to the National Safety Council's *Injury Facts,* 19,900 motor vehicle deaths occurred in 2003 as a result of collisions with other vehicles. Approximately 10,500 of these fatal collisions were angle collisions, 5,300 were head-on, 2,400 were rear-end, and 1,700 were sideswipes and other two-vehicle collisions.

Source: Fact Sheet on Driving Defensively, National Safety Council, www.nsc.org.

among other driving behaviors.[4] Speeding is especially dangerous; it is a major factor in most fatal crashes.[5] Speeding-related crashes decrease with driver age.[3] **Defensive driving** can help you reduce your risk of injury at the hands of people who drive improperly (see the box "Defensive Driving").

In addition to improper driving, factors contributing to motor vehicle crashes include driver inattention, aggressive driving, alcohol-impaired driving, and environmental hazards.

Driver Inattention

The National Highway Traffic Safety Administration (NHTSA) estimates that at least 25 percent of highway crashes involve some form of driver inattention.[6] Drivers under age 20 are the most likely to be involved in distraction-related crashes. Certain distractions are more prevalent in certain age groups. Adjusting the radio or CD player is a greater distraction among drivers under age 20. People age 20 to 29 are more likely to be distracted by young children, and those 65 and older are

most often distracted by objects and events outside the vehicle.[7] Talking on a cell phone is a major source of distraction, and some states and many countries have passed laws making it illegal to use a cell phone while driving; for more on this topic, see the box "Cell Phones and Driving Safety."

Drowsiness is a major source of driver inattention. As described in Chapter 6, driving while you are sleepy or drowsy can be as dangerous as driving under the influence of alcohol. Drowsiness reduces your awareness of your surroundings, impairs your judgment, and slows reaction time. Thirty-three percent of traffic accidents are associated with sleepiness, and fatigue is the leading cause of fatal crashes in people aged 18 to 25.[3,8]

Aggressive Driving

The NHTSA estimates that two thirds of all traffic fatalities are associated with overly aggressive driving behavior.[3] An aggressive driver is someone who tailgates, speeds, runs red lights, changes lanes without signaling, and makes illegal turns.

Challenges & Choices

Cell Phones and Driving Safety

Americans spend substantial amounts of time in their cars, and many try to optimize their use of this time by conducting business or keeping in touch with friends on their cell phones. Most people on the road have observed drivers who are distracted by talking on their cell phones drift across lanes on the highway, follow other cars too closely, or drive through stop signs or red lights. A study conducted at Aston University in the United Kingdom found that drivers talking on the phone did not perform as well as drivers who were not distracted by phone calls and that their performance did not return to normal for several minutes after hanging up. Using the phone per se was not what impaired performance so much as the degree to which the driver became involved in the call.

New York was the first state to ban the use of cell phones while driving; it has been joined by New Jersey and the District of Columbia as well as a number of local jurisdictions across the country. Several states have partial bans in place regarding cell phones (such as bans on use by bus drivers). Nearly 50 countries have bans as well, including Australia, France, Germany, India, Japan, and Russia. In Canada, the issue has been debated in Parliament, and bans are in effect in some parts of the country.

If you live in an area where it is legal to use cell phones while driving, the following recommendations will increase your safety:

- Familiarize yourself with how your cell phone works so you know its features when you need to use it while driving.

- Use the speed dial, redial, memory dial, and phone book features available on most cell phones.
- Use a hands-free device with a speaker phone or a headset.
- Tell the person you are speaking to that you are driving, and be prepared to end the call at any time.
- Don't place or answer calls in heavy traffic or hazardous weather conditions.
- Time your calls so you can make them when you are stopped.
- Never engage in stressful or emotional conversations on your cell phone while driving.
- Place your phone within easy reach in your car so you can grab it without taking your eyes off the road. If you get a call in heavy traffic or hazardous conditions, let it go to your voice mail.

It's Not Just Personal . . .

The NHTSA estimates that about 3 percent of people behind the wheel at any given moment during the day are talking on cell phones. As noted in the chapter, about a quarter of all motor vehicle crashes involve driver inattention.

Source: Cell Phones and Driving: A Prescription for Disaster, Smart Motorist, www.smartmotorist.com.

Aggressive driving can escalate into **road rage.**[9] This extreme form of aggressive driving may occur when a driver becomes enraged at another driver's poor driving behaviors, such as sudden merging or lane changing, or it may occur when one driver provokes another with a curse or gesture and the second driver retaliates. One or both drivers may take more aggressive actions, such as flashing bright lights, passing and cutting in, or attempting to damage the other's vehicle or physically injure the other driver. The irrational thoughts of a driver in the grip of road rage may last for minutes or hours. Road rage has been implicated in numerous fatal car crashes; people who experience this kind of uncontrolled anger need to seek help in managing their anger. (To measure your level of hostility on the road, see the Add It Up! feature at the end of this chapter.)

Alcohol-Impaired Driving

According to NHTSA, alcohol was involved in 41 percent of fatal car crashes and 69 percent of all crashes in 2002.

KEY TERMS

defensive driving Responsible driving that anticipates potential hazards and monitors changing environmental conditions.

road rage Extreme form of aggressive driving in which a driver becomes enraged at another driver's behaviors and one or both drivers take increasingly aggressive actions, such as passing and cutting in or attempting to physically injure the other driver.

Table 18.1	Blood Alcohol Concentrations and Fatal Motor Vehicle Crashes
Compared with drivers who have not consumed alcohol . . .	
If you drive with blood alcohol concentration (BAC) in this range:	**Then your chances of being killed in a single-vehicle crash increase by:**
0.02–0.04 percent	1.4 times
0.05–0.09 percent	11 times
0.10–0.14 percent	48 times
0.14 percent and above	380 times

Sources: "Alcohol and Health," 2000, National Institute on Alcohol Abuse and Alcoholism; "A Review of the Literature on the Effects of Low Doses of Alcohol on Driving-Related Skills," by H. Moskowitz and D. Fiorentino, April 2000, U.S. Department of Transportation.

Alcohol-related crashes cause an average of one death every 30 minutes and a nonfatal injury every 2 minutes. About 3 in 10 Americans are involved in an alcohol-related crash at some point in their lives. Nearly 40 percent of those killed in these crashes are people other than the drinking driver. The highest rate of alcohol-impaired driving occurs among males aged 17 to 34. Overall, 4 percent of men and 1 percent of women report that they have driven while impaired by alcohol. Rates appear to be higher among white men than among Hispanic and black men. Among people who binge drink, 14.6 percent say they have driven while impaired, a rate 30 times higher than the rate for non-binge drinkers.[2,3,10,11]

As discussed in Chapter 11, alcohol slows reaction time and impairs perception, information processing, judgment, memory, and motor coordination. Research has established that the risks of a motor vehicle crash and of a fatal crash increase as blood alcohol concentration (BAC) increases (Table 18.1). Data also show that the more demanding the driving task, the lower the BAC at which impairment begins.[10] These risks are even greater for drivers under age 21, who are likely to have less driving experience.

Again as discussed in Chapter 11, drinking and driving laws and penalties are set by the states, but the federal government uses its leverage to influence state legislation. In 1984 Congress passed the National Minimum Drinking Age Act, which required states to set the legal drinking age at 21 or risk losing federal funding. In 1995 Congress amended the act to encourage the states to pass legislation making it illegal for persons under 21 to drive after drinking alcohol and setting legal BAC limits of 0 to 0.02 percent for drivers under 21. By 1998 all states had complied with these zero tolerance limits for minors.[12] Public health

experts estimate that these laws have reduced alcohol-related crashes by 20 percent.[11]

By 2004, all but three states and the District of Columbia had set the legal BAC limit for adults at 0.08 percent. In Colorado, Delaware, and Minnesota, it is 0.10 percent. Forty-two states also have administrative license revocation laws, which allow a police officer or other law enforcement official to confiscate the license of a driver whose BAC exceeds the legal limit.[2] Research suggests that BAC limits work best when used in conjunction with administrative license revocation laws.[10]

Studies show that more than 90 percent of Americans favor the idea of using **designated drivers,**[10] individuals in a group who abstain from drinking alcohol on a particular occasion and drive for others who do not abstain. Whether this practice has reduced alcohol-related crashes is not clear, but it appears that the use of designated drivers is increasing.[12] Community campaigns have not only promoted the use of designated drivers but also encouraged individuals to take a bus or cab or walk when they have been drinking. Some clubs and lounges now have coin-operated breath-testing devices that estimate a person's BAC.

Many drugs other than alcohol impair the ability to drive safely. They include illicit drugs such as marijuana and heroin, prescription drugs, and over-the-counter drugs such as sleep aids. Driving safety requires mental alertness, clear vision, physical coordination, and the ability to react quickly. Any drugs that induce dizziness, light-headedness, nausea, drowsiness, fatigue, nervousness, or fuzzy thinking make driving dangerous. (For more on the special challenges faced by older adults, see the box "Older Adults and Safe Driving.") If you take any drugs that could impair driving, arrange to be picked up, use public transportation, or stay where you are until the drug effects wear off.

Environmental Hazards

Environmental hazards account for less than 5 percent of vehicle crashes, but when combined with human error, they account for 27 percent. Environmental hazards can be natural, such as snow, ice, wind, poor visibility, or glare, or of human origin, such as construction zones, broken-down cars on the side of the road, or drunk drivers. To reduce the number and lethality of injuries that occur as a result of environmental factors, states and local communities use such measures as ice-melting chemicals, crash cushions, breakaway signs and light poles, and median barriers and guard rails.[1]

Approaches to Motor Vehicle Safety

Motor vehicle safety is addressed by a variety of measures, including testing cars to make sure they meet NHTSA standards, designing effective restraint systems and

HIGHLIGHT ON HEALTH
Older Adults and Safe Driving

In 2003 about 15 percent of drivers were age 65 or older. By 2030, that number will increase to 20 percent, and more than 10 million drivers will be age 85 or older. Compared to younger age groups, drivers age 75 and older have more accidents per mile driven. It is likely that the higher number can be attributed to a subset of people with significant cognitive and physical impairments who overestimate their ability to drive safely.

A National Institute on Aging study estimated that Americans outlive their ability to drive by 6 to 10 years. Most older adults stop driving when they no longer feel they can drive safely. Some compensate by not driving in poor weather, at night, or for long distances. Others, however, are reluctant to limit their driving, no doubt because driving represents both real and metaphorical independence. Several approaches have been taken to address this problem. Some states require more frequent license testing for older adults. The American Association for Retired Persons and the American Automobile Association Safety Foundation for Traffic Safety offer driver safety programs for older people. Sometimes family physicians advise older adults or their adult children that they may no longer be able to drive safely. And on occasion, concerned family members may find it necessary to take away the older person's car keys.

Sources: "MIT Study: Older Drivers Know When to Slow Down," by F. Pope, July/August 2003, *AARP Bulletin*, pp. 11–12; "Risk to Self Versus Risk to Others: How Do Older Drivers Compare to Others on the Road?" by A. M. Dellinger, M. Kresnar, D. D. White, and M. Schgal, 2004, *American Journal of Primary Medicine, 26* (3), pp. 217–221.

increasing the likelihood that people will use them, and developing new safety technology.

NHTSA Standards

Crash worthiness is a measurement of how well a car performs in a crash in terms of damage to the car and other vehicles and injury to people.[13] All cars sold in the United States must pass a test that measures the effectiveness of the vehicle's structural design in preventing occupants from being ejected, trapped, burned, or crushed in a 30-mph (miles per hour) collision. The test also determines a vehicle's ability to absorb, control, or reduce crash impacts on occupants. The NHTSA estimates that a person's risk of death and severity of injury is reduced by 50 percent in vehicles that pass the test.[13]

Light trucks, vans, and sport utility vehicles (SUVs) have become popular choices of consumers in recent years, and questions have been raised about their safety in crashes. For more on this topic, see the box "SUVs, Light Trucks, and Crash Safety."

Restraint Systems

During a car crash, there are really two collisions. The first collision happens when one car hits another car or a structure. The **second collision** occurs when unbelted occupants are thrown against the windshield or other structures inside the car, such as the steering wheel, or against other passengers. Most injuries are incurred in the second collision.[1] The hard surfaces inside the car are potential sources of death during any crash, whether front, side, or rear impact.

Safety belts prevent at least 50 percent of serious injuries and reduce the risk of fatality by 45 percent for front seat passengers.[14] Safety belts also prevent ejection during a crash; in 2002, only 1 percent of passengers wearing safety belts were ejected, compared with 30 percent of passengers who weren't restrained. Because many people resisted using safety belts when they were first installed in cars, public information campaigns, incentive programs, and seat belt reminder systems in vehicles were introduced to encourage usage; most of these measures had little effect. Mandatory safety belt laws have proved more effective; today, 49 states and the District of Columbia have such laws in place (New Hampshire requires seat belt use by those under 18 only). Nationwide, seat belt use is estimated at 84 percent for occupants of vans and SUVs, 81 percent for occupants of passenger cars, and 69 percent for occupants of light trucks.[2]

KEY TERMS

designated driver A person in a group who abstains from drinking alcohol and drives for the others.

crash worthiness Measurement of the impact of car crashes on people and property.

second collision Impact of an unbelted occupant with the windshield, steering wheel, doors, dashboard, or other passengers after a collision with another vehicle or object (first collision).

HIGHLIGHT ON HEALTH

SUVs, Light Trucks, and Crash Safety

Because of their greater weight and height, sport utility vehicles (SUVs), minivans, and light trucks (or pickup trucks) cause significantly more damage to passenger cars in collisions than they sustain themselves. They are also responsible for many fatalities and serious injuries when they collide with passenger cars. Although SUVs, vans, and light trucks make up only 36 percent of all motor vehicles, they are involved in nearly 50 percent of fatal two-vehicle crashes that include passenger cars. Eighty percent of the people killed are occupants of the passenger cars. In any front-to-side crash between vehicles, the occupant of the vehicle hit is almost seven times more likely to be killed than the occupant of the vehicle that hits it. This likelihood increases 26 times when the vehicle that hits the other vehicle is an SUV or other light truck.

Although it is safer to be in an SUV or a light truck than a passenger car in a collision, the risks are reversed in the event of a rollover. A rollover is a dangerous single-car crash with a higher fatality rate than other types of crashes. In 2002, rollovers accounted for 33 percent of crash-related fatalities, even though they accounted for only 3 percent of all vehicle crashes. The average chance of a rollover is twice as high or higher for vans, light trucks, and SUVs as it is for passenger cars, according to NHTSA's rollover resistance rating system for 2001–2003 vehicles (see figure).

To minimize the risk of injury in a rollover, drivers of any vehicles, but especially drivers of SUVs, vans,

*if involved in a single-vehicle crash. 2001-2003 NCAP data

NHTSA's Rollover Resistance Rating System

and light trucks, should make sure all occupants wear seatbelts, avoid driving after consuming alcohol or drugs or when drowsy, adjust speed to road and weather conditions, avoid overcorrecting in frightening situations, maintain properly inflated tires and replace worn tires, and carry no more than the maximum safe load for the vehicle.

Sources: Rollover Rating System Administration: Vehicle Administration Class Comparison, National Highway Traffic Safety Association, www.safecar.gov; NCAP Frequently Asked Questions, National Highway Traffic Safety Association, New Car Assessment Program, www.nhtsa.dot.gov/cars; Testimony before the U.S. Senate Committee on Commerce, Science, and Transportation, by J. W. Runge, February 26, 2003, www.nhtsa.gov/dot.

Air bags—fabric cushions that instantly inflate during a collision—are a kind of **passive restraint** that protects front seat passengers from impact with the interior of the vehicle in a crash. The effectiveness of air bags at reducing fatalities over and above safety belts is estimated at 12 percent.[2] Generally, sensing devices in the dashboard inflate air bags at impacts of 12 mph or more. The bags deflate seconds after the impact. Front air bags do not protect occupants against side-impact collisions, which account for 30 percent of crash deaths, and cars are now being equipped with side-impact protection systems.[15]

Infants and children need to be secured in child seats placed in the back seat and anchored by the vehicle's safety belts. Child seats effectively protect small children from injuries that occur when children are thrown from the car or slammed into the car's interior during a crash. Infants should ride in carriers in which they are in a semi-reclining position facing the rear of the car. Infants and toddlers should not ride in the front seats of cars with air

bags, because air bags can deploy with enough force to cause severe head and neck injuries in very young children. For maximum protection, children aged 12 and under should always ride in the back seat. Injuries resulting from motor vehicle crashes are the leading cause of death for children ages 1 to 14.[3,15,16]

To assess the risks posed to motor vehicle safety by combinations of factors, see the box "Who Is Least Likely to Be Involved in a Motor Vehicle Crash?"

New Safety Technology

Automakers are continually developing new safety technology. New devices will include an intricate network of sensors embedded in bumpers, doors, and seats that anticipate a crash and direct the car's safety devices to work in harmony with one another. For example, to prevent neck injuries and broken ribs, air bags will fire at a precise velocity, or not at all, while safety belts retract to snug

Beating the Odds

Who Is Least Likely to Be Involved in a Motor Vehicle Crash?

The chances of being involved in a motor vehicle crash are influenced by a variety of factors, ranging from driving experience, to distractions inside and outside the car, to alcohol and drug use. Brief profiles of three individuals are presented here. Which one do you think is least likely to be involved in a motor vehicle crash?

Mariel is a 21-year-old college student who drives a 2003 compact car. She uses her car to drive around campus, and every two or three months she drives home to see her family, a 400-mile trip on a six-lane interstate highway. Mariel has a huge collection of CDs she listens to in the car, and she frequently uses her cell phone while driving. Because of her schedule, she is often sleep deprived and has nearly fallen asleep at the wheel on the interstate a few times. She usually makes the trip at night and frequently exceeds the speed limit. When the weather is bad or the highway is fogged in, she drives carefully. She always wears her seat belt.

Kalil is an 18-year-old high school student living in a mid-sized city. He took a driver ed course and has been driving for a year and a half. His parents gave him their 1998 Buick when they bought a new car, and he drives it to and from school. After school, Kalil and several of his friends usually go joy-riding around town, and on weekends, they often drive to parties and clubs. Kalil usually monitors his drinking when he is driving, but he has occasionally driven while intoxicated. His friends are often drunk and boisterous when riding in his car. Kalil always wears his seat belt and makes sure his passengers do too.

Dexter is a 35-year-old insurance salesman who travels extensively. He drives a company car equipped with a navigation system, AM/FM radio, CD player, hand-held cell phone, in-vehicle computer for message service, and fax machine. Dexter drinks moderately and does not smoke. His job is highly stressful, and he frequently feels frustrated, angry, and impatient with other drivers on the road. Because of the demands of the job, Dexter often drives when fatigued. He always wears his seat belt.

OLC Web site Visit the **Online Learning Center** at www.mhhe.com/teague1e for comments by the authors.

occupants into their seats and then, a fraction of a second later, slacken to enable them to "ride down the crash." Airbags that drop from the ceiling to protect the head will also be available.[13] Computer sensor devices will prevent tipovers and wheel spin by activating brakes together at one time and slowing the engine to prevent vehicle swerving or skidding.[17]

Emergency notification systems are being developed that will automatically call for help when an air bag deploys or allow drivers to call with the push of a button. The goal of these systems is to reduce the number of people who die from their crash injuries before they reach the hospital. Some systems will go even further by sending information that will help rescuers determine the type of assistance needed.[18]

Another invention is a lane-drifting system, which uses a camera linked to a computer that monitors the vehicle's distance to the left and right of lane markings. If the computer senses an unintended lane departure, whether from the driver falling asleep or fiddling with a CD player, it applies torque to the steering wheel to ease the vehicle back into the proper lane.[18]

Other developments include a system that uses forward-facing cameras in the vehicle's side-view mirrors to give drivers a 360-degree view of the road; a system that

uses lasers and radar to sense the cars ahead and brakes the car if it gets too close to other vehicles; electronic feelers that detect danger ahead and steer the vehicle out of harm's way; and intelligent highways that use global positioning satellites and road sensors to warn drivers of hazards in their path.[17]

Motorcycle Safety

Motorcyclists are about 5 times more likely than passenger car occupants to die in a motor vehicle crash and about 26 times more likely to be injured. In 2002 motorcycles made up 2 percent of all registered vehicles in the United States, but motorcycle crashes accounted for 9 percent of motor vehicle deaths. Contributing factors in these crashes were lack of proper training, distraction, alcohol, and environmental conditions (weather, roadway surface, equipment malfunction). However, the Motorcycle Safety

KEY TERMS

passive restraints   Safety devices that do not require vehicle occupants to engage them.

Pedestrian crosswalks are designed for safety, with low curbs to accommodate older adults and wheelchair users, but the timing of stoplights is often geared to our fast-paced society.

Foundation reports that about 65 percent of all collisions between motorcycles and other types of vehicles were precipitated by a vehicle operator other than the motorcyclist, usually because the driver failed to see the motorcycle. Wearing a helmet reduces a motorcyclist's risks of both fatal injury and traumatic brain injury. Despite these safety benefits, most motorcyclists choose not to wear helmets, unless state law requires it.[2,3,19–21]

Pedestrian Safety

Pedestrians account for about 13 percent of traffic-related deaths, second to vehicle occupants. On average, one pedestrian in the United States is killed every 109 minutes and one is injured each 7 minutes. About one out of every six pedestrian deaths occurs in a hit-and-run incident. About 45 percent of pedestrian deaths occur when pedestrians enter or cross streets, and 10 percent occur when pedestrians are walking in the roadway.[2,3,22,23]

The highest number of pedestrian deaths occurs among men aged 35–44, but the highest death rate per 100,000 people occurs among those aged 75 and older. The pedestrian fatality rate for men is about twice that for women, and the rate of nonfatal pedestrian injuries is also higher for men. The pedestrian fatality rate for African Americans is almost twice that for whites, and for American Indians and Native Alaskans it is nearly three times as high. Safety experts believe this difference can be partly attributed to the fact that members of these groups generally walk more than whites, because they own fewer cars. Children and older adults are also especially vulnerable to pedestrian deaths and injuries.[1–3]

Child Safety

Young children are curious and like to explore their environment; they are often unaware of potential dangers posed by running into a street, do not have accurate perception of vehicle distance and speed, and may not understand traffic signs and signals.[22] Parents can overestimate their children's ability to cross the street on their own. Because children are small, drivers often don't see them. Children aged 5 to 9 make up nearly 7 percent of all pedestrian deaths and injuries, and children aged 10 to 14 make up nearly 10 percent.[2] Schools and communities need to work together to provide traffic education programs and safe roads and streets to reduce pedestrian injuries and deaths among children.

Older Adult Safety

Although pedestrian deaths make up about one seventh of all traffic-related fatalities, almost one third of people age 70 or older killed in traffic are pedestrians.[23] Inadequate safety islands and traffic lights that do not allow enough time for older people to cross the street contribute to the risk for older adults. Other factors include declining vision and physical impairments in older people. To improve pedestrian safety, communities have introduced traffic-calming measures (speed bumps, lower speed limits), pedestrian crosswalk signs that display the number of seconds left on the red light, cameras that record vehicles that run red lights, and pedestrian safety education programs.[22]

RECREATIONAL SAFETY

Injuries occur in a wide variety of recreational activities and sports, including football, basketball, soccer, swimming, skateboarding, snowboarding, and many others. A new source of recreational injury is paintball. Between 1997 and 2001, nearly 12,000 people, almost all of them male, were treated in emergency rooms for paintball-related injuries. Recreational injuries among older adults are also increasing. Activities associated with injuries in this age group include bicycling, golfing, exercising (walking, running, taking exercise classes), snow skiing, and fishing.[2] In this section we consider bicycling, in-line skating and riding motorized scooters, water activities, and hunting.

Bicycle Safety

Collisions between bicycles and motor vehicles resulted in an estimated 700 deaths in 2003 and an estimated 28,000 nonfatal disabling injuries.[2] Emergency room visits for bicycle-related injuries were estimated at more than 520,000 in 2002. More than 90 percent of those killed in bicycle-related crashes are male. A successful bicycle safety program combines the use of safety equipment with injury-reducing behaviors. Three important considerations are making sure your bicycle fits you properly, wearing a helmet, and employing safe cycling practices.

The Right Fit

When your bicycle fits you properly, you are more comfortable and have more control. Several factors determine the appropriate fit.[1] One is the size of the bike and the height of the top tube from the ground. On a road bike, you should be able to straddle the bar with both feet flat on the ground and about a one-inch gap between your crotch and the bar. If this is not the case, the bike is too large or too small for you.

Another factor is the height of the seat. When you are cycling, your legs should be fully extended, but not overextended, at the bottom of the cycling stroke. Sit on your bike and completely extend one leg straight down while someone holds the bike for you. Make sure the heel of your foot reaches the pedal in its lowest position. If you have to stretch your toes or shift your weight to reach the pedals, the seat is too high.

A third factor is stem length, the distance from the front of the seat to the handlebars. If this distance is too long or too short, you will put excessive strain on your back or excessive weight on your hands and wrists. Stem length should be equal to the length of your arm from elbow to fingertips. Other factors in the right fit include seat angle (start with the seat level with the ground, then tip it up or down a few angles if you experience discomfort), seat fore and aft position (your knee should be above the pedal axle), and handlebar height (level with the seat). Different guidelines can apply for mountain bikes and other kinds of bikes. For the best fit, consult with the staff in a bike shop.

Bicycle Helmets

Head trauma is involved in most of the bicycle-related injuries and deaths that occur every year. Bicycle helmets are estimated to reduce the risk of head injury by 85 percent and the risk of brain injury by 88 percent. About 39 percent of adults and 69 percent of children under 16 wear bike helmets on a regular basis. Among those who don't wear helmets, reasons include cost, discomfort, and lack of knowledge about their effectiveness. Bicycle safety programs in elementary schools provide information for young cyclists and encourage helmet use, and 19 states, the District of Columbia, and many local communities have laws requiring the use of helmets.[2] For tips on buying a bicycle helmet, see the box "Choosing the Right Helmet."

Safe Cycling Practices

The biggest safety problem for bicyclists is making themselves visible to other vehicle operators. If you are a cyclist, your safety in traffic depends on your being visible, riding in a predictable manner, and knowing the rules of the road.[1] Reflective tape, brightly colored cycling clothes and safety vests, portable leg or arm lights, and headlights are effective for making riders visible. Air-powered horns can add another dimension to safety.

Bicycles are considered vehicles and must follow all traffic laws that apply to cars, including stopping at traffic lights and stop signs and signaling before turning. Obeying traffic laws also helps drivers of other vehicles anticipate your actions. Use bike lanes where they are available; otherwise, ride in the right lane of traffic along the line made by the right wheel of a vehicle. Watch for parked cars and people opening car doors. Know the local laws and regulations governing bicycle traffic.

In-Line Skating and Motorized Scooters

More than 250,000 in-line skaters a year are injured badly enough to seek treatment in hospital emergency departments.[3] Injuries to the wrist and head are the most common and often occur because the skater was not wearing proper safety gear. Skaters should always wear helmets, wrist guards, and elbow and knee pads; long pants and long-sleeved shirts are also recommended. Don't drink alcohol before skating; drinking appears to be a significant factor in injuries on college campuses.[1]

A relatively new source of injury is motorized scooters, two-wheel vehicles equipped with a gasoline engine or an electric motor and battery. The U.S. Consumer Product Safety Commission (CPSC) has reported a dramatic increase in scooter-related injuries, particularly in children under age 15.[24] Hand and arm fractures, cuts, bruises, and sprains are the most common injuries. Motorized scooters can roll downhill at dangerous speeds; most do not have brakes. Riding in wet conditions or when visibility is reduced can be especially hazardous.

The CPSC recommends that scooters be carefully maintained and routinely inspected to make sure nuts and bolts are securely fastened.[24] Riders should wear

Consumer Clipboard

Choosing the Right Helmet

Whether you are bicycling, skating, or skateboarding, you need to wear the right helmet to prevent head injury in case you fall or crash. The Snell Memorial Foundation, a nonprofit organization that tests and develops helmet safety standards, advises trying on several different helmets before purchasing one. Here are some tips for selecting the right one:

- Remember these four *s*'s: size, strap, straight, and sticker.

    Size: The helmet should sit comfortably on your head, fitting snugly but not squeezing your head. When the straps are fastened, you should not be able to pull it off or move it in any direction. Most helmets come with pads you can fasten inside the helmet to adjust the fit.

    Strap: Make sure the chin strap fits snugly and that the **V** in the straps meets under the ear.

Straight: Wear a helmet low on the forehead, about two finger widths above your eyebrows, and not tilted in any direction.

Sticker: Look for a manufacturer's sticker citing the U.S. Consumer Product Safety Commission standard. You can also look for independent certification by the Snell Foundation or the Safety Equipment Institute.

- Replace your helmet according to the helmet's instruction manual. Some helmets need to be replaced after a certain number of years or after you have been in a crash. Skateboarding helmets are designed for multiple knocks.

- Establish a "helmet habit." Children are more likely to wear helmets if their parents do and if they're introduced to them early. Always wear a helmet when participating in an activity that can cause head injury.

Source: Choose the Right Helmet for Your Favorite Summer Sport, National Safety Council, www.nsc.org.

---

helmets, knee and elbow pads, and sturdy shoes, and they should ride on smooth, paved surfaces. Some communities have laws against the use of motorized scooters by persons under the age of 16, and children under 12 should not ride them even if it is not illegal. If you are interested in a motorized scooter, check with local authorities about riding guidelines and restrictions.

Water Safety

Drowning is the second leading cause of death for children aged 1 to 14.[3] For children aged 1 to 4, between 60 and 90 percent of those who drown die in residential pools, half of them at the child's own home.[25] Children under age 1 often drown in bathtubs, toilets, or buckets.

Overall, about nine people drown every day in the United States; 80 percent of them are male. More than one third of adults are unable to swim the length of a pool 24 yards long. Women report less swimming ability than men, although fewer women drown. More than half of all drowning victims are white non-Hispanic males, although this group has the lowest drowning rate per 100,000 persons. African American males have the highest drowning rate per 100,000 persons, followed by non-Hispanic males of other races (for example, Asian, Pacific Islander, American Indian), Hispanic males, and non-Hispanic white males. The lowest drowning rate occurs among Hispanic females.[1-3]

Drowning and other water-related injuries occur not just when people are swimming but also when they are boating, water-skiing, and using personal watercraft.

Boating Safety

Nearly three fourths of boating-related deaths are due to drowning. Nine out of every 10 victims were not wearing life jackets, or **personal flotation devices (PFDs).** Most swimming-associated deaths occur in the late spring and summer months, when the weather is usually warm. Boating deaths, however, occur as early as March and as late as October, when water may be cold. Water temperature of less than 70° F can numb your arms and legs and make it difficult to hold on to objects. In cold water, people who are older or not physically fit are more susceptible to cardiac arrest. Cold water cools the body 25 times faster than air of the same temperature does, and hypothermia (loss of body temperature) can cause respiratory failure even if the person does not drown.[1,3,25]

If you are on a boat that turns over, stay with the boat, where you are more likely to be spotted and rescued, rather than trying to swim to shore. Good swimmers can usually swim up to 0.8 mile in 50° F water before hypothermia occurs. Poor swimmers may be able to swim only about 100 yards. A swimmer may not accurately estimate the distance to the shore, and wind and currents may make it difficult to reach land. If you are close to shore, however, and immediate rescue is unlikely, attempting to swim to shore may be your best option.[1]

Six of every 10 recreational boating deaths are associated with alcohol consumption.[25] Many states have laws covering intoxication by people operating boats that are comparable to those covering intoxication by drivers of motor vehicles. Operating any vehicle, including any boat, under the influence of alcohol or drugs is illegal under the criminal code in Canada.

Waterskiing and Personal Watercraft

Each year about 50 water-skiers die and about 25,000 are injured.[3] Most of these injuries occur when the skier falls into the water, comes in contact with the boat propeller, collides with an obstacle, or becomes entangled with the tow rope.[1] If you waterski, make sure you receive training, ski within your ability, learn water survival techniques, use a personal flotation device, and know how to swim.

Jet-skis, or wave runners—boats less than 12 feet long that are powered by an inboard engine and a jet pump mechanism—are popular personal watercraft. Deaths and injuries associated with these boats have more than doubled since their introduction in the mid-1980s.[26] Most

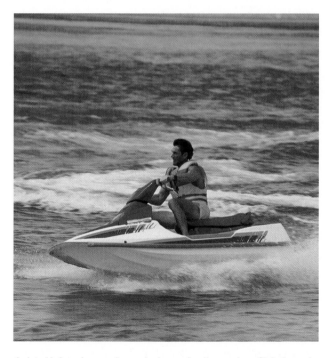

As jet-skis have become increasingly popular, the number of injuries and deaths associated with their use has climbed dramatically. Wearing a personal flotation device is a basic safety requirement for jet-skiing and many other water sports.

injuries involve blunt trauma to the legs, torso, or head. In some states, people under the age of 16 cannot legally operate a motorboat with more than 15 horsepower, including personal watercraft, unless supervised by a person on board who is 18 or older.

Personal flotation devices are essential protection for anyone participating in boating, waterskiing, or personal watercraft recreation. PFDs are made of buoyant material; various types have been designed for different watercraft. Check with your local jurisdiction for rules and regulations governing PFDs for your recreational activity.

Hunting Safety

Hunters who use firearms need to know the rules of gun use and storage to prevent unintentional injuries. If you hunt, never point a gun at anything but a hunting target, and never put your finger on the trigger until you are ready to fire. When you are walking, place your fingers on the outside of the trigger guard and point the barrel downward in front of you. Remove cartridges or shells from guns when crossing a fence, ditch, or stream. If you hunt in a group, walk or stand side by side with other hunters and designate a zone of fire for each hunter. Make sure you see your target clearly before firing, and unload your gun before getting into a vehicle.[1]

Nearly two thirds of unintentional injuries caused by firearms occur in the home.[27] Children in a home where guns are kept should be taught about their potential dangers and their proper use. Guns should be stored unloaded in a locked rack, cabinet, closet, or drawer well out of children's reach. Safety experts also recommend using a trigger lock, which prevents the trigger from being moved backward and discharging the gun. Some communities provide firearm storage, which is the safest option of all.

HOME SAFETY

Although more deaths occur each year in motor vehicle crashes than in any other category of unintentional injury, the highest number of injuries occurs in the home. In fact, nearly 40 percent of all disabling injuries occur in the home.[1] Home injuries and deaths occur primarily as a result of falls, fires, poisonings, and choking and suffocation. Figure 18.2 shows the number of deaths from these causes, along with deaths from motor vehicle crashes.

personal flotation device (PFD)   Life jacket worn while participating in water sports.

Figure 18.2   Leading causes of unintentional injury death by age, 2001. Source: *Injury Facts*, 2004, National Safety Council.

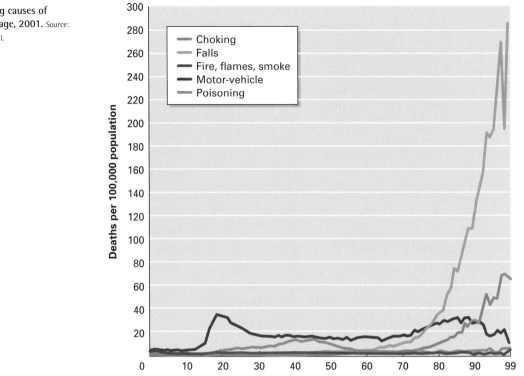

Falls

Falls are the most common cause of injury in the home. They are responsible for more open wounds, fractures, and brain injuries than any other cause of injury.[3] Falls are the most common cause of injury visits to the emergency room for two groups: young children and older adults.

Young Children and Falls

About 70 deaths occur each year when children fall out of windows; 25 percent of the children are 11 years of age or younger.[1] Other injuries occur when babies roll off beds or young children fall down stairs. Parents can lower the risk of fall-related injuries by supervising children, buying products that promote safety (such as nonslip rugs), and modifying the home (for example, installing gates at the tops of stairs and guards on windows).

Older Adults and Falls

Older adults have the highest rate of injury and death from falls of any age group. One of every three persons over age 65 falls each year, and two thirds of those who fall do so again within 6 months. Falls account for one third of the deaths from unintentional injuries among older adults.[2, 28,29] Older adults often suffer hip fractures when they fall and, because of poor healing, end up being confined to convalescent hospitals and nursing homes.

Older adults are more susceptible to falls than are younger people because of medical problems, changes in skeletal composition, poor balance, limited vision, muscular weakness, and medications.[29] Environmental factors like slippery floors, loose rugs, and poor lighting also play a role.[30] As the American population grows older, fall-related injuries are expected to increase. To make the home safer, older adults or their caregivers should make sure surfaces are clear of objects or conditions that could lead to a fall (for example, electrical cords inside, snow and ice outside); install hand rails and nonslip applications in bathtubs; and make sure rooms and stairways are well lit.

Fires

Of all fire-related deaths and injuries, 65 percent to 85 percent occur in homes. In 2003, 2,300 people in the United States died from fire, smoke inhalation, and injuries sustained during fires in the home.[2] More than 40 percent of the homes in which a fire fatality occurred did not have smoke detectors. Older adults are particularly at risk for injury and death in home fires; although they make up about 12 percent of the population, adults over 65 account for about 30 percent of all fire fatalities.[31]

Fires in the home are associated with smoking (especially smoking in bed), cooking, fireplaces and chimneys, electrical wiring and cords, and appliances, particularly electric heaters. You can reduce your risk of fire injury by changing careless behaviors, correcting faulty equipment, and having smoke detectors and fire extinguishers in your home. You can also improve your chances by having an emergency plan in place and knowing what to do in case of fire.

Smoke Detectors and Fire Extinguishers

Experts estimate that deaths from home fires could be reduced by 40 percent to 55 percent if smoke-sensing devices were installed in every home.[32] Your home should have at least one smoke detector on every level, placed on a ceiling or a wall 6 inches to 12 inches from the ceiling. Building codes in some local jurisdictions require a smoke alarm in every bedroom.

You can purchase battery-operated smoke detectors or models powered by household current, which are available with battery backup systems. If you have battery-powered detectors, replace the batteries every 6 months to 12 months. Some people remember to clean smoke detectors and change the batteries by doing it when they change their clocks to and from daylight savings time in the spring and fall. Because many people fail to replace old batteries, the more costly household-wired detectors are recommended.[1]

Home fire extinguishers are intended to knock down a fire long enough to allow the occupants to escape; most discharge their extinguishing agent for only about 30 seconds.[4] Use an extinguisher only on the type of fire for which it is designed; the wrong agent may intensify or spread a fire. A Class A fire consists of burning trash, wood, paper, or textile materials. Class B fires involve flammable products such as oil, gasoline, grease, paint, or alcohol. Class C fires involve electrical equipment. Many extinguishers contain a multipurpose dry chemical and are labeled ABC, meaning they can be used on any type of fire. They can be purchased in hardware stores.

Sprinkler systems are used in many commercial buildings, and most states have laws requiring sprinkler systems in newly constructed apartments, condominiums, and other multifamily dwellings.[32] Located in the ceilings of each room, the sprinklers activate at 160° F to 165° F. Sprinklers are now affordable for private homes.

In Case of Fire

Having an emergency plan will help you react quickly in case of fire. Make sure every room in your house has two escape routes, and designate a place away from the house where occupants or family members will meet once they are outside. The National Fire Protection Association recommends that families practice fire drills to make sure everyone, especially children, knows what to do in case of fire.

If a fire does occur in your home, leave the house as quickly as possible. Make sure that everyone gets out, and don't go back into the house once you are outside. If someone is missing when you get outside, tell the firefighters. If you are in a burning structure, avoid smoke inhalation by crawling along the floor toward a door or window, covering your mouth and nose with a wet cloth. If your clothes catch fire, drop to the ground and roll to extinguish the flames; do not run.

Poisonings

In 2003, there were 11,200 deaths from poisoning in the United States.[2] About half of all poisoning deaths are from drug overdoses, primarily illicit drugs like cocaine and heroin. Alcohol poisoning accounts for a small percentage of poisoning deaths, but it may be involved in poisoning deaths from other drugs. The death rate from poisoning is more than twice as high in males as in females.

Children are especially vulnerable to accidental poisoning in the home. The most common cause of poisoning in children is ingestion of household products, including cleaning products, furniture polishes, insecticides and herbicides, products containing lye or acids, and petroleum-based substances like kerosene, lighter fluid, turpentine, and solvents. All such products should be kept well out of the reach of children and stored in a locked cupboard or one with childproof safety latches. Federal law requires that many of these products be sold in containers with child-resistant caps.

Prescription and over-the-counter (OTC) drugs can be poisonous if taken in excess quantities or in improper combinations.[33] To help patients avoid medication errors, drug manufacturers now include patient package inserts (PPIs) with prescription drugs that provide information

Healthy People 2010

OBJECTIVE AREA *Injury and Violence Prevention*

- Reduce deaths caused by poisonings.

"Children are at significantly greater risk from poisoning death and exposure than adults because children are more likely to ingest potentially harmful chemicals. . . . Approximately 90 percent of all poison exposures occur at a residence."

"Among children aged 5 years and under [the majority] of poisoning exposures come from nonpharmaceutical products such as cosmetics, cleaning substances, plants, foreign bodies, toys, pesticides, and art supplies; [the remainder] come from pharmaceuticals. Immediately calling a poison control center can reduce the likelihood of severe poisoning, decrease the cost of a poisoning incident, and prevent the need for a hospital emergency department (ED) visit."

 For more information on Healthy People 2010 objectives, visit the Web site at www.healthypeople.gov.

 For more information on Canadian health objectives, visit the Health Canada Web site at www.hc-sc.gc.ca/english.

for the consumer, such as the purpose of the medication, possible side effects, drug interactions, and contraindications (conditions under which individuals should not take the drug). Pill boxes with a space for each day of the week are available to help patients take medications correctly. Pharmacists have begun taking a more active role in patient education as well.

To protect consumers against malicious tampering with products, the FDA requires tamper-resistant or tamper-evident packaging for all OTC drug products, along with a label informing consumers about this safety feature. Federal law requires that many OTC drugs be sold in containers with child-resistant closures,[34] although a patient may request an easy-open container.

Another poisoning hazard in the home is gases and vapors, such as carbon monoxide or natural gas. Carbon monoxide is a major component of motor vehicle exhaust; to avoid poisoning by this lethal gas, never leave your car engine running in a closed garage. Natural gas is used to operate many home appliances, such as furnaces, stoves, and clothes dryers. Although natural gas is odorless, producers add a gas with an odor so that leaks can be detected. If you smell gas, check to see if the gas is turned on but not lit on a stove burner or other appliance; if you cannot find the source of the leak, leave the area and call your utility company.

If you or someone you are with has been poisoned, seek medical advice and treatment immediately. If the skin has been exposed to a toxic substance, wash the area with soap and warm water. If the product contacted the eyes, flush them with warm water. If a poison has been ingested, do not induce vomiting unless instructed to do so. Some poisons cause more damage when vomited than they do in the stomach. Signs that a person has ingested or inhaled a poisonous substance include difficulty breathing or speaking, dizziness, unconsciousness, foaming or burning of the mouth, cramps, nausea, and vomiting.

In all cases of toxic contamination or poisoning, call 911, your local poison control center, or the national poison control hotline (1-800-222-1222). Be prepared to report the person's condition, age, and weight; the product consumed; and when the product was consumed. You may be instructed to administer first aid immediately. After administering first aid, you may need to take the person to the emergency room; if you do, take the poisonous substance with you.

Choking and Suffocation

About 3,000 deaths occurred from choking and suffocation in the United States in 2003.[35] Death rates for choking are highest in children under 4 years of age and adults over 65 years of age. Rates soar in adults over 75 years of age. Most choking emergencies occur when a piece of food or a swallowed object becomes lodged in the throat, blocking the tracheal opening and cutting the oxygen supply to the lungs. Muscles in the trachea may spasm and wrap tightly around the object.[1] Children are at risk for choking on small objects they put in their mouths or accidentally ingest, such as part of a toy or a balloon. Children under 3 should not play with toys with small parts; most toys sold in the United States have warning labels if they have small parts. Children can also choke on hard candies, raw carrots, popcorn, and other small, hard foods.

Older adults with poorly fitting dentures or missing teeth are at risk for choking because they may not adequately chew their food. Alcohol is a contributing factor to choking death, since it slows reflexes, desensitizes the back of mouth, and may cause a person to pay less attention to eating. The risk of choking can be reduced by cutting food into reasonably small pieces, chewing well, not rushing, and not talking or laughing while eating.

A person whose airway is obstructed may gasp for breath, make choking sounds, clutch the throat, or look flushed and strained. If a person's airway is only partially blocked, he or she may cough forcefully. Do not slap someone on the back if he or she is coughing; usually, the coughing will clear the obstruction. If the person continues to have difficulty breathing, coughing is shallow, the person is not coughing, or the person cannot talk or breathe, a rescue technique like the **Heimlich maneuver** is needed. See the box "The Heimlich Maneuver" to learn how to perform this technique to help a person who is choking.

Suffocation occurs when a person's air supply is cut off. The death rate for suffocation is highest in infants and small children. Infants sometimes suffocate when they become entangled in their crib bedding or when plastic materials cover their mouths and noses. Balloons and plastic bags pose a suffocation risk and should never be given to children.

Temperature-Related Injuries

Each year scores of people die from excessive heat, particularly older adults and people with weak hearts. The danger is highest for people 75 years of age and older. High temperatures can be exacerbated by high humidity, which prevents the evaporation of perspiration from the skin and makes it difficult for the body to control its core temperature. A temperature of 95° F combined with 75 percent humidity produces a heat index (the temperature the body feels) of 130° F, which can cause heatstroke, a life-threatening condition.[36] See Chapter 8 and Table 8.3 for more information on heatstroke and guidelines on how to treat it.

Temperatures inside vehicles can quickly reach dangerous levels. When the outside temperature is 93° F, the temperature inside a car can reach 125° F in 20 minutes, provided information on how to minimize this strain on the body. **Ergonomics** is the study of workplace design for the purpose of fitting environments to the physical and mental characteristics of the people who use them. Ergonomic principles can be used to create a workstation that minimizes your risk of strain or injury.

The main elements to consider are your chair, your desk, and the components of your computer. Adjust your chair so that your hips are slightly higher than your knees; this position pitches your pelvis slightly forward, allowing your back to maintain its natural curvature. A downward lip at the forward edge of the chair takes pressure off the back of your knees. If you don't have an adjustable chair, try putting some extra cushioning at the back of your chair to raise your hips slightly. Place your feet flat on the floor or on a foot rest slightly in front of your knees.

Place your monitor on your desk directly in front of you. If you place it to the side, you risk injuring your neck by continually turning your head to see the screen. (You should also protect your neck by using a headset when talking on the phone, rather than cradling the phone between your ear and your shoulder.) When you are sitting, you should be an arm's length from the monitor, about 2 feet to 2½ feet. Set the height of the monitor so your eyes are level with the top of the screen; you should be looking downward at the middle of the screen. If you wear reading glasses or bifocals, don't tip your head upward to read the screen.

Place the keyboard so the angle of your elbows is 90 degrees or greater and your wrists are in a neutral position, tilted neither up nor down. Your wrists, hands, and forearms should be parallel to the floor. If you have a keyboard tray, you may find it comfortable to tilt the back of the tray slightly down. You may also want to use a wrist support on the tray at the front of the keyboard, but resting your wrists on the support while you are typing is not recommended. Keyboards with separated sections for the right and left hands may also be helpful. The computer mouse should be at the same level as the keyboard. Ideal body position for computer use is shown in Figure 18.4.

When using the computer for long periods of time, take frequent breaks, getting up to stretch and move around. If you have a laptop computer, try to use it with separate components (monitor, keyboard, mouse) so you can adjust them to the right position. If you don't have separate components, it's even more important to take frequent breaks.

Excessive computer use can also affect your vision, causing eyestrain, irritated eyes, blurred vision, and headaches. Rest your eyes by refocusing them periodically, such as by looking at something in the distance. To relieve dry, irritated eyes, use lubricating eye drops and make sure air vents in the room are not directing air toward your eyes. Adjust window blinds and lighting to reduce excessive brightness in the room and **glare**, the reflection of light on a viewing surface. An antireflective shield

Figure 18.4   Ideal body position for computer use.

attached to your monitor can also reduce glare. To facilitate ease of reading, use black type on a white background whenever possible, and avoid extreme contrast on your screen.

Repetitive Strain Injuries

When motions and tasks are repeatedly performed in ergonomically incorrect ways, injuries to the soft tissues can occur that are known as **repetitive strain injuries.**

KEY TERMS

pulmonary resuscitation   Technique used to rescue a person who is not breathing; also known as mouth-to-mouth resuscitation or artificial respiration.

cardiopulmonary resuscitation (CPR)   Technique used when a person is not breathing and a pulse cannot be found; differs from pulmonary resuscitation by including chest compressions to restore heartbeat.

ergonomics   Study of workplace design for the purpose of fitting environments to the physical and mental characteristics of the people who use them.

glare   Reflection of light on a viewing surface.

repetitive strain injury   Injury to soft tissues that can occur when motions and tasks are repeatedly performed in ergonomically incorrect ways.

A common repetitive strain injury is **carpal tunnel syndrome (CTS),** the compression of the median nerve in the wrist caused by certain repetitive uses of the hands, including computer work. The median nerve is located inside a "tunnel" created by the carpals (wrist bones) and tendons in the hand. When the tendons become inflamed through overuse or incorrect use, they compress the median nerve. The symptoms of CTS are numbness, tingling, pain, and weakness in the hand, especially in the thumb and first three fingers. Symptoms are often worse at night, when pain can radiate up into the shoulder.

If untreated, CTS can damage the median nerve and the muscles at the base of the thumb. The first steps in addressing this condition are correcting ergonomic problems in the workstation, taking frequent breaks from repetitive tasks, and doing exercises that stretch and flex the wrists and hands. If symptoms persist, a physician may recommend a night splint that keeps the hand and wrist immobile during sleep to reduce inflammation of the tendons. Other treatments include injections of steroids to reduce inflammation and, in severe cases, surgery to reduce pressure on the nerve.[40]

NATURAL DISASTERS

A sudden event resulting in loss of life, severe injury, or property damage is typically defined as a **disaster.**[3] Disasters can be caused by humans, as in the case of terrorist attacks, or by natural forces. The greatest number of deaths from natural events in the United States occur as a result of floods, followed by tornadoes and lightning strikes. In this section we focus on three types of natural disasters: tornadoes, hurricanes, and earthquakes.

Tornadoes

A tornado is a violently rotating column of wind that extends to the ground. It usually lasts less than 10 minutes but can last more than an hour. The National Weather Service and the American Red Cross recommend that you have an emergency plan if you live in an area where tornadoes occur. If a tornado warning is given on television or the radio, go to a basement or an interior room on the first floor, such as a bathroom or closet. Cover yourself with a mattress or blanket for protection against flying glass. If you are in a mobile home, evacuation is advised. Highway overpasses are not a safe haven during a tornado.

Hurricanes

A hurricane is a tropical storm whose winds exceed 70 mph and spiral around a calm center, or eye. A hurricane may have a diameter of about 300 miles. Hurricanes can cause high tides called "storm surges," which are more dangerous than the wind and rain; they account for nearly 90 percent of hurricane-related deaths. These great domes of water, created by a combination of low pressure and high winds around the eye of the storm, may stretch 50 miles across and rise 20 feet above sea level. Breakers riding on top of the storm surge act as battering rams.[1]

As with tornadoes, the best way to avoid injury from a hurricane is to prepare. If you are in a coastal area, know how far you are from the beach and your elevation. Major hurricanes produce storm surges that can move inland more than 10 miles in low-lying areas. If a hurricane warning is issued, continue to listen to storm warning broadcasts; anchor outside objects; cover windows and glass with plywood; move valuable items upstairs; and store drinking water in jugs or bottles.[1] If you live on or near the beach or in a mobile home, you probably need to evacuate. If you stay, remain indoors in the center of your home, preferably in a closet or bathroom without windows.

Like individuals, emergency support agencies need to be well prepared to deal with hurricanes. When Hurricane Katrina hit New Orleans on August 29, 2005, emergency agencies, both federal and local, were not prepared to cope with a disaster of this magnitude. Even with adequate warning, the Federal Emergency Management Agency (FEMA) was slow to respond, and local support was quickly overwhelmed by the situation. As a result, many lives were lost and billions of dollars' worth of damaged occurred.

Earthquakes

An earthquake is a sudden movement of a portion of the earth's crust, accompanied by **seismic waves,** vibrations of the earth's surface. *Aftershocks,* earthquakes of lesser intensity, generally follow earthquakes. In a major earthquake, you may feel a rolling sensation accompanied by a rumbling sound, or you may feel a sudden, violent jolt followed by shaking of the land and buildings. The rolling and shaking can last from a few seconds to a few minutes. Most earthquake injuries and deaths are caused by collapsing walls and falling objects such as bookcases.[41]

To avoid injury during an earthquake, identify safe spots in your home, such as a sturdy table or desk that you can get under or an interior doorway that you can reach

KEY TERMS

carpal tunnel syndrome (CTS)   Compression of the median nerve in the wrist caused by certain repetitive uses of the hands.

disaster   Sudden event causing loss of life, severe injury, or property damage.

seismic waves   Vibrations of the earth's surface.

quickly. Stay away from chimneys, glass windows and doors, and furniture that could fall on you. If you are outdoors, move away from buildings and power lines. The National Center for Environmental Health (part of the CDC) provides detailed information on earthquake preparedness; see the Web Resources at the end of the chapter for the Web site address.

Earthquakes under the ocean are sometimes followed by tidal waves, or *tsunamis,* as was the case in the Indian Ocean on December 26, 2004. An estimated 250,000 people were killed when tides of 20 feet or more rushed onto the islands and low-lying areas of Indonesia, India, east Africa, and other countries bordering the ocean following the 8.7 magnitude earthquake. Early warning systems are under development in many of these countries to alert people so they can get to higher ground in the event of an earthquake and tsunami.

***

Unintentional injuries are among the most preventable health hazards you will encounter in your life. You can reduce your risk of injury by becoming more aware of dangerous situations, knowing your physical limitations, developing skills and strengths that lower your risks, and changing behaviors that increase your risks. For example, you can gather emergency supplies to use in case of an earthquake, check your bicycle helmet for signs of damage and replace it if necessary, never drive or let a friend drive under the influence of alcohol, and take a class in CPR. All such actions lower the likelihood that you or someone you love will become an unintentional injury statistic.

You Make the Call

Should Vehicles Be Equipped with In-Vehicle Internet Information Systems?

The BMW 745 sedan has more than 700 safety, communication, and entertainment features that the driver can control with buttons, switches, voice commands, and a joystick that operates a cursor on a dashboard screen. Cars now have built-in cell phones, global positioning navigation systems, DVD players, sensors that detect obstacles, cruise controls that display the distance of the car ahead, and in-dash cameras. Up to 80 percent of 2006 cars contain gadgets such as these; they are included not just in luxury vehicles but in mass market cars as well.

The National Highway Traffic Safety Administration (NHTSA) is concerned that these features and gadgets distract drivers and lead to more motor vehicle crashes, injuries, and deaths. The NHTSA is especially concerned that In-Vehicle Internet Information (IVI) systems will decrease driving safety. IVI systems enable drivers to access the Internet and e-mail services and to conduct business and use e-mail while they are driving.

Auto manufacturers and other supporters of IVI systems claim that IVI systems can assist drivers by enhancing vehicle control and enabling drivers and passengers to conduct business more efficiently. Digital maps and traffic updating, for example, will help drivers avoid roadwork delays, choose alternate routes, and, if they are delayed, communicate with their offices and participate in meetings and decision making from their cars. This ability will calm frazzled nerves and reduce aggressive driving by people rushing to get to work.

They also argue that IVI information and entertainment can combat driver drowsiness and fatigue and provide drivers with information about the area in which they are driving, such as the location of motels, restaurants, and gas stations. They point out that drivers with IVI systems will be able to report auto crashes, hazardous conditions, disabled vehicles, and medical emergencies to transportation system managers so that help can be dispatched more quickly and other drivers will be alerted to the danger. According to supporters of IVI systems, speech-activated devices will solve the problem of visual distraction.

The main concern of safety experts and other opponents of IVI systems is that they will make driving more dangerous for everyone on the road. The NHTSA estimates that driver error contributes to more than 90 percent of collisions, and driver inattention accounts for 25 percent of police-reported crashes. Speech-activated devices will not help, because the problem is cognitive inattention. Auditory interfaces have not proved effective in reducing distraction. Driver distraction will be particularly dangerous for younger drivers with less experience, who already have the highest rate of motor vehicle injury and death.

IVI systems will not assist traffic managers any more than cell phones do. Although cell phone users can increase road safety by reporting crashes and hazards, emergency response networks have been jammed when scores of drivers reported the same incident. Some cell phone users have gotten into crashes themselves because they were distracted by reporting traffic incidents. The same could be expected of IVI systems.

Auto makers are moving ahead with advanced technology devices for vehicles, and consumers are eager to have them, despite warnings by safety experts. Should vehicles be equipped with IVI systems? What do you think?

Pros

○ IVI systems improve the quality of life for commuters, allowing drivers to conduct business and keeping them informed and entertained.

○ IVI systems are good for the economy because they facilitate the conduct of business.

○ Drivers want the latest technology, and auto manufacturers are complying with their desires. Technological advances always precede safety controls; if communication and information devices in cars were restricted, innovation would be stifled.

○ IVI systems can increase highway safety because drivers are kept alert by information and entertainment and because they can report crashes and hazards.

Cons

○ IVI systems increase driver distraction, a major cause of fatal and nonfatal car crashes. To claim that a driver can focus on the road while surfing the Internet or sending e-mail is ridiculous.

○ The existence of new technology leads to the expectation that people will use it. People are already overworked and stressed out without additional demands being placed on them.

○ Claiming that auditory systems will prevent distraction is misleading. They may actually compel drivers to look more extensively at the IVI display.

○ Many countries and several states and localities have already banned the use of cell phones by drivers. The distraction caused by cell phones pales in comparison with the distraction caused by IVI systems.

○ The fact that drivers buy cars with these features and devices does not mean they are a good idea.

OLC Web site For more information about this topic, visit the Online Learning Center at www.mhhe.com/teaguele.

SOURCES: Data from "Enhanced Vehicle Safety ITS Integration," by B. H. Kantowitz, T. M. Granda, and M. J. Moyer, 1998, *Proceedings of the International Technical Conference on the Enhanced Safety of Vehicles*, NHTSA; *NHTSA Driver Distraction Research: Past, Present, and Future*, by T. R. Ranney, E. Mazzae, G. Riley, and M. J. Goodman, July 5, 2000, NHTSA, www-nrd.nhtsa.dot.gov; Alliance of Automobile Manufacturers, The Drowsy Driver Technology, www-nrd.nhtsa.dot.gov.

SUMMARY

• Unintentional injuries are the fifth leading cause of death for Americans. Public health experts avoid the word *accident* because it implies that injuries are unpreventable. Most injuries can be prevented by behavior changes and environmental modifications.

• The leading cause of unintentional injury death for Americans of all ages is motor vehicle crashes, followed by falls, poisoning, choking, and drowning. Causes of injury death vary by age group and ethnicity, but across the life span until age 80, more males than females die from unintentional injuries.

• Motor vehicle crashes account for 44 percent of unintentional injury deaths. Factors contributing to crashes include improper driving, driver inattention, aggressive driving, alcohol-impaired driving, and environmental hazards.

• Measures to improve motor vehicle safety include testing vehicles to ensure that they meet standards of crash worthiness set by the National Highway Traffic Safety Administration; designing effective restraint systems (seat belts, air bags, child seats) and developing means to ensure that drivers and occupants use them (primarily, laws); and developing new technology that integrates vehicle, driver, and road safety features.

• Motorcyclists are more likely to die or be injured in crashes than passenger car occupants. Two thirds of collisions involving motorcycles occur because the driver of the other vehicle didn't see the motorcyclist. Wearing a helmet significantly reduces the risk of head or brain injury.

• Pedestrians account for about 13 percent of traffic-related deaths. Children and older adults are especially vulnerable to pedestrian injury and death.

• Injuries are common in sports and recreational activities. On average, bicycle-related injuries account for hundreds of deaths, thousands of disabling injuries, and hundreds of thousands of emergency room visits every year. Three important components of bicycle safety are having a bike that fits, wearing a helmet, and following safe cycling practices and motor vehicle traffic laws.

• In-line skating and riding motorized scooters are associated with head, wrist, and arm injuries. Wearing protective equipment and riding on smooth paved surfaces can help prevent injuries.

• Drowning is a leading cause of death for children. More than one third of adults cannot swim 24 yards. Boating injuries and deaths result not just from drowning but also from hypothermia. Personal flotation devices are essential protection for anyone participating in boating, waterskiing, or personal watercraft use.

• Hunters need to know the rules of gun use and storage, which include storing guns unloaded in a locked container out of the reach of children or in a community storage facility.

- The highest number of injuries occurs in the home; leading causes of home injury and death are falls, fires, poisoning, and choking and suffocation.

- Falls are the most common reason for emergency room visits for children and older adults. Among older adults, falls account for one third of unintentional injury deaths; they often cause disabling hip fractures.

- Most fire-related injuries and deaths occur in the home; older adults are particularly at risk. Smoke detectors, fire extinguishers, and sprinkler systems greatly reduce the risk of injury and death. Having an emergency plan and practicing fire drills help people know what to do in case of fire.

- About half of all poisoning deaths occur from drug overdoses. Poisoning also occurs when children ingest household products and when people take medications and drugs improperly. Gases and vapors, such as carbon monoxide and natural gas, can also cause death.

- Choking is most common among children under 4 and adults over 75. It usually occurs when a piece of food or an object becomes lodged in the throat, obstructing the windpipe. The Heimlich maneuver is a rescue technique for someone who is choking. Suffo-

cation occurs when the air supply is cut off, such as by a plastic bag.

- Extremes of temperature can cause injury and death, and prolonged exposure to excessive noise can cause hearing loss.

- Individuals can learn how to provide emergency aid by taking a course in first aid and CPR.

- Work-related injuries and deaths have declined in the past 100 years but still affect more than a million workers annually.

- Back injuries are often associated with improper lifting techniques. Use of computers is associated with strain and injuries to the neck, back, hands, arms, and eyes. A computer workstation should be set up in accordance with ergonomic principles. Repetitive strain injuries, including carpal tunnel syndrome, result from the repeated performance of motions and tasks in ergonomically incorrect ways. They can be addressed by correcting problems in how the task is performed or how the workstation is configured, taking frequent breaks, doing exercises, and seeking medical treatment.

- Natural disasters include tornadoes, hurricanes, and earthquakes. The best way to avoid injury and death in a natural disaster is to be prepared and to know what to do when warnings are given.

REVIEW QUESTIONS

1. Why is the term *accident* no longer used to refer to unintentional injuries? What are some behaviors that can prevent unintentional injuries and deaths?

2. What are the five leading causes of unintentional injury death in the United States?

3. What age groups experience the highest number of motor vehicle deaths?

4. Describe several examples of improper driving and several examples of defensive driving.

5. What are two examples of driver inattention?

6. What is road rage?

7. What effects of alcohol make driving while intoxicated unsafe? What steps has the government taken to reduce drinking under the influence of alcohol by minors?

8. What are administrative license revocation laws?

9. What drug effects make driving dangerous?

10. What factors are considered in a test of a car's crash worthiness? How does the safety of SUVs and light trucks compare with that of passenger cars?

11. Describe how infant and child car seats should be placed and used.

12. Describe three examples of auto safety technology under development.

13. What factors contribute to the high risk of pedestrian injuries and deaths among older adults?

14. Why is it important to have a bicycle that fits you properly? What are the components of a proper fit?

15. What are the four *s*'s to consider when buying a bicycle helmet?

16. What are three factors that influence a bicyclist's safety in traffic?

17. What safety equipment is recommended for in-line skaters and people who ride scooters?

18. What dangers are associated with boating? What one behavior contributes to 60 percent of boating-related deaths?

19. What are the most commonly occurring unintentional injuries in the home?

20. What factors contribute to falls among older adults?

21. What are the most common causes of fires in the home? What behaviors promote fire safety?

22. What are the three types of fire, and why is it important to use the right kind of fire extinguisher?

23. What are three measures that have reduced the risk of poisoning by prescription and OTC medications?

24. What should you do in case of poisoning?

25. What are the signs that someone is choking? Describe the four steps of the Heimlich maneuver.

26. Describe the proper lifting technique to prevent back injury. What other factors contribute to back pain and injury?

27. Describe an ergonomically correct workstation setup for computer use.

28. What is carpal tunnel syndrome? How can it be treated?

29. What natural disaster causes the highest death toll in the United States?

30. What is the most dangerous aspect of a hurricane?

31. What are three safety measures to take in the event of an earthquake?

WEB RESOURCES

American Automobile Association Foundation for Traffic Safety: This organization offers educational materials for drivers, pedestrians, bicyclists, and others. Its Web site features FAQs, online quizzes on driving safety, and links to other resources. www.aaafts.org

American Red Cross: Highlighting news, safety tips, and disaster updates, this Web site features information on various emergencies, including blackouts, earthquakes, tornadoes, fires, floods, mudslides, and hurricanes. www.redcross.org

Consumer Information Center: The consumer help section of this Web site addresses a wide range of topics—from cars to health issues. It also offers contact information for corporations, manufacturers, federal agencies, Better Business Bureau offices, consumer organizations, and state resources. www.pueblo.gsa.gov

National Center for Environmental Health: This Web site provides practical information for all types of emergencies, including bioterrorism, chemical emergencies, natural disasters and severe weather, and radiation emergencies. www.cdc.gov/nceh

National Center for Injury Prevention and Control: This organization's Web site includes information on various injury-related topics, including falls, fires, and motor vehicles. Injury care information is also featured. www.cdc.gov/ncipc

National Highway Traffic Safety Administration: For information about traffic safety, news, vehicles and equipment, research, and laws and regulations, this organization is an authoritative resource. www.nhtsa.dot.gov

National Safety Council: This council publishes *Injury Facts,* an annual compilation of statistics on injuries. Its Web site features information on driving, ergonomics, falls, first aid, poison prevention, preparedness, and radon among other topics. www.nsc.org

U.S. Consumer Product Safety Commission: This government organization oversees the testing of products for safety and issues product recalls as necessary. Its publications include safety information for all-terrain vehicles, bicycle safety, child safety, poison prevention, and household products. www.cpsc.gov

REFERENCES

1. Bever, D. L. (1998). *Safety: A personal focus.* New York: WCB and McGraw-Hill.

2. National Safety Council. (2004). *Injury facts, 2004 edition.* Itasca, IL: Author.

3. Centers for Disease Control and Prevention, National Center for Injury Prevention and Control. *Injury fact book 2001–2002.* www.cdc.gov.

4. National Safety Council. What are the odds of dying? www.nsc.org.

5. National Highway Traffic Safety Administration. National survey of speeding and unsafe driving: Attitudes and behaviors. www.nhtsa.dot.gov.

6. National Highway Traffic Safety Administration. National survey of distracted and drowsy driving: Attitudes and behaviors. www.nhtsa.dot.gov.

7. Brown, T. L., Lee, S. D., Mcgehee, V., & Reyes, J. D. (2002). Collision warning timing, driver distraction and driver response to imminent rear-end collisions in a high-fidelity driver simulator. *Human Factors, 44* (2).

8. National Highway Traffic Safety Administration. Drowsy driving and automobile crashes. www.nhtsa.dot.gov.

9. Larson, J. (1999). *Road rage.* Tom Doherty Associates.

10. National Institute on Alcohol Abuse and Alcoholism. (2000). *Alcohol and health.* Washington, DC: U.S. Department of Health and Human Services.

11. Villareces, A., Cummings, P., & Koepsell, T. D. (2003). Association of alcohol-related laws with deaths due to motor vehicle and motorcycle crashes in the United States, 1980–1997. *American Journal of Epidemiology, 157* (2), 131–140.

12. Shults, R. A., et al. (2001). Task Force on Community Preventive Services. Reviews of evidence regarding interventions to reduce alcohol-impaired driving. *American Journal of Preventive Medicine, 21* (4 Suppl), 66–88.

13. U.S. Department of Transportation. (2004). U.S. DOT proposes tougher standard to protect occupants in side-impact crashes. Washington, DC: National Highway Traffic Safety Administration.

14. Cummings, P., & Rivera, F. P. (2004). Car occupant death according to the testimony use of other occupants: A matched cohort study. *Journal of the American Medical Association, 291* (3), 343–349.

15. Task Force on Community Preventive Services. (2001). Recommendations to reduce injuries to motor vehicle occupants: Increasing child safety seat use, increasing safety belt use, and reducing alcohol-impaired driving. *American Journal of Preventive Medicine, 21* (4 Suppl), 16–22.

16. National Highway Traffic Safety Administration. (2005, February). Child restraint use in 2004—Overall results. Washington, DC: U.S. Department of Transportation (DOT #8098 845).

17. Heisler, H. (2002). *Advanced vehicle technology* (2nd ed.). Woburn, MA: Butterworth-Heinemann.

18. Peraino, K. (2000, October 30). Safety first. *Newsweek,* 57–58.

19. Centers for Disease Control and Prevention. Motorcycle safety. U.S. Department of Health and Human Services. No. 29. www.cdc.gov.

20. Natalier, K. (2001). Motorcyclists' interpretation of risk and hazard. *Journal of Sociology, 37* (1), 65.

21. Motorcycle Safety Foundation. Riding gear. www.msfsa.org.

22. Retting, R. A., Ferguson, S. A., & McCarthy, A. T. (2003). A review of evidence-based traffic engineering measures to reduce pedestrian-motor vehicle crashes. *American Journal of Public Health, 93* (9), 1456–1462.

23. Office of Disease Prevention and Health Promotion. (2000, January). *Healthy people 2010.* Washington, DC: U.S. Department of Health and Human Services.

24. U.S. Consumer Product Safety Commission. Motorized scooter injuries climb. www.consumeraffairs.com.

25. Centers for Disease Control and Prevention. (2001). Drowning prevention. U.S. Department of Health and Human Services. www.cdc/gov/ncipe.

26. Ride smart: A rider's guide to personal watercraft. www.sacdelta.com.

27. National Rifle Association. NRA gun safety rules. www.nrahq.org.

28. Parra, E. K., & Stevens, J. A. (2001). *U.S. fall prevention programs for seniors: Selected programs using home assessment and home modification.* Atlanta, GA: Centers for Disease Control and Prevention, National Center for Injury Prevention and Control.

29. Casteel, C., Peek-Asa, O., Lacsamana, C., Vazquez, L., & Kraus, J. F. (2004). Evaluation of falls prevention program for independent elderly. *American Journal of Health Behavior, 28* (1), 551–560.

30. Becker, W. J. Preventing injuries from slips, trips and falls. Centers for Disease Control and Prevention. www.cdc.gov.

31. U.S. Fire Administration. www.usfema.org.

32. Davis, S. (2003, Fall). Fire stoppers. *Geico Direct,* 8–10.

33. Centers for Disease Control and Prevention. Poisoning prevention. U.S. Department of Health and Human Services. www.cdc.gov.

34. WebMD. (2003). Over-the-counter drug know-how. WebMD Public Information with the FDA. http://my.webmd.com.

35. Heimlich Maneuver Institute. How to do the Heimlich maneuver. www.heimlichinstitute.org.

36. Kilbourne, E. M. (2002). Heat-related illness: Current status of prevention efforts. *American Journal of Preventive Medicine, 22* (4), 328.

37. Mestel, R. (2000, April 13). Coping with a noisy world. *The Gazette,* Iowa City, IA, 1D.

38. The Arthritis Society. Chronic back injury. www.arthritis.ca.

39. Canadian Centre for Occupational Health and Safety. Back injury prevention. www.ccohs.ca.

40. Badia, A. Understanding carpal tunnel syndrome. www.ctsplace.com.

41. National Center for Environmental Health; Centers for Disease Control and Prevention. (2004). *Earthquakes: A prevention guide to promote your personal health and safety.* Atlanta, GA: Author.

Add It Up! ARE YOU AN AGGRESSIVE DRIVER?

The National Highway Traffic Safety Administration describes an aggressive driver as someone who "commits a combination of moving traffic offenses so as to endanger other persons or property." The NHTSA recommends avoiding the challenges and confrontations of such risk drivers. Do you ever exhibit any of the behaviors of an aggressive driver? To find out, answer yes or no to the following questions:

	Yes	No
1. Overtake other vehicles only on the left?	___	___
2. Avoid blocking passing lanes?	___	___
3. Yield to faster traffic by moving to the right?	___	___
4. Keep to the right as much as possible on narrow streets and at intersections?	___	___
5. Maintain appropriate distance when following other motorists, bicyclists, and motorcyclists?	___	___
6. Leave an appropriate distance between your vehicle and the one you have passed when cutting in after passing?	___	___
7. Yield to pedestrians?	___	___
8. Come to a complete stop at stop signs and before making a right turn on red?	___	___
9. Stop for red traffic lights?	___	___
10. Approach intersections and pedestrians slowly to show your intention and ability to stop?	___	___
11. Follow right-of-way rules at four-way stops?	___	___
12. Drive below posted speed limits when conditions warrant?	___	___
13. Drive at slower speeds in construction zones?	___	___

	Yes	No
14. Maintain speeds appropriate for conditions?	___	___
15. Use vehicle turn signals for all turns and lane changes?	___	___
16. Make eye contact and signal intentions when necessary?	___	___
17. Acknowledge intentions of others?	___	___
18. Use your horn sparingly around pedestrians, at night, and near hospitals?	___	___
19. Avoid unnecessary use of high-beam headlights?	___	___
20. Yield and move to the right for emergency vehicles?	___	___
21. Refrain from flashing headlights to signal a desire to pass?	___	___
22. Drive trucks at posted speeds and in the correct lanes, changing lanes at proper speeds?	___	___
23. Make slow U-turns?	___	___
24. Maintain proper speeds around roadway crashes?	___	___
25. Avoid returning inappropriate gestures?	___	___
26. Avoid challenging other drivers?	___	___
27. Try to get out of the way of aggressive drivers?	___	___
28. Refrain from using high occupancy vehicle or carpool lanes to pass vehicles?	___	___
29. Focus on driving and avoid distracting activities such as smoking, using a cell phone, reading, or shaving?	___	___

	Yes	No
30. Avoid driving when drowsy?	_____	_____
31. Avoid blocking the right-hand turn lane?	_____	_____
32. Avoid taking more than one parking space?	_____	_____
33. Avoid parking in a disabled space if you are not disabled?	_____	_____
34. Avoid letting your door hit the car parked next to you?	_____	_____
35. Avoid stopping in the road to talk with a pedestrian or other driver?	_____	_____
36. Avoid playing loud music that can be heard in neighboring cars?	_____	_____

Scoring

Count the number of no answers and use the following ranges to determine your level of hostility on the road.

1–3   Excellent. You are a responsible driver who behaves like an adult on the road.

4–7   Good. Pay attention to improving in your "no" areas.

8–11 Fair. You need to reevaluate your dangerous behaviors.

12+   Poor. You need to change your aggressive driving habits; you are endangering yourself and others.

SOURCE: National Highway Traffic Safety Administration, www.nhtsa.dot.gov.

CHAPTER 19

Environmental Issues: Making a Difference

DID YOU KNOW?

- When you take public transportation instead of driving your car, or when you put on a sweater instead of turning up the heat, you are contributing to the health of the planet by using less energy. Americans make up about 4.5 percent of the world's population, but they use about 24 percent of the world's energy resources, most of them fossil fuels—oil, coal, and gas.

- People sometimes experience nasal congestion, eye irritation, wheezing, and other symptoms when they are inside certain houses or buildings. In some cases, these symptoms are caused by chemical fumes seeping out of carpets, drapes, pressed-wood furniture, dry-cleaned clothes, and other home products. Levels of air pollution indoors can be higher and more hazardous than air pollution levels outdoors.

- The United States produces more pounds of garbage per person than any other country in the world, but it also has the highest rate of recycling of any country in the world. Americans recycle 28 percent of their waste, a rate that has doubled in the last 15 years.

OLC *Your Health Today* www.mhhe.com/teague1e

Go to the Online Learning Center for *Your Health Today* for interactive activities, quizzes, flashcards, Web links, and more resources related to this chapter.

Nowhere is the connection between personal health and the larger community more apparent than in the area of **environmental health.** In the context of the environment, our ability to achieve wellness depends not just on our own actions and those of our neighbors but also on the decisions of our national government and indeed the policies of peoples and nations around the world. When we look at environmental issues, we become aware that our lives are part of the intricate web of living organisms and nonliving natural resources that make the planet a single, vital ecosystem.

Only recently have people come to realize that the planet's resources are not infinite. We have also realized that many human activities have damaged the integrity of our ecosystem and threatened our own health. The possible enormity of this damage leaves many of us overwhelmed. A majority of environmental problems can be repaired, however, if individuals and societies recognize that resources are limited and if they take responsibility for protecting and preserving these resources.

The field of environmental health has traditionally been concerned with infectious diseases associated with contaminated water, food, waste, and other pollutants. Recently, the field has expanded to encompass pollutants that result from human and industrial activities and that cause chronic diseases and global environmental damage. In this chapter we focus mainly on the latter group of health threats. We look first at water and water quality, considering both the supply and the safety of this essential resource. We then turn to air and air quality, looking at air pollution as well as global problems such as the thinning of the ozone layer and global climate change. Next, we explore issues associated with the huge quantities of waste generated by humans and how this waste can be managed and reduced. We then consider threats to the world's ecosystems and biodiversity and problems associated with

the use of energy resources. We end with a look at an issue that underlies and amplifies all our environmental concerns—world overpopulation.

WATER AND WATER QUALITY

Although water is an abundant resource on earth, much of it is not suitable for drinking or other use by humans. Scientists estimate that only about 14 one-thousandths (0.014 percent) of the earth's water is readily available for human use.[1] Usable water supplies are further diminished by human activities that destroy or pollute natural ecological systems. In this section we look at our water supplies, threats to their safety, and what we can do to preserve and protect them.

Water Supplies and Shortages

The earth's supply of water is continuously collected, purified, and distributed in a natural process called the **water cycle** (Figure 19.1). Water is recycled 36,000 times faster than we can drink it, provided it is not polluted faster than it is replenished.[1] The water we use has two sources: surface water and groundwater. **Surface water** is precipitation that is stored in lakes, reservoirs, and wetlands (swamps, marshes, bogs) on the surface of the earth. It is renewed fairly rapidly in areas where precipitation occurs 12 to 20 days a year. **Groundwater** is precipitation that sinks into the ground. This water is stored in giant underground reservoirs called **aquifers** and slowly moves to areas where it is discharged, such as a stream, river, lake, or ocean, as part of the water cycle. Groundwater makes up 95 percent of the world's supply of freshwater.[2] In North America, about half of the drinking water comes from groundwater supplies.

Disposal of solid waste is an ongoing environmental challenge in the United States, where about 1,600 pounds of garbage per person are generated every year. Finding space for such waste is a reminder of the limits of the planet.

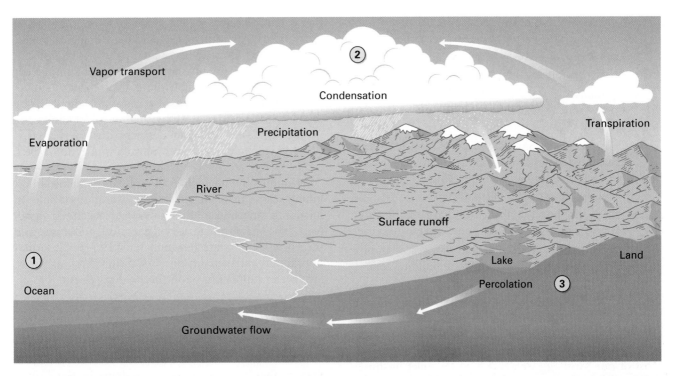

1. Oceans hold nearly 97 percent of the world's water. Ocean water evaporates into the air, is heated by the sun, condenses into clouds, and falls back to the earth. About 90 percent falls back into the ocean, and 10 percent falls on land.

2. More moisture accumulates in the air and clouds over land from evaporation of water in lakes, rivers, streams, and vegetation. Rain that falls on vegetated areas is absorbed in the soil. This water is slowly released in lakes and rivers and is used by plants.

3. Water not used by plants or carried into lakes or rivers slowly sinks into ground aquifers, giant underground reservoirs. The level of aquifers is called the water table. Water stored in aquifers slowly flows back into the ocean.

Figure 19.1   The water cycle.

Since 1900, the world use of water has increased nearly ninefold, and per person use has quadrupled. Withdrawal rates of surface water are projected to double in the next 20 years and exceed reliable sources in a growing number of areas. In the United States and Canada, water supplies are abundant, but much of our water is contaminated by industrial and agricultural wastes or is in the wrong place at the wrong time.[1,2] Conflicts between regions and states over water supplies have existed throughout U.S. history and are likely to intensify in the future, especially as people migrate and industries relocate to the West and Southwest.

In California, for example, two thirds of the state's precipitation falls in the northern part of the state, but half of the population lives in the Los Angeles basin, which receives only enough rain to support about 100,000 people. An acrimonious fight over water rights has been going on for more than a century among farmers, developers, environmentalists, city planners, public policy makers, and property owners. Solutions to water shortage problems include building dams and reservoirs to store surface water, transferring surface water from one area to another via pipelines and canals, withdrawing groundwater, converting salt water to freshwater, and adopting water conservation methods.[1]

Several water conservation measures can be adopted by communities to address water shortages. They include the following:[1,2]

- *Xeriscaping.* Replacement of green lawns in arid and semi-arid regions with vegetation adapted to a

KEY TERMS

environmental health   The area of health concerns that focus on the interactions of humans with all aspects of their environment.

water cycle   Natural process by which the earth's supply of water is continuously collected, purified, and distributed.

surface water   Precipitation stored in lakes, reservoirs, and wetlands (swamps, marshes, bogs) on the surface of the earth.

groundwater   Precipitation that sinks into the ground.

aquifers   Layer of permeable rock, sand, or gravel in the earth's crust that holds water.

dry climate reduces water use by 30 percent to 85 percent and sharply reduces water pollutants.

- *Drip irrigation.* Gardens and plants watered by drip irrigation systems effectively conserve water.
- *Ordinances.* Local laws requiring water conservation in water-short cities include water use bans, restrictions, and rationing.
- *Low-flow toilets.* Since 1994, all new toilets sold in the United States can use no more than 1.6 gallons per flush. A similar law (allowing (6 liters per flush) is in place in Ontario, Canada.
- *Water cost.* Local communities have significantly raised the price of water for home and business use.
- *Building codes.* Water-efficient fixtures or appliances may be required under local building codes.

Individuals also play an important role in water conservation. The per person use of drinking water is about 100 gallons per day in the United States and about 110 gallons per day in Canada.[2] In comparison, the per person per day use of drinking water in Nicaragua is 36 gallons.[1] Most of our "drinking water" is used for toilet flushing, bathing, cooking, lawn watering, clothes and dish washing, and cleaning. Communities also use about 35 gallons of water per person per day to support public activities, such as firefighting and park maintenance.[2] For tips on reducing your personal use of water, see the box "You Can Help Conserve Water."

Water Pollution

Water pollution is defined as any chemical, biological, or physical change in water quality that has a harmful impact on living organisms or makes water unsuitable for desired use.[3] The Environmental Protection Agency (EPA) claims that all but a few of the surface-water reservoirs in the United States are contaminated by discharge pollutants at specific locations through sewers, pipes, or ditches into bodies of surface water. Sources for these pollutants include factories, sewage treatment plants that remove some but not all pollutants, active and abandoned mines, oil spills, and agricultural feedlots. Runoff from large land areas such as croplands, golf courses, lawns, and parking lots also pollutes surface water.[1]

Cleaning up pollutants that reach aquifers lying deep in the ground is very difficult. The main sources of groundwater contamination are storage lagoons, septic tanks, landfills, hazardous waste dumps, and underground storage tanks filled with gasoline, oil, solvents, and hazardous waste. Such tanks can corrode and leak after 25 to 40 years. Groundwater is also contaminated when individuals dump or spill oil, gasoline, paint thinners, or other organic solvents onto the ground.[1,2]

The two basic types of water pollutants are biological and chemical. They can be ingested in drinking water, and they can also be absorbed through the skin or inhaled in water used for bathing or swimming. Biological pollutants include bacteria, viruses, and parasites; their health consequences are usually short-lived. A dangerous biological pollutant is cryptosporidium, a protozoan (single-celled organism) that causes a gastrointestinal disease called cryptosporidiosis. Young children, older adults, and people with immune system deficiency disorders are particularly vulnerable to cryptosporidium infection, which can be fatal.

Compared with biological pollutants, chemical pollutants can cause longer lasting health impairments, including cancer, liver and kidney damage, and birth defects. The main categories of chemical pollutants and their health effects are shown in Table 19.1. For information about water quality in your area, check with your local water supplier or public health department.[1,4]

Safe Drinking Water

Most public water suppliers deliver high-quality drinking water to millions of North Americans. There are more than 55,000 community water systems in the United States, and less than 9 percent of these systems report a violation of one or more health standards each year.[1]

In the United States, the Safe Drinking Water Act (SDWA) of 1974 established many health standards for drinking water. A 1996 amendment to this bill mandated that consumers receive more information about the quality of their drinking water supplies and about efforts by the state and local governments to protect these supplies. It also mandated that violations of health standards with the potential to cause serious health effects must be announced through the media within 24 hours.[2]

About 8 percent of people in the United States, primarily farmers and rural residents, rely on their own private drinking water supplies. Most of this water comes from wells, but some comes from streams and cisterns (water-holding tanks). Owners of private wells are not required to comply with EPA health standards, but people using private water supplies must take special precautions to ensure water safety.[1]

About 1 in 15 households in the United States use bottled water as the main source of drinking water.[2] Bottled water is sold in retail stores, and water dispensers and large bubble containers are delivered to businesses and homes under lease or purchase agreements. Bottled

KEY TERMS

water pollution   Any chemical, biological, or physical change in water quality that has a harmful impact on living organisms or makes water unsuitable for desired use.

Challenges & Choices

You Can Help Conserve Water

Americans use about 100 gallons of water per person a day for domestic purposes—drinking, cooking, washing laundry and dishes, bathing, and flushing toilets. This rate is three times the per capita average for the world as a whole. Here are some tips to help you conserve water:

Bathroom

About 65 percent of residential water is used in the bathroom. The toilet accounts for 40 percent of all water used in the home.

- Install a low-flow toilet, which saves about 30 gallons of water per day.
- Install water-saving showerheads and flow restrictors on all faucets. If you can fill a 1-gallon bucket in 15 seconds, you need a more efficient fixture.
- Turn off sink faucets when brushing your teeth, shaving, or washing. An open faucet sends about 7 gallons of water down the drain every minute.
- Repair leaks promptly. A faucet that leaks one drop a second can waste 200 gallons of water in a month. You can test for toilet leaks by adding a few drops of food coloring to the water in the toilet tank. If you have a leak, some color will show up in the toilet bowl within minutes.

Laundry

About 15 percent of residential water is used in the laundry room.

- When buying a new washing machine, purchase a front-loading machine that fills at different levels for loads of different sizes.
- Wash your clothes only when you have a full load. If you must wash small loads, select the lowest possible water-level setting.
- Buy appliances with an "energy star" label. An energy star washing machine can save up to 7,000 gallons of water a year.
- Check washing machine and hoses regularly for leaks.

Kitchen

About 10 percent of residential water is used for drinking and cooking.

- Run your dishwasher only when you have a full load. Use the short cycle and let your dishes air dry.
- If you wash your dishes by hand, do not let the water run continuously.
- Start a compost pile instead of using a garbage disposal. Garbage disposals and water softener systems use large amounts of water.
- Check regularly for faucet leaks.

Outdoors

About 10 percent of residential water is used outdoors. It takes 27,000 gallons of water a week to keep 1 acre of grass green.

- Water your lawn and plants early in the morning and in the evening, minimizing loss of water through evaporation in the midday heat.
- Install drip irrigation systems for gardens and flowerbeds.
- Landscape with native plants, which adapt to local annual precipitation.
- Wash your car using a bucket for soapy water; use the hose only for rinsing. If you use a commercial car wash, choose one that recycles water.

It's Not Just Personal . . .

The U.S. Geological Survey (www.usgs.gov) estimates that approximately 408 billion gallons of water per day were withdrawn for all uses in the United States in the year 2000. The largest uses were for thermoelectric power and irrigation, with California, Texas, and Florida accounting for about one fourth of all water withdrawals in that year.

Sources: *One Makes the Difference*, by J. B. Hill, 2002, New York: HarperCollins; *Living in the Environment*, by G. T. Miller, 2002, Belmont, CA: Wadsworth/Thomson Learning; U.S. Environmental Protection Agency. *Water on Tap: A Consumer's Guide to the Nation's Drinking Water*, Washington, DC: Office of Water, 1997.

water is just as vulnerable to contamination as tap water, however. Health experts estimate that about one third of bottled water is contaminated with bacteria.[1] Because bottled water is classified as food, it is regulated by the FDA. If you use bottled water, look for the trademark International Bottled Water Association (IBWA) for assurance of contaminant-free water.[2]

Although it is usually not necessary, some people install home water treatment devices to provide additional water safety or to improve water taste. These systems remove impurities from the water through mechanical or chemical filters or both. Home water treatment systems can be very expensive and are neither endorsed nor recommended by the EPA. A simpler and less expensive

Table 19.1	Major Categories of Water Pollutants That Affect Human Health	
Major Categories of Water Pollutants	**Major Human Sources**	**Human Health Effects**
Inorganic chemicals (acids, toxic metals, salts)	Industrial effluent, seepage from mines and lead pipes; fallout from leaded gasoline; runoff from pesticides; pesticide sprays; combustion of mercury-containing fossil fuel.	Skin cancers; abnormal skin pigmentation; cardiovascular disease; damage to nervous system, liver and kidneys.
Organic chemicals (cleaning solvents, petroleum products, plastics, pesticides, detergents)	Industrial effluent, household cleaners; surface runoff from yards and farms; dry-cleaning fluids; paint thinners.	Hepatitis; kidney failure; cancer; reproductive disorders; childhood leukemia; headaches.
Sediment (salt, silt)		Infectious diseases caused by bacteria, viruses, fungi carried in sediment.
Radioactive materials (radon, uranium, isotopes of iodine)	Nuclear power plants; nuclear weapons production; uranium mining; televisions; computers; electromagnetic fields; natural sources.	Cancer; genetic mutations; reproductive disorders; miscarriages.

Source: Data from *Living in the Environment*, by G. T. Miller, 2002, Belmont, CA: Wadsworth/Thomson Learning.

choice made by some consumers is a water filtering device that can be attached to a water pitcher.

In some older homes, contamination from lead water pipes or lead solder on pipes is a concern. Exposure to lead can cause serious health problems, especially in children. To minimize lead exposure, let the water run for a minute or so after turning on the tap; this can flush away lead that may have leached into the water.[2] Cold water is less likely to contain lead that has been leached from supply pipes, so use only cold water for cooking and preparing infant formula. Both lead water pipes and lead solder on pipes have been banned in the United States.

Ensuring a sustainable water supply for ourselves and future generations will require several strategies (see the box "Who Best Conserves Freshwater?"). Consumers and businesses need to use water-saving technologies; farmers and the agriculture industry need to develop ways to irrigate crops more efficiently; and government and policy makers must manage water basins and groundwater fairly and effectively. Such strategies are likely to be controversial and difficult to implement. Failure to address our water-related problems, however, will lead to economic and health problems, increased environmental degradation, and loss of biodiversity.

AIR AND AIR QUALITY

Like water, air is an essential resource that many of us take for granted until it becomes polluted and hazardous to our health.

Earth's Atmosphere

The atmosphere is the whole mass of air surrounding the earth. The innermost layer of atmosphere is called the *troposphere,* or lower atmosphere. This layer contains about 80 percent of the earth's air and extends 11 miles above sea level at the equator and about 5 miles above the poles. The second layer is the *stratosphere,* or upper atmosphere. It extends from 11 to 30 miles above Earth's surface. Ninety-nine percent of the air in the lower atmosphere consists of nitrogen (78 percent) and oxygen (21 percent). The remaining 1 percent consists of carbon dioxide, argon, and trace amounts of several other gases. Composition of gases in the upper atmosphere is similar except there is much less water vapor and much more ozone.[1]

The presence of certain gases in the lower atmosphere helps regulate the earth's temperature by trapping heat from the sun and preventing it from radiating back into space, a process called the **greenhouse effect.** Without the greenhouse effect, the surface of the earth would be much colder and less hospitable to life.[5] The two most important **greenhouse gases** are carbon dioxide and water vapor.

An important component of the upper atmosphere is **ozone,** an odorless, colorless gas composed of three atoms of oxygen. Ozone forms naturally in the upper atmosphere and provides a protective layer that shields us from the sun's harmful ultraviolet (UV) radiation waves. This shield prevents about 95 percent of the sun's UV rays from reaching the earth's surface.[6] Although it is protective in the upper atmosphere, ozone in the lower atmosphere is hazardous to health; ground-level ozone is discussed in the next section.

(a)

Pollutant: Particles
Today's Forecast: 130
Quality: Unhealthy for Sensitive Groups

People with heart or lung disease, older adults, and children are at risk.

Air Quality Index (AQI): Carbon Monoxide (CO)

Index Values	Levels of Health Concern	Cautionary Statements
0 - 50	Good	None
51 - 100*	Moderate	None
101 - 150	Unhealthy for Sensitive Groups	People with heart disease, such as angina, should reduce heavy exertion and avoid sources of CO, such as heavy traffic.
151 - 200	Unhealthy	People with heart disease, such as angina, should reduce moderate exertion and avoid sources of CO, such as heavy traffic.
201 - 300	Very Unhealthy	People with heart disease, such as angina, should reduce exertion and sources of CO, such as heavy traffic.
301 - 500	Hazardous	People with heart disease, such as angina, should reduce exertion and sources of CO, such as heavy traffic. Everyone else should reduce heavy exertion.

*An AQI of 100 for carbon monoxide corresponds to a CO level of 9 parts per million (averaged over 8 hours)

(b)

Figure 19.2   **The EPA's Air Quality Index.** *(a) A sample AQI report in a newspaper. (b) An AQI chart for carbon monoxide.* Source: *Air Quality Index: A Guide to Air Quality and Your Health,* U.S. EPA, 2004, www.epa.gov.

Ozone

As noted earlier, ozone in the upper atmosphere forms a protective shield against dangerous UV radiation from the sun, but at ground level, it is a hazard. Ozone is a highly reactive gas that is poisonous to most living organisms. It causes respiratory irritation, aggravates respiratory and heart disease, and damages the lungs. Physical activity or outdoor work requiring exertion and deep breathing results in deeper penetration of ozone in the lungs. For unknown reasons, about one in three people have an unusual susceptibility to ozone. Also at greater

risk are active children with respiratory disorders (such as asthma), adults with respiratory diseases (such as emphysema), and older adults (because respiratory function declines with age).[1,8]

Particulate Matter

Another hazardous component of air pollution is **particulate matter,** particles or droplets of dust, soot, oil, metals, or other compounds suspended in the air. The measurement unit for these particles is the micron (a human hair is about 70 microns in diameter), and the smaller the particle, the more likely it is to cause health damage. Scientists believe small particles that remain in the lungs for a long time irritate and damage alveoli, the tiny air sacs in the lungs.[1] Ultrafine particles may also trigger an immune system response that alters blood chemistry and blood pressure, contributing to heart disease and lung disease.[7]

Smog

One of the primary sources of outdoor air pollutants is **smog,** a mixture of pollutants in the lower atmosphere that makes the air hazy. There are two types of smog: industrial smog and photochemical smog. **Industrial smog** is caused primarily by the burning of large amounts of coal and oil for heating, manufacturing, and the production of electrical power.[3] This type of smog occurs mostly in cold weather and produces a low-lying layer of pollution close to the earth's surface. Industrial smog is no longer a major problem in most developed countries. Coal and heavy oil are burned only in large furnaces or boiler systems that maintain strict pollution control, and waste gases are removed via tall smokestacks that transfer pollutants to downwind areas. This type of smog is still very much a problem in developing countries, however.

Photochemical smog is the type of smog that sits as a thick haze over many cities in the summer. It forms when pollutants from motor vehicle exhaust, industry, and

KEY TERMS

particulate matter   Particles or droplets of dust, soot, oil, metals, or other compounds suspended in the air.

smog   Mixture of pollutants in the lower atmosphere that makes the air hazy.

industrial smog   Type of air pollution that forms mostly in cold weather and is caused primarily by burning large amounts of coal and oil.

photochemical smog   Type of air pollution that forms when pollutants from motor vehicle exhaust, industry, and other sources combine in the presence of sunlight and heat, producing ozone and more than 100 other chemicals.

Dense population, a climate that is sunny, warm, and dry, and fossil fuels from cars and factories together create photochemical smog. For older adults, children, and individuals with respiratory problems, this type of air pollution can be especially dangerous.

other sources combine in the presence of sunlight and heat, producing large amounts of ozone and more than 100 other chemicals. All modern cities have photochemical smog, but it is much more prevalent in sunny, warm, dry climates with high population density and high use of **fossil fuels** (oil, coal, and natural gas) in transportation and industry.

Photochemical smog problems can be amplified by a temperature inversion.[1] Under normal conditions, the air at the earth's surface is heated by the sun and rises to mix with cool air above it. Surface air is replaced by cooler air that in turn is heated and rises, creating a natural circulation process. In a **temperature inversion,** a warm layer of air moves in over a cooler layer, trapping it so the air cannot circulate. Pollutants at ground level can build up to dangerous levels if the inversion lasts more than a few days.

Some types of topography are particularly favorable to temperature inversions and photochemical smog. A town or city located in a valley surrounded by mountains is susceptible during cold and cloudy seasons because surrounding mountains block out the winter sun. Very large cities with mountains on three sides and the ocean on the other side, extensive automobile use, and a sunny climate with light winds have ideal conditions for temperature inversions and smog. These are the conditions that account for the very high level of photochemical smog in Los Angeles.

The Clean Air Act of 1990 required the EPA to set national emission standards for more than 100 different air pollutants. These standards have led to continued improvements in air quality by encouraging use of public transportation, non-gas-burning automobiles, the use of scrubbers to clean polluted air from smoke stacks, reduced use of fossil fuels, and increased use of renewable energy.[1] In addition, the 2002 Clear Skies Initiative amendment to the 1990 Clean Air Act set mandatory caps

that substantially reduce emissions of sulfur dioxide, nitrogen oxide, and mercury from coal-fired electric power generation.[9] Substantial reductions of ground-level ozone, photochemical smog, and acid deposition are expected by 2010. Individuals can also take steps to improve outdoor air quality; see the box "You Can Help Improve Outdoor Air Quality."

Acid Deposition and Precipitation

Another major source of outdoor air pollutants is **acid deposition,** which occurs when acidic pollutants drop out of the atmosphere onto the earth's surface. The two major pollutants involved in acid deposition are sulfur dioxide from coal-burning power plants and nitrogen dioxide from motor vehicle emissions. Acid deposition can be dry or wet. Dry deposition occurs when acidic gases and particulate matter are blown by winds onto buildings, homes, cars, and trees or washed from surface areas by rainstorms. Dry deposition causes damage to stone, metal, and paint and necessitates repair to public monuments and buildings totaling millions of dollars every year. Dry deposition accounts for nearly half of the acid deposition falling from the atmosphere.[10]

Wet deposition, or **acid precipitation,** occurs when acidic pollutants mix with moisture in the atmosphere and fall to earth as acid rain, snow, sleet, hail, or fog. This type of acid deposition has devastated lakes, streams, and forests in certain parts of the world, killing trees, fish, and aquatic wildlife. The pollutants in acid precipitation also cause respiratory problems in vulnerable individuals.

The degree of environmental damage from acid deposition depends on the ability of the soil to neutralize acid. Where soils are alkaline, such as in parts of the U.S. Midwest, there is less damage from acid precipitation. Where soils are neutral or acidic, as in the northwestern

Challenges & Choices

You Can Help Improve Outdoor Air Quality

Small changes in individual behaviors and lifestyles can add up to big changes in greenhouse gas emissions. If these small changes were multiplied by the 306 million people in North America or the 6 billion people worldwide, the effects could be enormous.

- Walk, bike, skate, carpool, or use public transportation instead of driving your car. Each gallon of gas used by a car contributes about 20 pounds of carbon dioxide to the atmosphere.

- Get regular tune-ups for your car. A well-running car produces about 475 fewer pounds of carbon dioxide than a poorly tuned car.

- Check your tires to make sure they are inflated to the right pressure. When tires are properly inflated, your car uses less gas.

- Make sure your car's air conditioner isn't leaking chemicals, and limit your use of it to only the hottest days.

- If you are buying a car, consider an electric or a hybrid car that does not rely heavily on gasoline. If you don't get a hybrid, look for a car that gets good gas mileage.

- Don't top off the tank when refueling your vehicle. Spilled fuel evaporates and contributes to air pollution.

- Turn down your home heating thermostat by at least 1 degree. You can cut energy consumption by as much as 10 percent for each degree.

- Buy the most energy-efficient homes, lights, and appliances available. Use compact fluorescent bulbs in lamps; they cost more than regular incandescent light bulbs but last much longer. Lighting accounts for about 20 percent of the total electricity used in the United States; refrigerators consume about 7 percent of total electricity.

- Turn down the thermostat on your water heater to between 110 and 120° F. Insulate hot water pipes. Hot water heaters consume about 20 percent of all energy used in a home.

- Keep houseplants to help clean the air in your home, and plant shade trees outside.

It's Not Just Personal . . .

The U.S. Environmental Protection Agency (www.epa.gov) notes that significant air pollution is transported between nations via weather changes. In the summer months, upper air winds allow for the transport of airborne pollutants to the United States from Mexico and Central America.

Sources: *Living in the Environment,* by G. T. Miller, 2002, Belmont, CA: Wadsworth/Thomson Learning; Clear Skies Initiative, U.S. EPA, www.epa.gov.

United States, northeastern North America, and many parts of Canada and Europe, damage is extensive. According to the EPA National Surface Water Survey of 9,000 lakes in the United States, many lakes in the upper Midwest and Northeast are threatened with excess acidity.[1]

The coal and automobile industries question the seriousness of the acid deposition problem in North America. They claim that there is no reliable evidence that levels of acid deposition have increased, that acid deposition causes serious health problems or environmental damage, or that coal and automobile emissions are a primary source of acid deposition.

Thinning of the Ozone Layer of the Atmosphere

Every spring and early summer, a massive "hole" appears in the ozone layer of the atmosphere over Antarctica. In 2000, this hole was three times the size of the continental United States.[11] This thinning of the ozone layer is caused

KEY TERMS

fossil fuels Oil, coal, and natural gas—fuels that were produced over the course of millions of years by the pressure and heat of the earth acting on the buried remains of plants and animals containing carbon; they are typically extracted from the earth by drilling.

temperature inversion Weather condition in which a warm layer of air moves in over a cooler layer, trapping pollutants in the air near the earth's surface.

acid deposition Depositing of acidic pollutants from the atmosphere on the earth's surface, in either dry or wet form.

acid precipitation Mixing of acidic pollutants in the atmosphere with moisture and their precipitation in the form of rain, snow, sleet, hail, or fog.

by **chlorofluorocarbons (CFCs),** chemicals used as coolants in refrigeration and air conditioning units, as propellants in aerosol sprays, as solvents in cleaning products, and as foaming agents in some rigid foam products.[12] When these chemicals are released or leak into the air, they slowly rise into the upper atmosphere, where chlorine atoms destroy ozone.

Without the protection of the ozone layer, humans are at risk for more severe sunburns, more skin cancers, more cataracts (clouding of the lens in the eye, causing blindness), and suppression of the immune system, which increases the risk for infectious diseases.[1,12] Estimates by the United Nations Environment Program predict that a 10 percent thinning of the ozone layer would cause an additional 300,000 cases of nonmelanoma skin cancer worldwide, 4,500 additional cases of malignant melanoma, and 1.5 million additional cases of cataracts annually.[1]

International agreements under the 1989 Montreal Protocol and subsequent treaties called for the reduction and eventual elimination of CFC production by 2000. This protocol is currently supported by 160 nations. However, because it takes CFCs 11 years to 20 years to reach the upper atmosphere, it will be at least 50 years before the ozone layer begins to recover.[1] In the meantime, the hole continues to grow. During certain times of the year, it extends into populated areas of South America and Australia, and people living there are advised to stay indoors during critical periods and wear sunscreen and hats when they go outdoors.

Global Warming

As noted earlier, the temperature of the earth's surface is regulated by a natural process called the greenhouse effect. For the past few hundred years, human activities have increased the amount of greenhouse gases in the lower atmosphere. These activities—burning fossil fuels, burning forests, cultivating cropland, raising cattle and other livestock on a mass basis, producing fertilizers, creating landfills—have significantly increased levels of carbon dioxide, methane, nitrous oxide, ozone, and other greenhouse gases. The intensification of the greenhouse effect has led to **global warming,** a gradual rise in the average temperature of the earth's surface.

According to the National Academy of Sciences, the surface temperature of the earth has risen 1.1–1.3° F in the past century, but research suggests that most global warming has taken place in the last 50 years. The 10 warmest years on record all occurred between 1985 and 2000; 1998 was the warmest year on record. Additional signs of global warming include melting of the ice caps and of glaciers, northward migration of some warm-climate fish, the bleaching of coral found in tropical areas, and the rise of sea levels by 4 to 8 inches over the past century. Scientists project that global temperatures could rise 1.0–4.5° F by 2050 and 2.2–10.0° F by the close of the 21st century.[1,12–15]

Predicted Effects of Global Warming

Agriculture, water resources, forests, wildlife, and coastal areas are all vulnerable to the effects of global warming and the climate changes it can cause. An increase in temperature of a few degrees could cause flooding in coastal cities as seas rise and affect the availability of fresh water by changing rates of precipitation and evaporation. Storms would become more frequent and intense, and some areas would receive more rain while others became drier. These changes would affect the kinds of food that could be grown and shift the nature of agriculture throughout the world. Crop damage could increase because agricultural pests and diseases flourish in warmer weather.[1,16,17] (For more on weather changes, see the box "El Niño and La Niña.")

Global warming is likely to have many adverse impacts on health, with significant loss of life. More frequent and severe heat waves would cause more heat-related deaths and illnesses. Air quality would decline, because pollution is worse in warmer weather. Older adults and people with cardiovascular and respiratory disorders would be particularly vulnerable to adverse health effects of global warming.[18,19]

What Can Be Done?

To address global climate change, 38 nations signed the Kyoto Protocol, a United Nations–sponsored international agreement, in 1997. The protocol called for nations to cut their emissions of greenhouse gases, particularly carbon dioxide, by about 5.2 percent below 1990 levels by 2012. This market-based treaty allows countries and private companies to trade and sell their greenhouse gas emission allowances to other countries and businesses. It also encourages private companies to develop new technologies that reduce greenhouse gas emissions.

The Kyoto Protocol was to take effect when ratified by 55 countries responsible for 55 percent of global greenhouse gas emissions. The United States signed the treaty in 1998 but withdrew in 2001, citing insufficiently conclusive evidence of global warming and potential strain on the economy, including probable job losses. Although 120 nations had signed the protocol by 2004, the nonparticipation of the United States, by far the greatest producer of greenhouse gases in the world, was a serious obstacle to its success. The United States has introduced its own emissions reduction plan for the nation, which calls for voluntary participation by all sectors of the economy. This plan was signed into law by the U.S. Senate in 2002.

Substantial reduction in carbon dioxide emissions will require massive changes in industrial processes, transportation, energy sources, and personal lifestyles.[3] Cost estimates to meet standards run into the billions of dollars, to be shouldered not just by businesses but also by consumers through higher car prices, higher gas prices, and costlier car maintenance to meet federal emission controls. One promising approach to the problem is the

HIGHLIGHT ON HEALTH
El Niño and La Niña

Every 2 to 7 years, the southern Pacific Ocean is affected by a climate pattern called El Niño (so named because it usually occurs around Christmas, the birthday of "El Niño," the Christ child). El Niño occurs when prevailing western winds cease or weaken and surface water off the coast of South America increases in temperature. This disruption in normal patterns causes widespread weather and climate changes, including increased rainfall and flooding in South America and the southern United States and drought in Indonesia and Australia.

If El Niño lasts 12 months or longer, it can cause severe weather changes over much of the planet, including heat waves, prolonged droughts, flooding, and violent storms. The 1997–98 El Niño was the strongest episode in the past 200 years; it occurred just 14 years after the second strongest, recorded in 1982–83. During these years, California was lashed by storms and mudslides, and countries in Africa experienced drought-related famines. Less strong episodes occurred in 1991–92, 1993, and 1994, an unusually frequent recurrence of this pattern.

La Niña is the counterpart of El Niño, bringing cooler temperatures to the southern Pacific and often occurring in the year following an El Niño episode.

Among the weather and climate effects of La Niña are more hurricanes in the Atlantic Ocean, colder winters in northeastern United States and Canada, warmer and drier conditions in the southwestern and southeastern United States, cooler and wetter winters in the Pacific Northwest, and conditions conducive to wildfires in Florida. A strong La Niña occurred in 1998–99, following the strong El Niño in 1997–98.

El Niño-related disasters like floods, droughts, and wildfires have caused thousands of deaths worldwide and billions of dollars' worth of damage. Advances in oceanographic and atmospheric monitoring systems have allowed scientists to predict these weather patterns more accurately, giving people a chance to prepare (for example, by planting drought-resistant crops). Some climate models suggest that global warming promotes more frequent occurrences of El Niño episodes, causing more unusual, violent, and destructive weather patterns around the world. Whether we are experiencing naturally occurring cycles or human-induced change remains to be seen.

Sources: What Is an El Niño? National Oceanic and Atmospheric Administration, U.S. Department of Commerce, www.pmel.noaa.gov; *Living in the Environment*, by G. T. Miller, 2002, Belmont, CA: Wadsworth/Thomson Learning; "Is El Niño Now a Man-Made Phenomenon?" by A. Galtie, 1999, *The Ecologist, 29* (2), 64–67.

promotion of hybrid gas-electric cars and cars with high fuel economy and low emissions. It has been estimated that hybrid gas-electric cars could reduce the pollution that causes global warming by at least one third.[20] Increasing fuel economy standards for new cars and light trucks to a combined 40 miles per gallon would eventually reduce carbon dioxide emissions by more than 650 million tons each year as these vehicles replace older models.[12]

At the same time, the sport utility vehicle trend needs to be reversed. Because of a loophole in the law, these fuel-inefficient vehicles do not have to meet the same energy efficiency standards as passenger cars. SUVs are responsible for a 20 percent increase in transportation-related carbon dioxide emissions from the early 1990s, when they made up 5 percent of U.S. cars, to 2003, when they accounted for nearly 55 percent.[12]

Although the vast majority of climate experts have concluded that global warming is a potentially significant problem, some scientists believe there is still insufficient research on natural climate variables that increase or decrease the average temperature of the earth's surface. They point out that computer models used to predict climate change are improving but are still not reliable.[1,12]

Businesses affected by the cost of reducing greenhouse gas emissions are hesitant to do so until consensus is reached by atmospheric scientists.

Indoor Air Pollution

Levels of air pollution indoors can be higher and more hazardous than levels of air pollution outside. On average, Americans spend between 80 and 90 percent of their time indoors.[21] Spending extensive time indoors magnifies health risks from indoor air pollutants, possibly to 50 times the health risks experienced outdoors. Eleven of the

KEY TERMS

chlorofluorocarbons (CFCs) Chemicals used as coolants, propellants, solvents, and foaming agents that destroy ozone in the upper atmosphere.

global warming Gradual rise in the average temperature of the earth's surface, believed to be caused by an increase in greenhouse gases in the lower atmosphere.

most common air pollutants are usually two to five times higher inside the home than outside.[1] The EPA estimates that exposure to indoor air pollutants causes 6,000 cases of cancer every year in the United States.[21]

Indoor air pollution can be more of a threat than outdoor air pollution for three reasons. First, the limited volume of air indoors causes higher concentrations of air pollutants per breath. Second, there is less exchange with fresh air indoors than outdoors. And third, elevated levels of humidity and dampness indoors are ideal environments for biological organisms, such as mold and mildew.[22]

Pollutants inside the home include allergens, such as dust mites and animal dander; mold and mildew; and chemicals, usually as fumes or vapors (Figure 19.3). You can reduce many of the biological pollutants (allergens, mold, bacteria) by keeping the house clean, keeping pets clean, washing bedding weekly, and maintaining the relative humidity between 30 and 50 percent. According to the EPA, the most dangerous indoor air pollutants are environmental tobacco smoke (discussed in Chapter 12), formaldehyde, radon, carbon monoxide, mold, and polybrominated diphenyl ethers.[21]

Formaldehyde

Formaldehyde is a colorless gas that is commonly used in the construction of household materials, such as furniture, drapes, and fiberboard. Vapors can seep out of these materials into the home. Daily exposures to this irritating gas can cause chronic breathing problems, dizziness, skin rash, headaches, sore throat, sinus infections, and eye irritation.[23]

Radon

Colorless, odorless, and tasteless, **radon** is a radioactive gas that occurs naturally in some soils, rocks, and building materials. It can seep into homes through dirt floors and cracks in foundations. When it becomes attached to dust particles, radon can be inhaled. It has been definitively linked to lung cancer but not other respiratory diseases, such as asthma.[24] Your chances of getting lung cancer from radon exposure depend on the level of radon in your home, the amount of time you spend in your home, and whether you are a smoker or an ex-smoker. Smokers and ex-smokers already have lung tissue damage that makes them more susceptible to radon-related lung cancer.[1]

The EPA recommends radon testing for all homes and for condominiums and apartments below the third-floor level of building complexes. Cracks in foundations should be sealed and fans installed to increase cross-ventilation.[24] If you are interested in finding a qualified radon professional, contact your state radon office or the National Environmental Health Association (NEHA).

Carbon Monoxide

As noted earlier, carbon monoxide is a colorless, odorless, tasteless gas produced by the incomplete burning of fuels

Healthy People 2010

OBJECTIVE AREA *Environmental Health*

• Reduce indoor allergen levels.

"Indoor allergens—such as from house dust mites, cockroaches, mold, rodents, and pets—can worsen symptoms of respiratory conditions, such as asthma and allergies. These allergens are an important public health issue because most people spend the majority of their time indoors, both at home and at work. In addition, effective methods to reduce exposure to some of these allergens exist (for example, placement of impermeable covers on mattresses and pillows reduces dust mite allergen exposures in beds)."

For more information on Healthy People 2010 objectives, visit the Web site at www.healthypeople.gov.

For more information on Canadian health objectives, visit the Health Canada Web site at www.hc-sc.gc.ca/english.

containing carbon. This gas impairs the transport of oxygen in the blood. Symptoms of carbon monoxide poisoning include mental confusion, irregular heartbeat, dizziness, blurred vision, mild nausea, and headache. Severe poisoning can cause seizures, coma, and death. Fetuses and very young children are especially vulnerable to the toxic effects of carbon monoxide.

High concentrations of carbon monoxide indoors are very dangerous. Gas stoves, space heaters, furnaces, fireplaces, wood-burning stoves, and cigarette smoke are common sources. Carbon monoxide detectors are widely available in stores, but they are not considered as reliable as smoke detectors because the technology is still developing. Preventing elevated levels of carbon monoxide is safer than relying on a detector, but if you decide to purchase a detector, look for certification by the American Gas Association and Underwriters Laboratories.[25] Purchase reliable brands and make sure your home is well ventilated. If you or family members experience symptoms of carbon monoxide poisoning, turn off combustion appliances and leave the contaminated area immediately. If the symptoms are serious, go to a hospital emergency center.

KEY TERMS

radon Radioactive gas that occurs naturally in some soils, rocks, and building materials and is hazardous to human health.

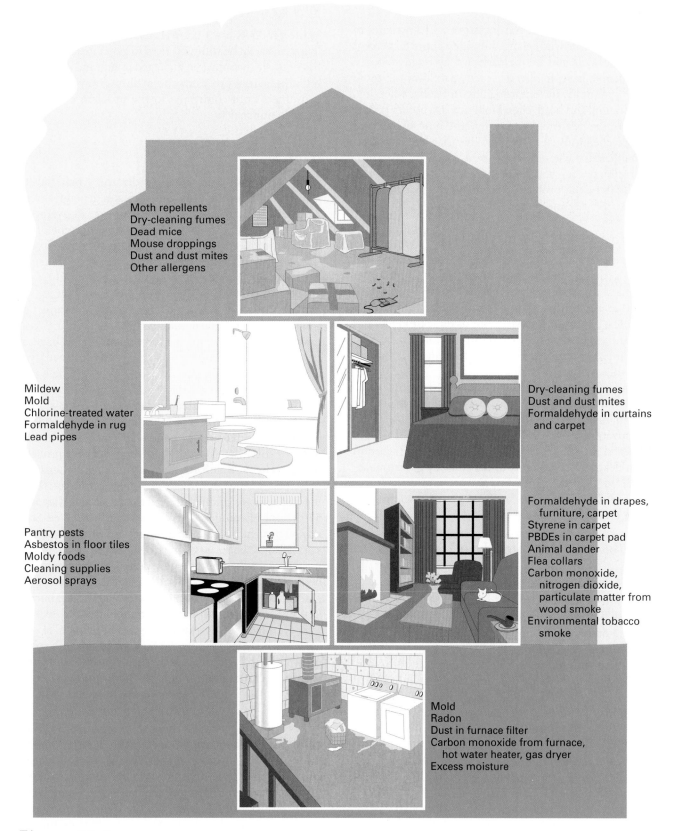

Moth repellents
Dry-cleaning fumes
Dead mice
Mouse droppings
Dust and dust mites
Other allergens

Mildew
Mold
Chlorine-treated water
Formaldehyde in rug
Lead pipes

Dry-cleaning fumes
Dust and dust mites
Formaldehyde in curtains
    and carpet

Pantry pests
Asbestos in floor tiles
Moldy foods
Cleaning supplies
Aerosol sprays

Formaldehyde in drapes,
    furniture, carpet
Styrene in carpet
PBDEs in carpet pad
Animal dander
Flea collars
Carbon monoxide,
    nitrogen dioxide,
    particulate matter from
    wood smoke
Environmental tobacco
    smoke

Mold
Radon
Dust in furnace filter
Carbon monoxide from furnace,
    hot water heater, gas dryer
Excess moisture

Figure 19.3   Common sources of indoor air pollution.

Mold

Molds are fungi; they need moisture and nutrients to thrive. Basements with relative humidity above 60 percent often have walls and floors blackened by mold colonies. Some people have an allergic reaction to airborne mold spores; symptoms include coughing, sneezing, wheezing, eye irritation, and headaches. Mold can also bother people without allergies; mold spores inflame lung tissues and produce chemicals called mycotoxins that are hazardous when inhaled. If you regularly sneeze, cough, or have trouble breathing when you are in certain parts of your home, mold may be the problem. You may need to consult an expert to identify and remove sources of mold.

Polybrominated Diphenyl Ethers (PBDEs)

PBDEs are flame retardant chemicals used in plastic and foam products, such as furniture cushions and carpet pads; hard casings for televisions, telephones, computers, and other electronic equipment; and insulation for cables and wires. PBDEs seep or leach out of these products and enter the environment, showing up in house dust, soil, and plants and animals. They have been found in human breast milk, tissue, and blood.

The major health concern is that PBDEs can accumulate in human tissue and may cause chromosome abnormalities. House dust can collect PBDEs at high concentration levels. Children who spend a lot of time at floor level are at greater risk for exposure by ingestion and inhalation.[24] PBDEs are under study by government-sponsored scientific endeavors, and some manufacturers of computers and office equipment have voluntarily stopped using them in their products.

"Sick Building" and "Sick House" Syndromes

Some newer buildings and houses are built to be airtight, with insulation and windows that prevent the flow of air in and out of the structure. This lack of ventilation prevents the diffusion of pollutants and moisture out of the building and allows a buildup of contaminants. Common sources of pollutants are carpets, furniture made from fiberboard, furnaces, fireplaces, and excessive moisture. Symptoms of "sick building" syndrome and "sick house" syndrome can include coughing, wheezing, congestion, dry or itchy skin, dizziness, nausea, headache, fatigue, difficulty concentrating, and eye, nose, or throat irritation.

In commercial buildings, solutions to the problem include identifying and removing the source of pollution, cleaning the air, and improving ventilation.[21] Several strategies can help in homes: replacing filters in furnaces, making sure fans and air conditioning units are clean and operating correctly, running the fan in the bathroom while showering, leaving windows open when new furniture, carpeting, or drapes are installed, and improving ventilation throughout the house.

WASTE MANAGEMENT

Waste products are a natural outcome of the process of living on earth, but humans tend to generate large quantities of waste that must be managed in safe and satisfactory ways. Industrial processes and a "throwaway" attitude by consumers both contribute to the problem of excessive waste in our society.

Solid Waste

Solid waste is any unwanted or discarded material that is not a liquid or gas. The United States generates nearly 12 billion tons of solid waste each year, an average of 97,000 pounds per person. Ninety-nine percent of this waste is produced by mining, oil and natural gas production, agriculture, and industrial activities. The remaining 1 percent is municipal solid waste, commonly called garbage and refuse, from businesses and homes. The United States leads the world in garbage production, generating about 1,600 pounds per person per year. Canada ranks third.[1,26] The main components of garbage are paper products (including packaging and junk mail), yard waste, plastics, metals, glass, and wood. Food waste is not a major contributor to garbage because most is processed in garbage disposals and directed into sewage systems.

Methods of managing solid waste have traditionally included burning, burying, and shipping wastes to other states or countries. Most of these methods were problematic and are now subject to numerous regulations. The principal method of dealing with solid waste today is burying it in sanitary landfills; this method is used to dispose of 54 percent of municipal solid waste in the United States and 80 percent in Canada.[1] **Sanitary landfills** are carefully selected sites where waste is buried, sometimes in plastic-lined containers or pits; they are designed to prevent leaching into water supplies and soil for at least 10 to 40 years.

A second method of dealing with solid waste is burning it in large city incinerators. Temperatures inside these incinerators exceed 1800° F, which prevents air pollution. In some cases, energy generated by the burning of refuse is sold as electricity to offset the cost of the incinerators, a waste management technique called waste-to-energy recovery.[1]

Hazardous Waste

Hazardous waste is any discarded solid or liquid material that meets one or more of four criteria: (1) the material contains a toxic, carcinogenic, or mutagenic compound at levels that exceed EPA safety standards (for example, solvents, pesticides); (2) it catches fire easily (for example, gasoline, oil-based paints); (3) it is reactive or unstable enough to explode or release toxic fumes (for example, chlorine, chlorine bleach); or (4) it corrodes metal containers (for example, drain cleaners, industrial cleaners).[1] The EPA estimates that 12 trillion tons of hazardous material

HIGHLIGHT ON HEALTH

Safety Advisory on Mercury in Fish

Mercury is a metal that can damage the brain and nervous system, causing such symptoms as impaired vision and hearing, tingling and numbness in the limbs, and mobility problems. Mercury consumed by pregnant women crosses the placental barrier and can damage the developing nervous system of the fetus. It has also been implicated as a carcinogen.

Today, mercury levels in more than 750,000 miles of river in the United States and 13 billion acres of lakes are high enough to pose health problems for fetuses and children. Much of it entered the environment from coal-burning power plants and mining operations. Mercury is very persistent in the environment and is metabolized very slowly when ingested. A person who has consumed mercury metabolizes 50 percent of it every 2 months; after 8 months, roughly 6 percent of the mercury will still be present in the person's body. If a woman consumes mercury and becomes pregnant, her fetus will be exposed to the toxin throughout the pregnancy.

Nearly all fish and shellfish contain traces of mercury, and some contain higher levels. For these reasons, the FDA and the EPA have issued advisories about fish consumption for women who are pregnant, considering pregnancy, or breast-feeding, and for young children. Individuals in these groups should not eat any shark, swordfish, king mackerel, or tilefish; these fish contain high levels of mercury. They can eat up to 12 ounces per week of fish and shellfish that are lower in mercury, such as shrimp, canned light tuna, salmon, pollock, and catfish. Only 6 ounces of this weekly allotment should be albacore tuna. They can also eat up to 6 ounces of fish caught in local waters if no safety advisories are issued, but no other fish should be eaten in the same week. Older children and adults may also want to limit their consumption of the fish with the highest mercury levels.

Sources: What You Need to Know About Mercury in Fish and Shellfish, U.S. EPA, www.epa.gov; *Risk: A Practical Guide for Deciding What's Really Safe and What's Really Dangerous in the World Around You,* by D. Ropeic and G. Gray, 2002, Boston: Houghton Mifflin.

are produced each year in the United States, about 44,000 pounds per person.[26] The top five chemical compounds of concern are arsenic, lead, mercury, vinyl chloride, and polychlorinated biphenyls, or PCBs (used to insulate electrical transformers). (See the box "Safety Advisory on Mercury in Fish.") Nearly 75 percent of the world's hazardous wastes is generated by the United States.[1]

Direct exposure to hazardous waste poses health hazards, whether it is touched, inhaled, or ingested. Safe handling measures have significantly reduced direct exposure to hazardous waste, but indirect exposure occurs when wastes leak from sanitary landfills and contaminate water supplies. Such leaks are suspected of causing cancer, respiratory diseases, neurological damage, developmental deficits, and other health problems in people in neighboring communities.

Today, federal laws drastically restrict the storage of hazardous waste in sanitary landfills.[26] Much of it is stored in ponds, pits, buildings, and specialized hazardous landfills or disposed of by injection into deep underground wells. Shipment of hazardous waste to disposal sites is also a concern. Each year there are about 13,000 crashes or incidents involving trucks and trains carrying hazardous waste. These incidents, on average, kill about 100 people, seriously injure 10,000 people, and require evacuation of more than 500,000 people from their communities.[1]

Household Hazardous Waste

Hazardous waste is also generated in the home. It is estimated that the average home accumulates about 100 pounds of household hazardous waste (HHW) annually.[26] This waste includes batteries, paints, cleaners, oils, and pesticides, often stored in closets, basements, and garages. These products pose serious health threats. Pesticides, for example, are responsible for an estimated 110,000 cases of poisoning every year as a result of misuse or unsafe storage, as well as about 20 deaths, mostly

KEY TERMS

solid waste Any unwanted or discarded material that is not a liquid or gas; garbage.

sanitary landfills Carefully selected sites where waste is buried, sometimes in plastic-lined containers or pits; they are designed to prevent leaching into water supplies and soil for at least 10 to 40 years.

hazardous waste Any discarded solid or liquid material that contains a toxic, carcinogenic, or mutagenic compound at levels that exceed EPA safety standards; catches fire easily; is reactive or unstable enough to explode or release toxic fumes; or corrodes metal containers.

HIGHLIGHT ON HEALTH
Alternatives to Household Pesticides

Americans use about 17 pounds of pesticides per person each year. About 21,000 different pesticide products are registered by the EPA. Pesticide use has increased more than 50-fold since 1950. Most of today's pesticides are 10 times more toxic than their pre-1950 predecessors. The EPA estimates that 84 percent of homes in the United States use some type of pesticide, such as pet flea collars and pest strips.

By definition, pests are a nuisance, whether flies in the kitchen, ants in the bathroom, rats in the attic, or fleas on pets. However, many chemical pesticides pose health hazards, including poisoning and increased risk of cancer, that are far more problematic than the pests themselves. Total elimination of pests is difficult or impossible, but pests can be controlled. An approach called Integrated Pest Management involves selecting the most effective and most economical control that also causes the least possible harm to humans and the environment. Sometimes, this might involve using a pesticide, but in many other cases, alternative controls can be found.

If you are faced with a pest infestation in your home or garden, try using natural chemicals and plant products instead of chemical pesticides. For example, you can discourage ants by sprinkling red pepper flakes or crushed mint leaves on their trails and wiping countertops with vinegar. Mosquitoes and flies are repelled by basil growing outside windows and doors, and mosquitoes are less likely to bite if you rub a bit of lime juice on your skin and avoid using scented soaps and lotions. Boric acid sprinkled under sinks and kitchen appliances and in closets and other warm, dark places reduces the appeal of these spots to insects, and desiccant powders sprinkled on carpets helps get rid of fleas. *A word of caution:* Some natural products, such as boric acid, are poisonous and should not be used in households with children or pets.

Besides natural products, you can use a biological control, such as a pest's natural predator, or a manual control, such as a flyswatter. Use organic farming techniques, such as raised beds and companion planting, to reduce the impact of garden pests on flowers and vegetables in home gardens. Biological and manual approaches eliminate the possibility that pests will develop genetic resistance to a control, and they are safe and usually longer lasting than chemical pesticides.

Prevention of pest infestations in the first place is also important. Different strategies are needed for indoor and outdoor pests. Indoor strategies include eliminating any sources of water that attract pests (for example, leaky faucets, damp materials), storing food in sealed containers and keeping your kitchen clean, emptying the garbage frequently, sealing cracks and other openings where pests could enter your home, and bathing pets frequently. Outdoor strategies include removing or destroying pest hiding places, such as woodpiles, thick vegetation, or fallen leaves or fruit; removing breeding sites, such as standing water; and maintaining your outdoor plants' health to reduce the need for pest control.

Source: *Living in the Environment,* by G. T. Miller, 2002, Belmont, CA: Wadsworth/Thomson Learning; Pesticides: Frequently Asked Questions, U.S. EPA, www.epa.gov; *Citizen's Guide to Pest Control and Pesticide Safety,* U.S. EPA (Publication No. 730-K-95-001), 1995.

among children. Farmworkers suffer the most from pesticide poisoning. About 25 farmworkers die each year in the United States, and nearly 300,000 suffer pesticide-related illness.[27] For ways to reduce the use of pesticides in the home, see the box "Alternatives to Household Pesticides."

Disposal of HHW is also a problem. When poured down drains or toilets, HHW can contaminate septic systems or wastewater treatment systems. When poured onto the ground or into storm drains, it can contaminate groundwater or flow to local lakes and streams. Improperly stored HHW poses a hazard to children and pets. Disposing of HHW in the trash not only causes environmental damage but poses a threat to the health of sanitation workers. Many communities offer special collection days for HHW or have permanent collection or exchange facilities available.

Medical Waste

The EPA has specific regulations pertaining to **medical waste,** any solid or liquid waste that is generated in the medical diagnosis, treatment, or immunization of human beings or animals. It includes used needles and syringes, used culture dishes and other glassware, discarded surgical gloves, blood and blood products, tissue samples, and any materials contaminated by contact with such products. The American Hospital Association estimates that the typical hospital generates 25 pounds of waste per day per patient bed. About 20 percent of this waste is considered infectious.[28] Medical waste disposal is strictly regulated by the states to prevent the spread of bloodborne pathogens and infectious disease. Public exposure to medical waste is very rare due to these regulations.

Radiation and Radioactive Waste

Low-level radiation is used in medical and dental procedures, such as chest X-rays, dental X-rays, nuclear medicine diagnosis, and radiation therapy. Although these uses have contributed to improvements in health in some areas, exposure to X-rays should be limited. Recently, concern has grown about other sources of low-level radiation, such as televisions, computer monitors, microwave ovens, and cell phones. These devices do emit low levels of radiation, but research has so far been inclusive on their health effects, if any.[1]

Disposal of radioactive waste is problematic. Waste with low levels of radioactivity, such as radioactive isotopes used in medicine, is often disposed of in landfills and near-surface burials, an approach that may lead to contamination of groundwater. High-level radioactive waste is generated by the production of nuclear weapons and the operation of nuclear power plants. This waste has to be sealed deep in mined geologic repositories in the earth.[1] A site in the Yucca Mountains of Nevada has been designed as a storage site for nuclear waste and will be opened for use sometime after 2010. High-level radioactivity is dangerous for tens of thousands of years; developing deposit sites that can offer this kind of protection is a challenge that has to be faced by the United States and other world powers.

Approaches to Waste Management: Recycling and More

Most citizens do not want landfills, incinerators, and hazardous waste repositories located in their communities. This understandable "not in my backyard" attitude frustrates waste management operators and government officials. Many citizens argue that the real problem is not where to dispose of waste but how to stop producing so much of it.[1]

Many communities have established recycling programs to help address the problem of excessive waste. **Recycling** is a circle, or loop, program in which materials that would otherwise be discarded are collected, sorted, cleaned, and processed into raw materials to make new products. Today, the United States has the highest recycling rate of any industrialized country. Americans recycle 28 percent of their waste, a rate that has doubled in the last 15 years.[1]

Methods of collection and processing recyclables vary from one community to the next. Many communities provide curbside pickup of paper, glass, metals, certain types of plastics, and yard material. In other communities, people take recyclable items to drop-off centers or sell them to buyback centers. Many states have deposit/refund programs to encourage recycling of beverage containers made of glass or aluminum. Communities with these laws report that 90 percent of glass and can beverage containers are returned.[29] Despite the popularity and success of recycling programs, they have their opponents; the issue of whether recycling makes sense is discussed in the You Make the Call feature at the end of the chapter.

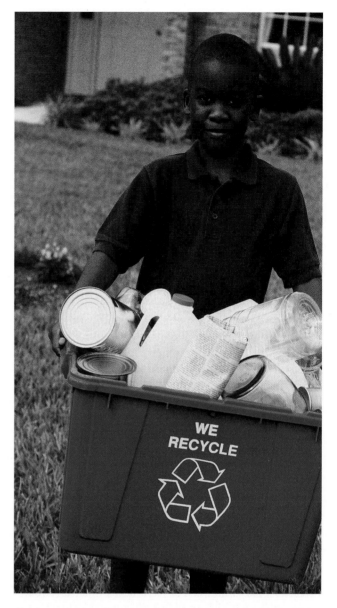

Many communities offer services for recycling of newspapers, cans and bottles, and yard waste. Customers pay a reasonable fee for this service, which may include the use of containers, and enjoy the convenience of having their recyclables picked up at their home.

Besides recycling household items, individuals can take many other actions to help control and prevent waste. These include buying recyclable, reusable, or compostable

KEY TERMS

medical waste   Any solid or liquid waste generated in the medical diagnosis, treatment, or immunization of human beings or animals.

recycling   Circle, or loop, program in which materials that would otherwise be discarded are collected, sorted, cleaned, and processed into raw materials to make new products.

products; composting yard trimmings; using rechargeable batteries; using reusable cloth bags for grocery shopping; reducing use of paper towels and other paper products; buying products with as little Styrofoam, cardboard, or paper packaging as possible; and stopping junk mail by contacting the Direct Marketing Association (see the Web Resources at the end of the chapter).

ECOSYSTEMS AND BIODIVERSITY

An **ecosystem** is an interconnected community of organisms living together in a physical environment as a balanced, mutually supportive system. A frog pond in a meadow is an ecosystem; so is our planet. **Biodiversity,** or biological diversity, is the variety of different animal and plant species on earth, numbering in the millions, and the genetic variation in their gene pools—the material used in the process of evolution when changing environmental conditions require that species adapt or die out.[3]

An ecologically and biologically diverse planet offers innumerable benefits to humans. Twenty-five percent of medicines used in North America are derived from natural substances contained in plants and animals.[30] Choices in food, fuel, and lumber are enhanced by the variety of life-forms on the planet. Wild areas provide abundant opportunities for recreation, retreat, and refreshment. Most importantly, natural ecosystems promote the health of the planet, playing a role in climate maintenance, water cycling, soil production, waste disposal, and pest control.

Unfortunately, human activities have significantly disrupted these ecosystems and caused a decline in biodiversity. Nearly 50 percent of the earth's land surface has been disturbed or degraded by human activities.[1] Forests, grasslands, and wetlands have been converted for urban expansion and agricultural, industrial, and recreational use. Every year, hundreds of plant and animal species become extinct, and thousands more are at risk of extinction. The processes involved in this pattern of disruption include deforestation, desertification, and loss of freshwater resources.

Deforestation

Deforestation is the removal of trees from a forested area without adequate replanting. When trees are cut down faster than they are replaced, forests become a nonrenewable resource. In the past 8,000 years, human activity has reduced the world's forests by about 46 percent, mostly in the past 3 decades.[1]

In North America, the size and health of forests have been slightly improved since 1920 by reforestation. Some ecologists believe, however, that replacing **old-growth forests** (those that have flourished for several hundred years without interference by human activities or natural disasters) with **second-growth forests** (those that have been replanted following human activities or natural disasters) causes an overall reduction in biodiversity. Others claim that national parks and forests, tree farms, and lumber companies' reforestation programs are sufficient to preserve forest biodiversity. Year-round recreational use of national forests, including use of snowmobiles and all-terrain vehicles, hiking, mountain biking, cross-country skiing, camping, swimming, and hunting, also threatens the natural habitats of animals and plants. Heavy use of national forests results in noise, litter, pollution, and vandalism.[1]

In tropical areas of the world—in Africa, Asia, and Central and South America—deforestation has resulted in significant declines in tropical forests. About 90 percent of forest loss is occurring in tropical forests. Although tropical forests make up only 6 percent of the world's land, they are home to between 50 and 90 percent of all terrestrial species. At present deforestation rates, 50 percent of tropical species could be extinct by 2042.[1,3,30] Such an extinction could carry a heavy price, because tropical plants play an important role in removing some of the excess carbon dioxide that human activity puts into the atmosphere.

Desertification

Another process of environmental degradation is **desertification,** the conversion of once fruitful land into infertile wasteland, or desert. A desert is a terrestrial region in which evaporation exceeds precipitation and the average annual precipitation is less than 10 inches.[31] Every day, an average of 40 square miles of land are turned into deserts by droughts in combination with human activities, such as livestock grazing, poor irrigation techniques, and overplanting of crops.[32] Unlike natural deserts, human-created deserts are associated with worldwide famines. Some scientists believe that global warming contributes to desertification, because climate change produces droughts in areas where adequate rainfall once fell.[1]

Loss of Freshwater Resources

Rivers, lakes, and wetlands occupy only about 1 percent of the earth's surface, but they provide trillions of dollars' worth of ecological and economic services. The causes of freshwater degradation and loss of biodiversity are the same as those of terrestrial ecosystems.[3] Freshwater species are actually more at risk of extinction than land-based species. Nearly half of all freshwater species are now threatened with extinction.[1]

Many rivers in North America are threatened by industrial, agricultural, and city wastes as well as disruption of water flow by dams, channelization, and diversion of water for agricultural irrigation. The National Wild and Scenic Rivers Act (NWSRA) of 1968 protects rivers with outstanding scenic, recreational, geological,

The vital role that wetlands play in the balance of ecosystems was not always recognized, and over the past 200 years the United States lost more than 50 percent of its wetlands through drainage, building, and agriculture. Today the slow process of reclaiming and preserving wetlands is under way.

wildlife, historical, or cultural values from development, but only 0.2 percent of the 3.5 million miles of waterways in the United States are protected by the NWSRA. Environmentalists have lobbied Congress to increase designated waterway lengths to 2 percent, a proposal opposed by many developers and some local communities.[1]

Lakes are threatened by acid precipitation and pollution, which kill plant and animal life. Sewage and agricultural runoff also pollute lakes and deplete oxygen in the water. Some lakes have shrunk or dried up when humans withdrew more water from them than could be replaced by rainfall. Another threat is the intentional or unintentional introduction of nonnative species of fish and other organisms into lakes, which disrupts the balance of the ecosystem and usually results in the extinction of native species.

Wetlands are vulnerable as well. Swamps, marshes, and bogs are vital ecological resources for wildlife and the environment. They provide breeding areas and habitats for wildlife, store enormous amounts of water, keep the water table high during droughts, and help prevent flooding.[33] Wetlands also act as natural purifiers by filtering out pollutants. Despite their vital ecological roles, wetlands are often viewed as wasteland and considered fair game for draining, building, and agriculture. They are also vulnerable to industrial and agricultural runoff and human sewage, all of which destroy animal and plant life. The U.S. Fish and Wildlife Service estimates that more than 50 percent of wetlands in the United States have been destroyed in the past 2 centuries.[1]

Protecting Ecosystems

Stringent federal and state protection of animal and plant habitats in forests, deserts, and wetlands is a component of sustainable land management programs. The United States has several laws in place protecting endangered species, and many species are protected by international agreements. Genetically improved trees and tree farms can be part of a successful forest management program. Business and industry can help preserve forests by recycling paper, using fiber that does not come from trees to make paper, and using wood efficiently.

Individuals can help preserve forests by reusing and recycling paper products, refusing to buy products or materials made from endangered or threatened species, purchasing wood products with the Good Wood Seal, and

KEY TERMS

ecosystem Interconnected community of organisms living together in a physical environment as a balanced, mutually supportive system.

biodiversity Variety of different animal and plant species on earth and the genetic variation in their gene pools.

deforestation Removal of trees from a forested area without adequate replanting.

old-growth forests Uncut or naturally regenerated forests that have not been seriously depleted by human activities or natural disasters for several hundred years.

second-growth forest Forests that have been replanted after an area has been cleared for human activities or devastated by a natural disaster such as fire, flood, or volcanic eruption.

desertification Conversion of once fruitful land into desert.

stopping junk mail. Individuals can also let their elected representatives know that they are in favor of environmental protections, and they can support groups taking action to preserve natural habitats.[34]

ENERGY RESOURCES

Although the United States contains 4.5 percent of the world's population, it uses 24 percent of the world's commercial energy. Energy use per person in North America is nearly 50 percent higher than that in Germany, France, Japan, or the United Kingdom and 100 times higher than that in India or China. Nonrenewable energy resources provide 91 percent of the commercial energy used in the United States, 84 percent of it from fossil fuels and 7 percent from nuclear power.[1] The United States used 20 million barrels of oil a day in 2004. Of this oil, 40 percent was consumed by passenger vehicles, 24 percent by industry, 12 percent by commercial and freight trucks, 7 percent by aircraft, and 6 percent in residential and commercial buildings.[20] Heavy dependence on oil, coal, and natural gas for energy is the primary cause of air pollution, water pollution, and global warming.

The United States has only 2 percent of world oil reserves and thus is heavily dependent on foreign oil to meet its energy needs.[20] In 2004, 55 percent of the oil consumed was imported, with 20 percent coming from countries in the Middle East. To increase energy independence, the petroleum industry and some government officials want to expand oil and gas drilling on public lands in the United States, including pristine wilderness areas and offshore coastal areas. They claim, for example, that more than 16 billion barrels of oil are available in the Arctic National Wildlife Refuge in Alaska, even though the

U.S. Geological Survey states that only 3.2 billion barrels can be profitably extracted from this area.[20] Drilling proponents also favor relaxing environmental protections such as those in the Clean Air Act of 1968.[1]

Environmentalists believe the solution lies not in the relentless pursuit of fossil fuels but in energy conservation. They argue that our efforts should focus on reducing the ecological effects of current energy practices, diminishing energy waste, and shifting toward renewable, nonpolluting energy sources such as water, wind, geothermal, and solar power.[1] When we conserve energy, they point out, we lower the demand on commercial energy sources, which in turn reduces the emission of air pollutants and greenhouse gases. Environmentalists also support improving fuel economy in motor vehicles and promoting hybrid gas-electric vehicles. Individuals, too, can take action to conserve energy resources and reduce pollution, as described earlier in the box "You Can Help Improve Outdoor Air Quality." To consider your own position on energy conservation and related issues, see the box "Environmental Activism: Where Do You Stand?"

WORLD POPULATION GROWTH

Overpopulation increases the severity of every environmental problem on our planet. The world's population grew slowly until about 1750, when living conditions began to improve as a result of the Industrial Revolution. Since then, it has grown exponentially (Figure 19.4). World population reached 1 billion in about 1800, 1.6 billion in 1900, 2 billion in 1930, and 3 billion in 1960. A billion people were added between 1960 and 1975 and another billion between 1975 and 1987.[35] By the year 2000, world population stood at 6.1 billion, and by 2005, it reached 6.5 billion. The United

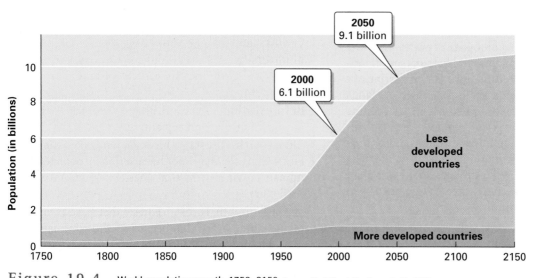

Figure 19.4   **World population growth, 1750–2150.** Sources: *World Population Prospects: The 2004 Revision,* United Nations Population Division, 2005, New York: United Nations; Human Population: Fundamentals of Growth, Population Reference Bureau, www.prb.org/; Historical Estimates of World Population, U.S. Census Bureau, 2005, www.census.gov.

Consumer Clipboard

Environmental Activism: Where Do You Stand?

Environmentalism is commonly defined as activism aimed at improving the environment through public education programs, advocacy, legislation, and treaties. There are thousands of nongovernmental organizations (NGOs) involved in the environmental movement, including such mainstream groups as the Sierra Club, Nature Conservancy, National Audubon Society, Worldwatch Institute, Natural Resources Defense Council, Greenpeace, Friends of the Earth, and Biodiversity Action Network. Any of these groups can be accessed on the Internet.

Mainstream environmental groups typically work within the political system. Much of environmental activism is focused on prevention or elimination of pollution and conservation of natural resources for future generations. Environmentalists often come into conflict with individuals and groups that have different priorities, such as economic interests, jobs, or property rights. For example, environmentalists seeking to preserve the habitat of the northern spotted owl, a threatened species living in old-growth forests in Oregon, were opposed by people who earned their livelihood in the lumber and logging industries. Such disputes are often settled in the courts, although decisions usually leave one or more parties dissatisfied.

Other environmental groups have aims similar to those of these mainstream organizations but use different means to achieve them. Radical environmentalists, eco-anarchists, and eco-terrorists believe that extreme methods must be used to disrupt the entrenched corporate interests that are damaging the environment. One such group is the Earth Liberation Front, which publishes the journal *EarthFirst!* This group asserts that it aims to speed the collapse of industry and un-

dermine the state, and it advocates such actions as attacking power lines, shooting out transformers, and sabotaging logging operations. Other actions undertaken by radical groups have included vandalizing and destroying utility bridges, ski lifts, construction equipment, power stations, SUV dealerships, and U.S. Forest Service facilities. Although mainstream environmental groups condemn any action that causes harm to humans, some of them have been tolerant of this kind of property destruction by radical groups.

Public polls suggest that the American people generally support environmental laws and regulations, but these polls also suggest that very few Americans consider the environment to be one of America's most pressing problems. This lack of deep conviction has opened the door to an anti-environmental movement that favors weakening or rolling back existing environmental protections and blocking any new laws or regulations. The growing momentum of this movement in turn fuels the radical branch of the environmental movement.

Most environmental issues are complex, controversial, and subject to distortion and polarization. In examining these issues and evaluating opposing views, you need to access a wide variety of sources, including environmental groups, business groups, government agencies, and scientific reports. Look for consensus statements by scientists working in a particular field of study, and seek information in different media, including magazines, newspapers, television, the Internet, government reports, and more. When you reach your own conclusions about a particular environmental issue, you have the option of providing support, whether financial, political, or activist, to the groups aligned with your position.

Sources: *Living in the Environment,* by G. T. Miller, 2002, Belmont, CA: Wadsworth/Thomson Learning; The Greenpeace Mission Statement, www.greenpeace.org.uk.

Nations predicts that world population will reach 9.1 billion by 2050 and stabilize at about 10 billion in 2200.[36] Much of the population growth will take place in the less developed countries of Africa, Asia, and Latin America.

How Many People Can the Planet Support?

The projected growth in the world's population has raised a vital question: How many people can the planet support?

The answer depends on whether we are talking about the number of people the earth can support at subsistence levels—referred to as **global carrying capacity**—or the

KEY TERMS

global carrying capacity   The number of people the earth can support at subsistence levels.

number the earth can support at an optimum standard of living—referred to as **cultural carrying capacity.** Subsistence living includes enough food, water, land, and energy to survive. An optimum standard of living includes the luxuries that are part of life in the developed world, such as plentiful food, indoor plumbing, cars, and air conditioning.

Analysts estimate that the global carrying capacity of the earth is 50 billion people,[37] but the cultural carrying capacity is much less. If luxuries are minimized, the cultural carrying capacity could be well above the population of 9 billion projected for 2050. If luxuries are maximized, it is probably lower than the current population of 6 billion. In other words, there are probably not enough resources, especially energy resources, to extend an optimum standard of living to everyone alive on the planet right now.

These global inequities may only be magnified in the future, with the world's 200-some nations coexisting in a finite global environment with very different standards of living. Currently, at least 2 billion people in the world are poorer than the 34 million people living below the official poverty line in the United States. This discrepancy increases by a million people every year.[1]

Approaches to Population Control

If standards of living are to be improved for all the people on the planet, population growth has to be slowed. Approaches to population control include extending **family planning** resources that help people make informed decisions about the number and spacing of their children to women and couples around the world; empowering women and increasing their access to educational and employment opportunities; reducing poverty and infant mortality and improving access to health care, all of which encourage parents to have fewer, healthier children; and offering incentives (such as salary bonuses, free education) and disincentives (such as higher taxes) to promote smaller families.

Family planning programs alone could have a significant effect if implemented in developing countries, according to the United Nations. If the global birth rate were reduced from 2.9 children per woman to 2.0 children per woman, the world's population could be stabilized at 7.8 billion in 2054 rather than the currently projected 9 billion.[38] The success of family planning programs in developing nations has been mixed, however. Minimal success has been attained in some very populous countries, including many countries in Africa and Latin America, primarily for cultural and religious reasons.[1]

***

Looking at environmental issues helps us recognize some of the features that characterize life: interdependence, diversity, adaptability, and limits. Acknowledging and honoring these characteristics can help us live in harmony with the environment. Americans leave a bigger ecological footprint on the earth—that is, we consume more resources, generate more pollution, and discard more wastes—than any other people in the world. Even though environmental health involves human activities all over the globe, each of us can take actions today to reduce the size of that footprint.

KEY TERMS

cultural carrying capacity   The number of people the earth can support at an optimum standard of living.

family planning   Informed decisions that individuals and couples make about the number and spacing of their children; most family planning programs provide information on birth control, birth spacing, breast-feeding, and prenatal care.

You Make the Call

Is Recycling Worth the Trouble?

In the 1960s and 1970s, many landfills around the country reached their capacity and closed, prompting a sense of crisis in many communities and an interest in developing long-term waste disposal plans. One of the proposed solutions was recycling, which grew in popularity as environmental awareness increased. In the 1970s and 1980s, recycling became a popular fund-raising activity for community groups, and the slogan "Recycling Pays" was used to encourage consumers to recycle. By the late 1980s, some states were setting up deposit/refund programs for beverage containers and passing other recycling laws; programs were becoming more formalized.

At the same time, recycling was becoming a victim of its own success: Supply exceeded demand for some recyclable materials, and the public was becoming aware that it cost money to recycle—sometimes more money than simply throwing something in the garbage. Costs of recycling included collection and processing of materials, promotion and administration of programs, capital investment in equipment and containers, labor costs, and the fees that are charged to process certain materials. In some cases, consumers objected to recycling practices, such as having to pay refundable deposits on beverages, and some retail merchants complained about having to store returned bottles and cans.

As costs increased and objections surfaced, questions arose about whether recycling was worth the time and money. Some people were concerned about reports that recycling sometimes increases rather than decreases pollution, and others wondered whether there even was a "garbage crisis." One commentator, writing in *The New York Times* in 1996, called recycling the U. S. public's "rite of atonement for the sin of excess."

Supporters of recycling assert that the point is not necessarily to save money but to save the planet. Recycling slows the filling of landfills and conserves natural resources. It is environmentally sound, whereas unlimited consumption and waste production are not. Supporters point to research showing that although recycling of some materials, such as newsprint, actually creates more pollution than processing virgin materials, the overall environmental advantages of recycling are beyond doubt. Even if landfills do not contain hazardous materials, they emit methane, a greenhouse gas, as waste decomposes. One expert states that U.S. landfills are one of the biggest contributors to global methane emissions. Supporters also point out that recycling can save money: Landfill and incineration fees are avoided; recycled products are sold; and recycled products cost less to produce than products made from virgin materials.

Recycling—a worthwhile endeavor or a waste of time and money? What do you think?

Pros

- There is a limit to the amount of land available for landfills, especially since no community wants a landfill in its back yard. Landfills are potentially dangerous (if they contain hazardous wastes) and produce methane, a greenhouse gas. Recycling reduces the amount of waste that has to be disposed of in landfills.

- Recycling reduces water pollution (for example, from paper mills) and air pollution (from methane gas and incinerators).

- Recycling conserves natural resources. Less land has to be allocated for landfills; less fuel is used to run incinerators; trees, forests, and habitats are preserved and biodiversity is protected.

- People throughout the world are interdependent; we need to be aware of our relationships and responsibilities to others. Recycling helps us reduce our impact on the global environment.

- Well-run recycling programs can make money.

Cons

- Recycling is not good business. In a capitalist economy, any program must prove its economic value, and recycling has not done that. It costs more to run recycling programs than to run a landfill.

- Landfills are the logical choice for garbage disposal; they are safe, cheap, and convenient. Most do not contain hazardous waste.

- Some forms of recycling actually cause pollution, as when newsprint is processed.

- Recycling programs allow people to delude themselves into thinking they are doing something for the environment, while actually they are still consuming goods, using energy, and creating waste at the same excessive levels.

OLC Web site For more information about this topic, visit the Online Learning Center at www.mhhe.com/teaguele.

SOURCES: "Let's Talk about Recycling: Is There Still a Garbage Crisis?" Passaic County, N. J., Office of Natural Resource Programs, 2004, www.passaiccountynj.org; "The Pros and Cons of Recycling," June 1997, *Environmental Health Perspectives, 105*(6).

SUMMARY

- The field of environmental health focuses on all the interactions human beings have with their environment; it includes not just agents that cause infectious diseases but pollutants that cause chronic diseases and damage the environment. Most of these pollutants arise from human activities.

- Only a small percentage of all the water on the planet is available for human use. Both communities and individuals can take steps to conserve water.

- Many water supplies, both surface and groundwater, are contaminated; pollutants can be biological (bacteria, parasites) or chemical (toxic metals, petroleum products, pesticides, radioactive materials).

- Most communities in the United States supply safe drinking water to residents; some people prefer bottled drinking water or have home water treatment systems.

- The atmosphere is the mass of air surrounding Earth, consisting of the lower atmosphere (troposphere) and upper atmosphere (stratosphere). Greenhouse gases trap some of the sun's heat and radiate it back to earth, warming the planet and regulating its temperature. Ozone forms a protective shield in the upper atmosphere against ultraviolet radiation from the sun.

- Six major air pollutants are carbon monoxide, sulfur oxides, nitrogen oxides, suspended particulate matter, ozone, and metal and metal compounds. They are hazardous to human health. The Environmental Protection Agency informs the public about air quality every day with a measure called the Air Quality Index.

- At ground level, ozone is a dangerous pollutant, as is particulate matter, tiny droplets or particles of dust, soot, oil, metals, or other compounds suspended in the air.

- Smog is a mixture of pollutants in the lower atmosphere that makes the air hazy. The less common type of smog, industrial smog, is caused primarily by the burning of coal and oil. Photochemical smog occurs in warm, sunny conditions when pollutants from motor vehicle exhaust, industry, and other sources combine in the presence of sunlight and heat.

- Smog is amplified when a blanket of warm air traps a layer of cold air next to the earth's surface so that pollutants cannot be dispersed by wind currents, a condition called a temperature inversion.

- Laws regulating pollution have substantially improved air quality over the last 15 years; individuals can contribute by such measures as driving less and buying energy-efficient vehicles.

- Acid deposition occurs when acidic chemicals in the air, especially sulfur dioxide and nitrogen dioxide, drop onto the earth's surface in either dry or wet form. Acid deposition damages buildings, kills vegetation and wildlife, and causes respiratory problems in vulnerable individuals.

- Thinning of the ozone layer of the atmosphere is occurring as a result of the destruction of ozone molecules by chlorofluorocarbons (CFCs), chemicals used in several industrial applications. Damage to the ozone layer increases human risks of skin cancer, cataracts, and other health problems.

- Greenhouse gases produced by human activities are amplifying the greenhouse effect, causing the temperature of the atmosphere to rise gradually, a condition referred to as global warming. An increase of only a few degrees could cause shifts in climate and weather around the world, affecting agricultural practices and human health.

- Indoor air pollution can be more hazardous than outdoor air pollution, primarily because there are more pollutants per breath indoors and they are more concentrated. Pollutants inside the home include allergens, such as dust mites and animal dander; mold and mildew; and chemicals. The most dangerous are environmental tobacco smoke, formaldehyde, radon, carbon monoxide, mold, and PBDEs.

- Huge amounts of solid waste are generated by human activity and require safe disposal. The two most common methods of disposal are burial in sanitary landfills and burning.

- Hazardous waste must be disposed of carefully so toxic chemicals do not enter the environment. The top five chemical compounds of concern are arsenic, lead, mercury, vinyl chloride, and polychlorinated biphenyls, or PCBs.

- Recycling helps to reduce the burden of solid waste, but in the long term, our society needs to produce less disposable material.

- Human activities like urban development and conversion of land for human use have led to the destruction of ecosystems and a loss of biodiversity worldwide. Processes involved in this pattern of disturbance include deforestation, desertification, and loss of freshwater resources.

- The United States uses about a quarter of the world's energy resources. Most energy comes from burning fossil fuels; a small percentage comes from nuclear power.

- Overpopulation magnifies the effect of all the environmental problems on the planet. The population of the world increased exponentially in the 20th century and is expected to reach 9 billion by 2050. The planet can support fewer than this number at the standard of living currently enjoyed by a small percentage of the population living in the developed countries of the world. If inequities are to be reduced, world population growth has to be slowed.

- Approaches to population control include extending family planning resources; empowering women; reducing poverty and infant mortality; and offering incentives and disincentives to promote smaller families.

REVIEW QUESTIONS

1. What were the traditional concerns of the field of environmental health? What additional concerns are now encompassed in this field?

2. What is the difference between surface water and groundwater? Which is the larger source of the world's drinking water?

3. Describe three water conservation measures that can be adopted by communities. Describe three actions individuals can take to conserve water.

4. What are the main sources of surface water pollution? What are the main sources of groundwater pollution?

5. What are the main components of the atmosphere? How are the lower atmosphere and the upper atmosphere different?

6. Describe the greenhouse effect.

7. Why is the ozone layer important?

8. What are the air pollutants of greatest concern and their sources? What is the AQI?

9. Why is ozone a problem at ground level? Why is particulate matter a problem?

10. Describe the difference between industrial smog and photochemical smog. How does a temperature inversion affect smog levels?

11. What are the major effects of acid deposition?

12. What is the "hole" in the ozone layer? What causes it, and why is it dangerous?

13. What are the human activities that have increased the amount of greenhouse gases in the atmosphere? What effect is this increase having?

14. What is the Kyoto Protocol?

15. Why is indoor air pollution more of a threat than outdoor air pollution? What are the main categories of indoor air pollutants?

16. Why is radon dangerous? What can you do about it?

17. What are the potential sources of carbon monoxide in the home?

18. How do mold and mildew affect health?

19. What are PBDEs? What are their sources, and why are they a concern?

20. What are the main sources of solid waste? What percentage is generated by nonindustrial businesses and homes?

21. What is hazardous waste? What are the most common toxic chemicals, and how do they get into the environment? How are they disposed of or treated?

22. How can individuals reduce the amount of waste they produce?

23. Why is loss of biodiversity a concern? What activities and processes are responsible for this loss?

24. Explain deforestation and desertification. Why are they concerns?

25. What measures can be taken to conserve energy resources?

26. Why is world population growth a concern? What approaches are being taken to slow the rate of growth?

WEB RESOURCES

CDC National Center for Environmental Health: This Web site provides information on environmental topics such as the elimination of chemical weapons, earthquakes, lead poisoning, and cancer clusters. The organization offers fact sheets, brochures, and other publications.
www.cdc.gov/nceh

The Direct Marketing Association: The organization's Web site offers a Consumer Assistance Guide that includes information on how to have your name removed from junk mail lists.
www.the-dma.org

Environmental Organization Web Directory: This search engine covers a wide range of environmental topics, including energy, forestry, pollution, recycling, and sustainable development.
www.webdirectory.com

Greenpeace: This organization works for new laws and policies to protect the environment. It includes information on how to get involved in environmental action at the local level.
www.greenpeaceusa.org

Natural Resources Defense Council: This Web site features weekly Web picks and a current legislative watch. Its Guide to Green Living includes ideas for green gifts, how to live green, and buying energy-efficient appliances.
www.nrdc.org

Scorecard: The Pollution Information Site: To find out how your community measures up to living in harmony with the environment, visit this Web site. It features a special focus on environmental burdens felt by different racial/ethnic and income groups at the community level.
www.scorecard.org

U.S. Environmental Protection Agency: The EPA site offers news and information on topics such as acid rain, environmental laws, hazardous waste, oil spills, ozone, radon, and wetlands. Click on "where you live," enter your zip code, and find out environmental information about your community.
www.epa.gov

U.S. Geological Survey: Focusing on the study of our landscape, natural resources, and natural hazards, USGS provides information on a variety of science topics, including climate, oceans and coastline, water resources, and plants and animals.
www.usgs.gov

World Watch Institute: This independent research organization focuses on critical global issues, looking for practical solutions. It offers a wide range of publications and online features on such topics as global security, population, and climate change.
www.worldwatch.org

World Wildlife Fund: This organization is dedicated to protecting endangered wildlife and preserving wild places. Its Global 200 is a scientific ranking of critical terrestrial, freshwater, and marine habitats that must be protected to preserve the "web of life."
www.wwfus.org

REFERENCES

1. Miller, G. T. (2002). *Living in the environment.* Belmont, CA: Wadsworth/Thomson Learning.

2. U.S. Environmental Protection Agency. Ground water: Drinking water: Frequently asked questions. www.epa.gov.

3. Gralla, P. (1994). *How the environment works.* Emeryville, CA: Ziff-Davis Press Books.

4. Hill, M. K. (2004). *Understanding environmental pollution: A primer.* Cambridge, UK: Cambridge University Press.

5. U.S. Environmental Protection Agency. Global warming: Fundamentals. www.epa.gov.

6. Weinhold, B. (2004). Weather warning: Climate change can be hazardous to your health. *Environmental Health Perspectives, 112* (3), A532–533.

7. Bernard, S. M., et al. (2001). The potential impacts of climate variability and change on air pollution–related health effects in the United States. *Environmental Health Perspectives, 109* (2), A199–209.

8. U.S. Environmental Protection Agency. Smog—who does it hurt? www.epa.gov.

9. U.S. Environmental Protection Agency. Clear skies initiative. www.epa.gov.

10. U.S. Environmental Protection Agency. (2002). Acid rain. www.epa.gov.

11. U.S. Environmental Protection Agency. Climate: Changing atmosphere/changing climate. www.epa.gov.

12. Natural Resources Defense Council. Global warming basics. www.nrdc.org.

13. Intergovernmental Panel on Climate Change. (2001). Summary for policymakers, *IPPC WGI Third Assessment Report.* Geneva.

14. Shepherd, A., Wingham, D. J., Mansley, J. A. D., & Corr, H. F. J. (2001). Inland thinning of Pine Island Glacier, West Antarctica. *Science, 291* (5505), 862–864.

15. Breslin, K. (2004). Hot new report on climate change. *Environmental Health Perspectives, 112* (3), A157.

16. U.S. Environmental Protection Agency. Global warming: Health impacts. www.epa.gov.

17. Epstein, P. R. (2000, August). Is global warming harmful to health? *Scientific American,* 50–57.

18. Gilbreath, J. (2004). Global warming kills. *Environmental Health Perspectives, 112* (3), A160.

19. Weinhold, B. (2004). Infectious disease: The human costs of our environmental errors. *Environmental Health Perspectives, 112* (3), A32–39.

20. Natural Resources Defense Council. Reducing America's energy dependence. www.nrdc.org.

21. U.S. Environmental Protection Agency. Indoor air facts no. 4 (revised): Sick building syndrome. www.epa.gov.

22. U.S. Environmental Protection Agency. (2003). *A brief guide to mold, moisture and your home.* Office of Air and Radiation. Environments Division. Washington, DC: Author: EPA publication 402-K-02-003.

23. The facts on formaldehyde. (2003, June 15). *Safety Compliance Letter,* 7.

24. Samet, J. M., & Spengler, J. D. (2003). Indoor environments and health: Making it to the 21st century. *American Journal of Public Health, 93* (9), 1489–1493.

25. U.S. Environmental Protection Agency. Protect your family and yourself from carbon monoxide poisoning. www.epa.gov.

26. U.S. Environmental Protection Agency. Household hazardous waste. www.epa.gov.

27. U.S. Environmental Protection Agency. Pesticides: Frequently asked questions. www.epa.gov.

28. U.S. Environmental Protection Agency. Medical waste. www.epa.gov.

29. U.S. Environmental Protection Agency. Recycling. www.epa.gov.

30. Chirian, A., & Bernstein, A. (2004). Embedded in nature: Human health and biodiversity. *Environmental Health Perspectives, 112* (1), A12–13.

31. McKenzie J. F., Pinger, R. R., & Kotecki, J. E. (2002). *An introduction to community health.* Boston: Jones & Bartlett.

32. Middledon, N. (2000). Shifting sands. *Geographical, 72* (4), 24–30.

33. Wilder, R. J., Tegner, M. J., & Dayton, P. K. (2000). Saving marine biodiversity. *Issues in Science and Technology, 15* (3), 57–64.

34. Hill, J. B. (2002). *One makes the difference: Inspiring actions that change our world.* New York: HarperCollins.

35. Population Reference Bureau. World population data sheets. www.prb.org.

36. United Nations Population Division. (2005). *World population prospects: The 2004 revision.* New York: United Nations.

37. Barrett, G. W., & Odum, E. P. (2000). The twenty-first century: The world at carrying capacity. *Bioscience, 50* (4), 363–368.

38. Worldwatch Institute. (2005). *Vital signs 2003: The trends that are shaping our future.* New York: W. W. Norton, 66–67.

Add It Up! IS YOUR LIFESTYLE ENVIRONMENTALLY FRIENDLY?

Do you have a lifestyle that promotes the health of the environment, or are you contributing to pollution and waste? Answer the following statements by indicating whether each one is true for you regularly, sometimes, or never.

	Regularly	Sometimes	Never
1. I keep my car in good operating condition and get oil or fluid leaks fixed immediately.	_____	_____	_____
2. I use mass transit, walk, or bike instead of using my car.	_____	_____	_____
3. I don't allow people to smoke in my home, and I make sure my home is well ventilated.	_____	_____	_____
4. I store and dispose of household cleaners, solvents, and pesticides properly.	_____	_____	_____
5. I recycle plastic, glass, aluminum cans, newspapers, and paper products.	_____	_____	_____
6. I turn off lights when leaving a room.	_____	_____	_____
7. I buy products with the least amount of packaging.	_____	_____	_____
8. I take my own cloth shopping bag to the grocery store instead of using the store's paper or plastic bags.	_____	_____	_____
9. I use rechargeable batteries and recycle those batteries after their useful life period.	_____	_____	_____
10. I use cloth dish towels and washable sponges rather than paper products.	_____	_____	_____
11. I avoid turning on my car air conditioner.	_____	_____	_____
12. I water my lawn and/or outdoor plants early in the morning or in the evening.	_____	_____	_____
13. I wear a sweater at home when it's cold rather than raise the thermostat.	_____	_____	_____
14. I do not let tap water run continuously when I shave and/or brush my teeth.	_____	_____	_____
15. I use compact fluorescent bulbs in lamps and lighting fixtures.	_____	_____	_____
16. I try to produce as little garbage as possible.	_____	_____	_____
17. I participate in community cleanup days.	_____	_____	_____
18. I read labels on household products and buy the least toxic ones available.	_____	_____	_____

527

	Regularly	Sometimes	Never
19. I run the washing machine and the dishwasher only with full loads.	_____	_____	_____
20. I write to my local and state elected officials to support environment-friendly legislation.	_____	_____	_____

Scoring

Give yourself 2 points for each activity you do regularly, 1 point for each activity you do sometimes, and 0 points for each activity you never do.

Interpretation

35–40	Very environmentally friendly. You are helping to heal the planet. Keep up the great work.
30–34	Above average. Your lifestyle contributes to a healthy environment.
25–29	Average. You are on the right track, but you can do more.
20–24	Below average. Look for ways to improve your record.
Under 20	Environmentally unfriendly. There are many changes you can make to develop a more environmentally friendly lifestyle.

PART 6

Protecting Your Health

Part 6 addresses health issues that affect most of us at some time during our lives—either personally or among our family and friends. Even when we're doing everything right to achieve good health, diseases do occur and we need to be prepared to deal with them. Infectious diseases can be as commonplace as the flu or as life-threatening as AIDS. Patterns of cardiovascular disease are changing—with a growing number of young people being affected by this disease and women and men dying of it in nearly equal numbers. A cure for cancer still eludes us, but researchers are putting together some important clues and helping cancer survivors live longer, fuller lives. Complementary and alternative medicine, once a target for criticism and even scorn, is gaining new respect and challenging us to rethink our approaches to health care.

THINK IT OVER

If you were faced with a diagnosis of AIDS, how would you react to this news?

Do you have a protection plan for your heart health?

Do you expect to see a cure for cancer in your lifetime?

Will complementary and alternative medicine ever gain the same degree of acceptance that conventional medicine holds?

CHAPTER 20

Infectious Diseases: Prevention and Management

DID YOU KNOW?

- Using antibacterial hand soap or household cleaner may kill some of the bacteria on your hands or in your kitchen, but these products may ultimately contribute to the growing incidence of antibiotic resistance. An estimated 50 percent to 60 percent of bacterial infections acquired in hospitals in the United States show resistance to at least one antibiotic. Some bacteria are resistant to all known antibiotics.

- Some of the childhood diseases that you were probably immunized against include measles, mumps, whooping cough, and polio. One that you may not have been immunized against is smallpox—vaccination against this disease ended in 1980, after smallpox was eradicated worldwide. Now, fears of a bioterrorist attack involving smallpox have sparked a debate about whether a smallpox vaccination program should be revived.

OLC *Your Health Today*   www.mhhe.com/teague1e

Go to the Online Learning Center for *Your Health Today* for interactive activities, quizzes, flashcards, Web links, and more resources related to this chapter.

The moment you enter the world, your body is colonized by millions of bacteria. Your whole life is shared with other organisms, some helpful and some harmful. The strongest influence on human evolution has been the microscopic world. Microorganisms have affected where, how, with whom, and how long we live. They have determined the outcomes of wars and attempts at colonization, and they have shaped the way populations have moved around the globe.

Prior to 1900 infectious diseases were the leading cause of death in the United States, with 30 percent of all deaths occurring among young children. Public health measures, vaccinations, and antibiotics are responsible for the reduction in the death rate from infectious diseases to about 2 percent by the end of the 20th century. Perhaps the greatest reductions in infectious diseases have come from improved sanitation and hygiene practices, especially clean water supplies. In recent years, however, death rates from infectious diseases have started to creep up again, as a result of new diseases such as HIV infection/AIDS and the reemergence of existing diseases once thought vanquished.

In this chapter we discuss the body's interactions with microorganisms, the ways it fights infections, and patterns of infectious diseases. We begin by examining the process of infection and the variety of disease-causing agents that can cause harm to human beings. We then consider the complex and amazing system that identifies, attacks, and fights off these disease-causing organisms, along with some steps we can take to keep the immune system healthy. We continue with a look at the technological and behavioral changes that underlie the shifting patterns of infection currently seen around the world, and we briefly discuss some of the new and reemerging diseases we now have to face. We then examine the major and minor sexually transmitted diseases, beginning with HIV infection/AIDS. We close with a very brief look at what we can do to maintain a healthy balance with the microscopic world.

THE PROCESS OF INFECTION

Microorganisms, the tiniest living organisms on earth, do what all living organisms do: eat, reproduce, and die. An **infection** occurs when part of a microorganism's life cycle involves you. An infection is considered an illness or disease if it interferes with your usual lifestyle or shortens your life.

Infections can result in different outcomes. Some infections cause a sudden illness with a high risk of death, such as infection with the Ebola virus. Some infections stimulate your body's immune response, causing the death of the microorganism, as occurs with the common cold virus. Still other infections may persist without signs of illness for years and yet be passed on to other people, as

is the case with the human immunodeficiency virus (HIV). Finally, some infections are walled off by the immune system, as in the case of tuberculosis, and held at bay for as long as the immune system is healthy.

The Chain of Infection

The **chain of infection** is the process by which an infectious agent, or **pathogen,** passes from one organism to another. Pathogens often live in large communities, called *reservoirs,* in soil or water or within organisms. Many pathogens cannot survive in the environment and require a living *host*. To cause infection, pathogens must have a *portal of exit* from the reservoir or host and a *portal of entry* into a new host (Figure 20.1). A pathogen can exit a host in respiratory secretions (coughing, sneezing); via feces, genital secretions, blood or blood products, or skin; or through an insect or animal bite. The pathogen enters the new host in similar ways: through skin-to-skin contact, genital-to-genital contact, inhalation of respiratory droplets, or exposure to blood products or insect or animal bites. If the transfer from host to host or reservoir to host is carried out by an insect or animal, that organism is said to be a **vector.**

Breaking or altering the chain of infection at any point can either increase or decrease the risk of infection. For example, chlorinating drinking water reduces the number of pathogens and the size of reservoirs; using condoms disrupts both the portal of exit and the portal of entry for infectious agents that may be present in semen or vaginal secretions; controlling mosquito populations eradicates vectors and disrupts a pathogen's mode of transmission. (See also the box "Hand Washing.")

The extent or spread of an infection depends on several factors, including the **virulence** (speed and intensity) of the pathogen, the mode of transmission, the ease of transmission, the duration of infectivity (how long a person with infection can spread it to other people), and the number of people an infected person has contact with while he or she is infectious. If an infected person does not transmit the infection to anyone else, that person's disease

KEY TERMS

infection Disease or condition caused by a microorganism.

chain of infection Process by which an infectious agent passes from one organism to another.

pathogen Infectious agent capable of causing disease.

vector Animal or insect that transmits a pathogen from a reservoir or an infected host to a new host.

virulence Speed and intensity with which a pathogen is likely to cause an infection.

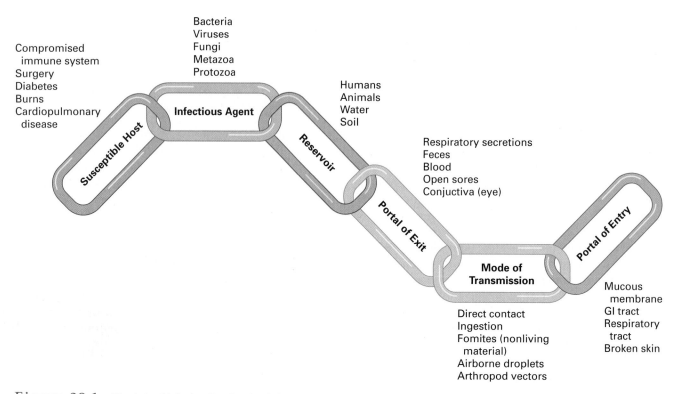

Figure 20.1 The chain of infection. *Breaking the chain at any point decreases the risk of infection.*

dies out. If the person transmits it to at least one other person, the infection continues. If the infection is transmitted to many people, an **epidemic** may occur.

Pathogens

Millions of different pathogens cause human infections, but they fall into several broad categories, of which viruses and bacteria are the most commonly known.

Viruses

Viruses represent some of the smallest pathogens. They are also among the most numerous; it is estimated that there are more different types of viruses than all other creatures combined.

Viruses consist of a genome (a genetic package of either DNA or RNA), a capsid (protein coat), and in some cases an outer covering or envelope. They are unable to reproduce on their own; they can replicate only inside another organism's cells. Viruses do not survive long outside of humans or other hosts. A virus infects a host cell by binding to its receptors and injecting its genetic material into the cell. Once inside, the virus can have a number of different effects. It can make many copies of itself, burst the cell, and release the copies to infect more cells. It can persist within the cell, slowly continuing to cause damage or becoming inactive and reactivating at a later time. Some viruses integrate themselves into a cell's DNA and

alter the growth pattern of the cells. This process can lead to the development of a tumor or cancer.[1]

A wide variety of viral illnesses affect humans. The common cold is caused by a corona virus that is spread from person to person via respiratory secretions. A cold is usually a 3- to 5-day self-limited illness marked by a runny nose, sneezing, coughing, and a low-grade fever. Influenza ("flu"), also spread by respiratory secretions, can last 7 to 10 days and has more severe symptoms, including diffuse body aches, coughing, and high fever. Influenza can be severe and require hospitalization; it can be life threatening for young children and older adults. Other viral diseases include warts (caused by the human papilloma virus and spread by skin-to-skin contact), hepatitis A and polio (both spread by fecal-oral contact), and rabies (spread by the bite of an infected animal).

Bacteria

Bacteria are single-celled organisms that can be found in almost all environments. They are classified based on shape (spherical, rodlike, spiral), the presence or absence of a cell wall, and growth requirements. Speed of replication varies from 20 minutes to 2 weeks. Some bacteria can enter a dormant or spore state in which they can survive for years.

Many bacteria inhabit a person harmlessly or helpfully and are considered part of the person's **normal flora.** Sometimes, bacteria that are normal in one body location

Consumer Clipboard

Hand Washing: Your First Defense Against Infection

As every first-year medical student learns, the most important thing you can do to prevent the spread of disease is to wash your hands. Throughout the average day, you can pick up germs from other people, from contaminated surfaces, or from animals and animal waste. If you don't wash your hands frequently, you're likely to transmit those germs to yourself whenever you touch your eyes, nose, or mouth. That's how colds are passed around so easily. More serious diseases, such as hepatitis A, meningitis, and infectious diarrhea, also can be transmitted through dirty hands.

It's especially important to wash your hands at these times:

- Before, during, and after you prepare food
- After handling uncooked foods such as raw meat, poultry, or fish
- Before you eat
- When your hands are dirty
- After blowing your nose, coughing, or sneezing
- After you use the bathroom
- After cleaning up a child who has used the bathroom
- When caring for someone who is sick

- When treating a cut or wound
- After handling an animal or animal waste
- After handling garbage

The Centers for Disease Control and Prevention recommends this method for correct handwashing:

- Place your hands together under water (warm water, preferably).
- Apply liquid or clean bar soap. Place the bar soap on a rack and let it drain.
- Rub your hands together vigorously for at least 20 seconds, scrubbing all surfaces, including wrists, palms, backs of hands, fingers, and under the fingernails.
- Rinse the soap from your hands.
- Dry your hands with a gentle patting motion, and throw away the disposable towel.
- If water is not available, use an alcohol-based product to keep your hands clean.

Since one out of three people don't wash their hands after using the restroom, handwashing is especially important when you're out in public.

Source: Data from "Handwashing," 2005, Centers for Disease Control and Prevention, www.cdc.gov.

---

are pathogens in another location, as when *Escherichia coli,* a bacterium that inhabits the large intestine and aids in digestion, enters the bladder, where it causes a bladder or urinary tract infection.

One kind of common bacterial infection is caused by *Staphylococcus aureus,* a bacterium found on the skin and in mucous membranes. It can cause problems if there is a change in the area it inhabits. For example, if a common cold virus causes swelling of the nasal passages, the small holes that drain the sinuses can become plugged. *S. aureus* can build up in the sinuses and cause a secondary bacterial sinus infection. A common scenario would be that after a week of cold symptoms, a person suddenly develops a higher fever, increased nasal discharge, and pain in the face. Antibiotics may be required to treat the infection.

Another bacterium commonly found on the skin is *Streptococcus;* it can cause an infection in the throat (strep throat), sinuses, ears, or lungs (pneumonia). A fatal form of meningitis (infection of the brain lining) is caused by the bacterium *Neisseria meningitidis;* symptoms include

fever, headache, and rash. Bacterial meningitis requires immediate treatment with antibiotics.

Some atypical bacteria have characteristics of both bacteria and viruses. For example, *Chlamydiae* and *Rickettsiae* have DNA or RNA (like bacteria), but they cannot survive independently of a host (like a virus). One strain of *Chlamydia* causes a sexually transmitted infection; another causes trachoma, an eye infection that leads to blindness. *Rickettsia* organisms cause Rocky Mountain

KEY TERMS

epidemic   Widespread outbreak of a disease that affects many people.

normal flora   Bacteria that live in or on a host at a particular location without causing harm and sometimes benefiting the host.

spotted fever, Q fever, and typhus. They spend most of their life cycle inside a host mammal (usually a small rodent) and are transferred via insects. Human beings are not part of the normal life cycle of *Rickettsia* organisms and usually serve as accidental hosts.[1]

Prions

Prions, the least understood infectious agents, are known to be responsible for the neurodegenerative disease bovine spongiform encephalopathy (BSE), or mad cow disease. The term *prion* was coined as a shortened form of *proteinaceous infectious particle*. Prions are believed to be made entirely of protein. They are found in brain tissue and appear to alter the function or shape of other proteins when they infect a cell, initiating a degeneration of brain function. Prions appear to spread by the ingestion of infected brain or nerve tissue.[1]

Fungi

A fungus is a single-celled or multicelled plant. Several kinds of fungi, including yeasts and molds, cause infection in human beings. Fungi reproduce by budding or by making spores; many fungal infections result from exposure to spores in the environment, such as in the soil or on tile floors. Except for tinea (ringworm) in children, fungal infections rarely spread from person to person.

Dermatophytes are a group of fungi that commonly infect the skin, hair, or nails; they are responsible for tinea, athlete's foot, and nail fungus. The yeast *Candida* may be part of a person's normal flora but can overgrow and cause a yeast infection in the vagina or mouth. Some fungal infections are acquired through inhalation of the spores from the soil, a common cause of pneumonia in Central America. All of the fungi can become serious infections in a person with a compromised immune system (for example, someone with HIV infection or AIDS, someone undergoing chemotherapy for cancer, or someone taking immunosuppressant drugs following an organ transplant).[1]

Helminths

Helminths, or parasitic worms, include roundworms, flukes, and tapeworms. They are large compared with other infectious agents, ranging in length from 1 centimeter to 10 meters. People usually become infected by accidentally ingesting worm eggs in food or water or by having the skin invaded by worm larvae. Worldwide, parasitic worms cause a huge disease burden. For example, hookworm, which attaches to the human intestine and causes blood loss, is a leading cause of anemia and malnutrition in developing countries.

Protozoa

Protozoa are single-celled animals; most can live independently of host organisms. Protozoal infection is a leading cause of disease and death in Africa, Asia, and Central

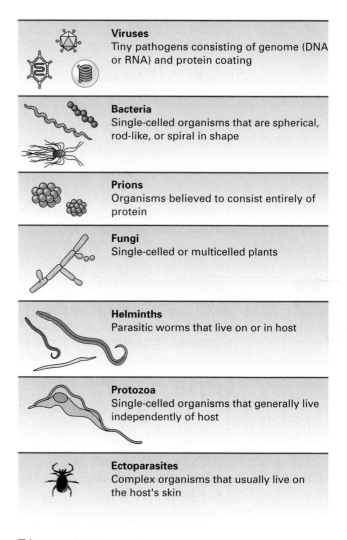

Figure 20.2   Main types of pathogens.

and South America. Infection may be transmitted by contaminated water, feces, or food, as is the case in the protozoal infections giardia, toxoplasmosis, and amebiasis; by air, as in *Pneumocystis carinii* pneumonia; or by a vector, such as the mosquito in the case of malaria.[1]

Ectoparasites

Ectoparasites are complex organisms that usually live on or in the skin, where they feed on the host's tissue or blood. They cause local irritation and are frequently vectors for serious infectious diseases. Examples are fleas, ticks, lice, mosquitoes, and scabies.[2]

The main types of pathogens are illustrated in Figure 20.2.

THE BODY'S DEFENSES

A single square inch of skin on your arm is home to thousands of bacteria. A sneeze projects hundreds of thousands of viral particles into the air. Bacteria can double in number every 20 minutes, and a virus can replicate thousands of times within a single human cell. Although you are substantially larger than microorganisms, you feel the power of their numbers each time you catch a cold.

Considering these facts, our ability to overcome invasion and survive infectious diseases is remarkable. Our bodies have defense mechanisms that recognize and protect us against foreign organisms and substances; they include external defenses (physical and chemical barriers) as well as the complex set of interacting processes organized as the immune system.

External Barriers

The skin is the first line of defense against infection. Most organisms cannot get through skin unless it is damaged, such as by a cut, burn, or infection, or if passage is aided by an insect bite or needle stick. Most portals of entry into the body, such as the mouth, lungs, nasal passages, and vagina, are lined with mucous membranes. Although these linings are delicate, mucus traps many organisms and prevents them from entering the body. Nasal passages and ear canals have hair that helps trap particles. The lungs are protected by the cough reflex and by cilia, tiny hairlike structures that rhythmically push foreign particles up and out. Damage to these physical barriers increases risk of infection. For example, tobacco, alcohol, and some illnesses can decrease the effectiveness of the cough reflex and the clearing of mucus from the body; burns and cuts compromise the integrity of the skin and allow entry by infectious agents.

If pathogens get past these barriers, they often encounter chemical defenses. Saliva contains special proteins that break down bacteria, and stomach acids make it difficult for most organisms to survive. The small intestine contains bile and enzymes that break down pathogens. The vagina normally has a slightly acidic environment, which favors the growth of normal flora and discourages the growth of other bacteria. The body protects pores and hair follicles in the skin by excreting fatty acids and lysozyme, an enzyme that breaks down bacteria and reduces the likelihood of infection. Some medications reduce the effectiveness of chemical barriers, as when medications for acid reflux decrease stomach acidity or antibiotics kill normal flora in the vagina and create conditions conducive to a yeast infection. The physical and chemical barriers to infection are illustrated in Figure 20.3.

The Immune System

The **immune system** is a complex set of cells, chemicals, and processes that protects the body against pathogens when they succeed in entering the body. The immune system is organized to fulfill three functions: recognize foreign particles or infectious organisms, attack and destroy these agents, and communicate with other parts of the immune system about when to begin and end an attack.

The immune system has two subdivisions: the innate immune system and the acquired immune system. These two overlap in many of their functions, and both operate largely through the action of white blood cells, but there are some key differences. The **innate immune system** is a rapid response designed to catch and dispose of foreign particles or pathogens in a nonspecific manner. The **acquired immune system** is a highly specialized response that recognizes specific targets.

The Innate Immune System

The body's initial reaction to tissue damage, whether it is due to trauma or infection, is an **acute inflammatory response,** a series of changes that increase the flow of blood and its cellular contents to the site. Signs of the inflammatory response are redness, warmth, pain, and swelling. The following molecular and cellular events occur when the innate immune system is activated:

- *Mast cells* located in the skin and around blood vessels release histamine and leukotrienes, proteins that increase blood flow, make blood vessels leaky, and call white blood cells to the area.
- If bacteria or fungi are present, the *complement cascade,* a series of proteins, is activated; these proteins can bind to the outside of bacteria or fungi and cause their death. They also promote further inflammation by binding to mast cells.
- *Acute phase proteins* circulate in the blood and remove material released by tissue damage; they also bind to bacteria and activate the complement cascade.
- *Cytokines* are chemicals that promote the inflammatory response, stimulate immune cell growth, signal movement of immune cells, inhibit the inflammatory response, and inhibit viral infection. The cytokines responsible for the antiviral effect are called interferons.
- *Neutrophils* and *macrophages* travel in the bloodstream to areas of infection or tissue damage.

(KEY) TERMS

immune system   Complex set of cells, chemicals, and processes that protects the body against pathogens when they succeed in entering the body.

innate immune system   Part of the immune system designed to rapidly dispose of pathogens in a nonspecific manner.

acquired immune system   Part of the immune system that recognizes specific targets.

acute inflammatory response   Series of cellular changes that bring blood to the site of an injury or infection.

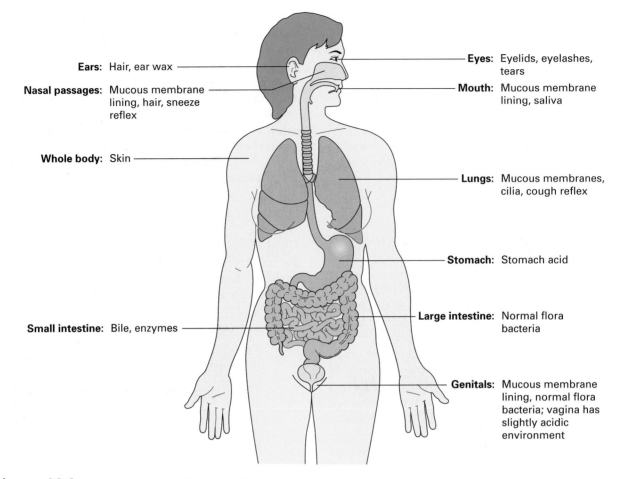

Ears: Hair, ear wax

Nasal passages: Mucous membrane lining, hair, sneeze reflex

Whole body: Skin

Small intestine: Bile, enzymes

Eyes: Eyelids, eyelashes, tears

Mouth: Mucous membrane lining, saliva

Lungs: Mucous membranes, cilia, cough reflex

Stomach: Stomach acid

Large intestine: Normal flora bacteria

Genitals: Mucous membrane lining, normal flora bacteria; vagina has slightly acidic environment

Figure 20.3 Physical and chemical barriers to infection.

These *phagocytes* ("cell eaters") are white blood cells that digest damaged cells and foreign particles or microorganisms and release chemical signals to call more white blood cells to the scene.

- *Dendritic cells*—white blood cells that reside in tissue and lymph nodes—recognize pathogens, take hold of them, and present them to the lymphocytes of the acquired immune system.

- *Natural killer cells* are white blood cells that destroy virus-infected cells or cells that have become cancerous.

The Acquired Immune System

Your acquired (or adaptive) immunity develops as you are exposed to potential infections, infections, and vaccinations. Each time the cells of the acquired immune system are exposed to a pathogen, they form a kind of memory of it and can mount a rapid response the next time they encounter it. The defining white blood cells of the acquired immune system are **lymphocytes,** which circulate in the bloodstream and lymphatic system. The lymphatic system is a network of vessels and organs

throughout the body that serves to move fluid from body tissues and clear infection. It includes the lymph nodes, spleen, and thymus.

If the lymphocytes encounter an **antigen** (a marker on the surface of a foreign substance), they rapidly duplicate and "turn on" their specific function. The two main types of lymphocytes are *T cells* (originating in the bone marrow and maturing in the thymus) and *B cells* (originating in the bone marrow). T cells monitor events that may be occurring inside the body's cells. If a cell is infected, molecules on its surface are altered that indicate it is now "nonself." *Helper T cells* "read" this message and trigger the production of killer T cells and B cells; helper T cells also enhance the activity of the cells of the innate immune system and of B cells once they are activated. *Killer T cells* attack and kill foreign cells and body cells that have been infected by a virus or have become cancerous. *Suppressor T cells* slow down and halt the immune response when the threat has been handled.

B cells monitor the blood and tissue fluids. When they encounter a specific antigen, they mature to become plasma cells that produce **antibodies**—proteins that circulate in

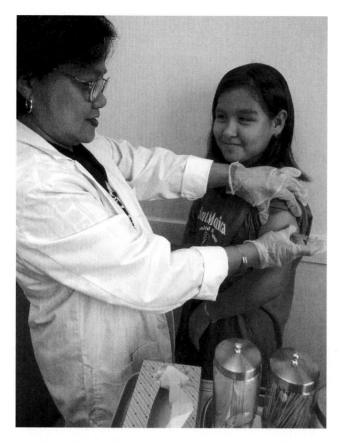

Although vaccination against childhood diseases is generally required by public schools in the United States, critics contend that this is not necessary. What are some arguments against vaccination?

the blood and bind to specific antigens, triggering events that destroy them. Antibodies may neutralize the pathogen just because they are bound to the antigen; they may signal other cells to destroy the organism that has the antigen on its outside; or they may activate the complement cascade system, which destroys the pathogen.

Immunization

Once a person has survived infection by a pathogen, he or she often acquires **immunity** to future infection by the same pathogen. The reason for this is that some B and T cells become *memory cells* when exposed to an infectious agent; if they encounter the same antigen in the future, they can respond rapidly, destroying the invader before it can cause illness. Immunization is based on this principle: The immune system is exposed to part of an infectious agent so that an immune response is triggered. On subsequent exposures, the immune system mounts a rapid response, preventing disease.

The concept of immunization was first introduced in 1796 by English physician Edward Jenner.[3] Jenner realized that people who had been infected with cowpox, a disease that causes mild illness in humans, seldom became ill or died when exposed to smallpox, a related but often fatal

disease. Jenner's observation led to the development of **vaccines,** preparations of weakened or killed microorganisms or parts of microorganisms that are administered to confer immunity to various diseases. Since 1900, vaccines have been developed for many infectious diseases, and significant reductions in death rates from these diseases have occurred.[4]

Vaccination serves two functions. The first is to protect an individual, frequently but not always a child, by stimulating an immune response. The second is to protect society by decreasing the incidence of diseases in a community. For example, widespread use of the smallpox vaccine has led to the elimination of naturally occurring smallpox worldwide. All future generations benefit from the earlier smallpox vaccination campaigns and no longer require vaccination themselves. Universal vaccination is controversial, however; for a discussion of the issues, see the You Make the Call feature at the end of the chapter.

Risk Factors for Infection

Your risk for infections depends on numerous factors. Some of them are within your control; others are beyond your individual control, but knowledge and awareness can help you reduce the likelihood that you will become seriously ill.

Controllable Risk Factors

You can reduce your risk of infection by adopting behaviors that support and improve the health of your immune system. One such behavior is eating a balanced diet, because poor nutrition is associated with a higher risk of infectious disease. Other behaviors that support a healthy immune system are exercising, getting enough sleep, and managing stress. Vaccination, when available,

KEY TERMS

lymphocytes   White blood cells that circulate in the blood stream and lymphatic system.

antigen   Marker on the surface of a foreign substance that identifies it to immune cells as "nonself."

antibodies   Proteins that bind to specific antigens and trigger events that destroy them.

immunity   Reduced susceptibility to a disease based on the ability of the immune system to remember, recognize, and mount a rapid defense against a pathogen it has previously encountered.

vaccines   Preparations of weakened or killed microorganisms or parts of microorganisms that are administered to confer immunity to various diseases.

Beating the Odds

Who Is Least Likely to Get an Infectious Disease?

Many factors contribute to the likelihood that a person will get an infectious disease. Among the most important are health-related behaviors that contribute to the strength of the immune system. Brief profiles of three individuals are presented here. Which one do you think is least likely to get an infectious disease?

Rachel is a 25-year-old graduate student at a university in the Northeast. She lives off campus with two friends and has a part-time job waiting tables at a small café. She is healthy, eats a balanced diet, and does not smoke. She dates several different men and is sexually active. Rachel had chicken pox as a child and has had all the recommended vaccinations for her age group, including those for meningococcal meningitis and hepatitis B. She plays ultimate frisbee with a club team, which practices for 2 hours outside three evenings a week. Despite frequent applications of mosquito repellent, she almost always comes home with 10 to 15 mosquito bites per practice.

Hannah is a 19-year-old college freshman. She lives in the dormitories with three roommates; recently they all got tattoos. Hannah is healthy but she has been eating more junk food since starting college. She has also found it difficult to make time for exercising and often does not get enough sleep. She feels stressed out most of the time. She is not sexually active but has been dating. Although she has had asthma since she was 9, Hannah smokes cigarettes when she goes out with friends on the weekend. She got all her vaccinations as a child, but she hates shots, so she declined vaccination for meningococcal meningitis.

Suzanne is a 30-year-old kindergarten teacher. She lives in a city with a large immigrant population, and quite a few of her students are first-generation Americans. She eats well, does not smoke, and exercises in a step aerobics class 4 days a week. She is sexually active and has been with her male partner for 6 months. Their use of condoms has been spotty. They are thinking about traveling over the summer; they would both like to visit China and Southeast Asia.

OLC Web site Visit the **Online Learning Center** at www.mhhe.com/teague1e for comments by the authors.

---

can boost your immune system and facilitate a quicker response to pathogens. Good hygiene practices like hand washing reduce the risk of many infections, and protecting your skin from damage keeps many pathogens out of your body. Avoiding tobacco and environmental tobacco smoke improves your defenses against respiratory illness.

Uncontrollable Risk Factors

Age plays a role in vulnerability to infection, with higher risks at both ends of the life span. Newborns and young children are at increased risk because they have not been exposed to many infections; pregnancy and breast-feeding confer **passive immunity**—a mother's antibodies can pass to the fetus or child to provide temporary immune protection. Children also have structural body differences that make infection more dangerous; for example, their airways are smaller and can be more easily blocked by an infection. Older people are at increased risk due to a gradual decline in the immune system that can occur with aging. Other factors that increase vulnerability include undergoing surgery, having a chronic disease such as diabetes, and being bed-bound.

Genetic predisposition may play a role in susceptibility to infectious disease. It is unclear why certain people develop an overwhelming, life-threatening illness when exposed to a pathogen while others develop only a mild fever. Certain sociocultural factors are associated with higher risk for infectious disease; in many situations, these are not controllable risk factors. Overcrowded living environments increase the risk for any infectious disease that is spread from person to person, such as tuberculosis. Poverty is associated with increased risk for many illnesses, probably owing to poor nutrition, stress, and lack of access to health care, among other factors. To evaluate risk factors for infection, see the box "Who Is Least Likely to Get an Infectious Disease?"

Disruption of Immunity

Because the immune system is so complex, it is occasionally subject to malfunctions. Two such disruptions are autoimmune diseases and allergies.

Autoimmune Diseases

Sometimes, a part of the body is similar enough to an antigen on a foreign agent that the immune system mistakenly identifies it as "nonself." Other times, the immune control system fails to turn off an immune response once an infection is over. In both cases, a process of self-destruction can ensue, causing damage to body cells and tissues. Autoimmune diseases vary in their effects, depending on which part of the body is seen as foreign. In rheumatoid arthritis the immune system can cause destruction of joints, kidneys, and other internal organs. In psoriasis, the immune system causes severe rashes and damage to internal organs. Other autoimmune diseases include multiple sclerosis, scleroderma, and lupus erythematosis. Genetics is known to play a role in some autoimmune diseases.[1] For unknown reasons, autoimmune diseases are more common in women than in men.

Allergies

Allergic reactions occur when the immune process identifies a harmless foreign substance as an infectious agent and mounts a full-blown immune response. Allergic responses to substances like pollen or animal dander, for example, may include a runny nose, watery eyes, nasal congestion, and an itchy throat. Asthma, a condition characterized by wheezing and shortness of breath, is caused by inflammation of the bronchial tubes and spasm of the muscles around the airways in response to an allergen or other trigger. **Anaphylactic shock** is a life-threatening systemic allergic response. Medications containing antihistamine can help relieve mild allergy symptoms; powerful drugs called steroids are sometimes used to decrease an immune response that has become chronic. Epinephrine (adrenaline) is used in an emergency situation to reduce the swelling associated with anaphylactic shock.

Immunity and Stress

As described in Chapter 5, stress can have a significant impact on the immune system. Short-term stress can actually enhance immune system functioning by activating the body's responses to stressors like puncture wounds, scrapes, and animal bites. Chronic, long-term stress, however, suppresses immune system functioning; the longer lasting the stress, the greater the negative effect on immune system functioning. Although the relationship between stress and immune system change has been verified by more than 300 studies conducted over the past 30 years, it is not clear that stress "causes" illness. Further research is needed to determine the exact nature of the relationship. You can support your immune system by practicing stress management and relaxation techniques, as described in Chapter 5.[5]

CHANGING PATTERNS IN INFECTIOUS DISEASE

In 1969 the surgeon general of the United States declared before Congress that it was time to close the book on infectious diseases.[6] Dramatic declines in the death rate from infectious diseases during the 20th century inspired this bold statement (Figure 20.4). Within a little more than 10 years, however, the first cases of what would soon

be identified as human immunodeficiency virus (HIV) infection were causing perplexity and alarm in hospitals in several U.S. cities. Since then, the appearance of other new infections, changes in patterns of infection, and the development of antibiotic resistance in many strains of bacteria have demonstrated that infectious diseases remain an important health concern.

Over the course of the 20th century, advances in technology and drugs have led not only to new treatments but also to new opportunities for infection. For example, the airplane has changed patterns of human travel, migration, and disease transmission, creating a global community for infectious diseases. Antibiotic drugs control infectious diseases, but they also create conditions for the development of resistant strains of microorganisms. In this section, we consider several such changes.

Technology-Related Changes that Affect Disease Transmission

Technological advances that have increased the ease with which infectious organisms can get from one person to another include blood banks and centralized food production.

Blood Products

Within the United States, 11 to 12 million units of blood are transfused each year, saving many lives. This lifesaving treatment can also serve as a vector for infectious organisms. If donated blood contains infectious agents, these pathogens readily infect the blood of the person receiving a transfusion. If the donated blood is administered to many people, the number of people exposed to a single person's infected blood can be very high.

Blood banks in the United States and Canada screen extensively for known infections; they are currently the safest they have ever been. New infections continually arise, however, and screening can start only after an infectious agent has been identified, as was the case for hepatitis C and HIV. Before 1992, for example, 80,000 people a year were infected with hepatitis C, a virus that attacks the liver, via blood transfusions. Blood banks in the United States have screened for hepatitis C since July 1992, and

KEY TERMS

passive immunity Temporary immunity with antibodies from an external source—such as passed from mother to child in breast milk.

anaphylactic shock Hypersensitive reaction in which an antigen causes an immediate and severe reaction that can include itching, rash, swelling, shock, and respiratory distress.

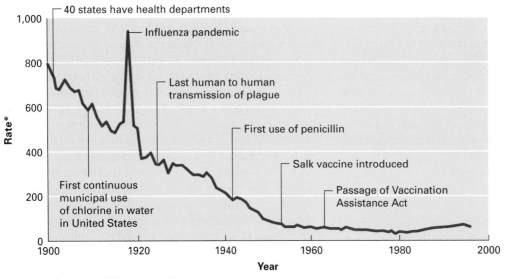

*Deaths per 100,000 population per year.

Figure 20.4   **Death rate from infectious diseases, United States, 20th century.** Sources: Adapted from "Achievements in Public Health, 1900–1999: Control of Infectious Disease," (MMWR serial online), 1999, *Morbidity and Mortality Weekly Report, 48* (29), p. 621, www.cdc.gov/mmwr; Trends in Infectious Disease Mortality in the United States during the 20th Century, by G. L. Armstrong, L. A. Conn, and R. W. Pinner, 1999, *Journal of the American Medical Association, 281*, pp. 61–66; "Water Chlorination Principles and Practices: AWWA Manual M20," American Water Works Association, 1973, Denver, CO: Author.

transmission of this disease through blood products is now estimated at only 1 case for every 103,000 units of blood transfused. Blood banks also routinely screen for HIV and for hepatitis B, another virus that attacks the liver; rates of transmission via blood transfusion are only 1 case in 677,000 units transfused for HIV and 1 case in 63,000 units transfused for hepatitis B.[7]

Blood products in developing countries are less safe. Many countries lack the resources to screen all blood for known infections or to use new or sterile equipment to administer blood products. Many countries also continue to pay blood donors for giving blood. Paid donors are less likely to answer screening questions about risk for infectious diseases honestly. The situation is especially serious in countries where questions about risk are the only screening mechanism.

Food Production and Distribution

For the most part, the days of backyard gardens, local butchers, and corner groceries are gone. Now we have oranges in Minnesota in December and fresh seafood in Iowa year round. Much of our food is grown in one part of the country or in a foreign country, shipped to a central processing plant, packaged, and then distributed to locations from coast to coast. This widespread distribution of food lowers some costs and makes production more convenient, but it also increases the risk that contaminated food will cause infectious diseases in many people.

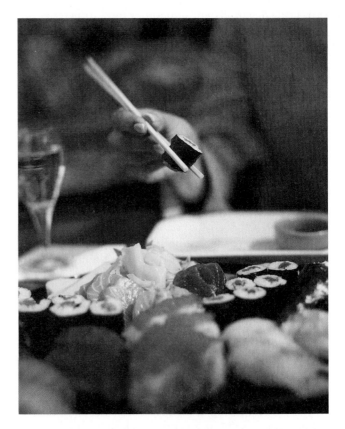

Fish caught in Nova Scotia may be sent to a food processing plant in the Midwest, where it is packaged and sent to various locations throughout the United States. By the time the fish reaches this sushi bar, there have been many chances for contamination.

One case of widespread illness occurred in fall 2003, when outbreaks of hepatitis A affected people living in Tennessee, North Carolina, Georgia, and Pennsylvania. Heptaitis A is a viral illness spread by fecal contamination; risk can be reduced by avoiding undercooked or raw foods. The 2003 outbreaks were all associated with the consumption of raw or undercooked green onions at restaurants. Some of the green onions were traced to a source in Mexico, and the U.S. Food and Drug Administration and the Centers for Disease Control and Prevention worked with Mexican authorities to reduce the risk of recurrence.[8]

Another case occurred in July 2002, when 18.6 million pounds of fresh and frozen ground beef were recalled by the U.S. Department of Agriculture. The recall was in response to 18 cases of *E. coli 0157* infection in Colorado and 8 cases in six other states. Although *E. coli* normally lives in the large intestine, the *0157* strain can cause bloody diarrhea, fevers, anemia, kidney failure, and even death.[9] *E. coli 0157* can be spread by fecal contamination of meats or vegetables. The outbreak was traced to the Omaha-based ConAgra Beef Company.

In December 2003, the first case of bovine spongiform encephalopathy (mad cow disease) in a slaughtered cow was reported in the United States. The prion responsible for mad cow disease is strongly associated with a variant form of Creutzfeldt-Jakob disease (vCJD) in humans, a progressive, fatal deterioration of brain function. A "classic" version of CJD leads to death at an average age of 68; the cause of this version is not known. The variant form of CJD leads to death at an average age of 28. The prion is spread by the ingestion of infected nerve or brain tissue.

Due to the seriousness of the consequences if the prion gets into the food supply, the United States has a targeted screening program to check slaughtered cattle for mad cow disease. Additionally, any cow that shows signs of weakness or neurological problems is slaughtered, and its brain is sent to a lab for testing; the animal may not be used in any products intended for human consumption. If mad cow disease is detected, a tracking system and investigation are deployed to identify other infected animals that may still be in the herd or in herds with whom the infected cow had contact.[10]

Behavior-Related Changes that Affect Disease Transmission

As people interact in different ways, changes in travel, in sexual behavior, and other behaviors can create situations where it is either easier or more difficult for infection-causing microorganisms to spread from one person to another.

Travel and Disease

Nothing has changed world patterns of disease more than automobiles and airplanes. When ships were the only means of crossing oceans, trips between continents took several weeks. A passenger who became infected before leaving on a trip usually showed symptoms before arriving at a distant port and could be quarantined (separated from others who were not infected) to control the spread of the disease. These days, people can reach almost any part of the world within 24 hours, carrying incubating infectious microorganisms with them.

The severe acute respiratory syndrome (SARS) outbreak in 2003 is an excellent example of how travel affects the spread of disease and how community efforts can control it. In March 2003, the World Health Organization activated a Global Outbreak Alert concerning an atypical pneumonia that was believed to have originated in southern China at the end of 2002. By February 2003 it had spread to Hong Kong, Vietnam, Singapore, Germany, and Canada. By the time the disease was contained in July 2003, there had been 8,098 probable cases and 774 deaths in 26 countries.

A team of 11 laboratories around the world identified the cause of SARS as a corona virus and one reason for its rapid spread as air travel. The virus is spread directly from person to person by coughing, sneezing, and skin contact. Airlines and travelers were alerted to the early symptoms, which consist of fever, body aches, and dry cough; these symptoms can progress fairly rapidly to a severe form of pneumonia. Travelers boarding planes that were departing from cities with SARS cases were screened for symptoms and in some cases prevented from traveling. If a traveler became ill in flight with symptoms suggestive of SARS, health officials boarded the plane on arrival to examine and possibly quarantine the individual. Travelers were advised to avoid cities with SARS cases, and many locales suffered financially until the advisory ended.

By July 2003, the last case of SARS caused by person-to-person transmission was believed to have been resolved. Countries around the world remain on alert for a recurrence, however, and have improved surveillance and preparedness as a result of their experience with this disease. New diseases—such as avian flu, also believed to have originated in Asia—will continue to arise and spread around the world as a result of air travel.[11]

Travelers also need to be alert to diseases they may encounter in other countries but do not occur in their home country. Particular care should be taken in selecting foods and drink in areas where hygiene and sanitation are inadequate. Undercooked or raw foods should be avoided; cooked foods should be eaten while still hot. In areas with inadequate water treatment, the safest option is to drink bottled beverages or to treat water before drinking, as noted in Chapter 7. Special vaccinations and medications are also recommended before and during travel in certain areas. See the Web Resources at the end of the chapter for sources of information about traveling to foreign countries.

Sexual Behavior and Disease

The major sexually transmitted diseases (STDs) are discussed later in this chapter; here, we consider the sexual behaviors that play a role in their transmission. STDs exit one host by excretion at a mucous membrane (such as the lining of the vagina or the opening of the penis) or from sores on the skin in the genital region, and they enter another host through similar mucosal surfaces. The key sexual behaviors known to be associated with STD transmission include partner variables, susceptible person variables, and sex act variables.

Partner variables that increase the risk of being exposed to an STD include the total number of sex partners a person has, how frequently he or she acquires new sex partners, and the number of concurrent sexual partners. Certain types of partners are associated with an increased risk of infection; the highest risks are associated with commercial sex workers (people who are paid to have sex) and unknown partners (for example, people picked up at bars or bath houses).[12]

Variables associated with increased susceptibility to infection if exposed to an STD include gender, age at first intercourse, and the general health of the susceptible person. Women are at greater risk than men due to anatomy (the larger mucosal surface of the vagina and the cervix in comparison to the penis). Young women are at particular risk because the cervix is more susceptible to infection in the first few years after the start of menstruation. The overall health of a person is important because it affects the strength of the immune response and the integrity of the mucosal surfaces. For instance, a person with one sexually transmitted infection may be more likely to contract a second infection, as discussed later in this chapter.

The sexual acts performed by a couple also affect how likely it is for an STD to be passed from one person to another. Nonpenetrative sex (fondling, mutual masturbation) has the lowest risk, followed in increasing order of risk by oral sex, penile-vaginal intercourse, and penile-anal intercourse. Other factors further increase or decrease the risk of transmission. The risk of exposure increases with the number of sexual acts. The amount of lubrication, either natural from foreplay or applied, affects risk, because abrasions to the mucosa make it easier for the STD to be transmitted. Forced sex or violent sex increases the risk of abrasions and of STD transmission. When used correctly, condoms decrease the risk of transmission of many STDs, but they are not 100 percent effective, and there is currently no data showing that they reduce the risk of transmission of the human papilloma virus, which causes genital warts and cervical cancer.[13]

Illicit Drug Use

When users of illicit drugs share needles and syringes, some blood from the first user is injected into the blood-stream of the next user, creating an effective means of transmitting bloodborne infections. Several viral infections, specifically HIV, hepatitis B, and hepatitis C, are easily transmitted through shared needles. We discuss HIV and hepatitis B later in the chapter; here, we consider hepatitis C.

All hepatitis viruses cause inflammation of the liver, with symptoms such as fatigue, weakness, loss of appetite, and jaundice (a yellow discoloring of the skin and eyes). Unlike hepatitis B, however, in which 60 percent to 70 percent of newly infected people become ill, only 20 percent to 30 percent of those with new hepatitis C infection have symptoms. Liver failure with initial hepatitis C infection is extremely rare, but the virus evades the immune system, so that 85 percent of infected people eventually develop chronic hepatitis. After about 20 years, the disease becomes more obvious and aggressive, and approximately 20 percent of people develop liver failure, scarring of the liver (cirrhosis), or liver cancer.

An estimated 3 million people are infected with hepatitis C in the United States and an estimated 170 million worldwide. Currently, there is no vaccine, and treatment—an intensive 6-month regimen of the drugs interferon and ribavirin—has only a 55 percent cure rate.[14] Thus, prevention is crucial.

Hepatitis C virus is not a highly infectious virus and requires introduction directly into the bloodstream for transmission. The virus was discovered in 1989, and a blood test was developed to detect infection. Before 1990, approximately 10 percent of blood transfusion recipients developed hepatitis, nearly always from hepatitis C virus. After blood banks started testing blood donors for hepatitis C virus, transfusion-related hepatitis C infection dropped. Most cases are now associated with the use of injection drugs (50–60 percent of cases) and high-risk sexual behavior (15–20 percent of cases). About 4 percent of cases occur when a health care worker is exposed to blood from an infected person; in the remaining cases, no risk factor can be identified.

Individuals reduce their risk of contracting hepatitis C by not using injection drugs and by limiting their number of sexual partners. Those who do use drugs should reduce their risk by not sharing needles or syringes or, at the very least, cleaning them after every use with bleach. People with hepatitis C should protect their remaining liver function by avoiding alcohol, limiting medications that affect the liver (such as acetaminophen), and getting vaccinated for hepatitis A and B. Communities can reduce the risk by establishing programs to link drug users with drug treatment programs and encouraging safe injection programs for addicts until they are able to receive treatment. Communities can also raise awareness about this asymptomatic disease and encourage individuals who have engaged in injection drug use to be tested for hepatitis C.[15]

Tattoos and Body Piercing

Nipple, nose, tongue, belly button, and genital piercings are popular today, as are tattoos decorating ankles, arms, or entire bodies, or marking gang membership. Health risks from piercing and tattooing are potentially serious. Tattoo and piercing artists have no licensing boards, no requirements for training, and no regulation of techniques. Most but not all reputable artists use sterile or new equipment for each tattoo or piercing. Equipment reuse carries a risk of transmitting HIV, hepatitis C, and other bloodborne infections. (See the Consumer Clipboard box in Chapter 10 for more information about tattooing and body piercing.)

Even with sterile equipment, piercing and tattooing break down the body's protective barriers against infection, increasing the risk of bacterial infections of the genitalia, tongue, nipple, or cartilaginous part of the ear. Health care providers are just starting to

Some individuals choose to have tattoos and body piercings to express their individuality or make a fashion statement. Since tattoo and piercing procedures are not regulated by health departments, the risk for transmission of infection through nonsterile conditions and equipment is high.

monitor disease transmission related to tattooing and body piercing, so the effects of this trend remain to be seen.[16]

Antibiotic Resistance

In 1928 British bacteriologist Alexander Fleming observed that a common mold, *Penicillium,* prevented the growth of bacteria. When penicillin, the first **antibiotic,** was isolated from this mold, it was declared a miracle drug. It was widely used during World War II and saved the lives of many wounded soldiers. By the 1950s, however, the bacterium *Staphlococcus aureus* was already showing signs of resistance to penicillin. A new antibiotic, methicillin, was introduced and proved effective. Since that time, hundreds of new antibiotics have been introduced to help treat infectious diseases.

The 21st century may mark the beginning of a postantibiotic era as **antibiotic resistance** grows (as well as antiviral and antifungal resistance). An estimated 50 percent to 60 percent of bacterial infections acquired in hospitals in the United States show less sensitivity to at least one antibiotic.[17] Some bacteria are resistant to all known antibiotics. Two factors are believed to account for bacterial resistance: the frequency with which resistant genes arise naturally among bacteria through mutation, and the extent of antibiotic use.

Resistant genes arise naturally because bacteria reproduce quickly, and mutations in their DNA occur frequently. Resistant genes can be passed from one bacterium to another in the form of plasmids, tiny loops of DNA that become incorporated in the recipient's DNA. Resistant genes can also be passed to bacteria by viruses.

The appearance of resistant genes in bacteria through mutation is amplified when a population of bacteria is exposed to an antibiotic. The most sensitive bacteria die quickly, while those with some resistance survive. Once the nonresistant bacteria are out of the way, the resistant bacteria have more space and food, and they quickly produce more resistant bacteria. Thus, frequent and widespread antibiotic use is accompanied by increased antibiotic resistance. Another way that resistance is promoted is through the action of antibiotics on the bacteria that are part of the normal flora. Antibiotics are nonspecific, so they kill helpful bacteria as well as pathogens and increase antibiotic resistance in helpful bacteria as well as in

KEY TERMS

antibiotic   Drug that works by killing or preventing the growth of bacteria.

antibiotic resistance   Lessened sensitivity to the effects of an antibiotic.

HIGHLIGHT ON HEALTH

Antibiotic Resistance

Have you ever pressured your physician to give you antibiotics when you have a stuffy nose, a sore throat, muscle aches, and a low-grade fever—symptoms of the common cold or the flu? Even though antibiotics are not effective against viral infections, physicians sometimes prescribe them when they are uncertain about a diagnosis, when patients request them, or when they don't have time to explain the difference between bacterial and viral infections. In fact, estimates are that up to 50 percent of the time that antibiotics are prescribed, they are not needed and do not alter the course of an illness. This is just one example of the misuse of antibiotics that is promoting antibiotic resistance.

Another example is that antibiotics, even when appropriately prescribed, are often not taken correctly. People routinely miss taking doses, or they stop taking an antibiotic in midcourse because they feel better. Both of these practices increase the likelihood that some bacteria will survive—the ones with the most resistance—and continue to reproduce.

Even though the presence of bacteria is normal and even beneficial, Americans are at war against bacteria. More than 700 antibacterial products, ranging from mattresses to soaps and household cleaners, have appeared on the market in the last 10 years. These products increase the risk that many harmless bacteria in the environment will develop resistance, which can then be passed to less common, disease-causing bacteria. Individuals who work in settings where antibiotic use is common, such as hospitals, day care settings, and nursing homes, can reduce their use of antibiotic products by frequent hand washing and the use of vaccines (when available).

When a child's immune system is developing normally, it appears to be strengthened by repeated exposure to common bacteria. If the environment is overly sterile, however, such immunity is not reinforced, and the child becomes vulnerable to infectious diseases. Some experts think that the increasing incidence of allergies in children is a result of the overuse of antibacterial soaps, wipes, and washes.

Some antibiotic use extends beyond the realm of the individual. An estimated 40 percent of the antibiotics used in the United States each year are related to agriculture—to increase the production of livestock or enhance crop production. When antibiotics are mixed in animal feed, the low dose and long-term exposure create the ideal setting for resistant bacteria to thrive. The World Health Organization has recognized this threat and recommends that antibiotics not be used in animal feed. Similarly, as fruit trees and other crops are sprayed with antibiotic agents, the antibiotics are often diluted and some of the solution is washed away. Again, the bacteria are exposed to a low level of antibiotic, promoting resistance.

As antibiotic resistance threatens the power of antibiotics, you can take steps to reverse this trend. These steps include taking antibiotic medications properly, limiting your use of antibacterial products, and choosing to purchase organic food.

Sources: Data from "Home Hygiene: A Risk Approach," by S. F. Bloomfield, 2003, *International Journal of Hygiene for Environmental Health, 206* (1), pp. 1–8; "Appropriate Antimicrobial Prescribing: Approaches That Limit Antibiotic Resistance," by R. Colgan, 2001, *American Family Physician, 64* (6), pp. 999–1004; "Antimicrobial Resistance: A Plan of Action for Community Practice," by T. M. Hooton, 2001, *American Family Physician, 63* (6), pp. 1087–1098.

pathogens. Such resistance can be passed on to pathogens during a subsequent infection.

One worrisome scenario involves *Staphylococcus aureus,* a bacterium that causes serious infections of the skin, sinuses, wounds, and blood. About 30 percent of *S. aureus* infections that arise in hospitals have developed resistance to many antibiotics, with the exception of an antibiotic called vancomycin. Some strains of a bacterium that is part of the normal intestinal flora, *Enterococcus faecali,* have developed resistance to vancomycin. Scientists fear that if *E. faecali* were to pass resistant genes to *S. aureus,* these staph infections would be untreatable by any antibiotics currently available.[17] For more on this troubling trend, see the box "Antibiotic Resistance."

Vaccine Controversies

Many of today's health care providers have never seen a case of measles, mumps, polio, diphtheria, or rubella. Childhood diseases that devastated previous generations have been largely eliminated by the widespread use of vaccines. As the diseases become less common, however, concern has grown about the vaccines themselves. Parents often complain about the number of shots recommended for infants, which can easily reach 17 by a child's first birthday. Recently, vaccination of infants for hepatitis B was temporarily suspended because of a fear that, because of the large number of shots, infants were receiving too much thimerosal, a mercury-containing preservative mixed with many vaccines. Routine hepatitis B vaccina-

Table 20.1	Risks From Disease vs. Risks From Vaccine: Measles-Mumps-Rubella (MMR) and Diphtheria-Tetanus-Pertussis (DTP)

Measles-Mumps-Rubella

Risk from Disease*
Measles	
Pneumonia:	1 in 20
Encephalitis:	1 in 2,000
Death:	1 in 3,000
Mumps	
Encephalitis:	1 in 300
Rubella	
Congenital Rubella Syndrome:	1 in 4 if woman infected during first trimester of pregnancy (<16 weeks)

Risk from MMR Vaccine*
Encephalitis or severe allergic reaction:	1 in 1,000,000

Diphtheria-Tetanus-Pertussis

Risk from Disease*
Diphtheria	
Death:	1 in 20
Tetanus	
Death:	3 in 100
Pertussis	
Pneumonia:	1 in 8
Encephalitis:	1 in 20
Death:	1 in 200

Risk from DTP Vaccine*
Continuous crying, then full recovery:	1 in 100
Convulsions or shock, then full recovery:	1 in 1,750
Acute encephalopathy:	0 to 10 in 1,000,000
Death:	None proven

*Risk expressed as number of adverse events per persons with disease or number of adverse events per vaccinated persons.

Source: National Immunization Program, 2004, Centers for Disease Control and Prevention.

tion has been reintroduced in a new formulation with less preservative.

Some people oppose vaccines because of their possible association with learning disabilities, autism, asthma, and sudden infant death. Large studies have confirmed some minor, short-term side effects of vaccines, such as local reactions, fever, discomfort, irritability, and, more rarely, allergic reactions, but they have not found any association with more serious conditions.[18]

Overall, vaccination is a vital part of disease prevention; risk from diseases is far greater than risk from vaccines (Table 20.1). New vaccines are constantly monitored when they are introduced, and efforts are continually under way to improve vaccine safety. As noted earlier, the controversy over vaccines is examined more fully in You Make the Call at the end of the chapter.

Reemerging and New Diseases

For a variety of reasons, several diseases that were thought to have been eliminated or controlled have reemerged in recent years. New diseases never seen before have also appeared, such as SARS. There are many such diseases; in this section we consider some of the most worrisome.

Tuberculosis

Worldwide, tuberculosis (TB) is the most common infectious disease, with approximately 30 percent of the world population infected.[19] It is caused by a mycobacterium, a subset of bacteria, and is spread primarily through aerosolized droplets coughed out of the lungs of an infected person and breathed in by another person. Once the mycobacterium is inhaled, a healthy immune system creates a wall around it and prevents it from growing or spreading. In this **latent infection,** the bacterium is in the body but not causing any signs of infection. About 5 percent to 10 percent of infected people develop the active disease at some point in their life, meaning that the bacterium is no longer controlled and can replicate, spread, and be transmitted to other people. Symptoms include cough, coughing up blood, fatigue, weight loss, night sweats, and fever. Active disease is more likely to develop if the immune system is not functioning well.

Tuberculosis has reemerged as a major health problem because of the rapid spread of HIV infection, which impairs the immune system. People with HIV/AIDS have a 30-fold increased risk of developing active tuberculosis.[20] Changes in population patterns have also influenced the spread of tuberculosis. As cities become larger and attract more people, tuberculosis spreads more easily and rapidly. Close living quarters vastly multiply the number of people who can be infected by a single person with active tuberculosis. In the United States, the people at highest risk for active tuberculosis are recent immigrants (particularly from Asia, Africa, Mexico, South America, and Central America), homeless people, prison populations, and HIV-infected people.[20]

The diagnosis of infection with TB is based on a tuberculin skin test known as a *ppd.* Latent TB infection is detected when someone has a positive skin test but a normal chest X-ray and no symptoms of active disease. Treatment is recommended for latent infection to reduce the risk of active disease. Active disease is diagnosed by a positive skin test, abnormalities on a chest X-ray and/or symptoms of disease. Treatment requires the combination of several antifungal antibiotics taken together over a period of 6 to 12 months. It is important that drug treatment is completed.

Drug-resistant tuberculosis is becoming a concern worldwide. The discipline required to take medication properly for 6 to 12 months is a barrier to effective treatment, and many people at risk for tuberculosis have additional barriers. Recent immigrants may have language barriers or fears of immigration services that may prevent them from seeking treatment. Homeless people often don't stay in one area for long and so may not follow up with the same health care provider for complete treatment. People with HIV may have complicated medication schedules that make it easy to forget the anti-tubercular drugs, or they may have interactions between medications that prevent them from taking a full course.

Public health departments play an important role in the treatment of tuberculosis. Tracking systems are in place to improve success for completion of treatment. Researchers are trying to develop simpler treatments, so that it will be easier to complete the course. New vaccines are being studied in an attempt to reduce the risk of infection and progression to active disease.[19]

Healthy People 2010

OBJECTIVE AREA *Immunization and Infectious Diseases*

- Reduce tuberculosis.

"The 1989 *Strategic Plan for the Elimination of TB in the United States* set a tuberculosis elimination goal of reducing TB to 1 new case per million by 2010. . . . However, in the mid-1980s the trend toward TB elimination was reversed, and drug-resistant strains emerged that were even more deadly. TB cases increased by 20 percent between 1985 and 1992. . . . From 1993 through 1998, new cases of TB again declined, although the resurgence and related outbreaks set back TB elimination efforts by about a decade. Elimination of TB depends on significant effort and cooperation between public and private health care providers and agencies at the Federal, State, and local levels."

For more information on Healthy People 2010 objectives, visit the Web site at www.healthypeople.gov.

For more information on Canadian health objectives, visit the Health Canada Web site at www.hc-sc.gc.ca/english.

Smallpox

Smallpox is a highly contagious viral disease transmitted through face-to-face contact or through exposure to body fluids. There are two forms of smallpox, both caused by the variola virus. Variola major causes high fever, muscle aches, and a rash that blisters and scabs. It has a fatality rate of nearly 30 percent; those who do not die are often permanently disfigured by pock marks on their skin. Variola minor is less common and has a fatality rate of 1 percent. In the 20th century alone, smallpox was responsible for the death of an estimated 300 million to 500 million people.

A worldwide vaccination program was undertaken by the World Health Organization beginning in 1967, and the last case of naturally occurring smallpox was reported in 1977. The eradication of smallpox is considered by some to be the single most important medical accomplishment of the 20th century. After the elimination of wild variola virus, vaccination for smallpox ceased. This would be the end of the story except that a few laboratories maintain stockpiles of the virus. Now, concern has arisen that variola virus could be used by terrorists in an attack.

Debate has arisen over whether large populations should be vaccinated against smallpox as protection against a possible bioterrorist attack. The vaccine causes

HIGHLIGHT ON HEALTH

An Influenza Pandemic: Could It Happen Again?

In 1918–1919, the infamous "Spanish flu" swept the globe, causing an estimated 50 million deaths. The world saw two more influenza pandemics—worldwide epidemics—in the 20th century: the "Asian flu" of 1957 and the "Hong Kong flu" of 1968. In each of these pandemics, serious illness and death were not limited to high-risk groups, such as older adults or infants; in fact, in 1918–1919, death rates were highest among healthy young adults. Today, people are asking if an influenza pandemic could happen again.

Two types of influenza virus, influenza A and influenza B, cause "flu" in humans. Influenza A is further divided into subtypes based on antigens on the surface of the virus, called H and N; subtypes are named according to these antigens, such as "H1N1." Like other viruses, the influenza virus is subject to frequent minor genetic changes—a phenomenon called antigenic drift—as well as infrequent, abrupt, major genetic change—called antigenic shift. When a slight change occurs, many people will have partial immunity from previous infection with a similar strain or vaccination. When a substantial change occurs, however, most people will have little or no immunity to the new strain.

An additional concern is that, although only three influenza A subtypes commonly infect humans (H1N1, H1N2, and H3N2), many others infect birds, pigs, horses, dogs, and other animals. Recently, outbreaks of avian (bird) influenza subtype H5N1 occurred in several Asian countries among domesticated birds, and hundreds of millions of birds died or were killed to control infection. Some humans were also infected, most from direct contact with poultry but a few apparently from contact with an infected person.

Because people have little or no immunity to the H5N1 virus, the risk of serious complications is high; in fact, in some areas nearly 50 percent of humans infected with H5N1 have died.

The fear is that the H5N1 virus could "jump" to humans—that is, that it could change such that it could easily infect people and easily spread by person-to-person contact (via droplets carried in coughs or sneezes). Such an antigenic shift could result in another influenza pandemic. Vaccination would not be effective in such a scenario. Each year, a new flu shot is developed in an attempt to respond to newer viral strains, but a major genetic shift is difficult to predict. Treatment of avian flu is also problematic, although some of the current antiviral medications are believed to be effective.

History suggests that it is only a matter of time before another influenza pandemic occurs. The virus would spread quickly around the world through international travel, leaving little time for preparation. A vaccine would not be available in the early stages. When vaccines and antiviral medications became available, there would not be enough for everyone, and decisions would have to be made about access. In some places quarantines might be imposed. All of these problems highlight the difficult issues involved in balancing the rights of individuals with society's role in serving the greater good.

While the public discussion continues, remember to practice basic good health habits: Avoid people who are sick, stay home when you are sick, wash your hands often, and take good care of your immune system. For more information on protecting yourself from influenza, visit the CDC Web site at www.cdc.gov/flu.

---

side effects and, in rare cases, severe complications.[21] At this point, smallpox vaccination is not available for the general public.

Pneumonia

Pneumonia—infection of the lungs or lower respiratory tract—is the leading cause of death due to infectious disease. Young children and older adults are at greatest risk for pneumonia; besides age, factors that increase risk include exposure to environmental pollutants and use of tobacco, alcohol, or drugs, all of which reduce the lungs' ability to clear infection. Close living situations, such as in college dorms or military barracks, can also increase the risk for pneumonia.

In general, viral pneumonia tends to be milder than bacterial pneumonia, but viral pneumonia caused by influenza can be serious and even deadly (see the box "An Influenza Pandemic: Could It Happen Again?"). Bacterial pneumonia caused by the organism *Streptococcus*

KEY TERMS

latent infection   Infection that is not currently active but could reactivate at a later time.

pneumoniae (sometimes called pneumococcal pneumonia) can also be dangerous, but it usually responds well to antibiotics. Either type of pneumonia can cause high fever, sharp chest pain, shortness of breath, and shaking chills. Vaccines are available for influenza and *S. pneumoniae*. The influenza vaccine is offered every fall; it has to be redesigned annually in an attempt to match the current strain of the virus. It is recommended for people over age 50, pregnant women, people with HIV/AIDS, and others at increased risk of pneumonia, such as those with sickle cell disease, diabetes, or alcoholism. The treatment for pneumonia depends on the organism responsible. Antiviral or antibiotic medicines can shorten the course of illness and reduce the risk of complications. If lab tests show that a case of pneumonia is viral, antibacterial antibiotics are not effective.

Whooping Cough

Whooping cough is the common name for an infection of the respiratory tract caused by the pertussis bacterium. It is highly contagious by inhaling respiratory droplets from an infected person's cough or sneeze. Initial infection may seem similar to a common cold, with nasal congestion, runny nose, mild fever, and a dry cough, but after one to two weeks, the coughing occurs in spells lasting a few minutes and ending in a "whooping" sound as the person gasps for air. Almost all infants and nearly half of older babies with pertussis require hospitalization. The illness is milder in older children, adolescents, and adults, but they can spread it to younger children. Whooping cough is treated with antibiotics, which may also be given to household members to decrease the spread of the disease. Reported cases of pertussis have increased 20-fold in the past 30 years. Most infants and young children are vaccinated against pertussis. However, immunity begins to wear off after 5 to 10 years, leaving many adolescents and adults susceptible to infection. In 2005, two new vaccines were approved as booster vaccines for teens and adults.[22]

Polio

Poliomyelitis is caused by the poliovirus and can lead to paralysis, permanent asymmetric weakness, or death. An effective vaccination campaign in the United States and many other countries has significantly reduced the incidence of polio, and in 1988, the World Health Organization pledged to eradicate the poliovirus by worldwide vaccination. In 2003, there were 784 reported cases of polio worldwide and only six countries where polio was endemic: Nigeria, India, Pakistan, Niger, Afghanistan, and Egypt. Ninety percent of cases were in Nigeria, India, and Pakistan.[23] Ongoing vaccination is important until complete eradication is attained to ensure the virus does not recur.

Ebola and Marborg Hemorrhagic Fevers

Ebola hemorrhagic fever is a severe, often fatal disease; it is caused by the Ebola virus. It was first recognized in 1976 and is believed to reside in an animal host, probably monkeys, in Africa. There have been sporadic outbreaks of Ebola in African countries, but no cases in humans have been reported in the United States, although monkeys at U.S. research facilities have been infected. The virus can be transmitted by contact with blood or secretions from an infected person.

The symptoms of Ebola hemorrhagic fever typically appear within 2 to 21 days of exposure. They include sudden onset of a fever, headache, and joint and muscle aches, followed by diarrhea, vomiting, stomach pain, and internal and external bleeding. There is no treatment, and supportive care during the disease course is all that can be offered. Early recognition and protective measures to prevent transmission to family members and caretakers are crucial to prevent the spread of the disease.[24]

Marborg hemorrhagic fever is caused by a virus in the same family as the Ebola virus. It has similar symptoms and sporadic outbreaks. In March 2005 an outbreak in Angola led to 117 deaths among 124 cases.[25]

West Nile Virus

West Nile virus was first identified in Uganda in 1937. Birds provide the reservoir for the virus, and mosquitoes are the vector that transmits the virus from birds to humans. West Nile virus causes severe inflammation of the spinal cord and brain and can lead to headache, fever, confusion, paralysis, and sometimes death.

West Nile virus probably arrived in the United States in 1999 in New York, carried by either an infected person or an infected mosquito. Since its arrival, it has spread across the United States; 2,470 people were diagnosed with West Nile viral infection and 88 deaths were attributed to the disease in 2004. The virus has been detected in humans or animals in all states except Washington, Alaska, and Hawaii.[26] Communities can address the problem posed by West Nile virus and other mosquito-borne diseases by educating the public about eliminating mosquito breeding grounds (standing water) and, in some cases, by spraying pesticides to eliminate inset populations. Individuals can protect themselves by using insect repellant containing DEET (N,N-diethyl-meta-toluamide); wearing long pants, long-sleeved shirts, and a hat when outdoors; and staying indoors during peak times of mosquito activity (early morning and early evening).

Hantavirus

Hantavirus causes hantavirus pulmonary syndrome, a rare but potentially lethal illness with a 37 percent fatality rate. The virus was first identified in the United States in 1993. The reservoir for hantavirus is the deer mouse; an infected

Table 20.2	Top Ten Infectious Diseases: Global Mortality
Condition	**Frequency ($\times$ 1,000)**
Pneumonia	4,400
Diarrhea	3,100
Tuberculosis	3,100
Malaria	2,100
AIDS	1,500
Hepatitis B	1,100
Measles	1,000
Neonatal tetanus	460
Pertussis	350
Worms	135

Source: Johns Hopkins Infectious Diseases, http://hopkins-id.edu.

mouse sheds virus in its stool, urine, and saliva. Humans become infected when they handle dry materials (such as soil) containing mouse droppings or urine and then inhale aerosolized particles from it. The disease became a concern when workers were excavating land for housing developments in previously undeveloped areas outside cities. Hantavirus cannot be spread from person to person.

The best way to protect against infection with hantavirus is rodent control. Individuals in areas where the virus is endemic should seal up any holes that allow rodents to enter the home. They should clean up sites that contain rodent droppings or nesting materials, wearing gloves and thoroughly wetting the area with a bleach solution afterwards. Campers and outdoor enthusiasts should take care not to disturb rodent burrows, nests, or dead animals.[27]

For a listing of the leading causes of death by infectious disease in the world, see Table 20.2.

SEXUALLY TRANSMITTED DISEASES

Sexually transmitted diseases (or sexually transmitted infections) are infections that are spread from one person to another through sexual contact. The best way to prevent infection with an STD is to abstain from intercourse and other intimate activities or to be in a mutually monogamous long-term relationship with an uninfected person. Condoms can prevent some but not all STD transmission.[13] Remember these ABCs of safer sex: Abstinence, Be faithful, Condom use.[28] Guidelines on talking to a partner about STDs and on protecting yourself from these widespread and potentially devastating infec-

tions are provided in Chapter 15. In this section we consider the most common and most serious STDs to which you might be exposed.

HIV/AIDS

Acquired immunodeficiency syndrome (AIDS) is caused by the human immunodeficiency virus (HIV). This new disease is taking a devastating toll worldwide. Reasons for its rapid progression to epidemic levels are that it often causes either no initial symptoms or symptoms that can be mistaken for the flu; it has a very long incubation period, so that people can be infected for months or years without knowing it and pass it on to multiple sex partners during that time; and the virus attacks the immune system, disabling and destroying the very cells that would otherwise protect the body against invading microorganisms.

At the end of 2003, an estimated 37.8 million people worldwide were infected with HIV, two thirds of them in sub-Saharan Africa and another 20 percent in Asia. In 2003 there were 4.8 million new infections and 2.9 million deaths. More than 20 million people have died from HIV/AIDS since the first case was diagnosed in 1981. The rates of infection vary significantly by country and even by region within countries. In some countries, the adult rate of infection is less than 2 percent; in others, such as Botswana and Swaziland, the rate is more than 35 percent. In sub-Saharan Africa, an estimated 12 million children have lost one or both parents to HIV/AIDS.[29]

In North America, an estimated 1 million people are living with HIV. In 2003 there were 44,000 new infections and 16,000 deaths. Of the people in the United States living with HIV, it is estimated that 25 percent of them are unaware that they are infected. The number of people living with HIV in North America is growing, owing to two factors: The number of new cases is increasing, and most infected people have access to antiviral medications that allow them to live longer with HIV.[30]

Course of the Disease

HIV-1 is the predominant strain in the United States and Canada. HIV-2, a different strain, is found primarily in Africa. Both viruses target the cells of the immune system, especially cells known as CD4 T cells and macrophages. Once inside these cells, the virus uses the host cell's DNA to replicate itself and disables the host cell so it cannot perform its normal function. During the initial infection with HIV, known as primary HIV infection, the virus replicates rapidly. Within 4 to 11 days of infection, several million viral copies may circulate in the bloodstream, more than at any other time during the natural course of infection. The immune system mounts a rapid response in an attempt to control and remove the virus, but HIV is able to mutate quickly and avoid complete eradication.

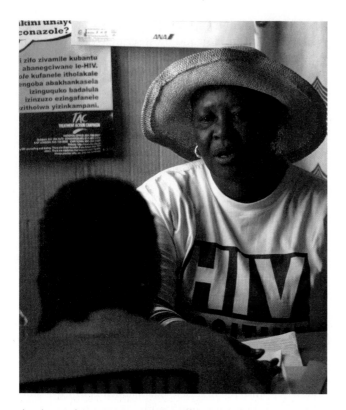

As advances in treatment approaches offer many individuals with HIV infection the chance for a reasonably good quality of life, affected people often take advantage of support groups as a resource for connection and hope.

Between 40 and 90 percent of people infected with HIV experience an illness during this acute infection phase, with such symptoms as fever, weight loss, fatigue, sore throat, lymph node swelling, night sweats, muscle aches, and diarrhea appearing 2 to 6 weeks after exposure. The symptoms may last for a few weeks and may be mistaken for other infections such as influenza, mononucleosis, or herpes.[31] (Since some of these symptoms are common, a person experiencing them should not assume they are signs of HIV infection; however, if at risk, he or she should get tested.)

After the early phase, the immune system and the virus come to a balance with the establishment of a *viral load set point,* a level of virus that continues to circulate in the blood and body fluids. During this phase, a person is asymptomatic and may remain so for 2 to 20 years. The virus continues to replicate, and the immune system continues to control it without completely removing it.

Eventually, the immune system is significantly weakened and can no longer keep up. This phase is signaled by a decreasing number of CD4 T cells and a diminishing ability of the person to fight **opportunistic infections** that someone with a healthy immune system would fight off. Common opportunistic infections are *Pneumocystis carinii* pneumonia, Kaposi's sarcoma (a rare cancer), and

tuberculosis. Opportunistic infections are the leading cause of death in people with HIV infection. A diagnosis of AIDS is given when the CD4 T cell count falls below a certain level (200 cells/ml) or when the person gets an opportunistic infection.

Methods of Transmission

HIV cannot survive long outside of a human host, and thus transmission requires intimate contact. The virus can be found in varying concentrations in an infected person's blood, saliva, semen, genital secretions, and breast milk. It usually enters a new host either at a mucosal surface or by direct inoculation into the blood. HIV is not transmitted through casual contact, such as by shaking hands, hugging, or a casual kiss, nor is it spread by day-to-day contact in the workplace, school, or home setting. Although HIV has been found in saliva and tears, it is present in very low quantities. It has not been found in sweat. Contact with saliva, tears, or sweat has not been shown to result in transmission of HIV.

Risk of HIV transmission is influenced by factors associated with the host (the already infected person), the recipient (the currently uninfected person), and the type of interaction that occurs between the host and recipient (behaviors). An important host factor is the level of virus circulating in the blood. High levels of circulating virus, such as during the initial infection stage, increase the risk of transmission. In addition, some people may have a higher viral load set point during the equilibrium period. Antiviral treatment (discussed in a later section) lowers the level of circulating virus and may reduce the risk of transmission.

Sexual Contact   The primary exposure risk for 70 percent of cases of HIV infection in the United States and for 68 percent of cases in Canada is sexual contact.[32,33] HIV can enter the body through the mucosa or lining of the vagina, penis, rectum, or mouth. If the mucosa is cut, torn, or irritated (as can happen with intercourse or if there is another STD), the risk increases. The sexual behaviors associated with transmission are receptive anal sex, insertive anal sex, penile-vaginal sex, and oral sex.

Although discussing HIV status with a potential sexual partner may be awkward, its importance cannot be overemphasized. As noted, the time of highest circulating virus is shortly after initial infection; the person may not have any symptoms and may not know he or she is infected. Also as noted, 25 percent of HIV-positive people in the United States do not know they are infected. Unless you have a conversation about whether your potential partner has been tested for HIV, what risky behaviors he or she has engaged in, and what other sexual partners he or she has been involved with, you do not know what your risk is in starting a sexual relationship.

Injection Drug Use   Injection drug use is reported as the method of HIV transmission by 20 percent of people with AIDS in Canada and 24 percent of people with AIDS in the United States. Another 4 percent and 5 percent, respectively, report both injection drug use and being a man who has sex with other men as combined risk factors. Individuals can reduce their risk of HIV infection by avoiding injection drug use. People who are already using drugs can reduce their risk by using sterile needles and not sharing needles with others. Communities can play a role in decreasing the spread of HIV by implementing needle exchange programs and ensuring adequate access to drug treatment programs.

Contact With Infected Blood or Body Fluids   HIV can be transmitted by direct contact with the blood or body fluids of an infected person. The risk of transmission again varies depending upon how much virus is in the body fluid, how much fluid gets onto another person, and where the fluid contacts the other person. If a small amount of infected blood gets onto the intact skin of another person, the risk of transmission is lower than if a large amount of blood gets onto the cut or scraped skin of another person.

The setting where this kind of transmission is most likely to occur is a health care setting. To reduce the risk of transmission of HIV, hepatitis B and C, and other blood-borne infections, the **universal precautions** approach has been instituted in these settings. Universal precautions include the use of gloves, gown, mask, and other protective wear (such as eyewear or face shields) in settings where someone is likely to be exposed to the blood or infected body fluids of another person. These precautions should be taken with every patient.[34]

Perinatal Transmission   Perinatal, or vertical, transmission—the transmission of HIV from an infected mother to her child—can occur during pregnancy, during delivery (when the fetus is exposed to the mother's blood in the birth canal), or after delivery (if the baby is exposed to the mother's breast milk). The risk of transmission from mother to child can be reduced through the use of antiretroviral medications during pregnancy and around the time of delivery. Infected mothers also reduce the risk to their babies by electing not to breast-feed.

In the United States and Canada, women are routinely offered HIV testing as part of prenatal care. If she tests positive, a woman is offered preventive therapy with antiretroviral medications to reduce her child's risk. In untreated women with HIV, approximately 30 percent of infants are infected; in treated women, less than 2 percent are infected.

Certain groups have higher rates of HIV infection than others do; see the box "Disproportionate Risk for HIV."

HIV Testing

The earlier HIV infection is recognized, the sooner treatment can begin, the longer the person is likely to remain symptom free, and the fewer people he or she is likely to expose to the virus. The only way to confirm HIV infection is by a laboratory test. The standard procedure in North America has been to screen the blood with an enzyme immune assay (EIA) or an enzyme-linked immunosorbent assay (ELISA) test. Both tests detect antibodies to HIV-1 and thus confirm infection only after the immune response has been activated. If the result is positive, a Western blot test is done to confirm the finding. The Western blot test also detects antibodies to HIV and can distinguish some other antibodies that might cause a false positive result on the earlier tests. A person with circulating antibodies is said to be HIV-positive.

It takes 1 to 2 weeks to get the results of an EIA or ELISA test. Several rapid tests are now available that allow a person to get results the same day. These tests are believed to be as accurate as the EIA or ELISA test, but their results must still be confirmed with a Western blot test. Because all these tests look for the immune response to HIV, they may not detect a recent infection. If the most recent potential exposure to HIV is within 3 months of testing, it is recommended that the test be repeated in 3 months. It is also possible to test for recent HIV infection by looking for the actual virus in the blood, through a viral load test. This test is used if HIV infection is suspected based on acute symptoms.

HIV testing requires a visit to a health care provider at this time. However, a home collection system called the Home Access Express HIV-1 test system has been approved by the FDA. The consumer buys the kit from a pharmacy, collects a small sample of blood at home from a finger prick, places the blood on a card, mails the card to a registered laboratory, and telephones for results. The FDA has not approved any home test kits in which the person determines the result him- or herself. Several of these kits are advertised but have not been shown to give consistent results. Consumers are warned against using them at this time.[35]

(KEY) TERMS

opportunistic infection   Infection that would be disposed of by a healthy immune system but that a weakened immune system cannot fight off.
universal precautions   Use of protective wear, such as gloves, gown, mask, and eyewear, in settings where someone is likely to be exposed to the blood or infected body fluids of another person.

HIGHLIGHT ON HEALTH
Disproportionate Risk for HIV

For a variety of reasons, certain groups have a disproportionately high risk of HIV:

- Men who have sex with men continue to be the group with the highest rates of HIV infection in North America. Male-to-male sexual contact is the exposure reported in 40 percent of AIDS cases. Recent studies suggest that rates of new infection in this population are rising, after a dramatic decline in the 1990s; this increase raises concern that individuals are no longer avoiding the riskiest sexual behaviors or taking necessary precautions. Men who have sex with men continue to be at risk for HIV and other sexually transmitted infections through unprotected receptive or insertive anal sex with casual partners or with partners of unknown status or with HIV-positive status.

- Minority populations bear a disproportionate burden in the HIV/AIDS epidemic. About 51 percent of reported AIDS cases in the United States occur among African Americans, even though they make up only about 12 percent of the total population. About 17 percent of AIDS cases occur among Hispanics, who make up about 13 percent of the population.

- Worldwide, 50 percent of the estimated 14,000 new infections a day in 2003 occurred in people aged 15 to 24. Youth are at increased risk because of risky sexual behaviors, substance use, and perceived lack of risk from HIV. Young people may also lack the power or skills to negotiate for safer sex.

- Of these same 14,000 new infections a day worldwide, 50 percent occur in women. The number of women living with HIV/AIDS is growing; their primary risk is heterosexual contact. In many countries in the world, women are infected by their husbands. In North America, rates of infection in women are increasing, again disproportionately affecting minority women. In the United States, 80 percent of HIV infections in women occur in African American and Hispanic women.

Sources: HIV/AIDS Update May 2004, Canada. www.hc-sc.gc.ca; HIV/AIDS Surveillance by Race and Ethnicity (through 2002), Centers for Disease Control and Prevention, www.cdc.gov; HIV/AIDS Among U.S. Women: Minority and Young Women at Continuing Risk, CDC Division of HIV/AIDS prevention, www.cdc.gov.

Medical and technological advances have made HIV testing easier and more convenient than in the past. There are several testing options, including rapid testing, and tests can be performed on urine or oral swabs as well as blood. If you have behavioral risks for HIV infection, you should consider getting tested.[36]

Management of HIV/AIDS

The development of new medications and improved understanding of the disease process have contributed to prolonged survival by some people infected with HIV. However, management of HIV/AIDS is complicated both for HIV-infected persons and for their health care providers. The benefits of medical treatment have been seen in the developed countries but have not reached the developing countries. A campaign called the 3 by 5 Initiative, undertaken by the World Health Organization and the UNAIDS organization, set a goal of providing effective treatment for HIV infection to 3 million people in developing countries by the year 2005. By December 2004, an estimated 700,000 people needing antiretroviral therapy had been reached. This represents only 12 percent of the estimated 5.8 million needing treatment.[37]

Antiretroviral Agents   The most important medications in HIV treatment are antiviral drugs—or, more accurately, antiretroviral drugs, since HIV is a type of virus called a retrovirus. Antiretroviral medications do not cure the infection, but they slow the rate at which the virus replicates and destroys the immune system, thus prolonging life and improving the quality of life for people who are HIV-positive. Four different categories of drugs are used against HIV: nucleoside reverse transcriptase inhibitors (NRTI), non-nucleoside reverse transcriptase inhibitors (NNRTI), protease inhibitors (PI), and fusion inhibitors (FI). Each functions in a different way to stop replication of HIV. Drugs within each category have slight differences in side effects, frequency of use, cost, and number of pills taken a day. These factors can be extremely important when a medication must be taken for years.

Drug Cocktails   HIV has an uncanny ability to develop drug resistance. On average, 10 billion viral particles are produced every day in an infected person, offering many opportunities for mutation and the development of resistance. If a single antiretroviral medication is used, resistant strains develop fairly quickly. To combat resistance, scientists have developed complicated drug combinations, called **drug cocktails,** that usually include a medication from two to four of the drug categories. It is less likely that a viral strain will develop several mutations allowing it to evade the combination of drugs than one or a few mutations allowing it to evade a single drug. However, the complexity, cost, and risk of side effects for the person taking the drugs are all increased.

New Treatment Possibilities   Since the identification of the virus, researchers have been attempting to develop a safe, effective, and inexpensive HIV vaccine, but the challenge is enormous. To develop a vaccine, scientists must be able to identify a part of the virus that could produce protective immunity if injected into a host. However, the immune system does not seem to be able to clear HIV and produce immunity; instead, the virus produces lifelong infection. Furthermore, the virus is a moving target; it mutates frequently and develops new strains rapidly. That said, more than 30 vaccine trials are under way around the world.[38]

Another avenue being pursued is the development of a **microbicide,** a compound or chemical in the form of a cream, gel, or suppository that would kill microorganisms and that could be applied topically to the vagina or rectum before intercourse, reducing the risk of STD transmission. Many such products are currently under study. Microbicides would offer an alternative to condoms and could be especially important to women. Condom use requires the cooperation of a woman's partner; microbicides can be used without the consent or cooperation of a partner and so could empower women and reduce their risk of infection.[39]

Other Major STDs

Sexually transmitted diseases are a major epidemic, especially among teenagers and young adults. The infections often go unnoticed, because most do not cause symptoms in early stages. They all can lead to significant health problems, and many can increase the risk of transmitting and acquiring HIV. Bacterial STDs can usually be treated effectively with antibiotics; viral STDs cannot be cured, but they can be managed. In this section we consider the most common major STDs.

Chlamydia

The most commonly reported bacterial STD, chlamydia is caused by the bacterium *Chlamydia trachomatis*. The rates of infection are increasing, with an estimated 2.8 million cases diagnosed annually in the United States. Add Health, a study that randomly tested a representative sample of men and women in the general population across the United States aged 18 to 26, revealed that 4.1 percent had chlamydia infections. Most of these people had no symptoms or at least did not have symptoms that were prompting them to seek treatment.[40]

Most people with chlamydia are not aware they are infected. The majority of infected women and up to 50 percent of infected men have no symptoms at all. If symptoms do develop, they occur about 1 to 3 weeks after exposure via vaginal, anal, or oral sex with an infected person. For women, symptoms could include a mild burning sensation with urination and a slight increase in vaginal discharge. Infected men may have a watery penile discharge, a burning sensation with urination, or pain and swelling in the scrotum. Untreated infection can persist for months or years and can lead to pelvic inflammatory disease in women (discussed later in this section). There is also an association between chlamydia infection and increased risk of HIV acquisition and transmission for both men and women. Chlamydia can be effectively treated with antibiotics; however, a person can be reinfected if reexposed. If there has been scarring of the fallopian tubes or other parts of the female reproductive system from pelvic inflammatory disease, that damage cannot be reversed.

Several tests have been developed to screen for chlamydia infection; they can be performed on urine or on a specimen collected from the penis or cervix. Routine screening of people with a high risk of infection is extremely important, given the lack of symptoms and the benefits of early treatment. Members of minority groups are at greater risk for chlamydia infection, as are people who live in regions of the United States with higher rates of infection, particularly the southern states. The primary risk factor appears to be age. Approximately half of all reported chlamydia cases occur in the 15-to-19-year-old age group, and another third occur in the 20-to-24-year-old age group.

Experts recommend that all sexually active women under age 25 be screened regularly for chlamydia, as should any women who are at increased risk because they have a new sexual partner, have multiple sexual partners, or are infected with another STD. There is a debate about whether it is cost effective to screen all sexually active men under age 25. Men should be aware that they can have no symptoms with this infection and should consider testing if they have a new sexual partner.[41]

KEY TERMS

drug cocktails   Complicated drug combinations used to overcome drug resistance in different strains of HIV.

microbicide   Compound or chemical in the form of a cream, gel, or suppository that would kill microorganisms and that could be applied topically to the vagina or rectum before intercourse, reducing the risk of STD transmission.

Gonorrhea

Gonorrhea is caused by the bacterium *Neisseria gonorrhoeae*. The Add Health study found that 0.43 percent of men and women ages 18 to 26 had gonorrhea but no symptoms.[40] As with chlamydia, the highest rates of gonorrhea infection occur in men and women aged 15 to 24 years.

In women, gonorrhea is usually asymptomatic. If women do develop symptoms, they usually occur at a late, severe stage when infection has caused pelvic inflammatory disease. The majority of men infected with gonorrhea eventually develop a penile discharge. Infection can also occur in the rectum or the throat in people who engage in anal or oral sex. Because men often (but not always) have symptoms, they usually notice the infection early and get treatment.

Several tests have been developed to screen and detect gonococcal infection in asymptomatic people and to confirm infection in people with symptoms suggestive of gonorrhea. The tests can be performed on samples taken from the throat, penis, anus, or vagina or on a urine sample. Regular screening is recommended for women at high risk of infection—those who are under 25 and have had two or more sex partners in the past year, who exchange sex for money or drugs, or who have a history of repeated episodes of gonorrhea. It is less clear if asymptomatic men should be screened, because most men eventually develop symptoms.

Gonorrhea is treated with antibiotics. Penicillin was the treatment of choice for many years, but because of widespread drug resistance, it has been replaced by a newer group of antibiotics called cephalosporin. The emergence of more resistant strains remains a concern. Reinfection can occur with repeat exposure.

Pelvic Inflammatory Disease

Pelvic inflammatory disease (PID) is an infection of the uterus, fallopian tubes, and/or ovaries. The infection occurs when bacteria from the vagina or cervix spread upward into the uterus and fallopian tubes. The bacteria involved are usually from STDs, such as chlamydia or gonorrhea, but they can be bacteria that are normally found in the vagina. PID occurs most commonly in women aged 15 to 25.

Symptoms of PID include fever, abdominal pain, pelvic pain, and vaginal bleeding or discharge. A woman experiencing any of these symptoms should see her health care provider. If PID is suspected, a combination of antibiotics is prescribed to cover gonorrhea, chlamydia, and vaginal bacteria. If symptoms are severe, hospitalization may be required. About 18 percent of women with PID develop chronic abdominal or pelvic pain that lasts more than 6 months.

PID can cause severe consequences and can be life threatening if untreated. Most of the long-term problems arise from scarring in the fallopian tubes, which increases the risk of ectopic pregnancy (a pregnancy that implants outside of the uterus) and infertility. Women with a history of PID have a 7- to 10-fold increased risk of ectopic pregnancy, and about 20 percent of women with PID will experience infertility. Regular screening for asymptomatic chlamydia infection in sexually active women under age 25 has been shown to reduce the risk of PID by detecting infection early.[42]

Human Papillomavirus

Human papillomavirus (HPV) is the most common STD in the United States. More than two dozen types of HPV infect the genital region. Some types are associated with genital warts, others with **cervical dysplasia** and cervical cancer in women. Four types of HPV account for approximately 80 percent of invasive cervical cancers. HPV is also associated with cancers at other body sites, including the vagina, vulva, anus, skin, throat, and penis.

Estimates are that 15 percent to 20 percent of the general population in the United States are infected with HPV. Rates of infection vary by age. A study of college-age women found HPV in 46 percent of the sample. As women get older, the rate of HPV infection declines, suggesting that the infection may spontaneously resolve with time. There is no treatment that eradicates or cures HPV infection, as is true of many viral infections.[43]

The most serious side effect of HPV infection is cervical cancer, which can occur in women in their 20s and 30s and at one time was a leading cause of cancer-related deaths in women. HPV infection progresses to cervical cancer usually over the course of many years, with low-grade lesions becoming high-grade lesions and then cancerous cells. The lesions can regress to less dangerous forms at any point in time, although this is less likely to occur farther along in the disease process. The Papanicolaou smear ("Pap" test) was introduced as a way to detect these early precursor cancer lesions, which can then be treated. Rates of cervical cancer and related deaths among women have dropped substantially since the introduction of the Pap test. This test is recommended for all sexually active women.

HPV is highly transmittable through penile-vaginal sex and anal sex. As noted earlier, condoms do not appear to reduce the risk of HPV transmission. However, condom use does appear to lead to a faster rate of regression of cervical lesions in an infected person.[13] Women who have sex with women should have regular Pap tests. Although they have lower HPV transmission rates than heterosexual women do, they are still at risk. Currently, women who have sex with women have Pap tests less frequently than heterosexual women do, often because of the misconception that they are not at risk for HPV.[44]

It appears that an effective vaccine for HPV may have been developed. Initial trials show that this vaccine can prevent HPV infection and the development of precursor cancer lesions. Although the vaccine is still experimental, larger trials are under way and it may be a reality before long.[45]

Genital Herpes

Genital herpes is caused by the herpes simplex virus (HSV), which has two strains, called HSV-1 and HSV-2. Both strains can infect the mouth, genitals, or skin. HSV-1 is often associated with lesions in and around the mouth (cold sores). This type of herpes is frequently acquired in childhood from nonsexual transmission, although up to 30 percent of genital herpes has been associated with HSV-1. The type more frequently associated with genital herpes is HSV-2.[46]

The first sign of herpes simplex infection is the appearance of small, painful ulcers or sores at the site where the person first contacted HSV, in or around the genitals or mouth. The initial illness can be quite severe, with fever and swelling of the lymph nodes. This acute stage may last from 7 to 10 days. The virus then becomes latent, remaining in the body and reactivating periodically with painful sores at the site of initial contact. The virus is shed or released even without evidence of a sore or an ulcer; an infected person can spread the infection to another even if there is no visible lesion.

Because there is no cure for HSV infection, prevention is particularly important. Condoms partially protect people against infection with HSV, but they are not 100 percent effective. Condoms must be used all the time and not just when a lesion is present. Several different vaccines for HSV are currently under study.[46] Antiviral medications are available that shorten the course of outbreaks and reduce their frequency. These medications may also reduce the risk of transmission to sexual partners.

Hepatitis

Hepatitis (inflammation of the liver) can be caused by several viruses, but the most common ones are hepatitis A, B, and C. We discussed hepatitis C earlier in the context of injection drug use, the most common route of acquiring the infection. There is debate over whether hepatitis C can be transmitted sexually. It does appear that sexual transmission can occur, but the virus is not efficient at getting from one person to another via this route.

Hepatitis A and B are both easily transmitted through sexual acts. Hepatitis A is transmitted through fecal-oral contact and can be spread through contact with contaminated food or water. The people at greatest risk for sexual transmission of hepatitis A are those who have oral-anal contact or penile-anal intercourse. About 4 weeks after exposure to the virus, hepatitis A causes a self-limited inflammation of the liver; symptoms include nausea,

vomiting, abdominal pain, and jaundice. The diagnosis is confirmed by a blood test for the virus. A safe and effective vaccine is available for hepatitis A and is recommended for men who have sex with men, illicit drug users, people with chronic liver disease, and the general population in areas that have high rates of hepatitis A or before travel to such areas.[47]

Most hepatitis B infections in the United States are sexually transmitted, although the infection can also be spread by exposure to infected blood. Worldwide, hepatitis B is a major cause of liver disease, liver failure, and liver cancer; unlike hepatitis A, it can cause chronic liver disease. The chance of developing chronic disease varies by age at the time of infection. An infant exposed to hepatitis B during delivery has a 90 percent chance of developing chronic disease; a child exposed before the age of 5 has a 60 percent chance; an adolescent or adult has a 2 to 6 percent chance. Chronic infection carries an increased risk of liver failure and liver cancer.

A safe and effective vaccine for hepatitis B is available, and universal vaccination of all children is recommended. Adolescents and adults who were not vaccinated in childhood and are sexually active should be vaccinated; some colleges encourage hepatitis B vaccinations for all entering students. (For more information on vaccinations recommended for adults, see the box "Vaccinations: Not Just for Kids.") Because of the risk of transmission by blood, hepatitis B vaccinations are currently required for all health care workers. In addition, all pregnant women are screened to determine whether their infants are at high risk of infection during delivery. High-risk infants can be vaccinated immediately after birth to further decrease risk of infection with hepatitis B during the birth process.[47]

Syphilis

Rates of syphilis, a disease caused by infection with the bacterium *Treponema pallidum*, decreased throughout the 20th century but began to increase slightly in 2001. Rates of infection vary significantly by population group and geographic region. New cases among women and non-Hispanic blacks continue to decrease, but rates among men who have sex with men are increasing. Rates among non-Hispanic blacks are 15 times higher than rates among non-Hispanic whites and account for 62 percent of cases. Historically, rates of syphilis have been high in the South, but they are decreasing in that region and increasing in the West and Northeast.[48]

 KEY TERMS

cervical dysplasia   Early changes in the cells of the cervix that can go on to become cancerous.

Challenges & Choices

Vaccinations: Not Just for Kids

You know that children should receive their regular recommended shots, but did you know that adults need shots too? Look over the following recommended adult vaccinations to see if you are up-to-date with your shots.

Varicella (chickenpox): Many adults have immunity to chickenpox from a childhood exposure. If you are not sure if you had this disease, see your physician to have your immune status checked with a blood test. If you don't show signs of immunity, you should get a vaccination. Chickenpox in adults can have serious complications.

Pneumococcal vaccine: Pneumococcal pneumonia can cause serious illness in older adults and people who are chronically ill. If you have a chronic illness, have had your spleen removed, have sickle cell disease, or are 65 years old or older, you should get a pneumococcal vaccination.

Tetanus: Tetanus, or lockjaw, is a potentially fatal disease caused by *Clostridium tetani,* an organism found in the soil that may enter the body through a puncture wound. Adults should have a booster shot every 10 years. If you are injured and your medical records don't show the date of your last tetanus vaccination, your physician may recommend the booster.

Influenza: Vaccination against influenza is recommended every year if you are 50 years old or older or if you have a medical condition that increases the risk of complications (for example, heart disease, lung disease, asthma, diabetes, pregnancy, immunosuppression). Because there are so many different strains of influenza virus, the vaccine is redesigned each year to target the strains that are expected to be most common.

Hepatitis B: Hepatitis B vaccination is recommended if you have multiple sexual partners (even if you have only one partner at a time), if you use intravenous drugs, if you are a health care worker, or if you have the potential for exposure to blood products.

Hepatitis A: Hepatitis A vaccination is recommended if you are traveling to an area where hepatitis A is common, such as Mexico, Central America, and South America, or if there is a local outbreak of the disease. Some authorities recommend vaccination for food service workers; if you work with food, check with your local health department for advice. Men who have sex with men are also at increased risk of hepatitis A and should be vaccinated.

Measles, mumps, and rubella: If you don't have a record of childhood measles or of measles vaccination, you should receive the measles, mumps, and rubella (MMR) vaccination. This vaccination is especially important if you are a woman of childbearing age, because rubella infection (German measles) during pregnancy can be devastating to a fetus. The MMR vaccination cannot be given during pregnancy, so women of childbearing age are advised to get it even if they are not currently planning to have a child.

Meningococcal vaccine: Meningococcal meningitis is a dangerous form of meningitis with symptoms of severe headache, high fever, stiff neck, and a rash. If you are living in close quarters, such as in a college dormitory, you should consider meningococcal vaccination.

Pertussis: Two new vaccines have been approved for use in adolescents and adults. They combine an acellular pertussis vaccine as part of the routine tetanus/diphtheria booster. The boosters offer extended protection against pertussis in adolescents and adults.

Other vaccinations: Other vaccines may be recommended if you plan on traveling to other countries. See your health care provider and visit the CDC Web site for travel advice.

It's Not Just Personal . . .

The dramatic success of the polio vaccine overshadows the fact that certain life-threatening diseases are still not under control. Malaria, for example, kills approximately 1.1 million people worldwide annually, most of them young children in sub-Saharan Africa. Despite many years of research and several promising leads, no effective vaccine for malaria has been developed to date. The reason comes down to money—or lack of it. Of the $56 billion spent on all biomedical research, only about $100 million has been directed toward malaria research.

Source: Data from Disease Information: Malaria, 2005, Global Alliance for Vaccines and Immunization. www.vaccinealliance.org.

Untreated syphilis progresses through several stages. In the first stage, called *primary syphilis,* a moist, painless sore called a *chancre* appears 10 days to 3 months after sexual contact with an infected person. The chancre is usually in the genital area, mouth, or anus and heals on its own within a few weeks. The primary stage can go unnoticed because the sore is painless. The second stage, *secondary syphilis,* occurs 3 to 6 weeks after the appearance of the chancre and is characterized by a skin rash that often involves the palms of the hands and soles of the feet. The rash can be accompanied by fever, fatigue, sore throat, joint pains, and a headache. Secondary syphilis also resolves without treatment, but it can recur over several years.

Many people then enter a period in which the syphilis is latent or inactive; the infected person is no longer contagious and may show no signs of disease. However, about a third of secondary syphilis cases progress to a final stage, called *tertiary syphilis,* many years after the initial infection. In this stage, the disease causes deterioration of the brain, arteries, bones, heart, and other organs, leading to dementia, ataxia (lack of coordination), and severe pain. Death can result from nervous system deterioration or heart failure. The treatment for syphilis in all stages is penicillin. However, in the late stages, organ damage cannot be reversed.[49]

A pregnant woman with active syphilis can transmit infection to her fetus, causing serious mental and physical problems. Infection with syphilis also increases the risk of transmitting and acquiring HIV infection. Screening for syphilis is recommended for all pregnant women at their initial prenatal care visit and for persons at increased risk for syphilis infection. This includes men who have sex with men, commercial sex workers, and anyone who tests positive for another STD, exchanges sex for drugs, or has sex with partners who have syphilis.[50]

Other STDs

Several other infections are transmitted sexually or involve the genital area. Most are treatable infections. While not all are sexually transmitted, we discuss them here because their symptoms can be confused with other sexually transmitted infections. They include trichomoniasis, bacterial vaginosis, candidiasis, urinary tract infection, and pubic lice and scabies.

Trichomoniasis

Trichomoniasis is caused by the protozoa *Trichomonas vaginalis* and is transmitted from person to person by sexual activity. Men infected with "trich" may have pain with urination or a watery discharge from the penis, but they usually have no symptoms. Infected women may experience vaginal soreness and itchiness, a frothy yellow-green vaginal discharge, and a musty, fishy vaginal odor. The di-

agnosis is confirmed by examination of the vaginal discharge under a microscope. Trichomoniasis is treated with the antibiotic metronidazole. Sexual partners of the infected person need to be contacted and treated to prevent the further spread and recurrence of the infection.[47]

Bacterial Vaginosis

Bacterial vaginosis (BV) is an alteration of the normal vaginal flora; lactobacillis, the usually predominant bacteria, is replaced with different bacteria, causing a vaginal discharge and unpleasant odor. It is not clear why women develop bacterial vaginosis. Although it is not considered an STD, women who have never had sex rarely experience the condition. Treatment of male partners does not alter the rate of recurrence for women.

BV is diagnosed by an evaluation of the vaginal flora under a microscope. Treatment is recommended not just because the symptoms are unpleasant but also because BV has been associated with increased risk of PID, complications in pregnancy, and transmission of HIV. The condition is treated with the same antibiotic that is used to treat trichomoniasis, metronidazole, which can be taken orally or vaginally.[47]

Candidiasis

Candidiasis is usually caused by the yeast *Candida albicans;* symptoms of yeast infection include vaginal discharge, itching, soreness, and burning with urination. About 75 percent of women have an episode of candidiasis during their lifetime. Yeast infections are not usually acquired through sexual intercourse, but they can be mistaken for an STD because the symptoms are similar. *C. albicans* can be a normal part of the vaginal flora and may overgrow in response to changes in the vaginal environment, such as when a woman takes antibiotics or if she has diabetes.

Candidiasis is treated by antifungal medications that can be taken orally as a pill or applied to the vagina as a tablet or cream. Several antifungal creams, such as miconazole or clotrimazole, are available over the counter. If a woman is unsure of the diagnosis, has recurrences, or is at risk for STDs, she should have the diagnosis confirmed by a health care provider before she treats herself.[47]

Urinary Tract Infection

Urinary tract infections and bladder infections are usually caused by the bacteria *E. coli,* although they can be caused by other bacteria. Women can develop urinary tract infections after intercourse if bacteria are pushed up into the bladder. Symptoms include pain or burning with urination, pain in the lower abdomen, urgency and frequency of urination, and, if the kidneys become involved, fever and pain in the back. Treatment includes increased fluids and antibiotics. For women, urinating after intercourse may reduce the risk of infection.

Pubic Lice and Scabies

Pubic lice and scabies are ectoparasites that can be sexually transmitted. Pubic lice (or "crabs") infect the skin in the pubic region and cause intense itching. Scabies can infect the skin on any part of the body and, again, cause intense itching. In adults, both pubic lice and scabies are most often sexually transmitted, but in children, scabies is usually acquired through nonsexual contact. Both infections are treated with a medicated cream or shampoo called permethrin or lindane. Bedding and clothing must be decontaminated to prevent reinfection, either by machine washing and drying or by enclosure in a plastic bag for at least 72 hours.[47]

PREVENTION AND TREATMENT OF INFECTIOUS DISEASES

Efforts to control and manage infectious diseases involve prevention, preparedness, surveillance, and treatment. *Prevention* includes vaccination, sanitation, and hygiene. *Preparedness* includes ongoing research into new vaccines, antibiotics, and lifestyle changes. *Surveillance* means maintaining strong public health organizations on local, regional, national, and international levels to keep a close watch on emerging and changing patterns of infection. *Treatment* consists of efforts by both the medical establishment and individuals to eliminate diseases once preventive measures have failed to ward them off.

There are many steps that you as an individual can take to help prevent the spread of infectious diseases. Here are a few:

- Support your immune system by eating a balanced diet, getting enough exercise and sleep, managing stress, not smoking, and adopting other practices that are part of a healthy lifestyle.

- Follow government recommendations for vaccinations for you and your children. If you are in a high-risk group, get a flu shot when it is offered in the fall.

- If you know you have been exposed to an infectious disease, take steps to minimize the chances that you will pass it on to someone else. For example, if you have a cold or the flu, follow good hygiene practices (for example, wash your hands frequently), stay home from work, and avoid crowded public places.

- Minimize your use of antibiotics: Don't buy antibacterial soaps, try to avoid meat or poultry from animals that have been fed antibiotics, and don't take antibacterial antibiotics for viral infections. When prescribed antibiotics for a bacterial infection, take them as directed and complete the full course of treatment.

- Practice the ABCs of safer sex. If you have been exposed to an STD, see your physician for testing and treatment, and tell any sexual partners that they have been exposed so that they can be treated too.

- If you are planning a trip to a new part of the country or a new country, consult a reliable source to learn what infectious diseases are common in that location and how you can decrease your risk of infection while visiting or living there.

- Participate in efforts to reduce the likelihood that new diseases will take hold in your community, such as by getting rid of any standing water in your yard where mosquitoes could breed.

Infectious diseases will always be part of human existence. We may discover treatments for some diseases, but new organisms are continually evolving, both independently and in response to human behaviors and activities. By being knowledgeable and vigilant, we can reduce their negative impact on our lives.

You Make the Call

Should Universal Vaccination Be Required?

Some of the decline in infectious disease mortality seen in the United States in the 20th century can be attributed to widespread vaccination campaigns, especially childhood vaccination programs carried out in schools and communities. All states currently require vaccinations for children attending public schools, with the exception of those children who have medical reasons not to be vaccinated. Most states do grant exemptions from

vaccination requirements for religious and philosophical reasons.

A movement against mandatory childhood vaccinations is gaining strength in the United States, and health care providers and public health officials are concerned. Most believe vaccination should continue to be required by law with few exemptions. Opponents argue that vaccination should be a matter of individual or parental choice.

Every vaccination poses some risk to the individual, but the disease that the vaccine protects against also carries a risk, usually a much greater one. The risk from the vaccine has to be balanced against the likelihood that the individual will be exposed to the disease and the likelihood that the disease will cause a significant health problem. Consider the case of pertussis, the bacterium that causes whooping cough. For adults, pertussis causes a bothersome cough, but for young children, it can cause a potentially life-threatening infection. An adult with pertussis can infect an infant, with devastating results. Vaccination against pertussis is recommended for all children starting at age 2 months, when the risk is highest for serious complications from the disease.

Vaccination programs work best if everyone vaccinates against diseases. When vaccination rates are high, the community develops "herd immunity"—that is, the whole group is protected even if some people are not vaccinated. There are no large reservoirs of the disease-causing organism, so it is simply less common. For herd immunity to be effective, most people need to be vaccinated. Some people consider it unfair when families refuse to have their own children vaccinated and instead rely on herd immunity, which requires that other members of the community take the individual risk associated with vaccination.

Some people also argue that because childhood diseases are now so rare in the United States, the risk of side effects from vaccination outweighs the risk of disease. Polio vaccination is an example of how a vaccine recommendation has changed because of the low prevalence of the disease. For many years, an oral vaccine was given against polio. In rare cases the oral vaccine caused vaccine-induced polio. It has been replaced by a safer injectable form of vaccine, even though the oral form was slightly more effective in triggering the desired immune response. Because there had not been a case of wild polio (polio not associated with vaccination) in the United States since the 1970s, authorities felt that any risk of vaccine-induced polio was too great.

At the same time, polio continues to be a threat in many countries in the world that are only a plane ride away from the United States. Today, no country can be totally isolated from vaccine-preventable diseases as long as those diseases continue to be present in other countries. The risk to individuals is ongoing.

Opponents of mandatory childhood vaccinations are also concerned with the rapidly increasing number of vaccinations recommended for children. Although the issues associated with the preservative thimerosal have been largely addressed, the number and complexity of vaccinations remain an issue. Opponents argue that too many vaccinations may stress the immune system to the point where it cannot respond properly to infectious agents normally encountered in the environment.

Public health officials think vaccination against childhood diseases should continue as long as the diseases appear anywhere in the world. Opponents disagree. What do you think?

Pros

- Vaccination decreases the risk that exposure to a pathogen will cause infection or disease in the vaccinated person; it is a highly successful health promotion measure for individuals, especially children. Even if a vaccinated person becomes infected with an organism, vaccination usually reduces the severity of the disease.
- Widespread vaccination shrinks the reservoir of infectious agents, protecting communities even if some individuals are not vaccinated. However, herd immunity is effective only if most people are vaccinated. A fully immunized population is the best way to promote health for all. As the percentage of vaccinated people declines, the risk of disease outbreaks and epidemics grows, as does the risk to vulnerable individuals, such as infants, pregnant women, and people with compromised immune systems.
- Even if a disease is rare in the United States, people can be exposed to it when traveling to other countries, or the pathogen may be carried here.
- Without vaccination, U.S. populations could become vulnerable to bioterrorist attacks with potentially dangerous infectious agents.

Cons

- Vaccinations can cause side effects, and the full range of potential side effects is sometimes unknown, especially with new vaccines.
- The increased number and complexity of recommended vaccinations increase the risk of exposure to preservatives and other vaccine components with unknown side effects.
- Parents should have the right to determine what medical treatments their children receive; health care decisions should not be dictated by the state.
- Many of the diseases for which we currently vaccinate are rarely found in the United States at this time. Thus, the risk of complications may be greater than the risk of exposure to disease.

SUMMARY

- An infection occurs when a microorganism invades a person's body, sometimes causing illness or death. The chain of infection is the process whereby a disease-causing agent, or pathogen, moves from one host to another. If many people are infected by the same pathogen at the same time, an epidemic may occur.

- Pathogens fall into several broad categories with similar characteristics. Viruses are some of the smallest pathogens; they can replicate only inside another organism's cells. Viral diseases include the common cold, influenza, and human papillomavirus, which causes genital warts and cervical cancer.

- Bacteria are single-celled organisms that come in a variety of shapes and cause such diseases as staphylococcus infections, strep throat, and chlamydia infection.

- Other pathogens include prions, identified as the infectious agent in mad cow disease; fungi, which cause such infections as ringworm, athlete's foot, and yeast infections; helminths (parasitic worms), which include tapeworm and hookworm; protozoa, which cause such infections as giardia, toxoplasmosis, and malaria; and ectoparasites, which include fleas, ticks, and lice.

- The body's defenses against disease consist of physical barriers (skin, mucous membranes); chemical barriers (saliva, stomach acid); and the immune system, the complex set of cells, chemicals, and processes that attack and destroy invading microorganisms.

- The innate immune system rapidly disposes of pathogens in a nonspecific way, through the action of phagocytes and other cells deployed during the acute inflammatory response. The acquired immune system is a set of specialized responses to specific targets; it develops as the individual is exposed to infections and vaccines. Plasma cells (a type of B cell) produce antibodies to destroy foreign substances; T cells work in a variety of ways to start, amplify, and end the immune response.

- Immunity is a reduced susceptibility to a disease based on the immune system's ability to remember, recognize, and mount a rapid defense against a pathogen it has previously encountered. Immunization and vaccination help prevent infection because of this ability. Vaccination protects both individuals and society.

- Healthy lifestyle behaviors like eating well, getting enough sleep, and managing stress support the immune system and reduce the risk of illness. Uncontrollable risk factors for infectious disease include age, genetic factors, and sociocultural factors.

- Autoimmune diseases occur when the immune system mistakenly identifies a part of the body as "nonself" and attacks it. Allergic reactions occur when the body identifies a harmless foreign substance, such as pollen, as an infectious agent and launches an immune response against it.

- Although infectious diseases are no longer the killers they once were, they remain an important concern, as demonstrated by the appearance of HIV and other new infections, changes in patterns of infection, and the development of antibiotic resistance in many strains of bacteria. These shifting patterns in infectious disease are related both to advances in technology and changes in human behavior. Technological advances include the development of blood banks and centralized food production and distribution; changes in human behavior include world travel, sexual behaviors, illicit drug use, and tattooing and piercing.

- Antibiotic resistance is increasing as a result of antibiotic misuse and overuse, not just by individuals and the medical establishment but also by the agriculture industry in livestock and crops.

- Although vaccines have been instrumental in controlling and eliminating infectious diseases, there is growing opposition to routine vaccination of all children for multiple diseases.

- Serious new diseases have appeared in recent years, and some dangerous old ones have reemerged. They include HIV infection, SARS, tuberculosis, smallpox, pneumonia, whooping cough, polio, Ebola and Marborg hemorrhagic fevers, West Nile virus, and hantavirus.

- HIV/AIDS is causing a worldwide epidemic, with the highest rates of infection and death in sub-Saharan Africa and Asia. In the United States, an estimated 25 percent of those who are HIV-positive do not know they are infected.

- The HIV virus attacks the cells of the immune system, using their DNA to replicate itself and spread. After the acute stage of HIV infection, which may or may not be marked by symptoms, the virus continues to inhabit the body for months or years, slowly destroying the immune system. People with HIV infection usually succumb to an opportunistic infection.

- HIV is transmitted in body fluids (semen, vaginal fluids) and blood via sexual contact; injection drug use; contact with blood or body fluids; and pregnancy, childbirth, and breast-feeding.

- HIV testing is becoming faster and more convenient. Infection is managed by antiretroviral drugs often combined in so-called drug cocktails; research on vaccines and microbicides is ongoing.

- Chlamydia, the most commonly reported STD, is caused by the bacterium *Chlamydia trachomatis*. Most infected women and about half of infected men have no symptoms.

- Gonorrhea is caused by the bacterium *Neisseria gonorrhoeae*. Most infected women have no symptoms, but many men do develop symptoms.

- Pelvic inflammatory disease is a painful infection of the female reproductive organs caused by a bacterial infection, usually chlamydia or gonorrhea, that can lead to sterility if not treated.

- Human papillomavirus is the most common STD in the United States. The virus causes genital warts and cervical cancer. Condoms do not seem to prevent the transmission of this virus. Women should be tested regularly for HPV and cervical cancer with a Pap test.

- Genital herpes, caused by the herpes simplex virus, causes painful lesions (sores) on the genitals. Once infected, a person carries the virus for life and can experience periodic outbreaks. The virus can be transmitted even when there are no active lesions.

- Hepatitis A, B, and C are caused by different strains of the hepatitis virus and cause inflammation of the liver. Hepatitis A is most often transmitted through fecal-oral contact via contaminated food or water. Hepatitis B is most often transmitted sexually; a safe and effective vaccine is available. Hepatitis C is usually transmitted by injection drug use.

- Syphilis, caused by the bacterium *Treponema pallidum,* has been increasing in incidence in recent years. The disease progresses through several stages and if untreated can eventually cause dementia and death.

- Other genital infections that are less serious but annoying include trichomoniasis, a protozoal infection; bacterial vaginosis; candidiasis, a yeast infection; bacterial urinary tract infections; and pubic lice and scabies (ectoparasites).

- Efforts to control infectious diseases focus on prevention, preparedness, surveillance, and treatment. Individuals can take many steps to reduce their risk of contracting an infectious disease.

REVIEW QUESTIONS

1. What measures are responsible for reduced death rates from infectious diseases over the past 100 years?

2. Describe the chain of infection. What are some ways to break the chain?

3. What factors influence the extent of an infectious disease?

4. Describe a virus and its effects when it invades a cell.

5. What are some examples of bacterial infections? What are their symptoms?

6. What disease is caused by a prion? What diseases are caused by fungi? By helminths? By protozoa? What are some ectoparasites?

7. Describe the body's physical barriers to infection. What are some chemical barriers?

8. What three functions is the immune system organized to fulfill? What are the two subdivisions of the immune system, and what is the difference between them?

9. What are some of the cellular and chemical actions that occur during the acute inflammatory response?

10. What function do B cells fulfill? What are the types of T cells, and what do they do?

11. How are T and B cells related to immunity? How do vaccines work? Why is it important for all or most members of a community to be vaccinated?

12. Name several behaviors that support a healthy immune system. What are some risk factors for infectious disease that you cannot control?

13. What is an autoimmune disease? What happens when you have an allergic reaction to a substance?

14. Why is it difficult to guarantee the safety of the blood supply? Why are blood products less safe in developing countries?

15. What is mad cow disease? What steps does the U.S. government take to protect the food supply from it?

16. How has air travel affected the transmission of infectious disease? What is SARS, and how was the 2002–2003 outbreak managed?

17. What are the variables that increase the risk of getting or transmitting an infectious disease by sexual contact?

18. Describe the course of hepatitis C. What is the most common means of transmission? What can individuals and communities do to reduce the risk of hepatitis C?

19. How does antibiotic resistance develop? What practices contribute to it?

20. How does the risk from infectious disease compare with the risk from vaccination? What is herd immunity?

21. Describe the course of tuberculosis. What factors contribute to its current reemergence? What are some barriers to treatment?

22. What factors contribute to the occurrence of an influenza pandemic?

23. What are the symptoms of pneumonia? Of whooping cough? Of Ebola hemorrhagic fever?

24. How is West Nile virus transmitted? How can it be prevented? How is hantavirus transmitted? How can it be prevented?

25. What are the ABCs of safer sex?

26. What characteristics of HIV infection have contributed to the rapid spread of the disease?

27. Describe the course of HIV infection. When is AIDS diagnosed? What is usually responsible for death?

28. Describe the means by which HIV can be transmitted. How can infection by each of these means be prevented?

29. Why is HIV infection treated with drug cocktails? What are the disadvantages of these treatments?

30. Why has it been difficult to develop a vaccine for HIV infection?

31. Describe the symptoms of the three major bacterial STDs. How are they treated? What causes pelvic inflammatory disease?

32. What diseases does human papillomavirus cause? What is the Pap test?

33. What are the symptoms of genital herpes? Why is it important for someone who has ever had herpes to always use a condom during sex?

34. What are the primary means of transmission for the three types of hepatitis? What different symptoms and conditions does each type cause?

35. Describe the disease course of syphilis. Why can it go undetected?

36. What causes trichomoniasis? What causes candidiasis? How is each of these infections treated?

37. List several measures that individuals can take to protect themselves from infectious diseases.

WEB RESOURCES

American Academy of Allergy, Asthma, and Immunology: This organization offers online tools that include a medication guide, a directory of allergists, and pollen count information. The Web site also features helpful tips, news, and other publications and resources.
www.aaaai.org

American Social Health Association: The ASHA Web site provides facts and answers about STDs, herpes blood tests, fact sheets, news, research, hotline information, and other resources.
www.ashastd.org

CDC National Center for Infectious Diseases Traveler's Health: This comprehensive Web site offers information on safe food and water, tips on traveling with children, travelers with special needs, illness and injury abroad, cruises, and air travel. Its Travel Notices section is updated regularly for health warnings and precautions.
www.cdc.gov/travel

CDC National Immunization Program: This organization offers a parent's guide to childhood immunizations, vaccine quizzes, vaccine requirements for travel, flu vaccine information, and a quick reference vaccine chart. Its publications include videos, slides, booklets, and American Indian and Alaska Native materials.
www.cdc.gov/nip

CDC National Prevention Information Network: This site focuses on prevention of HIV/AIDS, STDs, and tuberculosis.

Its many resources include information about HIV testing and statistics, organizations, and infectious diseases in the news.
www.cdcnpin.org

HIV InSite: Gateway to AIDS Knowledge: This organization looks at AIDS from a global perspective, offering research and news information about advances in knowledge about this disease, treatment approaches, and trends in spread of the disease.
http://hivinsite.ucsf.edu

National Foundation for Infectious Diseases: Publications offered by NFID include immunization guides, clinical updates, reports on special populations, and a newsletter. Its online fact sheets cover topics such as adult immunizations, foodborne diseases, herpes, and measles in adults.
www.nfid.org

National Institute of Allergy and Infectious Diseases: This organization provides publications on AIDS, allergies, asthma, hepatitis, Lyme disease, SARS, and West Nile virus. It also features links to information on clinical trials.
www.niaid.nih.gov

World Health Organization: Infectious Diseases: This site offers a comprehensive list of health topics that provide in-depth information on infectious diseases, including STDs. It also features links to other resources, such as journals and reports.
www.who.int/health-topics/idindex.htm

REFERENCES

1. Playfair, J., & Bancroft, G. (2004). *Infection and immunity* (2nd ed.). New York: Oxford University Press.

2. Mandell, G. L., Bennett, J. E., & Dolin, R. (2000). *Mandell, Douglas and Bennett's principles and practice*

of infectious diseases (5th ed.). Philadelphia: Churchill Livingstone.

3. Achievements in public health, 1900–1999: Impact of vaccines universally recommended for children—United States,

1990–1998. (1999). *Morbidity and Mortality Weekly Report, 48* (12), 243–248. www.cdc.gov/mmwr.

4. Frenkel, L. D., & Nielsen, K. (2003). Immunization issues for the 21st century. *Annals of Allergy and Asthma Immunology, 90* (6) (Suppl 3), 45–52.

5. Segerstrom, S. C., & Miller, G. E. (2004). Psychological stress and the human immune system: A meta-analytic study of 30 years of inquiry. *Psychological Bulletin, 130* (4), 601–630.

6. Eberhart-Phillips, J. (2000). *Outbreak alert: Responding to the increasing threat of infectious diseases.* Oakland, CA: New Harbinger Publications.

7. Glynn, S. A., et al. (2000). Trends in incidence and prevalence of major transfusion-transmissible viral infections in U.S. blood donors, 1991–1996. Retrovirus Epidemiology Donor Study (REDS). *Journal of the American Medical Association, 284,* 229–235.

8. Consumers advised that recent hepatitis A outbreaks have been associated with green onions. (2003, November 15). FDA Talk Paper. www.fda.gov.

9. Multistate outbreak of E. coli 0157:H7 infection associated with eating ground beef—United States June–July 2002. (2002). *Morbidity and Mortality Weekly Report, 51* (29), 637–639. www.cdc.gov/mmwr.

10. Bovine spongiform encephalopathy in a dairy cow—Washington state, 2003. (2004). *Morbidity and Mortality Weekly Report, 52* (53), 1280–1285. www.cdc.gov/mmwr.

11. SARS. (2004, May 19). World Health Organization-Western Pacific Region. www.wpro.who.

12. Holmes, K. K., et al. (Eds.). (1999). *Sexually transmitted diseases* (3rd ed.). New York: McGraw-Hill.

13. Holmes, K. K., Levine, R., & Weaver, M. (2004). Effectiveness of condoms in preventing sexually transmitted infections. Public Health Reviews. *Bulletin of the World Health Organization, 82* (6), 454–461.

14. Pearlman, B. L. (2004). Hepatitis C infection: A clinical review. *Southern Medical Journal, 97* (4), 364–373.

15. Seeff, L. B., & Hoofnagle, J. H. (2003). Appendix: The National Institute of Health Consensus Development conference—management of hepatitis C, 2002. *Clinical Liver Disease, 7* (1), 261–287.

16. Barnett, J. (2003). Health implications of body piercing and tattooing: A literature review. *Nursing Times, 99* (37), 62–63.

17. Jones, R. N. (2001). Resistance patterns among nosocomial pathogens: Trends over the past few years. *Chest, 119* (2 Suppl), 3975–4045.

18. Maldonado, Y. (2002). Current controversies in vaccination: Vaccine safety. *Journal of the American Medical Association, 288* (24), 3155–3158.

19. Fauci, A. (2004, April 18). The NIH response to emerging and re-emerging infectious diseases: Implications for global health. National Institute of Allergy and Infectious Diseases. www.niaid.nih.gov.

20. Lauzardo, M., & Ashkin, D. (2000). Phthisiology at the dawn of the new century: A review of tuberculosis and the prospects for its elimination. *Chest, 117* (5), 1455–1473.

21. Cono, J., Casey, C. G., & Bell, D. M. (2003). Smallpox vaccination and adverse reactions. *Morbidity and Mortality Weekly Report, 52* (RR04), 1–28. www.cdc.gov/mmwr.

22. First combination vaccine approved to help protect adolescents against whooping cough. (2005, May 3). FDA Talk Paper. U.S. Food and Drug Administration. Department of Health and Human Services. www.fda.gov.

23. Polio eradication. World Health Organization. www.polioeradication.org.

24. Ebola hemorrhagic fever. (2004, August 23). National Center for Infectious Diseases. Centers for Disease Control and Prevention. www.cdc.gov.

25. Marborg hemorrhagic fever in Angola-update 3. (2005, March 29). World Health Organization. www.who.org.

26. West Nile virus: Statistics, surveillance and control. (2004). Centers for Disease Control and Prevention. www.cdc.gov.

27. Hantavirus pulmonary syndrome—United States: Updated recommendations for risk reduction. (2002). *Morbidity and Mortality Weekly Report, 51* (RR09). www.cdc.gov/mmwr.

28. Shelton, J. D., et al. (2004). Partner reduction is crucial for balanced "ABC" approach to HIV prevention. *British Medical Journal, 328,* 891–893.

29. Report of the global AIDS epidemic: Executive summary June 2004. UNAIDS. www.unaids.org.

30. AIDS epidemic in high-income countries. (2004). UNAIDS Fact Sheet. www.unaids.org.

31. Kassutto, S., & Rosenberg, E. S. (2004). Primary HIV Type 1 infection. HIV/AIDS. *Clinical Infectious Disease, 38* (10), 1447–1453.

32. Cases of HIV infection and AIDS in the United States 2002. HIV/AIDS Surveillance Report, 14. Centers for Disease Control and Prevention. www.cdc.gov.

33. HIV/AIDS update May 2004, Canada. www.hc-sc.gc.ca.

34. Guidelines for the prevention of transmission of human immunodeficiency virus and hepatitis B virus to health care and public safety workers: A response to P.L. 100–607, the health omnibus program extension act of 1988. (1989). *Morbidity and Mortality Weekly Review Supplements, 38* (S-6), 3–37. www.cdc.gov/mmwr.

35. Testing yourself for HIV-1, the virus that causes AIDS. U.S. Food and Drug Administration. Department of Health and Human Services. www.fda.gov.

36. Revised guidelines for HIV counseling, testing and referral. (2001). *Morbidity and Mortality Weekly Report, 50* (RR19), 1–58.

37. "3 by 5" progress report. (2005, January 26). World Health Organization. www.who.org.

38. Garber, D. A., Silvestri, G., & Feinberg, M. B. (2004). Prospects for an AIDS vaccine: Three big questions, no easy answers. *The Lancet Infectious Diseases, 4,* 397–413.

39. Microbicides. HIV/AIDS. World Health Organization www.who.org.

40. Miller, W. C., et al. (2004). Prevalence of chlamydia and gonorrhea infection among 18–26 year old young adults in the U.S. *Journal of the American Medical Association, 291* (18), 2229–2236.

41. Screening for chlamydial infection: What's new from the third USPSTF. (2001, March). AHRQ Publication No. APPIP01-0010. Rockville, MD: Agency for Healthcare Research and Quality. www.ahrq.gov.

42. Beigi, R. H., & Wiesenfeld, H. C. (2003). Pelvic inflammatory disease: New diagnostic criteria and treatment. *Obstetrics and Gynecology Clinics of North America, 30* (4), 777–793.

43. Stoler, M. H. (2000). Human papillomaviruses and cervical neoplasia: A model for carcinogenesis. *International Journal of Gynecological Pathology, 19* (1), 16–28.

44. Marrazzo, J. M., et al. (2001). Papanicolaou test screening and prevalence of genital human papillomavirus among women who have sex with women. *American Journal of Public Health, 91* (6), 947–952.

45. Schreckenberger, C., & Kaufmann, A. M. (2004). Vaccination strategies for the treatment and prevention of cervical cancer. *Current Opinions in Oncology, 16* (5), 485–491.

46. Koelle, D. M., & Corey, L. (2003). Recent progress in herpes simplex virus immunobiology and vaccine research. *Clinical Microbiology Reviews, 16* (1), 96–113.

47. Sexually transmitted disease treatment guidelines 2002. (2002). *Morbidity and Mortality Weekly Report, 51* (RR-6). www.cdc.gov.

48. Primary and secondary syphilis—United States, 2000–2001. (2002). *Morbidity and Mortality Weekly Report, 51* (43), 971–973. www.cdc.gov/mmwr.

49. Syphilis. (2002). National Institute of Allergy and Infectious Disease. www.niaid.nih.gov.

50. Screening for syphilis infection. (2004). U.S. Preventive Services Task Force. www.ahrq.gov.

Add It Up! RATE YOUR HIV RISK

Many people think they can judge the likelihood that someone is infected with HIV by how the person looks or whether the person is in a high-risk group. In fact, risk is determined by behaviors, not appearance or membership in a group. Answer the following questions to find out whether your behaviors, past or present, have put you at risk for contracting HIV infection.

Your past behaviors

1. Did you receive a blood transfusion or other blood product before 1985?

2. Have you ever had sex?

3. Have you ever had sex with someone whose HIV status you didn't know?

4. Have you ever had sex while under the influence of drugs or alcohol?

5. Have you ever exchanged sex for drugs or money?

6. Have you ever had sex with a prostitute?

7. Have you had sex with more than one person during your lifetime?

8. Have you ever had unprotected sex (sex without a condom)?

9. Have you ever been the recipient in anal sex?

10. Have you ever had a sexual partner who has been the recipient in anal sex?

11. Have you ever had a sexually transmitted disease?

12. Have you ever had a genital injury (such as a tear or scrape) occur during sex?

13. Have you ever had an injection drug user as a sexual partner?

14. Have you ever used injection drugs?

15. Have you ever used the same needle that someone else used to inject drugs?

16. Have you ever worked in a health care setting?

17. Have you ever been exposed to someone else's blood or body fluids (such as vaginal secretions or semen)?

18. If so, did the fluid make contact with a break in your skin, with your eyes, or with mucous membranes (such as the mouth)?

19. Have you ever accidentally been stuck with a needle contaminated with someone else's blood?

Your current behaviors

1. Are you sexually active?

2. Do you have sex with partners whose HIV status you don't know?

3. Do you sometimes have sex while under the influence of alcohol or drugs?

4. Do you have sex with prostitutes?

5. Do you exchange sex for drugs or money?

6. Do you have sex with multiple partners (even if you tend to have only one partner at any given time)?

7. Do you ever have unprotected sex (sex without a condom)?

8. Are you the recipient in anal sex?

9. Do you have a sexual partner who has been the recipient in anal sex?

10. Do you have rough sex or sex without lubrication, so that genital injury could occur?

11. Do you have an injection drug user as a sexual partner?

12. Do you use injection drugs?

13. Do you share needles for injection drug use?

14. Do you work in a health care setting?

If you answered yes to more than three questions about your past behaviors, there is a possibility that you have been infected with HIV, and you should consider getting tested. If you answered yes to three or more questions about your current behaviors, you are putting yourself at risk for HIV infection. Although you can't eliminate all risk in life, you can improve your chances by practicing safer sex (using a condom), avoiding injection drug use, and using universal precautions if you work in a health care setting.

CHAPTER 21

Cardiovascular Disease: Risks, Prevention, and Treatment

DID YOU KNOW?

- Adopting healthy lifestyle habits now can lower your risk of cardiovascular disease later in life. Heart attacks and strokes usually occur in older adults, but the disease process that underlies them—commonly referred to as "hardening of the arteries"—often begins in early adulthood and even in adolescence.

- Protecting yourself from infectious diseases may lower your chances of having a heart attack one day. Researchers are investigating a variety of viruses and bacteria that may be implicated in cardiovascular disease, including the influenza virus and a strain of the *Chlamydia* bacterium. In the future, vaccines may have a role in protecting the heart from disease.

- You can control some risk factors for cardiovascular disease by maintaining a healthy body weight and getting regular exercise. Other risk factors are beyond your control; for example, your risk is higher if you are male or African American or if someone in your family has had a heart attack or stroke. The more noncontrollable risk factors you have, the more important it is for you to manage the risks you can control.

OLC *Your Health Today*   www.mhhe.com/teague1e

Go to the Online Learning Center for *Your Health Today* for interactive activities, quizzes, flashcards, Web links, and more resources related to this chapter.

Westerners have long considered the heart a vital organ, with a role in human affairs beyond its mere physical function. We think of it as the seat of emotions, the source of love, the metaphorical center of the person. But Westerners have also been interested in understanding how the heart works in the body. Physicians in ancient Greece recognized the heart as a muscle, and scientists during the Renaissance studied the anatomy of the heart and vascular system. In 1628, English physician William Harvey correctly described the circulation of the blood and the roles of the heart, lungs, veins, and arteries. Our understanding of the anatomy, the cellular features, and the diseases of the heart and blood vessels has continued to grow.

Despite this intensive study, not long ago people still believed that heart attacks and strokes were like bolts out of the blue—they happened without warning. Today, we know that heart attacks and strokes are the result of a disease process that began many years earlier, often in young adulthood. We also know that many behavior patterns contribute to cardiovascular disease, including tobacco use, physical inactivity, and poor diet. These patterns are the result of both individual choice and societal structure.

In this chapter we explore both cardiovascular health and cardiovascular disease. We begin with a look at the basics of heart structure and function. Next we consider the main types of cardiovascular disease and the many risk factors, both controllable and noncontrollable, that are associated with them. We then take a brief look at diagnosis and treatment, and we conclude with a discussion of steps that individuals can take to reduce their risk of premature death or disability from cardiovascular disease.

Aerobic exercise is an excellent way of developing good heart health. Swimming, running, and brisk walking are a few examples of aerobic activities that offer health benefits and can be incorporated into your daily schedule.

THE CARDIOVASCULAR SYSTEM

The **cardiovascular system** consists of a network of blood vessels (arteries, veins, and capillaries) and a pump (the heart) that circulate blood throughout the body. The heart is a fist-sized muscle with four chambers, the right and left atria and the right and left ventricles, separated from one another by valves. The right side of the heart is involved in **pulmonary circulation**—pumping oxygen-poor blood to the lungs and oxygen-rich blood back to the heart. The left side of the heart is involved in **systemic circulation**—pumping oxygen-rich blood to the rest of the body and returning oxygen-poor blood to the heart (Figure 21.1).

In pulmonary circulation, oxygen-poor (or deoxygenated) blood returning from the body to the heart enters the right atrium via large veins called the inferior and superior **vena cava.** After the right atrium fills, it contracts and moves the blood into the right ventricle. The right ventricle fills and contracts, moving the blood into the lungs via the right and left pulmonary arteries. The pulmonary artery branches into a network of smaller arteries and arterioles that eventually become the pulmonary capillaries. Capillaries are the smallest blood vessels; some capillary walls are only one cell thick, readily allowing the exchange of gases and molecules. In the interweaving network of capillaries, the red blood cells in the blood pick up oxygen and discard carbon dioxide, a waste product from the cells. The capillaries then unite and form venules, and venules join to become pulmonary veins. The pulmonary veins return oxygen-rich blood from the lungs to the left atrium of the heart.

In systemic circulation, the left atrium fills and contracts to move oxygen-rich blood into the left ventricle. The left ventricle fills, contracts, and moves oxygen-rich blood into the body via the **aorta,** the largest artery in the body. The aorta branches into smaller and smaller arteries, and eventually, oxygen-rich, nutrient-rich blood enters the capillaries located throughout the body. At these sites, red blood cells release oxygen and nutrients to the tissues and pick up carbon dioxide to be carried back to the lungs. The capillaries unite to form veins and eventually connect to the inferior and superior **vena cava,** which returns the oxygen-poor blood to the heart. The cycle then repeats.

Like other muscles of the body, the heart needs oxygen and nutrients provided by blood; the blood being pumped through the heart does not provide nourishment for the heart muscle itself. Two special medium-sized arteries, called **coronary arteries,** supply blood to the heart muscle. The main vessels are the right coronary artery and the left coronary artery, each distributing blood to different parts of the heart (Figure 21.2). The distribution of blood flow is important, because when a blood vessel is narrowed, the section of muscle that it supplies does not get enough blood.

The four chambers of the heart contract to pump blood in a coordinated fashion. The contraction occurs in response to an electrical signal that starts in a group of

Superior vena cava

Right pulmonary artery

Pulmonary trunk

Right atrium

Right pulmonary veins

Pectinate muscles

Pulmonary semilunar valve

Tricuspid valve

Right ventricle

Inferior vena cava

Aorta

Left pulmonary artery

Left pulmonary veins

Left atrium

Mitral (bicuspid) valve

Aortic semilunar valve

Left ventricle

Interventricular septum

Myocardium

Visceral pericardium

Figure 21.1   The heart, showing interior chambers, valves, and major arteries and veins.

cells called the **sinus node** in the right atrium. The signal spreads through a defined course leading first to contraction of the right and left atria, then to contraction of the right and left ventricles. The contraction and relaxation of the ventricles is what we feel and hear as the heartbeat. The contraction phase is called *systole* and the relaxation phase is called *diastole*.

CARDIOVASCULAR DISEASE

The leading cause of death in the United States, **cardiovascular disease (CVD)** accounts for 38 percent of all deaths. Approximately 1.4 million Americans die each year from various forms of this disease. Since 1900, CVD has been the leading cause of death in the United States, except for 1918, when infectious disease was the leading cause. The number of deaths from CVD has increased since 1900 because people are living longer and dying later, primarily from chronic diseases like CVD and cancer, which are caused, in part, by lifestyle factors. Some good news can be seen in the fact that the death rate from CVD for men has decreased over the past 30 years (Figure 21.3). The drop in the death rate is believed to be the result of lifestyle changes, improved recognition and treatment of risk factors, and improved treatment of disease. The drop in death rate has not been

KEY TERMS

cardiovascular system   The heart and blood vessels that circulate blood throughout the body.

pulmonary circulation   Pumping of oxygen-poor blood to the lungs and oxygen-rich blood back to the heart by the right side of the heart.

systemic circulation   Pumping of oxygen-rich blood to the body and oxygen-poor blood back to the heart by the left side of the heart.

vena cava   Largest veins in the body; they carry oxygen-poor blood from the body back to the heart.

aorta   Largest artery in the body; it leaves the heart and branches into smaller arteries, arterioles, and capillaries carrying oxygen-rich blood to body tissues.

coronary arteries   Medium-sized arteries that supply blood to the heart muscle.

sinus node   Group of cells in the right atrium where the electrical signal is generated that establishes the heartbeat.

cardiovascular disease (CVD)   Any disease involving the heart and/or blood vessels.

Figure 21.2   **Blood supply to the heart.** *The heart muscle is supplied with oxygen and nutrients via the coronary arteries.*

seen for women, and some reasons for this are discussed later in the chapter.[1]

Cardiovascular disease is a general term that includes heart attack, stroke, peripheral artery disease, congestive heart failure, and other conditions. The disease process underlying many forms of CVD is atherosclerosis (hardening of the arteries), which causes damage to the blood vessels.

Atherosclerosis

A progressive process that takes years to develop and starts at a young age, **atherosclerosis** is a thickening or hardening of the arteries due to the buildup of lipid (fat) deposits. Autopsies of people aged 15 to 35 who died from unrelated trauma show that some young people already have the beginnings of significant atherosclerosis.[2]

Atherosclerosis starts with the formation of a **fatty streak** in an artery. Fatty streaks consist of an accumulation of lipoproteins within the walls of an artery. A **lipoprotein** is a combination of proteins, phospholipids (fat molecules with phosphate groups chemically attached), and **cholesterol,** a type of fat that is essential in small amounts for certain body functions. Lipoproteins can be thought of as packages that carry fat molecules through the bloodstream. An artery wall has several layers, including an inside lining consisting of a single layer of endothelial cells and a layer behind this consisting of smooth muscle cells. When the inner lining of the wall is damaged (by tobacco smoke, high blood pressure, or infection, for example), creating a *lesion,* lipoproteins from

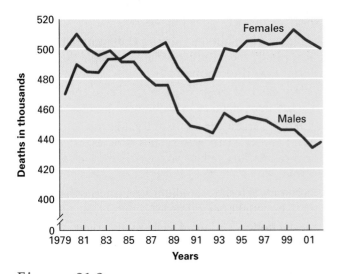

Figure 21.3   **Cardiovascular disease mortality trends for males and females, United States, 1979-2002.** Source: Centers for Disease Control and Prevention / National Center for Health Statistics, www.cdc.gov/nchs.

the blood can accumulate within the wall. Here, they can undergo chemical changes that trigger an inflammatory response, attracting white blood cells into the wall.

Once at the site, white blood cells take up the altered lipoproteins. Some white blood cells leave the site, cleaning lipids from the artery wall, but if blood lipoprotein levels are high, more lipoproteins continue to accumulate. Many of the white blood cells die within the lesion, forming a core of lipid-rich material. The accumulation of white blood cells stuffed with lipids creates a fatty streak.

The process may stop at this point, leaving a dynamic lesion that can still undergo repair. Other lesions develop further, with increased involvement of the artery's smooth muscle cells. Together with the white blood cells, smooth muscle cells release collagen and other proteins to form a **plaque,** an accumulation of debris that undergoes continuing damage, bleeding, and calcification. Plaques cause the artery wall to enlarge and bulge into the *lumen,* the channel through which the blood flows, slowing blood flow and reducing the amount of blood that can reach the tissue supplied by the artery. Plaques can also break off and completely block the artery, preventing any blood from flowing through (Figure 21.4).

Heart attacks, strokes, and peripheral vascular disease are all consequences of the narrowing of arteries caused by atherosclerosis. A diagnosis of one of these diseases suggests risks for the others. Atherosclerosis may also weaken an artery wall, causing a stretching of the artery known as an **aneurysm.** Aneurysms can rupture, tear, and bleed, causing sudden death.

Coronary Heart Disease

When atherosclerosis involves a coronary artery, the result is **coronary heart disease (CHD)** and, often, a heart attack. Coronary heart disease (also called coronary artery disease) is the leading form of CVD. An estimated 13 million Americans are living with CHD. Those who survive a heart attack are often left with damaged hearts and significantly altered lives.

Heart Attack and Angina

When a coronary artery becomes narrowed or blocked, the heart muscle does not get enough oxygen-rich blood, a condition called **ischemia.** If the artery is completely blocked, the person has a heart attack, or **myocardial infarction (MI).** The blockage may be caused by an atherosclerotic plaque that has broken loose or a blood clot (a **thrombus**) that has formed in a narrowed

| Damaged inner lining | Cholesterol-filled cells | Plaque and fatty deposits |

Figure 21.4   The process of atherosclerosis. *The process begins with damage to the lining of an artery and progresses to narrowing or blockage of the artery by fatty deposits and plaques.*

KEY TERMS

atherosclerosis   Thickening or hardening of the arteries due to the buildup of lipid (fat) deposits.

fatty streak   Accumulation of lipoproteins within the walls of an artery.

lipoprotein   Package of proteins, phospholipids (fat molecules with phosphate groups chemically attached), and cholesterol that transports lipids in the blood.

cholesterol   Type of fat that is essential in small amounts for certain body functions.

plaque   Accumulation of debris in an artery wall, consisting of lipoproteins, white blood cells, collagen, and other substances.

aneurysm   Weak or stretched spot in an artery wall that can tear or rupture, causing sudden death.

coronary heart disease (CHD)   Atherosclerosis of the coronary arteries.

ischemia   Insufficient supply of oxygen and nutrients to tissue, caused by narrowed or blocked arteries.

myocardial infarction (MI)   Lack of blood to the heart muscle with resulting death of heart tissue; often called a heart attack.

thrombus   Blood clot that forms in a narrowed or damaged artery.

HIGHLIGHT ON HEALTH
Signs of a Heart Attack

Recognizing the signs of a heart attack and getting treatment quickly are critical to survival. Although symptoms may vary, the following signs may indicate that a heart attack is occurring.

- *Chest discomfort.* Most heart attacks involve discomfort in the center of the chest that lasts more than a few minutes, or that goes away and comes back. It can feel like uncomfortable pressure, squeezing, fullness, or pain.
- *Discomfort in other areas of the upper body.* Symptoms can include pain or discomfort in one or both arms, the back, neck, jaw, or stomach.
- *Shortness of breath.* May occur with or without chest discomfort.

- *Other signs.* These may include breaking out in a cold sweat, nausea, or lightheadedness.

NOTE: Women are more likely to have nausea or pain in the upper abdomen than in the chest. They may also develop fatigue as the only symptom of a heart attack. Insomnia is another possible symptom in women.

If you or someone you are with experiences one or more of these symptoms, seek emergency medical treatment by calling 911 immediately.

Source: Data from American Heart Association, www.americanheart.org.

---

or damaged artery. The latter condition is called a **coronary thrombosis** and may cause sudden death. During a heart attack, the area of muscle supplied by the blocked coronary artery is completely deprived of oxygen. If blood flow is not quickly restored, that part of the heart muscle will die.

The severity of a heart attack is determined by the location and duration of the blockage. If the blockage occurs close to the aorta where the coronary arteries are just starting to branch, a large area of heart muscle is deprived of oxygen. If the blockage is farther out in a smaller coronary artery, the area of muscle supplied is smaller. The duration of the blockage is usually determined by the time between onset of symptoms and initiation of medical or surgical treatment to reopen the artery. Duration is directly dependent on how quickly a person recognizes the symptoms of a myocardial infarction and gets help.

A heart attack may occur when extra work is demanded of the heart, such as during exercise or emotional stress, or it may occur during light activity or even rest. A classic symptom of a heart attack is chest pain, often described as a sensation of pressure, fullness, or squeezing in the midportion of the chest. The pain can radiate to the jaw, shoulders, arms, or back (see the box "Signs of a Heart Attack"). For an unfortunate 20 percent of people who have a heart attack, sudden death may be the only sign of coronary artery disease. Not all symptoms occur in all cases. In fact, some people have a heart attack with no chest pain or just nausea or pain in the arm. The more symptoms a person has, the more likely it is that a heart attack is occurring.

When coronary arteries are narrowed but not completely blocked, the person may experience **angina**—pain, pressure, heaviness, or tightness in the center of the chest that may radiate to the neck, arms, or shoulders. Half of all heart attacks are preceded by angina. The difference between a heart attack and angina is that the pain of angina resolves, whereas the pain of a heart attack continues. Angina can be controlled with medical treatment. However, if angina is becoming more frequent or starting to occur with less exercise or at rest, it may mean that coronary artery disease is progressing, increasing the risk for a heart attack.

Many physical conditions can cause pain in the chest, including irritated esophagus, arthritis of the neck or ribs, gas in the colon, stomach ulcers, and gallbladder disease. Chest pain can also be caused by weight lifting or other heavy lifting or vigorous activity. If you are used to chest pain from any of these causes, you may be inclined to ignore angina or chest pain from a heart attack. Don't let complaisance or confusion delay your efforts to seek help if you experience the signs of a heart attack.

Arrhythmias and Sudden Cardiac Death

The pumping of the heart is usually a well-coordinated event, controlled by an electrical signal emanating from the sinus node in the right atrium, as described earlier. The sinus node establishes a rate of 60 to 100 beats per minute for a normal adult heart. The rate increases in response to increased demand on the heart, such as during exercise, and slows in response to reduced demand, such as during relaxation or sleep. If the signal is disrupted, it can cause an **arrhythmia,** or disorganized beating of the heart. The disorganized beating is usually not as effective at pumping blood.

An arrhythmia is any type of irregular heartbeat. It may be an occasional skipped beat, a rapid or slow rate, or an irregular pattern. Not all arrhythmias are serious or cause for concern. In fact, most people have occasional irregular heartbeats every day; some people do not even notice them. However, arrhythmia may cause noticeable symptoms, including palpitations, a sensation of fluttering in the chest, chest pain, light-headedness, shortness of breath, and fatigue.

Arrhythmias occur for a variety of reasons. The sinus node may be damaged and not produce a regular signal, or the normal electrical conduction course may be damaged, preventing the signal from traveling from the atria to the ventricles. Such damage can be the result of coronary artery disease; structural abnormalities of the heart (such as valve abnormalities or congenital heart disease); chemical imbalances; or the use of caffeine, alcohol, tobacco, cocaine, or medications, including some over-the-counter cold medications.

Some arrhythmias can also cause **sudden cardiac death,** an abrupt loss of heart function. Sudden cardiac death, or cardiac arrest, occurs when the electrical impulses controlling the heartbeat are disrupted and an arrhythmia called **ventricular fibrillation** results. The ventricles contract rapidly and erratically, causing the heart to quiver or "tremor" rather than beat. Blood cannot be pumped by the heart when the ventricles are fibrillating. Brain death starts to occur within 4 to 6 minutes of cardiac arrest. The condition is reversible in most people if they receive treatment with an electrical shock within minutes of the onset of ventricular fibrillation. The shock can restart the heart's normal rhythm. Every minute counts after cardiac arrest; each minute without appropriate emergency medical treatment results in an 8 percent to 10 percent reduction in chance of survival. About 335,000 Americans die each year from sudden cardiac death in emergency departments or before reaching the hospital.[1] Treatment may entail the surgical implanting of a pacemaker, an electrical device that establishes a regular heartbeat.

Response to sudden cardiac death provides an example of how communities can work together to improve health. The American Heart Association encourages federal, state, and local partners to strengthen each step in what they call the Chain of Survival:

- Early access to emergency medical services (by calling 911 in most areas)
- Early cardiopulmonary resuscitation (requiring that members of community are trained in CPR)
- Early defibrillation (requiring that proper automated external defibrillators be available and that people be trained to use them throughout the community)
- Early advanced cardiac care (requiring access to trained health professionals and equipment)

Stroke

When blood flow to the brain or part of the brain is blocked, the result is a **stroke,** or **cerebrovascular accident (CVA).** Stroke is the third-leading cause of death in the United States, after heart disease and cancer, and is a leading cause of severe, long-term disability. Eighty-eight percent of all strokes occur when the blood vessels to the brain become blocked, in the same way that a heart attack occurs when blood vessels to the heart are blocked. The blockage may be caused by a thrombus (a blood clot that stays where it is formed) or an **embolism** (a clot that travels from elsewhere in the body). These strokes are called **thrombotic strokes,** or **ischemic strokes.** The other 12 percent of strokes are **hemorrhagic strokes;** these occur when a blood vessel in the brain suddenly breaks open and bleeds. In hemorrhagic stroke, the bleeding is usually from a vessel that has been weakened by atherosclerosis or high blood pressure.[1]

As with the heart, different arteries supply different areas of the brain. Strokes may have a variety of symptoms, depending on the area of the brain involved. However, symptoms usually involve the sudden onset of neurological problems, such as headaches, numbness, weakness, or speech problems (see the box "Signs of a Stroke").

KEY TERMS

coronary thrombosis Blockage of a coronary artery by a blood clot that may cause sudden death.

angina Intermittent pain, pressure, heaviness, or tightness in the center of the chest caused by a narrowed coronary artery.

arrhythmia Irregular or disorganized heartbeat.

sudden cardiac death Abrupt loss of heart function caused by an irregular or ineffective heartbeat.

ventricular fibrillation Type of arrhythmia in which the ventricles contract rapidly and erratically, causing the heart to quiver or "tremor" rather than beat.

stroke or **cerebrovascular accident (CVA)** Lack of blood flow to the brain with resulting death of brain tissue.

embolism Blood clot that travels from elsewhere in the body.

thrombotic stroke or **ischemic stroke** Stroke caused by blockage in a blood vessel in the brain.

hemorrhagic stroke Stroke caused by rupture of a blood vessel in the brain, with bleeding into brain tissue.

HIGHLIGHT ON HEALTH

Signs of a Stroke

Neurological problems that have a sudden onset and are unremitting, especially if they involve only one side of the body, may be signs that a stroke is occurring or has occurred. Although some of the following symptoms may occur with other illnesses, such as migraine headache, the more symptoms there are, and the more severe they are, the more likely they are to be the result of a stroke.

- Sudden numbness or weakness of the face, arm, or leg, especially on one side of the body
- Sudden confusion, trouble speaking or understanding

- Sudden trouble seeing in one or both eyes
- Sudden trouble walking, dizziness, loss of balance or coordination
- Sudden, severe headache with no known cause

If you or someone you are with experiences one or more of these symptoms, seek emergency medical treatment by calling 911 immediately.

Source: Data from American Stroke Association, www.stroke.org.

A small percentage of people have **transient ischemic attacks (TIAs)** before having a stroke. Sometimes called "ministrokes," TIAs are periods of ischemia that produce the same symptoms as a stroke, but in this case the symptoms resolve within 24 hours with little or no tissue death. A TIA should be viewed as a warning sign of stroke. If untreated, 10 percent of people who have a TIA will have a stroke within a year that leads to permanent disability or death.[3] A person having symptoms of a stroke should get immediate medical care, whether the symptoms are caused by a TIA or a stroke.

Hypertension

Blood pressure is the pressure exerted by blood against the walls of arteries, and high blood pressure, or **hypertension,** occurs when the pressure is great enough to damage artery walls. Untreated high blood pressure can weaken and scar the arteries and makes the heart work harder, weakening it as well. Hypertension can cause heart attacks, strokes, kidney disease, peripheral artery disease, and blindness.[4]

Blood pressure is determined by two forces—the pressure produced by the heart as it pumps the blood and the resistance of the arteries as they contain blood flow. When arteries are already hardened by atherosclerosis, they are more resistant. Blood pressure is measured in millimeters of mercury and stated in two numbers, such as 120/80. The upper number represents **systolic pressure,** the pressure produced when the heart contracts; the lower number represents **diastolic pressure,** the pressure in the arteries when the heart is relaxed, between contractions. There is no definite line dividing normal blood pressure from high blood pressure, but categories have been established as guidelines on the basis of increased risk for CVD; see Table 21.1.

Hypertension is often referred to as the "silent killer," because it usually causes no symptoms. More than 65 million people in the United States (nearly one in three adults) and more than 1 billion people worldwide are estimated to have high blood pressure.[1] Although people are becoming more aware of this condition, 30 percent of people with high blood pressure do not know they have it. Of those who know they have the condition, only 59 percent are receiving treatment, and of those, only 34 percent are adequately treated. Thus, there is room for significant improvement by individuals and communities.[4]

In approximately 95 percent of cases, the cause of hypertension is unknown. In Western societies, aging seems to be a factor, but this is not the case in other cultures. Genetics plays a role in some cases. Other factors that contribute to elevated blood pressure include high salt consumption, use of alcohol, low potassium levels, physical inactivity, and obesity. Less frequently, medical conditions can cause hypertension. Women can develop

Table 21.1	Blood Pressure Guidelines	
Category	**Systolic**	**Diastolic**
Normal	Less than 120 *and*	Less than 80
Prehypertension	120–139 *or*	80–89
Hypertension		
Stage 1	140–159 *or*	90–99
Stage 2	160 and above *or*	100 and above

Source: "The Seventh Report of the Joint National Committee on Prevention, Detection, Evaluation and Treatment of High Blood Pressure," 2003, Bethesda, MD: National Heart, Lung, and Blood Institute, National Institutes of Health (NIH Publication No. 03-5233).

hypertension during pregnancy or while taking oral contraceptive pills; even children and adolescents occasionally develop hypertension, often as a result of underlying medical conditions or congenital problems.

Congestive Heart Failure

When the heart is not pumping the blood as well as it should, a condition known as **congestive heart failure** occurs. It can develop after a heart attack or as a result of hypertension, heart valve abnormality, or disease of the heart muscle. When the heart cannot keep up its regular pumping force or rate, blood backs up into the lungs, and fluid from the backed-up blood in the pulmonary veins leaks into the lungs. A person with congestive heart failure experiences difficulty breathing, shortness of breath, and coughing, especially when lying down. Blood returning to the heart from the body also gets backed up, causing fluid to leak into the ankles and legs and causing swelling of the lower legs. When blood fails to reach the brain efficiently, fatigue and confusion can result.

Approximately 5 million Americans live with congestive heart failure.[1] Symptoms can be treated with medications that help draw off extra fluid, decrease blood pressure, and improve the heart's ability to pump. Other factors that contribute to the development of congestive heart failure include cigarette smoking, high cholesterol, and diabetes; lifestyle changes such as weight loss, exercise, and smoking cessation can also reduce symptoms and the risk of disease progression. In some instances, surgery can be done to repair a heart valve or the damage incurred by coronary heart disease. In extreme cases, the only recourse may be a heart transplant.

Other Cardiovascular Diseases

Other conditions can affect the structure of the heart and blood vessels and their ability to function. Some of these conditions are congenital (present from birth), and others occur as progressive diseases.

Heart Valve Disorders

Four valves in the heart keep blood flowing in the correct direction through the heart (see Figure 21.1). A normally functioning valve opens easily to allow blood to flow forward but closes tightly to prevent blood from flowing backward. Sometimes a valve does not open well, preventing the smooth flow of blood, and sometimes a valve does not close tightly, allowing blood to leak backward. These problems can be caused by congenital abnormalities, rheumatic heart disease, or an aging-related degeneration process. When valves are not functioning normally, the flow of blood is altered and the risks of blood clots and infection increase. Often, the person experiences no symptoms; if symptoms do occur,

they can include shortness of breath, dizziness, fatigue, and chest pain.

The most common heart valve defect is **mitral valve prolapse** (the mitral valve separates the left atrium from the left ventricle). In this condition, the mitral valve billows backward and the edges do not fully close when the left ventricle contracts to move blood into the aorta, allowing blood to leak backward into the atrium. Mitral valve prolapse is common, affecting 5 percent to 10 percent of the population. It can occur at any age and affects both men and women; it is often detected when a physician hears a "click" or "murmur" in the heart beat. With certain types of mitral valve prolapse, individuals should take antibiotics before dental surgery and other procedures to reduce the risk of infection from bacteria introduced into the bloodstream by the procedure.

Rheumatic Heart Disease

A common cause of heart valve disorders and other heart damage is **rheumatic fever,** leading to **rheumatic heart disease**. In this disease, the heart is scarred following an infection with a strain of streptococcus bacteria (Group A streptoccocus, usually as strep throat). Symptoms of rheumatic fever include fever, joint pain, fatigue, and rash;

KEY TERMS

transient ischemic attack (TIA)   Period of ischemia that temporarily produces the same symptoms as a stroke.

blood pressure   Force exerted by the blood against artery walls.

hypertension   Blood pressure that is forceful enough to damage artery walls.

systolic pressure   Pressure in the arteries when the heart contracts, represented by the upper number in a blood pressure measurement.

diastolic pressure   Pressure in the arteries when the heart relaxes between contractions, represented by the lower number in a blood pressure measurement.

congestive heart failure   Condition in which the heart is not pumping the blood as well as it should, allowing blood and fluids to back up in the lungs.

mitral valve prolapse   Heart valve disorder in which the mitral valve, which separates the left ventricle from the left atrium, does not close fully, allowing blood to leak backward into the atrium.

rheumatic fever   Acute disease that can occur as a complication of an untreated strep throat infection.

rheumatic heart disease   Disease in which the heart is scarred following strep throat infection and rheumatic fever.

when the heart is affected, there can be congestive heart failure, valve dysfunction, or arrhythmia. Acute rheumatic fever can occur 2 to 3 weeks after a strep throat infection (although almost one in three people did not have a sore throat) and last weeks to months. Heart damage can occur over years. The condition is prevented by treating strep throat infections with antibiotics. Rheumatic fever often occurs in children, and worldwide it is a major cause of heart disorders. The incidence of rheumatic heart disease has declined significantly in developed countries, partly as a result of aggressive diagnosis and treatment of strep throat.

Congenital Heart Disease

A variety of structural defects that are present at birth can involve the heart valves, major arteries and veins in or near the heart, or the heart muscle. An abnormality can cause the blood to slow down, flow in the wrong direction, or not move from one chamber to the next. More than 35 types of heart defects have been described.[5] One of the more common defects is a **septal defect,** in which an extra hole in the heart allows blood to flow from one atrium to the other or one ventricle to the other. When there is a septal defect, poorly oxygenated blood from the

Congenital heart defects affect about 30,000 infants every year in the United States alone. Worldwide, these defects number in the millions.

body mixes with oxygenated blood from the lungs, resulting in lower oxygen supply to the body.

Approximately 36,000 babies are born with congenital heart defects each year in the United States. These defects are usually detected at birth or shortly thereafter. Some defects need to be corrected immediately; others can wait. Due to advances in diagnosis and medical and surgical treatments, there are more than 1 million adults in the United States living with congenital heart disease.[1]

Peripheral Vascular Disease

The result of atherosclerosis in the blood vessels of the arms or legs (more commonly, the legs), **peripheral vascular disease (PVD)** causes pain, aches, or cramping in the muscles supplied by a narrowed blood vessel. Although it is usually not fatal, PVD causes a significant amount of disability, limiting the activity level of many older people because of pain with walking. If circulation is severely limited by the ischemia, the affected leg or arm may have to be amputated. PVD affects 12 percent to 20 percent of older adults. It is a clue to advanced atherosclerosis and indicates the need for lifestyle change or medical treatment in order to reduce the risk of heart attack or stroke. Anyone who experiences unexplained pain in the legs or arms, especially if it is associated with exercise, should see a health care provider.

Cardiomyopathy

Deaths from **cardiomyopathy**—disease of the heart muscle—account for 1 percent of heart disease deaths in the United States, with the highest rates occurring among men and African Americans. The most common form of cardiomyopathy is *dilated cardiomyopathy,* an enlargement of the heart in response to weakening of the muscle. The cause is often unknown, although a virus is suspected in some cases. Other factors that can weaken the heart muscle are toxins (alcohol, tobacco, heavy metals, and some medications), drugs, pregnancy, hypertension, and coronary artery disease.

Another form is **hypertrophic cardiomyopathy,** an abnormal thickening of one part of the heart, frequently the left ventricle. The thickened wall makes the heart abnormally stiff, so the heart doesn't fill well. Although most people with hypertrophic cardiomyopathy have no symptoms, the condition can cause heart failure, arrhythmia, and sudden death. In fact, 36 percent of cases of sudden death in young competitive athletes are due to hypertrophic cardiomyopathy. The cause of the condition is unknown in about 50 percent of cases, but in the rest, there is a genetic link (see Chapter 2). Anyone with a family member who died suddenly from a heart attack or from an unexplained cause at a young age should be evaluated for signs of cardiomyopathy, as should anyone with a personal history of fainting or near fainting with exercise. Individuals with hypertrophic cardiomyopathy are advised to avoid vigorous exercise, so screening is essential for anyone who wants to participate in sports.

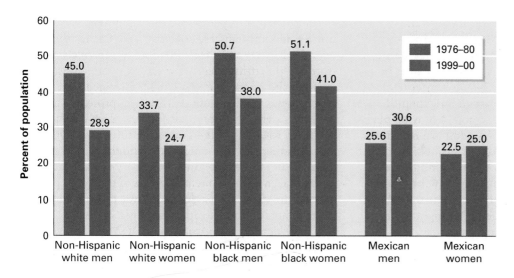

Figure 21.5 Age-adjusted prevalence trends for high blood pressure in Americans ages 20–74 by race/ethnicity, sex, and survey, National Health and Nutrition Examination Survey II (1976–1980) and IV (1999–2000).

Source: Centers for Disease Control and Prevention / National Center for Health Statistics, 2003, www.cdc.gov/nchs.

Data based on a single measure of blood pressure.

RISK FACTORS FOR CVD

A rapid increase in cardiovascular disease occurred in the United States in the 1930s, and by the late 1940s, CVD had become the leading cause of death. In an effort to understand this pattern, the U.S. Public Health Service joined with a group of researchers to look at differences between people who developed CVD and those who did not. This was the origin of the Framingham Heart Study, which began in 1948 and continues to this day.

The town of Framingham, Massachusetts, was chosen as the site of the study; 2,336 men and 2,873 women signed up to be studied longitudinally (followed over time). In the years since then, more participants have been added, including members of Framingham's minority communities. Every 2 to 4 years, participants in the study undergo extensive testing to evaluate their behaviors and health status. More than 50 years of study and the participation of more than 10,000 men and women have allowed researchers to identify multiple factors that alter the risk of cardiovascular disease.[6]

As discussed in Chapter 2, cardiovascular disease is a multifactorial disease, the result of genetic, environmental, and lifestyle factors interacting over time. Some factors are controllable, while others are not.

Major Controllable Risk Factors

Controllable risk factors are factors associated with CVD that can be reduced through individual behavior and/or community interventions. The six major controllable risk factors for CVD identified by the American Heart Association are tobacco use, hypertension, unhealthy blood cholesterol levels, physical inactivity, overweight, and diabetes.

Tobacco Use and CVD Risk

Tobacco use is the leading risk factor for all forms of CVD. Tobacco smoke functions in a variety of ways to increase risk. Components of tobacco smoke damage the inner lining of blood vessels, speeding up the development of

atherosclerosis. Toxins in tobacco smoke can stimulate the formation of blood clots in the coronary arteries and trigger spasms that close off the vessels. Smoking raises blood levels of LDL cholesterol ("bad" cholesterol) and decreases blood levels of HDL cholesterol ("good" cholesterol).[7] Exposure to environmental tobacco smoke (secondhand smoke) is also a risk factor for CVD; risk appears to be proportional to the amount of daily exposure. The risk for CVD decreases within a few years of quitting smoking.[8] For more on tobacco use and strategies for quitting, see Chapter 13.

Hypertension and CVD Risk

Hypertension increases the risk for heart attack, stroke, congestive heart failure, and kidney disease; the higher the blood pressure, the greater the risk. Hypertension makes the heart work harder to circulate the blood. The increased work may cause the heart to enlarge, which may lead to congestive heart failure. Hypertension can also cause damage to the lining of arteries, promoting atherosclerosis and causing blood vessel walls to weaken.

There are significant differences in the prevalence of high blood pressure across different minority populations (Figure 21.5). These differences were recently described in a study called REACH 2010, designed to

KEY TERMS

septal defect Congenital heart defect in which an extra hole allows blood to flow from one atrium to the other or one ventricle to the other.

peripheral vascular disease (PVD) Atherosclerosis in the blood vessels of the arms or legs.

cardiomyopathy Disease of the heart muscle.

hypertrophic cardiomyopathy Abnormal thickening of one part of the heart, frequently the left ventricle.

assess the health status of 1,000 people living in minority communities in the United States. The study found that among adult males, self-reported rates of high blood pressure were 46.5 percent for African Americans, 28.8 percent for Hispanics, 20.3 percent for Asian/Pacific Islanders, 40.5 percent for American Indians, and 32.5 percent for the general population of male minority group members. Among adult women, rates were 51.6 percent for African Americans, 27.2 percent for Hispanics, 20.2 percent for Asian/Pacific Islanders, 40.4 percent for American Indians, and 33.6 for the general population of female minority group members. These and other studies continue to highlight the need for increased awareness, screening, treatment, and prevention measures in minority communities.[9]

In African Americans, hypertension is not only more common; it also appears to follow a different course than it does in other groups. It develops earlier, is more severe, and is associated with more complications, such as heart attacks, stroke, and kidney failure. African Americans tend to excrete sodium (salt) at a slower rate than white Americans do, possibly making them more sensitive to dietary salt. This difference may contribute to the higher rate of stroke among African Americans. To date, there has not been a clear genetic explanation for the ethnic differences. Socioeconomic and behavioral factors may be involved as well, as discussed later in the chapter.[10]

Unhealthy Blood Cholesterol Levels and CVD Risk

Cholesterol plays such an important role in CVD that Healthy People 2010 objectives call for all Americans to know their cholesterol levels by age 20. Measures of cholesterol levels include measures of the two key subcategories of cholesterol, LDL and HDL, as well as total cholesterol, the combination of all the subcategories. Levels of total cholesterol are directly related to frequency of coronary heart disease; that is, as cholesterol levels rise, so does the incidence of coronary heart disease. The National Cholesterol Education Program (NCEP) recommends cholesterol testing every 5 years starting at age 20 with a blood test that measures total cholesterol, LDL cholesterol, HDL cholesterol, and triglycerides.

Cholesterol is a type of fat that is used in cell membranes, in some hormones, in brain and nerve tissue, and in bile acids to help digest fats. The body gets cholesterol in two ways: Some of it is manufactured in the liver, and the rest comes from food sources, primarily animal products such as meat, fish, eggs, and cheese. Although only food from animal sources contains cholesterol, food from both animal and plant sources can contain saturated fat, which the body uses to make cholesterol.

Because it is a fat, cholesterol cannot circulate in the blood in a free-floating state; it would bead up like cooking oil in water. Instead, it is combined with proteins and other molecules in packages called lipoproteins, as noted earlier. Lipoproteins are spherical and smaller than red blood cells; they are categorized into five main classes according to density (weight for size): chylomicrons, very-low-density lipoproteins (VLDLs), intermediate-density lipoproteins (IDLs), low-density liproproteins (LDLs), and high-density lipoproteins (HDLs). Each class plays a different role within the body. The roles of VLDLs and IDLs in atherosclerosis are unclear, and their levels are not usually measured. Chylomicrons carry dietary fats and can be taken up by white blood cells and become part of atherosclerotic deposits; this is one way that high levels of dietary fat contribute to atherosclerosis.

Low-density lipoproteins (LDLs)—"bad" cholesterol—are clearly associated with atherosclerosis. The higher the level of LDLs, the higher the risk of atherosclerosis. The level of LDLs in the blood is influenced by both diet and genetic factors. Three different LDL levels are recommended by the NCEP, depending on other risk factors. An LDL of less than 160 is recommended for people who have no risk factors or one other risk factor for coronary heart disease, such as tobacco use, hypertension, low HDL levels, family history of premature heart disease, or older age (older than 45 for men, older than 55 for women).[11] An LDL level of less than 130 is recommended for people with two or more other risk factors for coronary heart disease. An LDL level of less than 100 is recommended for people who already have coronary heart disease, other atherosclerotic disease, or diabetes. An LDL level of less than 70 is an alternative goal for people with a very high risk of CVD, such as those who have had a recent heart attack or stroke.[12] Recommended cholesterol levels are shown in Table 21.2.

High density lipoproteins (HDLs)—"good" cholesterol—consist mainly of protein and are the smallest of the lipoprotein particles. HDLs help to clear cholesterol from cells and atherosclerotic deposits and transport it back to the liver for recycling. Thus, they decrease blood levels of cholesterol and reverse the development of deposits and plaque. High HDL levels provide protection from CVD.

HDL levels are determined mainly by genetics, but they are influenced by exercise, alcohol, and estrogen. They are higher among African Americans and among women, especially before menopause, and they change little with age. The protective effect of HDL is quite significant: A 1 percent decrease in HDL level is associated with a 3 percent to 4 percent increase in heart disease.[11]

Physical Inactivity and CVD Risk

A sedentary lifestyle is another major risk factor for CVD, and regular physical activity reduces the risk of CVD and many cardiovascular risk factors, including high blood pressure, diabetes, and obesity. Physical activity conditions the heart, reduces high blood pressure, improves HDL cholesterol levels, helps maintain a healthy weight,

Table 21.2   Cholesterol Guidelines

Total cholesterol (mg/dl)

Less than 200	Desirable
200–239	Borderline high
240 or greater	High

LDL cholesterol (mg/dl)

Less than 100*	Optimal
100–129	Near or above optimal
130–159	Borderline high
160–189	High
190 or greater	Very high

HDL cholesterol (mg/dl)

Less than 40	Low (undesirable)
60 or greater	High (desirable)

Triglycerides (mg/dl)

Less than 150	Normal
150–199	Borderline high
200–499	High
500 or greater	Very high

*Achieving a goal of less than 70 is an option if there is a high risk for heart disease.

Source: Expert panel on detection, evaluation, and treatment of high blood cholesterol in adults, 2001, "Executive Summary of the Third Report of the National Cholesterol Education Program Expert Panel on Detection, Evaluation, and Treatment of High Blood Cholesterol in Adults." *Journal of the American Medical Association, 285* (19), pp. 2486–2497.

and helps control diabetes. Unfortunately, the majority of adults in the United States are not active at levels that can promote health. Only 45.4 percent of adult Americans report achieving the goal of 30 minutes of moderate intensity exercise most days of the week, or 20 minutes of vigorous exercise 3 or more days a week. One in four adults reports no leisure-time physical activity at all.[13] Exercise in children is especially important, because it is associated with lower blood pressure and weight control and because active children tend to become active adults.

Obesity and CVD Risk

Overweight and obesity are associated with increased risk for CVD and greater seriousness of the disease. Excess weight puts a strain on the heart and contributes to other risk factors, such as hypertension, high LDL levels, and diabetes. The association among all these risk factors is found across ethnic groups, including Mexican Americans, non-Hispanic African Americans, and non-Hispanic white Americans.[14]

As discussed in Chapter 9, body fat distribution also plays a role in CVD risk. People with central fat distribution—those who are apple-shaped, as suggested by an abdominal circumference of greater than 40 inches for men and greater than 35 inches for women—have a higher risk for diabetes, high blood pressure, and CVD. Weight loss of 10 percent to 15 percent for an overweight individual, if maintained, is associated with an improved cardiovascular risk profile.[15] Diet and exercise are recommended ways to reduce overweight and obesity, as discussed in Chapter 9.

Diabetes and CVD Risk

Diabetes is a metabolic disorder in which the production or use of insulin is disrupted. Insulin is a hormone that stimulates cells to take up the glucose circulating in the blood. In Type-1 diabetes, the pancreas is unable to produce insulin; thus, glucose cannot enter cells to be used for energy. This type occurs more often in young people. In Type-2 diabetes, either the pancreas does not produce enough insulin or the body cells are insulin resistant; again, cells cannot take up glucose for energy. This type of diabetes develops slowly, often in association with overweight. In the last decade, rates of Type-2 diabetes in overweight children have soared. In both types of diabetes, the levels of glucose that are circulating in the bloodstream rise, with consequences throughout the body, including damage to artery walls, changes in some components of the blood, and effects on organs. Blood vessels are particularly susceptible to atherosclerosis in a person with diabetes, and atherosclerosis occurs at an earlier age and is more extensive.

Both men and women with diabetes are at greater risk for CVD, but for women, the risk is even higher (three times the risk experienced by women without diabetes) than it is for men (twice the risk experienced by men without diabetes).[16] Another concern for people with diabetes is that their symptoms of heart attack may be different from the norm. They are more likely to have a "silent" heart attack without the typically experienced pain. Their only symptoms may be nausea, vomiting, sweating, or dizziness, any of which could easily be mistaken for another illness.

KEY TERMS

low-density lipoproteins (LDLs) "Bad" cholesterol; lipoproteins that accumulate in plaque and contribute to atherosclerosis.

high-density lipoproteins (HDLs) "Good" cholesterol; lipoproteins that help to clear cholesterol from cells and atherosclerotic deposits and transport it back to the liver for recycling.

diabetes Metabolic disorder in which the production or use of insulin is disrupted, so that body cells cannot take up glucose and use it for energy, and high levels of glucose circulate in the blood.

Beating the Odds

Who Is Least Likely to Have a Stroke?

Because atherosclerosis underlies several different forms of cardiovascular disease, the risk factors for stroke are the same as for coronary heart disease and heart attack. Some risk factors are genetic, some are environmental, and some are a function of behavior choices. Brief profiles of three individuals are presented here. Which one do you think is least likely to have a stroke?

Magda is a 32-year-old Caucasian woman who works as a software engineer in a high-tech computer company. She works 9-hour days but exercises at the gym on her lunch hour and rides her mountain bike on weekends. She has been trying to quit smoking for 6 months but has not been able to, partly because of job-related stress. She has been smoking half a pack a day since she was 18. She tends to eat a fairly high-fat diet, and she drinks moderately. Magda was born in Eastern Europe and adopted by her American parents when she was 2. Her blood pressure is 120/70 and her total cholesterol is 175.

Leonard is a 47-year-old African American man who drives a bus in a large city. His lifestyle is sedentary, and he con-siders his job stressful. He does not smoke or drink alcohol because of his religious beliefs. He has high blood pressure, which is controlled by medication. Leonard's father died of a stroke at the age of 54 and his mother has diabetes, so Leonard tries to follow a healthy diet, emphasizing leafy green vegetables, whole grains, monounsaturated fats, fruit, fish, and poultry. He seldom eats red meat and watches his salt consumption. Still, he is moderately overweight, and his physician recently told him he may be developing insulin resistance.

Juana is a 65-year-old Mexican American woman. She has always been active but is somewhat overweight. She does not smoke or drink, and her diet emphasizes chicken, fish, vegetables, beans, and rice, as well as pork and moderate amounts of saturated fat. Juana takes several medications for high blood pressure and high cholesterol. Her father had a heart attack when he was 60; her mother lived to be 90 but had a stroke at 75 and suffered mild speech impairment.

OLC Web site Visit the **Online Learning Center** at www.mhhe.com/teague1e for comments by the authors.

Contributing Risk Factors in CVD

Besides the six major controllable risk factors for CVD, other risk factors that can be controlled have been identified (see the box "Who Is Least Likely to Have a Stroke?") These factors contribute to risk, but their role is either slightly less than that of the major risk factors or has not been as clearly delineated yet.

High Triglyceride Levels

Triglycerides are blood fats like cholesterol; they are the most common form that fat takes in the body. They can be obtained from food or produced by the body from excess carbohydrates; they are packaged into lipoproteins and transported through the blood to fat cells, where they are stored for later use. A high level of blood triglycerides is a risk factor for CVD. Levels of less than 150 are desirable (see Table 12.2).[11] High triglyceride levels are associated with excess body fat, diets high in saturated fat and cholesterol, alcohol use, and some medical conditions, such as poorly controlled diabetes. The main treatment for high triglycerides is lifestyle modification, but medications can also be used.

High Alcohol Intake

The relationship between alcohol and CVD is complicated because different levels of alcohol consumption have dif-ferent effects. Heavy drinking, defined as more than three drinks per day, can damage the heart, increasing the risk of cardiomyopathy, some arrhythmias, and neurological complications. Light to moderate alcohol intake, defined as fewer than two drinks per day, appears to have a protective effect against heart disease and stroke, increasing HDL levels.[17] The benefit associated with light to moderate alcohol use is seen regardless of the beverage, which suggests that the protective factor is alcohol itself, rather than another substance in some beverages, such as the tannins in red wine. The disadvantages of alcohol consumption are that it may contribute to weight gain, higher blood pressure, and elevated triglycerides. The possible cardiovascular benefits have to be weighed against the disadvantages and potential harm associated with drinking.[16]

Psychosocial Factors

Five psychosocial factors have been studied that appear to play a role in the development and outcomes of CVD: personality, chronic stress, socioeconomic status, depression, and social support.

As described in Chapter 5, traits and behavior patterns associated with the so-called Type A personality—specifically, anger and hostility—have been shown to contribute to CVD risk. These feelings cause the release of stress hormones. When anger, hostility, and stress in general are persistent and pervasive, the continuous circulation of stress hormones in the blood increases blood pressure and heart rate and triggers the release of cholesterol and triglycerides into the blood. All these changes may promote the development of atherosclerosis and, for those with atherosclerosis, increase vulnerability to heart attack or stroke. Thus, anger, hostility, and chronic stress contribute to the risk for CVD.[18]

People with low socioeconomic status and low levels of educational attainment have a greater risk for heart attack, stroke, congestive heart failure, and hypertension. Income inequality in a country—the gap between the rich and poor—is directly related to national rates of death from CVD, coronary artery disease, and stroke.[19] Numerous factors may help explain the link between poverty and poor health. For example, poverty limits people's ability to obtain the basic requisites for health, such as food and shelter, as well as their ability to participate in society, which creates psychological stress. Poverty also limits access to health-related information, health care, medications, behavior change options, and physical activity.[1,18,20] In addition, racism, prejudice, and discrimination can act as psychosocial stressors and lead to increased risk of CVD.

Depression has a bidirectional relationship with CVD; that is, depression increases risk of CVD, and CVD increases risk of depression. Depression can play a role in all stages in the development of CVD. People who are depressed have a more difficult time choosing healthy lifestyle options, making lifestyle changes, initiating access to health care, and adhering to medication regimens. Early diagnosis and treatment of depression may help reduce risk of CVD in vulnerable individuals.[18]

People who lack social support or live in social isolation are at increased risk for many health conditions, including CVD. Strong social networks have been shown to decrease the risk of CVD, and social support, altruism, faith, and optimism are all associated with a reduced risk of CVD.[21,22] Thus, it appears that the strength of a person's relationships and the nature of his or her basic attitudes toward life play important roles in maintaining health and protecting against disease, as discussed in Chapter 4.

Possible Risk Factors in CVD

Factors that contribute to CVD are not fully understood, and some people with heart disease have none of the risk factors discussed so far. Researchers are constantly trying to identify additional risk factors; in this section we consider a few promising areas of ongoing research.

Lipoprotein(a)

A subgroup of LDL cholesterol, **Lipoprotein(a)** is similar to LDL but has an additional protein attached. Levels of

lipoprotein(a) are elevated in people with coronary heart disease. Experts think this type of LDL may increase blood clotting. Screening for lipoprotein(a) levels is possible, but whether screening will further identify people at risk for CVD beyond what can be learned from screening for LDLs is not clear. Steps that decrease LDL levels, such as dietary modifications and medications, also decrease levels of lipoprotein(a).[23]

Homocysteine

High blood levels of **homocysteine,** an amino acid, have been associated with increased risks of CVD. Homocysteine may damage the lining of blood vessels, leading to inflammation and atherosclerosis. Homocysteine is common in animal proteins, and blood levels are higher in people with diets high in animal protein and low in vitamin B_6, vitamin B_{12}, and folic acid (commonly found in fruits, vegetables, and grains). Both genetics and diet appear to play a role in setting homocysteine levels. Some experts recommend measuring homocysteine as a routine screening test for CVD risk; others have countered that there is no evidence showing that reducing homocysteine levels can reduce the risk of CVD. For now, testing remains controversial and has not become generally recommended. However, individuals can reduce their blood level of homocysteine by eating a diet rich in fruits, vegetables, and grains, especially grain products fortified with folic acid.

Metabolic Syndrome

A condition associated with a significantly increased risk of CVD and the development of Type-2 diabetes, **metabolic syndrome** is characterized by a combination of obesity, especially central obesity; elevated blood pressure; dyslipidemia (high triglycerides and low HDL cholesterol); and glucose intolerance, a pre-diabetes condition. It is estimated that 47 million adult Americans meet the criteria for diagnosis with metabolic syndrome. The prevalence varies by ethnic and racial group; for example,

KEY TERMS

triglycerides Blood fats similar to cholesterol.
lipoprotein(a) Subgroup of LDL cholesterol that is thought to increase blood clotting.
homocysteine Amino acid that circulates in the blood and may damage the lining of blood vessels.
metabolic syndrome Condition characterized by a combination of obesity, especially central obesity; elevated blood pressure; dyslipidemia (high triglycerides and low HDL cholesterol); and glucose intolerance, a pre-diabetes condition.

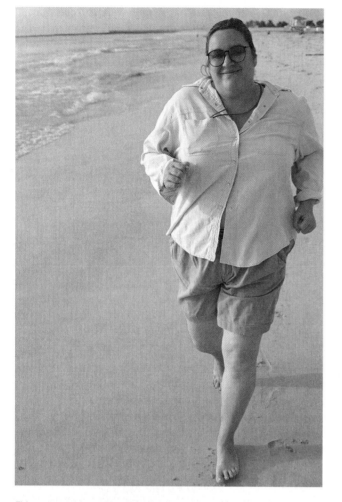

This woman carries excess weight in the center of her body, one characteristic of metabolic syndrome. When this factor is combined with high blood pressure, a high level of triglycerides, a low level of HDL (good) cholesterol, and glucose intolerance, the risk for cardiac disease and diabetes (Type-2) rises significantly.

prevalence is 21.6 percent in African Americans, 37 percent in Mexican Americans, and 23.8 percent in white Americans.[1] The causes are believed to be a combination of genetics and central obesity. Recommendations for metabolic syndrome include increasing physical activity, losing weight, and making dietary changes. Important dietary changes are decreasing total calories consumed; replacing refined carbohydrates with legumes, vegetables, and whole grains; and replacing saturated fats with monounsaturated fats, such as olive oil and canola oil (see Chapter 7).

Inflammatory Response and C-Reactive Protein

Inflammation is well established as a factor in all stages of atherosclerosis. Several blood test markers can be used to identify and measure an ongoing inflammatory response, and elevated levels of **C-reactive protein,** fibrinogen, and white blood cell count have all been associated with an increased risk of CVD. High levels of C-reactive protein are associated with increased risk for coronary heart disease in both men and women and have also been associated with more rapid progression of CVD.

Because the large studies of C-reactive protein have been conducted primarily with people of Northern European background, routine screening of all populations for C-reactive protein is not recommended at this time. Such screening may be helpful for people at moderate risk for CVD due to other risk factors. Statin medications, which are used to lower LDL cholesterol levels, have been shown to reduce C-reactive protein levels, but, again, it remains unclear whether these drugs should be used for elevated C-reactive protein independent of elevated cholesterol levels.[24]

Infectious Agents

Hard as it may be to believe, some heart disease may be caused by infectious agents. As we have seen, inflammation plays a role in atherosclerosis, and a common source of inflammation is infection. The first organism shown to have a potential role in CVD was *Chlamydia pneumoniae* (not the sexually transmitted strain of chlamydia). Researchers first noted a correlation between this type of chlamydia and atherosclerosis in 1988, when they found that 59 percent of arteries containing atherosclerotic plaques showed evidence of chlamydia, whereas only 3 percent of arteries without plaques showed such evidence. Cause and effect have not been completely determined, but initial studies on treatment with antibiotics suggest some benefit.[25]

Another study found a slightly increased risk of CVD in people with evidence of prior infection with *cytomegalovirus,* a common herpes virus that causes coldlike symptoms, but no increased risk associated with chlamydia, *Helicobacter pylori* (a bacteria associated with stomach ulcers), or hepatitis A.[26] Other studies suggest that the influenza virus may be linked with CVD, and vaccination against influenza has been associated with reduced risk of heart disease.[27] At this point, the jury is still out on which infectious organisms may play a role in CVD and how big that role may be. Antibiotics and antivirals are not being used to reduce the risk of CVD, but it may be that vaccination will offer this benefit in the future.

Fetal Origins

Research has shown a relationship between birth weight and risk of CVD, with lower birth weight associated with

KEY TERMS

C-reactive protein   Blood marker for inflammation that may indicate an increased risk for coronary heart disease.

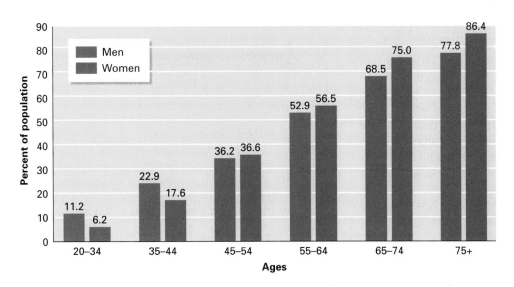

Figure 21.6   Prevalence of cardiovascular diseases in Americans age 20 and older by age and sex, National Health and Nutrition Examination Survey, 1999–2002. Source: Centers for Disease Control and Prevention/National Center for Health Statistics and National Heart, Lung, and Blood Institute (www.cdc.gov/nchs and www.nhlbi.gov).

These data include coronary heart disease, congestive heart failure, stroke, and hypertension.

higher risk.[28] This represents what is called a *programming phenomenon.* Tissues (in this case the heart muscle and blood vessels) may be damaged during sensitive stages of fetal development in a way that programs them to develop problems later in life. Fetal growth has been found to be associated with increased risk of other common adult health problems as well, such as hypertension and obesity.[29] Such findings further demonstrate the importance of providing healthy conditions for prenatal development (see Chapter 16).

Noncontrollable Risk Factors in CVD

Age, gender, ethnicity and race, family history, and, arguably, postmenopausal status are the noncontrollable risk factors for cardiovascular disease. Individuals with noncontrollable risk factors, especially, should choose healthy behaviors that do not promote CVD.

Age and CVD Risk

Age is probably the most important noncontrollable risk factor. The Framingham Study confirmed a progressive increase in CVD risk with each additional year of life, probably reflecting the progressive nature of atherosclerosis (Figure 21.6). There is a significant rise in deaths due to heart disease and stroke after age 65. Heart disease and stroke are responsible for 40 percent of deaths in people aged 65 to 74 and for 60 percent of deaths in people over age 85.[30] Age alone does not cause CVD, however; there is great variation in CVD among older people of the same age.

Gender and CVD Risk

Although heart disease is often thought of as a man's disease, CVD is the leading cause of death for both men and women. There are some differences between the sexes,

however. A 40-year-old man without evidence of heart disease has a 1 in 2 chance of developing CVD in his lifetime, whereas a 40-year-old woman has a 1 in 3 chance.[31]

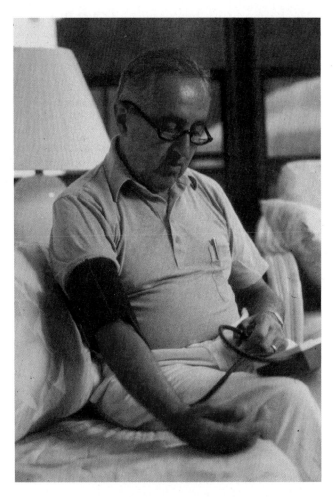

Although this man cannot control certain risk factors for cardiovascular disease, such as his age and gender, he follows a regimen that includes monitoring his blood pressure, following a heart-healthy diet, and taking long walks daily.

Women tend to develop heart disease about 10 years later than men, perhaps owing to the protective effect of estrogen before menopause. After age 50 (the average age of menopause), the difference in risk between men and women starts to decrease.

The death rates for CVD are higher in women, both African American and white American; this is true of heart attack, stroke, hypertension, and congestive heart failure. One reason for this is that women tend to be older and frailer when they develop heart disease and so are less likely to survive. Another reason is that women are more likely to have either no symptoms before a heart attack or symptoms that make the diagnosis of heart disease more confusing, such as stomach complaints. One study showed that women delay seeking treatment as much as 3.5 hours longer than men do. Because treatment is more effective the sooner it is started, this delay means that more damage occurs. A third reason is that health care providers may also delay treatment because they do not recognize the symptoms or are less likely to think about heart disease in women.[16]

Genetics and Family History and CVD Risk

Individuals who have a relative with a history of CVD have a higher risk of CVD themselves. The risk for heart attack appears to be greatest if a male relative had a heart attack before age 55 or a female relative had a heart attack before age 65. The risk for stroke is increased if a relative has had a stroke, regardless of age. High rates of CVD in a family may be related to genetics or lifestyle patterns or both; the genetic effect may act through elevated blood pressure or cholesterol levels. Most individuals with a family history of stroke or heart attack have at least one controllable risk factor, so they need to pay attention to areas of their lives where they can improve behavior patterns, such as diet or exercise. At the same time, individuals who do not have a family history of CVD should not ignore lifestyle factors. Many people with CVD have no family history of premature coronary artery disease.

Ethnicity and Race and CVD Risk

The frequency and severity of cardiovascular disease differs among different populations. African Americans have a higher risk of CVD and stroke than white Americans do, as well as higher rates of hypertension, obesity, and diabetes. Mexican Americans, American Indians, and native Hawaiians also have a higher risk of CVD than white Americans, along with higher rates of obesity and diabetes.

Recent improvements in cardiovascular health have not been shared evenly by all racial or ethnic groups. Although the death rate from heart attack has declined across all groups, it has declined less among minority groups and women. For example, since the 1980s, the

---

Healthy People 2010

OBJECTIVE AREA *Heart Disease and Stroke*

● Reduce coronary heart disease deaths.

"Heart disease and stroke share several risk factors, including high blood pressure, cigarette smoking, high blood cholesterol, and overweight. Physical inactivity and diabetes are additional risk factors for heart disease. The lifetime risk for developing CHD is very high in the United States. . . . A number of studies have shown that lifestyle interventions can help prevent high blood pressure and reduce blood cholesterol levels."

 For more information on Healthy People 2010 objectives, visit the Web site at www.healthypeople.gov.

For more information on Canadian health objectives, visit the Health Canada Web site at www.hc-sc.gc.ca/english.

---

death rate from heart attack has declined by 29 percent among white men and by 21.9 percent among African American men and 18.9 percent among American Indian men. Among women, the death rate has declined by 23.7 percent for white women and by 18.5 percent for African American women and 10.5 percent for American Indian women.[32] Several pathways may lead to these health disparities, including differences in such risk factors as hypertension, genetics, stress, and psychosocial factors.[33] Reducing these disparities is a major national health goal.

Postmenopausal Status and CVD Risk

Postmenopausal status is a risk factor for CVD. In the past there was debate as to whether it should be considered a controllable versus noncontrollable risk factor. The hormone estrogen has long been thought to protect premenopausal women from CVD. When levels of estrogen fall during menopause, levels of HDL also decline, and body fat distribution shifts to a more central distribution pattern, similar to the male pattern. For many years, medical practitioners prescribed hormone replacement therapy (HRT) for postmenopausal women to relieve the symptoms of menopause, lower the risk of osteoporosis (bone thinning), and reduce the risk of CVD. The belief in the benefits of estrogen was so strong that at one point, nearly one in three postmenopausal women was on HRT. As described in Chapter 15, research has now shown that HRT actually increases rather than decreases the risk of heart attack and stroke.[34,35] HRT is still prescribed as a treatment for the symptoms of menopause and prevention of osteoporosis, but these benefits must now be weighed against an individual woman's risk for CVD.

TESTING AND TREATMENT

People with no symptoms of CVD are usually not tested for evidence of disease; instead the focus is on screening for risk factors (hypertension, cholesterol levels, family health history, and so on). An exception is people in certain occupations, such as airline pilots or truck drivers, whose sudden incapacity would place other people at risk. Such individuals may be tested for asymptomatic CVD as part of an employment physical examination. People may also be screened for signs of CVD before surgery, and the American College of Sports Medicine recommends that an exercise stress test be performed on men older than age 40 and women older than age 50 if they are sedentary and about to begin an exercise program.

For people who do have symptoms suggestive of CVD, such as shortness of breath or angina with light activity, physical examination and diagnostic tests can help determine the presence of disease and the extent of the problem. If disease is present, a variety of steps can be taken, from lifestyle changes, to medication, to surgery.

Treatment for Heart Attack

When a heart attack occurs, emergency treatment is critical. Effectiveness of treatment depends on the time elapsed from the first symptoms to the beginning of treatment. The goal of treatment is to reestablish blood flow to the heart before the muscle is permanently damaged. Learn to recognize the signs of a heart attack or stroke, and call 911 or your local emergency services immediately if you or someone you are with has these symptoms. Don't delay—even 5 minutes can make a difference. An emergency medical technician (EMT) can monitor heart rhythm on the way to the hospital and stabilize the heart if there is an arrhythmia. Many EMTs are trained to give medications in the field, with physician telephone orders.

Diagnostic Testing

At the hospital, tests can be performed to see if the symptoms are due to a heart attack. An **electrocardiogram (EKG)**, a record of the electrical activity of the heart as it beats, can detect abnormal rhythms, inadequate blood flow (possibly due to heart attack or ischemia), and heart enlargement. Blood tests can be performed to detect proteins in the blood that are released by a damaged heart muscle. A variety of procedures allow visualization of the heart, heart valves, and any blocked or narrowed coronary arteries, including **echocardiograms** (using sound waves),

coronary **angiograms** (using a dye), computerized tomography (CT) scans, and magnetic resonance imaging (MRI).

Medical Management

If someone is having a heart attack, aspirin is often given immediately (even before diagnostic testing) to reduce the blood's ability to clot. Once a heart attack is diagnosed, the person may be given thrombolytic, or clot-busting, medications to dissolve clots, reopen coronary arteries, and restore blood flow to the heart muscle. Other medications can be given to improve blood flow and reduce the chest pain associated with a heart attack. Nitrates, such as nitroglycerine, relax blood vessels and can reduce pain and improve blood flow, and pain medications reduce the stress associated with pain. Other medications, such as beta-blockers, reduce the risk of another heart attack by slowing heart rate and lowering blood pressure.

Surgical Management

In some cases, physicians perform an **angioplasty** to reopen a blocked coronary artery. In this procedure, a balloon catheter (a thin plastic tube) is threaded into the narrowed area and inflated to stretch the vessel open again. A *coronary stent*, a springy framework that supports the vessel walls and keeps the vessel open, is often permanently placed in the artery to prevent it from closing again. Another surgical option is **coronary artery bypass grafting,**

KEY TERMS

electrocardiogram (EKG)   Record of the heart's electrical activity as it beats.

echocardiogram   Diagnostic test for a heart attack in which sound waves are used to visualize heart valves, heart wall movement, and overall heart function.

coronary angiogram   Diagnostic test for a heart attack in which a dye is injected into a fine catheter that is passed into the heart and X-rays are taken as the dye moves through the heart, showing any blocked or narrowed coronary arteries.

angioplasty   Procedure to reopen a blocked coronary artery, in which a balloon catheter (a thin plastic tube) is threaded into the narrowed area and inflated to stretch the vessel open again.

coronary artery bypass grafting   Surgical procedure in which a healthy blood vessel is taken from another part of the body and grafted to the coronary arteries to allow a bypass of blood flow around a narrowed vessel.

usually just called *bypass*. A healthy blood vessel is taken from another part of the body, usually the leg, and grafted to the coronary arteries to allow a bypass of blood flow around a narrowed vessel.

Treatment of Stroke

Before the 1990s, little could be done to alter the natural course of a stroke. Today, the same thrombolytic (clot-dissolving) medications that are used in heart attacks can be used to decrease the damage incurred by a stroke. As with heart attacks, the clot-dissolving medications work best when given as soon as possible after the onset of symptoms; in fact, they can be administered only within the first 3 hours of the onset of symptoms. Thus, it is critical that a person experiencing symptoms of a stroke receive medical care immediately.

Diagnostic Testing

At the hospital, a CT scan or an MRI can be used to generate images of the brain and blood flow and to determine whether a stroke has occurred. These tests can also show whether a stroke has been caused by a blockage or by a hemorrhage. Further testing may be done to find the source of the blockage. The carotid arteries, the large arteries on the sides of the neck that supply blood to the brain, are examined to see if they are blocked with atherosclerotic plaques. If so, part of the plaque may have broken off and become the source of an embolism blocking a blood vessel in the brain.

Management

If a stroke is found to be thrombotic (caused by a blockage) and there is no evidence of bleeding in the brain, thrombolytic medications can be administered to dissolve the clot and restore blood flow to the brain. Thrombolytic medications must not be given if the stroke is hemorrhagic, because they can cause increased bleeding. Aspirin and other anticlotting medications can be used after a thrombotic stroke to reduce the risk of another stroke. Control of blood pressure and other risk factors is important for all people who have a stroke, whether thrombotic or hemorrhagic.

Rehabilitation is a component of treatment for stroke. If an area of the brain is damaged or destroyed, the functions that were controlled by that part of the brain will be impaired. Rehabilitation consists of physical therapy (to strengthen muscles and coordination), speech therapy (to improve communication and eating), and occupational therapy (to improve activities of daily living and job retraining if appropriate). Progress and return of functions vary by individual. Some people recover fully within a few days to weeks, while others are left with long-term impairment.

PROTECTING YOURSELF FROM CVD

As scientists learn more about the progressive nature of cardiovascular disease, the significance of early prevention becomes clearer. The possible role of programming during fetal development shows that it is never too early to pay attention to diet, exercise, and avoidance of risk factors. Communities and society play a role in the prevention of CVD, through education, media campaigns, and screening programs. Individual behavior change is an important form of prevention. Adopting healthy lifestyle habits now, regardless of your age or current health status, is the best way to reduce your risk of developing cardiovascular disease in the future.

✴Eating for Heart Health

Diet and nutrition have been extensively studied and found to alter risk for heart disease and stroke. Diet also plays a role in controlling the major risk factors, such as diabetes, hypertension, and obesity. A diet that supports cardiovascular health emphasizes fruits, vegetables, whole grains, low-fat dairy products, fish, and lean meat and poultry. Several eating plans have been developed to promote heart health, including the 2005 *Dietary Guidelines for Americans,* described in Chapter 7, and the American Heart Association Dietary Guidelines, summarized in the box "Choosing a Heart-Healthy Diet."

As noted in Chapter 7, researchers have also been interested in the so-called Mediterranean diet because of the much lower rates of heart disease among people living in that part of the world. In addition to emphasizing other healthy components, the Mediterranean diet includes ample amounts of olive oil and margarine high in omega-3 fatty acids. Researchers believe that the emphasis on these kinds of fats, which may have an anti-inflammatory effect, may be the key factor in the protective effects of the diet. For more on the Mediterranean diet, see Chapter 7.

Another area of research focuses on micronutrients, some of which appear to play a role in cardiovascular health. Many micronutrients, especially antioxidants, are more plentiful in a diet that centers on plant products rather than animal products. Foods high in important antioxidants are brightly colored fruits and vegetables and nuts and seeds (see Chapter 7). Experts recommend that micronutrients be consumed in foods rather than in supplements.

One supplement that may be beneficial for some people with CVD is coenzyme Q_{10} (CoQ_{10}), an enzyme used by cells in energy production that may have a special role in the health of the heart muscle. Levels of CoQ_{10} are lower in some people with heart disease, and levels may decrease progressively with the severity of the disease. Supplementation may improve symptoms and survival rates for people with some forms of heart disease, although there is no general recommendation at this time.[36]

Challenges & Choices

Choosing a Heart-Healthy Diet

The American Heart Association encourages all Americans, young and old, to adopt a heart-healthy diet. AHA guidelines include the following recommendations:

- Eat a diet rich in fruits, vegetables, legumes (beans), whole grains, low-fat dairy products, fish, and lean meats and poultry.

- Consume less than 30 percent of total calories from fat and less than 10 percent of fat calories from saturated fats; if you have elevated LDL levels or other CVD risk factors, consume less than 7 percent of fat calories from saturated fats.

- Limit dietary cholesterol to no more than 300 mg per day; if you have elevated LDL levels or other CVD risk factors, limit dietary cholesterol to no more than 200 mg per day.

- Choose polyunsaturated and monounsaturated fats, such as those found in plant products, nuts, and olive oil, over the saturated fats found in animal products.

- Avoid consumption of trans fatty acids, which are found in foods containing partially hydrogenated vegetable oils, such as fried foods, margarines, and commercially baked goods.

- Limit salt intake to less than 2,400 mg per day.

- Maintain a healthy weight by limiting high-calorie foods with low nutritional quality.

It's Not Just Personal . . .

According to the American Heart Association, the incidence of heart disease in Mediterranean countries is lower than in the United States. Death rates are also lower. Although there is no single "Mediterranean" diet, the pattern of Mediterranean-style diets is often similar to the AHA dietary guidelines. The main difference is that Mediterranean diets often include a relatively high percentage of calories from fat.

Is there a cause-and-effect relationship between the Mediterranean-type diet and the lower incidence of cardiac disease in Mediterranean countries? It's possible, but lifestyle factors, such as physical activity and social support systems, may also play an important role. More studies are needed to make this relationship clearer.

Source: Data from the American Heart Association, www.americanheart.org.

Another type of supplementation, aspirin, has become a controversial approach to preventing heart disease (see the box "An Aspirin a Day?").

Other specific foods have been shown to alter cholesterol levels. Soy products and legumes, such as lentils and chickpeas, have both been shown to decrease LDL. Garlic appears to have a similar effect on total cholesterol, although fresh garlic (one to two cloves per day) is recommended over synthesized garlic capsules.[37] Foods rich in fiber also help reduce cholesterol levels; they include fruits, vegetables, oats, and barley.

Exercising Regularly

Exercise has an effect on many CVD risk factors. It has a direct conditioning effect on the heart, improving the health of the heart muscle and enhancing its ability to pump blood efficiently. Exercise helps in weight loss and weight-maintenance programs by increasing energy output. It also has more subtle effects, such as improving HDL levels and increasing the number of insulin receptors, which enhances the ability of people with diabetes to use insulin. The 2005 *Dietary Guidelines for Americans* recommends 30 minutes of moderate-intensity physical activity above usual activity on most days of the week to reduce the risk of chronic disease, including CVD. Even low-intensity activities, such as walking, gardening, or climbing stairs, can be helpful. See Chapter 8 for more information on exercising for health and fitness.

Avoiding Tobacco Use

Smoking is the leading preventable cause of CVD. It poses both an immediate hazard for heart attack and a long-term hazard for atherosclerosis. Because nicotine is so addictive, the best prevention is never to start smoking. If you do smoke, quitting now can significantly reduce your risk of developing CVD. See Chapter 13 for more information on tobacco use and strategies for quitting.

Controlling Blood Pressure

Regular screening for hypertension is recommended for individuals over age 18.[38] For anyone in the prehypertension or hypertension category, lifestyle changes are recommended, including weight reduction, dietary changes, low salt intake, physical activity, and moderate alcohol intake.[4] If lifestyle changes alone do not reduce blood

Consumer Clipboard

An Aspirin a Day?

Ten years ago, taking an aspirin a day to prevent a heart attack seemed like a good idea—as simple as taking a vitamin pill and an easy way to avoid a major health problem. More recently, however, studies have shown that this approach may not be advisable—at least not for everyone.

Early studies, which focused entirely or largely on men, found that aspirin does offer protection against heart attacks, and subsequent studies showed that even smaller doses of aspirin showed similar benefits. It was these studies that made aspirin therapy seem like a good approach to both consumers and health care professionals.

Yet recent studies tell a somewhat different story. The Women's Health Study, a 10-year study of healthy women over age 45, conducted by Brigham and Women's Hospital, was the first large clinical trial to look specifically at the effects of aspirin on women. Results showed that among women who took aspirin, the risk of all "cardiovascular events" taken together (heart attacks, strokes, and death from cardiovascular problems) was lower than it was for the placebo group, but the difference was not considered significant.

The women taking aspirin had approximately the same number of heart attacks as the participants taking the placebo. The surprising news was that the number of strokes in the aspirin group was 17 percent lower, which was considered significant. The aspirin takers had an especially low risk of ischemic stroke, the most common type, caused by a blood clot in an artery leading to the brain—24 percent lower than the placebo group. The risk of hemorrhagic stroke, the kind cause by bleeding, was slightly higher in the aspirin group, as expected, because aspirin reduces the blood's tendency to clot.

In the women who were 65 or older, aspirin takers had a 26 percent lower risk of a major cardiovascular problem than those who took placebos. Their risk of heart attack was 34 percent lower. As already known, women's risk of heart attack, compared to that of men, rises later in life, after menopause, most likely because of the loss of the protective effect of estrogen.

With this information, the American Heart Association offers guidelines for aspirin therapy but distinguishes between men and women in assessing level of risk for both heart attack and stroke.

- Aspirin therapy is recommended for patients who have had a heart attack, unstable angina, ischemic stroke (caused by blood clot), or transient ischemic attacks (TIAs or mini-strokes), if not contraindicated.

- Aspirin also helps prevent these events from occurring in people at high risk, such as those with high blood pressure, family history of heart disease, diabetes, smoking, and obesity.

- Adults, especially those over age 40 with two or more risk factors, should have their 10-year risk of coronary heart disease assessed with a multiple risk factor score every 5 years (or more often if risk factors change). Factors may include age, sex, smoking status, blood pressure, cholesterol levels, and diabetes.

- *Men* whose risk of heart disease in the next 10 years is at least 10 percent are considered candidates for aspirin therapy.

- *Women* should not be advised to take aspirin unless their 10-year risk is 20 percent (or if it is 10 percent and they have controlled high blood pressure).

- Don't start aspirin therapy without first consulting your physician. The risks vs. benefits vary for each person.

- If you are experiencing symptoms of a heart attack, call 911 immediately.

- If you are experiencing symptoms of a stroke, don't take an aspirin. Although most types of stroke are caused by blood clots, some are the result of ruptured blood vessels. Taking aspirin could make bleeding strokes more severe.

Sources: "Aspirin in Heart Attack and Stroke Prevention," 2005, American Heart Association, www.american.heart.org; "Aspirin Is Found to Protect Women from Strokes, Not Heart Attacks," *The New York Times*, March 8, 2005, p. D5.

pressure, medications are recommended. Hypertension can be controlled in most cases, but sometimes it takes lifestyle change plus two or more medications.

A diet known as Dietary Approaches to Stop Hypertension (DASH) has been shown to reduce elevated blood pressure. The diet is high in fruits, vegetables, and low-fat dairy products and low in saturated fat, cholesterol, and total fat. As discussed in Chapter 7, the 2005 *Dietary Guidelines for Americans* recommends the DASH diet, citing it as an eating plan that exemplifies the guidelines. The

Dietary Guidelines recommend a limit of 1,500 mg of sodium per day for individuals with hypertension, middle-aged and older adults, and African Americans.

Managing Cholesterol Levels

As noted earlier, the National Cholesterol Education Program recommends that all adults over age 20 have their cholesterol checked at least once every 5 years. If you find that your LDL cholesterol levels, in combination with other risk factors, put you at risk for CVD, your physician will work with you to develop an LDL goal and a plan for reaching it. Exercising, maintaining a healthy weight, and dietary changes, including reducing total and saturated fat intake and increasing dietary fiber, are first-line actions. However, as with high blood pressure, these changes may not be enough for some people and medication may be required. Some cholesterol-lowering drugs decrease cholesterol absorption from the diet; others decrease cholesterol synthesis by the liver. Taking medication to control cholesterol levels is complicated and should always be done under the guidance of a health care provider.

Controlling Diabetes

People with diabetes must control their blood glucose levels to reduce their risk of cardiovascular complications. For Type-1 diabetes, in which the pancreas produces no insulin, treatment requires lifelong self-administered in-sulin injections to maintain blood glucose levels as close to normal as possible. For Type-2 diabetes, in which body cells no longer respond well to insulin, exercise and weight loss are often enough to correct the condition without medication. When needed, pills can be taken to help improve the cellular response to insulin, or insulin injections may be given. People with diabetes also have to control their other CVD risk factors, such as high cholesterol levels, high triglyceride levels, and high blood pressure, all of which are more likely to occur in association with this disorder.[39]

Managing Stress and Improving Mental Health

Stress, anger, hostility, and depression can all contribute to CVD. If you frequently feel overwhelmed by negative feelings and moods, try some of the stress management and relaxation techniques described in Chapters 3, 4, and 5. You may want to increase your social support system by expanding your connections to family, friends, community, or church. You may want to simplify your schedule and slow down. Meditating can lower blood pressure and blood cholesterol levels, thereby slowing the process of atherosclerosis. Biofeedback may help reduce blood pressure. Hypnosis may be useful to help control hypertension and other chronic health problems.[40] Whatever approach you choose to manage stress and enhance your mental health, try to incorporate a daily practice into your life.

You Make the Call

Does Your Home Need an Automatic External Defibrillator?

Television shows like *ER* frequently depict physicians administering electric shocks to the chests of people who have suffered cardiac arrest. Most of these people have experienced an arrhythmia, usually from ventricular fibrillation. The electrical charge briefly stops the heart and allows it to restart in a normal rhythm.

Now the average layperson may have the opportunity to give the same kind of treatment if a family member is stricken at home. The Food and Drug Administration (FDA) recently approved over-the-counter sales of automatic external defibrillators (AED) for use in the home, and a spokesperson stated, "Soon AEDs will become as common in the home as fire extinguishers." Is this something you should have in your home?

Of the 235,000 people who experience an out-of-hospital cardiac arrest each year, only 5 percent survive. Survival is directly linked to the time it takes from the onset of a fatal arrythmia to the use of a defibrilla-tor to restart a normal rhythm. Survival decreases by 10 percent for every minute of delay. As mentioned in the chapter, the American Heart Association recommends a four-step "Chain of Survival" by witnesses or bystanders in the event of cardiac arrest: early access to emergency medical services (by calling 911), early CPR, early defibrillation, and early advanced cardiac care.

The use of home AED may reduce the time between arrest and defibrillation. AED devices have become easier to transport, easier to use, and cheaper, as manufacturers have tried to accommodate increased interest and need. Currently, an AED costs between $1,500 and $3,000. When applied correctly to the chest of someone experiencing cardiac arrest, it analyzes for arrythmia and prompts the user to deliver a shock if it is needed. Rapid use of an AED by a layperson requires knowledge of where the device is located and how to use it.

The Food and Drug Administration, which regulates defibrillators, has decided AEDs are safe enough for the general public to operate. The American Heart Association supported the recommendation that AEDs be sold over-the-counter but states that it lacks scientific evidence to recommend for or against the use of AEDs in the home. A large trial is currently underway to determine if early defibrillation by family members using an AED at home will increase survival.

Opponents of in-home use of AEDs state that the device is an expensive technology with a low likelihood of use. Although 335,000 sudden cardiac arrests occur each year, the chances are slim that one will occur in a home with an AED at a time when a family member is present who is trained to use it. Opponents argue that the money spent on an AED could be better used on preventive measures, such as joining an exercise facility. They also raise the concern that searching for the home AED may lead to a delay in calling 911, administering CPR, and getting the person to advanced cardiac care.

Are AEDs life savers or obstacles to survival? What do you think?

Pros

- Home automatic external defibrillators may reduce the time between onset of sudden cardiac arrest and restoration of a normal heart rhythm.
- AEDs are easily used by laypeople.
- The cost of AEDs is decreasing, and they are available over-the-counter for anyone to purchase.
- 335,000 people die each year from sudden cardiac arrest outside of the hospital or in the emergency department. Some of these people could be saved by increased access to AEDs.

Cons

- The cost of AEDs is still too high, given the low likelihood of use by any single purchaser.
- Home use of AEDs may delay access to emergency medical services and advanced cardiac care.
- There is no scientific evidence to suggest that increased access to AEDs in the home will reduce the number of people dying from sudden cardiac arrest.

OLC Web site   For more information about this topic, visit the Online Learning Center at www.mhhe.com/teague1e.

SOURCES: "American Heart Association Tells FDA Panel That Prescription Requirement Has No Effect on Safety of AEDs," by T. McRae and K. Kennai, *Advocacy News,* July 30, 2004, www.americanheart.org; "Automatic External Defibrillator," Heart Health Online, February 7, 2004, U.S. Food and Drug Administration, www.fda.gov/hearthealth; "Some Questions Remain About Home Use of Defibrillators" by R. Davis, *USA Today,* Sept 20, 2004, www.usatoday.com.

SUMMARY

- The cardiovascular system consists of a network of blood vessels (arteries, veins, and capillaries) and a pump (the heart) that circulate blood throughout the body. The heart is a four-chambered organ the size of a fist with two atria and two ventricles, separated by valves.
- The right side of the heart pumps blood to and from the lungs, and the left side of the heart pumps blood to and from the body.
- The heart muscle is supplied with blood via the coronary arteries.
- The heartbeat originates in the sinus node of the right atrium as an electrical signal that spreads first to the atria and then to the ventricles.
- Cardiovascular disease is the leading cause of death in the United States. The underlying disease process in many forms of CVD is atherosclerosis, a gradual thickening and hardening of the arteries due to a buildup in artery walls of fatty deposits known as plaques.
- Coronary heart disease occurs when the coronary arteries are damaged by atherosclerosis, leading to angina from narrowed arteries or myocardial infarction (heart attack) from blocked arteries. The longer the heart tissue is deprived of oxygen, the more damage is incurred.
- Sudden cardiac death can occur when a severe arrhythmia, or disruption of the electrical signal that controls the heartbeat, causes ventricular fibrillation, in which the ventricles quiver instead of beating. Cardiopulmonary resuscitation can help restart the heart, and defibrillators can restore normal beating.
- A stroke occurs when brain tissue is deprived of oxygen because of a blocked artery in the brain (a thrombotic, or ischemic, stroke) or when a blood vessel ruptures and leaks blood into brain tissue (a hemorrhagic stroke). Eighty-eight percent of strokes are thrombotic, and 12 percent are hemorrhagic. Transient ischemic attacks (TIAs) are "ministrokes" with temporary effects.
- Hypertension is a condition in which the force exerted by the blood against the artery walls is consistently great enough to damage the walls. It can lead to heart attack, stroke, and other forms of CVD. It has no symptoms and is known as a "silent killer."

- Congestive heart failure occurs when the heart fails to pump the blood forcefully or efficiently enough, and blood and fluid back up into the lungs.

- Other cardiovascular disorders include heart valve disorders, rheumatic heart disease, congenital heart disease, peripheral vascular disease, and cardiomyopathy.

- Risk factors for CVD can be controllable or noncontrollable. The six major controllable risk factors identified by the American Heart Association are tobacco use, hypertension, unhealthy blood cholesterol levels, physical inactivity, overweight, and diabetes.

- Tobacco use is the leading risk factor for all forms of CVD. Tobacco smoke damages artery walls, increases the formation of blood clots, triggers spasms that close blood vessels, raises levels of LDL cholesterol, and lowers levels of HDL cholesterol.

- Hypertension damages artery walls and makes the heart work harder to pump blood. Rates and severity of hypertension are higher among African Americans, for a variety of known and unknown reasons.

- Unhealthy blood cholesterol levels mean that levels of LDL cholesterol are high enough to contribute to the formation of atherosclerotic plaque and levels of HDL cholesterol are not high enough to provide the protective function of returning cholesterol to the liver.

- Physical inactivity is associated with overweight and obesity, hypertension, and diabetes; physical activity provides many cardiovascular benefits. Excess weight strains the heart and contributes to hypertension, diabetes, and high LDL cholesterol levels.

- Diabetes causes high levels of glucose to circulate in the blood, damaging artery walls and altering blood components.

- Contributing risk factors for CVD include high triglyceride levels; high alcohol intake; psychosocial factors, including anger, hostility, and chronic stress; low socioeconomic status; depression; and lack of social support.

- Possible CVD risk factors under investigation include lipoprotein(a), homocysteine, metabolic syndrome, C-reactive protein, infectious agents, and fetal programming.

- Noncontrollable risk factors for CVD include older age, male gender, a family history of CVD, being African American or a member of another minority group, and postmenopausal status.

- Asymptomatic people are usually not tested for CVD; people with symptoms may be tested and treated. A person having a heart attack requires emergency medical attention and transport to a hospital. At the hospital, diagnostic tests are performed and drugs are administered to break up a blood clot, improve blood flow, reduce pain, and reduce the likelihood of a repeat attack. In some cases, surgical procedures such as angioplasty or bypass surgery are performed.

- A person having a stroke requires emergency medical attention and transport to a hospital. Diagnostic testing will be done to determine the type of stroke that is occurring. A thrombotic stroke can be treated with drugs that break up the blood clot; a hemorrhagic stroke can be treated with drugs that lower blood pressure. Rehabilitation may be needed if impairment has occurred.

- Individual risk of CVD can be reduced by practicing healthy lifestyle habits. These include eating a heart-healthy diet, exercising regularly, avoiding tobacco use, having blood pressure checked regularly and controlling high blood pressure, having cholesterol levels checked regularly and controlling unhealthy cholesterol levels, controlling diabetes, and managing stress and improving mental health.

REVIEW QUESTIONS

1. Describe how blood circulates through the heart, from the heart to the lungs, and from the heart to the body.

2. What is the role of the coronary arteries? What is the role of the sinus node?

3. What explanations have been proposed for the drop in the CVD death rate for men in the past 30 years?

4. How can one disease process, atherosclerosis, be responsible for several different forms of CVD?

5. How is the inflammatory response involved in the process of atherosclerosis?

6. What is plaque? What role does it play in CVD?

7. What is ischemia? Why is it important to restore blood flow when an artery is blocked?

8. Describe the symptoms of a heart attack. How are men's symptoms different from women's?

9. What is an arrhythmia? What are some possible causes? What is ventricular fibrillation? How is it treated?

10. Explain the difference between a thrombotic and a hemorrhagic stroke. Which kind is more common?

11. Describe the symptoms of a stroke. How is a stroke different from a TIA?

12. What do the two numbers in a measure of blood pressure represent?

13. What is hypertension? What are some contributing factors and conditions?

14. What is congestive heart failure? What are some contributing factors and conditions?

15. What is mitral valve prolapse? What is a septal defect?

16. Why is it important to have a strep throat infection treated with antibiotics?

17. What is hypertrophic cardiomyopathy, and why should young athletes be screened for it?

18. How does tobacco use contribute to CVD?

19. What blood pressure levels are considered optimal? What factors may contribute to the higher rates of hypertension and stroke among African Americans?

20. Describe the actions of LDL and HDL cholesterol. What are healthy levels of total cholesterol, LDLs, and HDLs?

21. How do physical inactivity and overweight contribute to CVD?

22. What is the difference between Type-1 and Type-2 diabetes? How does diabetes contribute to CVD?

23. Describe how psychosocial factors may contribute to CVD.

24. What role may infectious agents play in CVD?

25. Describe five risk factors for CVD that cannot be controlled. What are some reasons for the higher death rate from CVD among women than among men?

26. How is a heart attack treated at the hospital? A thrombotic stroke? A hemorrhagic stroke?

27. Describe the components of a diet that promotes cardiovascular health. What are three examples of such a diet?

28. What are the screening recommendations for blood pressure? For cholesterol levels?

29. What are some ways to manage stress and promote mental health in the interest of reducing risk for CVD?

WEB RESOURCES

American Heart Association: This organization offers information on diseases and conditions that affect your heart, including a heart and stroke encyclopedia. The site also includes dietary and fitness advice for planning a healthier lifestyle.
www.americanheart.org

Centers for Disease Control and Prevention: A good resource for heart-related diseases and conditions, this site features health promotion activities for teens to older adults.
www.cdc.gov

HeartInfo—Heart Information Network: This site offers patient guides, FAQs, Ask the Doctor, and a heart encyclopedia. Animations include a demonstration of how a heart attack occurs.
www.heartinfo.org

National Heart, Lung, and Blood Institute: Besides information about many heart and vascular diseases and conditions, this site features health assessment tools and recipes for healthy eating.
www.nhlbi.nih.gov

National Institutes of Health: This site is a resource for wide-ranging information on health, including the heart and circulation. NIH's MEDLINEPlus offers more than 700 health topics, drug information, a medical encyclopedia, directories, and other resources.
www.nih.gov

National Stroke Association: This organization offers comprehensive information about stroke, including risks, symptoms, treatment approaches, and recovery and rehabilitation.
www.stroke.org

REFERENCES

1. American Heart Association. (2005). Heart disease and stroke statistics—2005 update. www.americanheart.org.

2. Strong, J. P. (1999). Prevalence and extent of atherosclerosis in adolescents and young adults: Implications for prevention from Pathobiological Determination of Atherosclerosis in Youth Study. *Journal of the American Medical Association, 281* (8), 727–735.

3. Solenski, N. J. (2004). Transient ischemic attacks: Part I. Diagnosis and evaluation. *American Family Physician, 69* (7), 1665–1679.

4. Seventh report of the Joint National Committee on Prevention, Detection, Evaluation and Treatment of High Blood Pressure. (2003). www.nhlbi.nih.gov.

5. National Heart, Lung and Blood Institute. (2004). Congenital heart disease. National Institutes of Health. www.nhlbi.nih.gov.

6. National Heart, Lung and Blood Institute. (1948). The Framingham Heart Study. National Institutes of Health. www.framingham.com/heart.

7. Villablanca, A. C., McDonald, J. M., & Rutledge, J. C. (2000). Smoking and cardiovascular disease. *Clinics in Chest Medicine, 21* (1), 159–172.

8. Ambrose, J. A., & Barva, R. S. (2004). The pathophysiology of cigarette smoke and cardiovascular disease: An update. *Journal of the American College of Cardiology, 43* (10), 1731–1737.

9. Liao, Y., et al. (2004). REACH 2010 surveillance for health status in minority communities—United States, 2001-2002. *Morbidity and Mortality Weekly Report, 53* (SS06), 1–36.

10. Watson, K. E., & Topol, E. J. (2004). Pathobiology of atherosclerosis: Are there racial and ethnic differences? *Reviews of Cardiovascular Medicine, 5* (Suppl 3), S14–S21.

11. Executive summary of the third report of the National Cholesterol Education Program Expert Panel on Detection, Evaluation, and Treatment of High Blood Cholesterol in Adults. (2001). *Journal of the American Medical Association, 285* (19), 2486–2497.

12. Grundy, S. M., et al. (2004). Implications of recent clinical trials for the National Cholesterol Education Program Adult Treatment Panel III guidelines. *Circulation, 110,* 227–239.

13. Prevalence of physical activity, including lifestyle activity among adults—United States, 2000-2001. (2003). *Morbidity and Mortality Weekly Report, 52* (32), 764–769.

14. Must, A., Spadano, J., Coakley, E. H., Field, A. E., Colditz, G., & Dietz, W. H. (1999). The disease burden associated with overweight and obesity. *Journal of the American Medical Association, 282,* 1523–1529.

15. Steinberger, J., & Daniels, S. R. (2003). Obesity, insulin resistance, diabetes and cardiovascular risk in children. AHA Scientific Statement. *Circulation, 107,* 1448.

16. Heim, L. J., & Brunsell, S. C. (2001). Heart disease in women. *Primary Care, 27* (3), 741–766.

17. Standridge, J. B., Zylstra, R. G., & Adams, S. M. (2004). Alcohol consumption: An overview of the benefits and risks. *Southern Medical Journal, 97* (7), 664–672.

18. Strike, P. C., & Steptoe, A. (2004). Psychosocial factors in the development of coronary artery disease. *Progress in Cardiovascular Diseases, 46* (4), 337–347.

19. Massing, M. W., et al. (2004). Income, income inequality and cardiovascular disease mortality: Relationship among county population of United States, 1985–1994. *Southern Medical Journal, 97* (5), 475–484.

20. Wong, M. D., Shapiro, M. F., Boscardin, W. J., & Ettner, S. L. (2002). Contribution of major diseases to disparities in mortality. *New England Journal of Medicine, 347* (20), 1585–1592.

21. Krantz, D. S., Sheps, D. S., Carney, R. M., & Natelson, B. H. (2000). Effects of mental stress in patients with coronary artery disease: Evidence and clinical implications. *Journal of the American Medical Association, 283,* 1800–1802.

22. O'Keefe, J. H., et al. (2004). Psychosocial stress and cardiovascular disease: How to heal a broken heart. *Comprehensive Therapy, 30* (1), 37–43.

23. Segrest, J. P. (2002). The role of non-LDL:non-HDL particles in atherosclerosis. *Current Diabetes Reports, 2* (3), 282–288.

24. Pearson, T. A., et al. (2003). Markers of inflammation and cardiovascular disease. *Circulation, 107,* 499.

25. Shor, A., & Phillips, J. I. (1999). *Chlamydia pneumoniae* and atherosclerosis. *Journal of the American Medical Association, 282,* 2071–2073.

26. Smieja, M., et al. (2003). Multiple infection and subsequent cardiovascular events in the Heart Outcome Prevention Evaluation (HOPE) Study. *Circulation, 107,* 251.

27. Madjid, M., Naghavi, M., Litovsky, S., & Casscells, S. W. (2003). Influenza and cardiovascular disease: A new opportunity for prevention and need for future studies. *Circulation, 108,* 2730–2736.

28. Morley, R. (2001). Fetal origins of adult disease. *Clinical and Experimental Pharmacology and Physiology, 28* (11), 962–966.

29. Ozanned, S. E., Fernandez-Twinn, D., & Hales, C. N. (2004). Fetal growth and adult diseases. *Seminars in Perinatology, 28* (1), 81–87.

30. Healthy People 2010. Cardiovascular Disease. Heart disease and stroke. National Center for Chronic Disease Prevention and Health Promotion. www.cdc.gov.

31. Lloyd-Jones, D. M., et al. (1999). Lifetime risk of developing coronary heart disease. *Lancet, 353,* 89–92.

32. Lillie-Blanton, M., et al. (2004). Disparities in cardiac care: Rising to the challenge of Healthy People 2010. *Journal of the American College of Cardiology, 44* (3), 503–508.

33. Wyatt, S. B., et al. (2003). Racism and cardiovascular disease in African Americans. *American Journal of the Medical Sciences, 325* (6), 315–331.

34. Hulley, S., et al. (1998). Randomized trial of estrogen plus progesterin for secondary prevention of coronary heart disease in postmenopausal women. Heart and Estrogen Replacement Study (HERS) research group. *Journal of the American Medical Association, 280* (7), 605–613.

35. Rossouw, J. E., et al. (2002). Risks and benefits of estrogen plus progestin in healthy postmenopausal women. *Journal of American the Medical Association, 288* (3), 321–333.

36. Warber, S. L., & Zick, S. M. (2001). Biologically based complementary medicine for cardiovascular disease help or harm? *Clinics in Family Practice, 3* (4), 945.

37. Yu, J. N. (2000). Hyperlipidemia. *Primary Care, 27* (3), 541–587.

38. U. S. Preventive Services Task Force. (2003). High blood pressure—Screening. www.ahrq.gov.

39. Nesto, R. W. (2004). Correlation between cardiovascular disease and diabetes mellitus: Current concepts. *American Journal of Medicine, 116* (Suppl5A), 11S–22S.

40. Barrows, K. A. (2002). Mind-body medicine. An introduction and review of the literature. *Medical Clinics of North America, 86* (1), 11–31.

Add It Up!

WHAT IS YOUR RISK FOR CORONARY HEART DISEASE?

The National Heart, Lung, and Blood Institute, a division of the National Institutes of Health, used data from the Framingham Heart Study to create an assessment that can be used to determine your risk of developing coronary heart disease in the next 10 years. Evaluate yourself on each of the risk factors (Steps 1–6), enter and add your points (Step 7),

and find out your risk (Step 8). You can compare your risk to that of a man or woman the same age as you with average and low risk (Step 9). If your risk is higher than you would like it to be, make sure you are practicing the healthy lifestyle habits described in the chapter.

Coronary Disease Risk Prediction Score Sheet for Women Based on Total Cholesterol Level

Step 1

Age	
Years	Points
30-34	−9
35-39	−4
40-44	0
45-49	3
50-54	6
55-59	7
60-64	8
65-69	8
70-74	8

-9

Step 2

Total Cholesterol				Key	
(mg/dl)	(mmol/L)	Points		Color	Risk
<160	≤4.14	−2		Green	Very low
160-199	4.15-5.17	0		White	Low
200-239	5.18-6.21	1		Yellow	Moderate
240-279	6.22-7.24	1		Rose	High
≥280	≥7.25	3		Red	Very high

Step 3

HDL - Cholesterol		
(mg/dl)	(mmol/L)	Points
<35	≤0.90	5
35-44	0.91-1.16	2
45-49	1.17-1.29	1
50-59	1.30-1.55	0
≥60	≥1.56	−3

Step 4

Blood Pressure					
Systolic (mmHg)	Diastolic (mmHg)				
	<80	<80	<80	<80	<80
<120	−3 pts				
120-129		0 pts			
130-139			0 pts		
140-159				2 pts	
≥160					3 pts

Note: When systolic and diastolic pressures provide different estimates for point scores, use the higher number.

Step 5

Diabetes	
	Points
No	0
Yes	4

Step 6

Smoker	
	Points
No	0
Yes	2

Risk estimates were derived from the experience of NHLBI's Framingham Heart Study, a predominantly Caucasian population in Massachusetts, USA.

Step 7 Sum from steps 1-6.

Adding Up the Points	
Age	_____
Total Cholesterol	_____
HDL Cholesterol	_____
Blood Pressure	_____
Diabetes	_____
Smoker	_____
Point Total	_____

Step 8 Determine CHD risk from point total.

CHD Risk	
Point Total	10 Yr CHD Risk
≤−2	1%
−1	2%
0	2%
1	2%
2	3%
3	3%
4	4%
5	4%
6	5%
7	6%
8	7%
9	8%
10	10%
11	11%
12	13%
13	15%
14	18%
15	20%
16	24%
≥17	≥27%

Step 9 Compare to women of the same age.

Comparitive Risk		
Age (years)	Average 10 Yr CHD Risk	Low* 10 Yr CHD Risk
30-34	<1%	<1%
35-39	1%	<1%
40-44	2%	2%
45-49	5%	3%
50-54	8%	5%
55-59	12%	7%
60-64	12%	8%
65-69	13%	8%
70-74	14%	8%

*Low risk was calculated for a woman the same age, normal blood pressure, total cholesterol 160-199 mg/dL, HDL cholesterol 55 mg/dL, non-smoker, no diabetes.

Coronary Disease Risk Prediction Score Sheet for Men Based on Total Cholesterol Level

Step 1

Age	
Years	Points
30-34	−1
35-39	0
40-44	1
45-49	2
50-54	3
55-59	4
60-64	5
65-69	6
70-74	7

Step 2

Total Cholesterol				Key	
(mg/dl)	(mmol/L)	Points		Color	Risk
<160	≤4.14	−3		Green	Very low
160-199	4.15-5.17	0		White	Low
200-239	5.18-6.21	1		Yellow	Moderate
240-279	6.22-7.24	2		Rose	High
≥280	≥7.25	3		Red	Very high

Step 3

HDL - Cholesterol		
(mg/dl)	(mmol/L)	Points
<35	≤0.90	2
35-44	0.91-1.16	1
45-49	1.17-1.29	0
50-59	1.30-1.55	0
≥60	≥1.56	−2

Step 4

Blood Pressure					
Systolic (mmHg)	Diastolic (mmHg)				
	<80	<80	<80	<80	<80
<120	0 pts				
120-129		0 pts			
130-139			1 pts		
140-159				2 pts	
≥160					3 pts

Note: When systolic and diastolic pressures provide different estimates for point scores, use the higher number.

Step 5

Diabetes	
	Points
No	0
Yes	2

Step 6

Smoker	
	Points
No	0
Yes	2

Risk estimates were derived from the experience of NHLBI's Framingham Heart Study, a predominantly Caucasian population in Massachusetts, USA.

Step 7 Sum from steps 1-6.

Adding Up the Points	
Age	_____
Total Cholesterol	_____
HDL Cholesterol	_____
Blood Pressure	_____
Diabetes	_____
Smoker	_____
Point Total	_____

Step 8 Determine CHD risk from point total.

CHD Risk	
Point Total	10 Yr CHD Risk
≤−1	2%
0	3%
1	3%
2	4%
3	5%
4	7%
5	8%
6	10%
7	13%
8	16%
9	20%
10	25%
11	31%
12	37%
13	45%
≥14	≥53%

Step 9 Compare to man of the same age.

Comparitive Risk		
Age (years)	Average 10 Yr CHD Risk	Low* 10 Yr CHD Risk
30-34	3%	2%
35-39	5%	3%
40-44	7%	4%
45-49	11%	4%
50-54	14%	6%
55-59	16%	7%
60-64	21%	9%
65-69	25%	11%
70-74	30%	14%

*Low risk was calculated for a man the same age, normal blood pressure, total cholesterol 160-199 mg/dL, HDL cholesterol 55 mg/dL, non-smoker, no diabetes.

CHAPTER 22

Cancer: Understanding a Complex Condition

DID YOU KNOW?

- Adding berries, grapes, oranges, carrots, and other brightly colored fruits and vegetables to your diet may help reduce your risk of cancer. Foods from plant sources are loaded with micronutrients and phytochemicals that may offer protection from cancer.

- If you patronize tanning salons, you are putting yourself at risk for both premature aging of your skin and skin cancer. The U.S. government includes exposure to radiation from the sun or artificial light sources on its list of known human carcinogens.

OLC *Your Health Today*   www.mhhe.com/teague1e

Go to the Online Learning Center for *Your Health Today* for interactive activities, quizzes, flashcards, Web links, and more resources related to this chapter.

Cancer, the second leading cause of death in the United States, has probably always been part of life. Human remains from thousands of years ago show evidence of cancer; the disease is found in all mammalian species and in many other organisms. Despite its ubiquity, cancer has long been shrouded in mystery, fear, and even shame. In the past, people with cancer often hid their diagnosis; the word *cancer* was not used even in obituaries. Today, with greater understanding of this complex condition, cancer patients have higher survival rates, better prospects for a cure, and more social support. Although there is still much to learn, there is cause for optimism.

In the United States, death rates from cancer declined by 1.5 percent per year every year from 1993 to 2001 in men and 0.8 percent per year every year from 1992 to 2001 in women. Still, the American Cancer Society projected an estimated 1.3 million new cancer cases in 2005 and more than 570,000 deaths from cancer, about 1,500 per day. Cancer causes about 23 percent of all deaths in the United States, with lung cancer the leading killer among both men and women. The four most common cancers—lung, colon, breast, and prostate—combined account for nearly half of all cancer deaths[1] (Figure 22.1).

In this chapter, we begin by considering exactly what cancer is and how it develops by looking at the rules for healthy cell growth and division and what happens when cells evade these rules. We then look at risk factors for cancers, along with protective actions that can be taken to reduce risk. We turn next to an examination of the most common cancers, considering signs and symptoms, early detection methods, and treatments. We then discuss screening tests and treatments, and we conclude with a look at some of the challenges of living with cancer.

WHAT IS CANCER?

Cancer is a condition characterized by the uncontrolled growth of cells. It develops from a single cell that goes awry, but a combination of events must occur before the cell turns into a tumor. The process by which this occurs is called **clonal growth,** the replication of a single cell such that it produces thousands of copies of itself in an uncontrolled manner. With 30 billion cells in a healthy person, the fact that one out of three people develops cancer is not surprising; what is surprising is that two out of three people do not.

Estimated New Cases*		Estimated Deaths	
Male	**Female**	**Male**	**Female**
Prostate 232,090 (33%)	Breast 211,240 (32%)	Lung & bronchus 90,490 (31%)	Lung & bronchus 73,020 (27%)
Lung & bronchus 93,010 (13%)	Lung & bronchus 79,560 (12%)	Prostate 30,350 (10%)	Breast 40,410 (15%)
Colon & rectum 71,820 (10%)	Colon & rectum 73,470 (11%)	Colon & rectum 28,540 (10%)	Colon & rectum 27,750 (10%)
Urinary bladder 47,010 (7%)	Uterine corpus 40,880 (6%)	Pancreas 15,820 (5%)	Ovary 16,210 (6%)
Melanoma of the skin 33,580 (5%)	Non-Hodgkin lymphoma 27,320 (4%)	Leukemia 12,540 (4%)	Pancreas 15,980 (6%)
Non-Hodgkin lymphoma 29,070 (4%)	Melanoma of the skin 26,000 (4%)	Esophagus 10,530 (4%)	Leukemia 10,030 (4%)
Kidney & renal pelvis 22,490 (3%)	Ovary 22,220 (3%)	Liver & intrahepatic bile duct 10,330 (3%)	Non-Hodgkin lymphoma 9,050 (3%)
Leukemia 19,640 (3%)	Thyroid 19,190 (3%)	Non-Hodgkin lymphoma 10,150 (3%)	Uterine corpus 7,310 (3%)
Oral cavity & pharynx 19,100 (3%)	Urinary bladder 16,200 (2%)	Urinary bladder 8,970 (3%)	Multiple myeloma 5,640 (2%)
Pancreas 16,100 (2%)	Pancreas 16,080 (2%)	Kidney & renal pelvis 8,020 (3%)	Brain & other nervous system 5,480 (2%)
All sites 710,040 (100%)	All sites 662,870 (100%)	All sites 295,280 (100%)	All sites 275,000 (100%)

*Excludes basal and squamous cell skin cancers and in situ carcinoma except urinary bladder.
Note: Percentage may not total 100% due to rounding.

Figure 22.1   Leading sites of new cancer cases and deaths, 2005 estimates. Source: American Cancer Society, Inc., Surveillance Research. Copyright American Cancer Society, Inc. www.cancer.org. Reprinted with permission.

Healthy Cell Growth

Healthy cells have a complicated system of checks and balances that control cell growth and division. From the start, beginning with the single-celled fertilized egg, cells develop in contact with other cells, sending and receiving messages about how much space is available for growth. Healthy cells in solid tissues (all tissues except the blood) require the presence of neighboring cells. This tendency to stick together serves as a safety mechanism, discouraging cells from drifting off and starting to grow independently.

Healthy cells divide when needed to replace cells that have died or been sloughed off. Each time a cell divides, there is a possibility that a mutation, an error in DNA replication, will occur (see Chapter 2). Mutations are always occurring randomly, but the risk of mutations is increased by exposure to certain substances, such as tobacco smoke, radiation, and toxic chemicals. Certain mutations may start the cell on a path toward cancer. Specific mechanisms are designed to correct genetic mutations and destroy cells with mutations.

As one mechanism, enzymes within the nucleus of each cell scan the DNA as it replicates, looking for errors. If an error is detected, the enzyme backtracks and repairs it. If too much DNA damage is detected and cannot be repaired, cells have a program for self-destruction, or cellular suicide. As another safety mechanism, cells are programmed to divide a certain number of times, and then they become incapable of further division. At this point, the cells die and the particular cell line (all the cells that originated from an initial cell) is lost, along with any mutations that might have occurred within it.

The immune system also helps to watch for cells that are not growing normally. Cancer cells often display an antigen, like a flag, on their cell surface; when the antigen is detected by the immune cells, the cell is labeled for destruction. If a cell has been infected by a cancer-causing virus, it also displays viral antigens on its surface, and again, the immune system labels and destroys it.

A special protective mechanism exists for certain cells called **stem cells.** These are cells that did not differentiate into specific cell types (for example, nerve cells, skin cells, bone cells) during prenatal development. Instead, they retain the ability to become different cell types, and they are capable of unlimited division. A small number of stem cells are present within most tissue types, where they are needed to replace lost or damaged cell lines. They are found in highest numbers within the skin, blood, lung lining, intestines, endocrine cells, and liver—all tissues with a high rate of turnover and replacement. Because stem cells do not have a predetermined number of cell divisions, they pose a risk for cancer. As a safety mechanism, they are physically located deep within tissues, where they are protected from factors that increase the risk of genetic mutations, such as exposure to the sun, chemicals, and irritation. Stem cells do have a system of self-destruction if they experience DNA damage or exposure to a toxin.

Cancer Cell Growth

Cancer starts from a single cell that undergoes a critical mutation, either as a result of an error in duplication or in response to a **carcinogen** or radiation. This **initiating event** allows a cell to evade one of the restraints placed upon healthy cells. To become a cancer, however, it must escape all the control mechanisms. Usually this process requires a series of 5 to 10 critical mutations within the cell's genetic material. It may take many years for these changes to progress to cancer, or they may never do so.

In time, perhaps a period of years, another mutation, such as one in an **oncogene** (a gene that drives cell growth regardless of signals from surrounding cells), may allow the cell line to divide forever rather than follow its preprogrammed number of divisions. A condition of cell overgrowth, called *hyperplasia,* develops at the site, and some cells may become abnormal, a condition called *dysplasia.* Eventually, a mass of extra tissue, a **tumor,** may develop.

A **benign tumor** grows slowly and is unlikely to spread. Benign tumors are dangerous if they grow in locations where they interfere with normal functioning and cannot be completely removed without destroying healthy tissue, as in the brain. A **malignant tumor** is capable of

KEY TERMS

cancer Condition characterized by the uncontrolled growth of cells.

clonal growth Process by which a single cell replicates such that it produces thousands of copies of itself in an uncontrolled manner.

stem cells Undifferentiated cells capable of unlimited division that can give rise to specialized cells.

carcinogen Cancer-causing substance or agent in the environment.

initiating event A critical mutation in a cell—either as a result of an error in duplication or in response to a carcinogen—that allows a cell to evade one of the restraints on growth and division placed on healthy cells.

oncogene Gene that drives a cell to grow and divide regardless of signals from surrounding cells.

tumor Mass of extra tissue.

benign tumor Tumor that grows slowly and is unlikely to spread.

malignant tumor Tumor that is capable of invading surrounding tissue and spreading.

Normal, healthy cells are bound by control mechanisms that guide their growth. Some cells undergo mutations, through errors in duplication or in response to a carcinogen, that allow them to avoid these controls and become cancerous, as shown here.

invading surrounding tissue and spreading. Malignant cells do not stick together as much as normal cells, and as the tumor grows, some cancer cells may break off, enter the lymphatic system or the bloodstream, and travel to nearby lymph nodes or to distant sites in the body. At a new site, the cancerous cell can grow and become a secondary tumor, or **metastasis.** When a cancer spreads from one part of the body to another, it is said to have *metastasized.* The terms *malignant cancer* and *neoplasia* are frequently used interchangeably with *cancer.*

Classifying Cancers

Cancers are classified according to the tissue in which they originate, called the *primary site.* If a cancer originates in the cells lining the colon, for example, it is considered colon cancer, even when it metastasizes to other, secondary sites. The most common sites of metastases are the brain, liver, and bone marrow. Occasionally, the primary site of a cancer cannot be determined. When a cancer is still at its primary site, it is said to be localized. When it has metastasized, it is referred to as invasive. The greater the extent of metastasis, the poorer the *prognosis* (likely outcome).

Tumors are *graded* on the basis of the degree to which the tumor cells resemble healthy cells of the same tissue type under the microscope. If they are very similar, they are considered well differentiated and low grade (grade I); if they are very different, they are considered poorly differentiated and high grade (grade IV). A poorly differen-

tiated, higher grade cancer grows more quickly, is more aggressive, and is more likely to metastasize.[2]

The *stage* of the disease is a description of how far the cancer has spread. Two systems of staging are used. In the first, there are five categories (stage 0, stage I, stage II, stage III, and stage IV). Stage 0 is also called "cancer *in situ,*" an early cancer that is present only in the layer of cells where it began. Stage I cancers are generally small and localized to the original site. Stage IV cancers have metastasized to distant sites. Stages II and III are locally advanced and may or may not involve local lymph nodes. Prognosis is related to the stage of a tumor but also depends on the kind of cancer. In the other staging system, called "TNM," tumors, nodes, and metastasis are rated based on size and extent of spread. Tumor size is rated from 0 to 4. A T1 tumor is a small local tumor that has not begun to invade local tissue, and a T4 tumor is a large tumor that has invaded surrounding structures. Nodes are rated in a similar way from 0 to 3. N0 means there is no lymph node spread, and N3 means extensive lymph node spread. Metastasis is either M0 (no metastases) or M1 (metastasis); so a cancer might be described as a T1, N2, M0 stage cancer. (For more on cancer terms, see the box "The Language of Cancer.")

Types of Cancer

Different tissues of the body have different risks for cancer, owing in part to their different rates of cell division. Four broad types of cancer are distinguished, based on the type of tissue in which they originate. **Carcinomas** arise from epithelial tissue, which includes the skin, the lining of the intestines and body cavities, the surface of body organs, and the outer portions of the glands. Epithelial tissue is frequently shed and replaced. From 80 to 90 percent of all cancers originate in epithelial tissues. **Sarcomas** originate in connective tissue, such as bone, tendon, cartilage, muscle, or fat tissues. **Leukemias** are cancers of the blood and originate in the bone marrow or the lymphatic system. **Lymphomas** originate in the lymph nodes or glands.

RISK FACTORS FOR CANCER

Can cancer be prevented? We have seen that because some cancers occur as a result of random genetic mutations, there is an element of chance in the development of the disease. Other cancers are associated with inherited genetic mutations. Still others occur as a result of exposure to carcinogens. Some such exposures can be limited by lifestyle behaviors, such as using sunscreen, but others are beyond individual control and require the involvement of local authorities, the larger society, or even the international community, as in the case of air pollution.

In this section, we consider several risk factors for cancer, as well as ways to reduce them or limit their

HIGHLIGHT ON HEALTH

The Language of Cancer

If you are around health professionals who are talking about cancer, or if you are reading news stories about the disease, you may encounter some unfamiliar terms. Here are a few that are commonly used.

Biopsy   The removal of a small sample of tissue for examination under a microscope to determine whether it contains cancerous cells. Some biopsies are done with a needle; others require surgery.

Cure   A term used cautiously with cancer. Even if a cancer seems to be gone, there may still be some cancer cells in the body, and these can multiply and cause a recurrence of the disease. The term *cure* is usually reserved for someone who has been cancer free for 5 years after the diagnosis.

Remission   A decrease in or disappearance of the signs and symptoms of cancer after treatment. Remission can be partial, meaning that some but not all signs of cancer have disappeared, or complete, meaning that all signs and symptoms of cancer have disappeared. The cancer may still be present, but no signs of it can be found in tests. Remission may last a few months or many years.

Recurrence or relapse   The return of a cancer after it had disappeared with treatment. It may recur at the same site or at a new location owing to metastases.

Incidence   The number of new cases of a disease that develop in a certain group of people in a set period of time.

Prevalence   The total number of people in a certain group with a disease at any one moment in time.

Morbidity   Relating to illness or disease; for example, the *morbidity rate* from cancer is the number of cases diagnosed within a set period (usually a year) per 100,000 people in a population.

Mortality   Relating to death; for example, the *mortality rate* from cancer is the number of people who die from cancer within a set period (usually a year) per 100,000 people in a population.

Prognosis   An assessment of the future course and outcome of a disease. Prognosis is based on knowledge of the disease course in other people and a particular patient's age, general health, and stage of disease.

Survival rate   The percentage of people who survive for a certain period of time after a diagnosis, usually given for 1 and 5 years. For example, the 5-year survival rate for prostate cancer is 98 percent, meaning that 98 percent of those diagnosed with this cancer will be alive in 5 years.

---

effect. Remember that risk factors are associated with a higher incidence of a disease but do not determine that the disease will occur. Some people without known risk factors develop cancer, and other people with multiple risk factors do not.

Family History

A family history of cancer increases an individual's risk. As described in Chapter 2, the risk is higher if the cancer occurred in a first-degree relative (parent or sibling) than in a second-degree relative (grandparent, aunt, uncle, or cousin). Risk also varies by the age of the family member at the time of diagnosis and the number of family members with a cancer diagnosis.

Certain cancers, such as breast cancer and colon cancer, appear to have a stronger familial link than other cancers do. Approximately 5 percent to 10 percent of women diagnosed with breast cancer have a hereditary form of the disease. Inherited alterations in the genes BRCA1 and BRCA2 (Breast Cancer 1 and Breast Cancer 2) are involved in many of these cases.[3] Approximately

25 percent of men and women diagnosed with colon cancer have a family history of colon cancer. Mutations have been identified to explain the increased risk for colon cancer in some families, but these account for only 5 percent to 6 percent of all colon cancer cases. If a family has two or more members with colon cancer, the possibility of an inherited genetic susceptibility is substantially higher.[4]

KEY TERMS

metastasis   Secondary tumor that appears when cancerous cells spread to other parts of the body.

carcinomas   Cancers that arise from epithelial tissue.

sarcomas   Cancers that originate in connective tissue.

leukemias   Cancers of the blood, originating in the bone marrow or the lymphatic system.

lymphomas   Cancers that originate in the lymph nodes or glands.

Challenges & Choices

Dietary Guidelines for Cancer Prevention

In extensive studies of the relationship between diet and cancer, the American Institute for Cancer Research (AICR) has concluded that there is no magic bullet—no single nutrient—that prevents cancer. Instead, protection comes from the collective impact of interacting factors—that is, from eating whole foods and a variety of foods, especially plant foods. These food sources contain vitamins, minerals, and thousands of phytochemicals, antioxidants, and other micronutrients believed to provide protection from cancer. The AICR strongly recommends a predominantly plant-based diet, citing the relationship between such a diet and a reduced risk of cancer.

In their "New American Plate" program, the AICR recommends that two thirds or more of each meal be made up of vegetables, fruits, beans, and whole grains (brown rice, kasha, whole wheat bread) and that one third or less be made up of animal protein (fish, chicken, meat, low-fat dairy products). The AICR suggests that people transition from traditional eating to the New American Plate as shown in the illustrations. The organization also recommends that people reduce portion sizes in order to manage weight.

Certain foods appear to be especially protective against cancer. They include beans, berries, cruciferous vegetables, dark green leafy vegetables, flaxseed, garlic, grapes and grape juice, green tea, soy products, tomatoes, and whole grains. Try to include some of these foods in your diet every week.

The AICR also offers the following Diet and Health Guidelines for Cancer Prevention:

1. Choose a diet rich in a variety of plant-based foods.
2. Eat plenty of vegetables and fruits.
3. Maintain a healthy weight and be physically active.
4. Drink alcohol only in moderation if at all.
5. Select foods low in fat and salt.
6. Prepare and store food safely.

And always remember . . . Do not use tobacco in any form.

It's Not Just Personal . . .

To reduce your cancer risk, increase not only the amount but also the diversity of fruits and vegetables in your diet. According to the AICR, there are between 150,000 and 200,000 edible plant foods in the world, and most Americans eat just three per day.

Source: *The New American Plate,* Rev. Ed., American Institute for Cancer Research, 2004, www.aicr.org/publications. Reprinted with permission from the American Institute for Cancer Research.

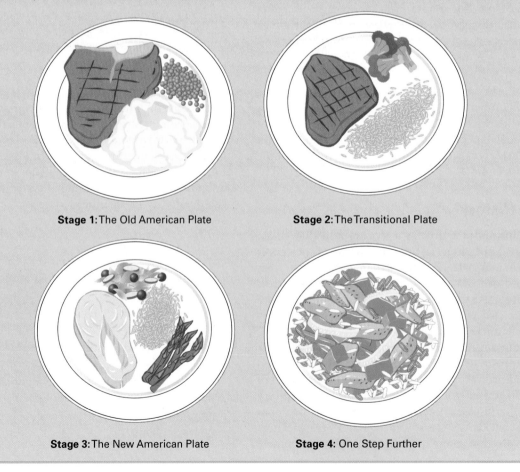

Stage 1: The Old American Plate

Stage 2: The Transitional Plate

Stage 3: The New American Plate

Stage 4: One Step Further

Examining your family health tree in consultation with your physician can help you understand whether you have an increased risk for any cancers. If you find that you do, making lifestyle adjustments that can reduce your risk and getting the recommended screening tests are especially important for you.

Lifestyle Factors

Most of the genetic mutations that eventually become cancer occur during an individual's lifetime, either as a mistake during cell division or in response to environmental factors, as noted earlier. Some environmental agents (carcinogens) have a direct impact on a cell, causing an initial genetic alteration that can lead to cancer. Other agents, called **cancer promoters,** have a less direct effect, enhancing the possibility that a cancer will develop if an initiating event has already occurred in a cell.

Tobacco Use and Cancer Risk

Tobacco use is the leading preventable cause of cancer in the United States. It is responsible for 30 percent of all cancer deaths and 87 percent of all lung cancer deaths.[5] Lung cancer occurs in smokers 20 times more often than in nonsmokers. Smokers are more likely to die from their lung cancer than nonsmokers—23 times more likely if they are men and 13 times more likely if they are women.

Tobacco use increases the risk of cancers of the mouth, throat, lung, and esophagus by direct exposure to the chemicals in tobacco smoke. It increases the risk of other cancers, including bladder, pancreas, stomach, liver, kidney, and bone-marrow cancers, because other chemicals from tobacco are absorbed into the bloodstream and travel to distant sites. Individual risk from tobacco use depends on the age at which the person starts smoking, the number of years the person smokes, the number of cigarettes smoked per day, and the type of cigarettes smoked, with higher tar content being more dangerous.[5] For more on tobacco use and strategies for quitting, see Chapter 13.

Dietary Patterns and Cancer Risk

For people who do not use tobacco products, nutrition and physical activity are the most significant contributors to cancer risk. Dietary patterns can be protective or harmful, depending on the choice of foods. Diets rich in fruits, vegetables, and whole grains appear to decrease the risk for many cancers, including lung, colon, rectal, breast, stomach, and ovarian cancer. Diets high in fiber appear to decrease the risk of colon cancer and possibly the risk of breast, rectal, pharyngeal, and stomach cancer.

Among the fruits and vegetables, those rich in caretenoids appear to confer additional benefits; these include dark yellow or orange vegetables and fruits (melon, carrots, sweet potatoes) and dark green leafy vegetables (broccoli, spinach, collard greens). Researchers have tried to determine exactly which components of the fruits and vegetables are beneficial, but studies have had mixed results. The National Cancer Institute recommends eating from 5 to 9 servings a day of fruits and vegetables in their National 5-a-Day for Better Health Program. See the box "Dietary Guidelines for Cancer Prevention" for more on this topic.

Diets high in fat have been associated with several types of cancer, including breast, colon, and prostate cancer. Eating red meat has been associated with an increased risk of cancer; the American Institute for Cancer Research recommends limiting consumption of red meat to 3 ounces per day. Grilling meat, poultry, and fish produces cancer-causing compounds, especially if fat drips onto hot coals, causing smoke and flare-ups. Measures that reduce this risk include trimming fat from meat, marinating or microwaving meat before grilling, and keeping meat portions small so they require a shorter time on the grill. Additionally, some foods contain toxins from the environment that may cause or promote cancer. Levels of toxins in food that are deemed safe are determined by government policies and regulations, so consumers have little or no control over this source of risk, except to follow the recommendations for food intake (such as limiting intake of fish caught in certain locations).

Overweight and Obesity and Cancer Risk

Studies have confirmed that being overweight or obese increases the risk of developing many types of cancer as well as the risk of dying from cancer once it occurs. Overweight and obesity not only make it harder to detect cancers at an early stage but also delay diagnosis and may make treatment more difficult. Although it is not clear how fat cells contribute to an increased risk of cancer, several pathways are possible. Fat cells produce hormones, some of which (such as estrogen) are linked to cancer. Fat cells may trigger an inflammatory reaction, alter insulin production, or release proteins that trigger cell growth, all of which may contribute to the development of cancer.

Physical Activity and Cancer Risk

Physical activity is associated with a reduced risk for colon cancer and probably a reduced risk for breast, prostate, and uterine cancers. Physical activity can help you maintain a healthy body weight and thus further reduce risk. It also alters body functions in a positive way; for example,

KEY TERMS

cancer promoters   Substances or agents in the environment that enhance the possibility that a cancer will develop if an initiating event has already occurred in a cell.

by increasing the rate that food travels through the intestines, it reduces the exposure of the bowel lining to potential carcinogens.[5] Appropriate exercise after a cancer diagnosis and during treatment can help people eat better, feel less tired, and recover faster.

Alcohol Consumption and Cancer Risk

Alcohol consumption of more than one serving a day for women and two servings a day for men increases the risk for cancers of the mouth, throat, esophagus, liver, and breast. The risk for liver cancer increases markedly with five or more drinks per day. Alcohol and tobacco used together amplify the risk for cancer and are associated with a greater risk than either one alone. On the other hand, red wine is under investigation for a potential beneficial role in reducing cancer risk.[6]

Environmental Factors

Some cancers are caused by exposure to carcinogens in the environment, but some exposures are more controllable than others, as noted earlier.

Ultraviolet Radiation

The type of radiation that comes primarily from the sun—ultraviolet (UV) radiation, and particularly ultraviolet B (UVB) rays—can damage DNA and cause skin cancer. The risk for the two milder forms of skin cancer, basal cell and squamous cell carcinomas, is cumulative; the more sun exposure over the years, the higher the risk. The risk for melanoma, the most dangerous form of skin cancer, appears to be related more to the timing and number of sunburns. Sunburns that occur during childhood seem to be the most dangerous, and the more sunburns, the greater the risk.

People who live in certain regions of the world have a higher risk of developing skin cancers because of their location close to the equator or in areas affected by the hole in the ozone layer of the atmosphere. As discussed in Chapter 19, the ozone layer, which protects the earth from the sun's damaging UV rays, is being disrupted by chemical pollution and is thinning over Antarctica and southern portions of the globe. Australia has one of the highest rates of skin cancer in the world, presumably because of this environmental condition. In 1981, a national campaign was initiated to slow rapidly rising skin cancer rates. The "Slip, Slap, Slop" campaign focused on three preventive measures: Slip into the shade, slap on a hat, and slop on some sunscreen. The increase in skin cancer rates has slowed as a result.

The Australian population supports this campaign, particularly focusing on children. At school, for example, children are not allowed outside for recess if they forget to bring a hat to wear.[7] In the United States, one in four parents still do not require their children to take

---

Healthy People 2010

OBJECTIVE AREA *Cancer*

- Reduce the rate of melanoma cancer deaths.

"Although the cause of melanoma is unknown, risk factors include a personal or family history of melanoma, the presence of atypical moles, a large number of moles, intermittent sun exposure, a history of sunburns early in life, freckles, and sun-sensitive skin (as measured by poor tanning ability and light skin, eye, or hair color). Evidence is insufficient to determine whether early detection through routine skin examination (self or physician) decreases the number of deaths from melanoma, but reduced ultraviolet exposure is likely to have a beneficial impact on the risk of melanoma and other skin cancers (basal and squamous cell skin cancers)."

For more information on Healthy People 2010 objectives, visit the Web site at www.healthypeople.gov.

For more information on Canadian health objectives, visit the Health Canada Web site at www.hc-sc.gc.ca/english.

---

any protective measures, and only one in three adolescents uses any sun protective wear, such as clothing, a hat, or sunscreen.[8]

Other Forms of Radiation

High-frequency ionizing radiation can also cause cancer; sources include occupational, environmental, and medical exposures. For example, underground uranium miners have high levels of lung cancer as a result of their exposure to radon. (As discussed in Chapter 19, radon is a naturally occurring radioactive gas in the ground in certain regions of the world; exposure increases the risk of lung cancer.) Residents in many parts of North America are exposed to low levels of radon in their homes, particularly homes with basements. In regions known to have high levels of radon in the ground, testing of homes is recommended, followed by the installation of a ventilation system if levels are found to be elevated.

Nuclear fallout is an environmental source of radiation. Survivors of atom bomb explosions and tests have high levels of cancer, particularly cancers of the bone marrow and thyroid. The nuclear reactors used in power plants have not been shown to emit enough ionizing radiation to place surrounding communities at risk. However, accidental releases of radioactive gases have occurred, and accidents at power plants, such as the one at Chernobyl in 1986, have contaminated land for miles around and caused an untold number of cancers in those exposed to radiation and radioactive debris.

Radiation is also used in medical settings. High-dose radiation is used to treat cancer, and this exposure can cause secondary cancers years later. Lower levels of radiation are used for diagnostic imaging, as in dental or chest X-rays. The lowest level of radiation needed to obtain clear images is used in these procedures, but the number of X-rays taken should be minimized as much as possible, particularly in children.[9]

Chemical Carcinogens

Several chemical substances in the environment have been clearly identified as carcinogens, such as dioxin, asbestos, and PCBs. Many others are released into the environment without clear evidence of their safety or toxicity. Your exposure to environmental carcinogens and cancer promoters varies, depending on where you live, where you work, what your hobbies and recreational activities are, and what you eat, among other factors. Some food additives are linked to cancer and should be consumed in small quantities; for example, the nitrites and nitrates used as preservatives in bacon, hot dogs, lunch meats, and beer can combine with other substances in the stomach to produce carcinogens. The greatest danger from the environment appears to result from occupational exposure to carcinogenic industrial products.

Infectious Agents

One risk from infectious disease occurs when a virus infects a cell and activates gene replication in order to produce copies of itself. Any time gene replication is activated, there is a chance of mutation. Another risk occurs when an infection causes a chronic irritation, prompting cell division and again increasing the chance of mutation.

Some viruses are known to cause cancer. The human papillomavirus (HPV) is linked to cancers of the cervix, anus, vagina, penis, and mouth.[10] The hepatitis B and C viruses are associated with liver cancer. Certain strains of Epstein-Barr virus, which causes mononucleosis, are associated with Hodgkins lymphoma, non-Hodgkins lymphoma, and some stomach cancers. Human immunodeficiency virus (HIV) suppresses the immune system and allows several types of cancer to develop. The only bacterium linked to cancer is *Helicobacter pylori,* which causes a chronic irritation of the stomach lining and is associated with stomach ulcers and an increased risk of stomach cancer.

Because you cannot eliminate all risk factors for cancer, you should get all the recommended cancer screening tests (discussed later in the chapter).

COMMON CANCERS

Since 1930 changes have occurred in the rates of different cancers in the United States (Figure 22.2). The most dramatic changes in overall rates can be seen for stomach, lung, and uterine cancers. A drop in mortality for stomach cancer occurred in both sexes early in the 20th century and is believed to be the result of changes in food processing. The dramatic increase in lung cancer for both sexes is believed to be the result of higher rates of smoking. Rates of smoking increased among women about 20 to 30 years after they increased in men, and there has been a corresponding increase in lung cancer among women; rates have just recently started to level off. The reduction in mortality from uterine cancer among women corresponds to the introduction of the Pap test to screen for cervical cancer (considered a form of uterine cancer).

In this section we consider some of the most common cancers. For each, we describe risk factors, signs and symptoms of the disease, screening tests and detection, and treatments.

Lung Cancer

The leading cause of cancer death for both men and women in the United States and the second most commonly diagnosed cancer is lung cancer. In 1987 lung cancer overtook breast cancer as the leading cause of cancer death for American women. The American Cancer Society (ACS) projected an estimated 172,570 new cases of lung cancer in 2005 and an estimated 163,510 deaths. The incidence rates are declining for men and have reached a plateau for women.[5]

The leading risk factor for lung cancer is the use of tobacco products in any form. Other risk factors are exposures to carcinogenic chemicals, arsenic, radon, asbestos, radiation, air pollution, and environmental tobacco smoke. Recently, experts determined that dietary supplements containing beta-carotene, a form of vitamin A, further increases the risk for lung cancer in people who smoke. Reducing risk factors, especially exposure to tobacco smoke and environmental tobacco smoke, is the first line of defense against this disease.

Signs and symptoms of lung cancer include coughing, blood-streaked sputum, chest pain, difficulty breathing, and recurrent lung infections. Unfortunately, symptoms do not appear in most people until the disease is advanced, a factor that frequently delays detection of the disease. There is currently no routine screening test for lung cancer, but both chest X-rays and a form of computerized tomography called *spiral CT* can detect early stage lung cancer. A large study called the National Lung Screening Trial is under way to determine whether screening high-risk, heavy smokers using these methods can improve survival.

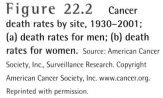

Figure 22.2 Cancer death rates by site, 1930–2001; (a) death rates for men; (b) death rates for women. Source: American Cancer Society, Inc., Surveillance Research. Copyright American Cancer Society, Inc. www.cancer.org. Reprinted with permission.

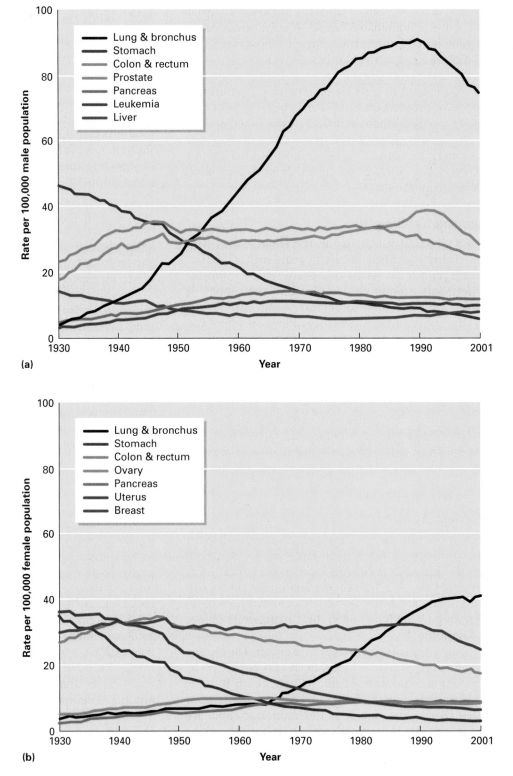

If symptoms suggest lung cancer and an abnormality is found on an X-ray or CT scan, the diagnosis is confirmed by a biopsy, performed either by surgery or by **bronchoscopy.** Survival and treatment depend upon the type of lung cancer and the stage of disease. People with small tumors that can be removed surgically have the best prognosis. For more advanced cancers or for people who are unable to tolerate surgery, radiation or a combination of radiation and chemotherapy is used. If the cancer has spread to distant sites, radiation and chemotherapy can be used for *palliative care* (care provided to give temporary relief of symptoms but not to cure the cancer). The 1-year survival rate for lung cancer is 42 percent, and 5-year survival rate is 15 percent.[5]

In the United States, lung cancer is the leading cause of cancer death for both men and women. It is also one of the most controllable types of cancer since the main risk factor is the use of tobacco products.

Colon and Rectal Cancer

The third leading cause of cancer death and the third most commonly diagnosed cancer is colon and rectal cancer (also called colorectal cancer). The ACS projected an estimated 145,290 new cases of colon and rectal cancer in 2005 and an estimated 56,290 deaths. During the 1990s, the incidence of colon and rectal cancer declined in the United States in both men and women, along with the number of deaths from the disease. The decrease is thought to be due to improved screening and treatment and the early detection and removal of **colon polyps.**[5]

The most important risk factor for colorectal cancer is age. More than 90 percent of colorectal cancers are diagnosed in people over age 50. A personal or family history of colon polyps or inflammatory bowel disease also increases risk, as does a family history of colorectal cancer, especially in a first-degree relative. Other factors associated with an increased risk for colon and rectal cancer include smoking, alcohol use, obesity, physical inactivity, a high-fat diet, and inadequate amounts of fruits and vegetables in the diet. Aspirin and hormone replacement therapy may reduce the risk for colon and rectal cancer.[11]

Warning signs of colorectal cancer include a change in bowel movements, change in stool size or shape, pain in the abdomen, or blood in the stool. The signs do not usually occur until the disease is fairly advanced. Screening tests are available that can enhance early detection of polyps or cancer. The **fecal occult blood test** detects blood mixed in stool. Polyps and early stage colon cancers can bleed trace amounts of blood, which can be detected with chemical reagents. The test is done at home and mailed or dropped off at the health care provider's office for testing. If blood is found in the stool, further diagnostic testing is done.

Two procedures can be done in the physician's office to examine the colon for polyps or early stages of cancer. A fiber-optic scope is inserted into the rectum and moved through the colon, allowing the health care provider to see the lining of the colon. In a **flexible sigmoidoscopy,** the lower third of the colon is examined, where the majority of colon cancers are found. In a **colonoscopy,** the entire colon is examined. If polyps are found, they can be biopsied or removed during these procedures. Another test is the **double-contrast barium enema,** in which contrast material is inserted through the rectum and X-rays are

(KEY) TERMS

bronchoscopy   Procedure in which a fiber-optic device is inserted into the lungs to allow the health care provider to examine lung tissue for signs of cancer.

colon polyps   Growths in the colon that may progress to colon cancer.

fecal occult blood test   A home test for blood in the stool, a sign of colon cancer.

flexible sigmoidoscopy   Procedure in which a fiber-optic device is inserted in the colon to allow the health care provider to examine the lower third of the colon for polyps or cancer.

colonoscopy   Procedure in which a fiber-optic device is inserted in the colon to allow the health care provider to examine the entire colon for polyps or cancer.

double-contrast barium enema   Test for colon cancer in which contrast material is inserted into the colon and X-rays are taken of the abdomen, revealing alterations in the lining of the colon if cancer is present.

Beating the Odds

Who Is Least Likely to Develop Breast Cancer?

There are many known risk factors for breast cancer, including age, family history, diet, weight, exposure to estrogen, and others. There are also ways to reduce the risk of developing the disease. Brief profiles of three women are presented here. Which one do you think is least likely to develop breast cancer?

Vicki is a 30-year-old Caucasian woman who has struggled with her weight since she was 12. Currently she is 60 pounds overweight and has a BMI of 29. Both of her parents are also overweight, and her mother had surgery for colon cancer 5 years ago. Vicki is an elementary school teacher and is active all day long, but she doesn't exercise regularly. She tries to eat a healthy diet with plenty of vegetables and fruits, but she has a weakness for rich desserts. She doesn't smoke. Vicki began menstruating when she was 10, and she has never been pregnant.

Esther is a 45-year-old Chinese American woman who has maintained a healthy weight all her life. She has two children, aged 10 and 3, and breast-fed both of them un-

til they were 9 months old. Esther eats a balanced diet and does not smoke, but she gets no exercise. She started menstruating at age 14. Her maternal grandmother was diagnosed with breast cancer at age 75, and her paternal grandfather died of prostate cancer. She is putting off getting her first mammogram.

Rachelle is a 34-year-old African American woman who works in the human resources department of a large company. She exercises regularly in the gym at work and eats a typical American diet, including fast food a few times a week and one or two beers most nights. She has been 20 pounds overweight since the birth of her son 5 years ago, whom she breastfed for 6 months. She started menstruating at age 12 and took birth control pills for 7 years in her 20s. Rachelle's mother was diagnosed with breast cancer at age 57 and is doing well following a mastectomy. Rachelle performs breast self-exams regularly and has talked with her physician about screening tests for breast cancer.

OLC Web site Visit the **Online Learning Center** at www.mhhe.com/teague1e for comments by the authors.

---

taken of the abdomen; if colon cancer is present, alterations in the lining of the colon can be seen.

The American Cancer Society recommends that people with average risk start colorectal cancer screening at age 50 with annual fecal occult blood testing. Also recommended is a flexible sigmoidoscopy or double contrast barium enema every 5 years or a colonoscopy every 10 years.[5] A new study suggests that colonoscopy is better than flexible sigmoidoscopy at detecting colon cancers in women, although the same effect is not seen in men.[12] For people with higher than average risk (for example, someone who has a close family member with colon cancer or polyps), earlier and more frequent screening may be recommended.[5]

Surgery is the most common treatment for colon and rectal cancer; it can cure the cancer if it has not spread. Chemotherapy and/or radiation are added if the cancer is large or has spread to other areas. The 1-year survival rate for all stages of colorectal cancer is 83 percent; the 5-year survival rate is 62 percent.

Breast Cancer

The second leading cause of cancer death in women and the most commonly diagnosed non-skin cancer in women is breast cancer. It was the leading cause of cancer death in women for many years, but it has been surpassed by lung cancer. The ACS projected an estimated 211,240 new cases

of breast cancer in 2005 and an estimated 40,410 deaths. Breast cancer occurs in men as well as women, but it is less common. There were an estimated 1,690 cases of breast cancer in men in the United States in 2005.[5]

There are both controllable and noncontrollable risk factors for breast cancer. Among the noncontrollable factors are early onset of menarche (first menstruation), late onset of menopause, family history of breast cancer in a first-degree relative, older age, and higher socioeconomic class. As mentioned earlier in this chapter and discussed in Chapter 2, two genes have been identified that are associated with an increased risk of breast cancer, called BRCA1 and BRCA2. Although inherited susceptibility accounts for only 5 percent of all breast cancer cases, having these genes confers a lifetime risk of developing the disease ranging from 35 to 85 percent. Some women with these genes choose to have their breasts and/or ovaries removed to lower their risk of developing breast or ovarian cancer. The estrogen-blocking drugs tamoxifen and raloxifene can also reduce risk.

Controllable risk factors for breast cancer that increase risk include never having children or having a first child after age 30, being obese after menopause, taking hormone replacement therapy, and drinking more than two alcoholic beverages a day. Breast-feeding, engaging in moderate or vigorous exercise, and maintaining a healthy body weight are all associated with decreased risk (see the box "Who Is Least Likely to Develop Breast Cancer?").

HIGHLIGHT ON HEALTH
Breast Self-Exam

Performing a monthly breast self-exam (BSE) can help you learn how your breasts normally feel so you can identify any changes that occur. Almost all women have some lumps and bumps in their breast tissue that change throughout the month. The best time to do your exam is a few days after your period when the breast tissue is least tender. If you no longer menstruate or have very irregular periods, do the exam on the same day every month.

If you choose to do a BSE, follow these steps:

- Lie down and put a pillow under your right shoulder. Place your right arm behind your head.

- Use the finger pads of your three middle fingers on your left hand to feel for lumps or thickening in your right breast. Use overlapping dime-sized circular motions of the finger pads to feel the breast tissue.

- Use three different levels of pressure—light, medium, and firm—to feel all the breast tissue. Use each pressure level to feel the breast tissue before moving on to the next spot. If you're not sure how hard to press, talk with your health care provider. A firm ridge in the lower curve of each breast is normal.

- Move around the breast in an up-and-down pattern starting at an imaginary line drawn straight down your side from the underarm and move across the breast to the middle of the chest (breast bone).

- Repeat the exam on your left breast, using the finger pads of the right hand and moving the pillow under your left shoulder.

- While standing in front of a mirror with your hands pressing firmly down on your hips, look at

(a)   (b)

your breasts for any changes of size, shape, contour, or dimpling. (Pressing down on your hips contracts the chest wall muscles and enhances any breast changes.)

- Examine each underarm while sitting up or standing and with your arm only slightly raised so you can easily feel in the area.

If you notice any change—such as the development of a lump or swelling, skin irritation or dimpling, nipple pain or retraction, redness or scaliness of the nipple or skin, or a discharge other than breast milk—see your health care provider right away for an evaluation. Most of the time, these changes are not cancer.

These BSE guidelines represent a change in previous recommendations, based on an extensive review of the medical literature and input from an expert advisory group.

Source: Copyright American Cancer Society, Inc., www.cancer.org. Reprinted with permission.

Early stages of breast cancer have no symptoms or symptoms that may be detected only by a mammogram. Symptoms of later stages include a persistent lump, swelling, redness, or bumpiness of the skin, and nipple discharge. Breast pain or tenderness is common in women without cancer and is usually not a cause for concern; more likely explanations are hormonal changes, infection, or breast cysts, which are rarely cancerous.

Breast cancer can be detected at an early stage by a mammogram, a low-dose X-ray of the breast. The effectiveness of mammography in detecting cancer depends on several factors, including the size of the cancer, the density of the breasts, and the skills of the radiologist. Although mammograms cannot detect all cancers, they

have been shown to decrease the number of women who die from breast cancer.[13] The American Cancer Society recommends annual mammograms for all women aged 40 and older.

Another screening technique for breast cancer is breast exam. The American Cancer Society recommends that women in their 20s and 30s have a clinical breast exam (CBE) performed by a health care provider every 2 to 3 years and that women over 40 have a breast exam performed by their health care provider annually near the time of their mammogram. The ACS also suggests that beginning in their 20s, women should be told about the benefits and limitations of performing a breast self-exam (BSE) every month (see the box "Breast Self-Exam"). The

ACS considers it acceptable for women to choose not to do self-exams or to do them only occasionally.

Any suspicious lumps, changes, or mammogram findings that are suggestive of cancer are typically followed by a biopsy so that cells or tissues can be evaluated under the microscope, the only way to make a definitive diagnosis. There are several noncancerous causes of lumps in the breast; in younger women, a lump is much more likely to be caused by a cyst or a benign tumor called a fibroadenoma. Other screening tools, including ultrasound and magnetic resonance imaging (MRI), are sometimes used to help determine whether a lump or abnormality is cancerous.

Surgery is usually the first line of treatment for breast cancer, either a lumpectomy (removal of a section of the breast around the cancer) or a mastectomy (removal of the entire breast). Lymph nodes under the arm on the affected side are often tested to determine whether the cancer has spread from the breast. Radiation, chemotherapy, and hormonal therapy are frequently used in the treatment of breast cancer.

The 5-year survival rate for all stages of breast cancer is 86.6 percent. For cancer that is localized (no lymph node involvement), it is 97 percent; for cancer that has spread regionally (only local lymph node involvement), it is 79 percent; and for cancer that has distant metastases, it is 23 percent.[5]

Prostate Cancer

The second most common cause of cancer death in men and the most commonly diagnosed cancer in men is prostate cancer. The ACS projected an estimated 232,090 new cases of prostate cancer in the United States in 2005 and an estimated 30,350 deaths.[5] The incidence of prostate cancer is significantly higher among African American men than Caucasian men, as is the death rate. The number of diagnosed cases of prostate cancer increased in the early 1990s, probably as a result of better screening. Death rates declined during the same period, although death rates for African American men remain twice as high as those for white men.[5]

The most important risk factor for prostate cancer is age. More than 70 percent of prostate cancer cases are diagnosed in men aged 65 and older. Other risk factors include a family history of prostate cancer, being African American, and possibly having a high-fat diet. The risk of dying from prostate cancer appears to increase with increasing body weight.

In its early stages, prostate cancer usually has no signs or symptoms. Advanced prostate cancer can be associated with difficulty urinating, pain in the pelvic region, pain with urination, or blood in the urine. These symptoms can also be caused by more common, noncancerous conditions, such as benign enlargement of the prostate gland and bladder infections.

Two tests are available to detect prostate cancer at an early, asymptomatic stage. One is a *digital rectal exam,* in which a health care provider inserts a gloved finger into the rectum and palpates the prostate gland. Prostate cancer usually occurs in the outer part of the gland and can often be detected by this exam. The other is the *prostate-specific antigen (PSA) test,* a blood test that detects levels of a substance made by the prostate (prostate-specific antigen) that are elevated when certain conditions are present, including benign prostate enlargement, infection, and prostate cancer. If PSA levels are elevated, a rectal ultrasound and prostate biopsy can be performed to assess and diagnose the cause. The American Cancer Society recommends that all men discuss with their health care professionals whether they should have a digital rectal exam and PSA screening annually starting at age 50; the ACS also recommends that African American men and men with a family history of prostate cancer begin having screening done at age 45.[5]

The routine use of PSA testing is controversial, because many prostate cancers progress slowly and would not cause symptoms before a man died of other causes. The difficulty of determining which prostate cancers are slow growing and which may progress more quickly complicates treatment decisions once a cancer has been detected. Treatments for prostate cancer can themselves cause problems, including erectile dysfunction and incontinence (inability to control the flow of urine). These side effects have to be balanced against the risk that the cancer will progress and spread.

Treatment for prostate cancer depends on the stage of the cancer and the man's age and other health conditions. In its early stages and in a younger man, prostate cancer is usually treated with surgery (removal of the prostate gland) and radiation, sometimes in combination with chemotherapy, radiation, and hormonal medication, which blocks the effects of testosterone and can cause tumors to shrink. Later stages are treated with chemotherapy, radiation, and hormonal medication. Radiation is sometimes administered by the implantation of radioactive seeds, which destroy cancer tissue and leave normal prostate tissue intact. The 5-year survival rate for all stages of prostate cancer is 98 percent. For cancers detected at local or regional stages, the 5-year survival rate is 100 percent. In studies that follow prostate cancer for more than 5 years, the survival rate decreases to 84 percent at 10 years and to 56 percent at 15 years.[5]

Cancers of the Female Reproductive System

Cancer can develop throughout the female reproductive system but occurs more frequently in the cervix, uterus, and ovaries.

Cancer patients and survivors join support groups for different reasons—to help them through a crisis, to learn how other people affected by cancer are coping with their situation, and to make plans for the future.

Cervical Cancer

The ACS projected an estimated 10,370 new cases of cervical cancer in 2005 and an estimated 3,710 deaths.[5] The incidence of this cancer and the number of related deaths have declined sharply in the past few decades as a result of improved detection and treatment of precursor lesions, primarily by means of the Papanicolaou (Pap) test.

As described in Chapter 20, cervical cancer is closely related to infection with the human papillomavirus (HPV) and possibly other sexually transmitted diseases like chlamydia. Risk factors include early sexual activity, multiple sex partners, cigarette smoking, and low socioeconomic status. Women who are overweight may be more likely to die from cervical cancer.

Cervical cancer develops at a specific site on the cervix, at the opening of the cervix into the vagina. In its early stages, it usually does not have any symptoms. Warning signs of more advanced cancer include abnormal vaginal discharge or abnormal vaginal bleeding, such as spotting between periods or spotting after sex. Pain in the pelvic region can be a late sign of cervical cancer. Early stages of cervical cancer can be detected by the Pap test, performed by a health care provider as part of a pelvic exam. A small sample of cells is collected from the cervix with a swab, placed on a slide, and examined under a microscope to detect any cells that have become precursor cells of cervical cancer.

Pap tests are good but not perfect; they occasionally give **false negatives** (they miss precursor lesions or cancer cells) or **false positives** (they identify cells as abnormal that are normal). A newer form of Pap test, called a liquid Pap, has been developed to try to decrease the number of false negatives and false positives. Cells are collected from the cervix with a swab, but instead of being placed on a slide, they are placed in liquid. When the liquid is processed, more cells are retained for examination under the microscope than with the conventional Pap test. The cells can also be tested for HPV. If abnormal cells—from a condition called **cervical dysplasia**—are found, a **colposcopy** can be performed. In this procedure, the health care provider uses a colposcope, a magnifying tool, to examine the cervix and identify abnormal areas, which can then be biopsied.

The American Cancer Society recommends that women start having Pap tests at age 21 or within 3 years of first sexual intercourse. Tests should be continued annually (conventional Pap test) or every 2 years (liquid Pap test). Beginning at age 30, women who have had three normal Pap tests in a row may decrease their screening to one every 2 or 3 years with either type of test.[5] As noted in Chapter 20, a vaccine for the types of HPV most associated with cervical cancer is under development. HPV is associated with at least 90 percent of cervical cancer cases,

KEY TERMS

false negative   A negative test result when a disease is actually present.

false positive   A positive test result when no disease is actually present.

cervical dysplasia   Abnormal cells on the cervix.

colposcopy   Procedure in which a health care provider uses a colposcope, a magnifying tool, to examine the cervix and identify abnormal areas.

so an effective vaccine could significantly reduce the incidence of this cancer.

Treatment for cervical cancer involves removing or destroying precursor cells. Several methods are available, including electrocoagulation (the destruction of tissue locally by intense heat), cryotherapy (the destruction of tissue locally by intense cold), and surgery. Invasive cervical cancer is treated with a combination of surgery, local radiation, and chemotherapy.

Uterine Cancer

Also called *endometrial cancer,* uterine cancer usually develops in the endometrium, the lining of the uterus. The ACS projected an estimated 40,880 new cases of uterine cancer in 2005 and an estimated 7,310 deaths.[5] Uterine cancer is diagnosed more often in Caucasian women than in African American women, but the death rate among African American women is nearly twice the rate among Caucasian women. African American women tend to have more advanced cancer when they are diagnosed, perhaps as a result of having less access to health care.

The risk for uterine cancer is related to a woman's exposure to estrogen, so risk factors include young age at menarche, late onset of menopause, irregular ovulation, infrequent periods, taking estrogen replacement therapy without the addition of other hormones, not having children, and obesity. Warning signs of uterine cancer include abnormal uterine bleeding (spotting between periods or spotting after menopause), pelvic pain, and low back pain. Pain is usually a late sign of uterine cancer.

Uterine cancer is frequently detected at an early stage in postmenopausal women because of vaginal bleeding. An endometrial biopsy is performed to collect cells and tissue from the uterus to determine whether the bleeding is due to cancer or a less serious condition. If uterine cancer is diagnosed, a hysterectomy—surgical removal of the uterus—is usually performed. Depending on the stage of cancer, other treatment methods may also be used, including radiation, chemotherapy, and hormonal therapy.

Ovarian Cancer

The leading gynecological cause of cancer death and the fourth overall cause of cancer death in women is ovarian cancer. The ACS projected an estimated 22,220 new cases of ovarian cancer in 2005 and 16,210 deaths.[5] Ovarian cancer has a low rate of survival because most cases are not diagnosed until they have spread beyond the ovaries. If ovarian cancer is diagnosed early, survival is as high as 95 percent. Thus, an important goal is to increase early diagnosis.[14] Between 90 and 95 percent of women with ovarian cancer have no risk factors. The strongest risk factor is a family history of ovarian

cancer in a first-degree relative. In families with a strong history of ovarian cancer, a genetic link involving the BRCA1 and BRCA2 genes can often be found. Women with either of these genetic mutations have a 40 percent to 60 percent chance of developing ovarian cancer. Other risk factors include not having children and a personal history of breast, colon, or endometrial cancer.

The early stages of ovarian cancer have very few signs or symptoms. At later stages, a woman may notice swelling of the abdomen, bloating, or a vague pain in the lower abdomen. Controllable factors associated with a reduced risk of ovarian cancer include the use of oral contraceptive pills, at least one full-term pregnancy, and having breast-fed. Avoidance of postmenopausal hormone replacement therapy may also reduce the risk of ovarian cancer.[15] For women at high risk of ovarian cancer, such as women with the BRCA1 or BRCA2 genetic mutations, removal of the ovaries decreases the risk of ovarian cancer.

The standard screening tool for ovarian cancer is the pelvic exam. Most women, as part of their annual checkup with a Pap test, undergo a "bimanual exam," in which the health care provider feels the uterus and ovaries with two gloved fingers in the vagina and a hand on the lower abdomen. The National Institutes of Health recommends this procedure as a yearly screening test. However, according to the U.S. Preventive Task Force, there are no strong data showing an improvement in early detection of ovarian cancer with this test, perhaps because the ovaries can be so hard to feel.

Several blood tests are also under investigation for ovarian cancer. A woman who has this cancer has higher than normal blood levels of two proteins, CA125 and lysophosphalidic acid, so they can be used as markers. Levels of these proteins can be elevated for other reasons, however, so they are not useful as a general screening tool for ovarian cancer. Another screening method is pelvic ultrasound, in which sound waves are used to visualize the ovaries and show whether they are enlarged or contain a mass. Again, this test can be effective at detecting ovarian cancers, but many abnormalities show up on ultrasound that are not cancer. A large study showed that if surgery were performed to evaluate masses revealed by ultrasound screening, only one case of ovarian cancer would be found for every 10 to 11 women screened.[14] In short, diagnosis and prevention of ovarian cancer remain a significant challenge.

Treatment for ovarian cancer depends on the stage at diagnosis. Typically, all or part of the ovaries, uterus, and fallopian tubes are surgically removed and the lymph nodes are biopsied to determine whether the cancer has spread. Chemotherapy and radiation may then be recommended. Treatment options currently under investigation include vaccinations, targeted drugs, and immunotherapy.[16]

Skin Cancer

Three forms of skin cancer exist: basal cell cancer, squamous cell cancer, and melanoma. More than 1 million cases of basal cell and squamous cell cancers occur each year in the United States. Most of these are curable, although both can be disfiguring and, if ignored, fatal. Melanoma is a less common but more serious form of skin cancer. The ACS projected an estimated 59,580 new cases of melanoma in 2005 and 7,770 deaths.[5] Skin cancers occur in all racial and ethnic groups, but they are more common in people with lighter skin colors.

Melanoma

Because it is capable of spreading quickly to almost any part of the body, melanoma is a particularly dangerous form of cancer. Rates of melanoma have been increasing since 1970, but mortality from this cancer has stabilized, probably owing to earlier detection.

The risk for melanoma is greatest for people with a personal history of melanoma, a large number of moles (especially if large or unusual in shape or color), or a family member with melanoma. Melanoma can occur on any part of the body, but it is directly related to sun exposure, especially intermittent, acute ultraviolet (UV) light exposure, as from exposure to sunlight (sunburns) or to UV light in tanning salons. Exposure during childhood or adolescence may be particularly dangerous. The risk appears to be higher in people who are fair-skinned and burn easily, and it increases with age.

Melanomas usually develop in pigmented, or dark, areas on the skin. Signs suggestive of melanoma are changes in a mole: a sudden darkening or change in color, spread of color outward into previously normal skin, an irregular border, pain, itchiness, bleeding, or crusting. You can monitor your skin for these signs by using the "ABCD" test for melanoma (Figure 22.3).

The most effective way to prevent melanoma is to avoid sun exposure, especially during childhood and adolescence. Recommended ways of achieving this goal, in order of importance, are staying out of the sun during midday (10:00 a.m. to 4:00 p.m.), wearing protective clothing (including a hat to shade the face and neck, long sleeves, and long pants), using sunscreen with a **sun protective factor (SPF)** of 15 or higher, and wearing sunglasses that offer UV protection. Parents should be particularly vigilant about protecting their children, because the risk appears to be greatest in childhood.

Early detection of skin cancer usually occurs as a result of individuals' monitoring their own skin and visiting a health care provider for evaluation of any changes or progressive growth. The American Cancer Society recommends that people have a skin exam (visual inspection of the skin all over the body) as part of a regular physical examination every 3 years between ages 20 and 40 and annually after age 40.

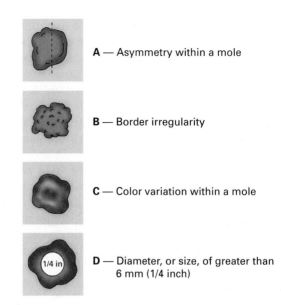

A — Asymmetry within a mole

B — Border irregularity

C — Color variation within a mole

D — Diameter, or size, of greater than 6 mm (1/4 inch)

Figure 22.3   The ABCD evaluation of moles for melanoma.

Treatment for melanoma begins with surgically excising (cutting out) and doing a biopsy of any suspicious lesions. If melanoma is confirmed, a larger area of surrounding skin is removed, which improves the chance of survival. The prognosis is based on the size and depth of the melanoma. Chemotherapy and immunotherapy can be added for advanced stages. The overall 5-year survival rate for melanoma is 90 percent; if the melanoma is diagnosed at an early stage, the 5-year survival rate is 97 percent.[5]

Basal Cell and Squamous Cell Carcinomas

Sun-exposed areas of the body are susceptible to basal cell and squamous cell cancers. People at high risk include those with fair skin; blonde, red, or light brown hair; blue, green, or hazel eyes; and freckles and moles. Other risk factors are cumulative sun exposure and age, with rates increasing after age 50. However, both types are increasing among younger people.

The signs of a basal cell cancer include new skin growth; a raised, domelike lesion with a pearl-like edge or border; or a sore that bleeds and scabs but never completely heals. The signs of a squamous cell cancer include a red, scaly area that does not go away; a sore that bleeds and does not heal; or a raised, crusty sore. Squamous cell

KEY TERMS

sun protective factor (SPF)   Measure of the degree to which a sunscreen protects the skin from damaging UV radiation from the sun.

cancers often develop from a precancerous spot called an actinic keratosis, a red, rough spot that develops in a sun-exposed area.

All forms of skin cancer have been associated with exposure to UV radiation in tanning beds, and in 2000, the U.S. Department of Health and Human Services added exposure to ultraviolet radiation from the sun or artificial light sources to its list of known human carcinogens. Tanning lamps emit mostly UVA radiation, a form of radiation less associated with skin cancer than is UVB radiation. However, UVA radiation is associated with more signs of skin aging, such as wrinkling and sagging. Furthermore, recent animal studies show a significant increase in skin cancer with exposure to UVA light, and human studies are starting to confirm the same.

Early detection of basal and squamous cell cancers involves monitoring the skin and having any persistent changes evaluated. The American Cancer Society recommends the same skin exams for these cancers as for melanoma. Treatment usually involves local removal and destruction of the cancer by surgery, heat, or freezing, with radiation therapy sometimes an option.[5]

Testicular Cancer

Although testicular cancer accounts for only 1 percent of all cancers in men, it is the most common malignancy in men 15 to 35 years of age. The ACS projected an estimated 8,010 new cases of testicular cancer in 2005 and an estimated 390 deaths.[5] The incidence of testicular cancer has nearly doubled worldwide over the past 40 years. It is not clear why this increase is occurring, but some researchers speculate that it could be due to fetal exposure to higher levels of estrogen during prenatal development as a result of environmental toxins.[17] Because of improved treatment methods, however, the survival rate has increased. Testicular cancer occurs nearly 4.5 times more often in white men in the United States than in African American men. Rates for men of Hispanic, Asian, and Native American backgrounds fall between those for white and African American men.[18]

The risk for testicular cancer is 3 to 17 times higher in men with a history of an undescended testicle (one of the testes fails to descend into the scrotum and is retained in the abdomen or inguinal canal). However, only 7 to 10 percent of men diagnosed with testicular cancer have a history of this condition. Other risk factors include a family history of testicular cancer, a personal history of testicular cancer in the other testicle, and abnormal development of the testes. The risk may be slightly higher in men with infertility or abnormal sperm.[18]

Warning signs of testicular cancer include a painless lump on the testicle and swelling or discomfort in the scrotum. Most testicular cancer is detected by an individual,

either unintentionally or during a testicular self-exam. Back pain and difficulty breathing can develop in the later stages after the cancer metastasizes.

For men who have a testicle that is undescended, a surgical procedure early in life can move the testicle into the scrotum. Whether this actually reduces the risk of cancer developing in the testis is unclear, but the repositioning allows for earlier detection of cancer if it does develop. The ACS recommends a testicular exam by a health care provider every 3 years for men over age 20 and annually after age 40. Men can also perform a self-exam, although there are no specific recommendations for how often it should be performed (see the box "Testicle Self-Exam"). If a lump is detected, an ultrasound is performed, and if the ultrasound suggests cancer, a biopsy is performed to confirm the diagnosis.

Testicular cancer is treated with surgery to remove the testicle; depending on the stage of disease, radiation or chemotherapy may be needed as well. Testicular cancer is highly treatable, with more than 90 percent of cases at all stages being cured. The cure rate approaches 100 percent if the cancer is diagnosed at an early stage. Even in a man with a late-stage diagnosis and extensive metastases, testicular cancer can be cured. International cycling champion Lance Armstrong, after being diagnosed at age 25 with advanced-stage testicular cancer with metastases to the brain and lungs, was successfully treated and went on to win the world's most prestigious cycling events.

Oral Cancer

Cancers that develop in the mouth or the pharynx (the back of the throat), which can involve the lips, tongue, gums, or throat, are classified as oral cancers. The ACS projected an estimated 29,370 new cases of cancers of the oral cavity and pharynx in 2005 and an estimated 7,320 deaths.[5] The rate of new cases has been declining since the 1970s, and death rates have also been declining. Oral cancers are more common in men than in women.

The major risk factor for oral cancers is tobacco use (smoking cigarettes, cigars, or a pipe or using smokeless tobacco); high levels of alcohol consumption also increase the risk. Early signs of oral cancer include a persistent sore in the mouth that does not heal or bleeds easily; a lump or bump that does not go away or that increases in size; or a patch of redness or whiteness along the gums or skin lining the inside of the cheeks. Late signs of oral cancer can include pain or difficulty swallowing or chewing.

Oral cancers are usually detected by a doctor or dentist, or the individual may report a sore that does not heal. A biopsy of any suspicious area is necessary to confirm the diagnosis. Treatment usually starts with surgery to

HIGHLIGHT ON HEALTH
Testicle Self-Exam

The testicle self-exam has not been studied enough to show whether it reduces the death rate from testicular cancer. For this reason, the American Cancer Society has not set a recommendation for this self-exam for the general population. Testicular cancer is often first detected by a man noticing a change in his own testicles, so some health providers do teach and recommend it.

If you decide to perform a self-exam, follow these steps:

- Stand in front of a mirror. Look for any changes or swelling on the skin of the scrotum.
- Examine each testicle with both hands. Place your index and middle fingers under the testicle with the thumbs placed on top. Roll the testicle gently between the thumbs and fingers. It's normal for one testicle to be slightly larger than the other.

- Find the epididymis, the soft, tubelike structure behind the testicle that collects and carries sperm. If you are familiar with this structure, you won't mistake it for a suspicious lump. Cancerous lumps usually are found on the sides of the testicle but also can appear on the front.

If you find a lump, see your doctor right away. Testicular cancer is highly curable, especially when it's detected and treated early. In almost all cases, testicular cancer occurs in only one testicle, and men can maintain full sexual and reproductive function with the other testicle.

---

remove as much as possible of the cancer, along with local radiation. If the cancer is advanced, chemotherapy can be added. The 5-year survival rate for all stages of oral cancer is 57 percent.

Leukemia

A group of cancers known as leukemia originate in the bone marrow or other parts of the body where white blood cells form. Leukemia is the overproduction of one type of white blood cell, which prevents the normal growth and function of other blood cells and can lead to increased risk of infection, anemia, and bleeding. Leukemias are considered either acute or chronic, depending on how quickly they progress. The ACS projected an estimated 34,810 new cases of leukemia in 2005 and an estimated 22,570 deaths.[5]

Risk factors include cigarette smoking and exposure to certain chemicals, particularly benzene, a chemical found in gasoline products and in cigarette smoke. Ionizing radiation can increase the risk for several types of leukemia; people who survive other cancers are at risk for developing leukemia as a result of radiation treatment. Infection with a virus, human T-cell leukemia/lymphoma virus (HTLV-1), can increase the risk of leukemia and lymphoma, another cancer of the white blood cells.

Symptoms of leukemia often occur because healthy white blood cells, red blood cells, and platelets are unable to perform their functions. Symptoms include fatigue, increased incidence of infection, and easy bleeding and bruising. Symptoms can appear suddenly in acute leukemia, but in chronic leukemia, they may appear gradually.

Because the symptoms are fairly nonspecific, early detection of leukemia can be challenging. There is no recommended screening test, but a health care provider can diagnose leukemia with a blood test or bone marrow biopsy if it is suggested by symptoms. The most effective treatment is chemotherapy. Supportive therapy can include blood transfusion, antibiotics, drugs to boost the function of healthy blood cells, and drugs to reduce the side effects of chemotherapy. Bone marrow transplantation can be effective for certain types of leukemia.

CANCER SCREENING

Early detection is the key to successful treatment of cancer, and **screening tests** are the key to early detection. Cancer screening involves trying to identify risk factors or undetected cancers in an asymptomatic person. An ideal screening test would always detect cancer at an early, treatable stage and never produce a false negative or false positive result. A false negative means that a cancer remains undetected and untreated.

KEY TERMS

screening test   Test given to a large group of people to identify a smaller group of people who are at higher risk for a specific disease or condition.

ACS Cancer Detection Guidelines

Regular physical exams should include examinations for cancers of the thyroid, oral cavity, skin, lymph nodes, testes, and ovaries. Special tests for certain cancer sites are recommended as outlined below.

Breast Cancer

- Yearly mammograms starting at age 40 and continuing for as long as a woman is in good health.
- Clinical breast exams (CBE) should be part of a periodic health exam, about every 3 years for women in their 20s and 30s and every year for women 40 and over.
- Women should report any breast change promptly to their health care providers. Breast self-exam (BSE) is an option for women starting in their 20s.
- Women at increased risk (those with family history, genetic tendency, past breast cancer) should talk with their doctors about the benefits and limitations of starting mammography screening earlier, having additional tests (such as breast ultrasound or MRI), or having more frequent exams.

Colon and Rectal Cancer

Beginning at age 50, both men and women at average risk should follow one of these five testing schedules:

- Yearly fecal occult blood test (FOBT)* or fecal immunochemical test (FIT)
- Flexible sigmoidoscopy every 5 years

- Yearly FOBT* or FIT plus flexible sigmoidoscopy every 5 years**
- Double-contrast barium enema every 5 years
- Colonoscopy every 10 years

All positive tests should be followed up with colonoscopy.

People should begin colorectal cancer screening earlier and/or undergo screening more often if they have any of the risk factors described in the chapter, such as a personal or family history of colon polyps or colon cancer; a personal history of chronic inflammatory bowel disease; or a family history of a hereditary colorectal cancer syndrome.

Cervical Cancer

- All women should begin cervical cancer screening about 3 years after they begin having vaginal intercourse, but no later than when they are 21 years old. Screening should be done every year with the regular Pap test or every 2 years using the newer liquid-based Pap test.
- Beginning at age 30, women who have had three normal Pap test results in a row may get screened every 2 to 3 years with either the conventional (regular) or liquid-based Pap test. Women who have certain risk factors such as diethylstilbestrol (DES) exposure before birth, HIV infection, or a weakened immune system owing to organ trans-

A false positive creates trauma for the person diagnosed and sometimes leads to unnecessary surgery. Unfortunately, no screening tests meet this ideal. The ACS screening recommendations for breast, colon, prostate, uterine, and cervical cancer were included in the discussions of these cancers and are summarized in the box "ACS Cancer Detection Guidelines." No screening recommendations exist for some cancers, including lung and ovarian cancers, because to date, no test has been shown to improve detection without increasing harm.

Genetic screening can also be done to assess cancer risk. At this time, it is being reserved for members of high-risk families, that is, families with multiple members with cancer. When families and individuals are identified as having a higher risk of cancer, increased cancer screening and lifestyle modifications can help to decrease mortality from certain cancers. Some genes are

associated with such a high risk of cancer that aggressive surgeries to prevent cancer are considered, as mentioned earlier.

CANCER TREATMENTS

Surgery is the oldest treatment for cancer; newer options include chemotherapy, radiation, biological therapies, bone marrow transplantation, and gene therapy.

Surgery

Surgery remains a mainstay in diagnosis and treatment of cancer. When a cancer is detected early and is small and localized, surgery can cure it, as when an *in situ* cancer of the breast is removed via a lumpectomy. Sometimes an organ affected by cancer can be removed plant, chemotherapy, or chronic steroid use should continue to be screened annually.

- Another reasonable option for women over 30 is to get screened every 3 years (but not more frequently) with either the conventional or liquid-based Pap test, *plus* the HPV DNA test.

- Women 70 years of age or older who have had three or more normal Pap tests in a row and no abnormal Pap test results in the last 10 years may choose to stop having cervical cancer screening. Women with a history of cervical cancer, DES exposure before birth, HIV infection, or a weakened immune system should continue to have screening as long as they are in good health.

- Women who have had a total hysterectomy (removal of the uterus and cervix) may also choose to stop having cervical cancer screening, unless the surgery was done as a treatment for cervical cancer or precancer. Women who have had a hysterectomy without removal of the cervix should continue to follow the guidelines above.

Endometrial (Uterine) Cancer

All women should be informed about the risks and symptoms of endometrial cancer and strongly encouraged to report any unexpected bleeding or spotting to their doctors. For women with or at high risk for hereditary nonpolyposis colon cancer (HNPCC),

annual screening should be offered for endometrial cancer with endometrial biopsy beginning at age 35.

Prostate Cancer

Both the prostate-specific antigen (PSA) blood test and digital rectal examination (DRE) should be offered annually, beginning at age 50, to men who have at least a 10-year life expectancy. Men at high risk (African American men and men with a strong family history of one or more first-degree relatives diagnosed at an early age) should begin testing at age 45. Men at even higher risk, due to multiple first-degree relatives affected at an early age, could begin testing at age 40; depending on the results of this initial test, further testing might be postponed until age 45.

Information should be provided to all men about what is known and what is uncertain about the benefits and limitations of early detection and treatment of prostate cancer so that they can make an informed decision about testing.

Men who ask their doctor to make the decision on their behalf should be tested. Discouraging testing is not appropriate, nor is not offering testing.

*For FOBT, the take-home multiple sample method should be used.

**The combination of yearly FOBT or FIT plus flexible sigmoidoscopy every 5 years is preferred over either of these options alone.

Source: American Cancer Society, www.cancer.org.

surgically without threatening life, as in the case of prostate or testicular cancer. Certain cancers are unlikely to spread widely, such as a basal cell carcinoma, and surgery often cures these cancers as well. If a cancer has spread, surgery may still be performed as part of the treatment.

Chemotherapy

Chemotherapy is a drug treatment administered to the entire body to kill any cancer cells that may have escaped from the local site to the blood, lymph system, or another part of the body. More than 50 chemotherapy medicines have been developed; different combinations are used for different cancers. All chemotherapeutic drugs operate by a similar mechanism—they interfere with rapid cell division. Because cancer cells divide more rapidly than normal cells, they are more vulnerable to destruction by chemotherapy than healthy cells.

Other normal tissues that divide rapidly are also harmed by chemotherapy, including the hair, stomach lining, and white blood cells. The timing and dosage must be carefully adjusted so the drugs kill cancer cells but do not damage normal cells beyond repair. Scientists are developing new chemotherapy techniques that focus on the features that make cancer cells unique. For instance, targeted chemotherapy drugs can distinguish antigen markers on the surface of cancer cells, so they can kill those cells with less harm to normal cells.

Radiation

Radiation causes damage to cells by altering their DNA; it can be used to destroy cancer cells with minimal damage to surrounding tissues. Radiation is a local treatment that can be used before or after surgery or in conjunction with chemotherapy. It can also be used to control pain in patients with cancer that cannot be cured.

Biological Therapies

Biological therapies enhance the immune system's ability to fight cancer (an approach called **immunotherapy**) or reduce the side effects of chemotherapy. One kind of immunotherapy is a vaccine that can be developed after a person has been diagnosed with a cancer. Administering the vaccine can boost the immune response to the cancer and may help prevent a recurrence. Vaccines for several types of cancers, including melanoma and cancers of the breast, colon, ovary, and prostate, are under investigation. Vaccines can also be used to prevent cancer, as in the case of the HPV vaccine for cervical cancer.

Medications can also be used to boost the immune response. Such drugs as interleukin-2, herceptin, and interferon-alpha are used to treat some cancers. Other medications improve the health of damaged immune system components by increasing the numbers of white blood cells, red blood cells, or platelets.[19]

Immunotherapy also includes boosting the immune system with social support, whether in the form of friends, family, or cancer support groups. Prolonged cancer survival is associated with good support systems and a positive outlook.

Bone Marrow Transplantation

Bone marrow transplantation was initially used for cancer of the white blood cells (leukemia, lymphoma). Now it is sometimes used for other cancers when healthy bone marrow cells are killed by high doses of chemotherapy. This treatment approach is controversial for some types of cancer because of complications from high-dose chemotherapy and the high risk of infection. Additionally, data have not conclusively shown a significantly improved survival rate for some cancers.

Gene Therapy and Genetic Testing

Gene therapy could be used in several different ways to improve cancer treatment. In theory, mutated genes could be replaced with functional genes, decreasing the risk that cancer will occur or stopping a cancer that has started to develop. Genes could be inserted into immune cells to increase their ability to fight cancer cells, or they could be inserted into the cancer cells themselves, causing them to self-destruct or making the cancer more susceptible to chemotherapy. The use of gene therapy for cancer treatment is still in the clinical trials stage at this time.[19]

Genetic testing may also become important in cancer treatment. It could allow physicians to predict more accurately how a cancer will behave, which chemotherapy drugs will work best against it, which patients will benefit from chemotherapy, and which patients can skip this treatment. Recent research in this area has had promising results.[20,21]

Complementary and Alternative Medicine

The role of complementary and alternative medicine (CAM) in cancer treatment is currently one of the most controversial areas in Western medicine. On the one hand, many CAM techniques are thought to enhance the immune system, helping the body fight cancer and improving response to treatment. On the other hand, some patients delay treatment with proven Western approaches because they focus exclusively on CAM approaches. For more on this topic and other aspects of CAM, see the box "Cancer Quackery" and Chapter 23.

Treatments on the Horizon: Clinical Trials

Studies designed by researchers and physicians to test different drugs and treatment regimens are known as **clinical trials.** Participants in clinical trials are patients with cancer who enroll both in the hopes of finding a better treatment for their own cancer and in the interest of furthering cancer research in general. Once enrolled in the study, participants are usually randomly assigned either to a group receiving a new drug or a group receiving the standard treatment. In rare situations, usually when there is no effective treatment, one group of patients may receive a placebo (a "sugar pill" that has no effect). If cancer is advancing in a patient who is receiving the placebo, he or she may be switched to the group receiving the drug. For more information about new and ongoing clinical trials in the United States, visit the Web site of the National Cancer Institute.

LIVING WITH CANCER

As a result of improved screening and treatment over the past 30 years, leading to higher survival rates, cancer is no longer seen as a death sentence; rather, it is seen, in many cases, as a chronic disease that can be managed. In the United States, the survival rate for all stages and types of cancer combined is 63 percent. Many cancers are now curable or controllable, and cancer survivors often return to a healthy life. An estimated 9.6 million people living in the United States have a history of cancer. Some are cancer free, others are undergoing treatment, and others are in remission.

As a chronic disease, however, cancer does change the way a person lives his or her life. Many issues and questions arise for people when they are living with a cancer

Consumer Clipboard

Cancer Quackery

Whether an individual has just been diagnosed with cancer, is undergoing treatment, or has been told "we've done everything we can for you," that person is a prime target for quackery. It's not always a dramatic case of a patient using his or her life savings for an unknown treatment or surgical procedure in another country. For many patients quackery works in different ways, but it still causes harm.

The direct results of quackery may involve unnecessary suffering, serious injury, or even death. At the extreme end, for example, cyanide poisoning from ingesting laetrile, electrolyte imbalance caused by coffee enemas, and brain damage from whole-body hyperthermia have all caused death in some patients.

Yet quackery can also cause harm in indirect ways—by causing patients to delay treatment or decide against having standard treatment. A newly diagnosed patient with cancer might read about a "natural cure" and try that method as a first step. By the time the person realizes that this approach isn't working, the cancer may have progressed greatly and conventional treatment may be less effective, or even ineffective.

Although the signs of quackery are varied, some examples involve the nothing-to-lose message ("You might as well try it—you're going to die anyway"), appeals to fear (chemotherapy is a toxic approach), and encouraging mistrust (the government and the medical profession are keeping information and effective therapies from patients). More subtle approaches include the following themes:

Health freedom. This message says that cancer patients should be free to choose whatever treatments they want. Government regulation is limiting the patients' choices and keeping them from helpful treatments. In reality, such regulation is a necessary safeguard and an important benefit to patients.

Detoxification of the body. This idea is that a body affected by cancer must be cleansed of "toxins" caused by the disease. Methods such as colon therapy, or colonic irrigation, are recommended to purify the body. However, there is no scientific evidence that this type of therapy is effective. In fact, colon therapy can cause infection, perforation, or even death.

Complementary and alternative therapies. Legitimate complementary and alternative therapies may be touted as "cures" for cancer. Many of these approaches are beneficial when used in conjunction with conventional therapy. For example, meditation, yoga, and massage therapy can be used to promote feelings of control and ease suffering in patients. However, they are not cures.

The American Cancer Society evaluates cancer methods by asking three questions:

- Has the method been objectively demonstrated in the peer-reviewed scientific literature to be effective?

- Has the method shown potential for benefit that clearly exceeds the potential for harm?

- Have objective studies been correctly conducted under appropriate peer review to answer these questions?

Sources: "Colon Therapy" and "Complementary and Alternative Therapies," American Cancer Society, www.cancer.org; "How Quackery Harms Cancer Patients" by W. T. Jarvis; and "Questionable Cancer Therapies" by S. Barrett and V. Herbert, www.quackwatch.com.

---

diagnosis, undergoing treatment, or becoming cancer survivors. For suggestions on dealing with some of these issues, see the box "Living With Cancer."

Important discoveries in the areas of cancer biology, genetics, screening, and treatment have transformed the face of cancer. Greater knowledge of risk factors has led to more effective prevention strategies. Mortality is declining, survival rates are rising, and the quality of life for those with cancer is improving. The future holds great promise for continuing progress.

KEY TERMS

immunotherapy Administration of drugs or other substances that enhance the ability of the immune system to fight cancer.

clinical trials Studies designed by researchers and physicians to test different drugs and treatment regimens.

Challenges & Choices

Living With Cancer

If you receive a diagnosis of cancer, many issues will come up that you probably have never had to deal with before. Here are some suggestions for managing this difficult time.

- Participate in decisions about your treatment and care to the extent possible for you. Maintaining a sense of control is associated with better health outcomes.

- Be an informed consumer. If you have questions for your physician, write them down and ask them at your next appointment. Find out information about the type of cancer you have if that is helpful to you.

- Make sure you are comfortable with your health care team; ideally, they will provide both technical expertise and emotional support.

- Consider how you will interact with family members, friends, and acquaintances—with whom will you share your diagnosis, and when? Who will provide you with the emotional support you need? Who will be able to help out with tasks such as accompanying or driving you to medical appointments?

- Consider your school or work obligations. You may have to take time off for treatment, and you may experience job discrimination. The Rehabilitation Act and the Americans with Disabilities Act are two federal laws that protect cancer patients. Your health insurance plan cannot drop you even if you leave your job, although your rates may go up and you will have to pay for it yourself.

- Be prepared for changes in your everyday routine; you may have to have daily treatments, or you may have to travel some distance for treatment. Many hospitals and communities have developed resources for families of cancer patients, such as Ronald McDonald houses for families of children with cancer. Find out about the resources available to you.

- Enlist support. A cancer support group can offer information, teach coping skills, and give you a place to voice your concerns and share your experiences. You can find support groups through your health care team, church, or community or on the Internet.

- Know what physical changes are likely to occur. For example, some cancer treatments have side effects that change how you feel on a daily basis; others change your appearance, as when chemotherapy causes hair loss. Your sense of identity may be affected, as you adapt to the loss of your health, of your precancer life, or of the integrity of your body (for example, if you have a breast removed or a limb amputated).

- If you have spiritual beliefs or practices, they can be an important part of life now. Research suggests that people with a sense of spirituality have a better quality of life while living with cancer than those who are not spiritual.

- Comply with follow-up recommendations. People with a history of cancer face the challenge of later developing a second cancer, as a result either of a genetic predisposition or of the cancer treatment itself. Survivors of childhood cancer are closely monitored to increase the likelihood that any second cancers will be detected early.

- Consult with your physician about the possibility of collecting and saving sperm and eggs before starting treatment if you are a young adult concerned about your future fertility.

- Know that palliative care, particularly hospice care, is available to you if you find you are facing incurable cancer. A team of physicians, nurses, social workers, and volunteers will work with you and your family to provide support for the physical, economic, emotional, and spiritual challenges of terminal cancer. The hospice philosophy views death as a natural part of life and emphasizes quality of life for the dying person and family members.

It's Not Just Personal . . .

Throughout the world, cancer support groups range from a dozen people who meet monthly in a cancer center to large online groups whose members log on any time to share their ups and downs. These groups may be organized in different ways—according to the type of cancer, the stage of cancer experience, or the coping skills needed. What they offer in common is a sense of togetherness and hope.

You Make the Call

Should Research on Embryonic Stem Cells Be Supported?

The issue of whether human embryonic stem cells should be used in research is a subject of heated public and private debate. Scientists believe that stem cells have the potential for a wide range of applications, including treatment and even cures for diabetes, many cancers, and neurological diseases such as Parkinson's disease and Alzheimer's disease. Yet, in 2001, President Bush announced restrictions on federal funding for stem cell research, limiting funds to research on certain embryonic stem cell lines that were already in existence (only lines that were created for reproductive purposes and no longer needed, and that were being used with the informed consent of the donors and with no financial inducements). Largely in response to the federal restrictions, California voters passed a controversial measure, Proposition 71, in November, 2004, approving $3 billion in bonds to fund stem cell research. A July 7, 2005, public opinion poll indicated that 58 percent of Americans support the use of embryonic stem cells in medical research and 63 percent favor a uniform national policy for research using embryonic stem cells.

What is involved in this controversial issue? As noted in the chapter, stem cells are undifferentiated cells with the potential for unlimited division. As such, they hold out the promise of repair or replacement for cells that have been damaged or are no longer functioning properly. Embryonic stem cells are derived from human embryos, most of which come from fertility clinics. In the course of in vitro fertilization and other fertility treatments, extra embryos are routinely created. Following fertilization, eggs are allowed to develop in culture for four to five days to the blastocyst stage (a ball of cells). After one or a few blastocysts are implanted in the woman's uterus, it is common practice to freeze the extras until the woman or the couple decides to use them (by implantation), donate them (for use by another infertile person), destroy them, or donate them for research purposes. If a person or couple elects to donate the embryo for research, cells from the center of the blastocyst are transferred to a culture dish and allowed to grow. The cells can yield millions of embryonic stem cells in culture, referred to as a stem cell line.

Stem cells can also be derived from adults. Such cells, which are present in many tissues and organs, can, in theory, divide indefinitely and differentiate into specialized cell types. Adult stem cells can be identified within tissues by special techniques, then collected and grown in culture. Adult stem cells differ in several ways from embryonic stem cells. Embryonic stem cells can differentiate into all cell types in the body, but adult stem cells are generally limited to the cell types of their tissue of origin and thus are less versatile. Embryonic stem cells can be grown rela-tively easily in culture, creating millions of cells; such large numbers may be needed for stem cell therapies. Adult stem cells are rare, their isolation is difficult, and they are more difficult to culture in large numbers. Many scientists believe embryonic stem cells have greater potential than adult stem cells do because of their greater versatility.

Opponents of embryonic stem cell research believe that it is immoral and unacceptable to destroy human embryos—potential human beings—in pursuit of any goal, no matter how noble. In announcing federal funding restrictions, President Bush stated, "This allows us to explore the promise and potential of stem cell research without crossing a fundamental moral line by providing taxpayer funding that would sanction or encourage further destruction of human embryos that have at least a potential for life." Federal policy allows funding for research using the 60 or so embryonic stem cell lines that were created prior to the announcement, because those embryos had already been destroyed, as well as research using adult stem cell lines.

Supporters argue that while embryos represent the potential for human life, there are people already alive who are suffering from diseases and who could benefit from this research. They point out that that according to most definitions, pregnancy begins when a blastocyst implants in the lining of the uterus, usually about a week after fertilization; until this point, the cluster of cells cannot really be considered potential human life. Proponents further claim that the existing embryonic stem cell lines are insufficient for the research that could be done, and they dispute the number of usable lines. They also point out that adult stem cells do not have the vast potential of embryonic stem cells.

In addition, supporters warn that without a nationally sanctioned embryonic stem cell research program, other countries will outpace the United States, making advances in medicine and technology and luring U.S. scientists to their labs. Already, scientists are leaving institutions in other states and moving to California to pursue their research. Finally, a nationally sanctioned research program would impose uniform standards on researchers who may be working now with few constraints.

Embryonic stem cell research might hold out hope for millions, but opponents question the moral and ethical cost. What do you think?

Pros

- Embryonic stem cell research may eventually lead to therapies that could be used to treat diseases that afflict millions of people.

○ Embryonic stem cells are derived from excess embryos created in the course of fertility treatment. Individuals must eventually decide the fate of their excess embryos, and many people are willing to donate them for research purposes. To be morally consistent, opponents should also oppose fertility treatments, including in vitro fertilization, which create the embryos that may be discarded or used in research.

○ Federally funded adult stem cell research has resulted in therapeutic treatments, and scientists believe embryonic stem cells hold even greater promise.

○ If federal funding is restricted, states and private organizations may proceed in a less regulated fashion.

Cons

○ Human life begins with conception; thus, embryos are human beings deserving of all the protections afforded infants, children, and adults.

○ There are already more than 60 human embryonic stem cell lines in existence, and federal funds can be used for research on these lines.

○ Adult stem cell lines have untapped potential and do not involve the moral dilemma associated with use of human embryos.

○ Current federal guidelines are intended to provide a uniform national policy.

○ If scientists are allowed to create new embryonic stem cell lines, there may be an incentive for the creation of embryos specifically for this purpose, perhaps for profit.

OLC Web site For more information on this topic, visit the Online Learning Center at www.mhhe.com/teague1e.

SOURCES: "Fact Sheet Embryonic Stem Cell Research," August 9, 2001, Office of the Press Secretary, www.whitehouse.gov/news/releases/2001; "Stem Cell Basics," June 10, 2004, National Institutes of Health, Department of Health and Human Services, http://stemcells.nih.gov; "Guidelines Released for Embryonic Stem Cell Research," National Academies, National Research Council, April 26, 2005, www.nationalacademies.org/news; "Californians Approve Stem Cell Research Funding," AP Press, November 2, 2004, www.usatoday.com/news.

SUMMARY

- Cancer, the second leading cause of death in the United States, is a condition characterized by the uncontrolled growth of cells.

- Healthy cells have a complicated system of checks and balances that control cell growth. Stem cells, which are capable of unlimited growth, are located deep within tissues to protect them from factors that might cause mutations.

- Cancer occurs when a critical mutation, called an initiating event, allows a cell to evade one of the restraints on growth. A series of 5 to 10 additional mutations can cause the cell to become cancerous and develop into a tumor, a mass of extra tissue.

- A benign tumor grows in one place and can interfere with normal functioning. A malignant tumor can invade neighboring tissue and metastasize to other parts of the body.

- When a cancer is still at its original site, it is called a localized cancer; when it has metastasized, it is called an invasive cancer. Tumors are graded by the degree to which they resemble healthy cells; the stage is a description of how far the cancer has spread.

- Four broad types of cancer are distinguished based on the type of tissue in which they originate. Carcinomas originate in epithelial tissue, sarcomas in connective tissue, leukemias in the bone marrow or lymphatic system, and lymphomas in the lymph nodes or glands.

- Risk factors include a family history of cancer, indicating a genetic predisposition; lifestyle factors, especially tobacco use, dietary patterns, overweight and obesity, physical inactivity, and excessive alcohol consumption; and environmental factors, including exposure to ultraviolet radiation and high-frequency ionizing radiation, chemical carcinogens, and infectious agents.

- Lung cancer is the leading cause of cancer death in both men and women and the second most commonly diagnosed cancer. The leading risk factor is tobacco use.

- Colon and rectal cancer is the third leading cause of cancer death in men and women and the third most commonly diagnosed cancer. Risk factors include age and a high-fat diet, among others.

- Breast cancer is the second leading cause of cancer death in women and the most commonly diagnosed cancer in women. Breast cancer has both controllable and non-controllable risk factors. Mammograms, self-exams, and clinical exams can all help detect breast cancer.

- Prostate cancer is the second leading cause of cancer death in men and the most commonly diagnosed cancer in men. The leading risk factor is age. Two screening tests, the digital rectal exam and the PSA blood test, can help detect prostate cancer.

- Cancers of the female reproductive tract include cervical cancer, uterine (endometrial) cancer, and ovarian cancer. Rates of cervical cancer have dropped sharply as a result of improved screening through the Pap test. Ovarian cancer is difficult to detect and is the fourth leading cause of cancer death in women.

- Two types of skin cancer, basal cell and squamous cell carcinomas, are curable if they are caught early. Melanoma is a dangerous form of skin cancer that usually begins in a mole and can quickly spread to almost any part of the body. All forms can be caused by sun exposure, and prevention involves protecting the skin from sources of ultraviolet radiation, including tanning salons.

- Testicular cancer is the most commonly diagnosed cancer in young men. This cancer is very treatable and can sometimes be cured even when it has metastasized.

- Oral cancers are most often caused by tobacco use, especially in combination with alcohol consumption.

- Leukemia is the overgrowth of one type of white blood cell, preventing other blood cells from functioning normally.

- Regular screening tests are recommended for breast, colon, and cervical cancers.

- Cancer treatments include surgery, chemotherapy, radiation, biological therapies, bone marrow transplantation, and gene therapy. Clinical trials are studies of new drugs and treatments.

- With a survival rate for all types of cancer combined at 63 percent, many people face the challenges involved in living with a cancer diagnosis, undergoing treatment, or becoming cancer survivors.

REVIEW QUESTIONS

1. Approximately what percentage of deaths are caused by cancer each year in the United States? What is the leading cause of cancer death?

2. What is clonal growth?

3. What are five safety mechanisms that regulate cell growth and division?

4. What are stem cells, and what safety mechanisms protect them from mutation?

5. What is an oncogene? What are hyperplasia and dysplasia?

6. What is the difference between a benign tumor and a malignant tumor?

7. What three characteristics determine the stage of a cancer?

8. What are the four broad types of cancers, and where do they originate?

9. Why do so many cancers arise in epithelial tissue?

10. Why does chance play a role in cancer?

11. What actions are suggested for people with an inherited susceptibility to cancer?

12. What lifestyle behaviors contribute the most to cancer risk?

13. How can tobacco use cause cancers of the pancreas, liver, or kidney?

14. What are some dietary strategies for preventing cancer? What is the "New American Plate"?

15. What are some possible pathways to cancer in people who are overweight or obese?

16. Describe four sources of radiation to which people may be exposed.

17. What are three ways infectious agents may increase the risk of cancer?

18. Why have rates of lung cancer been declining in men but only leveling off in women?

19. What are the risk factors for lung cancer? What are the signs and symptoms of this disease? What treatments are available?

20. What are the risk factors for colon cancer? What is the difference between sigmoidoscopy and colonoscopy?

21. What are the noncontrollable and controllable risk factors for breast cancer? What screening tests are available?

22. What two screening tests are available for prostate cancer? Why is routine blood testing for prostate cancer controversial?

23. Why have rates of cervical cancer declined in the last few decades? What are the symptoms of uterine cancer? Why is ovarian cancer so deadly?

24. What are the three forms of skin cancer, and which is the most dangerous form?

25. What are the warning signs of melanoma? What are the recommended ways of avoiding sun exposure?

26. What are the signs and symptoms of basal cell carcinoma? Of squamous cell carcinoma?

27. What are the risk factors for testicular cancer? What are the signs and symptoms?

28. What risk factors are associated with oral cancers? What are the signs and symptoms of these cancers?

29. Why is early detection of leukemia difficult? What treatments are available?

30. What are the three leading causes of cancer death in men? In women? What are the three most commonly diagnosed cancers in men? In women?

31. For which cancers are routine screening tests available?

32. How do chemotherapy drugs work? What are their side effects?

33. What are two biological therapies for cancer?

34. What are three possible ways that gene therapy might be used to treat or prevent cancer?

35. What are some questions and issues that people being treated with cancer or living with cancer have to face?

WEB RESOURCES

American Academy of Dermatology: Visit this site for information on sun protection, the different types of skin cancer, and finding a skin cancer screening site in your area. www.aad.org

American Cancer Society: The ACS site features topics such as learning about cancer, treatment options, treatment decision tools, clinical trials, and coping strategies. Its Statistics and Facts and Figures are valuable resources for health care consumers. www.cancer.org

American Institute for Cancer Research: This organization offers resources for cancer prevention, a free information program for cancer patients about living with cancer, and news about the latest advances in cancer research. www.aicr.org

Cancer News: Visit this site for news and information on cancer diagnosis, treatment, and prevention. Its Cancer Profiler shows the treatment options for different types of cancer. www.cancernews.com

Centers for Disease Control and Prevention: The cancer section of this site provides facts on all types of cancers. Its links lead to information on risk factors, prevention, survivorship, and statistics. www.cdc.gov

National Cancer Institute: This site offers a wide range of cancer information, including types, treatments, terminology, support and resources, screening and testing, statistics, and research. www.cancer.gov

National Coalition for Cancer Survivorship: This organization focuses on survivorship issues, such as palliative care and management of symptoms. It offers a cancer survival toolbox and a resource guide with links to other helpful sites. www.canceradvocacy.org

REFERENCES

1. American Cancer Society. Cancer statistics 2005. www.cancer.org.

2. American Joint Committee on Cancer. (2002). *AJCC cancer staging manual* (6th ed.). New York: Springer.

3. National Cancer Institute. Genetics of breast and ovarian cancer. U.S. National Institutes of Health. www.cancer.gov.

4. National Cancer Institute. Genetics of colorectal cancer. U.S. National Institutes of Health. www.cancer.gov.

5. American Cancer Society. (2004). *Cancer facts and figures 2004.* Atlanta, GA: Author.

6. National Cancer Institute. Cancer progress report—2003 update. http://progressreport.cancer.gov.

7. Marks, R. (1999). Two decades of the public health approach to skin cancer control in Australia: Why, how, and where we are now. *Australian Journal of Dermatology, 40* (1), 1–5.

8. American Cancer Society. Cancer prevention and early detection: Facts and figures 2004. www.cancer.org.

9. Wakeford, R. (2004). The cancer epidemiology of radiation. *Oncogene, 23* (38), 6404–6428.

10. National Cancer Institute. Human papillomaviruses and cancer. www.cancer.gov/cancer_information.

11. Giovannucci, E. (2002). Modifiable risk factors for colon cancer. *Gastroenterology Clinics of North America, 31* (4), 925–943.

12. Schoenfeld, P., et al. (2005). Colonoscopic screening of average-risk women for colorectal neoplasia. *New England Journal of Medicine, 352* (20), 2061–2068.

13. Fletcher, S. (2004). Screening for breast cancer. UptoDate ONLINE. http://patients.uptodate.com.

14. Paley, P. J. (2001). Screening for the major malignancies affecting women: Current guidelines. *American Journal of Obstetrics and Gynecology, 184* (5), 1021–1030.

15. Lacey, J. V., et al. (2002). Menopausal hormone replacement therapy and risk of ovarian cancer. *Journal of the American Medical Association, 288,* 334–341.

16. National Cancer Institute. Ovarian cancer. U.S. National Institutes of Health. www.cancer.gov.

17. Klotz, L. H. (1999). Why is the rate of testicular cancer increasing? *Canadian Medical Association Journal, 160* (2), 213–214.

18. National Cancer Institute. Testicular cancer. U.S. National Institutes of Health. www.cancer.gov.

19. National Cancer Institute. Types of treatment. U.S. National Institutes of Health. www.cancer.gov.

20. Couzin, J. (2004). Pharmacogenomics: Cancer sharpshooters rely on DNA tests for better aim. *Science, 305* (5688), 1222–1223.

21. Paik, S., et al. (2004). A multigene assay to predict recurrence of tamoxifen-treated, node negative breast cancer. *New England Journal of Medicine, 351* (27), 2817–2826.

Add It Up! ASSESSING YOUR RISK FACTORS FOR CANCER

The more risk factors you have for a particular cancer, the greater the likelihood that you will develop that cancer. In the lists below for six common cancers—lung, colon, breast, prostate, cervical, and melanoma—check any risk factors that apply to you. The more items you check, the more important it is that you adopt healthy lifestyle behaviors and have regular screening tests. There is no score.

Lung cancer risk factors

_____ Age greater than 40
_____ Family history of lung cancer
_____ Smoking cigarettes
_____ Smoking cigars
_____ Exposure to environmental tobacco smoke
_____ Exposure to air pollution
_____ Exposure to workplace chemicals
_____ Fewer than three servings of vegetables per day
_____ Fewer than three servings of fruit per day

Colon cancer risk factors

_____ Age greater than 50 (average age at diagnosis: 73)
_____ Family history of colon cancer
_____ Overweight
_____ More than one serving of red meat per day
_____ Fewer than three servings of vegetables per day
_____ More than one alcoholic drink per day
_____ Less than 30 minutes of physical activity per day
_____ Having inflammatory bowel disease for 10 years or more

Lower risk associated with:

- Taking a multivitamin with folate every day
- Taking birth control pills for at least 5 years
- Taking postmenopausal hormones for at least 5 years
- Taking aspirin regularly for more than 15 years
- Having regular screening tests

Breast cancer risk factors

_____ Age greater than 40 (average age at diagnosis: 62)
_____ Female sex
_____ Family history of breast cancer
_____ Jewish ethnicity, especially Ashkenazi descent
_____ Overweight
_____ Fewer than three servings of vegetables per day
_____ More than two alcoholic drinks per day
_____ Having had hyperplasia (benign breast disease)

Longer exposure to estrogen:

_____ Early age at menarche
_____ Older age at birth of first child
_____ Older age at menopause
_____ Fewer than two children
_____ Breast-feeding for less than one year combined for all pregnancies
_____ Currently taking birth control pills
_____ Taking postmenopausal hormones for 5 years or more

Prostate cancer risk factors

_____ Age greater than 55
_____ Family history of prostate cancer
_____ Five or more servings per day of foods containing animal fat
_____ Having had a vasectomy
_____ African American ethnicity

Lower risk associated with:

- Asian ethnicity
- At least one serving per day of tomato-based food

Cervical cancer risk factors

_____ Older age (average age at diagnosis: 47)
_____ Smoking cigarettes
_____ Having had sex at an early age
_____ Having had many sexual partners

_____ Having had an STD, especially HPV

_____ Having given birth to two or more children

Lower risk associated with:

- Using a condom or diaphragm on every occasion of sexual intercourse

- Having regular Pap tests

Melanoma risk factors

_____ Older age (average age at diagnosis: 57)

_____ Family history of melanoma

_____ Light-colored hair and eyes

_____ Having had severe, repeated sunburns in childhood

_____ Exposure to ultraviolet radiation

_____ Taking immunosuppressive drugs (for example, after organ transplant)

Lower risk associated with:

- Protecting the skin from the sun

- Regular self-examination of the skin

SOURCE: Adapted from "Your Disease Risk," Harvard Center for Cancer Prevention, www.yourdiseaserisk.harvard.edu.

CHAPTER **23**

Complementary and Alternative Medicine: Health Choices in a Changing Society

DID YOU KNOW?

- Do you practice meditation, deep breathing, progressive relaxation, yoga, or t'ai chi? If so, you are among the 62 percent of Americans who use some form of complementary and alternative medicine. Studies have found that many mind-body practices have positive effects on health.

- Pharmaceutical drugs undergo rigorous testing to demonstrate their safety and efficacy before they can be released for sale to consumers. Dietary supplements and herbal medicines are not required to meet this standard; they are simply subject to removal from the market if they prove harmful. Despite the different standards, there are as many safety concerns and risks associated with "natural" products as with drugs, if not more.

OLC *Your Health Today*   www.mhhe.com/teague1e

Go to the Online Learning Center for *Your Health Today* for interactive activities, quizzes, flashcards, Web links, and more resources related to this chapter.

If you catch a cold, do you drink chicken soup, take vitamin C and Echinacea, or get an acupuncture treatment? If you develop chronic lower back pain, do you start a regimen of stretching exercises, take pain medication, or see a chiropractor? Many options for health care are available in our society, and most people are aware of the different conventional health care providers they can consult, including physicians, psychologists, pharmacists, and so on. In the last 15 years, however, the use of **complementary and alternative medicine (CAM)** has grown dramatically. Some CAM practices have a degree of acceptance in conventional health care, such as chiropractic care and massage therapy; others, such as magnetic-field therapies and other forms of energy medicine, remain well outside the mainstream.

In this chapter we explore some of the practices, premises, therapies, and interventions that make up complementary and alternative medicine. We begin with a comparison of some of the underlying premises of Western conventional medicine with those of complementary and alternative medicine and a look at some facts about the use of CAM therapies. We then offer brief descriptions of several different categories of CAM practices, beginning with whole medical systems. We conclude the chapter with a consideration of the major three sectors of health care—conventional medicine, CAM, and self-care—and when and how to use each of them.

APPROACHES TO HEALTH CARE

As discussed in Chapter 1, health-related beliefs and practices are largely defined by a person's cultural background and context. In most industrialized countries, ideas about medicine are conditioned by the Western tradition; in other countries, different systems and sets of ideas have developed, in many cases over hundreds if not thousands of years. In recent years, some ideas and practices from other traditions have gained acceptance in Western medicine, as noted throughout this book. They include ideas about mind-body connections, the role of spirituality in wellness, and the importance of relationships and social support, among others.

In recognition of the interest in such ideas, Congress established the Office of Alternative Medicine in 1991 and expanded it into the National Center for Complementary and Alternative Medicine (NCCAM) in 1998. The NCCAM is an institute of the National Institutes of Health, which in turn is an agency of the U.S. Department of Health and Human Services. The goals of the NCCAM are to support the scientific investigation of complementary and alternative healing practices, to train researchers to explore these practices, and to disseminate authoritative information to the public and professionals. The NCCAM funds and conducts rigorous laboratory-based and clinical research projects and supports the integration of proven CAM practices into conventional medicine. In this way, the center acts as a clearinghouse for information about CAM and a bridge between the two traditions.

In this section we consider the features that have traditionally been part of Western medicine, and we contrast them with some of the features that characterize complementary and alternative medical practices. Remember that medical practices considered complementary or alternative in the United States may be, and in fact are likely to be, part of the mainstream medical system in other cultures.

Conventional Medicine

The term **conventional medicine** refers to the dominant health care system in the United States, Canada, and much of Europe and other parts of the developed world. Other terms for this system include *Western medicine, biomedicine,* and *allopathic medicine.*

Characteristics of Conventional Medicine

As discussed in Chapter 1, Western medicine has traditionally considered illness to be the result of pathogens like bacteria and viruses or organic changes in the body. Health is restored, according to this model, when a medical practitioner treats the illness with such means as drugs, vaccines, or surgery. Along with public health measures that improved the safety of the food and water supply, this medical intervention model has been highly successful in reducing the incidence of infectious diseases, enhancing quality of life, and lengthening life expectancy for people living in developed countries of the world.

Other characteristic ideas underlying conventional medicine include the following:

- The body is like a machine; it can be broken down into smaller parts that, in the case of illness, need to be fixed. The idea that the whole can be reduced to its parts—that the whole is not greater than the sum of its parts—is a way of thinking known as *reductionist.* The discovery of bacteria supported the search for isolated, external causes of disease and the tendency to treat diseases by destroying pathogens or limiting the damage they do.

- An illness is defined by a set of symptoms that are similar in everyone who has the illness. Thus, large populations can be treated the same way for a given disease, as in vaccination programs.

- Investigations into the causes of disease and treatments for them are conducted using the scientific method, which is based on empirical, observable evidence and controlled studies that can be verified and replicated by other researchers.

Conventional Health Care Providers

The practitioners of conventional medicine include an array of providers who often work side by side. Physicians

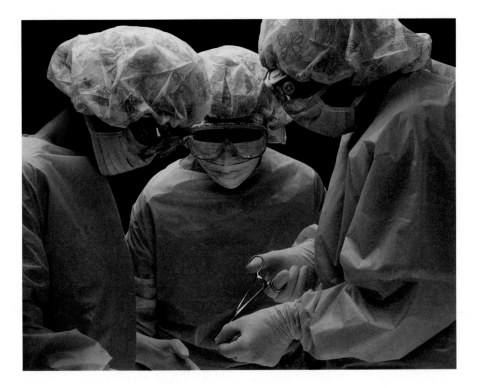

In conventional medicine, a team of health care providers, like this surgical team, work together in caring for the patient.

in conventional medicine hold an M.D. (medical doctor) or D.O. (doctor of osteopathy) degree. Physicians and other conventional providers often specialize in a specific part of the body: Cardiologists focus on the heart and blood vessels, neurosurgeons focus on brain surgery, orthopedists focus on bones and joints, and so on. Family physicians, pediatricians, and internists are considered generalists within conventional medicine. Other conventional providers include dentists, optometrists, podiatrists, and allied health care providers. This last category of trained professionals includes registered nurses, nurse practitioners, licensed vocational nurses, physician assistants, physical therapists, registered dietitians, nurse midwives, and medical assistants. Standards of practice and credentialing policies for providers are established by states and by professional medical associations.

Complementary and Alternative Medicine

As defined by the NCCAM, complementary and alternative medicine is "a group of diverse medical and health care systems, practices, and products that are not presently considered to be part of conventional medicine."[1] Note that practices considered complementary or alternative are "not presently" considered part of conventional medicine, but they may be in the future. As practices and approaches are studied and evaluated, they may be adopted into conventional medicine. In short, this highly fluid definition simply distinguishes CAM practices from the dominant health care system in the United States at the present time.

Complementary medicine is a group of practices used together with conventional medicine. The use of acupuncture to reduce pain after surgery would be considered a complement to conventional medicine. **Alternative medicine** is a group of practices used as an alternative to conventional medicine. The use of a special diet instead of chemotherapy as a treatment for cancer would be considered an alternative to conventional medicine. **Integrative medicine** combines conventional medicine and CAM

KEY TERMS

complementary and alternative medicine (CAM) As defined by the NCCAM, a group of diverse medical and health care systems, practices, and products that are not presently considered to be part of conventional medicine.

conventional medicine   The dominant health care system in the United States, Canada, and much of Europe and the rest of the developed world; also referred to as Western medicine, biomedicine, and allopathic medicine.

complementary medicine   Group of practices used together with conventional medicine.

alternative medicine   Group of practices used as an alternative to conventional medicine.

integrative medicine   Use of conventional medicine in combination with CAM practices that have been proven safe and effective.

HIGHLIGHT ON HEALTH

Domains of CAM and Representative Practices

Provider-based practices are indicated with an asterisk (*). Those without an asterisk can be performed without a provider.

Mind-Body Practices

Biofeedback*
Deep breathing
Guided imagery or visualization
Hypnosis*
Meditation
Prayer for health purposes
Progressive relaxation
T'ai chi
Yoga

Biologically Based Practices

Dietary supplements
Herbal medicines
Megavitamins

Manipulative and Body-Based Practices

Chiropractic care*
Massage therapy*
Rolfing*
Feldenkrais*

Energy Therapies

Magnetic-field therapies
Qigong
Reiki*

Whole Medical Systems

Homeopathy*
Naturopathy*
Ayurvedic medicine*
Traditional Chinese Medicine*
Acupuncture*

Source: National Center for Complementary and Alternative Medicine, www.nccam.nih.gov.

---

practices.[1] Sometimes a conventional health care provider and a CAM provider will work together to provide integrative medicine. At other times, a conventional provider will have training in certain CAM practices and integrate both forms of medicine. For example, some physicians and dentists obtain training in acupuncture and incorporate it into their medical or dental practices.[2]

Characteristics of Complementary and Alternative Medicine

CAM approaches encompass a vast array of practices that have developed in different cultures all over the world. Although they are extremely diverse, they have certain characteristics in common, including the following:

- The body is believed to have an inherent balance or ability to heal itself; treatments are aimed at restoring the balance or enhancing the body's self-healing capabilities.

- The whole person is treated, taking into account the physical, mental, emotional, and spiritual dimensions, rather than focusing on a particular part of the body or a specific pathogenic process.

- Each person is unique, so diagnosis and treatment are individualized. Symptoms of a cold in one person might require a different treatment than would similar symptoms in another person. The focus tends to be on the imbalance in a person that allows him or her to be susceptible to illness at this time rather than on the pathogen that might be causing illness in many people.

- Many practices use a complex combination of interventions, often involving the administration of many medications or medicinal substances at the same time, in addition to recommended behaviors, rather than a single intervention.[3,4]

Instead of taking allergy medication, this patient has chosen an alternative medicine approach that includes a special diet designed by a naturopath.

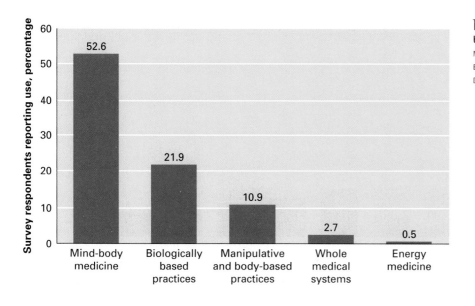

Figure 23.1   Use of CAM therapies, **by domain.** Source: "Complementary and Alternative Medicine Use Among Adults: United States, 2002," by P. Barnes, E. Powell-Griner, K. McFann, and R. Nahin, 2004, CDC Advance Data Report No. 343, www.nccam.nih.gov.

CAM Providers

Some CAM practices have well-established training programs with licensing and credentialing procedures similar to those in place for conventional providers. To become an acupuncturist in many states, for example, a person has to complete a rigorous course of training at a school of Chinese medicine and pass a state licensing exam or meet national certification requirements. Acupuncturists have to keep up to date by accumulating continuing education units, and they usually have to renew their licenses every 2 years. Other practices do not have standardized training programs, which can make it difficult for the consumer to evaluate a provider's background and competence.[2]

Classification and Use of CAM Practices

In an attempt to organize the diverse range of practices included in CAM, the NCCAM has identified four domains—mind-body interventions, biologically based therapies, manipulative and body-based therapies, and energy therapies—in addition to whole medical systems, which cut across the four domains and employ practices from some or all of them (see the box "Domains of CAM and Representative Practices").

In 2004 the NCCAM and the National Center for Health Statistics (NCHS) released the results of the National Health Interview Survey (NHIS), in which more than 30,000 Americans reported on their health-related behaviors, including their use of CAM. According to the survey, 62 percent of Americans report using some form of CAM when megavitamin therapy and prayer for health purposes are included. When these two interventions are excluded, 36 percent report using some form of CAM. The most commonly used domain of CAM is mind-body medicine when prayer for health reasons is included.

When prayer is not included, the use of biologically based or natural products (such as herbal remedies) is the most popular form of CAM (Figure 23.1).

CAM practices are more commonly used by women than by men and by people with higher educational levels. The use of CAM also varies by ethnic group (Figure 23.2). The condition for which CAM therapies are most frequently used is back pain, followed by colds and other kinds of body aches and pains. CAM therapies are also commonly used for anxiety and depression, stomach upset, headache, and insomnia (Figure 23.3).

Figure 23.2   Use of CAM therapies, by ethnicity and race.
Source: "Complementary and Alternative Medicine Use Among Adults: United States, 2002," by P. Barnes, E. Powell-Griner, K. McFann, and R. Nahin, 2004, CDC Advance Data Report No. 343, www.nccam.nih.gov.

Figure 23.3   Disease or condition for which CAM is most frequently used. Source: "Complementary and Alternative Medicine Use Among Adults: United States, 2002, by P. Barnes, E. Powell-Griner, K. McFann, and R. Nahin, 2004, CDC Advance Data Report No. 343, www.nccam.nih.gov.

Figure excludes the use of megavitamin therapy and prayer.

Factors considered important in the use of CAM are the desire of patients to be actively involved in their health care decisions, access to information about CAM on the Internet, and dissatisfaction with the limitations of conventional medicine in treating chronic conditions. For immigrant populations, the use of CAM in the United States is often a continuation of the medicine they practiced in their country of origin.[4]

WHOLE MEDICAL SYSTEMS

A whole medical system is a comprehensive group of practices based on a common philosophy. Some of the more widely known whole medical systems are Traditional Chinese Medicine; Ayurveda, a medical system developed in India; and two Western medical systems, homeopathy and naturopathy. Systems of folk medicine have developed in many cultures around the world, including Native American, African, and South American cultures.

Traditional Chinese Medicine

A well-developed medical system that has been in use in China for nearly 3,000 years, **Traditional Chinese Medicine (TCM)** focuses on maintaining or restoring the physical, mental, and spiritual well-being of the individual.[5] A basic concept is that good health stems from the free flow of **qi** (or **chi**), vital energy or life force, through the body. Qi moves through the body along several *meridians,* or pathways, each of which is linked with an internal organ or organ system. Illness occurs when the

flow of qi is blocked, usually as a result of an imbalance between yin and yang, two opposing but inseparable principles. *Yin* represents the inactive, internal, cold, and dark; *yang* represents the active, external, hot, and bright. Yin and yang are interdependent; each exists within the other, as can be seen in the yin-yang symbol (Figure 23.4). Good health requires balance and harmony between yin and yang; a deficiency or an excess of one or the other causes a disruption in the flow of qi, resulting in illness.[5]

Diagnosis in TCM involves evaluating an individual for signs of imbalance. Complexion, posture, body fluids, appearance of the tongue, and the quality of pulse in various locations of the body can all be used in diagnosis. The primary treatment methods are herbal medicines and acupuncture. Preventing illness in TCM involves maintaining a proper lifestyle, which includes eating a balanced diet, getting regular sleep, pursuing an active life, avoiding excessive stress, refraining from

Figure 23.4   Yin-yang symbol. *As indicated by the small circles within the larger symbol, the two forces are interdependent and exist within each other. Nothing is all black or all white.*

overindulgence in alcohol and sex, getting regular exercise, and protecting the body during harsh weather and seasonal changes.[6]

Herbal Medicine

Specific herbal remedies are believed to strengthen the blood, body, or organs that are imbalanced or weak. Different herbs have different actions and functions, but each one contains dozens of active compounds. Usually, several herbs are combined in a formula, and the proportions and dosage are adjusted to suit the characteristics of the particular patient. Chinese herbal remedies are difficult to evaluate or even analyze because of this variation. Herbal medicine is discussed more fully later in the chapter.

Acupuncture

Long, thin needles are inserted at certain points in the skin to stimulate the flow of qi in **acupuncture.** The acupuncturist assesses the individual by questioning, observing, and performing a physical exam that focuses on the tongue, pulse, and any painful trigger points, which correlate with pathways and organs that need rebalancing. Needles are inserted in a pattern that opens blockages and restores energy flow. Treatment usually takes about 30 minutes and may be repeated weekly for 5 to 10 sessions.[7] Practitioners may also use **moxibustion,** a treatment in which heat is applied to acupuncture points by burning an herb called moxa.

In the United States, acupuncture is used primarily to treat muscular problems. Limited studies indicate that acupuncture can help relieve both acute and chronic pain. It is also used to decrease nausea and vomiting during pregnancy and cancer treatment, and studies suggest it may be helpful in substance withdrawal and drug treatment programs.[7] Millions of Americans use acupuncture each year, with relatively few complications reported. The FDA requires that acupuncturists use sterile, disposable needles to reduce the risk of spreading infection from person to person. Some mild side effects sometimes occur, including sleepiness, fatigue, and pain at the needle site. Very rarely, life-threatening complications have occurred, including serious infection, shortness of breath, organ punctures, and spinal cord injuries.

Ayurveda

One of the oldest healing systems in the world, **Ayurvedic medicine** has been practiced in India for 5,000 years.[8] It emphasizes balance among the body, mind, and spirit and sets a goal of restoring harmony to the individual. Three energy sources, called *doshas,* are believed to be present within everyone and everything. *Vatta* is the energy of movement and consists of space and air. *Pitta* is the energy of metabolism and digestion and consists of fire and water. *Kapha* is the energy that forms body structure and holds cells together; it consists of earth and water.[9] Each person has a unique combination of the three doshas at birth. One or more can be dominant, and seven different combinations are possible. When your three doshas are in balance, you are in good health. When there is an imbalance in your doshas, your body is susceptible to disease. Even if you have a bacterial or viral infection, an Ayurvedic health provider will try to determine why you are susceptible to infection at this particular time.

Ayurvedic practitioners work by helping you align your individual lifestyle with your particular constitution

Complementary medicine is a treatment that is used in conjunction with conventional medicine. This woman is receiving an acupuncture treatment to enhance the effects of her medications for postoperative pain.

KEY TERMS

Traditional Chinese Medicine (TCM) Well-developed medical system originating in China; TCM's focus is on maintaining or restoring the physical, mental, and spiritual well-being of the individual.

qi (chi) Vital energy or life force, believed to flow through the body; a concept in TCM and other forms of CAM.

acupuncture Treatment method in TCM involving the insertion of long, thin needles at certain points in the skin to stimulate the flow of qi.

moxibustion Treatment in which heat is applied to acupuncture points by burning an herb called moxa.

Ayurvedic medicine Traditional medical system of India; its focus is on restoring balance among the body, mind, and spirit.

and health history. Assessment involves questioning and observation, especially of the pulse, tongue, eyes, and body fluids. Treatment options include dietary modification, exercises, yoga, meditation, massage, herbal tonics, and controlled breathing.[9]

There is no formalized Ayurvedic training or licensing system in the United States. Some U.S.- trained health care providers complete short courses in India or the United States and incorporate elements of Ayurvedic medicine in their practices.

Homeopathy

A set of principles developed by German chemist and physician Samuel Hahnemann in the 19th century are the basis for **homeopathy.** One principle of homeopathy is the law of similars, or "like cures like." According to this principle, a substance that causes disease in a healthy person can cure the same symptoms in a sick person. For instance, large doses of a plant bark called cinchona will cause a healthy person to develop a fever; homeopaths believe that if a person has a fever, taking a remedy made from diluted cinchona will help the person recover faster.[10]

A second principle of homeopathy is the principle of minimal dose. According to this principle, using the smallest possible dose will have the greatest effect. Homeopathic remedies are intended to encourage the body to heal itself; thus, a single small dose is often enough. Remedies are derived from many natural sources, including plants, animals, chemicals, metals, and minerals, and are made through a process called *succession,* a series of shaking and diluting. Solutions are often so diluted that no chemical evidence of the original substance remains.

The third principle of homeopathy is prescribing for the individual. According to this principle, every patient is unique. Treatment in homeopathy is prescribed based not only on the medical diagnosis but also on the specific patient's personality characteristics and emotional and physical responses.

Studying the effectiveness of this system in large groups of people is difficult because of the uniqueness of each individual treatment plan. The studies that have been conducted have had mixed results, with some showing no improvements and others showing benefits. Homeopathy may be beneficial in treating allergies, acute diarrhea in children, and arthritis and in reducing the duration of influenza.[11]

There does not appear to be significant risk associated with homeopathy. Some studies have shown minor, limited side effects, such as headaches, tiredness, and symptom aggravation, and some problems have arisen due to mislabeling of homeopathic products. The cost of homeopathic medications is typically less than that of pharmaceutical medications, but approximately $200 million is spent on homeopathic treatments each year in the United States.[10]

In Europe, homeopathy is practiced as a separate health profession, but in the United States, it is practiced as a subset of another profession. It is a standard component of naturopathy training; medical doctors, osteopaths, chiropractors, and acupuncturists sometimes take courses in homeopathy and integrate it into their practice.

Naturopathy

Like the other systems described in this section, **naturopathy** is a philosophy and way of life as much as a health system. Its main principle is that the body has the ability to heal itself, and its goal is to stimulate the body to do so, especially through nutrition. Health is believed to be the natural order if one lives wisely and simply. The focus of naturopathy is on cleansing and strengthening the body rather than on treating the symptoms of a specific illness.

Assessment may include interviewing, observation, evaluation of body fluids, hair analysis, and iridology (a detailed microscopic evaluation of the iris of the eye to aid in diagnosis of disease and illness). Treatments include a variety of noninvasive therapeutic practices, including dietary modification, nutritional supplementation, herbal remedies, hydrotherapy, massage and joint manipulation, homeopathy, acupuncture, biofeedback, stress reduction techniques, and lifestyle counseling.[12]

Several colleges of naturopathy now exist in the United States. Naturopaths complete a four-year training program and then take a licensing exam, although only some states currently license or regulate naturopaths.[2] Only scant data for evaluating naturopathy as a complete system of medicine are available.

Folk Medicine

Traditional healing systems, or **folk medicine,** flourished in all cultures long before the development of conventional Western medicine. The various forms of folk medicine that developed among the Native American tribes of North America are an example. A common thread in most forms of folk medicine is the integral relationship of humans with one another, the natural environment, and the spiritual world. Healing and spirituality merge; physical well-being is associated with spiritual balance and illness with imbalance.

Folk healers, whether called shamans, *curanderos,* or medicine men or women, are considered to have spiritual powers or ties to the supernatural. The ability to heal is seen as a gift, often passed down through several generations of the same family. In addition, through a process of observation or apprenticeship, the healer usually learns the medicinal uses of roots, herbs, and other plants.

In most folk medicine systems, illness can have internal or external causes. Internal causes are primarily negative thoughts about oneself or others or the breaking of

Beating the Odds

Who Is Least Likely to Develop Health Problems?

Both conventional medicine and CAM therapies have risks associated with them. Knowing the risks and taking steps to minimize danger are signs of an informed consumer. Brief profiles of three individuals are presented here. Which one do you think is least likely to develop health problems?

Paula is a 25-year-old graduate student in biochemistry. She has had problems with her weight since she was a teenager and currently has a BMI of 30. She has tried many diets and exercise plans with little success. Recently, she started seeing her family physician about her weight, and he is prescribing Meridia, a prescription weight loss drug. She also takes a weight loss supplement that she ordered from the Internet. It lists about 20 ingredients on the label but doesn't indicate what they do. She has not told her physician about the supplement.

Jack is a 27-year-old contractor who lifts weights as a hobby and has entered a few strength competitions. When he started having some problems with low back pain, he began seeing a chiropractor once a week for adjustments. The treatments seem to be helping with the pain. For the past year, Jack has also been taking megadoses of vitamins and a muscle-enhancing supplement. His girlfriend recently asked him what substances were in the supplement, and he could not tell her.

Wendy is a 37-year-old woman who has been trying to get pregnant for 5 years. She briefly tried fertility drugs, but she didn't like the side effects, and she and her husband were worried that they would have twins or triplets. A friend with a 6-month-old baby told her she got pregnant after being treated by a practitioner of Traditional Chinese Medicine, and Wendy started seeing him too. He gives her acupuncture treatments. He also suggested that she and her husband try yoga or t'ai chi to reduce stress. Wendy is optimistic that she will get pregnant soon.

OLC Web site Visit the **Online Learning Center** at www.mhhe.com/teague1e for comments by the authors.

---

taboos. External causes might be poisons, traumas, ghosts, witchcraft, or negative thoughts sent from another person. Although a causal agent may be external, individuals are more susceptible if there is an imbalance in their spirit. Techniques that aid in diagnosis and treatment include vision quests, dream interpretation, purification ceremonies, and the use of sweat lodges. Specific remedies may include prayer, healing touch, herbal teas, tinctures, charms, and healing rituals.[13]

DOMAINS OF COMPLEMENTARY AND ALTERNATIVE MEDICINE

The four categories of CAM identified by the NCCAM, as noted earlier, are mind-body practices, biologically based practices, manipulative and body-based practices, and energy therapies. (To assess your existing knowledge of CAM practices, see the box "Who Is Least Likely to Develop Health Problems?")

Mind-Body Practices

Mind-body practices are based on the premise that the mind influences the body in ways that can promote or detract from well-being. Perceptions, beliefs, and patterns of thinking can have a powerful effect on the immune system, endocrine system, cardiovascular system, digestive system, and other parts of the body. For example, as discussed in Chapters 5 and 21, chronic anger and hostility can cause the release of stress hormones, which can damage the lining of arteries and contribute to cardiovascular disease. Conversely, techniques that enhance stress management, relaxation, and coping skills are beneficial adjuncts to treatment for people with coronary heart disease and pain-related conditions such as arthritis.

Several mind-body practices have been described in this book in the context of mental health, spirituality, and

KEY TERMS

homeopathy Medical system based on a set of principles developed by Samuel Hahnemann in the 19th century; principles include the law of similars and the principle of minimal dose.

naturopathy Health system based on the principle that the body can heal itself if stimulated to do so, especially through nutrition.

folk medicine Traditional healing systems that flourished in all cultures before the development of conventional Western medicine.

stress management. They include deep breathing, prayer, meditation, progressive relaxation, visualization, yoga, and biofeedback. Many of these practices have health benefits. For example, mindfulness meditation has been shown to decrease chronic pain and anxiety and improve general psychological health when practiced as part of a stress reduction program.[14] Progressive relaxation has been found useful in reducing stress, tension, headaches, and sleep difficulties. Yoga may be beneficial for low back pain, hypertension, arthritis, and sleep difficulties and can improve coordination and flexibility.[15] Biofeedback has proved useful in treating headaches, low back pain, seizures, and incontinence.

The risk associated with mind-body therapies as an adjunct to conventional care is minimal. Most are inexpensive and relatively easy to learn, and they can be integrated into regular self-care. Many people have a daily mind-body practice. In this section we briefly consider two forms of mind-body medicine not previously discussed in this book, hypnosis and t'ai chi ch'uan.

Hypnosis

Hypnosis is the use of intentional relaxation and focusing exercises to produce an altered state of consciousness (a trancelike state) in which a person is more responsive to suggestion. When hypnosis is used for health purposes, the hypnotist makes suggestions that may help the person change behavior, such as quitting smoking. The person may find it easier to follow suggestions made during hypnosis but is not compelled to do so. Hypnosis is used as an adjunct to other therapies and may be practiced by many different kinds of practitioners, including family physicians, anesthesiologists, naturopaths, and psychologists. When hypnosis, visualization, and relaxation techniques are used before surgery, patients recover more quickly and have less pain.[16]

T'ai Chi Ch'uan

T'ai chi ch'uan, or **t'ai chi,** originated in China as a martial art and has developed into a system of slow, fluid movements through a series of meditative poses. As described in Chapter 5, it incorporates breathing, stretching, and stimulation of various organs and organ systems as identified in Traditional Chinese Medicine. In the United States, t'ai chi has evolved into a popular form of exercise that facilitates body awareness and the flow of energy. It is used to reduce stress; promote relaxation; and improve aerobic fitness, strength, flexibility, and coordination.

Preliminary studies suggest that practicing t'ai chi may improve physical functioning for older adults, improve blood circulation, reduce anxiety and depression, and increase bone density in women after menopause. There appear to be some minimal risks, particularly for people with balance problems, especially if the practice is initiated without proper training. Overall, however, these

are mild exercises that can be performed daily for 15 minutes to several hours and should be considered safe for most people. If you are interested in learning t'ai chi, the best approach is to look for a class with a qualified teacher at your school or community center.

Biologically Based Practices

Biologically based practices include the use of vitamins, minerals, dietary supplements, herbal remedies, functional foods, and dietary regimens. Conventional medicine emphasizes the importance of food and diet in health, as described throughout this book. CAM practitioners frequently incorporate diet into their treatments, but recommendations are usually based on the individual patient's makeup. Therapeutic diets often involve limiting or excluding certain foods, such as processed foods, refined sugars, or wheat products, for a set period of time. Dietary regimens are usually used as an adjunct or complement to other therapy.

Dietary Supplements

Dietary supplements include vitamins, minerals, herbs, enzymes, and metabolites. Both conventional and CAM practitioners recommend that adequate micronutrients be obtained from a balanced diet, but they occasionally recommend supplements in order to reach certain Recommended Daily Allowances (RDAs). CAM practitioners sometimes recommend high-dose supplementation or the use of megavitamins—taking vitamins well in excess of the RDAs. For example, megadoses of vitamin C (4 grams a day) are sometimes recommended to ward off the common cold. A large review of studies to date showed no effect if taken to prevent colds but did show a possible effect, at megadoses of 8 grams a day, in reducing the length and severity of a cold when taken at the onset of symptoms.[17] High doses of water soluble vitamins, such as vitamin C, B_3, and B_6, do not pose a significant risk if taken for short periods, but it is possible to overdose on the fat soluble vitamins (vitamins A, D, E, and K), even with a short course of treatment.

Supplementation of minerals and trace elements can also be part of CAM. For many minerals, there are no clearly established RDAs, and high dose supplementation for short periods is sometimes recommended by CAM practitioners. For example, zinc is believed to boost the immune system. Studies show that zinc lozenges and nasal sprays do shorten the course and severity of the common cold when treatment is started within 24 hours of the onset of symptoms.[18] High dose dietary supplementation should not exceed the upper limits of safety (ULs) established for some vitamins and minerals (see Chapter 7). When upper limits have not been established, harm may still result from high doses; thus, the best course is caution.

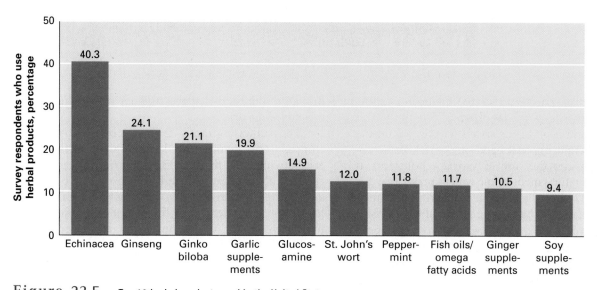

Figure 23.5   Top 10 herbal products used in the United States. Source: "Complementary and Alternative Medicine Use Among Adults: United States, 2002," by P. Barnes, E. Powell-Griner, K. McFann, and R. Nahin, 2004, CDC Advance Data Report No. 343, www.nccam.nih.gov.

Herbal Remedies

Herbal remedies, or **botanicals,** include a vast array of products derived from plants and other natural substances. They are a major part of all systems of folk medicine and the original source of many pharmaceutical drugs used today. For example, yams are a source of the estrogen used in birth control pills and hormone replacement therapy, and the heart medication digitalis comes from the foxglove plant. Pharmaceutical companies are engaged in an ongoing search for new sources of drugs in the natural world and in research aimed at identifying the active ingredients in known plant remedies.

Only a few herbal medicines have been investigated in controlled clinical studies. Although results have been mixed, some herbs show promise. Ginkgo biloba appears to slow the deterioration of brain function in people with Alzheimer's disease and ease the leg pain associated with peripheral vascular disease (narrowing of the blood vessels in the legs). St. John's wort appears to be beneficial for people with mild depression, and kava kava appears to be useful in treating anxiety.[19] Various forms of Echinacea stimulate the immune system, helping people with colds recover faster, and valerian may help people overcome insomnia. The top 10 herbal products used by adults in the United States are shown in Figure 23.5.

Many people assume that herbs are safe because they are "natural," but herbs can have powerful effects, sometimes adverse ones, and safety is a major concern in the use of herbal remedies. Under the Dietary Supplement and Health Education Act (DSHEA) of 1994, herbal medicines and dietary supplements are subject to less stringent regulations than pharmaceutical drugs (see the box "Regulation of Drugs vs. Regulation of Herbs"). When new pharmaceutical medications are produced, they must undergo rigorous tests for safety, efficacy, and side effects before the FDA will approve their release. The burden is on the manufacturer to prove the safety and efficacy of the product; drugs are considered "guilty until proven innocent." Dietary and herbal supplements are released to the market and then removed or banned only if they prove to be unsafe. The burden is on the public and the FDA to demonstrate that the product is not safe; these products are considered "innocent until proven guilty."

One safety issue is contamination. Herbal products have been found to contain lead, mercury, arsenic, bacteria, pesticides, and herbicides. Other problems can be caused if manufacturers substitute one plant species for another, as occurred in China when a plant substitution caused renal failure in 30 women taking an herbal

KEY TERMS

hypnosis   Use of intentional relaxation and focusing exercises to produce an altered state of consciousness in which a person is more responsive to suggestion.

t'ai chi (t'ai chi ch'uan)   System of slow, fluid movements through a series of meditative poses, incorporating breathing, stretching, and stimulation of various organs and organ systems.

herbal remedies (botanicals)   Products derived from plants and other natural substances, used to treat illness and promote health.

HIGHLIGHT ON HEALTH
Regulation of Drugs vs. Regulation of Herbs

Pharmaceutical drugs and herbal medicines follow very different routes to the pharmacy or the health food store, and if problems arise after they are on the market, different processes and outcomes can be expected. Consider the case of Vioxx, a nonsteroidal anti-inflammatory medication widely prescribed for chronic pain, especially the pain of arthritis. Although Vioxx was known to have some potential health risks, its benefits were thought to outweigh the risks. In September 2004, however, the FDA ordered the removal of Vioxx from the market after studies revealed that it caused a significantly increased risk of heart disease and stroke. Despite rigorous clinical trials, this risk had not become apparent until the drug was used for several years by the general population. The manufacturer pulled the drug from the market, and drugs from the same family were subjected to close scrutiny for similar problems.

A different scenario played out with ephedra, a stimulant used in Chinese medicine to treat asthma and other respiratory and lung conditions. Derived from the plant called Ma Huang in Chinese herbology, ephedra was included in many dietary supplements and herbal medicines, mainly for the purposes of losing weight and boosting athletic performance. It was known to increase blood pressure, cause heart arrhythmias, and have other effects on the cardiovascular system. After it was on the market for years, its use was associated with cases of heart attack, seizure, and stroke as well as numerous deaths. In April 2004, the FDA banned the sale of products containing ephedra, stating that its use posed "a significant and unreasonable risk to human health" and that the risks far outweighed the benefits of the drug.

The ban was promptly challenged by a Utah-based company that manufactured ephedra products. The company claimed that the FDA had not proven that ephedra actually caused the health problems or that adverse events occurred when the drug was taken at the low doses recommended by the manufacturer. A Utah judge agreed with the manufacturer and ruled that the FDA did not have the power to ban a dietary supplement based on weighing risks against benefits (a standard used for pharmaceutical drugs). The judge pointed out that the Dietary Supplement and Health Education Act of 1994 (DSHEA), under which the FDA is empowered to regulate herbs, was meant to protect the public's access to dietary supplements and herbal products. In passing this law, the judge said, Congress clearly meant to distinguish dietary supplements and herbal medicines from drugs and to define them as a subset of foods, which are presumed to be safe. The DSHEA does not require a manufacturer to show that a dietary supplement confers a benefit or to prove its safety, the judge pointed out; rather, the onus is on the FDA to show that it is unsafe. Products containing low doses of ephedra returned to the market and remain available today. In the meantime, the FDA is requesting an amendment to the DSHEA to make manufacturers of dietary supplements and herbal remedies demonstrate the safety of their products once a safety question has been raised.

Source: "Federal Court Weakens FDA Ephedra Ban," by D. Denoon, April 15, 2005, WebMD Medical News, www.webmd.com.

medication.[19] If you take any herbal products, purchase those made by reputable manufacturers.

Another issue is the lack of standardization in herbal remedies and associated variation in the quantity of active ingredient in a dose. For many herbs, the "correct" dose is unknown. There is also individual variation in response to herbs; in other words, two people might have different responses to the same herb. The lack of standardization also makes it difficult to compare the effects of herbal treatments with those of other medications.

A third issue is interaction of herbs with other drugs. For instance, Dong Quai, an herb sometimes used to treat menstrual cramps and menopausal symptoms, causes increased risk of bleeding in patients taking the blood-thinning drug coumadin. Licorice, an herb used for stomach problems, can cause extremely low levels of potassium in patients taking some blood pressure medications.[19] Inform your physician of any herbal medications you are taking, especially if you are also taking prescription drugs. Finally, there is little or no data on the use of herbs during pregnancy or breast-feeding. Given the lack of knowledge and the high potential risk to the unborn or nursing child, it is generally recommended that pregnant and nursing women not use herbal medicines.[19]

A traditional advantage of herbal medications has been that they are available at a lower cost than pharmaceutical medications. Herbal remedies are no longer part of the folk culture, however; they represent a multibillion-dollar

Healthy People 2010

OBJECTIVE AREA *Medical Product Safety*

- Increase the proportion of primary care providers . . . who routinely review with their patients aged 65 years and older . . . all new prescribed and over-the-counter medicines.

"Adults aged 65 years and older account for less than 15 percent of the population but they use about one-third of all retail prescriptions. This population also purchases at least 40 percent of all nonprescription medicines. Further, older adults are more likely to suffer from multiple chronic diseases and, as a result, may routinely visit multiple physicians, each of whom may be unaware of other medicines that have been prescribed. . . . Physicians [are urged] to incorporate medication reviews as part of routine office-based practice."

For more information on Healthy People 2010 objectives, visit the Web site at www.healthypeople.gov.

 For more information on Canadian health objectives, visit the Health Canada Web site at www.hc-sc.gc.ca/english.

industry. Sales of herbal remedies are doubling every 4 years, and herbs are moving into mainstream supermarkets and drugstores. The cost of drugs, including prescription, over-the-counter, and herbal medicines, is rising faster than any other health care cost. Because money spent in one area takes away from money spent in another, research needs to be continued on the efficacy and safety of herbal medicines and consumers need to make informed decisions about where to spend their medical dollars.[20]

Manipulative and Body-Based Practices

Manipulative and body-based practices focus on the body's structures and systems—the bones, joints, muscles, soft tissues, and circulatory system.[8] Practitioners use touch, pressure, manipulation, and other techniques to help the body overcome illness and heal itself.

Osteopathic Medicine

Osteopathic medicine has been so well integrated into mainstream practice that it is usually considered a form of conventional medicine rather than a form of CAM. **Osteopathy** is a health system developed in the United States at the end of the 19th century by physician Andrew Taylor Still. Through personal experience, Still came to believe that healing could be achieved through manipulation of the musculoskeletal system without the use of drugs. He believed that manipulation of the bones and muscles could improve blood circulation and balance the functioning of the nerves, thereby allowing the body to heal. The philosophy behind osteopathic medicine has changed slightly over time, but Still's original four principles remain the same: (1) the body is a whole unit; (2) the body is self-protecting and self-regulating; (3) structure and function are interrelated; and (4) treatment incorporates the first three principles.[21]

Osteopathic physicians receive a medical education comparable to that of conventional physicians and are subject to the same licensing regulations, but their training includes osteopathic manipulation techniques and their focus is on treating the whole person. Since the introduction of antibiotics in the 1940s, most osteopaths have included the use of drugs in their practice. In some settings, it can be difficult to distinguish osteopaths (D.O.s) from conventional physicians (M.D.s).

Chiropractic Medicine

Chiropractic medicine was developed by American physician Daniel David Palmer in the 1890s. Palmer believed that most illnesses were the result of **subluxation** of the spine—a misalignment, displacement, or dislocation of vertebrae in the spinal column. Such a misalignment interrupts the flow of energy and signals from the brain to the rest of the body, causing illness. Relocating the misaligned joints restores the balance of energy and health. Chiropractic care is based on four principles: (1) the nervous system influences all other body systems; (2) the human body has the ability to heal itself; (3) joint dysfunction may interfere with the ability of the nervous system to perform in an optimal fashion and may contribute

KEY TERMS

osteopathy Health system developed by Andrew Taylor Still that focuses on healing through manipulation of the musculoskeletal system; now considered a form of conventional medicine.

chiropractic medicine Health system developed by Daniel David Palmer that focuses on realigning dislocated vertebrae to restore the flow of energy from the brain to the rest of the body.

subluxation In chiropractic medicine, a misalignment, displacement, or dislocation of vertebrae in the spinal column.

to disease; and (4) the primary goal of treatment is to identify and treat joint dysfunction, thus allowing the body to heal.

Chiropractors receive their training in a 4-year program post-college at an accredited chiropractic college; upon completion of the program, they receive a Doctor of Chiropractic (D.C.) degree. Chiropractic medicine is licensed in all 50 states and the District of Columbia.[2] It is widely accepted as a form of manual healing; many health insurance plans cover chiropractic treatments.

Studies of the effectiveness of chiropractic have focused on its use in treating low back pain and neck pain. Some studies have shown it to be as effective as standard treatment for low back pain, and others have shown it to be more effective.[22] Other studies suggest a possible benefit in other painful conditions, such as fibromyalgia (a chronic pain condition), carpal tunnel syndrome, and osteoarthritis.[21] Like all treatments, chiropractic has some risks associated with it. Patients can experience mild discomfort, headache, and tiredness after treatment. Serious side effects are rare but can include paralysis and stroke.[22]

Massage Therapy and Bodywork

Massage therapy involves the application of pressure to the skin and muscles with the aim of increasing blood flow and inducing relaxation. Massage is believed to promote healing by boosting the immune system and stimulating the release of natural painkillers. It is part of many treatment modalities and has been shown to be beneficial for reducing anxiety, depression, and pain and improving immune function.[23]

There are more than 75 different types of massage. Swedish massage involves long smooth strokes and kneading motions along the skin, working all parts of the body. Deep tissue massage uses heavier strokes to reach muscles lying at a deeper level in the body. Shiatsu massage, or acupressure, involves pressure applied at acupuncture points to improve the flow of qi. Some limited studies of acupressure have shown it to be effective in reducing nausea, headaches, and some pain. It has been used in palliative care and may produce an improvement in energy level.[24]

Bodywork encompasses a number of physical healing methods. One form of bodywork, Rolfing, was developed in the 1950s by Ida Rolf. She believed that adhesions and scarring in the fascia (the soft tissue covering muscles) can restrict the body's ability to move smoothly, which in turn impairs emotional well-being. She developed a technique of applying deep pressure to the fascia with the thumbs, fingers, and elbows to release these adhesions. Typically, the client undergoes a series of sessions, and with each session, deeper pressure is applied, at times to the point of pain. Although there have been few studies of Rolfing, proponents claim that it can reduce chronic pain, improve posture and movement, and provide an improved sense of well-being.

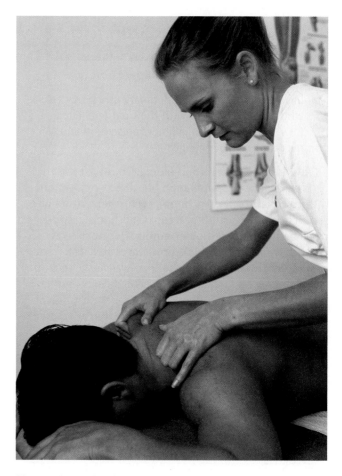

Massage therapy is believed to stimulate the release of natural pain-killers in the body as well as boost the immune system. It is used to relieve different types of pain, from sore muscles to depression.

Energy Therapies

Energy therapies are among the most controversial CAM practices. Their underlying idea is that humans are infused with energy and that this energy can be modified to influence health. As we have seen, many CAM practices include the idea that a disruption or imbalance of energy, whether called life force, vital energy, qi, dosha, or something else, is at the root of illness and that the restoration of balance promotes health.

Some forms of energy can be measured, and their use in treating illness is well incorporated into conventional medicine. Light therapy is used to treat seasonal affective disorder, a form of depression associated with low exposure to sunlight, and psoriasis, a skin condition. Electromagnets (magnets that pulsate in response to an intermittent electrical current) are used to treat nonhealing bone fractures (although magnetic-field therapies are not part of standard medical treatment). Other forms of energy cannot be measured by means currently available, and their use in treating illness is considered complementary or alternative. We consider here magnetic-field therapies, qigong, Reiki, and therapeutic touch.[25]

Magnetic-Field Therapies

Magnets produce a measurable energy called a magnetic field. They have long been used in attempts to treat pain, especially chronic pain, such as occurs in arthritis. It is estimated that Americans currently spend $500 million per year on magnets for pain.[26] There is no proven mechanism by which magnets might work, but some hypotheses are that they may affect cell function, alter blood flow to an area, affect how nerve cells respond to pain, or affect the production of immune cells.

Limited studies have been conducted on magnets, and their results have been mixed. If magnets are going to reduce pain, they usually do so in a week or two. Except for cost, there do not appear to be any significant risks associated with magnets, although they are not recommended for women who are pregnant or for people with an implanted medical device, such as a defibrillator or pacemaker.[27]

Qigong

A Chinese energy therapy, **Qigong** (pronounced "chi-kung") combines physical movement and breathing to enhance the flow of qi and boost immune functioning. Therapy can be administered by a practitioner, who redirects the patient's energy through light touch or massage, or the individual can practice self-healing Qigong by performing a series of movements and exercises. The exercises can be movement oriented, involving very slow, dancelike movements that are believed to promote energy balance and maintain suppleness, or they can be oriented more toward meditation and internal energy flow with minimal external movement. In China, Qigong is widely used in hospitals and clinics to treat asthma, arthritis, stress, allergies, hypertension, and chronic pain. Qigong providers are rare in the United States and Canada.

Therapeutic Touch and Reiki

Like many other CAM therapies, **therapeutic touch** is based on the idea that illness results from a disturbance in the flow of a person's life energy. Related to the ancient practice of "laying-on of hands," therapeutic touch involves a practitioner passing his or her hands over a patient's body to detect imbalances and redirect energy, thus promoting healing. Some studies have suggested that therapeutic touch can be effective in wound healing, osteoarthritis, migraine headaches, and anxiety.[25]

Reiki (pronounced "ray-kie") is a Japanese energy therapy in which the practitioner uses a number of different hand positions over the patient's body to channel and direct healing energy. Although Reiki has been used for thousands of years, there are few studies confirming its beneficial effects. It is being studied as an adjunct to treatment of fibromyalgia, heart disease, and cancer and in patients with AIDS.

MAKING INFORMED HEALTH CARE CHOICES

When you are sick, how do you know whether to see your regular health care provider, to seek out a complementary or alternative treatment, or to treat the illness yourself? In general, conventional medicine is highly effective in treating a wide range of illnesses, including infectious diseases and acute and chronic conditions like heart disease, diabetes, and cancer. CAM can be effective in such areas as boosting your immune system, improving energy levels, relieving pain, managing stress, and addressing other symptoms as described in this chapter. Self-care is probably the most commonly used health option. A view of these intersecting areas of health care is shown in Figure 23.6.

Evaluating CAM Choices

As the NCCAM advances in its mission of investigating CAM therapies in rigorous scientific studies, more information will emerge about the safety and efficacy of these practices. For now, if you are interested in using a CAM approach, you will need to educate yourself and make informed choices (see the box "Questions to Ask When Considering Health Care Choices"). The NCCAM recommends that you begin your investigation by consulting with your regular physician or health care provider to find out if there are conventional treatments that address your condition before trying CAM. It is especially important to discuss any CAM treatments you are considering with your physician if you take prescription medications, since drug interactions can be dangerous.

If your physician is knowledgeable about the CAM approach you are considering, he or she may be able to help you make a decision about using it. Otherwise, you may have to investigate it by yourself at the library or on the Internet. Remember to use reliable Web sites like those of major universities, the NCCAM, and the FDA, and look for government-sponsored clinical trials. Be

---

KEY TERMS

Qigong Chinese energy therapy that combines physical movement and breathing to enhance the flow of qi and boost immune functioning.

therapeutic touch Therapy in which a practitioner passes his or her hands over a patient's body to detect imbalances and redirect energy, thus promoting healing.

Reiki Japanese energy therapy in which the practitioner uses a number of different hand positions over the patient's body to channel and direct healing energy.

Figure 23.6   Sectors of health care. *Health care can be thought of as overlapping sectors in which individuals initiate their own health care or receive care from others.*

wary of commercial Web sites that want to sell you a product. Refer to Chapter 1 for guidelines on being an informed consumer of health care information.

Choosing Self-Care

As discussed in Chapter 1, self-care involves actions you take on behalf of your own health. It includes observing your own symptoms, gathering information and advice, making an informed decision, and then either treating yourself or seeking professional care. If you have symptoms that are severe, unusual, persistent, or recurrent, it is generally recommended that you see your health care provider.

If your symptoms don't meet these criteria, you may decide to choose self-care. Both conventional medicine and CAM recommend regular exercise, a balanced diet,

and adequate sleep as basic self-care behaviors. (See the box "Dietary Approaches to Self-Care" for information on nutritional approaches to consider.) Many forms of CAM involve such self-care practices as deep breathing, progressive relaxation, yoga, and other stress management techniques. You can also practice self-care by taking over-the-counter medications for such conditions as headache, backache, stomach upset, muscle or joint pain, mild infections, colds, and allergies, among others.

Influences on Health Care Choices

Ideas and beliefs about self-care and other health care choices are formed through a variety of influences, including interactions with family, friends, and health care providers; the media and the Internet; public health campaigns; and societal forces in general. For example,

Challenges & Choices

Questions to Ask When Considering Health Care Choices

When making health care decisions, you need to think about your options in terms of several different dimensions. The following areas are important to consider whether you are thinking about taking ibuprofen, seeing an acupuncturist, or having surgery.

- **Safety**   All activities have some risk associated with them. For example, the pain reliever Tylenol is sold over the counter and is safe for most people, but it can aggravate problems in people who have liver disease and can cause liver failure if taken in too high a dose. For any health care choice you are considering, ask whether the benefits outweigh the risks. What possible side effects are reported with the proposed diagnostic or treatment plan? How does this plan compare with other options? What risk is associated with not choosing another treatment option or with delaying another treatment?

- **Efficacy**   How likely are you to get a benefit from the treatment option? Are there studies or data confirming benefits? Have other options been shown to be beneficial? Evidence is available for some complementary and alternative treatments, but for others, you may have to base your decisions on other people's experience. The problem is that people respond differently to illness and to treatments. You might recover from a cold in 3 days after taking vitamin C and Echinacea, and your friend might take the same remedies but still have the cold for 10 days. You would not really know whether the vitamins and herbs shortened the course of the illness or not. It could be that you would have recovered in 3 days without any treatment and your friend would have been sick for 3 weeks if she had not taken the vitamins and herbs.

- **Cost**   How expensive is each option? Cost includes not just the dollar amount you pay but also the cost of any side effects that choice may cause, any cost associated with not making another choice, and time that you may gain or lose. For example, a person who delays surgery and chemotherapy for melanoma in order to try a less drastic alternative approach may have to pay a heavy cost in lost treatment time.

- **Qualifications of the provider**   How qualified is the health care provider? Find out about licensing requirements and other regulations in the field, and check your provider's background. Also find out whether your provider has a financial stake in the option he or she is recommending. If so, is that a source of bias in the advice you are receiving?

It's Not Just Personal . . .

Safety, efficacy, cost, and qualifications of the provider are universal health care issues. Yet every day people make health care choices in ways that are less than ideal. Someone who has been told by a friend that an over-the-counter product is "great" may not think about whether it's safe for her, considering that she takes several other medications. An individual who sees an ad for an herbal product that promises to relieve depression may try it without even checking on the claim. A person who can't afford health insurance may not get a refill on an expensive but necessary prescription. Someone with a life-threatening illness may choose a health care provider who is persuasive and confident but lacks certain credentials and has inadequate experience. To avoid such patterns, keep yourself well informed, think critically, and work with your health care provider as you make health care choices.

popular diets frequently arise almost overnight and are adopted by millions of people, only to fall into oblivion when they fail to deliver or sustain the promised weight loss. Most newspapers have health sections, and more than 50 consumer magazines about health care appear monthly.

A relatively new influence on how people define health and illness is **direct-to-consumer advertising.** In the past, pharmaceutical companies marketed their products primarily to health care providers, but in 1997, changes made by the FDA in advertising regulations allowed manufacturers to take their campaigns directly to

the public. Between 1996 and 2000, spending on direct-to-consumer advertising skyrocketed from approximately $790 million to $2.5 billion. The most heavily marketed

KEY TERMS

direct-to-consumer advertising   Marketing of products directly to consumers instead of to health care providers.

Consumer Clipboard

Dietary Approaches to Self-Care

The foundation of self-care through diet is a basic healthy eating plan. For most people, that means following the 2005 *Dietary Guidelines for Americans,* which highlight key areas and make recommendations for both the general population and specific groups, such as people over 50 and those who need to lose weight. The Guidelines recommend following the USDA Food Guide (MyPyramid) or the DASH Eating Plan.

Both of these healthy eating plans emphasize consuming nutrient-dense foods and beverages and limiting intake of saturated and trans fats, cholesterol, added sugars, salt, and alcohol. They also encourage the consumption of fruits and vegetables, whole grains, and fat-free or low-fat dairy products.

Putting these eating plans into practice starts with smart food shopping. This approach allows you to control what you're going to eat and what you're going to avoid. It also involves making use of food labels, which can be helpful in choosing healthy foods.

The next step is preparing your own meals as often as possible. This approach offers the control that makes good nutrition possible. You can avoid greasy and fatty foods and use "good" fats and bake or broil foods. You can also make fresh fruit desserts or low-fat, low-sugar treats.

Dining out does not have to be off limits. You just need to choose carefully—both where you eat and what you eat. In general, avoid eating at fast-food restaurants. Although they offer some decent choices, much of the food is salty, sugary, and fatty. At a regular restaurant, your choices are often wide and you can order foods to your specifications—without salt or with salad dressing on the side. You have to be assertive, though, and ask for these things.

For those following a vegetarian diet, careful planning is especially important. Although vegetarian eating is a healthy approach, vegetarians of all types need to be sure that they're getting enough protein and the necessary balance of all nutrients.

For individuals with high blood pressure, eating plans that involve no added salt, low-fat foods, and limited sweets and alcoholic beverages are recommended. For people with diabetes, the American Dietetic Association offers eating guidelines and cookbooks that feature sweet alternatives to regular desserts.

For people with special needs, such as cancer patients, an eating plan should be outlined in consultation with a nutritionist or other health care provider. Throughout chemotherapy, a nutrient-dense diet is often recommended because nutrients are not well absorbed by the body.

For individuals who are eating a well-balanced diet, dietary supplements usually are not necessary. There are exceptions, though, such as pregnant women, who need supplemental folic acid (to prevent neural tube defects in the developing fetus), and older adults, who may need extra calcium to maintain bone density.

Much of dietary self-care is based on common sense—following a sensible eating plan, paying attention to portion control, balancing calories in and out, and making moderate physical activity a part of your daily routine. It sounds easy, but it is a challenge for many people, as evidenced by the large number of overweight adults and children in the United States. For long-term success, nutrition experts recommend taking small steps over time to incorporate these changes into your lifestyle.

drugs are for allergies, cholesterol, depression, and pain. Drugs for hair loss, acne, erectile dysfunction, and sexual desire disorder in women are also commonly advertised.

Direct-to-consumer ads may educate consumers about new medications for health conditions, or they may motivate people to seek treatment for an untreated illness. Physicians report that they are prescribing drugs for patients who ask for them by name after seeing ads on television or in magazines. However, these ads are designed primarily to create feelings of inadequacy about having certain conditions and a sense of need for the advertised

product. Ad campaigns not only sell products but also help shape a society's views of health and illness, especially by medicalizing physical differences and personality traits. For example, a recent addition to the list of heavily advertised drugs is Propecia, a treatment for male baldness. In 1999, the year after Propecia was released, its manufacturer spent $100 million on direct-to-consumer advertising.[28] The message is that baldness is a health problem that needs to be fixed.

As in all decisions, it pays to use your critical thinking skills and to be an informed consumer of messages about health and illness. Quackery and fraud exist in all aspects of health care. Again, refer to Chapter 1 for guidelines on evaluating sources of health news and information.

Supporting Integrative Medicine

Many people believe that the future of health care lies in a convergence of conventional medicine and CAM practices. As noted earlier in the chapter, the use of mainstream medical therapies in combination with CAM therapies that have been shown to be safe and effective is known as integrative medicine. Proponents of integrative medicine suggest that it might provide more effective and comprehensive medical treatment for all.

Another benefit of integrative medicine might be a reduction in health care spending, which currently is spiraling out of control in the United States. In 2000, 13 percent of the U.S. gross domestic product (GDP) was spent on health care, compared to an average of 6 percent in other industrialized countries.[29] The cost of health care as a percentage of GDP is increasing faster than any other part of the economy. Recent tallies show that the total health care expenditure in the United States in 2000 was $1.25 trillion.[30]

At the same time, consumers are spending out-of-pocket money for CAM therapies. In 1997, the U.S. public spent $36–$47 billion on CAM. Of this amount, $12–$20 billion was paid to professional CAM health care providers and $5 billion was spent on herbal medicines.[8] These expenditures rival the out-of-pocket payments made for conventional treatments. Combining conventional medicine and CAM might be a way of consolidating some of this spending.

A key component in the future of integrative medicine is the work of the NCCAM in funding and conducting rigorous scientific studies of CAM therapies and in identifying the most cost-effective ways of maximizing health. Another key component of integrative medicine is the conventional medical system's primary care provider. Such providers are sometimes described as gatekeepers, meaning that they make decisions about who can see specialists and CAM providers, when they can see them, and for what conditions. A new role for the primary care provider might be that of pathfinder. In this role, providers might be expected to be knowledgeable about various CAM therapies, or they might be trained in certain CAM techniques. With this added knowledge and training, they would be better equipped to guide people through the increasingly complex medical systems that await the next generation of health care consumers.

As mentioned at the beginning of the chapter, many practices and ideas from complementary and alternative medicine are already being absorbed into conventional health care. They include the following:

- A focus on wellness as a positive, multidimensional state of being rather than simply the absence of pain or symptoms of disease
- Treatment of the whole person
- Interest in mind-body connections
- Acknowledgment of the role of spirituality in wellness
- The use of stress management techniques
- An emphasis on individual responsibility for health, especially in making daily decisions about nutrition, exercise, sleep, relationships, and other lifestyle behaviors

These are also some of the concepts incorporated in this book. They represent just a few of the basic premises that underlie the pursuit of personal health today and the range of choices available to you as you face the 21st century in a changing society.

You Make the Call

Should CAM Be Covered by Health Insurance?

If your primary care physician refers you to a specialist, such as an endocrinologist, a cardiologist, or an oncologist, your health insurance will very likely pay for your care. If your primary care physician were to refer you to a chiropractor, an acupuncturist, or a massage therapist, or if you decided to seek such treatment on your own, your visits might or might not be covered by your insurance. Should all health care options be equally accessible to consumers? Should insurance plans cover CAM practices the same way they cover conventional treatments? And who should decide what kind of practitioners people can see?

Proponents of health insurance coverage for CAM therapies point out that many of these practices have been in existence far longer than Western medicine. They have been developed to meet the health needs of people all over the world and have been proven safe and effective through time. Proponents note that CAM practices tend to be less invasive, less costly, and safer than conventional medicine; they also comment that conventional care tends to be directed toward the very sick and the elderly rather than toward the general population and that not enough attention is paid to disease prevention and health promotion.

CAM systems incorporate prevention into their underlying belief systems; by focusing on health promotion, they arguably decrease the cost and burden of chronic disease to individuals and society. Finally, proponents argue that by providing access to only one type of health care, insurance plans are not speaking to the needs of a diverse population.

Opponents point out that many health practices deemed useful in the past have been shown to have limited value; in time, they have been replaced by safer, more effective options. The fact that a practice is old and traditional does not necessarily mean that it has been proven by time. Opponents agree that prevention is important, but they point out that even well-supported, proven prevention practices that are recommended by conventional providers are not well used by the general population. Giving people additional choices will just increase confusion and create resistance to prevention practices that have clearly been proven beneficial, such as vaccinations and Pap tests.

Opponents also point out that although many alternative treatments appear to be relatively safe, they are not without risk. Due to the current lack of organization, licensing, and regulation of some CAM practitioners in the United States, some health care providers are inadequately trained and may cause harm to patients. Finally, although preventive practices may decrease the cost and burden of chronic disease, there is little evidence that patients receiving CAM care have lower health care costs. In fact, most patients receiving CAM care continue to receive conventional care; expanding insurance coverage may simply further increase health care spending in the United States.

Should health insurance cover CAM treatments? What do you think?

Pros

- CAM practices have been proven by time; they are less invasive, less costly, and safer than conventional medicine.
- CAM practices tend to focus on health promotion and prevention of illness for the whole population, whereas conventional medicine directs most of its attention to the very ill and elderly.
- Providing insurance coverage for both conventional and CAM practices promotes access to health care for a diverse population.

Cons

- Many CAM practices have not been proven safe or effective. Providing insurance coverage for unproven treatments may mislead consumers into thinking these treatments have more legitimacy than they do.
- Training and licensing are not regulated for many CAM providers, making it difficult or impossible to evaluate their qualifications and competence. Insurance coverage should not be extended to practitioners who may cause more harm than good.
- Adding CAM practices to insurance plans would complicate health services and may reduce the use of proven tests and treatments, such as Pap tests.
- The health care system is already financially overburdened; adding coverage for unproven practices just adds to the burden.

OLC Web site For more information about this topic, visit the Online Learning Center at www.mhhe.com/teaguele.

SUMMARY

- The use of practices and concepts from complementary and alternative medicine (CAM) has grown dramatically in the United States in the last 15 years. In recognition of this interest, Congress established the National Center for Complementary and Alternative Medicine (NCCAM) and charged it with investigating CAM therapies in rigorous scientific studies.

- Conventional medicine, also known as Western medicine, biomedicine, and allopathic medicine, is the dominant health care system in the United States, Canada, and much of Europe and other parts of the developed world. It operates on the premises that illness is caused by pathogens and organic changes in the body and can be treated with such interventions as drugs, vaccines, and surgery. Providers of conventional medicine include medical doctors, osteopathic doctors, and allied health care providers.

- Complementary and alternative medicine is a group of medical and health care systems, practices, and products that are not presently considered to be part of conventional medicine. These systems operate on the premise that health is a reflection of balance among the physical, mental, and spiritual dimensions of an individual and that an imbalance can lead to illness.

- Some but not all forms of CAM have standardized training and licensing requirements for practitioners.

- The NCCAM identifies four CAM domains—mind-body interventions, biologically based therapies, manipulative and body-based therapies, and energy therapies—in addition to whole medical systems, which employ practices from some or all of the domains.

- The most commonly used domain is mind-body medicine when prayer for health reasons is included. When prayer is not included, the use of biologically based or natural products is the most popular.

- Traditional Chinese Medicine (TCM) is a well-developed medical system that has been used in China for thousands of years. It is based on the premise that illness is the result of an imbalance in yin and yang, two opposing but interrelated principles, and a blockage of qi, vital energy, in the body. Its primary treatment methods are herbal medicine and acupuncture.

- Acupuncture is a treatment method in which long, thin needles are inserted at certain points in the skin to stimulate the flow of qi.

- Ayurveda is a traditional medical system that has been used in India for thousands of years. It seeks to restore harmony and balance to the individual through dietary modification, exercises, yoga, meditation, massage, herbal tonics, and controlled breathing.

- Homeopathy is a Western medical system based on the law of similars, the principle of minimal dose, and the idea of prescribing for the individual.

- Naturopathy is a Western medical system based on the idea that health is the natural order if the individual lives simply and wisely; treatments are aimed at strengthening the body, especially through nutritional modification.

- Folk medicine encompasses the traditional healing systems of all cultures before the advent of Western medicine. A common thread in most forms of folk medicine is a focus on the integral relationship of humans with one another, the natural environment, and the spiritual world.

- Mind-body practices are based on the premise that the mind influences the body in ways that can promote or detract from well-being. Mind-body therapies include deep breathing, prayer, meditation, progressive relaxation, visualization, yoga, biofeedback, hypnosis, and t'ai chi.

- Biologically based practices include the use of vitamins, minerals, dietary supplements, herbal remedies, functional foods, and dietary regimens to treat illness and promote health. Dietary supplements can include megadoses of vitamins and minerals. Herbal remedies, or botanicals, include a vast array of products derived from plants and other natural substances.

- Safety is a major concern in the use of herbal medicines. Safety issues include contamination, lack of standardization, interaction with other drugs, and use during pregnancy and breast-feeding.

- Manipulative and body-based practices focus on the body's structures and systems—the bones, joints, muscles, soft tissues, and circulatory system.

- Osteopathy, a form of conventional medicine, focuses on treating the whole person and on manipulating the musculoskeletal system to improve circulation and improve the functioning of nerves.

- Chiropractic is a system of healing based on the idea that illness occurs when vertebrae are misaligned or displaced, interrupting the flow of energy from the brain to the rest of the body. Treatment involves realigning displaced joints in the spine.

- Massage therapy involves the application of pressure to the skin and muscles with the aim of increasing blood flow and inducing relaxation. Rolfing is a form of bodywork in which deep pressure is applied to the fascia to loosen adhesions and improve emotional well-being.

- Energy therapies are based on the idea that humans are infused with energy and that this energy can be modified to influence health. Energy therapies include magnetic-field therapies, qigong, therapeutic touch, and Reiki.

- Conventional medicine, CAM, and self-care are three intersecting areas of health care. In choosing a CAM therapy, consumers need to consult with their conventional care physician, research the therapy, and use their critical thinking skills in evaluating its likely safety, efficacy, and cost as well as the qualifications of the CAM practitioner.

- Self-care includes actions individuals take on behalf of their own health, such as exercising, managing stress, and taking over-the-counter medications. If symptoms are severe, unusual, persistent, or recurring, professional care is advised.

- Influences on health care choices include family and friends, the media and the Internet, public health campaigns, and direct-to-consumer advertising.

- The future of health care may lie in integrative medicine, the use of mainstream medical therapies in combination with CAM therapies that have been shown to be safe and effective. Many ideas and practices from CAM have already been incorporated into Western medicine.

REVIEW QUESTIONS

1. Why did Congress establish the NCCAM? What are its goals?

2. Describe several characteristics and premises of conventional Western medicine. What are the benefits of this approach? What are the drawbacks?

3. What is integrative medicine?

4. Describe several characteristics and premises of complementary and alternative medicine. What are the benefits of this approach? What are the drawbacks?

5. What are the different categories of CAM practices? Which is the most frequently used? For what health problems do consumers most commonly use CAM treatments?

6. What is qi or chi? What do yin and yang represent?

7. What methods of prevention are recommended in TCM? What are the primary treatment methods?

8. What is the aim of an acupuncture treatment? What symptoms and conditions has acupuncture been shown to treat effectively?

9. If you have a cold, what will an Ayurvedic practitioner try to determine? What treatment methods are used in Ayurveda?

10. Describe the basic principles of homeopathy. What is meant by "like cures like"?

11. What are some of the assessment techniques used in naturopathy? What training do naturopaths receive?

12. What is the common thread in all folk medicines?

13. Explain the basic premise of mind-body medicine. What are some examples?

14. What herbal medicines have been found to have positive health effects?

15. How are drugs and herbal medicines regulated differently?

16. What safety concerns are associated with the use of herbal remedies?

17. How does the training of osteopathic doctors differ from that of medical doctors?

18. Describe the four principles of chiropractic care. What conditions can be effectively treated by this therapy?

19. What are the aims of massage therapy? Of Rolfing?

20. Why are energy therapies the most controversial of all forms of CAM? What are some accepted uses of energy in health care?

21. What condition are magnets most often used to treat? How are they hypothesized to work? What conditions are Qigong and Reiki usually used to treat?

22. What questions should the consumer consider when making health care choices?

23. How would you know you should seek professional care for a condition rather than treat yourself? What are three self-care behaviors?

24. What is the purpose of direct-to-consumer advertising? What are some of its effects?

25. Describe several practices and ideas from complementary and alternative medicine that have been incorporated into conventional medicine.

WEB RESOURCES

American Academy of Medical Acupuncture: This site provides information about acupuncture, including conditions appropriate for this method, FAQs, articles by physicians, and research. Look here for how to find a board-certified acupuncturist near you.
www.medicalacupuncture.org

American Chiropractic Association: This organization's site addresses what chiropractic is, its history, and misunderstandings about this approach. It offers information on back pain, chiropractic medicine, news, and current research on chiropractic.
www.amerchiro.org

American Medical Association: The AMA offers online news about health issues and publishes the authoritative *Journal of the American Medical Association* (JAMA). Its site offers many articles about complementary and alternative medicine and how it relates to conventional medicine.
www.ama-assn.org

American Osteopathic Association: This site explains what a D.O. is, including the required medical education, and discusses osteopathic terms and osteopathic manipulative treatment (OMT). It also addresses various health issues in terms of the osteopathic approach.
www.osteopathic.org

MayoClinic.com: The Mayo Clinic site offers interactive health tools, such as calculators and assessments, and features information on complementary and alternative medicine, including drugs and dietary supplements.
www.mayoclinic.com

National Center for Complementary and Alternative Medicine: This organization is a valuable resource for information on complementary and alternative medicine. Its site features understanding CAM, major areas of this approach, alerts and advisories, treatment information, dietary and herbal supplements, and clinical trials.
http://nccam.nih.gov

National Center for Homeopathy: Offering information on what homeopathy is, this site provides research supporting the

effectiveness of homeopathy and guides you in finding a homeopathic practitioner.
www.homeopathic.org

National Council Against Health Fraud: This organization addresses the need for consumers to have complete information about health care products and services to make informed decisions. Its consumer information sheets address a wide variety of topics, including complementary and alternative medicine. www.ncahf.org

Office of Dietary Supplements, National Institutes of Health: This site offers information on specific dietary supplements,

nutrient recommendations, and consumer safety. To help consumers make informed decisions, it features topics such as product claims and labeling.
http://dietary-supplements.info.nih.gov

Quackwatch: Operated by Stephen Barrett, M. D., Quackwatch works to combat health-related frauds, myths, fads, and fallacies. It distributes reliable health publications, reports illegal marketing, and assists with consumer protection lawsuits. www.quackwatch.com

REFERENCES

1. National Center for Complementary and Alternative Medicine (NCCAM). Get the facts: What is complementary and alternative medicine? www.nccam.nih.gov/health.

2. Eisenberg, D. M., et al. (2002). Credentialing complementary and alternative medical providers. *Annals of Internal Medicine, 137,* 965–973.

3. Jonas, W. B., & Levin, J. S. (Eds.) (1999). *Essentials of complementary and alternative medicine.* Philadelphia: Lippincott, Williams and Wilkins.

4. Barnes, P., Powell-Griner, E., McFann, K., & Nahin, R. (2004). Complementary and alternative medicine use among adults: United States, 2002. Centers for Disease Control and Prevention. *Advance Data from Vital and Health Statistics,* No. 243, 1–20.

5. Nestler, G. (2002). Traditional Chinese Medicine. *Medical Clinics of North America, 86* (1), 63–73.

6. Goldstein, M. (1999). Alternative health care: Medicine, miracle or mirage? Philadelphia: Temple University Press.

7. Nasir, L. S. (2002). Acupuncture. *Primary Care, 29* (2), 393–405.

8. National Center for Complementary and Alternative Medicine. www.nccam.nih.gov.

9. Chopra, A., & Doiphode, V. (2002). Ayurvedic medicine. *Medical Clinics of North America, 86* (1), 75–89.

10. D'Huyvetter, K., & Cohrssen, A. (2002). Homeopathy. *Primary Care, 29* (2), 407–418.

11. NCCAM. (2003). Research report: Questions and answers about homeopathy. Publication No. D183. www.nccam.nih.gov.

12. NCCAM. (2004). Whole medical systems: An overview. Publication No. D236. www.nccam.nih.gov.

13. Mehl-Madrona, L. E. (1999). Native American medicine in the treatment of chronic illness: Developing an integrated program and evaluating its effectiveness. *Alternative Therapies, 5* (1), 36–44.

14. Barrows, K. A., & Jacobs, B. P. (2002). Mind body medicine: An introduction and review of the literature. *Medical Clinics of North America, 86* (1), 11–31.

15. Garfinkel, M., & Schumacher, H. R. (2000). Yoga. *Rheumatic Diseases Clinics of North America, 26* (1), 37–53.

16. Astin, J. (2004). Mind-body therapies for the management of pain. *Clinical Journal of Pain, 20* (1), 27–32.

17. Douglas, R. M., et al. (2004). Vitamin C for preventing and treating the common cold. *Cochrane Data Base Systematic Review, 18* (4), CD000980.

18. Hulisz, D. (2004). Efficacy of zinc against common cold viruses: An overview. *Journal of the American Pharmacology Association, 44* (5), 594–603.

19. Ernst, E., & Pittler, M. H. (2002). Herbal medicine. *Medical Clinics of North America, 86* (1), 149–161.

20. Gruenwald, J., et al. (2004). PDR for herbal medicines (3rd ed.). Montvale, NJ: Thomson PDR.

21. Fiechtner, J. J., & Brodeur, R. R. (2002). Manual and manipulation techniques for rheumatic diseases. *Medical Clinics of North America, 86* (1), 91–103.

22. NCCAM. (2003). Research report: About chiropractic and its use in treating low back pain. Publication No. D196.

23. Field, T. (2002). Massage therapy. *Medical Clinics of North America, 86* (1), 163–171.

24. Aetna InteliHealth. (2003). Complementary and alternative medicine: Acupressure, shiatsu and tuina. www.intelihealth.com.

25. NCCAM. (2004). Backgrounder: Energy medicine: An overview. Publication No. D235.

26. Winemiller, M. H., et al. (2003). Effect of magnetic vs. sham-magnetic insoles on plantar heel pain: A randomized controlled trial. *Journal of the American Medical Association, 290* (11), 1474–1478.

27. NCCAM. (2004). Research report: Questions and answers about using magnets to treat pain. Publication No. D208.

28. Direct to consumer advertising: Finasteride for male pattern hair loss. (2001). *Therapeutics Letter.* www.ti.ubc.ca.

29. Anderson, G., et al. (May 2003). It's the prices, stupid: Why the United States is so different from other countries. *Health Affairs.*

30. Cowan, C., et al. (2002). The burden of health care costs. *Health Care Financing Review, 23* (3), 132–159.

Add It Up!

ARE YOU AN INFORMED CONSUMER OF HEALTH CARE?

Informed consumers share important information with their health care providers and don't hesitate to ask questions. Use the following checklists to make sure you are working effectively with your health care provider, whether a conventional provider or a CAM practitioner.

When seeing a health care provider, do you share the following information?

_____ I have allergies; I am allergic to _____.

_____ I am pregnant or trying to get pregnant.

_____ I am breast-feeding.

_____ I have other medical problems.

_____ I have other symptoms.

_____ I am taking other medications (prescription, over the counter, dietary supplements, herbal remedies).

_____ I am being treated, or plan to seek treatment, by another health care provider.

When seeing a CAM practitioner, do you ask the following questions?

_____ How does this treatment work?

_____ Will it be effective for my condition?

_____ Are there any scientific studies supporting the use of this treatment for my condition? Where can I read about them?

_____ What improvements can I expect to see and when?

_____ What risks are associated with the treatment?

_____ Does the treatment have side effects?

_____ How long will treatment last/how many treatments will I need?

_____ How much do treatments cost?

_____ Is this treatment covered by health insurance?

_____ What is your background in this type of therapy?

_____ Are providers in your field licensed or certified by the state or a professional organization?

_____ Is there a Web site I can visit for more information on this therapy?

When being given a prescription for a medication or an herbal remedy, do you ask the following questions?

_____ For what condition of mine are you prescribing this medicine?

_____ What is this medicine supposed to do?

_____ How do I take this medicine?

- What is the administration route?
- How much do I take?
- How often do I take it?
- At what time of the day?
- With meals or without food?
- How long should I take it?

_____ What should I do if I miss a dose?

_____ When will the medicine begin to work?

_____ How will I know if the medicine is working?

_____ What should I do if it doesn't seem to work?

_____ What side effects should I watch for?

- What should I do if they occur?
- How long will they last?
- How can I reduce the side effects?

_____ While using this medicine, should I avoid:

- Driving or operating machines?
- Drinking alcohol?
- Eating certain foods?
- Taking certain medications (prescription, over the counter, dietary supplements, herbal remedies)?

_____ Are there any other precautions?

_____ How should I store the medicine?

- At room temperature?
- In the refrigerator?
- Away from heat, sunlight, or humidity?

_____ Can I get refills? How many?

_____ Are there any special instructions about how to use this medicine?

When taking medication, do you follow these precautions?

_____ I take the medication exactly as directed.

_____ I do not share medications with anyone else, even if they have a similar condition.

_____ I do not leave my medications where children or pets can get them.

_____ I discard unused or expired medications.

_____ I know what to do in case of an overdose by myself or a child.

_____ I keep the telephone numbers of my health care provider and pharmacy handy.

_____ I keep the telephone number of the poison control center handy (800-222-1212).

SOURCE: Data from "Just Ask! A Dozen Questions to Help You Understand Your Medicines," U.S. Pharmacopeia, www.usp.org.

Photo Credits

Index

Boldface numbers indicate pages on which glossary definitions appear.

A